ENDOCRINOLOGY
ADULT AND PEDIATRIC

ENDOCRINOLOGY
ADULT AND PEDIATRIC   6TH EDITION

THE THYROID GLAND

Volume Editor

Leslie J. De Groot, MD
Research Professor
Cellular and Life Sciences
University of Rhode Island, Providence Campus
Providence, Rhode Island

ELSEVIER
SAUNDERS

1600 John F. Kennedy Blvd.
Ste 1800
Philadelphia, PA 19103-2899

Endocrinology, Adult and Pediatric: The Thyroid Gland

ISBN: 978-0-323-22153-5
POD ISBN: 978-0-323-24064-2

Content for this eBook is derived from a book that may have contained additional digital media. Media content is not included in this eBook purchase.

Library of Congress Cataloging-in-Publication Data
Endocrinology / senior editors, Leslie J. De Groot, J. Larry Jameson ; section editors Ashley Grossman ... [et al.].—6th ed.
      p. ; cm.
   Includes bibliographical references and index.
   ISBN-13: 978-1-4160-5593-9 (v.1& v.2 : hardback : alk. paper)
   ISBN-13: 978-9996074479 (v.1 : hardback : alk. paper)
   ISBN-10: 9996074471 (v.1 : hardback : alk. paper)
   ISBN-13: 978-9996074417 (v.2 : hardback: alk. paper)
   [etc.]
   1. Endocrine glands–Diseases. 2. Endocrinology. I. De Groot, Leslie J.   II. Jameson, J. Larry.
   [DNLM: 1. Endocrine System Disease. 2. Endocrine Glands. 3. Hormones. WK 140 E5595 2010]
   RC648.E458 2010
   616.4—dc22

Acquisitions Editor: Helene Caprari
Developmental Editor: Mary Beth Murphy
Publishing Services Manager: Anne Altepeter
Project Manager: Jennifer Nemec
Design Direction: Ellen Zanolle

Transferred to Digital Printing in 2013

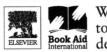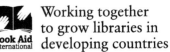

Senior Editors

J. Larry Jameson, MD, PhD

Professor of Medicine, Dean
Northwestern University Feinberg School of Medicine
Northwestern University
Chicago, Illinois

David de Kretser, AO, FAA, FTSE, MD, FRACP

Emeritus Professor
Monash Institute of Medical Research
Monash University
Clayton, Melbourne, Victoria, Australia

Ashley Grossman, BA, BSc, MD, FRCP, FMedSci

Professor of Neuroendocrinology
Endocrinology
St. Bartholomew's Hospital
London, United Kingdom

John C. Marshall, MD, PhD

Andrew D. Hart Professor of Internal Medicine
Director Center for Research in Reproduction
Department of Medicine
University of Virginia School of Medicine
Charlottesville, Virginia

Shlomo Melmed, MD

Senior Vice President, Academic Affairs and Dean of
the Faculty
Cedars Sinai Medical Center
Los Angeles, California

Leslie J. De Groot, MD

Research Professor
Cellular and Life Sciences
University of Rhode Island, Providence Campus
Providence, Rhode Island

John T. Potts, Jr, MD

Jackson Distinguished Professor of Clinical Medicine
Harvard Medical School;
Director of Research and Physician-in-Chief Emeritus
Department of Medicine
Massachusetts General Hospital
Boston, Massachusetts

Gordon C. Weir, MD

Head, Section on Islet Transplantation and Cell Biology
Diabetes Research and Wellness Foundation Chair
Joslin Diabetes Center;
Professor of Medicine
Harvard Medical School
Boston, Massachusetts

Harald Jüppner, MD

Professor of Pediatrics
Endocrine Unit and Pediatric Nephrology Unit
  Massachusetts General Hospital and Harvard Medical
  School
Boston, Massachusetts

Contributors

Erik K. Alexander, MD
Assistant Professor of Medicine
Department of Medicine
Brigham & Women's Hospital/Harvard Medical
  School
Boston, Massachusetts

Peter Angelos, MD, PhD, FACS
Professor and Chief of Endocrine Surgery
The University of Chicago
Chicago, Illinois

Rebecca S. Bahn, MD
Professor of Medicine
Endocrinology, Diabetes, Metabolism and
  Nutrition
Mayo Clinic
Rochester, Minnesota

John D. Baxter, MD
Senior Member, Co-Director
Diabetes Center
The Methodist Hospital Research Institute;
Chief of Endocrinology
The Methodist Hospital
Houston, Texas

Paolo Beck-Peccoz, MD
Professor of Endocrinology
Department of Medical Sciences, University of
  Milan
Fondazione Policlinico IRCCS
Milan, Italy

Manfred Blum, MD, FACP
Professor of Medicine and Radiology
Director, Thyroid Unit
Director, Nuclear Endocrine Laboratory
New York University School of Medicine
NYU Langone Medical Center
New York, New York

Steen J. Bonnema, MD, PhD
Associate Professor
Department of Endocrinology
Odense University Hospital
Odense, Denmark

Col. Henry B. Burch, MD
Chief, Endocrinology
Walter Reed Army Medical Center;
Professor of Medicine and Chair
Endocrinology Division Uniformed Services
  University of the Health Sciences
Washington, D.C.

V. Krishna Chatterjee, MD, FRCP
Professor of Endocrinology
Department of Medicine
Institute of Metabolic Science
University of Cambridge
Cambridge, United Kingdom

Luca Chiovato, MD, PhD
Professor of Endocrinology
University of Pavia
Head, Unit of Internal Medicine and
  Endocrinology
Fondazione Salvatore Maugeri IRCCS
Pavia, Italy

Daniel Christophe, PhD
Research Director FNRS and Professor of
  Molecular Biology at the ULB
Institut de Recherche Interdisciplinaire en Biologie
  Humaine et Moléculaire (IRIBHM)
Université Libre de Bruxelles (ULB)
Institut de Biologie et de Médecine Moléculaires
  (IBMM), Charleroi (Gosselies)
Brussels, Belgium

Mario De Felice, MD
Professor of Pathology
Department of Cellular and Molecular Biology and
  Pathology
University of Naples "Federico II";
Scientific Coordinator
Biogem

Leslie J. De Groot, MD
Research Professor
Cellular and Life Sciences
University of Rhode Island, Providence Campus
Providence, Rhode Island

Roberto Di Lauro, MD
Full Professor of Medical Genetics
Department of Cellular and Molecular Biology and
  Pathology
University of Naples "Federico II"
Naples, Italy

Jacques E. Dumont, MD, PhD
Honorary Professor
Iribhm
University of Brussels
Brussels, Belgium

Gianfranco Fenzi, MD, PhD
Professor of Endocrinology
Dipartimento di Endocrinologia e Oncologia
  Clinica
Università di Napoli "Federico II"
Napoli, Italy

David F. Gordon, PhD
Associate Professor
Department of Medicine/Endocrinology
University of Colorado Medical School
Aurora, Colorado

Valéria C. Guimarães, MD, PhD
Clinical Endocrinologist
Endocrinology
ENNE
Brasília-DF, Brazil

Mark Gurnell, PhD, FRCP
University Lecturer in Endocrinology
Institute of Metabolic Science and Department of
  Medicine
University of Cambridge
Cambridge, United Kingdom

Laszlo Hegedüs, MD, PhD, DMSc
Professor, University of Southern Denmark in
  Odense
Department of Endocrinology and Metabolism
Odense University Hospital, and University of
  Southern Denmark
Odense, Denmark

**Georg Hennemann, MD, PhD, FRCP,
FRCPE**
Professor of Medicine and Endocrinology
Department of Internal Medicine
Medical Center Spijkenisse
The Hague, The Netherlands

J. Larry Jameson, MD, PhD
Professor of Medicine, Dean
Northwestern University Feinberg School of
  Medicine
Northwestern University
Chicago, Illinois

Edwin L. Kaplan, MD
Professor of Surgery, Section of General Surgery
Department of Surgery
The University of Chicago
Chicago, Illinois

Meyer Knobel, MD
Associate Professor of Endocrinology, Thyroid Unit
Division of Endocrinology, Department of Internal
  Medicine
University of São Paulo Medical School
São Paulo, SP, Brazil

Knut Krohn, PhD
Head of DNA Technologies
IZKF Leipzig
University of Leipzig, Medical Faculty
Leipzig, Germany

John H. Lazarus, MD, FRCP, FACE, FRCOG
Professor of Clinical Endocrinology
Centre for Endocrine and Diabetes Sciences
Cardiff School of Medicine
Cardiff, Wales, United Kingdom

Diana L. Learoyd, MBBS, PhD, FRACP
Associate Professor
Department of Endocrinology
Royal North Shore Hospital and Sydney Medical
  School
University of Sydney
St. Leonards, New South Wales, Australia

Paolo Emidio Macchia, MD, PhD
Assistant Professor
Dipartimento di Endocrinologia ed Oncologia
    Molecolare e Clinica
Università degli Studi di Napoli "Federico II"
Napoli, Italy

Carine Maenhaut, PhD
Assistant Professor
Institute of Interdisciplinary Research (IRIBHM)
Faculty of Medicine
Free University of Brussels
Brussels, Belgium

Susan J. Mandel, MD, MPH
Professor of Medicine and Radiology
Division of Endocrinology, Diabetes, and
    Metabolism
University of Pennsylvania School of Medicine
Philadelphia, Pennsylvania

Stefania Marchisotta, MD
Post-Doc in Endocrinology
Internal Medicine, Endocrinology and Metabolism
    and Biochemistry
University of Siena
Siena, Italy

Michele Marinò, MD
Assistant Professor of Endocrinology
Department of Endocrinology and Metabolism
University of Pisa
Pisa, Italy

Geraldo Medeiros-Neto, MD, MACP
Senior Professor of Endocrinology, Thyroid Unit
Division of Endocrinology, Department of Internal
    Medicine
University of São Paulo Medical School
São Paulo, Brazil

Furio Pacini, MD
Professor of Endocrinology and Metabolism
Department of Internal Medicine, Endocrinology
    and Metabolism and Biochemistry
University of Siena
Siena, Italy

Ralf Paschke, MD, DMsc
Professor
Medical Department
Leipzig University
Leipzig, Germany

Kevin Phillips, PhD
Research Scientist
Diabetes Research Center
The Methodist Hospital Research Institute
Houston, Texas

Aldo Pinchera, MD
Professor of Endocrinology
University of Pisa,
Chief, Division of Endocrinology
University Hospital of Pisa
Pisa, Italy

Samuel Refetoff, MD
Frederick H. Rawson Professor in Medicine
Medicine, Pediatrics, and Genetics
The University of Chicago
Chicago, Illinois

E. Chester Ridgway, MD, MACP
Frederic Hamilton Professor of Medicine, Senior
    Associate Dean for Academic Affairs, Vice Chair
Department of Medicine
University of Colorado Denver School of Medicine
Aurora, Colorado

Bruce Robinson, MD, MSc, FRACP
Professor and Dean
Sydney Medical School
University of Sydney
Sydney, New South Wales, Australia

Pierre P. Roger, PhD
Senior Research Associate
Institute of Interdisciplinary Research (IRIBHM)
Université Libre de Bruxelles
Brussels, Belgium

Mary H. Samuels, MD
Professor of Medicine
Division of Endocrinology, Diabetes and Clinical
    Nutrition
Oregon Health and Science University
Portland, Oregon

Virginia D. Sarapura, MD
Associate Professor of Medicine
Department of Medicine, Division of
    Endocrinology
University of Colorado Health Sciences Center
Aurora, Colorado

Donald L. St. Germain, MD
Professor
Department of Medicine and Physiology
Dartmouth Medical School
Lebanon, New Hampshire;
Director
Maine Medical Center Research Institute,
Associate Vice President of Research
Maine Medical Center
Scarborough, Maine

Jim Stockigt, MD, FRACP, FRCPA
Professor of Medicine
Monash University,
Consultant Endocrinologist
Epworth Hospital,
Emeritus Consultant Endocrinologist
Alfred Hospital
Melbourne, Australia

Lyndal J. Tacon, MBBS, FRACP
Department of Endocrinology, Royal North Shore
    Hospital
Cancer Genetics Unit, Kolling Institute of Medical
    Research
Sydney, Australia

Gilbert Vassart, MD, PhD
Professor
IRIBHM
Faculty of Medicine
Free University Brussels
Brussels, Belgium

Theo J. Visser, PhD
Professor
Department of Internal Medicine
Erasmus MC
Rotterdam, The Netherlands

Paul Webb, PhD
Research Scientist/Associate Member
Center for Diabetes Research
The Methodist Hospital Research Institute
Houston Texas

Anthony P. Weetman, MD, DSc
Professor of Medicine
Department of Human Metabolism
University of Sheffield
Sheffield, United Kingdom

Roy E. Weiss, MD, PhD
Rabbi Esformes Professor
Chairman (interim), Department of Medicine
Chief, Section of Adult and Pediatric
    Endocrinology, Diabetes, Metabolism and
    Hypertension
The University of Chicago
Chicago, Illinois

**Wilmar M. Wiersinga,
    MD, PhD, FRCP (London)**
Professor of Endocrinology
Department of Endocrinology and Metabolism
Academic Medical Center
University of Amsterdam
Amsterdam, The Netherlands

Preface

The sixth edition of *Endocrinology, Adult and Pediatric,* starts a new and exciting project! Our text has witnessed many changes during its nearly 40-year history and multiple editions. The guiding principle has always been to provide a comprehensive and authoritative source covering the practice of clinical endocrinology, and to offer our readers coverage of the patho-physiology, patho-biochemistry, and patho-immunology behind the clinical process. We grew to three lengthy volumes, and then decided to streamline into two volumes. We added major coverage of pediatric endocrinology and cardiovascular endocrinology. With the fifth and sixth editions we added web-based versions and periodic chapter updates.

And now in response to reader interest, we offer our material rearranged for readers with selective interests: thyroid disease, diabetes mellitus and obesity, reproductive endocrinology, etc. The current volume contains all of the 25 chapters on thyroid function, thyroid testing, and diagnosis and treatment that are found in the sixth edition of our two-volume textbook. It is available at modest cost, through the miracles of the digital age and contemporary on-demand printing. If you are primarily, or especially, interested in thyroid problems, you will have access to all of the top-flight authors and top-flight chapters, without the need to carry your two-volume set—or your computer—with you. This smaller volume might even be suitable for reading at the beach, depending, of course, on competing views.

So read on and enjoy this slimmed-down version of *Endocrinology, Adult and Pediatric: Thyroid Disease.*

Leslie J. De Groot, MD

Contents

Chapter 1

ANATOMY AND DEVELOPMENT OF THE THYROID

MARIO DE FELICE and ROBERTO DI LAURO

Anatomy of the Thyroid Gland

GROSS ANATOMY

The thyroid gland was first described by Galen (130–210 AD) in his work "De Voce." The gland was named *thyroid* by Thomas Whorton (1614–1673) because of its proximity to the thyroid cartilage.[1] Despite its name (*thyreòs* in Greek means "shield"; also the German name *Schilddrüse* means "shield gland"), the characteristic shape of the thyroid, consisting of two lateral lobes connected by a narrow isthmus, is more reminiscent of a butterfly or a capital *H* than a shield (Fig. 1-1). The lateral lobes are 3 to 4 cm long and 15 to 20 mm wide and are located between the larynx and the trachea medially and the carotid sheath and the sternomastoid muscles laterally. The upper pole of the lobes reaches the level of the thyroid cartilage, while the lower pole reaches tracheal ring V-VI. The isthmus is 12 to 20 mm long, 20 mm wide, and crosses the trachea between ring I and II.

In a normal adult, the entire gland is approximately 6 to 7 cm wide, 3 to 4 cm long, and its weight ranges between 15 and 25 g. The thyroid is generally asymmetrical, the right lobe being even twice as large as the left and extending higher and lower in the neck than the left lobe. Interestingly, in patients with dextrocardia, the size of the lobes is reversed, suggesting that the asymmetry of the thyroid lobes could be connected to the position of the heart.[2] A thin connective capsule encloses the thyroid. Fibrous septa are occasionally detached from this capsule and penetrate into the parenchyma to produce an incomplete lobulation. This inner capsule is connected to an outer capsule (also called the *false capsule* of the thyroid) that is continuous with the pretracheal fascia. Blood vessels, the parathyroids, and the recurrent laryngeal nerves are located in the space between the two capsules and are in close contact with the thyroid—the parathyroids on the posterior surface of the gland and the recurrent laryngeal nerves just medial to the lateral lobes.

BLOOD SUPPLY

The thyroid is a highly vascularized organ with four arteries providing the gland with an abundant blood supply. Frequent anastomoses among these blood vessels and an arteriolar network are present on the surface of the gland; from this network, small arteries branch out and enter deeply into the tissue. The capillaries are localized in the interfollicular connective tissue, forming a basketlike network that surrounds each follicle. The capillary endothelial cells are fenestrated, like those of other endocrine glands. Each fenestration is about 50 nm in diameter. Stimulation with thyroid-stimulating hormone (TSH) increases the number and density of fenestrations.[3] The veins emerge from the thyroid parenchyma and form a plexus of three groups of veins: the superior, middle, and inferior thyroid veins.

LYMPHATICS

A rich plexus of lymphatic capillaries surrounds the thyroid follicles and communicates with small lymphatic vessels found in the interlobular connective tissue. These deep blood vessels give

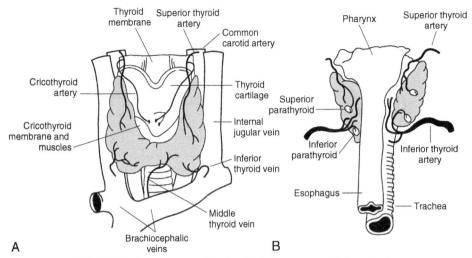

FIGURE 1-1. Gross anatomy of the thyroid. **A,** Anterior view. **B,** Posterior view.

rise to a surface network of lymphatics that drain into several groups of nodes. The uppermost group of nodes is situated just above the thyroid isthmus and is a systematic group consisting of one to five nodes called the *Delphian nodes*.[2] These are readily felt when involved in cancer or Hashimoto's thyroiditis. Other more variable groups of nodes in the thyroid area include the pretracheal nodes below the isthmus, those on the thyroid surface, and a last group found along the lateral vein, the recurrent laryngeal nerve, or along the carotid sheath.

INNERVATION

Thyroid innervation is very poor compared to that of other endocrine glands.[3] The innervation of the thyroid is provided by sympathetic, parasympathetic, and peptidergic fibers, although few fibers enter the gland.[4,5] Both sympathetic and parasympathetic fibers extend throughout the tissue among the follicles in close relation to the follicular cells or around blood vessels.

The regulator peptides detected in the thyroid are produced by both neural crest–derived parafollicular cells and intrathyroid peptidergic nerve fibers.[6,7] Some neuropeptides, such as the vasoactive intestinal peptide (VIP), neuropeptide Y,[8] substance P, or galanin, are exclusively produced in the nerve fibers distributed throughout the thyroid.[9] Presumably, these neuropeptides regulate follicular cell functions via a paracrine pathway.

ANATOMIC VARIANTS

The anatomic variants most frequently described in healthy individuals are caused by defects in the regression of the thyroglossal duct. This group of anomalies is generally characterized by the presence of an accessory lobe (pyramidal lobe) attached to the upper part of the isthmus of the thyroid (15% of the population).[2] The pyramidal lobe is a rostral-directed stalk that results from the retention and growth of the caudal end of the thyroglossal duct. Other anomalies are associated with a defective atrophy of the duct. In some instances, the entire thyroglossal duct persists as an epithelial cord connecting the foramen cecum of the tongue to the larynx; in other cases, remainders of the duct form isolated or multiple cysts along the line of descent of the duct. Persistent portions of the thyroglossal duct may differentiate into thyroid tissue and form structures called *accessory thyroids*. The presence of accessory thyroids in addition to a normally located gland is characteristic of this anomaly.

A different developmental defect results in the formation of an ectopic thyroid gland (see "Ectopic Thyroid" later in this chapter). The other frequent anatomic variant (5% of the population) is a thyroid gland that has not developed as a unique mass[2] but has the posterior part split into two distinct globes of thyroid tissue. Other anatomic anomalies are rare and found in less than 1% of healthy individuals. These variants include the absence of the isthmus (the thyroid consists of two independent lateral lobes, a physiologic condition in nonmammalian vertebrates[10]) or the absence of a significant portion of a lateral lobe, frequently the lower half of the left lobe.

The Thyroid Follicle

The thyroid gland displays a peculiar, highly-organized architecture characterized by the presence of spheroidal structures known as *follicles*. The follicles are supported by an interfollicular extracellular matrix and a capillary network. Thyroid follicles are composed of a single layer of epithelial cells (thyroid follicular cells) that surround a closed cavity (follicular lumen) filled with colloid, a concentrated solution of thyroglobulin.[11] The follicle has been defined as the "morphofunctional unit" of the thyroid.[12] As described later, thyroid follicular cells express a specific set of genes whose protein products perform functions which are essential for thyroid hormone biosynthesis. However, it is the follicular organization that, together with the polarity of the follicular cells, allows the biochemical steps required for thyroid hormone biosynthesis to occur as a functional chain of events (secretion of proteins in the follicular lumen as exocrine cells do; reabsorption and hydrolysis of proteins; release of hormones into blood by endocrine secretion[13]). The follicular architecture is absolutely required for thyroid function. In both mice[14] and humans,[15] T_4 is detected only after the differentiation of the follicles.

The follicular cell separates the follicular lumen (where hormone synthesis begins and pre-formed hormone is stored) from the bloodstream, from where iodide has to be uploaded and where hormones will be released at the end of the process. Follicular cells have a specific structural polarity established by molecular mechanisms that create specialized regions in the plasma membrane and cytoplasm.[16,17] The surface of the cells is divided into two functionally distinct but physically contiguous regions: an apical and a basolateral domain. The apical domain faces the follicle lumen and displays a differentiated tissue-specific organization that is characterized by the presence of apical microvilli, pseudopods, and by the localization of thyroperoxidase (TPO),[18] Na^+ or Cl^- channels,[19,20] pendrin,[21] and dual oxidase (Duox).[22] The basal domain faces the extracellular matrix and is characterized by the expression of sodium/iodide symporter (NIS),[23] Na^+/K^+ adenosine triphosphatase (ATPase),[24] epidermal growth factor (EGF),[25] and TSH receptors (TSHR).[26] Junctional complexes between cells separate the apical and basal domains to prevent the mixing of the proteins that are sorted asymmetrically. Thyroid hormone synthesis requires basal to apical transport of iodide and thyroglobulin.[27] Conversely, hormone secretion is based on apical to basal transport of thyroglobulin. In addition, follicular size is controlled by a bi-directional ion transport system. The basal cell plasma membrane is structurally and functionally connected by integrins to the basal lamina surrounding the follicle.[28,29] The basal lamina consists of laminin, type IV collagen, and fibronectin[30,31]; a very thin connective space—less than 2 μm wide—separates the basal lamina from the endothelial capillary cells.

In the follicles, thyroid cells form a barrier between the extrafollicular space and the lumen. A tight barrier is critical because it promotes cell polarity, guarantees efficient transport, and prevents passive back-diffusion.[32] The strong intercellular adhesion is mediated by a junctional complex that consists of tight junctions (zonula occludens), adherens junctions, and desmosomes. The three different types of cell junctions present an apical-to-basal distribution. In fact, the tight junctions are located close to the apical border of the cells, followed by the adherens junctions (located immediately below the tight junctions), and finally by the desmosomal junctions, which are positioned below the adherens junctions and occur on the plasma membrane. The anchoring junctions connect the cytoskeleton of a cell to the cytoskeleton of its neighbor or to the extracellular matrix. All these adhesion structures present the same overall organization: adhesive transmembrane proteins linked to the cytoskeleton by cytosolic adapter proteins.

Among the different types of cell junctions, the tight junctions are the structures that seal cells together. Tight junctions control the permeability of the paracellular space and define the boundary between the apical and basolateral domain of the follicular plasma membrane. They appear as a complex network of anastomosing fibrils consisting of junctional proteins responsible for cell-cell contact. This macromolecular complex interacts with different cellular structures. The major transmembrane proteins in a tight junction are occludin and claudins. The cytoplasmic portion of these proteins interacts with intracellular peripheral membrane proteins, such as ZO-1 and ZO-2,[33] which link the junction to the microfilaments. The microtubules can also be functionally linked to the tight junctions via cytoskeletal-associated proteins[34] such as cingulin, 7H6 antigen, and actin.

The epithelial adherens junctions, which as already said are located below the tight junctions, are formed by transmembrane adhesion proteins that belong to the cadherins family (cadherins and transmembrane Ca^{++}-dependent adhesion molecules). In the thyroid tissue, as well as in other epithelial tissues,[35] E-cadherin accumulates in adherens junctions and plays a crucial role in the induction of these stable adhesions, forming homophilic contacts between neighboring cells. E-cadherin is linked to an intracellular anchor protein, catenin, which in turns binds to the actin cytoskeleton. The catenins participate in intracellular signal

transduction pathways,[36] creating a functional bridge that couples physical adhesion to intracellular signaling events.

Desmosomal junctions, another type of anchoring junction, are the third type of junction present in epithelia. The transmembrane proteins found in desmosomal junctions are the desmogleins and desmocollins, members of the cadherins superfamily.[37] The cytoplasmic tails of these adhesion proteins bind intracellular proteins (plakoglobin, desmosplakin), which in turn bind to the intermediate cytoskeleton filaments. These protein-protein interactions lead to the formation of a network through the tissue that connects different adjacent cells.[38]

Follicular cells in the epithelia communicate via gap junctions.[39] Gap junctions are formed by channel-forming proteins (connexins). These channels allow inorganic ions and other small water-soluble molecules to pass directly from the cytoplasm of one cell to another, coupling the cells both electrically and metabolically.

Primary cultures of porcine thyroid follicular cells provided a useful in vitro model to understand the mechanisms leading to folliculogenesis. Follicular cells freshly isolated from pig thyroid glands and cultured in the absence of TSH aggregate only transiently.[40] In the presence of TSH, these cells assemble epithelial junctions, polarize, and organize themselves into follicle-like structures in which apical poles of cells delineate a lumen cavity. The first and essential step for in vitro folliculogenesis is cell aggregation mediated by E-cadherin. During the first few hours in culture, E-cadherin expression increases in the lateral cell surface and accumulates in the subapical regions, where the adherens junctions will be assembled.[41] ZO-1 and Na^+/K^+ ATPase are expressed. The earliest stage of cell-surface differentiation is marked by the redistribution of these two proteins: ZO-1 is recruited around the future pole of the cell, and ATPase is confined to the basal-lateral cell surface. At this stage, apical domain–associated proteins are detected in intracellular vacuoles that later fuse with the cell surface at the nascent apical pole. The follicular lumen is generated in two different steps, both of which are consequences of the polarized phenotype of thyroid cells. The first step is triggered by the lack of adhesive properties of the apical cell surface. The second step, which is required for the control of follicular size, is driven by a bi-directional ion transport system that secrets Cl^- in a basal-to-apical direction and, conversely, absorbs Na^+ in an apical-basal direction.[12]

The formation and maintenance of follicle-like structures in cultured porcine thyroid cells is dependent on TSH. In the absence of TSH or cyclic adenosine monophosphate (cAMP) stimulators, follicles undergo a morphologic conversion: thyroid cells spread and form epithelial monolayers.[42] The activation of the ERK kinase signaling pathway is involved in this conversion. TSH, acting through its second messenger cAMP, inhibits ERK activation and represses the epithelial conversion.[43] In addition, TSH modulates other steps required to maintain follicle organization.[44] Stimulation of cAMP/PKA stabilizes E-cadherin-dependent cell-cell adhesions[45] and inhibits the production of thrombospondin 1, a matricellular protein which acts as a negative modulator of cell-cell adhesion, thereby inhibiting the dissociation of tight and adherens junctions.[46] Furthermore, TSH down-regulates the expression of TGF-β1,[47] which induces the loss of epithelial polarization.[48] TSH might also control follicular lumen generation because chloride channels, located at the apical pole, are regulated by cAMP.[49]

One limitation of the data on follicle formation from in vitro studies is that it cannot be directly extrapolated to comprehend tissue follicles in vivo. Follicles in the thyroid gland are surrounded by a basal lamina, which is absent in cultured follicles.[41] Furthermore, cultured follicles invert their polarity and manifest a dramatic change in functional properties unless they are cultured with a gel consisting of extracellular matrix proteins.[50] In addition, TSH is not required for the formation of follicles in vivo, since folliculogenesis is not affected in mutant mice with impaired TSH/TSHR signaling (see heading "TSHR").

The Thyroid Cells

In addition to the stromal component, the thyroid gland is composed of three epithelial cell populations (the thyroid parenchyma) of different embryologic origin: (1) the follicular cells, the largest population, which surround the follicular lumen and are responsible for thyroid hormone synthesis; (2) the parafollicular C cells, devoted to calcitonin production; and (3) the epithelial cells, vestiges of the ultimobranchial body.

THYROID FOLLICULAR CELLS

When observed under the light microscope, thyroid follicular cells (TFCs) show a neutrophilic cytoplasm, a basal nucleus, and para-aminosalicylic acid (PAS)-positive vacuoles (phagosomes).[51] Follicular cells appear as cuboidal epithelial cells whose height is approximately 15 μm. Cells become flatter (squamous) or higher (columnar) depending on whether or not they undergo TSH stimulation.

Electron microscopy (Fig. 1-2) reveals the characteristic features of cells actively engaged in protein synthesis.[52] The rough endoplasmic reticulum and the Golgi apparatus are the dominant organelles in the cell. The apical surface of the cell is covered with thin microvilli or pseudopods that protrude into the follicular lumen. A distinctive feature of follicular cells engaged in protein synthesis is the presence of several vesicles

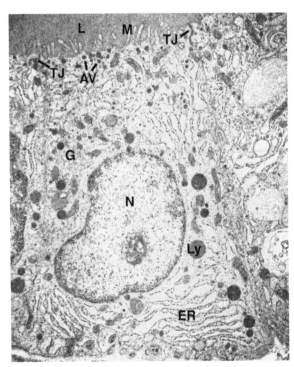

FIGURE I-2. Electron micrograph of a rat follicular cell. *AV,* Apical vesicles; *ER,* endoplasmic reticulum; *G,* Golgi apparatus; *L,* lumen; *Ly,* lysosome; *M,* microvilli; *N,* nucleus; *Tg,* thyroglobulin; *TJ,* tight junction. (Courtesy Professor L. Nitsch.)

localized in the apical or subapical cytoplasm. The smaller (150 to 200 nm) vesicles are exocytotic vesicles containing newly synthesized thyroglobulin. The fusion of these vesicles with the apical plasma membrane leads to the delivery of thyroglobulin into the follicle lumen. TPO and hydrogen peroxide–producing enzymes are localized to the luminal side of the follicular cell membrane,[18] thus allowing the iodination process to occur. The larger vesicles (500 to 4000 nm) are filled with dense material called *colloid droplets* that are the result of the uptake of the iodinated thyroglobulin stored in the follicular lumen. TSH induces the uptake of thyroglobulin from the follicle lumen, increasing the number of colloid droplets.[53] The reabsorption of the colloid involves a macropinocytosis mechanism whose first step is the formation of pseudopods at the apical pole. The pseudopods close, and a portion of the colloid is internalized into the cell.[54]

At the molecular level (Fig. 1-3), a follicular cell can be identified by the presence of a specific set of proteins—and corresponding mRNAs—indispensable for its specialized functions.[55] Among such proteins, thyroglobulin (Tg) and TPO are remarkably specific, being detectable exclusively in thyroid follicular cells. Other proteins, such as TSHR, NIS, pendrin, and Duox, though expressed in thyroid follicular cells, are also present in other tissues. The exclusive or prevalent expression of genes necessary for thyroid hormone biosynthesis in thyroid follicular cells appears to be due to a combination of transcription factors unique to this cell type.[55] These transcription factors (Nkx2-1/Ttf-1, Pax8, Foxe1) have subsequently been found to be important in controlling not only the differentiation but also the morphogenesis of the gland. The molecular features and the functions of these factors will be described further on (see "Molecular Genetics of Thyroid Gland Development").

C CELLS

C cells represent the other endocrine cellular type present in the thyroid gland of mammals. They synthesize and secrete calcitonin,[56] a polypeptide hormone involved in calcium metabolism. In lower vertebrates, C cells form an organ called the *ultimobranchial gland* that is separate from the thyroid gland. Quail chick chimera experiments have demonstrated that C cells of avian species derive from neural crest cells,[57] which during embryonic development colonize the ultimobranchial body, a transient organ in mammals, to finally disperse into the thyroid gland.[58]

C cells are known as *parafollicular cells* because of their distribution among follicular cells. However, in spite of their name, not all C cells are located between follicular cells and the basement membrane (a real parafollicular position); they are also found among the follicles (interfollicular) or in an intrafollicular position. In fact, C cells are found dispersed as individual cells in small groups closely associated to follicular cells, and in more complex structures consisting of both follicular and C cells. The number of parafollicular cells in the thyroid differs among species.[59] In humans, the number of C cells decreases with age: the neonatal thyroid has 10 times more C cells than the adult thyroid, where they are fewer than 1% of the follicular cells. These cells are usually distributed in the upper two thirds of the lateral lobe in intrafollicular and parafollicular positions.[60]

C cells are characterized by clear cytoplasm and small, compact nuclei. Electron microscopy reveals that these cells contain cytoplasmic secretory granules 100 to 200 nm in diameter.[61] At the molecular level, C cells are identified by the presence of calcitonin. The *calcitonin/calcitonin gene-related peptide (CGRP)* gene encodes four proteins: calcitonin, CGRP, katacalcin

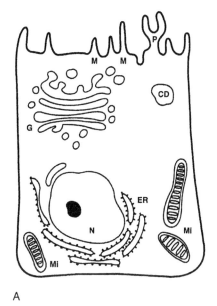

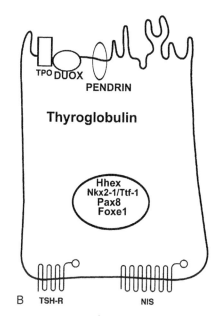

FIGURE I-3. Thyroid follicular cell. **A,** Schematic structural representation. **B,** Schematic molecular representation. *CD,* Colloid droplets; *ER,* endoplasmic reticulum; *G,* Golgi apparatus; *M,* microvilli; *MI,* mitochondrion; *N,* nucleus; *P,* pseudopod.

I and katacalcin II. The splicing of the first three exons to the fourth gives rise to an mRNA that encodes for a protein precursor which is subsequently processed to give calcitonin and a peptide, katacalcin I. CGRP and katacalcin II are the products of alternative splicing and are by far less abundant than calcitonin in C cells. CGRP is a 37-amino-acid vasoactive peptide with unknown effect on calcium metabolism.[62] Interestingly, C cells, although different from follicular cells in function and embryologic derivation, express Nkx2-1/Ttf-1,[63] which is a distinctive marker of thyroxine-producing cells. Nkx2-1/Ttf-1 is also present in immature C cells, in the migrating ultimobranchial body, and in the cells of the fourth pharyngeal pouch.[14,64,65]

Parafollicular cells share several biological features with other neuroendocrine cells that originate from the neural crest. Indeed, parafollicular cells express neuroendocrine markers such as neurospecific enolase and chromogranin A and a large number of regulatory peptides and their receptors,[66] including somatostatin, serotonin, cholecystokinin$_2$-receptor (CCK$_2$R), gastrin releasing peptide, thyrotropin-releasing hormone (TRH), and helodermin. Whether different subpopulations of parafollicular cells synthesize different sets of regulatory factors has not yet been demonstrated. However, there is some evidence of functional heterogeneity within mammalian parafollicular cells.[7] In neonatal rats, 90% of calcitonin-producing cells coexpress somatostatin, while in adults this factor is detected in only 1% of parafollicular cells.[66] Also, in humans calcitonin and somatostatin are co-localized in few parafollicular cells.[67] However, somatostatin is detected in almost all C-cell carcinomas in rats.[66] Similarly, in many human medullary thyroid carcinomas, C cells can express somatostatin.[68] The functional relevance of the production of these regulatory peptides by C cells is still unclear. These biologically active peptides might regulate thyroid function in a paracrine pathway, because parafollicular cells are distributed among follicular cells and often tightly adhered to them. Somatostatin, calcitonin, CGRP, and katacalcin inhibit thyroid hormone secretion, while gastrin-releasing peptide and helodermin stimulate this process.[7] The expression of CCK$_2$R, which binds cholecystokinin and gastrin,[69] and the observation that

gastrin induces calcitonin secretion suggest an interrelationship between calcium homeostasis and gastrointestinal hormones. In addition, the presence of CCK$_2$ in thyroid tissues allows one to hypothesize that CCK$_2$ and its receptor are both involved in an autocrine loop required for C-cell function.[69]

ULTIMOBRANCHIAL BODY–DERIVED EPITHELIAL CELLS

In addition to the common thyroid follicles, other epithelial structures are evident in the mammalian thyroid. These structures, described as a "second kind of thyroid follicles,"[70] rarely display a clear follicular organization. The finding that the second kind of thyroid follicles are absent in the avian thyroid (where ultimobranchial bodies never merge with the thyroid) has suggested that these structures represent remnants of the ultimobranchial body of endodermal origin.[71]

In humans, ultimobranchial-body remnants known as *solid cell nests* (SCN)[72] are frequently present in the thyroid gland and are preferentially located in the middle and upper third of the lobes.[72] SCN appear as para- or intrafollicular clusters and cords of epithelial cells clearly separated from the follicles by a basal lamina.

SNC are composed of two cell types: C cells and "main" cells, the most important cell population of these structures. The presence of C cells is consistent with the common ultimobranchial derivation of both SNC and C cells. In most cases, the SNC are found mixed with another structure known as a *mixed follicle,* in which follicular cells and main cells underline a lumen filled with colloid-like material.[72,73] Main cells, polygonal in shape, show squamoid features, with oval nuclei and eosinophilic cytoplasm lacking intercellular bridges. The molecular phenotype of main cells is peculiar. These cells express p63,[73] Bcl2 and telomerase.[74] They do not express markers of differentiation such as Nkx2-1/ Ttf-1, Tg, calcitonin, and CGRP. It is worth noting that recent studies in mouse embryos have revealed that Nkx2-1/Ttf-1– negative, p63-positive cells are present both in the epithelium of the fourth pharyngeal pouch and in the ultimobranchial body, confirming the SNC are ultimobranchial-body remnants.[64] The presence in the main cells of both telomerase and p63, a transcription factor present in basal/stem cells of several multilayered epithelia and absent in differentiated cells, has suggested the hypothesis that these cells could be a source of multipotent cells able to differentiate towards either Tg- or calcitonin-producing cells. In addition, it has been suggested that main cells could be the cells of origin of a subset of papillary thyroid carcinoma.[75]

Development of the Thyroid Gland

The adult thyroid gland in mammals is assembled from two different embryologic structures. This composite origin reflects the dual endocrine function of the gland. The thyroglobulin-producing follicular cells derive from a small group of endodermal cells of the primitive pharynx (the thyroid anlage). The calcitonin-producing parafollicular cells are neural crest–derived cells from the ultimobranchial bodies. The ultimobranchial bodies are transient embryonic structures originated from the fourth pharyngeal pouch. The thyroid anlage and the ultimobranchial bodies migrate from their original sites, reach their final position anterior to the trachea, and fuse to form the definitive thyroid gland. The thyroid follicles derive from the thyroid anlage cells, while the C cells are scattered within the interfollicular space. After this early ontogenetic phase, the thyroid begins to function at a basal level; subsequent differentiation of the hypothalamic nuclei and the organization of the pituitary-portal vascular system guarantee the maturation of the thyroid-system function.[76]

Data on thyroid organogenesis in humans are scarce and in many cases based on out-of-date reports. In contrast, the morphogenesis and differentiation of the thyroid have been extensively studied in animal models, mostly in the mouse and rat. Studies on patients affected by congenital hypothyroidism with thyroid dysgenesis have confirmed that identical genetic mechanisms are involved in thyroid organogenesis, both in humans and in mice. Furthermore, the recent introduction of zebrafish as a model for the analysis of thyroid development confirmed that the molecular pathways involved in the formation of the thyroid and in the differentiation of follicular cells are essentially conserved among all vertebrates.

Here we will describe in detail the morphologic and molecular aspects of thyroid development in mice (summarized in Fig. 1-4). These data can reasonably be extended to humans; the known relevant differences will be highlighted.

SPECIFICATION OF THE THYROID FOLLICULAR CELLS: THE THYROID ANLAGE

Gastrulation involves dramatic changes in the overall structure of the embryo, converting it into a complex three-dimensional structure. The anterior and posterior endoderm invaginates, forming two pockets which extend and fuse, generating a primitive gut tube that runs along the anterior-posterior axis of the embryo. The foregut is the most anterior (cranial) region of this tube. The endoderm of the foregut gives rise to a number of cell lineages which eventually form the epithelial components of thyroid, thymus, lungs, stomach, liver, and pancreas. All organs derived from the gut tube undergo a rather similar process. First, a restricted group of cells differentiate from their neighbors, as can be visualized both by the appearance of specific molecular markers (usually transcription factors) and by the almost simultaneous appearance of a multilayered structure. Subsequently, all organs undergo a morphogenetic process that entails, depend-

ing on the organ, proliferation, branching morphogenesis, and/or migration or a combination of these processes. Finally, each organ forms a specific cellular organization that is directly correlated to the organ function (i.e., follicular organization in the case of the thyroid). The first differentiation step in this process will be called throughout this chapter *specification*, even though the term usually refers to a reversible process; in the case of all organs derived from the gut, it is at present unknown whether the first differentiation event is either reversible or irreversible.

While the inductive mechanisms by which endodermal cells produce liver, pancreas, and lung cell lineage begin to be detailed, the events that commit a group of multipotent endodermal cells to a thyroid fate are almost unknown. The first morphologic consequence of thyroid specification is the appearance of the thyroid anlage (also called *thyroid placode*). In the mouse (19.5-day-long gestation) it is visible at embryonic day (E)8 to 8.5 and in humans at E22.[77] In both the species, the thyroid anlage appears as a midline endodermal thickening in the ventral wall of the primitive pharynx caudal to the region of the first branchial arch that forms the tuberculum impar[78] (see Fig. 1-4). The cells of the thyroid anlage simultaneously express four transcription factors: Hhex,Nkx2-1/Ttf-1, Pax8 and Foxe1.[79] This unique molecular signature hallmarks these cells, which can be defined as the *precursors* of the TFCs.

The genetic program directing the specification of thyroid precursor cells is rather obscure. Any genes relevant in the patterning process of the foregut, such as *Nodal*, members of the *Gata* family, or *Sox* genes could play a role in thyroid specification. As yet, there have been no reports of either cell-fate mapping studies or genetically modified mice clarifying the early steps of the thyroid specification. Actually, mouse embryos carrying targeted inactivation of genes involved in foregut patterning usually show developmental arrest at stages that preclude the assessment of the thyroid anlage. In zebrafish, Bon and Gata5, two transcription factors that are downstream effectors of Nodal activity, seem to be specifically involved in the commitment of thyroid fate. Indeed, in the absence of these factors, endodermal cells form a reduced gut tissue but do not contribute to the thyroid.[80]

The study of the developing thyroid in mice has shown that at E8.5, the earliest identifiable thyroid anlage appears in close apposition to the aortic sac, the cardiac region that gives rise to the embryonic heart outflow and pharyngeal arteries. This observation suggests that short-range inductive signals from cardiac mesoderm or from the endothelial lining of the aortic sac could have an inductive role to specify undifferentiated endodermal cells towards a thyroid fate. In mice, alterations in the foregut have been observed as a consequence of an impaired heart development[81]; furthermore, it has been reported that signals from cardiac tissue adjacent to the endodermal layer are crucial in the early stages of liver, pancreas, and lung development.[82-84]

Data obtained from zebrafish are proving invaluable for the study of thyroid specification. The close association between thyroid anlage and aortic sac is maintained also in zebrafish.[85] In this species it has been demonstrated that in the absence of the basic Helix-loop-helix (bHLH) transcription factor Hand2, expressed in the cardiac mesoderm surrounding the site of initiation of thyroid development, the endoderm appears to be normal, but thyroid precursor cells are not present. Experiments strongly suggest both that Hand2 has a non–cell-autonomous role in thyroid specification and that FGF proteins participate in this pathway.[85] Interestingly, in mice it has been proved that FGF signals are required for correct thyroid development, but the

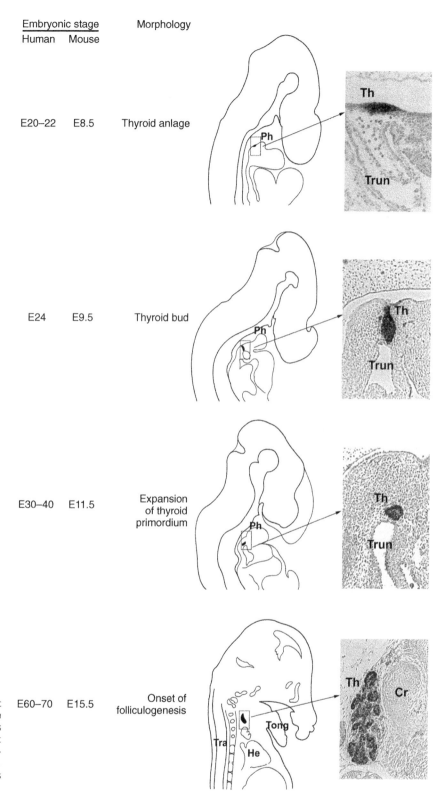

FIGURE 1-4. Thyroid development. In the *middle* is a schematic representation of the different steps of thyroid organogenesis in mouse embryos; on the *left*, the correspondent embryonic stages (*E*, embryonic day) in mice and humans are indicated; on the *right* relevant sagittal sections of mouse embryos stained with an anti-Nkx2-1/Ttf-1 are shown. *Cr*, Cricoid cartilage; *He*, heart; *Ph*, pharynx; *Th*, thyroid; *Tong*, tongue; *Tra*, trachea; *Trun*, truncus arteriosus.

role of these factors in thyroid specification has never been demonstrated.[86]

Consistent with the hypothesis of a role of cardiac tissue in thyroid development are the findings that cardiac malformations represent the most frequent birth defects associated with thyroid dysgenesis in humans,[87] and DiGeorge syndrome is characterized by both congenital heart defects and an increased risk of congenital hypothyroidism.[88]

EARLY STAGES OF THYROID MORPHOGENESIS: BUDDING, MIGRATION, AND LOBULATION OF THE THYROID PRIMORDIUM

After the specification stage, the developing thyroid undergoes very rapid changes in its appearance. In mice, by E8.5 the thyroid anlage first appears as a multilayered epithelium. Shortly after, it forms a bud that, evaginating from the floor of the pharynx, invades the surrounding mesenchyma as an endodermal extro-flexion close to the aortic sac. In these early stages of morphogenesis, the expansion of the thyroid primordium does not seem to be due to the proliferation of cells of the primitive thyroid anlage; indeed, these cells show a very low cell proliferation rate as compared to that of the cells of the surrounding endoderm. Other cells from the pharyngeal endoderm could be recruited into the developing thyroid, thus contributing to the increase of the number of thyroid progenitor cells.[89] At E10.5, the thyroid bud has a flask-shaped structure still connected to the floor of the pharynx by a thin cord, the thyroglossal duct, a transient narrow channel. One day later, the thyroid bud is visible as a caplike shape that has migrated caudally into the mesenchyme, losing all connections with the floor of the pharynx (see Fig. 1-4). At this stage, the developing thyroid begins to expand laterally, the first step of the process that eventually leads to the formation of the two lobes. At E12.5, the thyroid primordium appears as an elongated structure, extended laterally, in contact with the third pharyngeal arch arteries that will participate in the formation of the definitive carotid vessels.

By E13, the thyroid bud continues its downward relocation into the mesenchyme and approaches the ultimobranchial bodies that are accomplishing their ventro-caudal migration from the fourth pharyngeal pouch. By E13.5, the developing thyroid, already formed by rudimental lobes connected by a thin central portion, reaches its definitive pretracheal position where it merges with the ultimobranchial bodies containing the precursors of C cells derived from the neural crest.[78] Once the gland reaches its final location, the two rudimentary paratracheal lobes expand, and by E15 and 16, the thyroid gland assumes its definitive shape (see Fig. 1-4). In the last stages of thyroid organogenesis, the gland increases further in size, probably due to the high proliferation of TFCs.

In humans, as described in mice, at an early stage of embryonic life, the thyroid anlage appears as a bud invading the mesenchyma at E26; in a few days it appears as a migrating primordium, connected to the pharynx by the thyroglossal duct that disappears around E37. At this stage, the thyroid bud acquires a bilobed shape. The developing thyroid merges with the ultimobranchial bodies by the sixth week and reaches its final position in front of the trachea around the seventh week.[90]

The translocation of TFC precursors to reach the sublaryngeal position is a process that lasts for almost 4 days in the mouse embryo and almost 4 weeks in the human embryo. Budding and translocation from the gut tube is a developmental process shared by many endoderm-derived organs.[91] In the case of the thyroid, since the definitive location is rather distant from the site of primitive specification, this process mostly involves active migration of the precursors, even if other morphogenetic events occurring in the neck region and in the mouth[92] could contribute to the definitive location of the thyroid. The molecular mechanisms involved in the movement of the thyroid primordium are still a matter of debate. In many processes of embryogenesis, such as gastrulation, neural-crest migration, and heart formation, cell migration is involved. However, in these processes, migrating cells lose the epithelial phenotype and acquire mesenchymal features.[93] This phenomenon, called *epithelial-mesenchymal transition*, is hallmarked by an increased expression of N-cadherin and the down-regulation of E-cadherin. In contrast, TFC precursors seem to use a different and yet unidentified pathway to move, because they maintain their epithelial phenotype throughout the entire translocation process and never acquire a mesenchymal identity.[94] The expression of transcription factors such as either Hhex or Pax8 or Nkx2-1/Ttf-1 is not sufficient for

thyroid migration, while Foxe1 plays a crucial role because the presence of this factor in the thyroid bud is required to allow the cells to move.[79,95]

The genetic basis of the formation of two symmetrical lateral lobes (lobulation) is beginning to be understood. When the lobulation process begins at E11.5, the developing thyroid is in contact with the third pharyngeal arch arteries that will participate in the formation of the definitive carotid vessels located most closely to the mature thyroid lobes. Signals originating from adjacent vessels or factors regulating vasculogenesis could instruct the process of lobulation by non–cell-autonomous mechanisms. The study of animal models seems to confirm this hypothesis. Mice deficient in either Shh (a key regulator of embryogenesis)[96] or TBX (a factor regulated by Shh itself)[88] display a disturbed morphogenetic patterning of vessels adjacent to the developing thyroid. In these mutated embryos, as a consequence of the absence of caudal pharyngeal arch arteries, the thyroid bud is never in close contact with vessels, and the lobulation process is impaired. The thyroid fails to separate into two distinct lobes, maintaining the shape of a single tissue mass throughout development. In line with these findings is the observation that thyroid dysgenesis is not uncommon in patients affected by DiGeorge syndrome,[97] characterized by congenital anomalies of the heart and great vessels. However, the inductive signals from adjacent tissues must interact with events restricted to the thyroid cells to accomplish the lobulation process. Indeed, thyroid hemiagenesis is very frequent in mice double heterozygous for the null allele of *Nkx2-1/Ttf-1* and *Pax8*, genes expressed in thyroid precursor cells and absent in other structures close to the developing thyroid.[98]

LATE STAGES OF THYROID MORPHOGENESIS: FUNCTIONAL DIFFERENTIATION AND HISTOGENESIS

When the thyroid primordium reaches the sublaryngeal position, TFC precursors accomplish their functional differentiation. Notably, the normal final location of thyroid follicular cells in front of the trachea is not an essential requirement for functional differentiation, since an ectopic, sublingual thyroid expresses thyroglobulin in both human patients[99] and mutated mice.[95]

The functional differentiation of TFCs is hallmarked by the expression of a series of proteins essential for thyroid hormone biosynthesis, such as Tg, TPO, TSHR, NIS, Duox, and pendrin. This program requires almost 3 days, between E14 and E16.5, and results in the differentiation of the thyroid primordium in a functional thyroid gland that is able to produce and release hormones. *Tg* and *Tshr* genes are expressed by E14[100]; TPO and NIS, the two key enzymes involved in the process of Tg iodination appear between E15 and E15.5,[101] probably because their expression is absolutely dependent on the pathway activated by the binding of TSH to its receptor, TSHR.[101] Duox appears at E15.5[102] and finally, thyroxine by E16.5.[14]

Alongside functional differentiation, the thyroid gland accomplishes its peculiar histologic organization. An inductive role of the stromal component surrounding follicular cells can be hypothesized in histogenesis. Accordingly, follicular cells, when explanted from a developing chick thyroid, can organize a correct histologic pattern in vitro only if co-cultured in the presence of fibroblasts obtained from the capsule of a thyroid gland.[103] By E15.5, TFCs start to form small rudimentary follicles, as revealed by the expression of ZO-1, a tight-junction marker. At E16.5, the gland displays an evident follicular organization. The histogenesis is complete in late fetal life between E17 and E18: the thyroid parenchyma is organized into small follicles surrounded by a capillary network, enclosing thyroglobulin in their lumen.[89] At birth, the thyroid gland is able to produce and release thyroid hormones, though the regulation of its growth and function by the hypothalamic-pituitary axis is fully active only after birth.[104]

The molecular mechanisms involved in the differentiation of the human thyroid are not much different from those found in mice. Functional differentiation of TFCs requires almost 3 weeks. It begins after the developing thyroid is located in front of the trachea, at E48, when TFCs express Tg and TSHR; T_4 synthesis is detected at the 10th week.[90] In humans, the establishment of the characteristic histologic organization lasts several weeks and can be divided into three phases: the precolloid, the beginning colloid, and the follicular growth, which occur at 7 to 10, 10 to 11, and after 11 weeks of gestation, respectively.[76] In the precolloid phase, small intracellular canaliculi develop as an accumulation of colloid material. These small canaliculi enlarge, and the colloid organizes itself into extracellular spaces. In the last phase, primary follicles are clearly visible, and the fetal thyroid is able to concentrate iodide and synthesize thyroid hormones. The human thyroid continues to expand until term, and contrary to mice, the hypothalamic-pituitary-thyroid axis starts functioning at mid-gestation.

It is widely accepted that thyroglobulin-producing cells are derived from the endodermal cells of the thyroid anlage. However, the thyroid is assembled from both thyroid anlage and ultimobranchial bodies. Because of this composite origin, the question arises whether the neural crest–derived cells of ultimobranchial bodies (fated to become calcitonin-producing parafollicular cells) could also differentiate towards thyroglobulin-producing cells. In fish, amphibians, and birds, Tg- and calcitonin-producing cells are found in separate gland organs. In addition, lineage studies in zebrafish suggest that ultimobranchial bodies do not contribute to the development of the thyroid, which derives completely from the endodermal cells of the thyroid anlage.[105]

In mammals, where endodermal cells from thyroid anlage and ultimobranchial bodies merge in the definitive gland, the contribution of the different cell lineages to the TFC population is still controversial. In the past, embryologists considered the ultimobranchial bodies as the lateral anlage of the thyroid, whose cells were fated to differentiate towards the typical follicular cells and become a definitive component of the mature gland.[106] This hypothesis is consistent with the report of patients displaying thyroid tissue in the submandibular region and no detectable thyroid tissue in the normal median position.[107] Furthermore, structures appearing as colloid-containing follicles have been observed in ultimobranchial bodies which fail to fuse with the thyroid bud (persistent ultimobranchial body).[108] Data suggesting that thyroid follicular cells could originate from ultimobranchial bodies are supported by the study of some murine models displaying persistent ultimobranchial bodies.[109-112] In mice, the size of the follicular thyroid appears smaller than would be expected if only cells contributed by ultimobranchial bodies were missing. However, it is worth noting that the expression of follicular cell-specific genes (such as Tg or TPO) in the ultimobranchial bodies has not been described. Thus, there is no conclusive evidence that these cells can differentiate in cells producing thyroid hormones.

ULTIMOBRANCHIAL BODIES DEVELOPMENT

In vertebrates, calcitonin-producing cells differentiate from the ultimobranchial body, a structure that derives from the fourth pharyngeal pouch. The ultimobranchial body is a definitive organ in all vertebrates except in placental mammals, where it is an embryonic transient structure fated to join the medial thyroid bud.

By E10 in mice, the fourth pharyngeal pouch is evident for the first time. It appears as a lateral extroflexion of the primitive foregut expressing both the transcription factor Islet1 (Isl)[113] and protein gene product (PGP)9.5.[114,115] Shortly after, the caudal portion of the pouch grows, and at E11.5 the fourth pharynx-branchial duct is pinched off, forming an ultimobranchial body primordium visible as an ovoid vesicle with a lumen lined by a columnar epithelium identified by the simultaneous presence of Isl1, PGP9.5, and Nkx2-1/Ttf-1.[64,114,115] By E11.5 ultimobranchial body primordia migrate, and at E13 they appear as solid clusters of cells in contact with the midline primordium of the thyroid. By E14.5, ultimobranchial body cells begin to disperse within the thyroid parenchyma, and 1 day later only remnants of ultimobranchial bodies can be distinguished in the thyroid gland. C cells complete their differentiation program through the expression of a series of proteins according to a precise temporal pattern: the basic helix-loop-helix transcription factor Mash1 is expressed by E12.5; the neuronal markers TuJ1, CGRP, and somatostatin by E14.5. One day later, the expression of Mash1 disappears, and calcitonin-producing cells can be detected between follicular cells. During the late stages of thyroid morphogenesis, the expression of Isl1 decreases,[113] while calcitonin-producing cells gradually increase in number.[114,115]

In humans, the development of ultimobranchial bodies is similar to that of mice. At E24 the ultimobranchial body primordia appear as an outpouching of the ventral component of the fourth pharyngeal pouch. At this stage, the primordium of parathyroid IV is visible as a dorsal evagination of the same pouch. Some authors describe a transient fifth pouch as the endodermal origin of the ultimobranchial body.[116] Probably the shape of the ultimobranchial body anlage itself, which appears as an incomplete pouch, has generated these different interpretations. By E35 the ventral extroflexion is a long-necked flask still attached to the pharynx; a few days later, the ultimobranchial body primordium loses its connection with the pharyngeal cavity, starts its migration, and at E40 reaches the posterior surface of the median thyroid. A connective layer separates these two buds, which display a different histologic organization: the lateral bud is composed of a compact mass of cells, while the median bud is composed of interconnecting sheets of epithelium. Finally, at E55 the ultimobranchial bodies are incorporated with the lateral lobes of the thyroid, and the cells from both structures mix with each other.

The genetic mechanisms that allow the developing thyroid and ultimobranchial body to recognize each other and fuse are beginning to be understood. Ultimobranchial bodies are absent in Splotch mutant mice,[117] a strain characterized by an impaired migration of neural crest cells due to a loss-of-function mutation in Pax3, a gene expressed in the migrating neural crest cells.[118] The absence of ultimobranchial bodies is also reported in Pax9 null mice.[119] Pax9 is expressed in the entire pharyngeal endoderm and has been reported to be involved in the regulation of epithelial-mesenchymal interactions that are crucial for the correct morphogenesis of both teeth[119] and thymus.[120] Ultimobranchial body defects have been reported in mice carrying mutations in Hox3 paralog genes. In Hoxa-3 null mice,[110] the migration of neural crest cells is not impaired and C cells differentiate correctly, but their number is significantly reduced. In many cases, ultimobranchial bodies fail to fuse with the thyroid bud and remain as bilateral vesicles composed exclusively of calcitonin-producing cells (persistent ultimobranchial bodies). The phenotype appears more severe in mice carrying various mutant combinations in *Hoxa3* and its paralogs *Hoxb3* and *Hoxd3*.[111] These data indicate that *Hox3* paralogs do not play a direct role in the migration and differentiation of C cells but control the correct development of the ultimobranchial body and its fusion to the ventral thyroid primordium. Another gene, *Eya1*, expressed in the pharyngeal arches mesenchyme and in the endoderm pouches, could control the interactions between ultimobranchial bodies and the thyroid primordium. Indeed, mice in which the *Eya1* gene has been inactivated show fewer calcitonin-producing cells and persistent ultimobranchial bodies.[112] Thus both Hoxa3 and Eya1 seem to control the merging of ultimobranchial bodies and thyroid primordium, a step in thyroid gland organogenesis that only occurs in mammals. Recently it has been demonstrated that Nkx2-1/Ttf-1is required for the survival of ultimobranchial body cells during migration, but it is not necessary for ultimobranchial body formation.[64] Nkx2-1/Ttf-1 functions are in part dosage sensitive. Indeed, *Nkx2-1/Ttf-1[+/-]* mice display an abnormal fusion of the ultimobranchial bodies with the thyroid diverticulum. Ultimobranchial body cells are incompletely incorporated into the thyroid parenchyma and remain at the dorsal part of the thyroid lobe.[64] A phenotype similar to that has been reported in mice defective for *Hox3* genes.

DIFFERENTIATION OF C CELLS

It is generally accepted that C-cell precursors do not originate from the endodermal epithelium of the pouches but derive from the cells of the neural crest that, during early development, colonize the ventral part of the fourth pharyngeal pouches. The ontogenesis and differentiation of C cells were initially studied in birds, using quail chick chimeras as models.[57] The analysis of this model demonstrated that avian C-cell precursors, derived from the neural crest, colonize the ultimobranchial bodies. Neural crest cells originate early in embryonic life at the boundary between neural and non-neural ectoderm. The cells undergo an epithelial-mesenchymal transition, delaminate from the neural tube, migrate, and reach different areas of the embryo, where they differentiate into a variety of cell types. In birds, C-cell precursors probably originate from the vagal region of the neural crest that also gives rise to serotonergic enteric neurons. Indeed, mature C cells and serotonergic enteric neurons share some biochemical and morphologic features.[121]

In birds, the thyroid diverticulum does not fuse with the ultimobranchial bodies, which remain as distinct glands,[122] but in mammals, the thyroid primordium and ultimobranchial bodies merge in the definitive thyroid gland. Experimental transplantation and ablation studies in mice[123] suggest that precursors of C cells colonize the mesenchyme of the fourth pharyngeal pouch around E9 to E9.5 and a day later are localized in the endodermal layer of the pouch. However, no experimental evidence of the neural crest origin of these cells is available. Recently, fate-mapping techniques using neural crest–specific transgenes have challenged the ectodermal origin of C cells in mice,[114] and it has been proposed that these cells can be derived from the endodermal epithelium of the fourth pharyngeal pouch. Consistent with this hypotheses are the findings that precursors of C cells express Isl1, a gene expressed along the endoderm and absent in neural crest cells.[113]

The genetic pathway controlling the differentiation of C cells is unknown. It is worth noting that expression of neuronal genes (such as TuJ1, CGRP, and somatostatin) in precursor C cells follows the expression of Mash1.[114,115] This gene is involved in the differentiation of autonomic neurons.[124] The relevance of Mash1 for C-cell differentiation is confirmed by the finding that

Mash1 null mutant mice lack thyroid C cells.[115] These mutant mice show a normal formation and migration of ultimobranchial bodies, but precursor C cells degenerate before they become differentiated C cells. It has been suggested that the transmembrane receptor tyrosine kinase Ret could also be involved in C-cell differentiation. Indeed, Ret is expressed in precursors of C cells at early stages of development, and the expression of this receptor continues in adult C cells. The role of Ret in the development of C cells has not yet been elucidated. At E18, calcitonin-producing cells are present in the thyroid of *Ret* null mouse embryos, even though the number is reduced compared to a wild type thyroid. These data suggest that only a subgroup of C cells (or their progenitor) require Ret/GDNF signaling to differentiate or to survive.[125]

Molecular Genetics of Thyroid Gland Development

ANIMAL MODELS

The discovery of transcription factors, which regulate the expression of follicular cell-specific genes in the mature thyroid and are also expressed in the thyroid primordium, offered a useful tool to explore the genetic basis of the developmental process of the thyroid gland. At E8.5 epithelial cells fated to become thyroid follicular cells are unequivocally individualized in the endodermal layer of the primitive pharynx. These cells are characterized by the expression of Nkx2-1/Ttf-1,[100] Foxe1,[126] Pax8,[127] and Hhex.[128] Although these transcription factors are also expressed in other embryonic tissues, the coexpression of all four is only seen in the presumptive thyroid anlage when the thickening of proliferating cells appears in the midline of the floor of the primitive pharynx. When the thyroid diverticulum forms and begins its migration, only the thyroid primordium still expresses Nkx2-1/Ttf-1, Foxe1, Pax8 and Hhex, while the thyroglossal duct does not.[100] These four factors remain expressed and are a hallmark of differentiated thyroid follicular cells (Table 1-1). Their expression is down-regulated only after transformation of the cells.[129] The hypothesis that the expression of these four factors is required at early stages of thyroid morphogenesis has been confirmed by studies on both animal models and patients affected by thyroid dysgenesis.[86,130] However, the presence of these genes is not sufficient to guarantee a correct organogenesis of the gland. Mutations in other genes, both thyroid-enriched and ubiquitous, have been demonstrated to impair the development of the thyroid. Here we summarize what we know at the moment about the molecular genetics of thyroid development, mainly as deduced by the phenotype of knockout animals.

Nkx2-1/Ttf-1

Nkx2-1/Ttf-1 (formerly TTF-1, for thyroid transcription factor 1, or T/EBP) is a transcription factor that recognizes and binds to specific DNA sequences via a 61-amino-acid long DNA binding domain called a *homeodomain*. The homeodomain sequence is conserved from the fruit fly to humans. Nkx2-1/Ttf-1 was initially identified in a rat thyroid cell line[131] as a nuclear protein able to bind to specific sequences in the *Tg* promoter. The corresponding cDNA was subsequently cloned, and comparative sequence analyses demonstrated that Nkx2-1/Ttf-1 has a considerable degree of homology to the *Drosophila* NK-2 class of homeodomain proteins.

Table 1-1. Expression of Relevant Genes and Capacity to Produce Thyroid Hormones at Different Stages of Thyroid Development in Mice

	Controller Genes		Functional Differentiation			
	Nkx2-1/Ttf-1					
	Foxe1					
	Pax8					
Embryonic Day	*Hhex*	*Ffgr2*	Tg, Tshr	TPO, NIS	Duox	Thyroid Hormones
E8.5	+	−	−	−	−	−
E11.5	+	+	−	−	−	−
E14-14.5	+	+	+	−	−	−
E15-15.5	+	+	+	+	−	−
E15.5-16	+	+	+	+	+	−
E16.5	+	+	+	+	+	+

Nkx2-1/Ttf-1 is a member of the Nkx2 class of transcription factors and is encoded by a single gene whose official name is *Nkx2-1* in mice and *NKX2-1* in humans, located on chromosome 12 and on chromosome 14q13,[132] respectively. The gene is formed by at least three exons that express multiple transcripts.[133,134] The most abundant is the shorter isoform, a 2.3-kilobase (kb) mRNA which encodes a 42-kD protein 371 amino acids long in humans.[135] In the lung, a longer protein has also been detected; however, the biological relevance of the various proteins is unclear. Functional studies have determined that the homeodomain is responsible only for the binding to DNA,[136] while the transactivating activity resides in two domains, N and C, localized at the NH_2 and COOH ends of the protein, respectively.[137] These two domains appear redundant in in vitro assay but could have different functions in vivo. In fact, a number of interactors of Nkx2-1/Ttf-1 have been identified that bind specifically to either the N or C domain. Nkx2-1/Ttf-1 is phosphorylated in several serine residues.[138] This posttranslation modification could regulate Nkx2-1/Ttf-1 activity. Indeed, a mouse model harboring an unphosphorylated *Nkx2-1/Ttf-1* allele shows impaired differentiation of both thyroid and lung.[139]

The expression pattern of Nkx2-1/Ttf-1 has been exhaustively studied in rodents. Nkx2-1/Ttf-1 is expressed in the thyroid, lung, and brain. In mouse embryos, Nkx2-1/Ttf-1 is detected in the developing thyroid as soon as the thyroid anlage is visible (E8.5).[100] Interestingly, Nkx2-1/Ttf-1 is present also in the epithelial cells of the four pharyngeal pouches forming the ultimobranchial body.[64] In the adult thyroid, Nkx2-1/Ttf-1 maintains its expression in both follicular and parafollicular C cells.[63] During embryonic life, Nkx2-1/Ttf-1 is detected in the epithelial cells of the developing trachea and lungs; in adults, it is present in bronchiolar epithelial Clara cells and in type II alveolar cells. As for the brain, Nkx2-1/Ttf-1 is expressed in some areas of the developing diencephalon, such as the hypothalamic areas and the infundibulum from which the neurohypophysis develops.[100] Nkx2-1/Ttf-1 expression in adult hypothalamus is faint but is up-regulated before the onset of puberty.[140] In human embryos, the expression pattern of Nkx2-1/Ttf-1 is not different from that of mice except that Nkx2-1/Ttf-1 is not detected in the fourth pharyngeal pouch.[77]

Gene targeting experiments have allowed in vivo study of the role of this transcription factor. In the absence of Nkx2-1/Ttf-1, newborn mice immediately die at birth and are characterized by impaired morphogenesis of both lung and brain and lack of thyroid and the entire pituitary[141] (Fig. 1-5). In *Nkx2-1/Ttf-1* null newborns, the lungs appear as dilated saclike structures without normal pulmonary parenchyma[141]; furthermore, the trachea has a reduced number of cartilage rings and is not separated from

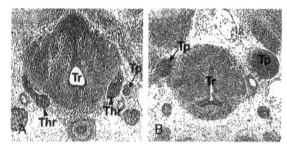

FIGURE 1-5. Thyroid gland phenotype in *Nkx2-1/Ttf-1* mouse embryos. Transversal sections of E13 wt **(A)** and *Nkx2-1/Ttf-1*$^{-/-}$ **(B)** mouse embryos stained with hematoxylin/eosin. In *Nkx2-1/Ttf-1* null embryos, the thyroid primordium is absent. *Thr,* Thyroid; *Tr,* trachea; *Tp,* Thymic primordium. (From Kimura S, Hara Y, Pineau T et al: The T/ebp null mouse: Thyroid-specific enhancer-binding protein is essential for the organogenesis of the thyroid, lung, ventral forebrain, and pituitary. Genes Dev 10:60–69, 1996.)

the esophagus.[142] In the case of the brain, alterations in the ventral region of the forebrain are evident.[143] In addition, both neurohypophysis and anterior hypophysis are absent. As a consequence of the lack of signals from the pituitary, the morphogenesis of adrenal glands is impaired too.[141]

In *Nkx2-1/Ttf-1* null embryos, the thyroid anlage forms in its correct position, but at an early stage, the morphogenesis of the gland is impaired. The thyroid primordium by E10 is hypoplastic; subsequently it undergoes degeneration probably due to apoptosis.[144] The ultimobranchial bodies undergo the same process; they form but degenerate by E12.[64] Hence, Nkx2-1/Ttf-1 is dispensable for the initial commitment of both follicular and parafollicular thyroid cells. However, both cell types that will form the thyroid gland require Nkx2-1/Ttf-1 for their survival. In the absence of this transcription factor, no thyroid rudiment is detectable. The genetic pathways defective in *Nkx2-1/Ttf-1* null embryos have been only partially elucidated. In the case of the developing thyroid, we know that Nkx2-1/Ttf-1 is part of a network that includes Pax8, Hhex, and Foxe1. Actually, the expression of these factors is slightly (Pax8) or strongly (Hhex and Foxe1) reduced in the absence of Nkx2-1/Ttf-1.[79]

We do not know which genes are controlled by Nkx2-1/Ttf-1 factor in the thyroid primordium. A detailed analysis of the phenotype of other tissues, such as lung and brain, reveals that when Nkx2-1/Ttf-1 is absent, the expression of Bmp4, a TGF-β-related peptide growth factor that is required for the proximal-distal patterning of the lung bud, is abolished.[142] In *Nkx2-1/Ttf-1* null embryos, Fgf8 is down-regulated in the infundibulum of the pituitary, probably causing the regression of the pituitary primordium in these embryos.[145] These data indicate that both in the lung and in the pituitary, signaling molecules that are important for a further specification of preformed structures are controlled by Nkx2-1/Ttf-1. A similar role could be hypothesized also for the developing thyroid. The finding that Fgfr2 is expressed in the thyroid bud suggests that Nkx2-1/Ttf-1 could regulate the survival of the precursor thyroid cells through an Fgf-dependent mechanism.[86]

In *Nkx2-1/Ttf-1* null mice, the thyroid primordium disappears before TFC precursors accomplish their differentiation. For this reason, information on the function of this factor in differentiated TFC is scarce. A mutated mouse in which *Nkx2-1/Ttf-1* has been disrupted only in the thyroid gland in the middle of organogenesis presents a variable phenotype: either the thyroid follicles appear atrophic, or the thyroid shows a reduced number of dilated follicles.[146] This indicates the requirement of Nkx2-1/Ttf-1 in adult life to maintain the follicular structure of the gland.

Other studies on culture cell lines can offer data on the role of Nkx2-1/Ttf-1 in terminal differentiated cells. In the promoters of thyroid-specific or enriched genes, such as *Tg, TPO, Tshr* and *NIS*, consensus sequences recognized by Nkx2-1/Ttf-1 have been identified. Nkx2-1/Ttf-1 has also been shown to be able to bind in vitro to its own 5′-flanking region.[147] In both *Tg* and *TPO* proximal promoters, multiple Nkx2-1/Ttf-1 binding sites are present, and transfection assays have demonstrated that binding of Nkx2-1/Ttf-1 to these sites leads to the activation of *Tg* or *TPO* promoters.

Pax8

Pax8 (paired box gene 8) is a member of a family of transcription factors characterized by the presence of a 128-amino-acid domain that recognizes and binds to specific DNA sequences. This DNA binding domain is called a *paired domain* because it was first identified in the *Drosophila* segmentation gene as paired. Pax8 was identified in the mouse as a protein expressed in the developing thyroid gland.[127] Further studies demonstrated that the Pax8 paired domain recognizes and binds to a single site present in the *Tg* and in *TPO* promoters.[148]

The gene encoding Pax8 is located on chromosome 2 in mice,[89,127] and the human orthologue, *PAX8*, is located on chromosome 2q12-q14.[149] It consists of 12 exons[150] that encode for different alternative spliced transcripts,[151] at least six different transcripts in the mouse and five in humans. All the isoforms generated share the paired domain located near the amino terminus and differ in their carboxy-terminal regions. Pax8a, the most abundant protein isoform, is 457 amino acids long in mice[127] and 450 amino acids long in humans.[152]

Pax8 is expressed in kidney, in the nervous system, and in the thyroid.[127] At an early stage in the developing kidney, Pax8 is expressed in the nephrogenic cord and in mesonephric tubules; then it is present in the cortex of the metanephros. In the adult kidney, Pax8 is clearly detected in the medullar zone. In embryos, Pax8 is transiently expressed in the myelencephalon, through the entire length of the neural tube, otic vesicle, and at the midbrain-hindbrain boundary[127] but is no longer detected by E12.5. As for the thyroid, Pax8 is expressed in the thyroid follicular cells and in their precursors from the early stages of gland morphogenesis.

Recently it has been reported that Pax8 is expressed in the uterine epithelium, the luminal epithelium of the oviduct, and vagina in 3-week-old as well as sexually mature female mice.[153,154] In males, a strong Pax8 mRNA expression was observed in the epithelium of the epididymis.[155] In humans, PAX8 is detected in the developing thyroid, kidneys, otic vesicle, and central nervous

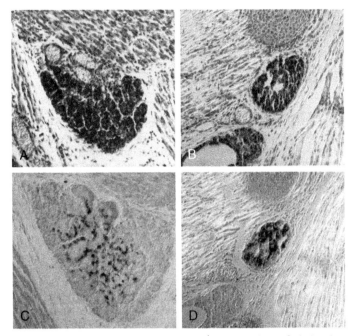

FIGURE 1-6. Thyroid gland phenotype in *Pax8⁻/⁻* mouse embryos. Sagittal sections of E18 wt **(A, C)** and *Pax8⁻/⁻* **(B, D)** mouse embryos stained with hematoxylin/eosin **(A, B)** and anticalcitonin-specific antibody **(C, D)**. The thyroid gland of *Pax8⁻/⁻* embryos is smaller than that of wt and composed almost wholly of C cells. (From Mansouri A, Chowdhury K, Gruss P: Follicular cells of the thyroid gland require *Pax8* gene function. Nat Genet 19:87–90, 1998.)

system at E32[77] and in both luminal and glandular epithelium of the endometrium.[154]

Studies in cultured thyroid cells[156,157] have suggested that Pax8 synthesis is regulated by TSH by a cAMP-mediated mechanism. However, mutated mice in which the TSH/TSHR signaling is abolished do not show a reduced expression of Pax8.[101]

Analysis of *Pax8⁻/⁻* mice[65] (Fig. 1-6) offers the unique possibility of studying the in vivo role of this transcription factor. *Pax8* null pups are born without any apparent brain or kidney defects. On the contrary, the thyroid appears as a rudimental structure lacking thyroid follicular cells, composed almost completely of calcitonin-producing C cells. The animals are affected by a severe hypothyroidism, show growth retardation, and die within 2 to 3 weeks after birth. The administration of thyroxine to these mice leads to their survival. However, in T₄-treated female *Pax8⁻/⁻* animals, the development of the reproductive system is severely affected: the uterus appears as remnants of myometrium lacking endometrial structures, and the vaginal opening does not occur at all.[154]

In *Pax8* null embryos, the thyroid anlage is correctly formed, evaginates from the endoderm, and begins to migrate into the mesenchyme. However, by E11 the thyroid bud is much smaller compared to that of a wild-type. In addition, in the absence of Pax8, other transcription factors such as Foxe1 and Hhex are down-regulated in the precursors of thyroid cells.[79] At E12.5, thyroid follicular cells are not detectable.[65] During morphogenesis, Pax8 holds a specific upstream role in the genetic regulatory cascade which controls thyroid development; it is required for the survival of the thyroid precursor cells and to maintain the tissue-specific gene expression program. In particular, Foxe1 seems to be tightly regulated by Pax8, which is necessary for the onset of its expression.[79]

In *Pax8* null mice, mature TFCs are absent, making it difficult to reveal the role of this factor in the control of adult thyroid function. All the available data on Pax8 functions in differentiated cells come from studies on cell lines in culture. Functional assays have demonstrated that Pax8 is required to activate the *TPO* promoter and to a lesser extent the *Tg* promoter[148] and *NIS* enhancer.[158] In addition, Pax8 is able to bind in vitro to the 5′-flanking region of *Foxe1* and *Duox* genes.[147] Pax8 activates the expression of the endogenous genes encoding Tg, TPO, and NIS at their chromosomal locus.[159] These data suggest that Pax8 has an important role in the maintenance of functional differentiation in thyroid cells.[159]

Pax8 and Nkx2-1/Ttf-1 are coexpressed only in thyroid cells. This finding has suggested some interaction between these two factors. In fact, coimmunoprecipitation experiments in thyroid cells have shown that Nkx2-1/Ttf-1 and Pax8 form a protein complex in vivo. Furthermore, Nkx2-1/Ttf-1 and Pax8 also have functional interactions, since the two factors cooperate in a synergistic manner in activating *Tg* promoter.[160]

Foxe1

Foxe1 (formerly called *TTF-2* for thyroid transcription factor 2) was originally identified as a thyroid-specific nuclear protein that can bind to a sequence present on both *Tg* and *TPO* promoters under insulin, insulin-like growth factor 1 (IGF-1), or TSH stimulation.[161] Subsequently, rat *Foxe1* cDNA was cloned, allowing characterization of the salient features of this protein.[126] Foxe1 belongs to the winged helix/forkhead family of transcription factors characterized by a 100 amino acid–long DNA binding domain[162] homologous to that of the *Drosophila* forkhead gene.[163] The official name for the genetic locus encoding this transcription factor is *Foxe1* in mice (located on chromosome 4[126]) and *FOXE1* in humans (located on chromosome 9q22[95,164]). *Foxe1* is an intronless gene coding for a 42 kD protein that is phosphorylated.[165] The protein contains an alanine stretch of variable length. In humans, the most frequent *FOXE1* allele contains 14 alanine residues and is 371 amino acids long.[166]

Like Nkx2-1/Ttf-1 and Pax8, Foxe1 is detected in the thyroid primordium, and its expression is maintained in TFCs during all stages of development and in adulthood. However, during embryonic life, Foxe1 has a wide domain of expression. Indeed, at early stages of development, Foxe1 is detected in the endodermal epithelium lining the primitive pharynx, the arches and the foregut and, transiently, in Rathke's pouch. Subsequently, Foxe1 is expressed in tissues which are developed from the pharynx and pharyngeal arches: thyroid, tongue, epiglottis, palate, choanae and esophagus. In addition, Foxe1 is also detected in the whiskers and hair follicles which derive from the ectoderm.[165] Studies in mutant mice have shown that Foxe1 is tightly regulated in the thyroid bud by Pax8 and in the pharyngeal cells by Shh.[79] In humans, FOXE1 is expressed in the thyroid, foregut, embryonic thymus,[77] in the outer follicular hair sheath, and the seminiferous tubules of prepubertal testis.[167]

Analysis of *Foxe1* null mice (Fig. 1-7) revealed the role of this transcription factor during thyroid development. Targeted inactivation of *Foxe1* showed that homozygous *Foxe1−/−* mice are born at the expected Mendelian ratio but die within 48 hours of birth. These mice display a severe cleft palate, probably responsible for the perinatal death, an absent thyroid or ectopic thyroid, lack of thyroid hormones and elevated TSH levels in the bloodstream.[95] The early stages of thyroid morphogenesis, when the thyroid anlage is the formed, are not affected in *Foxe1−/−* embryos. However, at E10, thyroid precursor cells are still on the floor of the pharynx in *Foxe1* null embryos, whereas in wild-type embryos the thyroid primordium begins to descend towards its final loca-

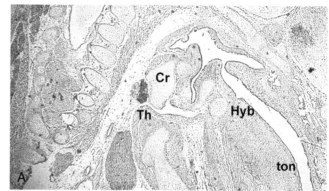

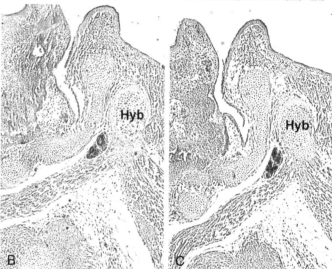

FIGURE 1-7. Thyroid gland phenotype in *Foxe1−/−* mouse embryos. Sagittal sections of E15.5 *Foxe1+/−* **(A)** and *Foxe1−/−* **(B, C)** embryos stained with an anti-Nkx2-1/Ttf-1 **(A, B)** or antithyroglobulin **(C)** antibody. The thyroid gland of *Foxe1−/−* embryo is in a sublingual position. *Cr,* Cricoid cartilage; *Hyb,* hyoid bone; *Th,* thyroid; *ton,* tongue. (From De Felice M, Ovitt C, Biffali E et al: A mouse model for hereditary thyroid dysgenesis and cleft palate. Nat Genet 19:395–398, 1998.)

tion. At later stages of development, in the absence of Foxe1, thyroid follicular cells either disappear or form a small thyroid remnant still attached to the pharyngeal floor. In this case, the cells are able to complete their differentiation program, as tested by their ability to synthesize thyroglobulin. These data indicate that during embryonic life, Foxe1 has a specific role in controlling the migration of thyroid follicular cell precursors, most likely by controlling the expression of target genes required for the migration process, but this is not relevant for the specification and differentiation of the thyroid anlage. In addition, Foxe1 could be involved in the survival of TFCs, since in many *Foxe1* null embryos, the thyroid primordium disappears.[79,95]

Since *Foxe1* null newborns die at birth, conditional knockout mice are necessary to the study of the functions of this gene in the physiology of the gland during adulthood. Functional studies in cell culture systems have shown that Foxe1 can act as a promoter-specific transcriptional repressor through a repression domain located at the carboxy terminus of the protein.

In differentiated thyroid cell lines, the transcription of the *Foxe1* gene is under the tight control of TSH and cAMP as well as that of insulin and IGF-1.[126,168] These data suggest that Foxe1 plays an important role in controlling the interactions between hormone signaling pathway and thyroid specific gene expression. In the developing thyroid these controls do not seem to be effective, since in mutated mice which lack TSH, growth hormone (GH), and IGF-1, the expression of Foxe1 is not affected.[101]

Hhex

Hhex (formerly known as *Hex* for hematopoietically expressed homeobox or *Prh* for proline-rich homeobox) is a homeodomain-containing transcription factor that was first identified in multipotent hematopoietic cells.[169] It was successively demonstrated that Hhex is expressed in other tissues, including the thyroid.[128]

Hhex is encoded by a gene called *Hhex* in mice and *HHEX* in humans, located on chromosome 19 and chromosome 10q23.32, respectively. The gene has 4 exons and codes for a protein 270 amino acids long. *Hhex* is an orphan homeobox-containing gene because the sequence of its homeodomain responsible for binding to DNA shows some differences with respect to other homeodomains.[169] Outside the homeodomain, Hhex contains an N-terminal proline-rich region and a C-terminal acid region. These two regions are probably involved in repressing the transcription of the target genes.

In mouse embryos, Hhex is expressed very early in the primitive and then in the definitive endoderm. At E7.0, Hhex is detected in the developing blood islands, in the ventral foregut endoderm at E8.5, and in the endothelium of the developing vasculature and heart at E9.0. Hhex is an early marker of thyroid cells, since it is already expressed in the thyroid anlage at E8.5[128] at the same stage in which Nkx2-1/Ttf-1, Foxe1, and Pax8 are detected. In the adult, in addition to the thyroid, Hhex expression is maintained in liver and lungs.

The analysis of mutated mice has revealed that this factor is absolutely necessary in many developmental processes. *Hhex*[-/-] embryos die at mid-gestation (between E13.5 and E15.5) and show severe defects in liver, forebrain, heart, and thyroid morphogenesis.[170,171] In *Hhex* null embryos, thyroid precursor cells are present and express Nkx2-1/Ttf-1, Pax8, and Foxe1 until E9. At E10, the thyroid primordium is composed of a few cells which express neither Nkx2-1/Ttf-1 nor Foxe1 nor Pax8.[170] Hence, Hhex guarantees the survival of TFC precursors and maintains the expression of Foxe1, Nkx2-1/Ttf-1, or Pax8. However, in the absence of either Nkx2-1/Ttf-1 or Pax8, the expression of Hhex is down-regulated.

As for Nkx2-1/Ttf-1, Pax8, and Foxe1, a conditional knockout mouse will be a useful tool to elucidate the role of Hhex in the adult thyroid gland. Studies in differentiated thyroid cells suggest that the network ruling Hhex and the other thyroid-specific transcription factors is complex. Hhex seems to be regulated by Nkx2-1/Ttf-1,[172] and the overexpression of Hhex partly inhibits *Tg* promoter activity. These data are consistent with the hypothesis that Hhex is a transcriptional repressor in thyroid cells as reported in other systems.[173]

Fgfr2

Fgfr2-IIIb (fibroblast growth factor receptor 2, isoform IIIb) is a tyrosine kinase receptor present in many types of epithelial cells. This receptor is recognized and activated by specific peptide growth factors (Fgf1, Fgf3, Fgf7 and Fgf10) expressed in the mesenchyme.[174] Interactions of Fgfr2 with its cognate ligands mediate epithelium-mesenchyme cross-talk and are involved in important processes of organogenesis.[174] The relevance of Fgfr2/Fgf interaction in thyroid morphogenesis is demonstrated by the absence of the thyroid gland in mutant mice expressing a soluble dominant negative form of Fgfr2-IIIb[175] and in mice deficient for this isoform.[176] The stage at which thyroid morphogenesis is first

impaired has not been elucidated yet. Since Fgfr2 is expressed in the thyroid primordium starting at E11.5, it is possible that Fgfr2/Fgf signaling is required after budding for the progression of the differentiation programs.

Nkx2-5, Nkx2-6, and Nkx2-3

Nkx2-5 is present in the ventral region of the pharynx and in the thyroid anlage by E8.5[177]; however, after E11.5, the expression of *Nkx2-5* is no longer detected in the thyroid bud.[178] In *Nkx2-5*[-/-] embryos, thyroid morphogenesis occurs, but the thyroid bud appears to be smaller than that of wild-type embryos.[178] It is not possible to study the role of this factor in differentiated thyroid morphogenesis, because *Nkx2-5*[-/-] embryos die at an early stage of development.

Other genes of the *Nkx2* family are present in the primitive pharynx and the thyroid anlage. *Nkx2-6* is transiently expressed in the endodermal layer of the midline region of the pharynx at E8.5.[177] *Nkx2-3* is strongly expressed in the developing thyroid and disappears at birth.[177] However, neither *Nkx2-6*[179] nor *Nkx2-3* null mice show any apparent thyroid phenotype.[89,177]

TSHR

TSHR (thyroid-stimulating hormone receptor), a member of the family of G protein–coupled receptors,[180] is encoded by the gene *Tshr* in mice and *TSHR* in humans, located on chromosome 12 and on chromosome 14q31, respectively. The gene, formed by 10 exons, is translated into a protein 765 amino acids long, expressed on the basolateral membrane of TFCs and in a few other tissues. The binding of TSH to TSHR triggers a signaling pathway that regulates many functions of the thyroid gland in postnatal life. Here we describe the role of the TSH/Tshr pathway during thyroid organogenesis.

In the mouse embryo, TSHR is detected in TFC precursors between E14 and 14.5,[100,181] when the developing thyroid has reached its final position and *Tg* is expressed. At later stages of development, *Tshr* expression increases and remains expressed in adult life.

The availability of mice that carry mutations in the *Tshr* gene allowed elucidation of the role of TSH/TSHR signaling during embryonic life.[101] Both *Tshr*[hyt/hyt] (carrying a loss-of-function mutation in the *Tshr* gene[182]) and *Tshr*[-/-] adult mice[183] display a severe hypothyroidism with an hypoplastic thyroid. During embryonic life, in the absence of a functional TSHR, the developing thyroid does not show any alterations in either size or histologic structure. However, the expression of both *TPO* mRNA and NIS is strongly down-regulated.[101] Thus, TSH/TSHR signaling is required to complete the differentiation program of the thyroid follicular cell. However, the TSH-induced cAMP pathway is not involved in controlling the growth of the embryonic gland, while this pathway is the main regulator of the growth of the adult thyroid. Other growth factors expressed during embryogenesis, such as IGF-1 or EGF, able to promote the growth of thyroid cells in culture, could also be involved in controlling the proliferation of immature thyroid cells. It is worth noting that the requirements for the growth of the embryonic thyroid seem to be different between mouse and human; in the latter, TSH/TSHR signaling during fetal life is necessary for the development of thyroid.[104]

Hoxa3, Eya1, and Tbx

Hoxa3 belongs to the Hox family of transcription factors characterized by the presence of a homeodomain as the DNA binding domain. These factors regulate the regionalization of the

Table 1-2. Currently Available Mouse Models of Thyroid Dysgenesis and Summary of Known and Potential Genes Involved in the Pathogenesis of the Disease

Stage of Morphogenesis Impaired	Thyroid Phenotype Expected	Mouse Model	Other Candidate Genes	Genetic Defect in Human Diseases
Formation of thyroid anlage	Agenesis	Not available	Unknown genes responsible for specification	Unknown
Translocation of thyroid bud	Ectopic thyroid	Foxe1 knockout	Genes controlled by Foxe1	Unknown
Survival and expansion of immature thyroid cells	Athyreosis	Foxe1 knockout Nkx2-1/Ttf-1 knockout Pax8 knockout Fgf10 knockout Fgfr2 knockout Hhex knockout	Genes controlled by Nkx2-1/Ttf-1, Foxe1, Pax8 and Hhex	FOXE1 mutations
Expansion of differentiated thyroid cells	Hypoplasia	Tshr knockout Tshr$^{hyt/hyt}$ mouse Tshr$^{dw/dw}$ mouse	TSH-induced genes	PAX8 mutations* NKX2-1/TTF-1 mutations* TSHR mutations TSH-induced genes
Interactions with ultimobranchial body	Hypoplasia	ET-1 knockout Hoxa3 knockout Eya1 knockout Pax3 knockout (splotch) Tbx knockout	Other Hox genes	Unknown

*In humans, unlike mice, the abnormal phenotype is detected in heterozygotes.

embryo along its major axes and are also involved in the morphogenesis of several structures. Hoxa3 is expressed in the pharynx, in the developing thyroid, and in the mesenchymal, endodermal, and neural crest–derived cells of the fourth pharyngeal pouch.[110]

Mice in which Hoxa3 has been disrupted lack the thymus and parathyroid and show persistent ultimobranchial bodies and variable thyroid anomalies,[109,110] including hypoplasia, hemiagenesis, reduction of the number of follicular cells, and absence of isthmus. The thyroid phenotype is exacerbated in mice carrying various mutant combinations in Hoxa3 and its paralogs Hoxb3 and Hoxd3.[111] It is thought that the impaired organogenesis of the thyroid is secondary to defects in the ultimobranchial bodies. This hypothesis is confirmed by other findings. Mice deprived of Eya1—a transcription factor expressed in the ultimobranchial bodies but not in the developing thyroid—display a thyroid phenotype that is almost identical to that displayed in Hoxa3 mutants.[112] Furthermore, mice carrying mutations in Pax3[117] or Endothelin-1,[184] both molecules implicated in the development of neural crest–derived structures, show a defective thyroid organogenesis. Finally, in Tbx null embryos, the ultimobranchial bodies fail to develop, and the thyroid gland appears as a hypoplastic single-tissue mass.[88] Tbx is a transcription factor expressed in the non–neural crest mesoderm and endoderm of the pharyngeal arches but not in thyroid precursor cells. It is worth noting that hypothyroidism is detected in a number of patients affected by velocardiofacial syndrome/DiGeorge syndrome, which is most likely associated with haploinsufficiency of the Tbx1 gene.[185] Taken together, these observations suggest a relevant role for non–cell-autonomous factors in thyroid development.

INSIGHTS FROM HUMAN DISEASES

In 85% of congenital hypothyroidism (CH) cases, the most frequent endocrine disorder in newborns, the condition is due to thyroid dysgenesis (TD). The term thyroid dysgenesis indicates an ectopic or hypoplastic thyroid as well as the absence of thyroid (thyroid agenesis or athyreosis).[186] In addition, the term also includes thyroid malformations, such as hemiagenesis, which are not associated with apparent thyroid dysfunction.[187] Thyroid

dysgenesis is due to anomalies during gland organogenesis: defects in growth and/or differentiation of the thyroid primordium can result in an absent or hypoplastic thyroid; an impaired migration of thyroid precursor cells causes an ectopic gland.

The study on the molecular genetics of thyroid dysgenesis seems to be a useful tool in the elucidation of the mechanisms underlying thyroid development, since in many cases it has confirmed data obtained in animal models and has provided new insights into thyroid morphogenesis and differentiation.[86,90,188] Here we will focus on genes known (or candidate) to be responsible for this phenotype (Table 1-2). The mutations thus far identified in patients with congenital hypothyroidism associated with TD account only for a very small number of cases. However, these cases could be much more frequent than hitherto identified because mutations which might arise in specific regulatory elements were not searched for in the published studies.

Agenesis and Athyreosis

Both athyreosis and agenesis indicate the absence of thyroid tissue. However, agenesis should be used to define the absence of the gland due to a defective initiation of thyroid morphogenesis.[86] The term athyreosis indicates a dysgenesis characterized by the disappearance of the thyroid due to alterations in any step following the specification of the thyroid anlage. In several patients with athyreosis, the presence of cystic structures (probably resulting from the degeneration of TFC clusters[189]) suggests that thyroid specification was not impaired in these subjects.

At the moment, there are no animal models that display a bona fide agenesis. Indeed, gene-targeting experiments have demonstrated that Nkx2-1/Ttf-1, Foxe1, Pax8, and Hhex play no role in the thyroid anlage specification, which forms correctly in embryos deprived of any of these proteins. Agenesis could be due to defects in genes involved in the early regionalization of the endoderm, including the genes controlling the onset of NKX2-1/TTF-1, FOXE1, PAX8, and HHEX. However, the relevance of these genes in congenital hypothyroidism is difficult to demonstrate, since mutations in genes that are widely expressed in the endoderm at early stages of development could cause embryo-lethal phenotypes and/or many additional defects. On the contrary, the knockout mice described in the previous section are good models of athyreosis. In these mutants, the morphogenesis of the gland begins, but the thyroid bud disappears, probably owing to a defective survival program or to the proliferation of the precursors of the follicular cells. Absence of the thyroid has been described in patients with CH associated with mutations in either *FOXE1* or *PAX8* genes.

FOXE1 and Thyroid Dysgenesis

Homozygous loss-of-function mutation in the *FOXE1* gene was first reported[190] in two siblings affected by syndromic congenital hypothyroidism characterized by athyreosis, cleft palate, bilateral choanal atresia, and spiky hair (Bamforth-Lazarus syndrome[191]). After this report, a different mutation in *FOXE1* has been recorded in two siblings with athyreosis and a less severe extrathyroidal phenotype.[192] A third loss-of-function mutation within the *FOXE1* forkhead domain has been described[193] in a child displaying CH with eutopic thyroid tissue and extrathyroidal defects. The variable thyroid phenotype displayed by patients carrying *FOXE1* mutations could be due to different effects of the various mutations. The phenotype is consistent with the expression domain of *FOXE1* and partially overlaps that displayed by *Foxe1* null mice. However, in mice, the absence of this factor causes either athyreosis or defects in thyroid migration, whereas in humans, *FOXE1* mutations associated with an ectopic thyroid have not been described.

Ectopic Thyroid

The ectopic thyroid is a consequence of an impaired thyroid bud migration. More than 50% of patients affected by CH show an ectopic thyroid, but to date no known genes have been associated with this dysgenesis.[194] Familial cases of TD have been described, in which affected members show either ectopic thyroid or athyreosis.[195] This observation raises the possibility that athyreosis and thyroid ectopy have a common underlying mechanism. This hypothesis is consistent with the data from mice lacking the Foxe1 protein, which show either ectopy with a very small thyroid or no thyroid at all.[95]

Recently, four subjects affected by CH with TD-carrying heterozygous mutations in the *NKX2-5* gene have been described. In three out of the four patients, the presence of an ectopic thyroid suggests that *NKX2-5* mutations might have a specific pathogenic role in this thyroid malformation.[178]

Hypoplasia

About 5% to 17% of cases of CH are associated with a hypoplastic thyroid, that is, a gland containing a reduced number of follicular cells. Thyroid hypoplasia is probably a genetically heterogeneous disorder and could be a consequence of alterations in any of the steps that control the expansion and/or survival of thyroid cells during organogenesis.

Genes involved in early stages of development (*NKX2-1/TTF-1*, *FOXE1*, *PAX8*, and *HHEX*) as well as in the late steps (*TSHR*) could be good candidates for this dysgenesis. Indeed, mutations in *NKX2-1/TTF-1*, *PAX8*, or *TSHR* genes have been found in patients with CH associated with hypoplasia.

PAX8 and Thyroid Dysgenesis

Mutations in the DNA binding domain of the *PAX8* gene have been found in sporadic and familial cases of CH with TD.[196-200] Patients show a variable phenotype ranging from mild to severe hypoplasia of the thyroid in the presence of elevated levels of TSH in the bloodstream. Since the phenotype shows discrepancy even in familial cases in which related individuals carry the same

mutation, effects of other modifier genes could be hypothesized. In two patients, renal hemiagenesis has been reported.[199]

Affected individuals are heterozygous for the mutations, and in the familial cases, the mode of inheritance is dominant. Thus in humans, both *PAX8* alleles are necessary for correct thyroid morphogenesis, and a reduced dosage of the gene product (haploinsufficiency) causes dysgenesis; in contrast, *Pax8*⁺/⁻ mice display a normal phenotype.[65] The reason for this discrepancy is unknown.

NKX2-1/TTF-1 and Thyroid Dysgenesis

Heterozygous point mutations or chromosomal deletions in the *NKX2-1/TTF-1* locus have been found in patients affected by a complex syndrome characterized by thyroid alterations, choreoathetosis, and lung abnormalities.[201-206]

All affected individuals are heterozygous for the mutations. The dominant effect of *NKX2-1/TTF-1* mutations in humans could be due to a haploinsufficiency. Accordingly, in mice Nkx2-1/Ttf-1 functions are partially dosage-sensitive. Functional studies have revealed that *Nkx2-1/Ttf-1*⁺/⁻ mice present decreased coordination and mild hyperthyrotropinemia.[204,206] *NKX2-1/TTF-1*⁺/⁻ subjects display a highly variable thyroid phenotype. In many patients, thyroid alterations have not been reported; in other cases, patients show elevated TSH levels with mild or severe hypoplasia of the gland. There is no clear correlation between the phenotype severity and the type of mutations. In addition, a variable phenotype has also been reported in the same familial cluster. As in the case of *PAX8* disease, other modifier genes could be responsible for the incomplete penetrance and variability of the phenotype.

TSHR and Thyroid Dysgenesis

Almost 40 years ago, Stanbury[207] hypothesized that TSH unresponsiveness could cause CH without goiter. However, mutations in the *TSHR* gene were identified 15 years ago[208] and shown to be responsible for TD-associated congenital hypothyroidism. Among the molecular defects causing TD, mutations in the *TSHR* gene represent the most frequent find. Patients affected with CH show increased TSH secretion and mild or severe thyroid hypoplasia.[209] In many cases, the thyroid size appears normal, and only an asymptomatic hyperthyrotropinemia characterizes these individuals. Athyreosis or ectopic thyroid have never been found in patients carrying *TSHR* mutations. These observations confirm that the TSHR-induced pathway is not involved in the early stages of thyroid development. All the affected individuals are homozygous or compound heterozygous for loss-of-function mutations. Consistently in the familial forms, the disease is inherited as an autosomal recessive trait.

Phylogenesis of the Thyroid Gland

The morphologic bases of thyroid function are the same in all vertebrates, as reflected by the conserved follicular structure throughout vertebrate evolution. On the contrary, the gross anatomy of the thyroid gland appears different among vertebrate classes.[10] In placental mammals and in some reptiles, the thyroid is composed of two lobes connected by an isthmus which crosses the trachea. In nonplacental mammals, birds, and amphibians, the thyroid consists of two isolated lobes. In cartilaginous fish and in some teleosts (mostly marine ones), the thyroid is massed into a compact organ. In the remaining marine and almost all freshwater teleosts, the thyroid consists of nonencapsulated follicles scattered in the subpharyngeal connective tissue.[122] Often heterotopic follicles are found in nonpharyngeal areas such as kidneys, heart, esophagus, or spleen in these animals. Interestingly, the ability of thyroid cells to proliferate in these ectopic areas has been shown to be genetically controlled in platyfish, and low iodine intake represents a strong inductive stimulus towards this condition.[210] Even though iodine-concentrating activity and iodoamino acid production are ancient phenomena that have also been described in nonvertebrate animals, only cyclostomes (such as the lamprey) have a bona fide thyroid characterized by follicles scattered in the subpharyngeal connective tissue.

The ontogeny of the thyroid follows the same pattern in all vertebrates, including teleosts[211]: the thyroid anlage arises from an outpouching of the primitive pharynx, migrates caudally, and reaches its definitive position. The development of the thyroid in cyclostomes follows a different pattern from that used by the higher vertebrates. Thyroid follicles of the adult lamprey derive from the endostyle, an organ present only during larval life. In the larval lamprey, at the early stages of development, the endostyle forms as a ciliated groove in the ventral part of the pharynx. During development the groove becomes a cylinder and then a complex structure connected to the pharyngeal cavity by the ductus hypobranchialis.[212] The epithelium of the endostyle differentiates into different types of cells, a group of which displays the ability to trap iodine, peroxidase activity, and expression of thyroxine.[213] These cells are fated to become "typical" follicular cells only after metamorphosis.[214]

A structure similar to the lamprey endostyle is present in the ventral pharynx of protochordates such as cephalochordates (amphioxus) and urochordates (such as ascidians). This organ, which is also called the *endostyle*, is composed of different cell types, the major part of which are involved in the food-capturing process.[212] More than a century ago, the homology between the cyclostome endostyle and the thyroid suggested the hypothesis that the endostyle of protochordates was a primitive antecedent of the vertebrate thyroid gland.[215,216] This hypothesis, based on morphologic observation, has gained support from the presence of iodine trapping,[217] thyroperoxidase activity,[218] and *Ci-Duox* (the *Ciona* homolog vertebrate Duox) in a group of cells of the endostyle of protochordates. Thus, these cells can be considered "protothyroid" cells.[212] The molecular mechanisms involved in the differentiation of thyroid cells of mammals are conserved throughout the evolution of protochordates to vertebrate chordates. In urochordates (*Ciona intestinalis*), the group of cells that express the *TPO* homologs[219] also express *Ci-FoxE* (*Foxe1*) homolog[220] but not *Ci-Nkx2-1/Ttf-1*.[221,222] On the contrary, in amphioxus, both *Nkx2-1/Ttf-1* and *TPO* homologous genes are coexpressed in the same cells of the endostyle,[218] while the *Foxe1* homolog *Amphi-FoxE4* is not detected in the endostyle but in another pharyngeal-derived structure.[223] These data suggest that during the evolution of protochordates, a group of genes whose function was to contribute to the specification of the anterior part of the gut were selected as part of the genetic program that leads to thyroid specification.

REFERENCES

1. Werner S: Historical resume. In Ingbar SH, Braverman LE, editors: The Thyroid, Philadelphia, 1986, Lippincott, pp 3–6.
2. Netter FH: Anatomy of the thyroid and parathyroid glands. In The CIBA Collection of Medical Illustrations, vol 4, Summit, NJ, 1965, CIBA Pharmaceutical Products, pp 41–70.
3. Fujita H: Functional morphology of the thyroid, Int Rev Cytol 113:145–185, 1988.
4. Romeo HE, Gonzalez Solveyra C, Vacas MI, et al: Origins of the sympathetic projections to rat thyroid and parathyroid glands, J Auton Nerv Syst 17:63–70, 1986.
5. Cauna N, Naik N: The distribution of cholinesterases in the sensory ganglia of man and some mammals, J Histochem Cytochem 11:129–138, 1963.
6. Sundler F, Grunditz T, Hakanson R, et al: Innervation of the thyroid. A study of the rat using retrograde tracing and immunocytochemistry, Acta Histochem Suppl 37:191–198, 1989.
7. Sawicki B: Evaluation of the role of mammalian thyroid parafollicular cells, Acta Histochem 97:389–399, 1995.
8. Grunditz T, Hakanson R, Rerup C, et al: Neuropeptide Y in the thyroid gland: neuronal localization and enhancement of stimulated thyroid hormone secretion, Endocrinology 115:1537–1542, 1984.
9. Ahrèn B: Regulatory peptides in the thyroid gland—a review on their localization and function, Acta Endocrinol 124:225–232, 1991.
10. Gorbman A, Bern HA: Thyroid gland. In Gorbman A, Bern HA, editors: A Textbook of Comparative Endocrinology, New York, 1962, Willey, pp 99–173.
11. Mauchamp J, Mirrione A, Alquier C, et al: Follicle-like structure and polarized monolayer: role of the extracellular matrix on thyroid cell organization in primary culture, Biol Cell 90:369–380, 1998.
12. Yap AS, Stevenson BR, Armstrong JW, et al: Thyroid epithelial morphogenesis in vitro: a role for butamide-sensitive Cl⁻ secretion during follicular lumen development, Exp Cell Res 213:319–326, 1994.
13. Romagnoli P, Herzog V: Transcytosis in thyroid follicle cells: regulation and implications for thyroglobulin transport, Exp Cell Res 194:202–209, 1991.

14. Meunier D, Aubin J, Jeannotte L: Perturbed thyroid morphology and transient hypothyroidism symptoms in *Hoxa5* mutant mice, Dev Dyn 227:367–378, 2003.
15. Shepard T: Onset of function in the human fetal thyroid: biochemical and radioautographic studies from organ culture, J Clin Endocrinol Metab 27:945–958, 1987.
16. Drubin DG, Nelson J: Origins of cell polarity, Cell 84:335–344, 1996.
17. Matter K, Mellman I: Mechanism of cell polarity: sorting and transport in epithelial cells, Curr Opin Cell Biol 6:545–554, 1994.
18. Ekholm R: Biosynthesis of thyroid hormones, Int Rev Cyt 120:243–288, 1990.
19. Bourke JR, Sand O, Abel KC, et al: Chloride channels in the apical membrane of thyroid epithelial cells are regulated by cyclic AMP, J Endocrinol 147:441–448, 1995.
20. Bourke JR, Abel KC, Huxham GJ, et al: Sodium channel heterogeneity in the apical membrane of porcine thyroid epithelial cells, J Endocrinol 149:101–108, 1996.
21. Royaux IE, Suzuki K, Mori A, et al: Pendrin, the protein encoded by the Pendred syndrome gene (PDS), is an apical exchanger of iodide in the thyroid and is regulated by thyroglobulin in FRTL-5 cells, Endocrinology 141:839–845, 2000.
22. De Deken X, Wang D, Many MC, et al: Cloning of two human thyroid cDNAs encoding new members of the NADPH oxidase family, J Biol Chem 275:23227–23233, 2000.
23. Paire A, Bernier-Valentin F, Selmi-Ruby S, et al: Characterization of the rat thyroid iodide transporter using anti-peptide antibodies, J Biol Chem 272:18245–18249, 1997.
24. Gerard C, Gabrion J, Verrier B, et al: Localization of the Na⁺/K⁺-ATPase and of an amiloride sensitive Na⁺ uptake on thyroid epithelial cells, Eur J Cell Biol 38:134–141, 1985.
25. Westermack K, Westermack B, Karslsson A, et al: Localization of epidermal growth factor receptors on porcine thyroid follicle cells and receptor regulation by thyrotropin, Endocrinology 118:1040–1046, 1986.

26. Costagliola S, Rodien P, Many MC, et al: Genetic immunization against the human thyrotropin receptor causes thyroiditis and allows production of monoclonal antibodies recognizing the native receptor, J Immunol 160:1458–1465, 1998.
27. Ericson L: Exocytosis and endocytosis in the thyroid follicle cell, Mol Cell Endocrinol 22:1–24, 1981.
28. Lohi J, Leivo I, Franssila K, et al: Changes in the distribution of integrins and their basement membrane ligands during development of human thyroid follicular epithelium, Histochem J 29:337–345, 1997.
29. Vitale M, Casamassima A, Illario M, et al: Cell-to-cell contact modulates the expression of the beta1 integrins in primary cultures of thyroid cells, Exp Cell Res 220:124–129, 1995.
30. Burgi-Saville ME, Gerber H, Peter HJ, et al: Expression patterns of extracellular matrix components in native and cultured normal human thyroid tissue and in human toxic adenoma tissue, Thyroid 7:347–356, 1997.
31. Andre F, Filippi P, Feracci H: Merosin is synthesized by thyroid cells in primary culture irrespective of cellular organization, J Cell Sci 107:183–193, 1994.
32. Gumbiner B: Cell adhesion: the molecular basis of tissue architecture and morphogenesis, Cell 84:345–357, 1996.
33. Denker BM, Nigam S: Molecular structure and assembly of the tight junction, Am J Physiol 274:1–9, 1998.
34. Yap AS, Stevenson BR, Abel KC, et al: Microtubule integrity is necessary for the epithelial barrier function of cultured thyroid cell monolayers, Exp Cell Res 218:540–545, 1995.
35. Boller K, Vestweber D, Kemler R: Cell-adhesion molecule uvomorulin is localized in the intermediate junctions of adult intestinal epithelial cells, Cell Biol 100:327–332, 1985.
36. Kemler R: From cadherins to catenins: cytoplasmic protein interactions and regulation of cell adhesion, Trends Genet 9:317–321, 1993.
37. Buxton RS, Magee A: Structure and interactions of desmosomal and other cadherins, Semin Cell Biol 3:157–167, 1992.

38. Kowalczyk AP, Bornslaeger EA, Norvell SM, et al: Desmosomes: intercellular adhesive junctions specialized for attachment of intermediate filaments, Int Rev Cytol 185:237–302, 1999.

39. Munari-Silem Y, Rousset B: Gap junction-mediated cell-to-cell communications in endocrine glands-molecular and functional aspects: a review, Eur J Endocrinol 135:251–264, 1996.

40. Yap AS, Manley S: Contact inhibition of cell spreading: a mechanism for the maintenance of thyroid cell aggregation in vitro, Exp Cell Res 208:121–127, 1993.

41. Yap AS, Stevenson BR, Keast JR, et al: Cadherin-mediated adhesion and apical membrane assembly define distinct steps during thyroid epithelial polarization and lumen formation, Endocrinology 136:4672–4680, 1995.

42. Yap AS, Manley SW: Thyrotropin inhibits the intrinsic locomotility of thyroid cells organized as follicles in primary culture, Exp Cell Res 214:408–417, 1994.

43. Yap AS: Initiation of cell locomotility is a morphogenetic checkpoint in thyroid epithelial cells regulated by ERK and PI3-kinase signals, Cell Motil Cytoskeleton 49:93–103, 2001.

44. Yap AS, Abel KC, Bourke JR, et al: Different regulation of thyroid cell-cell and cell-substrate adhesion by thyrotropin, Exp Cell Res 202:366–369, 1992.

45. Nilsson M, Fagman H, Ericson L: Ca^{2+}-dependent and Ca^{2+}-independent regulation of the thyroid epithelial junction complex by protein kinases, Exp Cell Res 225:1–11, 1996.

46. Pellerin S, Croizet K, Rabilloud R, et al: Regulation of the three-dimensional organization of thyroid epithelial cells into follicle structures by the matricellular protein, thrombospondin-1, Endocrinology 140:1094–1103, 1999.

47. Gartner R, Schopohl D, Schaefer S, et al: Regulation of transforming growth factor beta 1 messenger ribonucleic acid expression in porcine thyroid follicles in vitro by growth factors, iodine, or delta iodolactone, Thyroid 7:633–640, 1997.

48. Toda S, Matsumura S, Fujitani N, et al: Transforming growth factor beta 1 induces a mesenchyma-like cell shape without epithelial polarization in thyrocytes and inhibits thyroid folliculogenesis in collagen gel culture, Endocrinology 138:5561–5575, 1997.

49. Paire A, Bernier-Valentin F, Rabilloud R, et al: Expression of alpha- and beta subunits and activity of Na^+K^+-ATPase in pig thyroid cells in primary culture: modulation by thyrotropin and thyroid hormones, Mol Cell Endocrinol 146:93–101, 1998.

50. Tacchetti C, Zurzolo C, Monticelli C, et al: Functional properties of normal and inverted rat thyroid follicles in suspension culture, J Cell Physiol 126:93–98, 1986.

51. Halmi N: Anatomy and histochemistry. In Ingbar SH, Braverman LE, editors: The Thyroid, Philadelphia, 1986, Lippincott, pp 24–36.

52. Fujita H: Fine structure of the thyroid gland, Int Rev Cytol 40:197–280, 1975.

53. Engstrom G, Ericson L: Effect of graded dose of thyrotropin on exocytosis and early phase of endocytosis in the rat thyroid, Endocrinology 108:399–405, 1981.

54. Bernier-Valentine F, Kostrouch Z, Rabilloud R, et al: Analysis of the thyroglobulin internalization process using in vitro reconstituted follicles: evidence for a coated vesicle-dependent endocytic pathway, Endocrinology 129:2194–2201, 1991.

55. Damante G, Tell G, Di Lauro R: A unique combination of transcription factors controls differentiation of thyroid cells, Prog Nucleic Acid Res Mol Biol 66:307–356, 2001.

56. Pearse A: The cytochemistry of the thyroid C cells and their relationship to calcitonin, Proc Roy Soc Biol 164:478–487, 1966.

57. Le Douarin N, Fontaine J, LeLievre C: New studies on the neural crest origin of the avian ultimobranchial glandular cells. Interspecific combinations and cytochemical characterization of C cells based on the uptake of biogenic amine precursors, Histochemie 38:297–305, 1974.

58. Pearse AG, Caralheira A: Cytochemical evidence for an ultimobranchial origin of rodent thyroid C cells, Nature 214:929–930, 1967.

59. Martin-Lacave M, Conde E, Montenero C, et al: Quantitative changes in the frequency and distribution of the C-cell population in the rat thyroid gland with age, Cell Tissue Res 270:73–77, 1992.

60. Wolfe HJ, DeLellis RA, Voelkel EF, et al: Distribution of calcitonin-containing cells in the normal neonatal human thyroid gland: a correlation of morphology with peptide content, J Clin Endocrinol Metab 41:1076–1081, 1975.

61. Neve P, Wollman S: Fine structure of ultimobranchial follicles in the thyroid gland of the rat, Anat Rec 171:259–272, 1971.

62. Minvielle S, Giscard-Dartevelle S, Cohen R, et al: A novel calcitonin carboxyl-terminal peptide produced in medullary thyroid carcinoma by alternative RNA processing of the calcitonin/calcitonin gene-related peptide gene, J Biol Chem 266:24627–24631, 1991.

63. Suzuki K, Kobayashi Y, Katoh R, et al: Identification of thyroid transcription factor-1 in C cells and parathyroid cells, Endocrinology 139:3014–3017, 1998.

64. Kusakabe T, Hoshi N, Kimura S: Origin of the ultimobranchial body cyst: T/ebp/Nkx2.1 expression is required for development and fusion of the ultimobranchial body to the thyroid, Dev Dyn 235:1300–1309, 2006.

65. Mansouri A, Chowdhury K, Gruss P: Follicular cells of the thyroid gland require *Pax8* gene function, Nat Genet 19:87–90, 1998.

66. Martin-Lacave I, Rojas F, Bernabe R, et al: Comparative immunohistochemical study of normal, hyperplastic and neoplastic C cells of the rat thyroid gland, Cell Tissue Res 309:361–368, 2002.

67. Kameda Y, Oyama H, Endoh M, et al: Somatostatin immunoreactive C cells in thyroid glands from various mammalian species, Anat Rec 204:161–170, 1982.

68. Neonakis E, Thomas GA, Davies HG, et al: Expression of calcitonin and somatostatin peptide and mRNA in medullary thyroid carcinoma, World J Surg 18:588–593, 1994.

69. Blaker M, de Weerth A, Schulz M, et al: Expression of the cholecystokinin 2-receptor in normal human thyroid gland and medullary thyroid carcinoma, Eur J Endocrinol 146:89–96, 2002.

70. Wollman SH, Neve P: Postnatal development and properties of ultimobranchial follicles in the rat thyroid, Anat Rec 171:247–258, 1971.

71. Calvert R: Structure of rat ultimobranchial bodies after birth, Anat Rec 181:561–580, 1974.

72. Harach H: Solid-cell nests of the thyroid, J Pathol 155:191–200, 1988.

73. Reis-Filho JS, Preto A, Soares P, et al: p63 expression in solid-cell nests of the thyroid: further evidence for a stem cell origin, Mod Pathol 16:43–48, 2003.

74. Preto A, Cameselle-Teijeiro J, Moldes-Boullosa J, et al: Telomerase expression and proliferative activity suggest a stem cell role for thyroid solid cell nests, Mod Pathol 17:819–826, 2004.

75. Burstein DE, Nagi C, Wang BY, et al: Immunohistochemical detection of p53 homolog p63 in solid cell nests, papillary thyroid carcinoma, and Hashimoto's thyroiditis: a stem cell hypothesis of papillary carcinoma oncogenesis, Hum Pathol 35:465–473, 2004.

76. Fisher DA, Dussault JH, Sach J, et al: Ontogenesis of hypothalamic-pituitary-thyroid function and metabolism in man, sheep and rat, Recent Prog Hormone Res 33:59–116, 1976.

77. Trueba SS, Auge J, Mattei G, et al: PAX8, TITF1 and FOXE1 gene expression patterns during human development: new insights into human thyroid development and thyroid dysgenesis associated malformations, J Clin Endocrinol Metab 90:455–462, 2004.

78. Kaufman MH, Bard J: The thyroid. In Kaufman MH, Bard J, editors: The Anatomic Basis of Mouse Development, San Diego, 1999, Academic Press, pp 165–166.

79. Parlato R, Rosica A, Rodriguez-Mallon A, et al: An integrated regulatory network controlling survival and migration in thyroid organogenesis, Dev Biol 276:464–475, 2004.

80. Elsalini OA, von Gartzen J, Cramer M, et al: Zebrafish Hhex, Nk2.1a, and Pax2.1 regulate thyroid growth and differentiation downstream of nodal-dependent transcription factors, Dev Biol 263:67–80, 2003.

81. Cai CL, Liang X, Shi Y, et al: Isl1 identifies a cardiac progenitor population that proliferates prior to differentiation and contributes a majority of cells to the heart, Dev Cell 5:877–889, 2003.

82. Kumar M, Melton D: Pancreas specification: a budding question, Curr Opin Genet Dev 13:401–407, 2003.

83. Lammert E, Cleaver O, Melton D: Role of endothelial cells in early pancreas and liver development, Mech Dev 120:35–43, 2003.

84. Serls A, Doherty S, Parvatiyar P, et al: Different thresholds of fibroblast growth factors pattern the ventral foregut into liver and lung, Development 132:35–47, 2005.

85. Wendl T, Adzic D, Schoenebeck JJ, et al: Early developmental specification of the thyroid gland depends on han-expressing surrounding tissue and on FGF signals, Development 134:2871–2879, 2007.

86. De Felice M, Di Lauro R: Thyroid development and its disorders: genetics and molecular mechanisms, Endocr Rev 25:722–746, 2004.

87. Olivieri A, Stazi MA, Mastroiacovo P, et al: A population-based study on the frequency of additional congenital malformations in infants with congenital hypothyroidism: data from the Italian Registry for Congenital Hypothyroidism (1991–1998), J Clin Endocrinol Metab 87:557–562, 2002.

88. Fagman H, Liao J, Westerlund J, et al: The 22q11 deletion syndrome candidate gene Tbx1 determines thyroid size and positioning, Hum Mol Genet 16:276–285, 2007.

89. Fagman H, Andersson L, Nilsson M: The developing mouse thyroid: embryonic vessel contacts and parenchymal growth pattern during specification, budding, migration, and lobulation, Dev Dyn 235, 2006.

90. Polak M, Sura-Trueba S, Chauty A, et al: Molecular mechanisms of thyroid dysgenesis, Horm Res 62:14–21, 2004.

91. Hogan B, Zaret K: Development of the endoderm and its tissue derivatives. In Rossant J, editor: Mouse Development: Patterning, Morphogenesis, and Organogenesis, New York, 2002, Academic Press, pp 301–310.

92. Hilfer SR, Brown JW: The development of pharyngeal endocrine organs in mouse and chick embryos, Scan Electron Microsc 4:2009–2022, 1984.

93. Thiery JP, Sleeman J: Complex networks orchestrate epithelial-mesenchymal transitions, Nat Rev Mol Cell Biol 7:131–142, 2006.

94. Fagman H, Grande M, Edsbagge J, et al: Expression of classical cadherins in thyroid development: maintenance of an epithelial phenotype throughout organogenesis, Endocrinology 144:3618–3624, 2003.

95. De Felice M, Ovitt C, Biffali E, et al: A mouse model for hereditary thyroid dysgenesis and cleft palate, Nat Genet 19:395–398, 1998.

96. Fagman H, Grande M, Gritli-Linde A, et al: Genetic deletion of sonic hedgehog causes hemiagenesis and ectopic development of the thyroid in mouse, Am J Pathol 164:1865–1872, 2004.

97. Burke BA, Johnson D, Gilbert EF, et al: Thyrocalcitonin-containing cells in the DiGeorge anomaly, Hum Pathol 4:355–360, 1987.

98. Amendola E, De Luca P, Macchia PE, et al: A mouse model demonstrates a multigenic origin of congenital hypothyroidism, Endocrinology 146:5038–5047, 2005.

99. Hartzband PI, Diehl DL, Lewin KJ, et al: Histological characterization of a lingual mass using thyroglobulin immunoperoxidase staining, J Endocrinol Invest 7:221–223, 1984.

100. Lazzaro D, Price M, De Felice M, et al: The transcription factor TTF-1 is expressed at the onset of thyroid and lung morphogenesis and in restricted regions of the foetal brain, Development 113:1093–1104, 1991.

101. Postiglione MP, Parlato R, Rodriguez-Mallon A, et al: Role of the thyroid-stimulating hormone receptor signaling in development and differentiation of the thyroid gland, Proc Natl Acad Sci U S A 99:15462–15467, 2002.

102. Milenkovic M, De Deken X, Jin L, et al: Duox expression and related H_2O_2 measurement in mouse thyroid: onset in embryonic development and regulation by TSH in adult, J Endocrinol 192:615–626, 2007.

103. Hilfer SR, Stern M: Instability of the epithelial-mesenchymal interaction in the eight-day embryonic chick thyroid, J Exp Zool 178:293–305, 1971.

104. De Felice M, Postiglione MP, Di Lauro R: Mini review: thyrotropin receptor signaling in development and differentiation of the thyroid gland: insights from mouse models and human diseases, Endocrinology 145:4062–4067, 2004.

105. Alt B, Reibe S, Feitosa NM, et al: Analysis of origin and growth of the thyroid gland in zebrafish, Dev Dyn 235:1872–1883, 2006.

106. Weller G: Development of the thyroid, parathyroid and thymus glands in man, Contrib Embryol 24:93–140, 1933.

107. Kumar R, Gupta R, Bal CS, et al: Thyrotoxicosis in a patient with submandibular thyroid, Thyroid, 363–365, 2000.

108. Harach H: Thyroglobulin in human thyroid follicles with acid mucins, J Pathol 164:261–263, 1991.

109. Chisaka O, Musci TS, Capecchi MR: Developmental defects of the ear, cranial nerves and hindbrain resulting from targeted disruption of the mouse homeobox gene Hox-1.6, Nature 355:516–520, 1992.

110. Manley NR, Capecchi M: The role of Hoxa-3 in mouse thymus and thyroid development, Development 121:1989–2003, 1995.

111. Manley NR, Capecchi M: Hox group 3 paralogs regulate the development and migration of the thymus, thyroid, and parathyroid glands, Dev Biol 195:1–15, 1998.

112. Xu PX, Zheng W, Laclef C, et al: Eya1 is required for the morphogenesis of mammalian thymus, parathyroid and thyroid, Development 129:1033–1044, 2002.

113. Westerlund J, Andersson L, Carlsson T, et al: Expression of Islet1 in thyroid development related to budding, migration, and fusion of primordia, Dev Dyn 237:3820–3829, 2008.

114. Kameda Y, Nishimaki T, Chisaka O, et al: Expression of the epithelial marker E-cadherin by thyroid C cells and their precursors during murine development, Histochem Cytochem 55:1075–1088, 2007.

115. Kameda Y, Nishimaki T, Miura M, et al: Mash1 regulates the development of C cells in mouse thyroid glands, Dev Dyn 236:262–270, 2007.

116. Merida-Velasco JA, Garcia-Garcia JD, Espin-Ferra J, et al: Origin of the ultimobranchial body and its colonizing cells in human embryos, Acta Anat 73:325–330, 1989.

117. Franz T: Persistent truncus arteriosus in the Splotch mutant mouse, Anat Embryol 180:457–464, 1989.

118. Epstein JA, Li J, Lang D, et al: Migration of cardiac neural crest cells in Splotch embryos, Development 127:1869–1878, 2000.

119. Neubüser A, Peters H, Balling R, et al: Antagonistic interactions between FGF and BMP signaling pathways: a mechanism for positioning the sites of tooth formation, Cell 90:247–255, 1997.

120. Hetzer-Egger C, Schorpp M, Haas-Assenbaum A, et al: Thymopoiesis requires Pax9 function in thymic epithelial cells, Eur J Immunol 32:1175–1181, 2002.

121. Clark MS, Lanigan TM, Page NM, et al: Induction of a serotonergic and neuronal phenotype in thyroid C-cells, J Neurosci 15:6167–6178, 1995.

122. Gorbman A: Comparative anatomy and physiology. In Ingbar SI, Braverman LE, editors: The Thyroid, Philadelphia, 1986, Lippincott, pp 43–52.

123. Fontaine J: Multistep migration of calcitonin cell precursors during ontogeny of the mouse pharynx, Gen Comp Endocrinol 37:81–92, 1979.

124. Guillemot F: Analysis of the role of basic-helix-loop-helix transcription factors in the development of neural lineages in the mouse, Biol Cell 84:3–6, 1995.

125. Lindahl M, Timmusk T, Rossi J, et al: Expression and alternative splicing of mouse Gfra4 suggest roles in endocrine cell development, Mol Cell Neurosci 522–533, 2000.

126. Zannini M, Avantaggiato V, Biffali E, et al: TTF-2, a new forkhead protein, shows a temporal expression in the developing thyroid which is consistent with a role in controlling the onset of differentiation, EMBO J 16:3185–3197, 1997.

127. Plachov D, Chowdhury K, Walther C, et al: Pax8, a murine paired box gene expressed in the developing excretory system and thyroid gland, Development 110:643–651, 1990.

128. Thomas PQ, Brown A, Beddington R: Hex: a homeobox gene revealing peri-implantation asymmetry in the mouse embryo and an early transient marker of endothelial cell precursors, Development 125:85–95, 1998.

129. Francis-Lang H, Zannini MS, De Felice M, et al: Multiple mechanisms of interference between transformation and differentiation in thyroid cells, Mol Cell Biol 12:5793–5800, 1992.

130. De Felice M, Di Lauro R: Murine models for the study of thyroid gland development, Endocr Dev 10:1–14, 2007.

131. Civitareale D, Lonigro R, Sinclair AJ, et al: A thyroid-specific nuclear protein essential for tissue-specific expression of the thyroglobulin promoter, EMBO J 8:2537–2542, 1989.

132. Guazzi S, Price M, De Felice M, et al: Thyroid nuclear factor 1 (TTF-1) contains a homeodomain and displays a novel DNA binding specificity, EMBO J 9:3631–3639, 1990.

133. Lonigro R, De Felice M, Biffali E, et al: Expression of thyroid transcription factor 1 gene can be regulated at the transcriptional and posttranscriptional levels, Cell Growth Differ 7:251–261, 1996.

134. Hamdan H, Liu H, Li C, et al: Structure of the human Nkx2.1 gene, Biochim Biophys Acta 1396:336–348, 1998.

135. Ikeda K, Clark JC, Shaw-White JR, et al: Gene structure and expression of human thyroid transcription factor-1 in respiratory, J Biol Chem 270:8108–8114, 1995.

136. Damante G, Di Lauro R: Several regions of Antennapedia and thyroid transcription factor 1 homeodomains contribute to DNA binding specificity, Proc Natl Acad Sci U S A 88:5388–5392, 1991.

137. De Felice M, Damante G, Zannini MS, et al: Redundant domains contribute to the transcriptional activity of thyroid transcription factor 1 (TTF-1), J Biol Chem 270:26649–26656, 1995.

138. Zannini MS, Acebron A, Felice MD, et al: Mapping and functional role of phosphorylation sites in the thyroid transcription factor 1 (TTF-1), J Biol Chem 271:2249–2254, 1996.

139. De Felice M, Silberschmidt D, DiLauro R, et al: TTF-1 phosphorylation is required for peripheral lung morphogenesis, perinatal survival, and tissue-specific gene expression, J Biol Chem 278:35574–35583, 2003.

140. Lee BJ, Cho GJ, Norgren RB Jr, et al: TTF-1, a homeodomain gene required for diencephalic morphogenesis, is postnatally expressed in the neuroendocrine brain in a developmentally regulated and cell-specific fashion, Mol Cell Neurosci 17:107–126, 2001.

141. Kimura S, Hara Y, Pineau T, et al: The T/ebp null mouse: thyroid-specific enhancer-binding protein is essential for the organogenesis of the thyroid, lung, ventral forebrain, and pituitary, Genes Dev 10:60–69, 1996.

142. Minoo P, Su G, Drum H, et al: Defects in tracheo-esophageal and lung morphogenesis in Nkx2.1(–/–) mouse embryos, Devel Biol 209:60–71, 1999.

143. Sussel L, Marin O, Kimura S, et al: Loss of Nkx2.1 homeobox gene function results in a ventral to dorsal molecular respecification within the basal telencephalon: evidence for a transformation of the pallidum into the striatum, Development 126:3359–3370, 1999.

144. Kimura S, Ward JD, Minoo P: Thyroid-specific enhancer-binding protein/transcription factor 1 is not required for the initial specification of the thyroid and lung primordia, Biochimie 81:321–328, 1999.

145. Takuma N, Sheng HZ, Furuta Y, et al: Formation of Rathke's pouch requires dual induction from the diencephalon, Development 125:4835–4840, 1998.

146. Kusakabe T, Kawaguchi A, Hoshi N, et al: Thyroid-specific enhancer-binding protein/NKX2.1 is required for the maintenance of ordered architecture and function of the differentiated thyroid, Mol Endocrinol 20:1796–1809, 2006.

147. D'Andrea B, Iacone R, Di Palma T, et al: Functional inactivation of the transcription factor Pax8 through oligomerization chain reaction, Mol Endocrinol 20:1810 1824, 2006.

148. Zannini MS, Francis-Lang H, Plachov D, et al: Pax-8, a paired domain-containing protein, binds to a sequence overlapping the recognition site of a homeodomain and activates transcription from two thyroid-specific promoters, Mol Cell Biol 12:4230–4241, 1992.

149. Stapleton P, Weith A, Urbanek P, et al: Chromosomal localization of 7 Pax genes and cloning of a novel family member, Pax-9, Nature Genet 3:292–298, 1993.

150. Okladnova O, Poleev A, Fantes J, et al: The genomic organization of the murine Pax 8 gene and characterization of its basal promoter, Genomics 15:452–461., 1997.

151. Poleev A, Wendler F, Fickenscher H, et al: Distinct functional properties of three human paired-box-protein, PAX8, isoforms generated by alternative splicing in thyroid, kidney and Wilms' tumors, Eur J Biochem 228:899–911, 1995.

152. Poleev A, Fickenscher H, Mundlos S, et al: *PAX8*, a human paired box gene: isolation and expression in developing thyroid, kidney and Wilms' tumors, Development 116:611–623, 1992.

153. Ferretti E, Arturi F, Mattei T, et al: Expression, regulation, and function of paired-box gene 8 in the human placenta and placental cancer cell lines, Endocrinology 146:4009–4015, 2005.

154. Mittag J, Winterhager E, Bauer K, et al: Congenital hypothyroid female Pax8-deficient mice are infertile despite thyroid hormone replacement therapy, Endocrinology 148:719–725, 2007.

155. Wistuba J, Mittag J, Luetjens CM, et al: Male congenital hypothyroid Pax8–/– mice are infertile despite adequate treatment with thyroid hormone, J Endocrinol 192:99–109, 2007.

156. Fabbro D, Pellizzari L, Mercuri F, et al: Pax-8 protein levels regulate thyroglobulin gene expression, J Mol Endocrinol 21:347–354, 1998.

157. Van Renterghem P, Vassart G, Christophe D: Pax 8 expression in primary cultured dog thyrocyte is increased by cyclic AMP, Biochim Biophys Acta 1307:97–103, 1996.

158. Ohno M, Zannini MS, Levy O, et al: The paired-domain transcription factor Pax8 binds to the upstream enhancer of the rat Sodium/Iodide symporter gene and participates in both thyroid-specific and cyclic-AMP-dependent transcription, Mol Cell Biol 19:2051–2060, 1999.

159. Pasca di Magliano M, Di Lauro R, Zannini MS: Pax8 has a key role in thyroid cell differentiation, Proc Natl Acad Sci U S A 97:13144–13149, 2000.

160. Di Palma T, Nitsch R, Mascia A, et al: The paired domain-containing factor Pax8 and the homeodomain-containing factor TTF-1 directly interact and synergistically activate transcription, J Biol Chem 278:3395–3402, 2003.

161. Santisteban P, Acebron A, Polycarpou-Schwarz M, et al: Insulin and insulin-like growth factor 1 regulate a thyroid-specific nuclear protein that binds to the thyroglobulin promoter, Mol Endocrinol 6:1310–1317, 1992.

162. Kaestner KH, Lee KH, Schlondorff J, et al: Six members of the mouse forkhead gene family are developmentally regulated, Proc Natl Acad Sci U S A 90:7628–7631, 1993.

163. Lai E, Prezioso VR, Tao WF, et al: Hepatocyte nuclear factor 3 alpha belongs to a gene family in mammals that is homologous to the *Drosophila* homeotic gene forkhead, Genes Dev 5:416–427, 1991.

164. Chadwick BP, Obermayr F, Frischau A: FKHL15, a new human member of the forkhead gene family located on chromosome 9q22, Genomics 41:390–396, 1997.

165. Dathan N, Parlato R, Rosica A, et al: Distribution of the Titf2/Foxe1 gene product is consistent with an important role in the development of foregut endoderm, palate, and hair, Dev Dyn 224:450–456, 2002.

166. Macchia PE, Mattei MG, Lapi P, et al: Cloning, chromosomal localization and identification of polymorphisms in the human thyroid transcription factor 2 gene (TITF2), Biochimie 81:433–440, 1999.

167. Sequeira M, Al-Khafaji F, Park S, et al: Production and application of polyclonal antibody to human thyroid transcription factor 2 reveals thyroid transcription factor 2 protein expression in adult thyroid and hair follicles and prepubertal testis, Thyroid 13:927–932, 2003.

168. Ortiz L, Zannini MS, Di Lauro R, et al: Transcriptional control of the forkhead thyroid transcription factor TTF-2 by thyrotropin, insulin and insulin-like growth factor 1, J Biol Chem 272:23334–23339, 1997.

169. Crompton MR, Bartlett TJ, MacGregor AD, et al: Identification of a novel vertebrate homeobox gene expressed in haematopoietic cells, Nucleic Acids Res 20:5661–5667, 1992.

170. Martinez Barbera JP, Clements M, Thomas P, et al: The homeobox gene Hex is required in definitive endodermal tissues for normal forebrain, liver and thyroid formation, Development 127:2433–2445, 2000.

171. Hallaq H, Pinter E, Enciso J, et al: A null mutation of Hhex results in abnormal cardiac development, defective vasculogenesis and elevated Vegfa levels, Development 131:5197–5209, 2004.

172. Puppin C, D'Elia AV, Pellizzari L, et al: Thyroid-specific transcription factors control Hex promoter activity, Nucleic Acids Res 31:1845–1852, 2003.

173. Tanaka T, Inazu T, Yamada K, et al: DNA cloning and expression of rat homeobox gene, Hex, and functional characterization of the protein, Biochem J 339:111–117, 1999.

174. De Moerlooze L, Spencer-Dene B, Revest J, et al: An important role for the IIIb isoform of fibroblast growth factor receptor 2 (FGFR2) in mesenchymal-epithelial signalling during mouse organogenesis, Development 127:483–492, 2000.

175. Celli G, LaRochelle WJ, Mackem S, et al: Soluble dominant-negative receptor uncovers essential roles for fibroblast growth factors in multi-organ induction and patterning, EMBO J 17:1642–1645, 1998.

176. Revest JM, Spencer-Dene B, Kerr K, et al: Fibroblast growth factor receptor 2-IIIb acts upstream of Shh and Fgf4 and is required for limb bud maintenance but not for the induction of Fgf8, Fgf10, Msx1, or Bmp4, Dev Biol 231:47–62, 2001.

177. Biben C, Wang CC, Harvey RP: NK-2 class homeobox genes and pharyngeal/oral patterning: Nkx2-3 is required for salivary gland and tooth morphogenesis, Int J Dev Biol 46:415–422, 2002.

178. Dentice M, Cordeddu V, Rosica A, et al: Missense mutation in the transcription factor NKX2-5: a novel molecular event in the pathogenesis of thyroid dysgenesis, J Clin Endocrinol Metab 91:1428–1433, 2006.

179. Tanaka M, Yamasaki N, Izumo S: Phenotypic characterization of the murine Nkx2.6 homeobox gene by gene targeting, Mol Cell Biol 20:2874–2879, 2000.

180. Parmentier M, Libert F, Maenhaut C, et al: Molecular cloning of the thyrotropin receptor, Science 246:1620–1622, 1989.

181. Brown RS, Shalhoub V, Coulter S, et al: Developmental regulation of thyrotropin receptor gene expression in the fetal and neonatal rat thyroid: relation to thyroid morphology and to thyroid-specific gene expression, Endocrinology 141:340–345, 2000.

182. Stuart A, Oates E, Hall C, et al: Identification of a point mutation in the thyrotropin receptor of the hyt/hyt hypothyroid mouse, Mol Endocrinol 8:129–138, 1994.

183. Marians RC, Ng L, Blair HC, et al: Defining thyrotropin-dependent and independent steps of thyroid hormone synthesis by using thyrotropin receptor-null mice, Proc Natl Acad Sci U S A 99:15776–15781, 2002.

184. Kurihara Y, Kurihara H, Maemura K, et al: Impaired development of the thyroid and thymus in endothelin-1 knockout mice, J Cardiovasc Pharmacol 26:13–16, 1995.

185. Liao J, Kochilas L, Nowotschin S, et al: Full spectrum of malformations in velo-cardio-facial syndrome/DiGeorge syndrome mouse models by altering Tbx1 dosage, Hum Mol Genet 13:1577–1585, 2004.

186. Fisher DA, Klein A: Thyroid development and disorders of thyroid function in the newborn, New Engl J Med 304:702–712, 1981.

187. Maiorana R, Carta A, Floriddia G, et al: Thyroid hemiagenesis: prevalence in normal children and effect on thyroid function, J Clin Endocrinol Metab 88:1534–1536, 2003.

188. Van Vliet G: Development of the thyroid gland: lessons from congenitally hypothyroid mice and men, Clin Genet 63:445–455, 2003.

189. Marinovic D, Garel C, Czernichow P, et al: Additional phenotypic abnormalities with presence of cysts within the empty thyroid area in patients with congenital hypothyroidism with thyroid dysgenesis, J Clin Endocrinol Metab 88:1212–1216, 2003.

190. Clifton-Bligh RJ, Wentworth JM, Heinz P, et al: Mutation of the gene encoding human TTF-2 associated with thyroid agenesis, cleft palate and choanal atresia, Nat Genet 19:399–401, 1998.

191. Bamforth JS, Hughes IA, Lazarus JH, et al: Congenital hypothyroidism, spiky hair, and cleft palate, J Med Genet 26:49–60, 1989.

192. Castanet M, Park SM, Smith A, et al: A novel loss-of-function mutation in TTF-2 is associated with congenital hypothyroidism, thyroid agenesis and cleft palate, Hum Mol Genet 11:2051–2059, 2002.

193. Baris I, Arisoy AE, Smith A, et al: A novel missense mutation in human TTF-2 (FKHL15) gene associated with congenital hypothyroidism but not athyreosis, J Clin Endocrinol Metab 91:4183–4187, 2006.

194. Grueters A, Krude H, Biebermann H: Molecular genetic defects in congenital hypothyroidism, Eur J Endocrinol 151:U39–U44, 2004.

195. Gagne N, Parma J, Deal C, et al: Apparent congenital athyreosis contrasting with normal plasma thyroglobulin levels and associated with inactivating mutations in the thyrotropin receptor gene: are athyreosis and ectopic thyroid distinct entities? J Clin Endocrinol Metab 83:1771–1775, 1998.

196. Congdon T, Nguyen LQ, Nogueira CR, et al: A novel mutation (Q40P) in PAX8 associated with congenital hypothyroidism and thyroid hypoplasia: evidence for phenotypic variability in mother and child, J Clin Endocrinol Metab 86:3962–3967, 2001.

197. Komatsu M, Takahashi T, Takahashi I, et al: Thyroid dysgenesis caused by PAX8 mutation: the hypermutability with CpG dinucleotides at codon 31, J Pediatr 139:597–599, 2001.

198. Macchia PE, Lapi P, Krude H, et al: PAX8 mutations associated with congenital hypothyroidism caused by thyroid dysgenesis, Nat Genet 19:83–86, 1998.

199. Meeus L, Gilbert B, Rydlewski C, et al: Characterization of a novel loss of function mutation of PAX8 in a familial case of congenital hypothyroidism with in-place, normal-sized thyroid, J Clin Endocrinol Metab 89:4285–4291, 2004.

200. Vilain C, Rydlewski C, Duprez L, et al: Autosomal dominant transmission of congenital thyroid hypoplasia due to loss-of-function mutation of PAX8, J Clin Endocrinol Metab 86:234–238, 2001.

201. Doyle DA, Gonzalez I, Thomas B, et al: Autosomal dominant transmission of congenital hypothyroidism, neonatal respiratory distress, and ataxia caused by a mutation of NKX2-1, J Pediatr 145, 2004.

202. Iwatani N, Mabe H, Devriendt K, et al: Deletion of NKX2.1 gene encoding thyroid transcription factor 1 in two siblings with hypothyroidism and respiratory failure, J Pediatr 137:272–276, 2000.

203. Krude H, Schutz B, Biebermann H, et al: Choreoathetosis, hypothyroidism, and pulmonary alterations due to human NKX2-1 haploinsufficiency, J Clin Invest 109:475–480, 2002.

204. Moeller LC, Kimura S, Kusakabe T, et al: Hypothyroidism in thyroid transcription factor 1 haploinsufficiency is caused by reduced expression of the thyroid-stimulating hormone receptor, Mol Endocrinol 17:2295–2302, 2003.

205. Moya CM, Perez de Nanclares G, Castano L, et al: Functional study of a novel single deletion in the TITF1/NKX2.1 homeobox gene that produces congenital hypothyroidism and benign chorea but not pulmonary distress, Clin Endocrinol Metab 91:1832–1841, 2006.

206. Pohlenz J, Dumitrescu A, Zundel D, et al: Partial deficiency of thyroid transcription factor 1 produces predominantly neurological defects in humans and mice, J Clin Invest 109:469–473, 2002.

207. Stanbury JB, Rocmans P, Buhler UK, et al: Congenital hypothyroidism with impaired thyroid response to thyrotropin, N Engl J Med 279:1132–1136, 1968.

208. Sunthornthepvarakui T, Gottschalk ME, Hayashi Y, et al: Brief report: resistance to thyrotropin caused by mutations in the thyrotropin-receptor gene, N Engl J Med 332:155–160, 1995.

209. Park SM, Chatterjee VK: Genetics of congenital hypothyroidism, J Med Genet 42:379–389, 2005.

210. Eales J: Thyroid functions in cyclostomes and fishes. In Barrington E, editor: Hormones and Evolution, New York, 1979, Academic Press, pp 341–436.

211. Wendl T, Lun K, Mione M, et al: Pax2.1 is required for the development of thyroid follicles in zebrafish, Development 129:3751–3760, 2002.

212. Ericson LE, Fredriksson G: Phylogeny and ontogeny of the thyroid gland. In Greer M, editor: The Thyroid Gland, New York, 1990, Raven, pp 1–35.

213. Kluge B, Renault N, Rohr KB: Anatomical and molecular reinvestigation of lamprey endostyle development provides new insight into thyroid gland evolution, Dev Genes Evol 215:32–40, 2005.

214. Wright GM, Youson JH: Transformation of the endostyle of the anadromous sea lamprey, *Petromyzon marinus L.*, during metamorphosis. I. Light microscopy and autoradiography with ^{125}I1, Gen Comp Endocrinol 30:243–257, 1976.

215. Müller W: Ueber die Hypobranchialrinne der Tunicaten und deren Vorhandensein bei Amphioxus und den Cyklostomen, Jena Z Med Naturw 7:327–332, 1873.

216. Dohrn A: Thyroidea bei Petromyzon, Amphioxus und den Tunicaten, Mitt Zool Stat Neapel 6:49–92, 1885.

217. Dunn A: Properties of an iodinating enzyme in ascidian endostyle, Gen Comp Endocrinol 40:484–493, 1980.

218. Ogasawara M: Overlapping expression of amphioxus homologs of the thyroid transcription factor 1 gene and thyroid peroxidase gene in the endostyle: insight into evolution of the thyroid gland, Dev Genes Evol 210:231–242, 2000.

219. Ogasawara M, Di Lauro R, Satoh N: Ascidian homologs of mammalian thyroid peroxidase genes are expressed in the thyroid-equivalent region of the endostyle, J Exp Zool 285:58–69, 1999.

220. Ogasawara M, Satou Y: Expression of FoxE and FoxQ genes in the endostyle of Ciona intestinalis, Dev Genes Evol 213:416–419, 2003.

221. Ristoratore F, Spagnuolo A, Aniello F, et al: Expression and functional analysis of Cittf1, an ascidian NK-2 class gene, suggest its role in endoderm development, Development 126:149–159, 1999.

222. Ogasawara M, Shigetani Y, Suzuki S, et al: Expression of thyroid transcription factor-1 (TTF-1) gene in the ventral forebrain and endostyle of the agnathan vertebrate, *Lampetra japonica*, Genesis 30:51–58, 2001.

223. Yu JK, Holland LZ, Jamrich M, et al: AmphiFoxE4, an amphioxus winged helix/forkhead gene encoding a protein closely related to vertebrate thyroid transcription factor-2: expression during pharyngeal development, Evol Dev 4:9–15, 2002.

Chapter 2

THYROID-STIMULATING HORMONE: Physiology and Secretion

DAVID F. GORDON, VIRGINIA D. SARAPURA, MARY H. SAMUELS, and E. CHESTER RIDGWAY

Ontogeny of TSH-Producing Thyrotrope Cells
TSH Subunit Genes
Biosynthesis of TSH
TSH Secretion
Regulation of TSH Biosynthesis
Regulation of TSH Secretion
Action of TSH
TSH Measurements
Disorders of TSH Production

Thyroid-stimulating hormone (TSH) is a glycoprotein produced by the thyrotrope cells of the anterior pituitary gland. TSH, luteinizing hormone (LH), and follicle-stimulating hormone (FSH), as well as chorionic gonadotropin (CG) in the placenta, consist of a heterodimer of two noncovalently linked subunits, α and β. The α subunit is common to all four glycoproteins, whereas the β subunit is unique to each and confers specificity of action. Each TSH subunit is encoded by a separate gene and is coordinately transcribed and regulated mainly by thyroid hormone inhibition. Production of bioactive TSH involves a process of co-translational glycosylation and folding that enables combination between the nascent α and β subunits. TSH is stored in secretory granules and is released into the circulation in a regulated manner responsive mainly to the stimulatory effect of hypothalamic thyrotropin-releasing hormone (TRH). Circulating TSH binds to specific cell-surface receptors on the thyroid gland, where it stimulates the production of thyroid hormones, L-thyroxine (T_4) and L-triiodothyronine (T_3), which act on multiple organs and tissues to modulate many metabolic processes, resulting in a feedback inhibition of TSH output. The introduction of sensitive TSH assays has allowed accurate measurement of the level of circulating TSH and has led to the recognition of abnormal production of TSH related to abnormal function of the thyroid gland and reflecting a wide spectrum of metabolic derangements.

Ontogeny of TSH-Producing Thyrotrope Cells

Thyrotropes make up only 5% of pituitary cells in the anterior pituitary and are solely responsible for synthesizing TSH. The distinct cell types of the anterior pituitary are defined by the hormone they produce and include thyrotropes (TSH), gonadotropes (LH, FSH), corticotropes (adrenocorticotropic hormone [ACTH]), somatotropes (growth hormone [GH]), and lactotropes (prolactin [PRL]). Cell fate mapping demonstrated that the anterior pituitary develops from Rathke's pouch, an invagination of oral ectoderm that directly contacts the hypothalamus[1] at embryonic day 9.5 (e9.5). Pituitary organogenesis involves progenitor cells and their differentiation by signals that regulate proliferation, lineage commitment, and terminal differentiation.[2] The key genes initiating and controlling these developmental pathways include transcription factors, secreted signaling molecules, and receptors. Distinct cell lineages emerge as a result of signaling gradients of transcription factors formed in a spatially and temporally specific manner.[3]

The glycoprotein hormone α–subunit (αGSU) is the first pituitary hormone gene expressed during development[4] at e10.5. Wnt5a and BPM4, which are expressed in the adjacent neuroepithelium, provide the initial signals followed by expression of Hesx1, Ptx1/2, and Lhx3/4.[5] TSHβ expression begins in the rostral tip of the pituitary at e12.5 and correlates with thyrotrope embryonic factor (TEF).[6] By birth, TSHβ expression in the rostral tip has disappeared and another population of thyrotropes arises by e15.5 in the caudomedial region, following expression of Pit-1 (POU1F1), a pituitary-specific transcription factor.[7] Both Pit-1 and TSHβ subunit expression are present in the wild-type but not in the Snell dwarf mouse, which has a mutation of the Pit-1 gene.[8] These data suggest that the second population of thyrotropes, associated with Pit-1, is likely the source of mature thyrotropes. Pit-1 expression depends on the transient expression of Prophet of Pit-1 (Prop1) along with Atbf1.[9]

A zinc finger transcription factor, Gata2, plays a critical role in thyrotrope differentiation.[3] Gata2 is transcribed in the developing anterior pituitary as early as e10.5 and persists in an expression pattern coincident with the glycoprotein hormone α-subunit. Gata2 binds and transactivates the αGSU promoter[10] and acts synergistically with Pit-1 to activate the TSHβ gene.[11] A ventral-dorsal gradient of Gata2 occurs early in development: the intermediate cells that express both Gata2 and Pit-1 develop into thyrotropes. The in vivo function of Gata2 in pituitary development has been examined by targeted inactivation of Gata2 in a transgenic mouse model using Cre recombinase directed by the αGSU promoter/enhancer.[12] When Gata2 is ablated, mice have a decreased thyrotrope cell population at birth and lower levels of circulating TSH and FSH when adults. These studies showed that Gata2 is important for optimal thyrotrope and gonadotrope function but not for cell fate.

A recent study has uncovered the existence of an adult population of multipotent stem cells in the adult pituitary[13,14] that are distinct from the embryonic precursor cells. These nestin- and Sox2-containing stem cells reside in a localized niche within the periluminal region of the gland, have the capacity to expand into all of the terminally differentiated pituitary cell types after birth, and may contribute to pituitary tumors.[13]

TSH SUBUNIT GENES

The TSH α and β subunits are encoded by separate genes located on different chromosomes. Thyrotrope cells are believed to contain specific transcription factors that bind to the regulatory regions of the genes and interact with ubiquitous factors to initiate transcription. Extensive biochemical studies show that activation and/or repression of these genes within thyrotropes is fundamentally determined by modifications of the chromatin state at each gene. Following an activating (TRH) or inhibitory (T₃) stimulus, factors bind to the promoter, recruit specific chromatin-modifying enzymes, and initiate transcription when the gene is accessible or silence it when inaccessible to the transcriptional machinery.

TSHβ Subunit Gene Structure

The human TSHβ subunit gene has been isolated and characterized.[15] This single-copy gene is 4527 base pairs (bp) in size, and is located on the short arm of chromosome 1.[16] The gene structure consists of three exons and two introns (Fig. 2-1, *top panel*). The first exon has 37 bp and contains the 5′-untranslated region of the gene. It is separated from the second exon by a large first intron of 3.9 kb. The coding region of the gene is contained within the second (163 bp) and third (326 bp) exons, which are separated by a 0.45 kb intron, while the 3′-untranslated region is contained within the third exon.

DNA sequences close to the transcriptional start site in the promoter of the TSHβ gene contain elements responsible for initiating transcription and regulating expression. A consensus TATA box is located 28 bp upstream of the transcriptional start site and is important for positioning RNA synthesis. Progressive 5′ deletions of the mouse TSHβ promoter linked to a luciferase reporter following expression in thyrotrope cells defined the *cis*-acting sequences required for expression to the first 270 bp of the promoter.[17,18] Although these sequences defined the minimal promoter, other studies have shown that enhancer sequences located more than 6 kb upstream are also required for

TSHβ -Subunit Gene

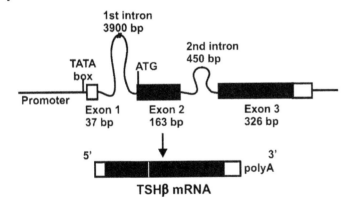

α-Subunit Gene

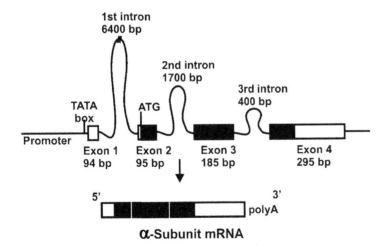

FIGURE 2-1. Structural organization of the human TSH subunit genes and mRNAs. The two panels show the TSHβ *(top)* and α subunit *(bottom)* genes. Shown are the relative locations and sizes of the exons and introns. Untranslated regions are shown as *open boxes*, and protein coding regions are shown in *black boxes*. The TATA box important for positioning the RNA transcriptional start is located in the promoter close to exon 1. Following transcription, introns are spliced out, exons precisely joined, and a polyA tail added to the 3′ end of the mature mRNA.

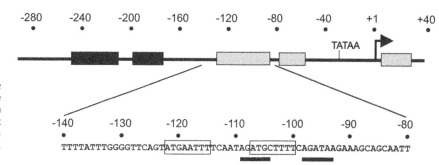

FIGURE 2-2. Functionally important regions of the TSHβ gene promoter. *Top,* Schematic showing regions *(shaded boxes)* of the TSHβ promoter that interact with transcription factors present in thyrotrope cells. *Below,* The DNA sequence of a key region that is critical for high level of TSHβ expression in thyrotropes. Within this region, Pit-1 sites are boxed, and sites interacting with Gata2 are underlined.

the promoter to express in pituitary thyrotropes in transgenic mice.[19]

Promoter deletion studies have demonstrated that the mouse TSHβ promoter from −271 to −80 is sufficient to confer thyrotrope-specific activity,[17] and thyrotrope transcription factors can bind to the proximal promoter.[20] Within this broad area, four regions of protein interaction have been identified using nuclear extracts from thyrotrope cells.[18] Two factors, Pit-1, a homeodomain factor, and Gata2, a zinc finger transcription factor, can bind to TSHβ promoter sequences from −135 to −88[21] (Fig. 2-2). Both factors can bind independently to the promoter, form a heteromeric complex with DNA, physically interact with each other, and functionally synergize to activate TSHβ promoter activity. Recently, an additional transcription factor, TRAP220 (Med1, PBP), was shown to be recruited to the TSHβ proximal promoter, where it was shown to play a role in transcriptional activation.[22]

TRAP220 was originally defined as part of a transcriptional mediator complex that interacts with hormone-occupied thyroid/steroid hormone receptors.[23] Mice with a single copy of this gene were hypothyroid with reduced levels of pituitary TSHβ transcripts.[24] TRAP220 is recruited to the TSHβ gene by virtue of its physical interaction with both Pit-1 and Gata2, since the protein itself does not bind DNA. Co-transfections in nonpituitary cells showed that Pit-1, Gata2, or TRAP220 alone could not stimulate the TSHβ promoter. However, maximal activity resulted when all three factors were expressed. Interaction studies showed that all three factors interact with each other in vivo and in vitro. The regions of interaction were important for maximal function. Chromatin immunoprecipitation demonstrated in vivo occupancy on the proximal TSHβ promoter.[22] Thus, the TSHβ gene is activated by a unique combination of transcription factors present in pituitary thyrotropes, including those that act via binding to the proximal promoter, as well as others that are recruited to the promoter via protein-protein interactions.

α Subunit Gene Structure

The human glycoprotein hormone α subunit gene is located on chromosome 6 at position 6q12-q21.[25] It is present as a single copy gene that is 9635 kb in size and contains four exons and three introns and contains a consensus TATA box located 26 bp upstream of the transcriptional start site.[26] The first exon (94 bp) contains 5′-untranslated sequences and is separated from the second exon by a 6.4 kilobase (kb) intron. The second exon contains 7 bp of 5′-untranslated sequence and 88 bp of the coding region. The coding sequence continues in the third (185 bp) and fourth (75 bp) exons, and the 3′-untranslated region (220 bp) is contained within the fourth exon (Fig. 2-1, *bottom panel*).

The α subunit gene is expressed in thyrotropes, gonadotropes, and placental cells but is differentially regulated. Cell-specific expression in each cell type is dependent on different regions of the promoter. Whereas the region downstream of −200 is sufficient for placental expression,[27] gonadotropes require sequences between −225 and −200,[28] and regions farther upstream appear to be critical for thyrotrope expression.[29] Transgenic mouse studies have shown 480 bp of the mouse α subunit 5′-flanking DNA could target transgenic expression to both gonadotropes and thyrotropes.[30] A region from −225 to −200 that binds steroidogenic factor 1 appears to be critical for gonadotrope expression,[31] but not for thyrotrope expression.[32] Another important sequence involves the pituitary glycoprotein hormone basal element, extending from −342 to −329, that is critical for both thyrotrope and gonadotrope expression.[33] The element interacts with P-LIM, a pituitary-specific LIM-homeodomain transcription factor that is important for other pituitary cells.[34] Several sequences within the region from −480 to −300 appear to be important for mouse α subunit expression in thyrotropes but not gonadotropes.[29] Among these is the sequence from −434 to −421, which interacts with the developmental homeodomain transcription factor Msx1.[35] Other sequences within the 480 bp promoter have been found to interact with the pituitary-specific homeodomain factor Ptx-1, and a synergism between Ptx-1 and P-LIM, mediated by the co-activator C-LIM, has been described.[36] Recent studies with the mouse promoter in transgenic mice showed that an upstream DNA element located between −4.6 and −3.7 kb further enhanced expression in both thyrotropes and gonadotropes, and contained consensus binding sites for Gata, SF1, Sp1, ETS, and bHLH factors, which suggests cooperativity between factors binding both to proximal *cis*-acting elements and to the distal enhancer.[37]

BIOSYNTHESIS OF TSH

The intact TSH molecule is a heterodimeric glycoprotein with a molecular weight of 28 kDa that is composed of the noncovalently linked α and β subunits. The common α subunit contains 92 amino acids, and the specific TSHβ subunit has 118 amino acids. TSH biosynthesis and secretion by thyrotrope cells of the anterior pituitary are precisely regulated events. This section examines our understanding of the biosynthesis of TSH, including the processes of transcription, translation, glycosylation, folding, combination, and storage.

Transcription of TSH Subunit Genes

The DNA information contained in the TSHβ and α subunit genes is transcribed into a precursor RNA by a complex of enzymes, as directed by their respective promoters in the presence of both ubiquitous and specific transcription factors. The transcribed RNAs undergo a precise series of splicing events at the exon-intron junctions that lead to the production of the mature messenger RNA (mRNA) that then exits the nucleus and is translated to protein in the cytoplasm prior to posttranslational modification, subunit association, storage, and finally secretion. Transcription of the TSHβ and α subunit genes is coordinated under the influence of physiologic regulators, the most important of which are T_3 and TRH.

Translation of TSH Subunits

The next steps in TSH biosynthesis are summarized in Fig. 2-3.[38] The mRNAs for the TSHβ and α subunits are independently translated by ribosomes in the cytoplasm. The first peptide sequences consist of "signal" peptides of 20 amino acids for TSHβ and 24 amino acids for α.[39] These signal peptides are hydrophobic, allowing insertion through the lipid bilayer of the membrane of the rough endoplasmic reticulum. Translation into TSHβ and α pre-subunits continues into the lumen of the rough endoplasmic reticulum, and cleavage of the signal peptide occurs before translation is completed. This results in the formation of a 118 amino acid TSHβ subunit[40] and a 92 amino acid α subunit. Cleavage of TSHβ to a protein of 112 amino acids appears to be an artifact of purification. Synthesis of recombinant TSHβ subunit has resulted in two products of 112 and 118 amino acids, both of which are similarly active in vitro.[41]

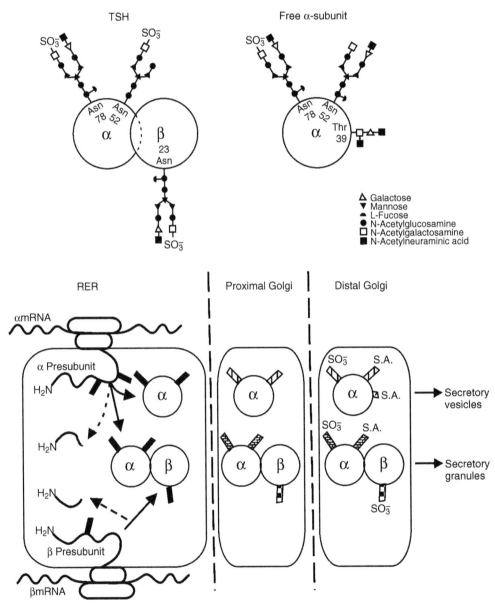

FIGURE 2-3. *Top panel,* Oligosaccharide chains of thyroid-stimulating hormone (TSH). Shown are typical oligosaccharide chains present on the TSH heterodimer and the free α subunit. Glycosylated asparagine (Asp) and threonine (Thr) residues are indicated. Symbols represent the oligosaccharide chain residues as indicated in the key. *Bottom panel,* Biosynthesis of thyroid-stimulating hormone (TSH). Schematic shown includes the processes of translation and glycosylation within the rough endoplasmic reticulum (RER) and Golgi apparatus, divided into proximal and distal. Cleavage of the aminoterminal (H_2N) signal peptide and early addition of high mannose chains *(black boxes),* as well as the combination of α and β subunits, occur in the RER. In the proximal Golgi, oligosaccharide chains are modified *(shaded boxes),* and the final steps of sulfation and sialation occur in the distal Golgi apparatus. (From Weintraub BD, Gesundheit N: Thyroid-stimulating hormone synthesis and glycosylation: clinical implications. Thyroid Today 10:1–11, 1987.)

Glycosylation of TSH

Glycosylation of TSH has a significant impact on its biological activity.[42] The TSHβ subunit has a single glycosylation site, the asparagine residue at position 23, whereas the α subunit is glycosylated in two sites, the asparagine residues at positions 52 and 78[43] (see Fig. 2-3). Excess free α subunit is glycosylated at an additional site, the threonine residue at position 39.[44] This residue is located in a region believed to be important for combination with the TSHβ subunit. It is not known whether glycosylation at this residue is a regulated step that inhibits combination with the TSHβ subunit, or whether it occurs in excess free α subunits because this site is exposed.

Extensive studies on the processes of TSH subunit glycosylation have been carried out. Glycosylation of the TSHβ and α subunits begins before translation is completed (co-translational glycosylation), and addition of the second oligosaccharide in the α subunit occurs after translation is completed (posttranslational glycosylation). The first step in this process involves the assembly of a 14-residue oligosaccharide, (glucose)3-(mannose)9-(N-acetylglucosamine)2 on a dolichol-phosphate carrier. This oligosaccharide then is transferred to asparagine residues by the enzyme olygosaccharyl transferase, which recognizes the tripeptide sequence (asparagine)-(X)-(serine or threonine).[45] This mannose-rich oligosaccharide is progressively cleaved in the rough endoplasmic reticulum and Golgi apparatus. An intermediate with only six residues is produced and then other residues are added, resulting in complex oligosaccharides.[46] The residues added include N-acetylglucosamine, fucose, galactose, and N-acetylgalactosamine. Oligosaccharides before the six-residue intermediate are termed high mannose and are sensitive to endoglycosidase H, which releases the oligosaccharide from the protein, whereas the intermediate and complex oligosaccharides are endoglycosidase H resistant. Complex oligosaccharides usually consist of two branches (biantennary), but sometimes three or four branches are seen, as are hybrid oligosaccharides consisting of one complex and another high-mannose branch. Sulfation and sialation occur late in the pathway, within the distal Golgi apparatus. Sulfate is bound to N-acetylgalactosamine residues, and sialic acid, or its precursor N-acetylneuraminic acid, is bound to galactoside residues.[47] Thus, activation of the enzymes sulfotransferase and N-acetylgalactosamine transferase may involve important regulatory steps that affect the ratio of sulfate to sialic acid. As demonstrated with LH, it appears that sulfation increases and sialylation decreases the bioactivity of TSH,[47] because the exclusively sialylated recombinant glycoprotein produced in Chinese hamster ovary cells has been found to have attenuated activity in vitro.[48]

Processing of complex oligosaccharides appears to occur at a slower rate for secreted glycoproteins, such as TSH, when compared with that for nonsecreted glycoproteins. For example, after an 11 minute pulse labeling with [35S]methionine and a 30 minute chase, only a few α subunits were endoglycosidase H resistant, and only 76% reached this stage after an 18 hour chase.[49] Secretion was observed after a 60 minute chase, and the secreted products—TSH, free α subunit but no free β subunit—had mostly complex oligosaccharides associated with them.[43] It may be important to note that many of the studies described were carried out in thyrotropic tumor tissue obtained from hypothyroid mice, and glycosylation may differ in the euthyroid as compared with the hypothyroid state. In addition, differences between species have been noted, such as the human TSH may contain more sialic acid than the bovine TSH.[40]

Folding, Combination, and Storage of TSH

Elucidation of the crystal structure of human CG (hCG)[50] allowed the construction of a model of human TSH, as supported by other evidence.[51,52] This model has greatly facilitated the interpretation of structure-function studies of the protein backbone. However, crystallization was achieved only with partly deglycosylated hCG, so it is likely that the conformation of the glycosylated protein may differ to some extent, although nuclear magnetic resonance studies suggest that the α subunit carbohydrate moieties project outward and may be freely mobile.[53] Nevertheless, this model predicts that the tertiary structure of each TSH subunit consists of two hairpin loops on one side of a central knot formed by three disulfide bonds and a long loop on the opposite side. In this tertiary structure, the glycoprotein hormones share features in common with transforming growth factor β, nerve growth factor, platelet-derived growth factor, vascular endothelial growth factor, inhibin, and activin, all of which are now grouped in the family of "cystine knot" growth factors.[54]

Folding of nascent peptides begins before translation is completed. It has been shown that proper folding is dependent on glycosylation, because the drug tunicamycin, which prevents the initial oligosaccharide transfer to the asparagine residue, results in a peptide that does not fold properly and is degraded intracellularly.[55] Site-directed mutagenesis of a single glycosylation site also disrupted processing and decreased TSH secretion in transfected Chinese hamster ovary cells.[56] Folding is a critical step that allows correct internal disulfide bonding, which stabilizes the tertiary structure of the protein, allowing subunit combination.

Combination of TSH β and α subunits begins soon after translation is completed in the rough endoplasmic reticulum and continues in the Golgi apparatus.[43] Subunit combination then accelerates and modifies oligosaccharide processing of the α subunit.[57] In fact, studies have suggested that the conformation of the α subunit differs after combination with each type of β subunit,[58] and this may affect subsequent processing. The rate of combination of TSHβ and α subunits has been examined in mouse thyrotropic tumors. After a 20 minute pulse labeling with [35S]methionine, 19% of TSHβ subunits were combined with α subunits, and this percentage increased to 61% after a additional 60 minute chase incubation.[43] Recent studies have shown that the combination of the TSHβ and α subunits, as is also the case with other glycoprotein hormones, occurs after "latching" of the disulfide "seatbelt" of the β subunit, with subsequent "threading" of loop 2 and the attached oligosaccharide of the α subunit beneath that "seatbelt."[59]

The sequence of the TSHβ subunit from amino acid 27 to 31 (CAGYC) is highly conserved among species and is thought to be important for combination with the α subunit. In a case of congenital hypothyroidism, a point mutation in the CAGYC region (see "Disorders of TSH Production") results in the synthesis of altered TSHβ subunits that are unable to associate with α subunits, with consequent lack of intact TSH production.[60] A lack of free circulating TSHβ subunit was also observed, suggesting that combination with α subunit is necessary for TSHβ subunit secretion. This phenomenon was also demonstrated in studies where synthesis of wild-type recombinant TSHα subunit was carried out in the presence or absence of recombinant β subunit.[61] Using site-directed mutagenesis, another study showed that a mutation at residue 25 in the glycosylation recognition site, which substitutes a serine for a threonine, does not alter glycosylation but decreases TSH production by 70%, possibly because of disruption of the nearby CAGYC region.[62]

After TSH and free α subunit are processed in the distal Golgi apparatus, they are transported into secretory granules or vesicles.[63] The secretory granules constitute a regulated secretory pathway, mainly influenced by TRH and other hypothalamic factors. These granules contain mostly TSH, whereas free α subunit is contained in the secretory vesicles that constitute a nonregulated secretory pathway.

TSH SECRETION

In healthy humans, the production rate of TSH is between 100 and 400 mU/day.[64,65] The distribution space of TSH is slightly greater than the plasma volume. In euthyroid subjects, the half-life of TSH in plasma is approximately 50 minutes, with a plasma clearance rate of approximately 50 mL/min. In hypothyroid subjects, TSH secretion rates increase by 10 to 15 times normal rates, and the clearance rate decreases slightly. In hyperthyroid subjects, TSH secretion is suppressed, and metabolic clearance is accelerated.

Ontogeny of TSH Levels

At 8 to 10 weeks of gestation in the human, TRH is measurable in the hypothalamus, with progressive increases in TRH levels until term. By 12 weeks of gestation, immunoreactive TSH cells are present in the human pituitary gland,[66] and TSH is detectable in the pituitary and the serum.[67,68] Serum and pituitary TSH levels remain low until week 18, when TSH levels increase rapidly, followed by increases in serum T_4 and T_3 concentrations. Fetal serum TSH and T_4 concentrations continue to increase between 20 and 40 weeks of gestation. Pituitary TSH begins to respond to exogenous TRH early in the third trimester, and negative feedback control of TSH secretion develops during the last half of gestation and the first 1 to 2 months of life.[69]

An abrupt rise in serum TSH levels occurs within 30 minutes of birth in term infants. This is followed by an increase in serum T_3 concentrations within 4 hours and a lesser increase in T_4 levels within the first 24 to 36 hours. The initial increase in serum TSH levels appears to be stimulated by cooling in the extrauterine environment. Serum TSH levels fall to the adult range by 3 to 5 days after birth, and serum thyroid hormone levels stabilize by 1 to 2 months. Serum TSH levels in healthy premature infants (less than 37 weeks gestational age) are highly variable but tend to be lower at birth compared with those of term infants. TSH levels decrease slightly during the first week of life, followed by a gradual increase to normal term levels. Serum TSH levels are even lower in ill premature infants but rise toward normal levels during recovery.[70,71]

Patterns of TSH Secretion

TSH is secreted from the pituitary gland in a dual fashion, with secretory bursts (pulses) superimposed upon basal (apulsatile) secretion (Fig. 2-4, *upper panel*). Basal TSH secretion accounts for 30% to 40% of the total amount released into the circulation, and secretory bursts account for the remaining 60% to 70%. TSH pulses occur approximately every 2 to 3 hours, although considerable variability is noted among individuals.[72] TSH pulses appear to directly stimulate T_3 secretion from the thyroid gland, as cross-correlation analysis has shown that a free T_3 peak occurs between 0.5 and 2.5 hours after a TSH peak. However, changes in free T_3 levels from nadir to peak are only 11% of mean free T_3 levels, probably because T_3 has a long serum half-life, and most T_3 does not arise from the thyroid gland.[73]

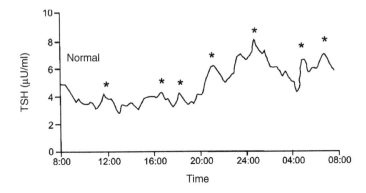

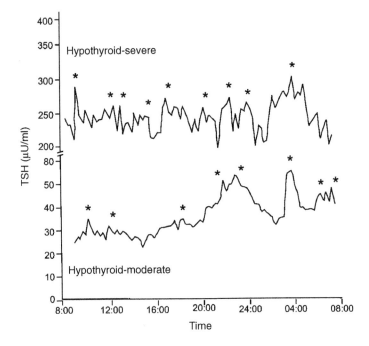

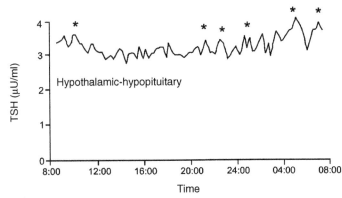

FIGURE 2-4. Serum thyroid-stimulating hormone (TSH) levels measured every 15 minutes in a healthy subject *(upper panel)*, in two subjects with primary hypothyroidism *(middle panel)*, and in a subject with hypothyroidism due to a craniopharyngioma *(lower panel)*. Significant TSH pulses were located by cluster analysis, a computerized pulse detection program, and are indicated by asterisks. (Data from Sarapura VD, Samuels MH, Ridgway EC: Thyroid-stimulating hormone. In: Melmed S [ed]: The Pituitary, 2nd ed. Blackwell Science, Malden, MA, pp 187–229, 2002.)

In healthy euthyroid subjects, TSH is secreted in a circadian pattern, with nocturnal levels increasing to up to twice daytime levels[72] (Fig. 2-4, *upper panel*). Peak TSH levels occur at between 2300 and 0500 hours in subjects with normal sleep-wake cycles, and nadir levels occur at about 1100 hours. The TSH circadian rhythm is not present in infants younger than 4 weeks old but emerges between 1 and 2 months of life and is well established in healthy children.[74] The circadian variation in TSH levels is due to increased mass of TSH secreted per burst at night, as well as slightly increased frequency of bursts and more rapid increase to maximal TSH secretion within a burst.[72] The nocturnal increase in TSH levels can precede the onset of sleep, and sleep deprivation enhances TSH secretion. Therefore, in contrast to other pituitary hormones with a circadian variation, the nocturnal rise in TSH levels is not sleep entrained. Instead, a sleep-related inhibition of TSH release is of insufficient magnitude to counteract the nocturnal TSH surge.

Subjects with mild primary hypothyroidism retain the nocturnal rise in TSH levels, and patients with severe primary hypothyroidism have markedly increased TSH pulse amplitude throughout the day with loss of circadian variation in TSH levels (Fig. 2-4, *middle panel*).[72] L-Thyroxine therapy reestablishes the normal TSH circadian variation. In contrast, patients with hypothalamic-pituitary causes of hypothyroidism secrete less TSH over a 24 hour period, with loss of the nocturnal TSH surge in pulse amplitude[75] (Fig. 2-4, *lower panel*). A similar pattern of reduced 24 hour TSH secretion occurs in critical illness.[76]

The origin of pulsatile and circadian TSH secretion is not known. Thyroid hormones alter TSH pulse amplitude but have little effect on pulse frequency, and therefore are unlikely to participate in TSH pulse generation. The TSH pulse generator may reside in the hypothalamus, with TRH neurons acting in concert to stimulate a burst of TSH secretion from the pituitary gland. However, constant TRH infusions do not change TSH pulse frequency in humans, which casts doubt on this theory.[77] Dopamine suppresses TSH pulse amplitude but does not alter TSH pulse frequency, and therefore dopamine does not appear to control pulsatile TSH secretion. A diurnal variation in the activity of anterior pituitary 5'-monodeiodinase in the rat may control circadian TSH secretion.[78] However, this has not been confirmed in the human.

Physiologic serum cortisol levels may control circadian TSH secretion, although cortisol does not appear to affect TSH pulse frequency. When subjects with adrenal insufficiency were studied under conditions of glucocorticoid withdrawal, daytime TSH levels were increased, and the usual TSH circadian rhythm was abolished. When these subjects were given physiologic doses of hydrocortisone in a pattern that mimicked normal pulsatile and circadian cortisol secretion, daytime TSH levels were decreased, and the normal TSH circadian rhythm was reestablished. Hydrocortisone infusions at the same dose given as pulses of constant amplitude throughout the 24 hour period also decreased 24 hour TSH levels, but no circadian variation was noted.[79] Similarly, when healthy subjects were given metyrapone (an inhibitor of endogenous cortisol synthesis), TSH levels increased during the day, leading to abolition of the usual TSH circadian variation.[80] These data suggest that the normal early morning increase in endogenous serum cortisol levels decreases serum TSH levels and leads to the observed normal circadian variation in TSH.

REGULATION OF TSH BIOSYNTHESIS

TSH biosynthesis is regulated by coordinated signals from the central nervous system and feedback from the peripheral circulation. The most important positive input for TSH biosynthesis is hypothalamic TRH, and the most powerful negative regulators are circulating thyroid hormone levels. However, additional hypothalamic factors and circulating hormones have important modifying effects. Most of these factors have independent effects on the biosynthesis of the two subunits of TSH.

Hypothalamic Regulation of TSHβ Subunit Biosynthesis

Thyrotropin-releasing hormone (TRH) is a tripeptide that is secreted from the hypothalamus and transported to the pituitary via the hypothalamic-hypophyseal portal system; it is a major activator of TSH production with a significant three- to fivefold increase in the transcription of both TSHβ and α subunit mRNAs.[81] TRH from maternal or fetal sources is not required for normal thyrotrope development during ontogeny, and TRH-deficient mice are not hypothyroid at birth. However, TRH is required for the postnatal maintenance of TSH activation.[82]

TRH binding to its receptor initiates a cascade of intracellular events. In GH$_3$ cells, the TRH-receptor complex interacts with a guanine nucleotide binding regulatory protein (G) that then binds and activates GTP(G'). G' binds to phospholipase C (C) and activates it (C'). C' catalyzes the hydrolysis of phosphatidylinositol 4,5 bisphosphate, which results in the formation of two intracellular "second messengers," inositol triphosphate (InsP$_3$) and 1,2-diacylglycerol (1,2-DG). InsP$_3$ diffuses from the cell-surface membrane to the endoplasmic reticulum, where it causes the release of sequestered Ca^{2+}. This activates the movement of secretory granules to the cell surface and their exocytosis. Simultaneous with these events is a parallel activation of protein kinase C by 1,2-DG, which also leads to phosphorylation of proteins involved in exocytosis. TRH has been shown to stimulate a nuclear protein, Islet-brain-1 (IB1)/JIP-1, in the anterior pituitary gland and in cultured rat GH$_3$ cells[83] and has been implicated in the action of TRH in stimulating the TSHβ gene in thyrotropes. Studies in somatomammotrope cells, where TRH stimulates prolactin production, have suggested that phosphatidylinositol, protein kinase C, and calcium-dependent pathways may be involved,[84] although TRH stimulation of the TSHβ subunit promoter may be mediated by AP1.[85]

Two TRH-response regions are located from −128 to −61 and from −28 to +8 of the human TSHβ promoter.[86] The upstream region contains binding sites for the pituitary-specific transcription factor, Pit-1, suggesting a role for this or a similar factor in the regulation of the TSHβ subunit gene by TRH. In the rat TSHβ subunit gene, responsiveness to TRH has been localized to regions upstream of −204, where Pit-1 binding sites are also found.[87] Furthermore, it has been shown that both protein kinase C and protein kinase A pathways can phosphorylate Pit-1 at two sites in response to phorbol esters and cyclic adenosine monophosphate (cAMP),[88] thus altering the binding to Pit-1 transactivation elements on the human TSHβ gene.[89]

Dopamine acting via DA2 dopamine receptors inhibits TSHα and β subunit gene transcription by decreasing the intracellular levels of cAMP.[81] Studies of the TSHβ subunit gene have localized two regions of the promoter necessary for cAMP stimulation, from −128 to −61 bp and from +3 to +8 bp. The upstream region coincides with the TRH-responsive region and contains Pit-1 binding sites. The downstream region resides within the regions responsive to T$_3$ (+3 to +37) and TRH (−28 to +8). The downstream region also overlaps with an AP1 binding site (−1 to +6). The sequence from −1 to +6 appears to cooperate with Pit-1 in mediating responses to cAMP and TRH.[85] Thus, multiple interactions between transcription factors and hormonal regulators appear to converge on sequences close to the transcriptional start site.

Peripheral Regulation of TSHβ Subunit Biosynthesis

Thyroid hormone is thought to act predominantly through a classical TR-mediated genomic model. T_4 serves as a minimally active prohormone that is converted into a metabolically active T_3 via a family of tissue deiodinases, termed D1, D2, and D3. These selenoprotein enzymes are membrane bound and can activate or inactivate substrate in a time- and tissue-specific manner.[90] D2 is the major T_4-activating deiodinase. It is present on the endoplasmic reticulum close to the nucleus and produces 3,5,3′-triiodothyronine (T_3) through the removal of an iodine residue from the outer ring of thyroxine. D2 activity is rapidly lost in the presence of its substrate T_4 by a ubiquitin proteasomal mechanism.[91] Rat pituitary thyrotropes coexpress D2 RNA and protein, and both are increased in hypothyroidism. Murine thyrotropes in TtT-97 tumors or the TαT1 cell line have extremely high levels of D2, which accounts for the sustained production of T_3 by thyrotropes even in the presence of supraphysiologic T_4 levels. Serum TSH levels in normal mice are suppressed by administration of T_4 or T_3, although only T_3 was effective in the mouse with targeted disruption of the D2 gene. The observed phenotype of pituitary resistance to T_4 demonstrated the critical importance of D2 in controlling negative thyroid hormone regulation of TSH in thyrotropes.

T_4 can also act, in some cases, via nongenomic mechanisms that do not involve classical nuclear TR mechanisms. T_4 can bind to a cell-surface integrin $\alpha V\beta 3$ receptor followed by activation of a mitogen-activated protein kinase cascade, which transduces the signal into a complex series of cellular and nuclear actions. These nongenomic hormone actions are likely to be contributors to basal rate setting of transcription of some genes, and they may control complex cellular events.[92]

TSHβ and α subunit gene transcription rates are markedly inhibited by treatment with triiodothyronine (T_3). Studies using mouse TtT-97 thyrotropic tumors have demonstrated that suppression of TSHβ and α subunit mRNA transcription rates measured by nuclear run-on assays is evident by 30 minutes after treatment and is maximal by 4 hours.[93] This effect was seen in the presence of the protein synthesis inhibitor cycloheximide, indicating that it did not require an intermediary protein. Other studies using mouse and rat pituitaries along with mouse thyrotropic tumors have demonstrated that steady-state mRNA levels of TSHβ and α subunits are dramatically decreased by T_3[94] (Fig. 2-5). The mechanism of action of T_3 involves interaction with nuclear receptors that act mainly at the transcriptional level. The transcriptional response to T_3 is proportional to the nuclear receptor occupancy,[95] and the time course of T_3 nuclear binding and that of transcriptional inhibition are also in agreement[96] (see Fig. 2-5).

The T_3 inhibitory effect on the TSHβ gene requires ligand-occupied T_3 receptor (TR), specifically the TRβ1 or TRβ2 isoform, because patients with thyroid hormone resistance and inappropriate secretion of TSH have abnormalities only in the TRβ, not the TRα, gene.[97] TRβ interacts with specific cis-acting DNA sequences close to the transcriptional start. T_3 response elements have been reported to be located between +3 and +37 of the human TSHβ gene.[98] Two T_3 receptor binding sites, from +3 to +13 and from +28 to +37, may mediate T_3 inhibition. T_3 responses can be mediated through receptor monomers, homodimers, or heterodimers involving retinoid X receptors (RXR).[99] An RXR selective ligand was shown in vitro to inhibit TSHβ expression in TtT-97 thyrotropic tumor cells[100] and in cultured TαT1 thyrotropes.[101] This finding has been confirmed in vivo and

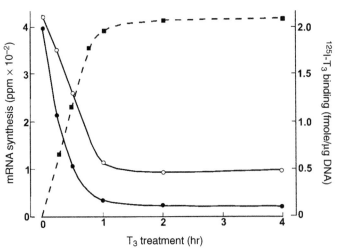

FIGURE 2-5. The effect of thyroid hormone on the transcription of the thyroid-stimulating hormone (TSH)β *(black circles)* and α subunit *(white circles)* genes. Murine thyrotropic tumor explants were incubated for up to 4 hours with 5 nmol T_3 for transcription measurements or with 5 nmole $^{125}I\,T_3$, with or without 1000-fold excess of unlabeled T_3 for binding measurements. Transcription rates were measured in pools of isolated nuclei. An inverse relationship has been noted between T_3 binding and TSHβ and α subunit mRNA synthesis. (Data from Shupnik MA, Ridgway EC: Triiodothyronine rapidly decreases transcription of the thyrotropin subunit genes in thyrotropic tumor explants. Endocrinology 117:1940–1946, 1985.)

resulted in central hypothyroidism (low T_4 and low TSH) in cancer patients treated with the retinoid bexarotene.[102] The RXR-selective retinoid (LG 268) decreased circulating TSH and T_4 levels in mice with marked lowering of pituitary TSHβ mRNA without decreasing TRH, suggesting a direct effect on thyrotropes.[101]

Other, more recent studies have disputed the requirement of the negative response element located in exon 1 of the human gene, because its deletion did not eliminate T_3 suppression of TSHβ promoter activity in a reconstitution system.[103] These studies showed that liganded TRβ can associate with Gata2 in vitro and in vivo via direct interaction between the zinc fingers of Gata2 and the DNA binding domain of TRβ. In addition, T_3-occupied TR can physically interact with TRAP220.[24] Thus, it is likely that interference with the transactivation function of the Pit-1/Gata2/TRAP220 complex on the proximal TSHβ promoter plays an important role in T_3 negative regulation.

Abundant information exists as to the mechanisms involved in gene stimulation by T_3. Generally, TRs bind to cis-acting DNA response elements (TRE) in the absence of ligand, interact with a family of nuclear receptor corepressor molecules that recruit histone deacetylases, and locally modify chromatin structure to result in repression of the target gene.[104] In the presence of T_3, the corepressor complexes rapidly dissociate and are replaced by coactivator complexes that bind to TRs and increase histone methylation and acetylation locally on the chromosomal DNA, which unwinds the chromatin into an open configuration.[105] Other activating transcription factors such as TRAP220 are then recruited to the TR via protein-protein interactions, which then activate RNA polymerase II–mediated transcription.

In contrast, the molecular mechanisms involved in negative T_3 regulation, such as the TSH subunit genes, have not been well characterized. Liganded TRβ has been reported to recruit histone deacetylase 3 and reduce histone H4 acetylation that modifies histones, resulting in a fully repressed chromosomal state of the TSHβ gene.[103] Several recent studies have demonstrated the requirement of an intact DNA binding domain of TRβ in the negative regulation of the TSHβ gene in vitro[106] and in vivo.[107] In one study, a combination of Pit-1 and Gata2 activated a human TSHβ (−128/+37) reporter construct along with vectors containing TRβ1 constructs in the absence or presence of T_3. These investigators found that unliganded TRβ1 did not stimulate promoter activity, whereas a mutation lacking the N-terminus and DNA binding domain of TRβ1 lost the ability of T_3-treated cells to negatively regulate TSHβ promoter activity. This demonstrated the importance of various modular domains that constitute the molecular structure of TRs. Moreover, using a gene targeting approach in transgenic mice and replacing the wild-type TRβ gene with a mutant that abolished DNA binding in vitro did not alter ligand and cofactor interactions.[107] Homozygous mutant mice demonstrated central thyroid hormone resistance with 20-fold higher serum TSH in the face of two- to threefold higher T_3 and T_4 levels, which were similar to those of TRβ homozygous null mice.

Although thyrotrope cells contain all TRs—TRα1, TRβ1, and TRβ2, as well as non-T_3 binding variant α2[108]—it is TRβ2 that is expressed predominantly in the pituitary and in T_3-responsive TRH neurons[109] and is most critical for the regulation of TSH.[110] Moreover, TRβ2-deficient mice had a phenotype consistent with pituitary resistance to thyroid hormone, with increased TSH and thyroid hormone levels, even in the presence of TRβ1 and TRα1, showing the lack of compensation between TR isoforms.[111] However, TRβ1 and TRα1 still may play a role, in that they are able to form heterodimers with TRβ2. Heterodimers of a TR and a TR accessory protein, such as RXR, may also bind to DNA,[112] constituting heterodimeric complexes that may have different affinities for specific DNA sequences and different functional activities. A particular RXR isoform, RXRγ1, is uniquely expressed in thyrotropes and appears to mediate the inhibition by 9-cis-retinoic acid through a region extending from −200 to −149 of the mouse TSHβ subunit promoter, an area upstream and distinct from that mediating negative regulation by thyroid hormone.[100] Other proteins that interact with TR include the coactivators, such as the glucocorticoid receptor interacting protein-1 (GRIP-1) and the steroid receptor coactivator-1 (SRC-1),[113] and corepressors, such as the silencing mediator for retinoid receptors and thyroid hormone receptors (SMRT) and the nuclear receptor corepressor (NCoR).[114] These coactivators and corepressors modulate the effects of many members of the steroid-thyroid hormone receptor superfamily. Their role in the regulation of TSH subunit promoters by thyroid hormone remains to be elucidated in detail.

Studies with genetic knockout mouse models in which both TRH and TRβ genes were removed have recently showed an unexpected dominant role for TRH in vivo in regulating the hypothalamic-pituitary-thyroid axis. It appears that the presence of both TRβ and TRH is necessary for a normal thyrotroph response during hypothyroidism, suggesting that unliganded TRβ stimulates TSH subunit gene expression.[115]

Posttranscriptional effects of T_3 have also been described. T_3 decreases the half-life of TSHβ subunit mRNA and decreases the size of the poly(A) tail.[116] The shortening of the poly(A) tail is thought to cause mRNA instability. Leedman et al. showed that T_3 increased the binding of an RNA-binding protein present in rat pituitary to the 3′-untranslated region of the rat TSHβ mRNA[117] and also induced a shortening of the poly(A) tail of the mouse TSHβ mRNA from 160 to 30 nucleotides.[118]

Steroid hormones, specifically glucocorticoids, inhibit TSH production, but TSH subunit mRNA levels do not change sig-

nificantly.[119] Their major effect may be seen at the secretory level. Estrogens mildly reduce both α and TSHβ subunit mRNA in hypothyroid rats compared with euthyroid controls.[120] In this study, estrogen also abolished the early rise in subunit mRNA levels seen following T_3 replacement. Testosterone has been shown to increase TSHβ subunit mRNA in castrate rat pituitary and mouse thyrotropic tumor.[121]

Leptin and neuropeptide Y have opposite effects on TSH biosynthesis. Leptin is the product of the *ob* gene, which is found mainly in adipose tissue and regulates body weight and energy expenditure.[122] Neuropeptide Y (NPY) is a neuropeptide that is synthesized in the arcuate nucleus of the hypothalamus and plays many roles in neuroendocrine function.[123] In dispersed rat pituitary cells, leptin stimulated and NPY inhibited TSHβ mRNA levels in a dose-related manner.[124] In contrast, both agents increased α subunit steady state mRNA levels.

Hypothalamic Regulation of α Subunit Biosynthesis

TRH stimulates α subunit biosynthesis through a novel mechanism. A CRE-binding protein that binds to the region from −151 to −135 of the human α subunit promoter appears to be important for TRH regulation, as well as a Pit-1–like protein that binds to a more distal region from −223 to −190.[125] The CRE of the human glycoprotein hormone α subunit gene promoter consists of an 18 bp repeat and extends from −146 to −111.[126] The mechanisms involved in TRH stimulation of the α subunit gene appear to involve two transcription factors, P-Lim and CREB binding protein (CBP). When stimulated with TRH, both of these factors transcriptionally cooperate to activate α subunit promoter activity caused by direct protein-protein interactions.[127] Both of these factors synergistically activated the α subunit gene promoter during TRH stimulation and interact in a TRH-dependent manner. P-Lim binds to the α subunit promoter directly, but CBP does not possess a DNA binding domain, so it must be recruited to the promoter via interaction with another factor. The P-Lim/CBP binding is formed in a TRH signaling-specific manner, in contrast to forskolin, which mimics protein kinase A signaling and dissociates both the binding and the transcriptional synergy. α subunit gene expression in thyrotropes is inhibited by dopamine in coordination with expression of the TSHβ subunit gene. Its action is mediated by decreases in intracellular cAMP levels.

Peripheral Regulation of α Subunit Biosynthesis

Thyroid hormone inhibition of α subunit gene transcription is observed in thyotropes in coordination with that of the TSH β subunit. The T_3 response element of the human α subunit gene promoter has been reported to be located from −22 to −7.[128] Similar to the TSHβ subunit gene, the T_3 response elements of human and of mouse[129] and rat[130] genes are located close to the transcriptional start. T_3 inhibition may be mediated by different isoforms of the T_3 receptor[131] in combination with the corepressors SMRT and NCoR.[132] Studies have suggested that mutations of the T_3 response element of the human α subunit promoter that eliminate TR binding do not abrogate the inhibitory effect of T_3, suggesting that protein-protein interactions may be more important than protein-DNA binding.[133]

Steroid hormone regulation of α subunit gene transcription is probably of limited importance. Androgen inhibition and androgen receptor (AR) binding have been localized to a region from −120 to −100. Negative regulation by estrogen was described in the gonadotropes of transgenic mice expressing a reporter gene under the control of both human and bovine promoters, but no binding of these regions to the estrogen receptor (ER) was detected, suggesting an indirect effect.[134] However, other studies using rat somatomammotropes have found positive regulation by estrogen localized to the proximal 98 bp of 5′-flanking DNA of the human α subunit gene and binding of the ER to the T_3 response element from −22 to −7.[135] Transcriptional inhibition by glucocorticoids may be mediated by binding of the glucocorticoid receptor to sequences between −122 and −93 of the human α subunit gene.[136] However, no direct binding was detected in other studies, suggesting that the GR inhibits transcription by interfering with other transactivating proteins.[137]

Regulation of TSH Glycosylation

Glycosylation is a regulated process that is primarily modulated by TRH and thyroid hormone.[138] Primary hypothyroidism[139] and TRH administration[140] have been found to increase oligosaccharide addition, which results in an increased bioactivity of TSH.[141] The same was noted in patients with resistance to thyroid hormone. TSH glycosylation patterns were found to differ in several pathologic states such as central hypothyroidism, TSH-producing pituitary adenomas, and euthyroid sick syndrome.[142] Also observed were changes in the sulfation and sialylation of the oligosaccharide residues, which modulate bioactivity.[139,143,144] Recently, thyroid hormone was shown to increase TSH bioactivity, and this was correlated with decreased sialylation.[145]

REGULATION OF TSH SECRETION

As with biosynthesis, TSH secretion is a result of complex interactions between central and peripheral hormones (Fig. 2-6).

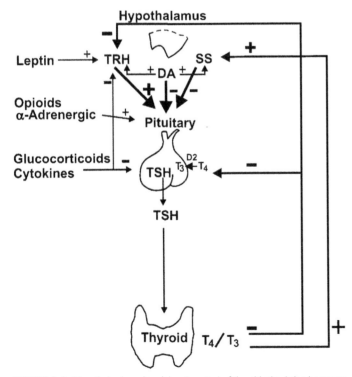

FIGURE 2-6. Hypothalamic and peripheral control of thyroid-stimulating hormone (TSH) secretion. Positive and negative stimuli are indicated at various levels within the hypothalamic-pituitary-thyroid axis. T_4, thyroxine; T_3, triiodothyronine; *TRH*, thyrotropin-releasing hormone; *SS*, somatostatin; *DA*, dopamine; D_2, deiodinase type II.

Hypothalamic Regulation of TSH Secretion

TRH directly affects TSH secretion in vivo and in vitro at concentrations that exist in the pituitary portal blood.[146] Immunoneutralization of TRH in animals leads to a decline in thyroid function,[147] and TRH knockout mice have a reduced postnatal TSH surge, followed by impaired baseline thyroid function with a poor TSH response to hypothyroidism. Lesions of the paraventricular nucleus (PVN) decrease circulating TRH and TSH levels in normal or hypothyroid animals and cause hypothyroidism[148] and electrical stimulation of this area causes TSH release. Although baseline levels of TSH are reduced in animals with lesions of the PVN, TSH levels still show appropriate responses to changes in circulating thyroid hormone levels. Thus, TRH likely determines the set point of feedback control by thyroid hormones.

Acute intravenous administration of TRH to human subjects causes a dose-related release of TSH from the pituitary. This occurs within 5 minutes and is maximal at 20 to 30 minutes. Serum TSH levels return to basal levels by 2 hours. More prolonged (2 to 4 hour) infusions of TRH lead to biphasic increases in serum TSH levels in humans and animals.[149] The early phase may reflect release of stored TSH, and the later phase may reflect release of newly synthesized TSH. Interpretation of TSH responses to even more prolonged TRH infusions is complicated by the increase in serum T_3 levels, with feedback to suppress further TSH release.[77] Continuous TRH administration in vitro also causes desensitization of TSH responses, which may further explain decreased TSH levels with long-term TRH exposure.[150]

Somatostatin (SS) in humans and animals inhibits basal and TRH-stimulated TSH secretion in vivo and in vitro at concentrations that exist in the pituitary portal blood.[151] In the hypothalamus, the highest concentrations of SS occur in the anterior paraventricular region.[152] From this region, axonal processes of SS-containing neurons project to the median eminence. Animals that have undergone sectioning of these fibers have depletion of SS content of the median eminence and increased serum TSH levels.[153] Similarly, immunoneutralization of SS in animals increases basal TSH levels and TSH responses to TRH.[154] In humans, SS infusions suppress TSH pulse amplitude, slightly decrease TSH pulse frequency, and abolish the nocturnal TSH surge.[155] Thus, TSH secretion probably is regulated through a simultaneous dual-control system of TRH stimulation and SS inhibition from the hypothalamus.

SS binds to specific, high-affinity receptors in the anterior pituitary gland. Five subtypes of the SS receptor (SST1 through SST5) have been identified,[156] and SST1 and SST5 have been localized to thyrotropes.[157] Binding of SS to its receptor inhibits adenylate cyclase via the inhibitory subunit of the guanine nucleotide regulatory protein, which lowers protein kinase A activity[156] and decreases TSH secretion. SS may also exert some effects by cAMP-independent actions on intracellular calcium levels. Hypothyroidism reduces the efficacy of SS in decreasing TSH secretion in vitro, which is reversed by thyroid hormone administration.[158] Additional studies in mouse thyrotropic tumors indicate that both SST1 and SST5 are markedly downregulated in hypothyroidism and are induced by thyroid hormone.[157] Although short-term infusions of SS lead to pronounced suppression of TSH secretion in humans, long-term treatment with SS or its analogues does not cause hypothyroidism.[159] This probably reflects compensatory mechanisms in the thyroid hormone feedback loop. GH deficiency is associated with increased TSH responses to TRH, and GH administration decreases basal and

TRH-stimulated TSH secretion,[160] possibly owing to GH stimulation of hypothalamic SS release.

Dopamine also inhibits basal and TRH-stimulated TSH secretion in vivo and in vitro at concentrations that exist in the pituitary portal blood.[161,162] Exogenous dopamine antagonists, including those that do not penetrate the blood-brain barrier, increase TSH levels.[163] In humans, dopamine infusions rapidly suppress TSH pulse amplitude, do not affect TSH pulse frequency, and abolish the nocturnal TSH surge[155]; administration of a dopamine antagonist has the opposite effect.[164] Dopamine also has direct effects on hypothalamic hormone secretion that may indirectly affect TSH secretion. For example, dopamine and dopamine-agonist drugs stimulate both TRH and SS release from rat hypothalami.[165]

In the hypothalamus, dopamine is secreted by neurons in the arcuate nucleus.[166] From the arcuate nucleus, neuronal processes project to the median eminence. Dopamine acts by binding to type 2 dopamine receptors (DA_2) on thyrotrope cells.[167] This leads to inhibition of adenylate cyclase, which decreases the synthesis and secretion of TSH. In addition, TSH may downregulate its own release through the induction of DA_2 receptors on thyrotrope cells.[168] The inhibitory effects of dopamine on TSH secretion vary according to sex steroids, body mass, and thyroid status. Dopamine antagonist drugs cause greater increases in serum TSH levels in women than in men. Recent studies show that obesity is associated with enhanced TSH secretion, which may be mediated via blunted central dopaminergic tone.[169] Dopamine inhibition of TSH release is greater in patients with mild hypothyroidism than in normal subjects, although subjects with severe hypothyroidism may be less responsive.[170] Although short-term infusions of dopamine lead to pronounced suppression of TSH secretion, long-term treatment with dopamine agonists does not cause hypothyroidism. This probably reflects compensatory mechanisms in the thyroid hormone feedback loop.

Adrenergic effects have also been reported in vivo and in vitro. α-Adrenergic activation stimulates TSH release directly from the rat pituitary gland at physiologic concentrations of catecholamines.[171] α-Adrenergic agonists stimulate TSH release in rats, and blockade of norepinephrine synthesis or treatment with adrenergic receptor blockers decreases TSH levels.[166,172] It is unclear whether these effects are mediated via changes in TRH and/or SS levels. In humans, data regarding adrenergic effects on TSH secretion are limited. α-Adrenergic blockade diminishes serum TSH responses to TRH.[173] However, administration of epinephrine does not alter TRH-stimulated TSH secretion.[174] These data suggest that endogenous adrenergic pathways do not have a major role in TSH secretion. Noradrenergic stimulation of TSH secretion is mediated by high-affinity $α_1$-adrenoreceptors linked to adenylate cyclase.[173] Therefore, dopamine and epinephrine appear to exert opposing actions on thyrotropes through opposite effects on cAMP generation.

Opioid administration to rats suppresses basal or stimulated TSH levels, and the opioid receptor antagonist naloxone reverses these effects.[175] Acute opiate administration in humans may slightly stimulate TSH levels, and acute naloxone administration has little effect.[176] In contrast to these acute studies, when naloxone is given over 24 hours, 24 hour TSH secretion decreases, primarily owing to a decrease in nocturnal TSH pulse amplitude.[177] TSH responses to TRH are also decreased. Serum T_3 levels are decreased as well, suggesting that the magnitude of TSH suppression is sufficient to affect thyroid gland function. These findings suggest that endogenous opioids may play a role in tonic stimulation of TSH secretion.

Peripheral Regulation of TSH Secretion

Thyroid hormone directly blocks pituitary secretion of TSH.[178] Acute administration of T_3 suppresses TSH levels within hours, and chronic administration leads to further suppression. Slight changes in serum thyroid hormone levels within the normal range alter basal and TRH-stimulated TSH levels, confirming the sensitivity of the pituitary gland to thyroid hormone feedback. Thyroid hormones alter tonic TSH secretion and TSH pulse amplitude without affecting pulse frequency, because subjects with primary hypothyroidism have a near-normal number of TSH pulses, and T_4 replacement leads to a decrease in TSH pulse amplitude without much change in pulse frequency.[72]

In addition to direct effects on TSH secretion, thyroid hormones have other actions that affect TSH secretion. At the pituitary level, thyroid hormones decrease the number of TRH receptors[179] and stimulate the activity of the pituitary TRH-degrading enzymes,[180] which act in concert to decrease TRH stimulation of TSH secretion. At the hypothalamic level, TRH mRNA levels in the PVN are increased in hypothyroidism and are reduced by T_3 and T_4.[181] Hypothalamic SS content is decreased in hypothyroid rats and is restored by T_3 treatment. Finally, T_3 directly stimulates SS release from hypothalamic tissue.[182] These combined effects of thyroid hormones on TRH and SS decrease TRH release from the hypothalamus and indirectly decrease TSH secretion.

Glucocorticoids at pharmacologic doses or high endogenous cortisol levels (Cushing's syndrome) suppress basal TSH levels, blunt TSH responses to TRH, and diminish the nocturnal TSH surge in humans and animals.[183,184] In healthy subjects, infusions of hydrocortisone that increase serum cortisol to levels seen in mild to moderate stress suppress 24 hour TSH secretion.[185,186] Glucocorticoid-induced changes in TSH levels are due to decreased TSH pulse amplitude without alteration in TSH pulse frequency, with more profound suppression of nocturnal TSH secretion and abolition of the TSH surge.

Physiologic glucocorticoid levels also affect TSH secretion.[79,80] Untreated patients with adrenocortical insufficiency can have elevated serum TSH levels that resolve with steroid replacement. Complimentary studies of metyrapone (an inhibitor of cortisol synthesis) administration to healthy subjects confirm that endogenous cortisol levels suppress TSH secretion, and physiologic hydrocortisone replacement in patients with adrenal insufficiency decreases daytime TSH levels back to those seen in healthy subjects.

Glucocorticoid suppression of TSH levels may occur directly at the pituitary gland. Animal studies suggest that glucocorticoids exert direct effects on thyrotropes to impair TSH secretion, although these appear to be highly dependent on dose and time course of administration.[187,188] It does not appear that glucocorticoids directly affect TSH gene transcription. In humans, TSH pulse frequency is maintained during glucocorticoid administration, TSH pulse amplitude is reduced, and TSH responses to exogenous TRH are attenuated, suggesting a direct effect on TSH secretion. In addition to direct pituitary effects, it appears that glucocorticoids may have hypothalamic actions that affect TSH levels. Dexamethasone increases hypothalamic TRH levels, and circulating TRH levels are decreased.[189] Reports that the proposed consensus sequence for glucocorticoid receptor binding is present in the 5'-flanking region of the TRH gene also support these data.[190]

Patients with Cushing's syndrome or subjects receiving prolonged courses of glucocorticoids may have low serum T_4 and

TSH levels. Whether such patients have true hypothyroidism, or whether they should be treated with thyroid hormone, is unclear; however, patients with acute or chronic illnesses and similar abnormalities in thyroid hormone levels do not appear to benefit from thyroid hormone therapy.

Leptin is primarily a product of adipocytes, although it is also located in thyrotrophs. It regulates food intake and energy expenditure, decreasing acutely with fasting in animals and humans.[191-193] Exogenous leptin administration to fed rats raises serum TSH levels, probably by increasing TRH gene expression and TRH release. Similarly, leptin administration to fasted rats or humans reverses fasting-induced decrements in TSH levels, also by increasing TRH gene expression and release. This suggests that fasting-related reductions in leptin levels play a role in suppressing TSH secretion. However, immunoneutralization of leptin increases TSH levels; therefore endogenous leptin may inhibit TSH release, at least in rats. In healthy subjects, leptin and TSH have coordinated pulsatility and circadian rhythms in plasma, with a nadir in the late morning and a peak in the early morning; however, leptin-deficient subjects have disorganized pulsatile and circadian rhythms.

Sex steroids may account for higher serum and pituitary TSH concentrations in male compared with female rats. In addition, TSH content is reduced by castration and is restored by androgen administration.[121] Testosterone administration to castrated male or female rats increases basal and TRH-stimulated serum TSH levels.[194] In contrast, androgen administration to intact female rats does not alter serum or pituitary levels of TSH.[195] Estrogen administration to euthyroid rats does not alter serum TSH levels. In euthyroid humans, most studies suggest that changes in endogenous or exogenous sex steroid levels do not affect basal or TRH-stimulated TSH levels.[196] No significant gender difference in the basal mean and pulsatile secretion of TSH or in the TSH response to TRH has been noted.[197] Therefore, sex steroids do not appear to play a major regulatory role in TSH secretion in humans.

Cytokines are circulating mediators of the inflammatory response that are produced by many cells and have systemic effects on the hypothalamic-pituitary-thyroid axis. Administration of tumor necrosis factor (TNF) or interleukin-6 (IL-6) decreases serum TSH levels in healthy human subjects, and TNF and interleukin-1 (IL-1) decrease TSH levels in animals.[198-200] Administration of some of these cytokines may mimic the alterations in thyroid hormone and TSH levels seen in acute nonthyroidal illness. In rats, TNF reduces hypothalamic TRH content and pituitary TSH gene transcription. IL-1 stimulates type II 5′-deiodinase activity in rat brain, which may decrease TSH secretion by increasing intrapituitary T_3 levels.

Autocrine and paracrine peptides may alter regulatory pathways within the pituitary gland for TSH secretion, acting in concert with the central and peripheral factors described above.[201] Peptides that have been implicated in this role include neurotensin, opioid-related peptides, galanin, substance P, epidermal growth factor (EGF), fibroblast growth factor (FGF), IL-1, and IL-6. Of particular interest is neuromedin B, a mammalian peptide that is structurally and functionally related to the amphibian peptide bombesin.[202] Neuromedin B is present in high concentrations in thyrotrope cells, with levels that change according to thyroid status. Administration of neuromedin B to rodents decreases TSH levels, and intrathecal administration of neuromedin B antiserum increases TSH levels. Therefore, neuromedin B appears to act as an autocrine factor that exerts a tonic inhibitory effect on TSH secretion. Additional data suggest that neuromedin B may modulate the action of other TSH secretagogues and release inhibitors, including TRH and thyroid hormones.

ACTION OF TSH

TSH acts on the thyroid gland by binding to the TSH receptor. An excellent review of this subject has been published recently.[203] The TSH receptor is located on the plasma membranes of thyroid cells and consists of a long extracellular domain, a transmembrane domain, and a short intracellular domain. The entire extracellular domain and parts of the transmembrane domain of the TSH receptor contribute to TSH binding.

Determinants of TSH Binding

Specificity of TSH binding is conferred by the TSH β subunit. It appears that amino acid residues from 58 to 69, within the βL3 loop, and from 88 to 105, in the "seatbelt" region of the TSH β subunit,[204] play an important role in binding to and activating the TSH receptor. The carboxylterminal end of the TSH β subunit contains multiple lysine residues (positions 101, 107, and 110) and a cysteine at position 105, all of which are critical for the ability to bind to the receptor.[205] Congenital hypothyroidism due to biologically inactive TSH was found to result from a frameshift mutation with loss of β-cysteine105[206] (see "Disorders of TSH Production"). Several regions of the α subunit are also important for TSH activity, particularly the residues α11-20 and α88-92.[51,56,207] In addition, the oligosaccharide chain at position α-asparagine52 plays an important role in both binding affinity and receptor activation. A mutant TSH lacking the α-asparagine52 oligosaccharide showed increased in vitro activity, although this same mutation had the opposite effect on CG binding to its native receptor.[56] However, such a mutation also increased TSH clearance and this decreased in vivo activity. In addition, the oligosaccharide chains on the TSH subunits are critically important for signal transduction.[42,208] In this regard, the α subunit oligosaccharides are important for all the pathways activated by the receptor, whereas the TSHβ subunit oligosaccharide influences only the adenylate cyclase pathway.[209] The mechanism by which the oligosaccharides influence signal transduction is not known. A model for the action of the glycoprotein hormones has been proposed that suggests a role for the oligosaccharides in directly modulating the influx of calcium into the target cell.[210]

Effects of TSH on the TSH Receptor

TSH has been shown to inhibit the expression of the rat TSH receptor by stimulating cAMP production.[211] TSH receptor desensitization also has been described both in vivo and in vitro, whereby prior TSH stimulation leads to a 30% to 70% decrease in the subsequent cAMP response to TSH stimulation.[212] Recent studies using recombinant TSH receptor have shown that desensitization does not occur when the receptor is expressed in nonthyroidal cells, suggesting that this phenomenon requires a cell-specific factor.[213]

Actions of TSH on the Thyroid Gland

The effects of TSH on the thyroid gland include changes in thyroid gland growth, cell morphology, iodine metabolism, and synthesis of thyroid hormone. The TSH receptor is coupled to the G_s protein cascade, and binding of TSH activates adenylate cyclase to produce cAMP.[214,215] The G_q/phospholipase C/inositol phosphates/Ca^{2+} pathway is also activated[216] and appears to play a role, particularly in regulating iodination.[217] TSH is also able to signal through the JAK/STAT[218] and mTOR/S6K1[219] pathways, with important roles in thyroid cell growth. The end point of TSH action is the production of thyroid hormone by the thyroid gland. The process begins with thyroglobulin gene transcription, which in itself is able to occur independently of TSH.[220] However, the transcriptional rate and possibly the mRNA stability are increased by TSH.[221] TSH regulates the expression and activation of Rab5a and Rab7, which are rate-limiting catalysts of thyroglobulin internalization and transfer to lysosomes.[222] TSH stimulates iodide uptake and organification, then acts on the iodinated thyroglogulin stored in the luminal colloid and stimulates its hydrolysis, resulting in release of the constituent amino acids, including the iodotyronines T_3 and T_4.

Extrathyroidal Actions of TSH

The ocurrence of precocious puberty in cases of severe juvenile primary hypothyroidism[223] has suggested that high levels of TSH are able to cross-activate the gonadotropin receptors. This interaction has now been demonstrated using recombinant human TSH, which has been found to be capable of activating the FSH[224] but not the CG/LH receptor.[225]

Expression of thyrotropin receptor has been reported in the brain[226] and pituitary gland.[227] In the brain, both astrocytes and neuronal cells were found to express TSH receptor mRNA and protein[226] and to stimulate arachidonic acid release and type II 5′-iodothyronine-deiodinase activity.[228] In the pituitary gland, the TSH receptor was localized to folliculo-stellate cells and may be involved in paracrine feedback inhibition of TSH secretion, which also may occur in response to TSH receptor autoantibodies.[227]

Expression of both TSH and its receptor has been reported in lymphocytes[229] and erythrocytes,[230] and this has led to speculation that TSH may have other nonclassic functions. The TSH receptor also was found to be expressed in adipocytes[231] and to stimulate proliferation and inhibit differentiation of preadipocytes in vitro.[232] TSH activated the nuclear factor-κB (NF-κB) pathway to induce the release of interleukin-6 (IL-6).[233] Direct effects of TSH were described in bone,[234] where it modulates tumor necrosis factor α (TNFα)[235] and receptor activator of NF-κB ligand (RANKL)[236] production to decrease osteoclast differentiation. More studies are needed to determine the physiologic significance of the extrathyroidal effects of TSH, as this may affect the safety of future treatment modalities for thyroid cancer that may attempt to target radioisotopes to the TSH receptor.[237]

TSH MEASUREMENTS

In 1926, Uhlenhuth discovered a substance in the anterior pituitary that stimulated thyroid cells, but it was not until the 1960s that TSH was purified from pituitary glands, and in 1963 the first antibodies against TSH were developed.[238,239] This provided the key reagents for measuring TSH in blood using immunologic techniques. Accurate and specific measurements of serum TSH concentrations have become the most important method for diagnosing and treating the vast majority of thyroid disorders. Initially, the radioimmunoassays were very insensitive and could detect only high levels seen in primary hypothyroidism.[240] Modifications subsequently led to improved sensitivity and specificity, enabling TSH levels as low as 0.5 to 1.0 mU/L to be detected.[241] These were called "first-generation assays." One hundred percent of primary hypothyroid subjects had elevated TSH levels, but these "first-generation assays" could not accurately quantitate values within the normal range, and considerable overlap with the values found in euthyroid and hyperthyroid subjects was noted.[242] Monoclonal antibody technology was applied to TSH after the first such antibody was reported in 1982.[243] This new method allowed two or more antibodies with precise epitope specificity to be used in sandwich-type assays that subsequently

were called immunometric assays.[244,245] One or more of the monoclonal antibodies are labeled and are called the "signal antibodies." The signal may be isotopic, chemiluminescent, or enzymatic. Another monoclonal antibody with completely different epitope specificity is attached to a solid support and is called the "capture antibody." All antibodies are used in excess, and therefore all TSH molecules in a sample are captured and the signal generated is directly proportional to the level of TSH.

These modifications in the measurement of TSH resulted in important changes. First, the assays were highly specific with no cross-reaction to the other human glycoprotein hormones. Second, 100% of euthyroid controls have detectable and quantifiable levels of TSH residing within a normal range of approximately 0.5 to 5 mU/L. Third, little or no overlap in TSH values is seen in patients with hyperthyroidism compared with euthyroid controls. The degree to which a given assay can separate undetectable TSH levels found in hyperthyroid subjects from normal values in euthyroid controls has improved steadily.[246] These improvements have resulted in progressively lower functional detection limits, defined as the lowest TSH value detected with an interassay coefficient of variation ≤20%. Thus, first-generation assays (usually radioimmunoassays) have functional detection limits of 0.5 to 1.0 mU/L, second-generation assays 0.1 to 0.2 mU/L, third-generation assays 0.01 to 0.02 mU/L, and fourth-generation assays 0.001 to 0.002 mU/L. At the present time, the most sensitive commercially available TSH assays are third-generation assays.

Although the population normal range for serum TSH levels is broad, within an individual subject TSH levels are regulated more tightly around an endogenous set point (Fig. 2-7). In a recent study of monthly sampling over a year in healthy euthyroid subjects, the significant difference in serum TSH levels on repeated testing was only 0.75 mU/L, far less than the population normal range.[247] It is not clear what determines this individual set point, although studies of monozygotic and dizygotic twins suggest that it is primarily genetically determined.[248] Genetic

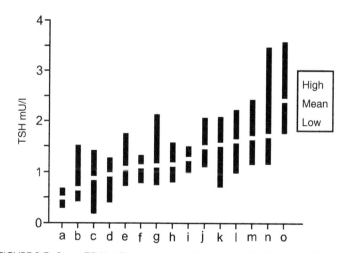

FIGURE 2-7. Serum TSH in 15 normal subjects taken monthly for 12 months. Each *black bar* represents the highest to lowest monthly TSH measurement, and *white rectangles* indicate individual mean values. Participants are sorted by increasing mean values (a through o). Laboratory reference range for TSH was 0.3 to 5.0 mU/L. Large differences were seen between individual set points, and unpredictable differences were seen in variations within individuals for the TSH assays. (Data used and figure revised from Andersen S, Pedersen KM, Bruun NH, Laurberg P: Narrow individual variations in serum T[4] and T[3] in normal subjects: a clue to the understanding of subclinical thyroid disease. J Clin Endocrinol Metab 87:1068–1072, 2002.)

analysis has revealed a number of significant linkage peaks, but no single gene appears to have a major regulatory influence, and regulation of the TSH set point is likely polygenic.[249,250] The main environmental factor that affects TSH levels in healthy euthyroid subjects appears to be iodine intake.[251]

Free TSH β and α Subunit Measurements

TSHβ and α subunits were purified in 1974 from human TSH, and specific antibodies to them developed.[252] Radioimmuno-assays were developed first, and then immunometric assays for the free α subunit. In general, free TSHβ levels are detectable only in primary hypothyroidism and therefore are of limited utility. Free α subunit levels have been useful in the evaluation of pituitary and placental disease. Free α subunit is detectable and measurable in both euthyroid and eugonadal human subjects.[253] Elevated values of free α subunit are found in the sera of patients with TSH-secreting or gonadotropin-secreting pituitary tumors[254-256] or choriocarcinoma,[257] and with a variety of nonpituitary and nonplacental malignancies, including cancers of the lung, pancreas, stomach, prostate, and ovary.[258-260]

Provocative Testing of TSH

TRH directly stimulates TSH biosynthesis and secretion. Given intravenously, intramuscularly, or orally, TRH causes a reproducible rise in serum TSH levels in euthyroid subjects.[261] The test is performed by giving 200 to 500 μg of TRH intravenously and measuring TSH at 0, 20 to 30, 60, 120, and 180 minutes after injection. In euthyroid subjects, an immediate release of TSH rises to peak levels approximately 20 to 30 minutes after TRH injection, usually reaching values fivefold to 10-fold higher than basal. With the use of third- and fourth-generation assays across a wide spectrum of normal and abnormal basal TSH levels, the increase in TSH after TRH stimulation has been between 2.8- and 22.9-fold[246] (Fig. 2-8). In hyperthyroid subjects, the undetectable basal serum TSH levels correlate with absent TSH responses to TRH. Patients with low basal serum TSH levels secondary to pituitary insufficiency (secondary hypothyroidism) or hypotha-

lamic disease (tertiary hypothyroidism) have absent or attenuated TSH responses to TRH.[262] In contrast, patients with elevated TSH levels due to primary hypothyroidism have exuberant responses to TRH stimulation. However, elevated TSH levels in patients with pituitary TSH-secreting tumors respond less than twofold to TRH stimulation.[254]

Drugs and TSH Levels

Among the most common causes of abnormal TSH levels are pharmacologic interventions that alter TSH production.[263] These can be divided into those that directly affect hypothalamic-pituitary function, those that affect thyroid gland function, and those that alter the distribution of thyroid hormones between free and protein-bound thyroid hormones in plasma.

Decreased Serum TSH: Drugs That Decrease Hypothalamic-Pituitary TSH Production

Clinically, the most important drug that results in decreased serum TSH levels is exogenously administered thyroid hormone. Twenty to thirty percent of patients treated with thyroid hormone have low serum TSH levels, most fitting the diagnostic criteria for subclinical hyperthyroidism. Similarly, thyroid hormone analogues such as 3,5,3′-triiodothyroacetic acid (TRIAC) have the same potential, and the future pharmacologic development of thyroid hormone analogues with increased affinity to the TRβ receptor isoforms will have the capacity to suppress TSH secretion. These compounds decrease TSHβ gene transcription. An interesting variation has been the discovery that RXR analogues such as Bexaroten, used in the treatment of cutaneous lymphoma, can decrease TSHβ transcription, serum TSH, and T_4 levels with resultant central hypothyroidism. High doses of glucocorticoids may decrease serum TSH levels through a similar mechanism. Drugs that act at a nongenomic level to decrease TSH production are somatostatin and its analogues and dopamine and its analogues, including bromocriptine, carbergoline, piribidil, levodopa, and lisuride. It is interesting to note that although these drugs acting nongenomically can acutely decrease TSH production, chronic administration usually results in compensatory mechanisms that prevent the development of clinical hypothyroidism. Growth hormone administration stimulating insulin-like growth factor (IGF)-1 production may decrease TSH levels by stimulating endogenous hypothalamic somatostatin production. Exogenous leptin administration can suppress hypothalmic TRH production. Cytokine administration (interferon and interleukins) commonly suppresses TSH levels and has been thought to mediate this action through stimulation of endogenous glucocorticoids. However, a novel alternative mechanism postulates that cytokines stimulate hypothalamic NF-κB production, and this protein directly increases deiodinase 2 gene transcription in astrocytes, leading to increased T_4 to T_3 conversion, TRH suppression, and central hypothyroidism.

Finally, serotonin antagonists (cyproheptadine), antidepressants of the selective serotonin reuptake inhibitor (SSRI) class (sertraline and fluoxetine), histamine receptor blockers (cimetidine), benzodiazepines, and α-adrenergic blocking drugs all have been reported to lower TSH levels, presumably by suppressing hypothalamic-pituitary TSH production.

Drugs That Increase Thyroid Hormone Production

Iodine and iodine-containing drugs such as amiodarone, many x-ray contrast agents, and antiseptics can increase thyroid gland production, particularly in susceptible individuals with nodular thyroid disease. Some of the most challenging cases of iodine-

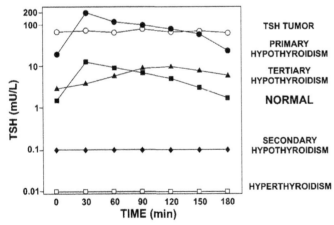

FIGURE 2-8. TSH responses to thyrotropin-releasing hormone (TRH) stimulation in patients with a variety of thyroid disorders compared with normal subjects. Serum samples of TSH were collected every 30 minutes for 3 hours. Subjects with different disorders are indicated on the right. Patients with TSH tumors, secondary hypothyroidism, and hyperthyroidism fail to respond normally to TRH stimulation. Patients with primary hypothyroidism have exuberant responses, whereas those with tertiary (hypothalamic) hypothyroidism have attenuated and delayed responses to TRH stimulation. (Data from Sarapura VD, Samuels MH, Ridgway EC: Thyroid-stimulating hormone. In: Melmed S [ed]: The Pituitary, 2nd ed. Blackwell Science, Malden, MA, pp 187–229, 2002.)

induced thyrotoxicosis involve the chronic administration of amiodarone. The resulting high levels of thyroid hormones suppress TSH production. Human chorionic gonadotropin (hCG) used in pharmacologic amounts also has the potential to increase thyroid gland hormone synthesis, because this hormone has 1% of the bioactivity of TSH against the TSH receptor. Increases in FT4 and resulting decreases in TSH levels in the first trimester of pregnancy are thought to be mediated by this mechanism; clearly, thyrotoxicosis in hydatidiform tumors is the result of very high levels of hCG.

Drugs That Increase Free Thyroid Hormones in Plasma

Salicylates and antiepileptic drugs such as Dilantin have long been known to compete with the binding of thyroid hormones to their binding proteins. They do not result in a higher free fraction of T_4 and T_3, nor do they suppress TSH biosynthesis. Drugs in the fenamate class of nonsteroidal antiinflammatory drugs such as fenoclofenac may also disrupt the normal partition of free T_4 by interfering with T_4 transport into cells that express the organic anion-transporting polypeptide 1C1, OATP1C1.[264] This transporter has very high specificity for T_4 and is found at the blood-brain barrier. Such a mechanism theoretically could increase free T_4. Heparin has a lypolytic action, resulting in increased free fatty acids, which also can displace thyroid hormones from binding proteins; this agent can cause spuriously elevated free T_4 during dialysis assays.

Increased Serum TSH: Drugs That Increase Hypothalamic-Pituitary TSH Production

Sustained increases in TSH production by direct stimulation of the hypothalamus or the pituitary are very unusual. TRH administration is the most potent but can be completely attenuated by subsequent rises in circulating thyroid hormones. Drugs from the opioid class, including morphine, apomorphine, heroin, buprenorphine, and pentazocine, all have been associated with increases in TSH levels. Theophylline and amphetamines, including ephedrine, may directly stimulate hypothalamic TRH or pituitary TSH production. Dopamine receptor antagonists domperidone, sulphuride, and metoclopramine decrease dopaminergic tone and thereby tonic suppression of TSH. Certain neuroleptics, haloperidol and chlorpromazine, have transiently increased TSH levels. Decreases in circulating glucocorticoids secondary to inhibition of adrenal gland hormone synthesis can cause high TSH levels. These drugs include aminoglutethimide, ethionamide, ketoconazole, and mitotane.

Drugs That Decrease Thyroid Hormone Production

Drugs that directly inhibit the thyroid gland, thereby increasing TSH levels, are perhaps the most important pharmacologic causes of high TSH levels. The antithyroid drugs propylthiouracil and methimazole directly inhibit thyroid hormone synthesis, thereby increasing TSH levels. All of the iodine-containing drugs and supplements can inhibit thyroid hormone production and release in susceptible individuals, particularly those with autoimmune thyroid disease. Lithium can have a similar sustained effect. Perchlorate, as a competitive inhibitor of iodine uptake by the thyroid gland, has been suspected to be a "thyroid gland disruptor" in contaminated water supplies and is certainly used in the therapy of severe hyperthyroidism.

Drugs That Decrease Free Thyroid Hormones in Plasma

Administration of estrogen has been reported to transiently decrease free thyroid hormones owing to increases in serum thyroxine binding globulin and increased TSH levels. One of the most common ways that drugs increase TSH levels is by blocking levothyroxine absorption from the intestine in patients taking this drug for hypothyroidism. Antacids and drugs that decrease gastric acid secretion inhibit thyroid hormone absortion. Iron and calcium to a lesser extent bind levothyroxine in the intestine and prevent its absorption. Drugs that block bile acid reabsorption such as cholestyramine and colestipol also inhibit levothyroxine uptake in the gut.

DISORDERS OF TSH PRODUCTION

Disorders in the hypothalamus, pituitary, and thyroid gland can alter TSH secretion. Advances in knowledge of the genetic and molecular regulation of TSH production have provided insights into many of the causes of abnormal TSH secretion.

Hypothalamic Disorders

The hypothalamus is the source of three important molecules that regulate TSH secretion: TRH, dopamine, and somatostatin. TRH is the only positive regulator of TSH production from the hypothalamus. Structural abnormalities in the hypothalamus have resulted in clinical hypothyroidism, which presumably is due to decreased or defective TRH production (Table 2-1). Exogenous administration of TRH to patients with hypothalamic hypothyroidism can restore serum thyroid hormone levels toward normal, resulting in clinical improvement.[265] Hypothalamic disease has not been reported to elevate endogenous SS or dopamine, resulting in decreased TSH and hypothalamic hypothyroidism. However, administration of GH has been associated with this syndrome,[160] presumably by stimulating hypothalamic SS production or enhancing the conversion of T_4 to T_3, both of which may result in decreased TRH production. In contrast, acute exogenous administration of both dopamine and somatostatin can decrease TSH production. It is therefore paradoxical that chronic administration of dopamine agonists or somatostatin analogues does not produce central hypothyroidism. It is likely that the exquisite sensitivity of TSH production to small changes in thyroid hormone levels may result in a correction for alterations induced by these analogues. As was outlined earlier, leptin derived from fat cells does circulate in plasma and has a variety of effects on the hypothalamus, one of which is to increase TRH production.

The serum levels of TSH in hypothalamic hypothyroidism may be low, normal, or even minimally elevated.[262] The paradoxical finding of low serum thyroid hormone levels in associa-

Table 2-1. Causes of Hypothalamic Hypothyroidism

Neoplasia	Pituitary adenoma
	Craniopharyngioma
	Dysgerminoma
	Meningioma
Infiltrative	Sarcoidosis
	Histiocytosis X
	Eosinophilic granuloma
Trauma	Radiation
	Head injury
	Postsurgical
Infection	Tuberculosis
	Fungus
	Virus
Vascular	Stalk interruption
Congenital	Midline defects
	Rathke's pouch cysts

tion with normal or elevated basal TSH levels suggests that circulating TSH in hypothalamic hypothyroidism is biologically defective.[265] In fact, TRH deficiency has been associated with differences in glycosylation patterns of the TSH molecule, which result in decreased TSH receptor binding and activation. The 24 hour secretory profile of TSH in patients with hypothalamic hypothyroidism is also abnormal.[75] The frequency of TSH pulses is the same as for euthyroid controls, but the amplitude of the pulses is decreased, particularly at nighttime, resulting in loss of the normal nocturnal surge (see Fig. 2-4, *bottom panel*).

Pituitary Disorders: Congenital TSH Deficiency

Increases or decreases in pituitary TSH production can result directly from abnormalities in the pituitary due to congenital or acquired causes. Congenital hypothyroidism due to decreased TSH production generally is inherited as an autosomal recessive disorder, and affected individuals have severe mental and growth retardation. The molecular basis for isolated TSH deficiency has usually involved mutations in the TSHβ gene (Table 2-2). For example, a single base substitution in one family at nucleotide position 145 of the TSHβ gene altered the CAGYC region,[266] a critically important contact point for the noncovalent combination of the TSHβ and α subunits. In other kindreds, a single base substitution introduced a premature stop codon, resulting in a truncated TSHβ subunit, which included only the first 11[267] amino acids. Another type of mutation involves a nonsense 25 amino acid protein that results from mutation of a donor splice site and a new out-of-frame translational start point.[268] In other cases, the disorder involves the production of biologically inactive TSH with loss of cysteine105 that disrupts the disulfide bridge formation important in "seatbelt" stability[269,270] and is perhaps the most common of the TSHβ mutations; the less common mutation at cysteine85 disrupts the cysteine knot that is important for heterodimer formation and TSH receptor binding,[268,271] resulting in a similar phenotype, except that in some cases circulating TSH was detectable.

A more common cause of congenital TSH deficiency arises not as the result of a mutation in the TSHβ gene, but rather following defective production of a key transcription factor necessary for TSHβ gene expression. This occurs in combined pituitary hormone deficiency (CPHD), in which subjects have congenital hypothyroidism and growth retardation secondary to TSH, GH, and prolactin deficiencies.[272,273] The genes for all three of these proteins are dependent on the pituitary-specific transcription factor Pit-1 for their expression. Mutations in the coding region of the *Pit-1* gene alter the function of the Pit-1 protein or completely disrupt its structure. The absence of Pit-1 prevents normal pituitary development, resulting in hypoplasia of the pituitary. In heterozygotes, in which a normal allele is present, the abnormal Pit-1 protein can bind to DNA but may not be able to effect transactivation, interfering with the function of the normal Pit-1 (dominant negative mechanism). It is interesting to note that a similar combined hormone deficiency syndrome has been reported in two murine models in which the *Pit-1* gene is defective: a point mutation found in the Snell dwarf (dw)[8] and a major deletion in the Jackson dwarf (dwJ).[274]

An even more frequent cause of CPHD has been delineated by the discovery of a pituitary-specific transcription factor called "prophet of Pit-1" (PROP-1). This factor is a paired-like homeodomain protein in which a mutation in the murine species causes the Ames dwarf (df) mouse phenotype.[275] Subsequently, patients with CPHD were found to have mutations in the *PROP-1* gene.[276,277] More than 50% of families with CPHD have been shown to contain mutations in the *PROP-1* gene,[278] far exceeding the prevalence of mutations in the *Pit-1* gene as a cause for CPHD. The mutations all are found in the homeodomain part of the molecule. It is interesting to note that the phenotype of patients with *PROP-1* mutations includes deficiencies not only of GH, prolactin, and TSH, but also of LH and FSH. Furthermore, the development of hormone deficiencies may not be neonatal but rather may occur progressively up to the age of adolescence. ACTH deficiency has been reported as a late consequence in CPHD.[279]

Table 2-2. Congenital Hypothyroidism: Isolated TSHβ Defects

	I	II	III	IV	V	VI
Inheritance syndrome	Autosomal recessive Cretinism	Autosomal recessive Cretinism	Autosomal recessive Cretinism	Autosomal recessive Cretinism	Autosomal recessive Cretinism	Autosomal recessive Cretinism, with phenotypic variability
Serum T$_4$	↓	↓	↓	↓	↓	↓
Serum TSH	None detected	None detected	Normal, ↓ or none	↓ or none	None detected	↓
Response to TRH	None detected	None detected	Impaired or none	Impaired or none	None detected	Impaired or none
Nucleotide change	Exon 2, Missense, G85A	Exon 2, Nonsense, G34T	Exon 3, Deletion, T313del	Exon 3, Nonsense, C145T	Exon 3, Missense, T256C	Intron 2 donor splice site variant IVS2 + 5G→A
Protein defect	G29R Altered CAGYC region, No combination with α	E12 X Premature stop (βL1 loop region) Truncated TSHβ (11 amino acids)	C105Vfs114X Altered seat-belt region and frameshift with premature stop codon (114 amino acids)	Q49X Truncated TSHβ (48 amino acids)	C85R Unstable or no combination with α	Nonsense protein of 25 amino acids
Reported cases	5 families in Japan[60,266]	2 families in Greece[284]	Over 10 families, in Brazil,[206] Germany,[271,288-291] Belgium,[292] Switzerland,[269] Argentina,[293] Portugal,[288] France,*[269] and USA[270,294]	Families in Egypt,[285] Turkey,[286] Greece,[286] and France*[288]	One case in Greece[286]	3 families in Turkey[285,287]

*Compound heterozygosity for T313del (C105Vfs114X) and C145T (Q49X) in one infant.

Pituitary Disorders: Acquired TSH Deficiency

The acquired causes of pituitary TSH deficiency generally relate to destructive processes in the anterior pituitary or hypothalamus. These can include infiltrative or infectious disorders, compression secondary to neoplastic processes, or active ischemic and hemorrhagic processes involving the pituitary gland. The most common cause of acquired pituitary TSH deficiency is neoplastic destruction or compression of normal anterior pituitary cells by a primary pituitary neoplasm, a craniopharyngioma, or infiltrating metastatic disease to the pituitary. Likewise, these same processes can extend into the hypothalamus, thus interrupting normal TRH production. In acquired pituitary TSH deficiency, multiple pituitary deficiencies are concomitantly associated; acquired isolated TSH deficiency is rarely, if ever, seen. When hypothyroidism is due to a pituitary disorder, the disease is called secondary hypothyroidism, and when it is due to a hypothalamic disorder (see "Hypothalamic Disorders"), it is called tertiary hypothyroidism. Most patients with acquired pituitary TSH deficiency have symptoms of hypothyroidism, as well as symptoms of LH, FSH, GH, and usually ACTH deficiency. Serum free T_4 and T_3 levels are low in association with a low or low/normal basal TSH level. The distinction between secondary and tertiary hypothyroidism can be challenging. A completely absent TSH and prolactin response to TRH favors secondary hypothyroidism, whereas a mildly elevated basal prolactin level (due to disrupted hypothalamic dopamine production) and normal or elevated basal TSH levels (with subnormal bioactivity) favor tertiary hypothyroidism.

Pituitary Disorders: Increased Pituitary TSH Production

Most cases of elevated serum TSH levels are a result of primary thyroidal disease, not primary pituitary disease. However, two important causes of elevated TSH levels originating from pituitary disorders have been described.

TSH-Secreting Pituitary Tumors

TSHomas are rare neoplasms of the anterior pituitary. They account for less than 1% of all pituitary tumors.[280] Patients have high levels of thyroid hormones in association with normal or high levels of TSH. Tumor cells are highly differentiated but synthesize the α subunit in excess of the TSHβ subunit.[254] This phenomenon is useful in that a molar ratio of α subunit:TSH (ng/mL divided by μU/mL multiplied by 10) of greater than 1 supports the diagnosis of a TSH-secreting pituitary tumor when found in a hyperthyroid and eugonadal patient. For example, if such a patient had a TSH of 10 μU/mL and a free α subunit of 3 ng/mL, the calculated ratio would be 3. Because menopausal women have high gonadotropins and high free α subunit levels, use of this calculated ratio in a hyperthyroid patient would not accurately reflect free α subunit coming from thyrotrope cells. TSH-secreting tumors fail to respond to TRH stimulation and suppression by dopamine (Fig. 2-9). Another characteristic of these tumors is their failure to respond to thyroid hormone by the normal negative feedback of thyroid hormone on TSH production. In contrast, inhibition of TSH release in response to SS is preserved in these tumors (see Fig. 2-9).

Thyroid Hormone Resistance Syndromes (RTH)

Another pituitary gland disorder resulting in elevated levels of serum TSH is thyroid hormone resistance (RTH).[281,282] In 1967, Refetoff et al.[283] were the first to describe three siblings who were clinically euthyroid or hypothyroid with goiters, stippled epiphyses, and deaf mutism. Each of the children had elevated levels of protein-bound iodide, which subsequently were shown to be associated with high serum total and free thyroid hormone levels, elevated TSH levels, and peripheral tissue responses that were refractory not only to the endogenous high levels of thyroid hormone, but also to exogenously administered supraphysiologic levels of thyroid hormone.[281] RTH was found to be linked to the TRβ gene locus on chromosome 3 and then was localized to point mutations in the 9th and 10th exons of the TRβ gene, which encode for the T_3 binding and adjacent hinge domains. These mutations usually disrupt normal T_3 binding without altering DNA binding. RTH without TRβ mutations occurs in about 15% of cases. Because most cases of RTH are heterozygotes and are inherited as autosomal dominant traits, only half of their

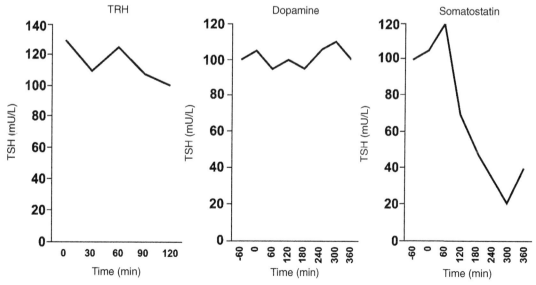

FIGURE 2-9. A patient with a TSH tumor fails to respond to TRH stimulation (500 μg intravenously) and dopamine suppression (4 μg/min for 4 hours). In contrast, TSH secretion is significantly suppressed by somatostatin (500 μg bolus followed by 250 μg/min for 4 hours). (Data from Sarapura VD, Samuels MH, Ridgway EC: Thyroid-stimulating hormone. In: Melmed S [ed]: The Pituitary, 2nd ed. Blackwell Science, Malden, MA, pp 187–229, 2002.)

TRβ receptors are abnormal. TRα gene mutations have not been reported in RTH. An overwhelming majority of mutations are single nucleotide substitutions, which change a single amino acid or introduce a stop codon. Since 1967 over 1000 cases of RTH belonging to 372 families have been identified.[282-294] Mutations have been found in 343 of these families, and many families have the same mutation, because only 124 different mutations have been identified.

REFERENCES

1. Kouki T, Imai H, Aoto K, et al: Developmental origin of the rat adenohypophysis prior to the formation of Rathke's pouch, Development 128:959–963, 2001.
2. Zhu X, Gleiberman AS, Rosenfeld MG: Molecular physiology of pituitary development: signaling and transcriptional networks, Physiol Rev 87:933–963, 2007.
3. Dasen JS, O'Connell SM, Flynn SE, et al: Reciprocal interactions of Pit1 and GATA2 mediate signaling gradient-induced determination of pituitary cell types, Cell 97:587–598, 1999.
4. Voss JW, Rosenfeld MG: Anterior pituitary development: short tales from dwarf mice, Cell 70:527–530, 1992.
5. Treier M, Gleiberman AS, O'Connell SM, et al: Multistep signaling requirements for pituitary organogenesis in vivo, Genes Dev 12:1691–1704, 1998.
6. Drolet DW, Scully KM, Simmons DM, et al: TEF, a transcription factor expressed specifically in the anterior pituitary during embryogenesis, defines a new class of leucine zipper proteins, Genes and Development 5:1739–1753, 1991.
7. Simmons DM, Voss JW, Holloway JM, et al: Pituitary cell phenotypes involve cell-specific Pit-1 mRNA translation and synergistic interactions with other classes of transcription factors, Genes and Development 4:695–711, 1990.
8. Camper SA, Saunders TL, Katz RW, et al: The Pit-1 transcription factor gene is a candidate for the murine snell dwarf mutation, Genomics 8:586–590, 1990.
9. Qi Y, Ranish JA, Zhu X, et al: Atbf1 is required for the Pit1 gene early activation, Proc Natl Acad Sci U S A 105:2481–2486, 2008.
10. Steger DJ, Hecht JH, Mellon PL: GATA-binding proteins regulate the human gonadotropin alpha-subunit gene in the placenta and pituitary gland, Mol Cell Biol 14:5592–5602, 1994.
11. Gordon DF, Woodmansee WW, Black JN, et al: Domains of Pit-1 required for transcriptional synergy with GATA-2 on the TSH beta gene, Mol Cell Endocrinol 196:53–66, 2002.
12. Charles MA, Saunders TL, Wood WM, et al: Pituitary-specific gata2 knockout: effects on gonadotrope and thyrotrope function, Mol Endocrinol 20:1366–1377, 2006.
13. Gleiberman AS, Michurina T, Encinas JM, et al: Genetic approaches identify adult pituitary stem cells, Proc Natl Acad Sci U S A 105:6332–6337, 2008.
14. Fauquier T, Rizzoti K, Dattani M, et al: SOX2-expressing progenitor cells generate all of the major cell types in the adult mouse pituitary gland, Proc Natl Acad Sci U S A 105:2907–2912, 2008.
15. Wondisford FE, Radovick S, Moates JM, et al: Isolation and characterization of the human thyrotropin beta-subunit gene: Differences in gene structure and promoter function from murine species, J Biol Chem 263:12538–12542, 1988.
16. Dracopoli NC, Rettig WJ, Whitfield GK, et al: Assignment of the gene for the beta subunit of thyroid-stimulating hormone to the short arm of human chromosome 1, Proc Natl Acad Sci U S A 83:1822–1826, 1986.
17. Wood WM, Kao MY, Gordon DF, et al: Thyroid hormone regulates the mouse thyrotropin beta subunit gene promoter in transfected primary thyrotropes, J Biol Chem 264:14840–14847, 1989.
18. Haugen BR, McDermott MT, Gordon DF, et al: Determinants of thyrotrope-specific TSH-beta promoter activation: Cooperation of Pit-1 with another factor, J Biol Chem 271:385–389, 1996.
19. Camper SA, Saunders TL, Kendall SK, et al: Implementing transgenic and embryonic stem cell technology to study gene expression, cell-cell interactions and gene function, Biol Reprod 52:246–257, 1995.
20. Wood WM, Ocran KW, Kao MY, et al: Protein factors in thyrotropic tumor nuclear extracts bind to a region of the mouse thyrotropin beta-subunit promoter essential for expression in thyrotropes, Molecular Endocrinology 4:1897–1904, 1990.
21. Gordon DF, Lewis SR, Haugen BR, et al: Pit-1 and GATA-2 interact and functionally cooperate to activate the thyrotropin beta-subunit promoter, J Biol Chem 272:24339–24347, 1997.
22. Gordon DF, Tucker EA, Tundwal K, et al: 2006 MED220/thyroid receptor-associated protein 220 functions as a transcriptional coactivator with Pit-1 and GATA-2 on the thyrotropin-beta promoter in thyrotropes, Mol Endocrinol 20:1073–1089, 2006.
23. Yuan CX, Ito M, Fondell JD, et al: The TRAP220 component of a thyroid hormone receptor-associated protein (TRAP) coactivator complex interacts directly with nuclear receptors in a ligand-dependent fashion, Proc Natl Acad Sci U S A 95:7939–7944, 1998.
24. Ito M, Yuan CX, Okano HJ, et al: Involvement of the TRAP220 component of the TRAP/SMCC coactivator complex in embryonic development and thyroid hormone action, Mol Cell 5:683–693, 2000.
25. Naylor SL, Chin WW, Goodman HM, et al: Chromosomal assignment of genes encoding the alpha and beta subunits of glycoprotein hormones in man and mouse, Somat Cell Genet 9:757–770, 1983.
26. Fiddes JC, Goodman HM: The gene encoding the common alpha subunit of the four human glycoprotein hormones, J Mol Appl Genet 1:3–18, 1981.
27. Jameson JL, Jaffe RC, Deutsch PJ, et al: The gonadotropin alpha-gene contains multiple protein binding domains that interact to modulate basal and cAMP-responsive transcription, J Biol Chem 263:9879–9886, 1988.
28. Horn F, Windle JJ, Barnhart KM, et al: Tissue-specific gene expression in the pituitary: the glycoprotein hormone alpha-subunit gene is regulated by a gonadotrope-specific protein, Mol Cell Biol 12:2143–2153, 1992.
29. Sarapura VD, Strouth HL, Wood WM, et al: Activation of the glycoprotein hormone alpha-subunit gene promoter in thyrotropes, Mol Cell Endocrinol 146:77–86, 1998.
30. Kendall SK, Gordon DF, Birkmeier TS, et al: Enhancer-mediated high level expression of mouse pituitary glycoprotein hormone alpha-subunit transgene in thyrotropes, gonadotropes, and developing pituitary gland, Molecular Endocrinology 8:1420–1433, 1994.
31. Barnhart KM, Mellon PL: The orphan nuclear receptor, steroidogenic factor-1, regulates the glycoprotein hormone alpha-subunit gene in pituitary gonadotropes, Molecular Endocrinology 8:878–885, 1994
32. Wood WM, Dowding JM, Sarapura VD, et al: Functional interactions of an upstream enhancer of the mouse glycoprotein hormone alpha-subunit gene with proximal promoter sequences, Mol Cell Endocrinol 142:141–152, 1998.
33. Roberson MS, Schoderbek WE, Tremml G, et al: Activation of the glycoprotein hormone alpha-subunit promoter by a LIM-homeodomain transcription factor, Mol Cell Biol 14:2985–2993, 1994.
34. Sheng HZ, Zhadanov AB, Mosinger B, et al: Specification of pituitary cell lineages by the lim homeobox gene Lhx3, Science 272:1004–1007, 1996.
35. Sarapura VD, Gordon DF, Strouth HL, et al: Msx1 is present in thyrotropic cells and binds to a consensus site on the glycoprotein hormone alpha-subunit promoter, Molecular Endocrinology 11:1782–1794, 1997.
36. Bach I, Carriere C, Ostendorff HP, et al: A family of LIM domain-associated cofactors confer transcriptional synergism between LIM and Otx homeodomain proteins, Genes and Development 11:1370–1380, 1997.
37. Wood WM, Dowding JM, Gordon DF, et al: An upstream regulator of the glycoprotein hormone alpha-subunit gene mediates pituitary cell type activation and repression by different mechanisms, J Biol Chem 274:15526–15532, 1999.
38. Weintraub BD, Gesundheit N: Thyroid-stimulating hormone synthesis and glycosylation: clinical implications, Thyroid Today 10:1–11, 1987.
39. Fiddes JC, Talmadge K: Structure, expression and evolution of the genes for the human glycoprotein hormones, Recent Prog Horm Res 40:43–78, 1984.
40. Pierce JG, Parsons TF: Glycoprotein hormones: Structure and function, Annu Rev Biochem 50:465–495, 1981.
41. Takata K, Watanabe S, Hirono M, et al: The role of the carboxyl-terminal 6 amino acid extension of human TSH-β subunit, Biochem Biophys Res Commun 165:1035–1042, 1989.
42. Thotakura NR, LiCalzi L, Weintraub BD: The role of carbohydrate in thyrotropin action assessed by a novel method of enzymatic deglycosylation, J Biol Chem 265:11527–11534, 1990.
43. Magner JA, Weintraub BD: Thyroid-stimulating hormone subunit processing and V combination in microsomal subfractions of mouse pituitary tumor, J Biol Chem 257:6709–6715, 1982.
44. Parsons TF, Bloomfield GA, Pierce JG: Purification of an alternative form of the α-subunit of the glycoprotein hormones from bovine pituitaries and identification of its O-linked oligosaccharides, J Biol Chem 258:240–244, 1983.
45. Behrens NH, Leloir LF: Dolichol monophosphate glucose: an intermediate in glucose transfer in liver, Proc Natl Acad Sci USA 66:153–159, 1970.
46. Kornfeld R, Kornfeld S: Assembly of asparagine-linked oligosaccharides, Annu Rev Biochem 54:631–664, 1985.
47. Magner JA: Thyroid Stimulating Hormone: Biosynthesis, Cell Biology, and Bioactivity, Endocrine Rev 11:354–385, 1990.
48. Thotakura NR, Desai RK, Bates LG, et al: Biological activity and metabolic clearance of a recombinant human thyrotropin produced in Chinese hamster ovary cells, Endocrinology 128:341–348, 1991.
49. Weintraub BD, Stannard BS, Meyers L: Glycosylation of thyroid-stimulating hormones in pituitary cells: Influence of high mannose oligosaccharide units on subunit aggregation, combination, and intracellular degradation, Endocrinology 112:1331–1345, 1983.
50. Lapthorn AJ, Harris DC, Littlejohn A, et al: Crystal structure of human chorionic gonadotropin, Nature 369:455–461, 1994.
51. Szkudlinski MW, Teh NG, Grossmann M, et al: Engineering human glycoprotein hormone superactive analogs, Nat Biotechnol 14:1257–1263, 1996.
52. Fairlie WD, Stanton PG, Hearn MTW: The disulphide bond structure of thyroid-stimulating hormone β-subunit, Biochem J 314:449–455, 1996.
53. Weller CT, Lustbader J, Seshadri K, et al: Structural and conformational analysis of glycan moieties in situ on isotopically 13C,15N-enriched human chorionic gonadotropin, Biochemistry 35:8815–8823, 1996.
54. Sun PD, Davies DR: The cystine-knot growth factor superfamily, Ann Rev Biophys Biomol Struct 24:269–291, 1995.
55. Weintraub BD, Stannard BS, Linnekin D, et al: Relationship of glycosylation to de novo thyroid-stimulating hormone biosynthesis and secretion by mouse pituitary tumor cells, J Biol Chem 255:5715–5723, 1980.
56. Grossmann M, Szkudlinski MW, Tropea JE, et al: Expression of human thyrotropin in cell lines with different glycosylation patterns combined with mutagenesis of specific glycosylation sites. Characterization of a novel role for the oligosaccharides in the in vitro and in vivo bioactivity, J Biol Chem. 270:29378–29385, 1995.
57. Magner JA, Papagiannes E: Structures of high-mannose oligosaccharides of mouse thyrotropin: differential processing of α- versus β-subunits of the heterodimer, Endocrinology 120:10–17, 1987.

58. Weiner RS, Dias JA: Biochemical analyses of proteolytic nicking of the human glycoprotein hormone α-subunit and its effect on conformational epitopes, Endocrinology 131:1026–1036, 1992.

59. Xing Y, Myers RV, Cao D, et al: Glycoprotein hormone assembly in the endoplasmic reticulum; I. The glycosylated end of human alpha-subunit loop 2 is threaded through a beta-subunit hole, J Biol Chem 279:35426–35436, 2004.

60. Hayashizaki Y, Hiraoka Y, Endo Y, et al: Thyroid-stimulating hormone (TSH) deficiency caused by a single base substitution in the CAGYC region of the β-subunit, EMBO J 8:2291–2296, 1989.

61. Matzuk MM, Kornmeier CM, Whitfield GK, et al: The glycoprotein hormone α-subunit is critical for secretion and stability of the human thyrotropin β-subunit, Mol Endocrinol 2:95–100, 1988.

62. Lash RW, Desai RK, Zimmerman CA, et al: Mutations of the human thyrotropin β-subunit glycosylation site reduce thyrotropin synthesis independent of changes in glycosylation status, J Endocrinol Invest 15:255–263, 1992.

63. Kelly RB: Pathways of protein secretion in eukaryotes, Science 230:25–32, 1985.

64. Odell WD, Utiger RD, Wilber JF, et al: Estimation of the secretion rate of thyrotropin in man, J Clin Invest 46:953–959, 1967.

65. Ridgway EC, Weintraub BD, Maloof F: Metabolic clearance and production rates of human thyrotropin, J Clin Invest 53:895–903, 1974.

66. Baker BL, Jaffe RB: The genesis of cell types in the adenohypophysis of the human fetus as observed with immunocytochemistry, Am J Anat 143:137–149, 1974.

67. Fisher DA, Polk DH: Development of the thyroid, Ballieres Clin Endocrinol Metab 3:67–80, 1989.

68. Fisher DA, Klein AH: Thyroid development and disorders of thyroid function in the newborn, N Engl J Med 304:702–711, 1981.

69. Roti E: Regulation of thyroid stimulating hormone (TSH) secretion in the fetus and neonate, J Endocrinol Invest 11:145–155, 1988.

70. Adams LM, Emery JR, Clark S, et al: Reference ranges for newer thyroid function tests in premature infants, J Pediatr 126:122–127, 1995.

71. Van Wassenaer AG, Kolk JH, Dekker FW, et al: Thyroid function in very preterm infants: influences of gestational age and disease, Pediatr Res 42:604–609, 1997.

72. Samuels MH, Veldhuis JD, Henry P, et al: Pathophysiology of pulsatile and copulsatile release of thyroid-stimulating hormone, luteinizing hormone, follicle-stimulating hormone, and α-subunit, J Clin Endocrinol Metab 71:425–432, 1990.

73. Russell W, Harrison RF, Smith N, et al: Free triiodothyronine has a distinct circadian rhythm that is delayed but parallels thyrotropin levels, J Clin Endocrinol Metab 93:2300–2306, 2008.

74. Mantagos S, Koulouris A, Makri M, et al: Development of thyrotropin circadian rhythm in infancy, J Clin Endocrinol Metab 74:71–74, 1992.

75. Samuels MH, Lillehei K, Kleinschmidt-Demasters BK, et al: Patterns of pulsatile pituitary glycoprotein secretion in central hypothyroidism and hypogonadism, J Clin Endocrinol Metab 70:391–395, 1990.

76. Van Den Barghe G, de Zegher F, Veldhuis JD, et al: Thyrotropin and prolactin release in prolonged critical illness: dynamics of spontaneous secretion and effects of growth hormone-secretagogues, Clin Endocrinol (Oxf) 47:599–612, 1997.

77. Samuels MH, Henry P, Luther M, et al: Pulsatile TSH secretion during 48-hour continuous TRH infusions, Thyroid 3:201–206, 1993.

78. Murakimi M, Tanaka K, Greer MA: There is a nyctohumeral rhythm of type II iodothyronine 5′-deiodinase activity in rat anterior pituitary, Endocrinology 123:1631–1635, 1988.

79. Samuels MH: Effects of variations in physiological cortisol levels on thyrotropin secretion in subjects with adrenal insufficiency: a clinical research center study, J Clin Endocrinol Metab 85:1388–1393, 2000.

80. Samuels MH: Effects of metyrapone administration on thyrotropin secretion in healthy subjects—a clinical research center study, J Clin Endocrinol Metab 85:3049–3052, 2000.

81. Shupnik MA, Greenspan SL, Ridgway EC: Transcriptional regulation of thyrotropin subunit genes by thyrotropin-releasing hormone and dopamine in pituitary cell cultures, J Biol Chem 261:12675–12679, 1986.

82. Shibusawa N, Yamada M, Hirato J, et al: Requirement of thyrotropin-releasing hormone for the postnatal functions of pituitary thyrotrophs: ontogeny study of congenital tertiary hypothyroidism in mice, Mol Endocrinol 14:137–146, 2000.

83. Abe H, Murao K, Imachi H, et al: Thyrotropin-releasing hormone-stimulated thyrotropin expression involves islet-brain-1/c-Jun N-terminal kinase interacting protein-1, Endocrinology 145:5623–5628, 2004.

84. Shupnik MA, Weck J, Hinkle PM: Thyrotropin (TSH)-releasing hormone stimulates TSH beta promoter activity by two distinct mechanisms involving calcium influx through L type Ca2+ channels and protein kinase C, Mol Endocrinol 10:90–99, 1996.

85. Kim MK, McClaskey JH, Bodenner DL, et al: An AP-1-like factor and the pituitary-specific factor Pit-1 are both necessary to mediate hormonal induction of human thyrotropin beta gene expression, J Biol Chem 268:23366–23375, 1993.

86. Weintraub BD, Wondisford FE, Farr EA, et al: Pre-translational and post-translational regulation of TSH synthesis in normal and neoplastic thyrotrophs, Horm Res 32:22–24, 1989.

87. Shupnik MA, Rosenzweig BA, Showers MO: Interactions of thyrotropin-releasing hormone, phorbol ester, and forskolin-sensitive regions of the rat thyrotropin-beta gene, Mol Endocrinol 4:829–836, 1990.

88. Kapiloff MS, Farkash Y, Wegner M, et al: Variable effects of phosphorylation of Pit-1 dictated by the DNA response elements, Science 253:786–789, 1991.

89. Steinfelder HJ, Radovick S, Wondisford FE: Hormonal regulation of the thyrotropin beta-subunit gene by phosphorylation of the pituitary-specific transcription factor Pit-1, Proc Natl Acad Sci U S A 89:5942–5945, 1992.

90. St Germain DL, Galton VA: The deiodinase family of selenoproteins, Thyroid 7:655–668, 1997.

91. Bianco AC, Salvatore D, Gereben B, et al: Biochemistry, cellular and molecular biology, and physiological roles of the iodothyronine selenodeiodinases, Endocr Rev 23:38–89, 2002.

92. Davis PJ, Leonard JL, Davis FB: Mechanisms of nongenomic actions of thyroid hormone, Front Neuroendocrinol 29:211–218, 2008.

93. Shupnik MA, Chin WW, Habener JF, et al: Transcriptional regulation of the thyrotropin subunit genes by thyroid hormone, J Biol Chem 260:2900–2903, 1985.

94. Shupnik MA, Ridgway EC: Thyroid hormone control of thyrotropin gene expression in rat anterior pituitary cells, Endocrinology 121:619–624, 1987.

95. Shupnik MA, Ardisson LJ, Meskell MJ, et al: Triiodothyronine (T3) regulation of thyrotropin subunit gene transcription is proportional to T3 nuclear receptor occupancy, Endocrinology 118:367–371, 1986.

96. Shupnik MA, Ridgway EC: Triiodothyronine rapidly decreases transcription of the thyrotropin subunit genes in thyrotropic tumor explants, Endocrinology 117:1940–1946, 1985.

97. Refetoff S: Resistance to thyroid hormone, Curr Ther Endocrinol Metab 6:132–134, 1997.

98. Bodenner DL, Mroczynski MA, Weintraub BD, et al: A detailed functional and structural analysis of a major thyroid hormone inhibitory element in the human thyrotropin beta-subunit gene, J Biol Chem 266:21666–21673, 1991.

99. Glass CK, Rosenfeld MG: The coregulator exchange in transcriptional functions of nuclear receptors, Genes Dev 14:121–141, 2000.

100. Haugen BR, Brown NS, Wood WM, et al: The thyrotrope-restricted isoform of the retinoid X receptor (gamma 1) mediates 9-cis retinoic acid suppression of thyrotropin beta promoter activity, Molecular Endocrinology 11:481–489, 1997.

101. Sharma V, Hays WR, Wood WM, et al: Effects of rexinoids on thyrotrope function and the hypothalamic-pituitary-thyroid axis, Endocrinology 147:1438–1451, 2006.

102. Sherman SI, Gopal J, Haugen BR, et al: Central hypothyroidism associated with retinoid X receptor-selective ligands, N Engl J Med 340:1075–1079, 1999.

103. Matsushita A, Sasaki S, Kashiwabara Y, et al: Essential role of GATA2 in the negative regulation of thyrotropin beta gene by thyroid hormone and its receptors, Mol Endocrinol 21:865–884, 2007.

104. Ordentlich P, Downes M, Evans RM: Corepressors and nuclear hormone receptor function, Curr Top Microbiol Immunol 254:101–116, 2001.

105. Liu Y, Xia X, Fondell JD, et al: Thyroid hormone-regulated target genes have distinct patterns of coactivator recruitment and histone acetylation, Mol Endocrinol 20:483–490, 2006.

106. Nakano K, Matsushita A, Sasaki S, et al: Thyroid-hormone-dependent negative regulation of thyrotropin beta gene by thyroid hormone receptors: study with a new experimental system using CV1 cells, Biochem J 378:549–557, 2004.

107. Shibusawa N, Hashimoto K, Nikrodhanond AA, et al: Thyroid hormone action in the absence of thyroid hormone receptor DNA-binding in vivo, J Clin Invest 112:588–597, 2003.

108. Wood WM, Ocran KO, Gordon DF, et al: Isolation and characterization of mouse complementary DNAs encoding alpha and beta thyroid hormone receptors from thyrotrope cells: the mouse pituitary specific beta-2 isoform differs at the amino terminus from the corresponding species from rat pituitary tumor cells, Molecular Endocrinology 5:1049–1061, 1991.

109. Hodin RA, Lazar MA, Wintman BI, et al: Identification of a thyroid hormone receptor that is pituitary-specific, Science 244:76–79, 1989.

110. Langlois MF, Zanger K, Monden T, et al: A unique role of the beta-2 thyroid hormone receptor isoform in negative regulation by thyroid hormone. Mapping of a novel amino-terminal domain important for ligand-independent activation, J Biol Chem 272:24927–24933, 1997.

111. Abel ED, Kaulbach HC, Campos-Barros A, et al: Novel insight from transgenic mice into thyroid hormone resistance and the regulation of thyrotropin, J Clin Invest 103:271–279, 1999.

112. Hallenbeck PL, Phyillaier M, Nikodem V: Divergent effects of 9-cis-retinoic acid receptor on positive and negative thyroid hormone receptor-dependent gene expression, J Biol Chem 268:3825–3828, 1993.

113. Weiss RE, Xu J, Ning G, et al: Mice deficient in the steroid receptor co-activator 1 (SRC-1) are resistant to thyroid hormone, EMBO J 18:1900–1904, 1999.

114. Tagami T, Gu WX, Peairs PT, et al: A novel natural mutation in the thyroid hormone receptor defines a dual functional domain that exchanges nuclear receptor corepressors and coactivators, Mol Endocrinol 12:1888–1902, 1998.

115. Nikrodhanond AA, Ortiga-Carvalho TM, Shibusawa N, et al: Dominant role of thyrotropin-releasing hormone in the hypothalamic-pituitary-thyroid axis, J Biol Chem 281:5000–5007, 2006.

116. Krane IM, Spindel ER, Chin WW: Thyroid hormone decreases the stability and the poly(A) tract length of rat thyrotropin beta-subunit messenger RNA, Molecular Endocrinology 5:469–475, 1991.

117. Leedman PJ, Stein AR, Chin WW: Regulated specific protein binding to a conserved region of the 3′-untranslated region of thyrotropin beta-subunit mRNA, Mol Endocrinol 9:375–387, 1995.

118. Staton JM, Leedman PJ: Posttranscriptional regulation of thyrotropin beta-subunit messenger ribonucleic acid by thyroid hormone in murine thyrotrope tumor cells: a conserved mechanism across species, Endocrinology 139:1093–1100, 1998.

119. Ross DS, Ellis MF, Milbury P, et al: A comparison of changes in plasma thyrotropin beta- and alpha-subunits, and mouse thyrotropic tumor thyrotropin beta- and alpha-subunit mRNA concentrations after in vivo dexamethasone or T3 administration, Metabolism 36:799–803, 1987.

120. Ahlquist JA, Franklyn JA, Wood DF, et al: Hormonal regulation of thyrotrophin synthesis and secretion, Horm Metab Res Suppl 17:86–89, 1987.

121. Ross DS: Testosterone increases TSH-beta mRNA, and modulates alpha-subunit mRNA differentially in mouse thyrotropic tumor and castrate rat pituitary, Horm Metab Res 22:163–169, 1990.

122. Friedman JM, Halaas JL: Leptin and the regulation of body weight in mammals, Nature 395:763–770, 1998.

123. Fekete C, Kelly J, Mihaly E, et al: Neuropeptide Y has a central inhibitory action on the hypothalamic-pituitary-thyroid axis, Endocrinology 142:2606–2613, 2001.

124. Chowdhury I, Chien JT, Chatterjee A, et al: Effects of leptin and neuropeptide-Y on transcript levels of thy-

rotropin beta and common alpha subunits of rat pituitary cells in vitro, Life Sci 75:2897–2909, 2004.
125. Kim DS, Yoon JH, Ahn SK, et al: A 33 kDa Pit-1-like protein binds to the distal region of the human thyrotrophin alpha-subunit gene, J Mol Endocrinol 14:313–322, 1995.
126. Deutsch PJ, Jameson JL, Habener JF: Cyclic AMP responsiveness of human gonadotropin-alpha gene transcription is directed by a repeated 18-base pair enhancer, J Biol Chem 262:12169–12174, 1987.
127. Hashimoto K, Zanger K, Hollenberg AN, et al: cAMP response element-binding protein-binding protein mediates thyrotropin-releasing hormone signaling on thyrotropin subunit genes, J Biol Chem 275:33365–33372, 2000.
128. Chatterjee VK, Lee JK, Rentoumis A, et al: Negative regulation of the thyroid-stimulating hormone alpha gene by thyroid hormone: receptor interaction adjacent to the TATA box, Proc Natl Acad Sci U S A 86:9114–9118, 1989.
129. Sarapura VD, Wood WM, Gordon DF, et al: Thyrotrope expression and thyroid hormone inhibition map to different regions of the mouse glycoprotein hormone alpha-subunit promoter, Endocrinology 127:1352–1361, 1990.
130. Burnside J, Darling DS, Carr FE, et al: Thyroid hormone regulation of the rat glycoprotein hormone alpha-subunit gene promoter activity, J Biol Chem 264:6886–6891, 1989.
131. Sarapura VD, Wood WM, Bright TM, et al: Reconstitution of triiodothyronine inhibition in non-triiodothyronine responsive thyrotropic tumor cells using transfected thyroid hormone receptor isoforms, Thyroid 7:453–461, 1997.
132. Tagami T, Madison LD, Nagaya T, et al: Nuclear receptor corepressors activate rather than suppress basal transcription of genes that are negatively regulated by thyroid hormone, Mol Cell Biol 17:2642–2648, 1997.
133. Madison LD, Ahlquist JA, Rogers SD, et al: Negative regulation of the glycoprotein hormone alpha gene promoter by thyroid hormone: mutagenesis of a proximal receptor binding site preserves transcriptional repression, Mol Cell Endocrinol 94:129–136, 1993.
134. Keri RA, Andersen B, Kennedy GC, et al: Estradiol inhibits transcription of the human glycoprotein hormone alpha-subunit gene despite the absence of a high affinity binding site for estrogen receptor, Mol Endocrinol 5:725–733, 1991.
135. Yarwood NJ, Gurr JA, Sheppard MC, et al: Estradiol modulates thyroid hormone regulation of the human glycoprotein hormone alpha subunit gene, J Biol Chem 268:21984–21989, 1993.
136. Akerblom IE, Slater EP, Beato M, et al: Negative regulation by glucocorticoids through interference with a cAMP responsive enhancer, Science 241:350–353, 1988.
137. Chatterjee VK, Madison LD, Mayo S, et al: Repression of the human glycoprotein hormone alpha-subunit gene by glucocorticoids: evidence for receptor interactions with limiting transcriptional activators, Mol Endocrinol 5:100–110, 1991.
138. Persani L: Hypothalamic thyrotropin-releasing hormone and thyrotropin biological activity, Thyroid 8:941–946, 1998.
139. Persani L, Borgato S, Romoli R, et al: Changes in the degree of sialylation of carbohydrate chains modify the biological properties of circulating thyrotropin isoforms in various physiological and pathological states, J Clin Endocrinol Metab 83:2486–2492, 1998.
140. Taylor T, Weintraub BD: Altered thyrotropin (TSH) carbohydrate structures in hypothalamic hypothyroidism created by paraventricular nuclear lesions are corrected by in vivo TSH-releasing hormone administration, Endocrinology 125:2198–2203, 1989.
141. Menezes-Ferreira MM, Petrick PA, Weintraub BD: Regulation of thyrotropin bioactivity by thyrotropin-releasing hormone and thyroid hormone, J Endocrinol 118:2125–2130, 1986.
142. Papandreou MJ, Persani L, Asteria Ronin C, et al: Variable carbohydrate structures of circulating thyrotropin as studied by lectin affinity chromatography in different clinical conditions, J Clin Endocrinol Metab 77:393–398, 1993.
143. Trojan J, Theodoropoulou M, Usadel KH, et al: Modulation of human thyrotropin oligosaccharide structures—enhanced proportion of sialylated and terminally galactosylated serum thyrotropin isoforms in subclinical and overt primary hypothyroidism, J Endocrinol 158:359–365, 1998.
144. Persani L, Ferretti E, Borgato S, et al: Circulating thyrotropin bioactivity in sporadic central hypothyroidism, J Clin Endocrinol Metab 85:3631–3635, 2000.
145. Oliveira JHA, Barbosa ER, Kasamatsu T, et al: Evidence for thyroid hormone as a positive regulator of serum thyrotropin bioactivity, J Clin Endocrinol Metab 92:3108–3113, 2007.
146. Sheward WJ, Harmar AJ, Fraser HM, et al: TRH in rat pituitary stalk blood and hypothalamus. Studies with high performance liquid chromatography, Endocrinology 113:1865–1869, 1983.
147. Fraser HM, McNeilly AS: Effect of chronic immunoneutralization of thyrotropin-releasing hormone on the hypothalamic-pituitary thyroid axis, prolactin and reproductive function in the ewe, Endocrinology 111:1964–1971, 1982.
148. Aizawa T, Green M: Delineation of the hypothalamic area controlling thyrotropin secretion in the rat, Endocrinology 109:1731–1738, 1981.
149. Chan V, Wang C, Yeung TT: Thyrotropin, α and β-subunits of thyrotropin and prolactin response to four hour constant infusions of thyrotropin releasing hormone in normal subjects and patients with pituitary-thyroid disorders, J Clin Endocrinol Metab 49:127–133, 1979.
150. Sheppard MC, Shennan KI: Desensitization of rat anterior pituitary gland to thyrotrophin releasing hormone, Endocrinology 101:101–105, 1984.
151. Vale W, Brazeau P, Rivier C, et al: Somatostatin, Recent Prog Horm Res 31:365–397, 1975.
152. Reichlin S: Somatostatin, N Engl J Med 309:1495–1501, 1983.
153. Urman S, Critchlow V: Long-term elevations in plasma thyrotropin, but not growth hormone, concentrations associated with lesion-induced depletion of median eminence somatostatin, Endocrinology 112:659–664, 1983.
154. Arima A, Schally AV: Increase in basal and thyrotropin-releasing hormone stimulated secretion of thyrotropin by passive immunization with antiserum to somatostatin, Endocrinology 98:1069–1075, 1976.
155. Samuels MH, Henry P, Ridgway EC: Effects of dopamine and somatostatin on pulsatile pituitary glycoprotein secretion, J Clin Endocrinol Metab 74:217–222, 1992.
156. Reisine T, Bell GI: Molecular biology of the somatostatin receptors, Endocrine Rev 16:427–442, 1995.
157. James RA, Sarapura VD, Bruns C, et al: Thyroid hormone-induced expression of specific somatostatin receptor subtypes correlates with involution of the TtT-97 murine thyrotrope tumor, Endocrinology 138:719–724, 1997.
158. Ridgway EC, Klibanski A, Martorana MA, et al: The effect of somatostatin on the release of thyrotropin and its subunits from bovine anterior pituitary cells in vitro, Endocrinology 112:1937–1942, 1983.
159. Page MD, Millward ME, Taylor A, et al: Long-term treatment of acromegaly with a long-acting analogue of somatostatin, octreotide, Q J Med 74:189–201, 1990.
160. Lippe BM, Van Herle AJ, La Franchi SH, et al: Reversible hypothyroidism in growth hormone-deficient children treated with human growth hormone, J Clin Endocrinol Metab 40:612–618, 1975.
161. Ben-Johnson N, Oliver C, Weiner HJ, et al: Dopamine in hypophyseal portal plasma of the rat during the estrous cycle and throughout pregnancy, Endocrinology 100:452–458, 1977.
162. Cooper DS, Klibanski A, Ridgway EC: Dopaminergic modulation of TSH and its subunits: in vivo and in vitro studies, Clin Endocrinol (Oxf) 18:265–272, 1983.
163. Pourmand M, Rodriguez-Arnao MD, Weightman DR, et al: Domperidone: a novel agent for the investigation of anterior pituitary function and control in man, Clin Endocrinol (Oxf) 12:211–215, 1980.
164. Samuels MH, Kramer P: Effects of metoclopramide on fasting-induced TSH suppression, Thyroid 6:85–89, 1996.
165. Lewis BM, Dieguez C, Lewis MD, et al: Dopamine stimulates release of thyrotrophin-releasing hormone from perfused intact rat hypothalamus via hypothalamic D2 receptors, J Endocrinol 115:419–424, 1987.
166. Morley JE: Neuroendocrine control of thyrotropin secretion, Endocrine Rev 2:396–436, 1981.
167. Foord SM, Peters JR, Dieguez C, et al: Dopamine receptors on intact anterior pituitary cells in culture: functional association with the inhibition of prolactin and thyrotropin, Endocrinology 112:1567–1571, 1983.
168. Foord SM, Peters JR, Dieguez C, et al: TSH regulates thyrotroph responsiveness to dopamine in vitro, Endocrinology 118:1319–1324, 1985.
169. Kok P, Roelfsema F, Frolich M, et al: Spontaneous diurnal thyrotropin secretion is enhanced in proportion to circulating leptin in obese premenopausal women, J Clin Endocrinol Metab 90:6185–6191, 2005.
170. Scanlon MF, Chan V, Heath M, et al: Dopaminergic control of thyrotropin, α-subunit and prolactin in euthyroidism and hypothyroidism: dissociated responses to dopamine receptor blockade with metoclopramide in euthyroid and hypothyroid subjects, J Clin Endocrinol Metab 53:360–365, 1981.
171. Klibanski A, Milbury PE, Chin WW, et al: Direct adrenergic stimulation of the release of thyrotropin and its subunits from the thyrotrope in vitro, Endocrinology 113:1244–1250, 1983.
172. Krulich L, Mayfield MA, Steele MK, et al: Differential effects of pharmacological manipulations of central β1- and β2-adrenergic receptors on the secretion of thyrotropin and growth hormone in male rats, Endocrinology 35:139–145, 1982.
173. Zgliczynski S, Kaniewski M: Evidence for β-adrenergic receptor mediated TSH release in men, Acta Endocrinol (Copenh) 95:172–179, 1980.
174. Rogol AD, Reeves GD, Varma MM, et al: Thyroid stimulating hormone and prolactin response to thyrotropin-releasing hormone during infusion of epinephrine and propranolol in man, Neuroendocrinology 29:413–420, 1979.
175. Howlett TA, Rees LH: Endogenous opioid peptides and hypothalamo-pituitary function, Ann Rev Physiol 48:527–536, 1986.
176. Morley JE, Baranetsky NG, Wingert TD, et al: Endocrine effects of naloxone-induced opiate receptor blockade, J Clin Endocrinol Metab 50:251–257, 1980.
177. Samuels MH, Kramer P, Wilson D, et al: Effects of naloxone infusions on pulsatile thyrotropin secretion, J Clin Endocrinol Metab 78:1249–1252, 1994.
178. Larsen PR: Thyroid-pituitary interaction, N Engl J Med 306:23–32, 1982.
179. Hinkle PM, Goh KBC: Regulation of thyrotropin-releasing hormone receptors and responses by L-triiodothyronine in dispersed rat pituitary cell cultures, Endocrinology 110:1725–1731, 1982.
180. Ponce G, Charli JL, Pasten JA, et al: Tissue-specific regulation of pyroglutamate aminopeptidase II activity by thyroid hormones, Neuroendocrinology 48:211–214, 1988.
181. Kakucska I, Rand W, Lechan RM: Thyrotropin-releasing hormone gene expression in the hypothalamic paraventricular nucleus is dependent upon feedback regulation by both triiodothyronine and thyroxine, Endocrinology 130:2845–2850, 1992.
182. Berelowitz M, Maefa K, Harris S, et al: The effect of alterations in the pituitary-thyroid axis on hypothalamic content and in vitro release of somatostatin-like immunoreactivity, Endocrinology 107:24–29, 1980.
183. Brabant G, Brabant A, Ranft U, et al: Circadian and pulsatile thyrotropin secretion in euthyroid man under the influence of thyroid hormone and glucocorticoid administration, J Clin Endocrinol Metab 65:83–88, 1987.
184. Bartalena L, Martino E, Petrini L, et al: The nocturnal serum thyrotropin surge is abolished in patients with adrenocorticotropin (ACTH)-dependent or ACTH-independent Cushing's syndrome, J Clin Endocrinol Metab 72:1195–1199, 1991.
185. Samuels MH, Luther M, Henry P, et al: Effects of hydrocortisone on pulsatile pituitary glycoprotein secretion, J Clin Endocrinol Metab 78:211–215, 1994.
186. Samuels MH, McDaniel PA: Thyrotropin levels during hydrocortisone infusions that mimic fasting-induced cortisol elevations—a clinical research center study, J Clin Endocrinol Metab 82:3700–3704, 1997.
187. Pamenter RW, Hedge GA: Inhibition of thyrotropin secretion by physiological levels of corticosterone, Endocrinology 106:162–166, 1980.

188. Mitsuma T, Nogimori T: Effects of dexamethasone on the hypothalamic-pituitary-thyroid axis in rats, Acta Endocrinol (Copenh) 100:51–56, 1982.

189. Mitsuma T, Hirooka Y, Nogimori T: Effects of dexamethasone on TRH and TRH precursor peptide (lys-arg-gln-his-pro-gly-arg-arg) levels in various rat organs, Endocrine Regulations 26:29–34, 1992.

190. Lee S, Sevarino K, Roos BA, et al: Characterization and expression of the gene encoding rat thyrotropin-releasing hormone (TRH). Ann NY Acad Sci 553:14–28, 1989.

191. Ortiga-Carvalho TM, Oliveira KJ, Soares BA, et al: The role of leptin in the regulation of TSH secretion in the fed state: in vivo and in vitro studies, J Endocrinol 174:121–125, 2002.

192. Schurgin S, Canavan B, Koutkia P, et al: Endocrine and metabolic effects of physiologic r-metHuLeptin administration during acute caloric deprivation in normal-weight women, J Clin Endocrinol Metab 89:5402–5409, 2004.

193. Mantzoros CS, Ozata M, Negrao AB, et al: Synchronicity of frequently sampled thyrotropin (TSH) and leptin concentrations in healthy adults and leptin-deficient subjects: evidence for possible partial TSH regulation by leptin in humans, J Clin Endocrinol Metab 86:3284–3291, 2001.

194. Farbota L, Hofman C, Oslapas R, et al: Sex hormone modulation of serum TSH levels, Surgery 102:1081–1087, 1987.

195. Ahlquist JAO, Franklyn JA, Ramsden DB, et al: Regulation of α and thyrotropin-β subunit mRNA levels by androgens in the female rat, J Mol Endocrinol 5:1–6, 1990.

196. Erfurth EM, Ericsson UB: The role of estrogen in the TSH and prolactin responses to thyrotropin-releasing hormone in postmenopausal as compared to premenopausal women, Horm Metab Res 24:528–531, 1992.

197. Franklyn JA, Ramsden DB, Sheppard MC: The influence of age and sex on tests of thyroid function, Ann Clin Biochem 22:502–505, 1985.

198. Hermus RM, Sweep CG, van der Meer MJ, et al: Continuous infusion of interleukin-1 induces a nonthyroidal illness syndrome in the rat, Endocrinology 131:2139–2146, 1992.

199. Van der Poll T, Romijn JA, Wiersinga WM, et al: Tumor necrosis factor: a putative mediator of the sick euthyroid syndrome in man, J Clin Endocrinol Metab 71:1567–1572, 1990.

200. Torpy DJ, Tsigos C, Lotsikas AJ, et al: Acute and delayed effects of a single-dose injection of interleukin-6 on thyroid function in healthy humans, Metabolism 47:1289–1293, 1998.

201. Pazos-Moura CC, Ortiga-Carvalho TM, Gaspar de Moura E: The autocrine/paracrine regulation of thyrotropin secretion, Thyroid 13:167–175, 2003.

202. Oliveira KJ, Ortiga-Carvalho TM, Cabanelas A, et al: Disruption of neuromedin B receptor gene results in dysregulation of the pituitary-thyroid axis, J Mol Endocrinol 36:73–80, 2006.

203. Farid NR, Szkudlinski MW: Minireview: structural and functional evolution of the thyrotropin receptor, Endocrinology 145:4048–4057, 2004.

204. Grossmann M, Szkudlinski MW, Wong R, et al: Substitution of the seat-belt region of the thyrotropin (TSH)-β subunit with the corresponding regions of the choriogonadotropin or follitropin confers luteotropic, but not follitropic, activity to chimeric TSH, J Biol Chem 272:15532–15540, 1997.

205. Leinung MC, Bergert ER, McCormick DJ, et al: Synthetic analogs of the carboxyl-terminus of β-thyrotropin: the importance of basic amino acids in receptor binding activity, Biochemistry 31:10094–10098, 1992.

206. Medeiros-Neto G, Herodotou DT, Rajan S, et al: A circulating biologically inactive thyrotropin caused by a mutation in the β subunit gene, J Clin Invest 97:1250–1256, 1996.

207. Grossmann M, Szkudlinski MW, Tropea JE, et al: Expression of human thyrotropin in cell lines with different glycosylation patterns combined with mutagenesis of specific glycosylation sites: characterization of a novel role for the oligosaccharides in the in vitro and in vivo bioactivity, J Biol Chem 270:29378–29385, 1995.

208. Szkudlinski MW, Thotakura NR, Weintraub BD: Subunit-specific functions of N-linked oligosaccharides in human thyrotropin: role of terminal residues of α- and

209. Thotakura NR, Desai RK, Szkudlinski MW, et al: The role of the oligosaccharide chains of thyrotropin α- and β-subunits in hormone action, Endocrinology 131:82–88, 1992.

210. Renwick A, Wiggin P: An antipodean perception of the mode of action of glycoprotein hormones, FEBS Lett 297:1–3, 1992.

211. Akamizu T, Ikuyama S, Saji M, et al: Cloning, chromosomal assignment, and regulation of the rat thyrotropin receptor: expression of the gene is regulated by thyrotropin agents that increase cAMP levels, and thyroid autoantibodies, Proc Natl Acad Sci U S A 87:5677–5681, 1990.

212. Field JB, Dekker A, Titus G, et al: In vitro and in vivo refractoriness to thyrotropin stimulation of iodine organification and thyroid hormone secretion, J Clin Invest 64:265–271, 1979.

213. Chazenbalk GD, Nagayama Y, Kaufman KD, et al: The functional expression of recombinant human thyrotropin receptors in non-thyroidal eukaryotic cells provides evidence that homologous desensitization to thyrotropin stimulation requires a cell-specific factor, Endocrinology 127:1240–1244, 1990.

214. Wolff J, Jones AB: The purification of bovine thyroid plasma membranes and the properties of membrane-bound adenyl cyclase, J Biol Chem 246:3939–3947, 1971.

215. Yamashita K, Field JB: Preparation of thyroid plasma membranes containing TSH-responsive adenyl cyclase, Biochem Biophys Res Commun 40:171–178, 1970.

216. Philip NJ, Grollman EF: Thyrotropin and norepinephrine stimulate the metabolism of phosphoinositides in FRTL-5 thyroid cells, FEBS Lett 202:193–196, 1986.

217. Grasberger H, Van Sande J, Mahameed AH-D, et al: A familial thyrotropin (TSH) receptor mutation provides in vivo evidence that the inositol phosphates/Ca2+ cascade mediates TSH action on thyroid hormone synthesis, J Clin Endocrinol Metab 92:2816–2820, 2007.

218. Park ES, Kim H, Suh JM, et al: Involvement of JAK/STAT (Janus kinase/Signal transducer and activator of transcription) in the thyrotropin signaling pathway, Mol Endocrinol 14:662–670, 2000.

219. Brewer C, Yeager N, Di Cristofano A: Thyroid-stimulating hormone-initiated proliferative signals converge in vivo on the mTOR kinase without activating AKT, Cancer Res 67:8002–8006, 2007.

220. Marians RC, Ng L, Blair HC, et al: Defining thyrotropin-dependent and -independent steps of thyroid hormone synthesis by using thyrotropin receptor-null mice, Proc Natl Acad Sci U S A 99:15776–15781, 2002.

221. Tosta Z, Chabaud O, Chebath J: Identification of thyroglobulin mRNA sequences in the nucleus and cytoplasm of cultured thyroid cells: a fast transcriptional effect of thyrotropin, Biochem Biophys Res Commun 116:54–61, 1983.

222. van den Hove M-F, Croizet-Berger K, Tyteca D, et al: Thyrotropin activates guanosine 5'-diphosphate/guanosine 5'-triphosphate exchange on the rate-limited endocytic catalyst, Rab5a, in human thyrocytes in vivo and in vitro, J Clin Endocrinol Metab 92:2803–2810, 2007.

223. Barnes ND, Hayles AB, Ryan RJ: Sexual maturation in juvenile hypothyroidism, Mayo Clin Proc 48:849–856, 1973.

224. Anasti JN, Flack MR, Froelich J, et al: A potential novel mechanism for precocious puberty in juvenile hypothyroidism, J Clin Endocrinol Metab 80:276–279, 1995.

225. Nagayama Y, Yamasaki H, Takeshita A, et al: Thyrotropin binding specificity for the thyrotropin receptor, J Endocrinol Invest 18:283–287, 1995.

226. Crisanti P, Omri B, Hughes EJ, et al: The expression of thyrotropin receptor in the brain, Endocrinology 142:812–822, 2001.

227. Prummel MF, Brokken LJS, Meduri G, et al: Expression of the thyroid-stimulating hormone receptor in the folliculo-stellate cells of human anterior pituitary, J Clin Endocrinol Metab 85:4347–4353, 2000.

228. Saunier B, Pierre M, Jacquemin C, et al: Evidence of cAMP-independent thyrotropin effects on astroglial cells, Eur J Biochem 218:1091–1094, 1993.

229. Peele ME, Carr FE, Baker JR, et al: TSHβ subunit gene expression in human lymphocytes, Am J Med Sci 305:1–7, 1993.

230. Balzan S, Nicolini G, Forini F, et al: Presence of a functional TSH receptor on human erythrocytes, Biomedicine and Pharmacotherapy 61:463–467, 2007.

231. Endo T, Ohta K, Haraguchi K, et al: Cloning and functional expression of thyrotropin receptor cDNA from fat cells, J Biol Chem 270:10833–10837, 1995.

232. Haraguchi K, Shimura H, Kawaguchi A, et al: Effects of thyrotropin on the proliferation and differentiation of cultured rat preadipocytes, Thyroid 9:613–619, 1999.

233. Antunes TT, Gagnon AM, Langille ML, et al: Thyroid-stimulating hormone induces interleukin-6 release from human adipocytes through activation of the nuclear factor-κB pathway, Endocrinology 149:3062–3066, 2008.

234. Bassett JHD, Williams GR: Critical role of the hypothalamic-pituitary-thyroid axis in bone, Bone 43:418–426, 2008.

235. Hase H, Ando T, Eldeiry L, et al: TNFα mediates the skeletal effects of thyroid-stiumlating hormone, Proc Natl Acad Sci U S A 103:12849–12854, 2006.

236. Martini G, Gennari L, De Paola V, et al: The effects of recombinant TSH on bone turnover markers and serum osteoprotegerin and RANKL levels, Thyroid 18:455–460, 2007.

237. Morris JC: Structure and function of the TSH receptor: its suitability as a target for radiotherapy, Thyroid 7:253–258, 1997.

238. Uhlenhuth E, Schwartzbach S: The anterior lobe of the hypophysis as a control mechanism of the function of the thyroid gland, Br J Exp Biol 5:1–5, 1927.

239. Bakke JL, Lawrence N, Arnett F, et al: The fractionation of exogenous and endogenous thyroid-stimulating hormone from human and rat plasma and tissues, J Clin Endocrinol Metab 21:1280–1289, 1961.

240. Odell WD, Wilber JF, Utiger RD: Studies of thyrotropin physiology by means of radioimmunoassay, Recent Prog Horm Res 23:47–78, 1967.

241. Ridgway EC, Weintraub BD, Cevallos JL, et al: Suppression of pituitary TSH secretion in the patient with a hyperfunctioning thyroid nodule, J Clin Invest 52:2783–2792, 1973.

242. Ridgway EC: Thyrotropin radioimmunoassays: Birth, life and demise, Mayo Clin Proc 63:1028–1034, 1988.

243. Ridgway EC, Ardisson LJ, Meskell MJ, et al: Monoclonal antibody to human thyrotropin, J Clin Endocrinol Metab 55:44–48, 1982.

244. Odell WD, Griffin J, Zahradnik R: Two-monoclonal-antibody sandwich-type assay for thyrotropin, with use of an avidin-biotin separation technique, Clin Chem 32:1873–1878, 1986.

245. Van Heyningen V, Abbott SR, Daniel SG, et al: Development and utility of a monoclonal-antibody-based, highly sensitive immunoradiometric assay of thyrotropin, Clin Chem 33:1387–1390, 1987.

246. Spencer CA, Schwarzbein D, Guttler RB, et al: Thyrotropin (TSH)-releasing hormone stimulation test responses employing third and fourth generation TSH assays, J Clin Endocrinol Metab 76:494–498, 1993.

247. Andersen S, Pedersen KM, Bruun NH, et al: Narrow individual variations in serum T(4) and T(3) in normal subjects: a clue to the understanding of subclinical thyroid disease, J Clin Endocrinol Metab 87:1068–1072, 2002.

248. Hansen PS, Brix TH, Sørensen TI, et al: Major genetic influence on the regulation of the pituitary-thyroid axis: a study of healthy Danish twins, J Clin Endocrinol Metab 89:1181–1187, 2004.

249. Panicker V, Wilson SG, Spector TD, et al: Genetic loci linked to pituitary-thyroid axis set points: a genome-wide scan of a large twin cohort, J Clin Endocrinol Metab 93:3519–3523, 2008.

250. Arnaud-Lopez L, Usala G, Ceresini G, et al: Phosphodiesterase 8B gene variants are associated with serum TSH levels and thyroid function, Am J Hum Genet 82:1270–1280, 2008.

251. Guan H, Shan Z, Teng X, et al: Influence of iodine on the reference interval of TSH and the optimal interval of TSH: results of a follow-up study in areas with different iodine intakes, Clin Endocrinol (Oxf) 69:136–141, 2008.

252. Kourides IA, Weintraub BD, Levko MA, et al: α and β subunits of human thyrotropin: purification and devel-

opment of specific radioimmunoassays, Endocrinology 94:1411–1421, 1974.

253. Kourides IA, Weintraub BD, Ridgway EC, et al: Pituitary secretion of free α and β-subunit of human thyrotropin in patients with thyroid disorders, J Clin Endocrinol Metab 40:872–885, 1975.

254. Kourides IA, Ridgway EC, Weintraub BD, et al: Thyrotropin-induced hyperthyroidism: use of α and β-subunit levels to identify patients with pituitary tumors, J Clin Endocrinol Metab 45:534–543, 1977.

255. Ridgway EC, Klibanski A, Ladenson PW, et al: Pure α-secreting pituitary adenomas, N Engl J Med 304:1254–1259, 1981.

256. Klibanski A, Deutsch PJ, Jameson JL, et al: Luteinizing hormone-secreting pituitary tumor: biosynthetic characterization and clinical studies, J Clin Endocrinol Metab 64:536–542, 1987.

257. Blackman MR, Weintraub BD, Rosen SW, et al: Human placental and pituitary glycoprotein hormones and their subunits as tumor markers: a quantitative assessment, J Natl Cancer Inst 65:81–93, 1980.

258. Kahn CR, Rosen SW, Weintraub BD, et al: Ectopic production of chorionic gonadotropin and its subunits by islet cell tumors: a specific marker for malignancy, N Engl J Med 197:565–569, 1977.

259. Rosen SW, Weintraub BD, Aaronson SA: Nonrandom ectopic protein production by malignant cells: direct evidence in vitro, J Clin Endocrinol Metab 50:834–841, 1980.

260. Blackman MR, Weintraub BD, Rosen SW, et al: Comparison of the effects of lung cancer, benign lung disease, and normal aging on pituitary-gonadal function in men, J Clin Endocrinol Metab 66:88–95, 1988.

261. Faglia G: The clinical impact of the thyrotropin-releasing hormone test, Thyroid 8:903–908, 1998.

262. Sarapura VD, Samuels MH, Ridgway EC: Thyroid-stimulating hormone. In Melmed S, editor: The Pituitary, ed 2, Malden, MA, 2002, Blackwell Science, pp 187–229.

263. Watanabe S, Hayashizaki Y, Endo Y, et al: Production of human thyroid-stimulating hormone in Chinese hamster ovary cells, Biochem Biophys Res Commun 149:1149–1155, 1989.

264. Heuer H, Visser TJ: Minireview: Pathophysiological importance of thyroid hormone transporters, Endocrinology 150:1078–1083, 2009.

265. Beck-Peccoz P, Amr S, Menezes-Ferreira NM, et al: Decreased receptor binding of biologically inactive thyrotropin in central hypothyroidism: effect of treatment with thyrotropin-releasing hormone, N Engl J Med 312:1085–1090, 1985.

266. Hayashizaki Y, Hiraoka Y, Tatsumi K, et al: DNA analyses of five families with familial inherited thyroid stimulating hormone (TSH) deficiency, J Clin Endocrinol Metab 71:792–796, 1990.

267. Borck G, Topaloglu AK, Korsch E, et al: Four new cases of congenital secondary hypothyroidism due to a splice site mutation in the thyrotropin-β gene: phenotypic variability and founder effect, J Clin Endocrinol Metab 89:4136–4141, 2004.

268. Sertedaki A, Papadimitriou A, Voutetakis A, et al: Low TSH Congenital Hypothyroidism: Identification of a novel mutation of the TSH β-subunit gene in one sporadic case (C85R) and of mutation Q49stop in two siblings with congenital hypothyroidism, Pediatr Res 52:935–940, 2002.

269. Deladoey J, Vuissoz J-M, Domene HM, et al: Congenital secondary hypothyroidism due to a mutation C105Vfs114X thyrotropin-β mutation: genetic study of five unrelated families from Switzerland and Argentina, Thyroid 13:553–559, 2003.

270. McDermott MT, Haugen BR, Black JN, et al: Congenital isolated central hypothyroidism caused by a "hot spot" mutation in the thyrotropin-β gene, Thyroid 12:1141–1146, 2002.

271. Vuissoz J-M, Deladoey J, Buyukgebiz A, et al: New autosomal recessive mutation of the TSH-β subunit gene causing central isolated hypothyroidism, J Clin Endocrinol Metab 86:4468–4471, 2001.

272. Rogol AD, Kahn CR: Congenital hypothyroidism in a young man with growth hormone, thyrotropin, and prolactin deficiencies, J Clin Endocrinol Metab 39:356–363, 1976.

273. Wit JM, Drayer NM, Jansen M, et al: Total deficiency of GH and prolactin and partial deficiency of thyroid stimulating hormone in two Dutch families: a new variant of hereditary pituitary deficiency, Horm Res 32:170–177, 1989.

274. Behringer RR, Mathews LS, Palmiter RD: Dwarf mice produced by genetic ablation of growth hormone expressing cells, Genes & Dev 2:453–461, 1988.

275. Sornson MW, Wu W, Dasen JS, et al: Pituitary lineage determination by the Prophet of Pit-1 homeodomain factor defective in Ames dwarfism, Nature 384:327–333, 1996.

276. Wu W, Cogan JD, Pfaffle RW, et al: Mutations in PROP-1 cause familial combined pituitary hormone deficiency, Nature Genet 18:147–149, 1998.

277. Fluck C, Deladoey J, Rutishauser K, et al: Phenotypic variability in familial combined pituitary hormone deficiency caused by a PROP-1 gene mutation resulting in the substitution of Arg→Cys at codon 120 (R120C). J Clin Endocrinol Metab 83:3727–3734, 1998.

278. Deladoey J, Fluck C, Buyukgebiz A, et al: "Hot spot" in the PROP1 gene responsible for combined pituitary deficiency, J Clin Endocrinol Metab 84:1645–1650, 1999.

279. Lamesch C, Neumann S, Pfäffle R, et al: Adrenocorticotrope deficiency with clinical evidence for late onset in combined pituitary hormone deficiency caused by a homozygous 301–302delAG mutation of the PROP1 gene, Pituitary 5:163–168, 2002.

280. Beck-Peccoz P, Persani L: Thyrotroinomas, Endocrinol Metab Clin North Am 37:123–134, 2008.

281. Refetoff S, Weiss RE, Usala SJ: The syndromes of resistance to thyroid hormone, Endocrine Rev 14:348–399, 1993.

282. Refetoff S: Resistance to thyroid hormone: one of several defects causing reduced sensitivity to thyroid

hormone, Nat Clin Pract Endocrinol Metab 4:1, 2008.

283. Refetoff S, DeWind LT, DeGroot LJ: Familial syndrome combining deaf-mutism, stippled epiphyses, goiter, and abnormally high PBI: possible target organ refractoriness to thyroid hormone, J Clin Endocrinol Metab 27:279–294, 1967.

284. Dacou-Voutetakis C, Feltquate DM, Drakopoulou M, et al: Familial hypothyroidism caused by a nonsense mutation in the thyroid-stimulating hormone β-subunit gene, Am J Hum Genet 46:988–993, 1990.

285. Bonomi M, Proverbio MC, Weber G, et al: Hyperplastic pituitary gland, high serum glycoprotein hormone α-subunit, and variable circulating thyrotropin (TSH) levels as hallmark of central hypothyroidism due to mutations of the TSHβ gene, J Clin Endocrinol Metab 86:1600–1604, 2001.

286. Sertedaki A, Papadimitriou A, Voutetakis A, et al: Low TSH congenital hypothyroidism: Identification of a novel mutation of the TSH β-subunit gene in one sporadic case (C85R) and of mutation Q49stop in two siblings with congenital hypothyroidism, Pediatr Res 52:935–940, 2002.

287. Pohlenz J, Dumitrescu A, Aumann U, et al: Congenital secondary hypothyroidism caused by exon skipping due to a homozygous donor splice site mutation in the TSHβ-subunit gene, J Clin Endocrinol Metab 87:336–339, 2002.

288. Karges B, LeHeup B, Schoenle E, et al: Compound heterozygous and homozygous mutations of the TSHβ gene as a cause of congenital central hypothyroidism in Europe, Horm Res 62:149–155, 2004.

289. Doeker BM, Pfaffle RW, Pohlenz J, et al: Congenital central hypothyroidism due to a homozygous mutation in the thyrotropin β-subunit gene follows an autosomal recessive inheritance, J Clin Endocrinol Metab 83:1762–1765, 1998.

290. Brumm H, Pfeufer A, Biebermann H, et al: Congenital central hypothyroidism due to homozygous thyrotropin beta 313deltaT mutation is caused by a founder effect, J Clin Endocrinol Metab 87:4811–4816, 2002.

291. Partsch CJ, Riepe FG, Krone N, et al: Initially elevated TSH and congenital central hypothyroidism due to a homozygous mutation of the TSH beta subunit gene: case report and review of the literature, Exp Clin Endocrinol Diabetes 114:227–234, 2006.

292. Heinrichs C, Parma J, Scherberg NH, et al: Congenital central hypothyroidism caused by a homozygous mutation in the TSH-beta subunit gene, Thyroid 10:387–391, 2000.

293. Domene HM, Gruneiro-Papendieck L, Chiesa A, et al: The C105fs114X is the prevalent thyrotropin beta-subunit gene mutation in Argentinean patients with congenital central hypothyroidism, Horm Res 61:41–46, 2004.

294. Felner EI, Dickson BA, White PC: Hypothyroidism in siblings due to a homozygous mutation of the TSH-beta subunit gene, J Pediatr Endocrinol Metab 17:669–672, 2004.

Chapter 3

THYROID REGULATORY FACTORS

JACQUES E. DUMONT, CARINE MAENHAUT, DANIEL CHRISTOPHE, GILBERT VASSART, and PIERRE P. ROGER

Four major biological variables are regulated in the thyrocyte as in any other cell type: function, cell size, cell number, and differentiation. The first three variables are quantitative, and the latter is qualitative. In this chapter, we consider the factors involved in these controls in physiology and in pathology, the main regulatory cascades through which these factors exert their effects, and the regulated processes, which are function, prolif-eration and cell death, gene expression, and differentiation. Whenever possible, we describe what is known in humans.

Thyroid Regulatory Factors

IN PHYSIOLOGY

The two main factors that control the physiology of the thyroid after embryogenesis are the requirement for thyroid hormones and the supply of its main and specialized substrate iodide (Table 3-1). Thyroid hormone plasma levels and action are monitored by the hypothalamic supraoptic nuclei and by the thyrotrophs of the anterior lobe of the pituitary, where they exert a negative feedback through T_3 receptor β. In normal rats, serum thyroid-stimulating hormone (TSH) levels are inversely related to thyrocyte sensitivity to TSH.[1] The corresponding homeostatic control is expressed by TSH (thyrotropin). The TSH receptor is also stimulated by a new, different natural hormone cloned by homology, thyrostimuline. The physiologic role of this protein is unknown, but its level is not controlled by a thyroid hormone feedback, and it does not participate in the homeostatic control of the thyroid.[2] Iodide supply is monitored in part indirectly as a substrate for the synthesis of thyroid hormones and therefore through its effects on the plasma level of thyroid hormones, but mainly in the thyroid itself, where it depresses various aspects of thyroid function and the response of the thyrocyte to TSH. These two major physiologic regulators control the function and size of the thyroid: TSH positively, iodide negatively.[3-6] In mice embryo, other unknown factors control differentiation and organ growth which takes place normally until birth in the absence of TSH receptor.[7,8] In humans, in whom birth occurs later in development, homozygous inactivating mutations of the TSH receptor in familial congenital hypothyroidism were found to be associated with a very hypoplastic thyroid gland.[9] Although the thyroid contains receptors for thyroid hormones, and a direct effect of these hormones on thyrocytes would make sense,[10] as yet little evidence has indicated that such control plays a role in physiology.[11] However, expression of dominant-negative thyroid hormone receptors in mice represses PPARγ expression and induces thyroid tumors in thyroid.[12] The role of increased TSH plasma level in this induction is not defined. Luteinizing hormone (LH) and human chorionic gonadotropin (hCG) at high levels

Table 3-1. Thyroid Regulatory Factors

	Function	Differentiation	Proliferation
SPECIFIC			
PHYSIOLOGIC			
TSH	↗	↗	↗
Thyrostimuline	↗	↗	↗
LH, hCG (high levels)	↗	↗	↗
I⁻	↘	?	↘
T₃ T₄	?	?	↘?
PATHOLOGIC			
TSAb	↗	↗	↗
TBAb	↘	?	↘
NONSPECIFIC			
PHYSIOLOGIC			
Hydrocortisone	0	↗	0
IGF I	?	↗	↗
EGF	↘/0	↘	↗
FGF	?	↘/0	↗
TGF-β	?	↘/0	↘
Norepinephrine	↗	0	0
PGE	↗	0	0
ATP bradykinin TRH	↗↘	?	?
PATHOLOGIC			
IL-I	↘	↘	↘
TNF	↘	↘	↘
IFN-γ	↘	↘	↘

↗, Stimulation; ↘, inhibition: *0*, no effect; *EGF*, epidermal growth factor; *FGF*, fibroblast growth factor; *hCG*; human chorionic gonadotropin; *IFN*, interferon; *IGF*, insulin-like growth factor; *IL*, interleukin; *LH*, luteinizing hormone; *PGF*, prostaglandin F; *T₃*, triiodothyronine; *T₄*, thyroxine; *TBAb*, thyroid-blocking antibody; *TGF*, transforming growth factor; *TRH*, thyrotropin-releasing hormone; *TSAb*, thyroid-stimulating antibodies.

activate the TSH receptor and thus directly stimulate the thyroid. This effect accounts for the depression of TSH levels and sometimes elevated thyroid activity at the beginning of pregnancy.[13-15]

The thyroid gland is also influenced by various other nonspecific hormones.[16] Hydrocortisone exerts a differentiating action in vitro.[17] Estrogens affect the thyroid by unknown mechanisms, directly or indirectly, as exemplified in the menstrual cycle, in pregnancy, and in the higher prevalence of thyroid tumors and other pathologies in women. Growth hormone (GH) induces thyroid growth, but its effects are thought to be mediated by locally produced somatomedins (insulin-like growth factor 1 [IGF-1]). Nevertheless the presence of basal TSH levels might be a prerequisite for the growth-promoting action of IGF-1, because a GH replacement therapy did not increase thyroid size in patients deficient for both GH and TSH.[18] Conversely, TSH does not induce the proliferation of human thyrocytes in the absence of IGF-1 or high levels of insulin. The anomalously low endemic goiter prevalence among pygmies living in iodine-deficient areas,[19] a population genetically resistant to IGF-1, is also compatible with an in vivo permissive effect of IGF-1 and IGF-1 receptor on TSH mitogenic action. In dog and human thyroid primary cultures, the presence of insulin receptors strictly depends on TSH, suggesting that thyroid might be a more specific target of insulin than generally considered.[20,21] Effects of

locally secreted neurotransmitters and growth factors on thyrocytes have been demonstrated in vitro and sometimes in vivo, and the presence of some of these agents in the thyroid has been ascertained. The set of neurotransmitters acting on the thyrocyte and their effects vary from species to species.[3,22] In human cells, well-defined, direct but short-lived responses to norepinephrine, ATP, adenosine, bradykinin, and thyrotropin-releasing hormone (TRH) have been observed.[3,23,24] Growth-factor signaling cascades demonstrated in vitro can exert similar effects in vivo. In nude mice, the injection of epidermal growth factor (EGF) promotes DNA synthesis in thyroid and inhibits iodide uptake in xenotransplanted rat[25] and human thyroid tissues.[26] By contrast, the injection of fibroblast growth factor (FGF) induces a colloid goiter in mice, with no inhibition of iodide metabolism or thyroglobulin and thyroperoxidase mRNA accumulation.[27] These effects are exact replicas of initial observations from the dog thyroid primary culture system[28] and other thyroid primary culture systems.[29-32] EGF and FGF have since been reported to be locally synthesized in the thyroid gland, as a possible response to thyroxine and TSH,[33] respectively. Their exact role as autocrine and/or paracrine agents in the development, function, and pathology of the thyroid gland of different species has yet to be clarified.[34,35] Transforming growth factor beta (TGF-β) constitutes another category of cytokines that are growth factors produced locally by thyrocytes and influence their proliferation and the action of mitogenic factors.[34,36] TGF-β inhibits proliferation and prevents most of the effects of TSH and cAMP in human thyrocytes in vitro.[37,38] TGF-β is synthesized as an inactive precursor which can be activated by different proteases produced by thyrocytes. TGF-β expression is up-regulated during TSH-induced thyroid hyperplasia in rats, suggesting an autocrine mechanism limiting goiter size.[39] Also present in the thyroid are activin A and bone morphogenic peptide (BMP), which are related to TGF-β and inhibit thyrocyte proliferation in vitro.[40] Unlike TGF-β, they are directly synthesized in an active form. Elements of a Wnt/β catenin signaling pathway (Wnt factors, Frizzled receptors, and disheveled isoforms) have been identified in human thyroid and thyroid cancer cell lines.[41] The eventual role in vivo in humans of most of these factors remains to be proved and clarified.

IN PATHOLOGY

Mutated, constitutively active TSH receptors and Gₛ proteins cause thyroid autonomous adenomas.[42,43] Mutations which confer to the TSH receptor a higher sensitivity to LH/hCG cause hyperthyroidism in pregnancy.[44,45] Pathologic extracellular signals play an important role in autoimmune thyroid disease. Thyroid-stimulating antibodies (TSAbs), which bind to the TSH receptor and activate it, reproduce the stimulatory effects of TSH on the function and growth of the tissue. Their effects on cAMP accumulation are slower and much more persistent than those of TSH.[46] Their abnormal generation is responsible for the hyperthyroidism and goiter of Graves' disease. Thyroid-blocking antibodies (TBAbs) also bind to the TSH receptor but do not activate it and hence behave as competitive inhibitors of the hormone. Such antibodies are responsible for some cases of hypothyroidism in thyroiditis. Both stimulating and inhibitory antibodies from mothers with positive sera induce transient hyperthyroidism or hypothyroidism in newborns.[4] The existence of thyroid growth immunoglobulins has been hypothesized to explain the existence of Graves' disease with weak hyperthyroidism and prominent goiter. The thyroid specificity of such immunoglobulins would imply that they recognize thyroid-specific targets.

This hypothesis is now abandoned.[47-49] Discrepancies between growth and functional stimulation may instead reflect kinetics or cell intrinsic factors. Local cytokines have been shown to influence, mostly negatively, the function, growth, and differentiation of thyrocytes in vitro and thyroid function in vivo. Because they are presumably secreted in loco in autoimmune thyroid diseases, these effects might play a role in the pathology of these diseases, but this notion has not yet been proved.[3,16] Moreover, in selenium deficiency, secretion of TGF-β by macrophages has been implicated in the generation of thyroid fibrosis[50] and the pathogenesis of thyroid failure in endemic cretinism. The overexpression of both FGF and FGF receptor 1 in thyrocytes from human multinodular goiter might explain their relative TSH independence.[51] On the other hand, the subversion of tyrosine kinase pathways similar to those normally operated by local growth factors (i.e., the activation and thyrocyte expression of Ret[52] and TRK,[53] the overexpression of Met/HGF receptor, sometimes in association with hepatocyte growth factor (HGF),[54] or erbB/EGF receptor in association with its ligand, TGF-α[55]) can be causally associated with TSH-independent thyroid papillary carcinomas. An autocrine loop involving IGF-2 and the insulin receptor isoform-A is also proposed to stimulate growth of some thyroid cancers.[56] Thyroid cancer cells often escape growth inhibition by TGF-β.[57]

Regulatory Cascades

The great number of extracellular signals acting through specific receptors on cells in fact control a very limited number of regulatory cascades. We will first outline these cascades, along with the signals that control them, and then describe in more detail the specific thyroid cell features: controls by iodide and the TSH receptor.

THE CYCLIC ADENOSINE MONOPHOSPHATE CASCADE

The cyclic adenosine monophosphate (cAMP) cascade in the thyroid corresponds, as far as it has been studied, to the canonic model of the β-adrenergic receptor cascade[4] (Fig. 3-1). It is activated in the human thyrocyte by the TSH and the β-adrenergic and prostaglandin E receptors. These receptors are classical seven-transmembrane receptors controlling transducing guano-

sine triphosphate (GTP)-binding proteins. Activated G proteins belong to the G_s class and activate adenylyl cyclase; they are composed of a distinct α_s subunit and nonspecific β and γ monomers. Activation of a G protein corresponds to its release of guanosine diphosphate (GDP) and binding of GTP and to its dissociation into α_{GTP} and βγ dimers; α_{sGTP} directly binds to and activates adenylyl cyclase. Inactivation of the G protein follows the spontaneous, more or less rapid hydrolysis of GTP to GDP by α_s GTPase activity and the reassociation of α_{GDP} with βγ. The effect of stimulation of the receptor by agonist binding is to increase the rate of GDP release and GTP binding, thus shifting the equilibrium of the cycle toward the α_{GTP} active form. Unless constrained in a multiprotein complex, one receptor can consecutively activate several G proteins (hit-and-run model). A similar system negatively controls adenylyl cyclase through G_i. It is stimulated in the human thyroid by norepinephrine through α_2-receptors and moderately by the TSH receptor. Adenosine at high concentrations directly inhibits adenylyl cyclase. The thyroid contains mainly three isoforms of adenylyl cyclase: III, VI, and IX.[58] The cAMP generated by adenylyl cyclase binds to the regulatory subunit of protein kinase A (PKA) that is blocking the catalytic subunit and releases this now-active unit. The activated, released catalytic unit of protein kinase phosphorylates serines and threonines in the set of proteins containing accessible specific peptides that it recognizes. These phosphorylations, through more or less complex cascades, lead to the observed effects of the cascade. Two isoenzymes (I, II) of cAMP-dependent kinases have been found, the first of which is more sensitive to cAMP; as yet no clear specificity of action of these kinases has been demonstrated. In the case of the thyroid, this cascade is activated through specific receptors, by TSH in all species, and by norepinephrine receptors and prostaglandin E in humans, with widely different kinetics: prolonged for TSH and short lived (minutes) for norepinephrine and prostaglandins.[59] Other neurotransmitters have been reported to activate the cascade in thyroid tissue, but not necessarily in the thyrocytes of the tissue.[24] Besides PKA, cAMP activates EPAC (exchange protein directly activated by cAMP) or Rap guanine nucleotide exchange factor 1 (GEF1) and the less abundant GEF2, which activates the small G protein Rap.[60] It does so in the thyroid.[61] However, despite high expression of EPAC1 in thyrocytes and its further increase in response to TSH, all the physiologically relevant cAMP-dependent functions of TSH studied in dog thyroid cells,

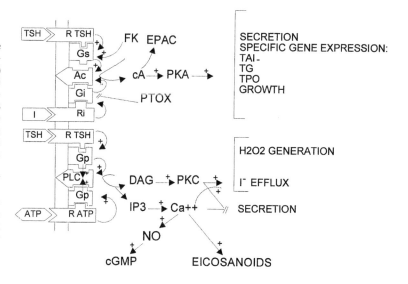

FIGURE 3-1. Regulatory cascades activated by thyroid-stimulating hormone (TSH) in human thyrocytes. In the human thyrocyte, H_2O_2 (H2O2) generation is activated only by the phosphatidylinositol 4,5-bisphosphate (PIP_2) cascade—that is, by the Ca^{2+} (Ca++) and diacylglycerol (DAG) internal signals. In dog thyrocytes, it is activated also by the cyclic adenosine monophosphate (cAMP) cascade. In dog thyrocytes and FRTL-5 cells, TSH does not activate the PIP_2 cascade at concentrations 100 times higher than those required to elicit its other effects. *Ac,* Adenylate cyclase; *cA,* 3′, 5′-cAMP; *cGMP,* 3′, 5′-cyclic guanosine monophosphate; *FK,* forskolin; G_i, guanosine triphosphate (GTP)-binding transducing protein inhibiting adenylate cyclase; G_q, GTP-binding transducing protein activating PIP_2 phospholipase C; G_s, GTP-binding transducing protein activating adenylate cyclase; *I,* extracellular signal inhibiting adenylate cyclase (e.g., adenosine through A_i receptors); IP_3, myoinositol 1,4,5-triphosphate; *EPAC,* cAMP-dependent Rap guanyl nucleotide exchange factor; *PKA,* cAMP-dependent protein kinases; *PKC,* protein kinase C; *PLC,* phospholipase C; *PTOX,* pertussis toxin; *R ATP,* ATP purinergic P_2 receptor; *R TSH,* TSH receptor; *Ri,* receptor for extracellular inhibitory signal I; *TAI,* active transport of iodide; *TG,* thyroglobulin; *TPO,* thyroperoxidase.

including acute regulation of cell functions (including thyroid hormone secretion) and delayed stimulation of differentiation expression and mitogenesis, are mediated only by PKA activation.[61] The role of the cAMP/EPAC/Rap cascade in thyroid thus remains largely unknown. Activation of PKA inactivates small G proteins of the Rho family (RhoA, Rac1, and Cdc42), which reorganizes the actin cytoskeleton and could play an important role in stimulation of thyroid hormone secretion and induction of thyroid differentiation genes.[62] Of the other known possible effectors of cAMP, cyclic guanosine monophosphate (cGMP)-dependent protein kinases are present in the thyroid but cyclic nucleotide–activated channels have not been looked for.

In the thyrocyte, the cAMP cascade is controlled by several negative feedbacks, including the direct activation by phosphorylation of phosphodiesterases and the induction of several proteins inhibiting the cascade.[63]

The thyrocyte is very sensitive to small changes in cAMP concentrations; a mere doubling of this concentration is sufficient to cause maximal thyroglobulin endocytosis.[64]

THE CALCIUM–INOSITOL 1,4,5-TRIPHOSPHATE CASCADE

The calcium (Ca^{2+})–inositol 1,4,5-triphosphate (IP_3) cascade in the thyroid also corresponds, as far as has been studied, to the canonic model of the muscarinic or α_1-adrenergic receptor–activated cascades. It is activated in the human thyrocyte by TSH—through the same receptors that stimulate adenylyl cyclase—and by ATP, bradykinin, and TRH through specific receptors. In this cascade, as in the cAMP pathway, the activated receptor causes the release of GDP and the binding of GTP by the GTP-binding transducing protein (G_q, G_{11}, G_{12}), and their dissociation into α_q and $\beta\gamma$. In turn, α_{GTP} then stimulates phospholipase C. The TSH receptor activates G_s and G_q, with a higher affinity for G_s.[65,66] Phospholipase C hydrolyzes membrane phosphatidylinositol 4,5-bisphosphate (PIP_2) into diacylglycerol and IP_3. IP_3 enhances calcium release from its intracellular stores, followed by an influx from the extracellular medium. The rise in free ionized intracellular Ca^{2+} leads to the activation of several proteins, including calmodulin. The latter protein in turn binds to target proteins and thus stimulates them (e.g., cyclic nucleotide phosphodiesterase and, most importantly, calmodulin-dependent protein kinases). These kinases phosphorylate a whole set of proteins exhibiting serines and threonines on their specific peptides and thus modulate them and cause many observable effects of this arm of the cascade. Calmodulin also activates constitutive nitric oxide (NO) synthase in thyrocytes. The generated NO itself enhances soluble guanylyl cyclase activity in thyrocytes and perhaps in other thyroid cells and thus increases cGMP accumulation.[67] Nothing is yet known about the role of cGMP in the thyroid cell.

Diacylglycerol released from PIP_2 activates protein kinase C, or rather the family of protein kinases C, which by phosphorylating serines or threonines in specific accessible peptides in target proteins causes the effects of the second arm of the cascade.[68] It inhibits phospholipase C or its G_q, thus creating a negative feedback loop. In the human thyroid, the PIP_2 cascade is stimulated through specific receptors by ATP, bradykinin, TRH, and TSH.[24,66,69,70] The effects of bradykinin and TRH are very short lived. Acetylcholine, which is the main activator of this cascade in the dog thyrocyte, is inactive on the human cell, although it activates nonfollicular (presumably endothelial) cells in this tissue.[24]

OTHER PHOSPHOLIPID-LINKED CASCADES

In dog thyroid cells and in a functional rat thyroid cell line (FRTL5), TSH activates PIP_2 hydrolysis weakly and at concentrations several orders of magnitude higher than those required to enhance cAMP accumulation. Of course, these effects have little biological significance. However, at lower concentrations in dog cells, TSH increases the incorporation of labeled inositol and phosphate into phosphatidylinositol. Similar effects may exist in human cells, but they would be masked by the stimulation of the PIP_2 cascade. They may reflect increased synthesis, perhaps coupled to and necessary for cell growth.[71]

Diacylglycerol can be generated by other cascades than the classic Ca^{2+}-IP_3 pathway. Activation of phosphatidylcholine phospholipase D takes place in dog thyroid cells stimulated by carbamylcholine. Because it is reproduced by phorbol esters (i.e., by stable analogs of diacylglycerol), it has been ascribed to phosphorylation of the enzyme by protein kinase C, which would represent a positive feedback loop.[72] Although such mechanisms operate in many types of cells, their existence in human thyroid cells has not been demonstrated.[73]

Release of arachidonate from phosphatidylinositol by phospholipase A_2 and the consequent generation of prostaglandins by a substrate-driven process are enhanced in various cell types through G protein–coupled receptors, by intracellular calcium, or by phosphorylation by protein kinase C. In dog thyroid cells, all agents enhancing intracellular calcium concentration, including acetylcholine, also enhance the release of arachidonate and the generation of prostaglandins. In this species, stimulation of the cAMP cascade by TSH inhibits this pathway. In pig thyrocytes, TSH has been reported to enhance arachidonate release. In human thyroid, TSH, by stimulating PIP_2 hydrolysis and intracellular calcium accumulation, might be expected to enhance arachidonate release and prostaglandin generation, but such effects have not yet been proved.

REGULATORY CASCADES CONTROLLED BY RECEPTOR TYROSINE KINASES

Many growth factors and hormones act on their target cells by receptors that contain one transmembrane segment. They interact with the extracellular domain and activate the intracellular domain, which phosphorylates proteins on their tyrosines. Receptor activation involves in some cases a dimerization and in others a conformational change of a preexisting dimer. The first step in activation is protein-tyrosine phosphorylation, followed by binding of various protein substrates on tyrosine phosphates containing segments of the receptor. Such binding through src homology domains (SH2) leads to phosphorylation of these proteins on their tyrosines. In turn, this phosphorylation causes sequential activation of the *ras* and *raf* proto-oncogenes, mitogen-activated protein (MAP) kinase kinase, MAP kinase, and so on, on the one hand, and phosphatidylinositol-3-kinase (PI-3-kinase), protein kinase B (PKB), and TOR (target of rapamycin) on the other hand. The set of proteins phosphorylated by a receptor defines the pattern of action of this receptor. In thyroids of various species, insulin, IGF-1, EGF, FGF, HGF, but not platelet-derived growth factor activate such cascades.[74,75] In the human thyroid, effects of insulin, IGF-1, EGF, FGF, but not HGF have been demonstrated.[3,21,51,76-78] TGF-β, acting through the serine threonine kinase activity of its receptors and its phosphorylated protein targets (Smad), inhibits proliferation and specific gene expression in human thyroid cells.[37,38,79] TSH and cAMP do not activate either the MAPK-ERK nor the

JUNK and p38 phosphorylation pathways in dog and human thyroids.[75]

CROSS-SIGNALING BETWEEN THE CASCADES

Calcium, the intracellular signal generated by the PIP_2 cascade, activates calmodulin-dependent cyclic nucleotide phosphodiesterases and thus inhibits cAMP accumulation and its cascade.[80] This activity represents a negative cross-control between the PIP_2 and the cAMP cascades. Activation of protein kinase C enhances the cAMP response to TSH and inhibits the prostaglandin E response, which suggests opposite effects on the TSH and prostaglandin receptors.[81] No important effect of cAMP on the PIP_2 cascade has been detected. On the other hand, stimulation of protein kinase C by phorbol esters inhibits EGF action.

Cross-signaling between the cyclic AMP pathway and growth factor–activated cascades have been observed in various cell types.[82,83] In ovarian granulosa cells, FSH (through cAMP) activates MAP kinases and the PI3 kinase pathway.[84] In FRTL5, but not in WRT cell lines, TSH (through cAMP) activates MAP kinase; in WRT cells but not in PCCl3 cells, TSH and cAMP activate PKB.[85,86] Such cross signalings have not been observed in human or dog thyroid cells. Ras, MAPK, p38, Jun kinase and ERK5, as well as PI3 kinase and PKB, are not modulated by cAMP.[74,75,87,88]

Other growth-activating cascades have been little investigated in the thyroid. In dog and human cells, TSH or cAMP have no effect on STAT phosphorylations (i.e., on the Jak-STAT pathways). The nuclear factor κB (NF-κB) pathway has not yet been investigated in thyroid cells.

Specific Control by Iodide

Iodide, the main substrate of the specific metabolism of the thyrocyte, is known to control the thyroid. Its main effects in vivo and in vitro are to decrease the response of the thyroid to TSH, to acutely inhibit its own oxidation (Wolff-Chaikoff effect), to reduce its trapping after a delay (adaptation to the Wolff-Chaikoff effect), and at high concentrations to inhibit thyroid hormone secretion (Fig. 3-2). The first effect is very sensitive inasmuch as small changes in iodine intake without any other changes (e.g., thyroid hormone levels) are sufficient to reset the thyroid system at different serum TSH levels, which suggests that in physiologic conditions, modulation of the thyroid response to TSH by iodide plays a major role in the negative feedback loop.[5,89] Iodide in vitro has also been reported to inhibit a number of metabolic steps in thyroid cells.[90,91] These actions might be direct or indirect as a result of an effect on an initial step of a regulatory cascade. Certainly, iodide inhibits the cAMP cascade at the level of G_s or cyclase and the Ca^{2+}-PIP_2 cascade at the level of G_q or phospholipase C; such effects can account for the inhibition of many metabolic steps controlled by these cascades.[92,93] In one case in which this process has been studied in detail, the control of H_2O_2 generation (i.e., the limiting factor of iodide oxidation and thyroid hormone formation), iodide inhibited both the cAMP and the Ca^{2+}-PIP_2 cascades at their first step but also the effects of the generated intracellular signals cAMP, Ca^{2+}, and diacylglycerol on H_2O_2 generation.[94]

The mechanism of action of iodide on all the metabolic steps besides secretion fits the "XI" paradigm of Van Sande.[95] These inhibitions are relieved by agents that block the trapping of iodide (e.g., perchlorate) or its oxidation (e.g., methimazole)—the Van Sande criteria. The effects are therefore ascribed to one

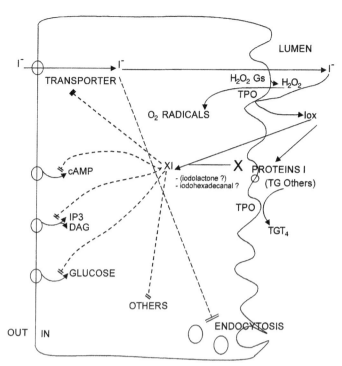

FIGURE 3-2. Effects of iodide on thyroid metabolism. All inhibitory effects of iodide, except in part the inhibition of secretion, are relieved by drugs that inhibit iodide trapping (e.g., perchlorate) or iodide oxidation (e.g., methimazole). Three possible mechanisms corresponding to this paradigm are outlined: generation of O_2 radicals, iodination of target proteins, and synthesis of an XI compound. Any of these mechanisms could account for the various steps ascribed to XI inhibition by I⁻ *(indicated by slashes)*.

or several postulated intracellular iodinated inhibitors called *XI*. The identity of such signals is still unproved. At various times, several candidates have been proposed for this role, such as thyroxine, iodinated eicosanoids (iodolactone),[96] and more plausibly iodohexadecanal.[97] The latter, the predominant iodinated lipid in the thyroid, can certainly account for the inhibition of adenylyl cyclase and of H_2O_2 generation.[97-99] It should be emphasized that iodination of the various enzymes, as well as a catalytic role of iodide in the generation of O_2 radicals (shown to be involved in the toxic effects of iodide), could account for the Van Sande criteria with no need for the XI paradigm.[95,100] With regard to thyroid secretion, its inhibition by iodide in patients treated with antithyroid drugs suggests a direct, XI-independent effect.

Apart from its inhibitory effects, iodide also activates H_2O_2 generation and thus protein iodination in the thyroid of some species including humans. This effect is also inhibited by inhibitors of thyroperoxidase transport and can be classified as an XI effect. It has physiologic sense as it links the generation of H_2O_2 to the availability of the cosubstrate iodide.

In dogs in vivo, iodide at moderate doses decreases cell proliferation and the expression of TPO and NIS mRNA but not the synthesis or secretion of thyroid hormone. The down-regulation of NIS explains the adaptation to the Wolff-Chaikoff effect.[101]

The Thyroid-Stimulating Hormone Receptor

STRUCTURE OF THE PROTEIN

The β subunits of glycoprotein hormones, to which TSH belongs, are encoded by paralogous genes displaying substantial sequence

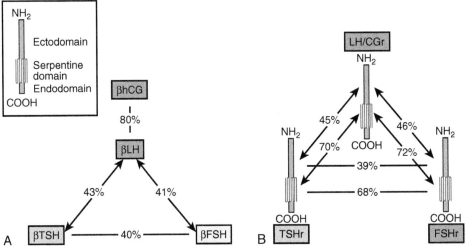

FIGURE 3-3. Both the glycoprotein hormone receptors **(A)** and the beta subunits of glycoprotein hormones **(B)** are encoded by paralogous genes. Sequence identities are indicated, separately for the ectodomains and serpentine domains of the three receptors, and for the β subunits of the four hormones. The pattern of shared similarities suggests coevolution of the hormones and the ectodomain of their receptors, resulting in generation of specificity barriers. The high similarity displayed by the serpentine portions of the receptors is compatible with a conserved mechanism of intramolecular signal transduction. (Data from Vassart G, Pardo L, Costagliola S: A molecular dissection of the glycoprotein hormone receptors, Trends Biochem Sci 29:119–126, 2004.)

similarity (Fig. 3-3). The corresponding receptors, FSHR, LH/CGR and TSHR, are members of the rhodopsin-like G protein–coupled receptor family. As such, TSHR contains a "serpentine" portion with seven transmembrane helices with many (but not all) of the sequence signatures typical of this receptor family. In addition, and a hallmark of the subfamily of glycoprotein hormone receptors, it contains a large (about 400 residues) aminoterminal ectodomain responsible for the high affinity and selective binding of TSH.[102-104] The higher-sequence identity of the serpentine portions of glycoprotein hormone receptors (about 70%), when compared with the ectodomains (about 40%, see Fig. 3-3), suggested early that the former are interchangeable modules capable of activating the G proteins (mainly $G_{\alpha s}$) after specific binding of the individual hormones to the latter.[4] Contrary to other rhodopsin-like GPCRs, binding of the hormones to their ectodomains can be observed with high affinity in the absence of the serpentine.[105] The intramolecular transduction of the signal between these two portions of the receptors involves mechanisms specific to the glycoprotein hormone receptor family (see later). The relatively high sequence identity between the hormone-binding domains of the TSH and LH/CG receptors opens the possibility of spillover phenomena during normal or, even more so, molar or twin pregnancies, when hCG concentrations are several orders of magnitude higher than TSH. This provides an explanation to cases of pregnancy hyperthyroidism.[15,15]

The TSHR contains six sites for N-glycosylation, of which four have been shown to be effectively glycosylated.[105] The functional role of the individual carbohydrate chains is still debated. It is likely that they contribute to the routing and stabilization of the receptor through the membrane system of the cell.

Alone among the glycoprotein hormone receptors, the TSHR undergoes cleavage of its ectodomain, severing it from the serpentine domain.[106] This phenomenon has been related to the presence in the TSHR of a 50-amino-acid "insertion" for which there is no counterpart in the FSHR or LH/CGR. The initial cleavage step, by a metalloprotease, takes place around position 314 (within the 50-amino-acid insertion), followed by nibbling of the aminoterminal extremity of the serpentine-containing

portion.[107,108] The aminoterminal and serpentine portions of the resulting dimer remain bound to each other by disulphide bonds. The functional meaning of this TSHR-specific posttranslational modification remains unclear. Whereas all wild-type TSHR at the surface of thyrocytes seem to be in cleaved form, it has been shown that noncleavable mutant constructs are functionally undistinguishable from cleaved receptors when expressed in transfected cells.[106] Noteworthy, when transiently or permanently transfected in nonthyroid cells, the wild-type human TSHR is present at the cell surface as a mixture of monomer and cleaved dimer. The cleavage and shedding of the ectodomain from a portion of the mature receptors has been related to the triggering or maintenance of autoimmunity in Graves' disease.[109,110]

The TSH receptor is specifically inserted into the basolateral membrane of thyrocytes. This phenomenon involves signals encoded in the primary structure of the protein, as it is conserved when the receptor is expressed in the MDCK cell, a polarized cell of nonthyroid origin.[111]

The possibility that TSHR are present at the cell surface as "dimers of cleaved dimers" has recently been raised following demonstration that most rhodopsin-like GPCRs do dimerize[112] (see following).

THE TSH RECEPTOR GENE

The gene coding for the human TSH receptor has been localized on the long arm of chromosome 14 (14q31).[113,114] It spreads over more than 60 kb and is organized into 10 exons displaying an interesting correlation with the protein structure.[104] The extracellular domain is encoded by a series of 9 exons, each of which corresponds to one or an integer number of leucine-rich repeat (LRR) motifs. The C-terminal half of the receptor containing the C-terminal part of the ectodomain and the serpentine domain is encoded by a single large exon. This finding is reminiscent of the fact that many G protein–coupled receptor genes are intronless. A likely evolutionary scenario derives from this gene organization[115]: the glycoprotein hormone receptor genes would have evolved from the condensation of an intronless classic G protein–coupled receptor with a mosaic gene encoding a protein with

LRRs. Triplication of this ancestral gene and subsequent divergence led to the receptors for LH/CG, FSH, and TSH. The existence of 10 exons in both the TSH and FSH receptor genes (as opposed to the 11-exon LH/CG receptor), suggests the following phylogeny: one ancestral glycoprotein hormone receptor duplicating in the LH receptor and in the ancestor of TSH and FSH receptor, which lost one intron. The latter would later duplicate yielding the TSH and FSH receptors.

The gene promoter has been cloned and sequenced in humans and rats.[115,116] It has characteristics of "housekeeping" genes in that it is GC-rich and devoid of TATA boxes; in the rat it was shown to drive transcription from multiple start sites.[116]

Expression of the TSH receptor gene is largely thyroid specific. Constructs made of a chloramphenicol acetyltransferase reporter gene under control of the 5′ flanking region of the rat gene show expression when transfected into FRTL5 cells and FRT cells but not into nonthyroid HeLa or a rat liver cell line (BRL) cells.[116] However, TSH receptor mRNA has been clearly demonstrated in fat tissue of the guinea pig[117] and following differentiation of preadipocytes into adipocytes.[118,119] Functional significance in man of reports showing its presence in lymphocytes, extraocular tissue, and recently in cartilage and bone requires additional studies.[109,120]

Recently, functional expression of the TSH receptor has been demonstrated in pars tuberalis of the pituitary in quails and ependymal cells in mice, in relation with the control of photoperiodic behavior.[118,119,121,122] No extrapolation of these studies to man has been attempted yet. Expression of the TSH receptor in thyroid cells is extremely robust. It is moderately up-regulated and down-regulated by TSH in vitro[123] and down-regulated by iodide in vivo.[101]

FUNCTIONAL ASPECTS

Recognition of the Receptor by TSH

The three-dimensional structures are available for hCG and FSH,[124-126] which allows accurate modelization of TSH on these templates. The crystal structure of the human FSHR-FSH complex[127] has confirmed that the ectodomain of glycoprotein hormone receptors belongs to the family of proteins with LRRs, as was previously suggested by sequence analysis and homology modeling.[128] The concave inner surface of the receptor (Fig. 3-4A) is an untwisted, noninclined β sheet formed by ten LRRs. Whereas the N-terminal portion of the β sheet (LRR1-7) is nearly flat, the C-terminal portion (LRR7-10) has the horseshoe-like curvature of LRR proteins. The crystal structure of part of the TSHR ectodomain in complex with a thyroid-stimulating autoantibody has recently been obtained.[129] Notably, both the structure of the ectodomain of TSHR and the receptor-binding arrangements of the autoantibody are very similar to those reported for the FSHR-FSH complex. The ectodomain of glycoprotein hormone receptors also contains, downstream of the LRR region, a cysteine cluster domain of unknown structure (the hinge region), involved in receptor inhibition/activation and containing sites for tyrosine sulfation important for hormone binding (see later).

Extensive amino acid substitutions by site-directed mutagenesis of the X_i residues in the LRR portion of the TSHR for their counterparts in the LH/CGR have been performed.[130] Exchanging eight amino acids of the TSHR for the corresponding LH/CGR residues resulted in a mutant displaying a sensitivity to hCG matching that of the wild-type LH/CGR. Surprisingly, while gaining sensitivity to hCG, the mutant kept a normal sensitivity

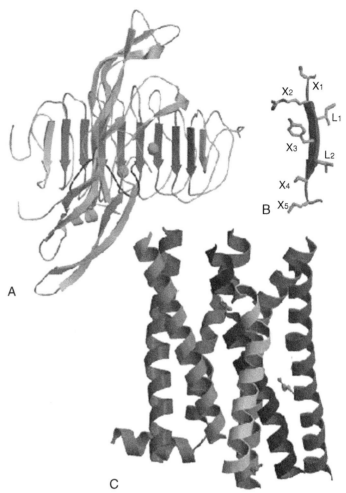

FIGURE 3-4. Schematic representation of the hormone receptor complex. **A,** General view of the follicle-stimulating hormone receptor (FSHR)-FSH crystal structure as a template to model the interaction between TSH and the TSH receptor 129. The concave inner surface of the receptor, formed by the β sheets of 10 leucine-rich repeats (LRRs), 2 through 9 (downward arrows), contact the middle section of the hormone molecule, both the C-terminal segment of the α subunit and the "seat-belt" segment of the β-subunit. **B,** Each LRR is composed of the X_1-X_2-L-X_3-L-X_4-X_5 residues (where X is any amino acid, and L is usually Leu, Ile, or Val), forming the central X_2-L-X_3-L-X_4, a typical β strand, while X_1 and X_5 are parts of the adjacent loops. **C,** Molecular model of the transmembrane domain of the TSH receptor, constructed from the crystal structure of bovine rhodopsin 123. The crystal structure of the $β_2$-adrenergic receptor bound to the partial inverse agonist, carazolol, has been published.[356] The structure of both rhodopsin and the $β_2$ receptor are similar at the transmembrane domain. (Adapted from Caltabiano G, Campillo M, De Leener A et al: The specificity of binding of glycoprotein hormones to their receptors, Cell Mol Life Sci 65:2484–2492, 2008.)

to TSH, making it a dual-specificity receptor. It is necessary to exchange 12 additional residues to fully transform it into a bona fide LH/CGR.[130] From an evolutionary point of view, these observations indicate that nature has built recognition specificity of hormone-receptor couples on both attractive and repulsive residues, and that residues at different homologous positions have been selected to this result in the different receptors.

Inspection of electrostatic surface maps of models of the wild-type TSH and LH/CG receptors and some of the mutants is revealing in this respect.[130,131] The LH/CGR displays an acidic groove in the middle of its horseshoe, extending to the lower part of it (corresponding to the C-terminal ends of the β strands). Generation of a similar distribution of charges in the dual-specificity and reverse-specificity TSHR mutants suggests that

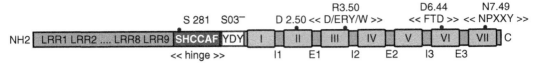

FIGURE 3-5. Linear representation of the TSH receptor. Sequence signatures common to all rhodopsin-like GPCRs and sequence signatures specific to the glycoprotein hormone receptor gene family are both implicated in activation of GPHRs. Key residues are indicated *(dots)* as well as conserved motifs: SO3⁻ stands for posttranslational sulfation of the indicated tyrosine residues. The *black boxes* stand for transmembrane helices and I1-I3, E1-E3, for intracellular and extracellular loops, respectively. (Adapted from Vassart G, Pardo L, Costagliola S: A molecular dissection of the glycoprotein hormone receptors, Trends Biochem Sci 29:119–126, 2004.)

this is important for hCG recognition. A detailed modelization of the interactions between TSH and the ectodomain of its receptor has been realized.[131]

In addition to the hormone-specific interactions genetically encoded in the primary structure of glycoprotein hormones receptors and their ligands, the importance of nonhormone-specific ionic interactions has been demonstrated, involving sulfated tyrosine residues present in the ectodomains of all three receptors.[132,133] Sulfation in the TSHR takes place on both tyrosine residues of a conserved Tyr-Asp-Tyr motif located close to the border between the ectodomain and the first transmembrane helix (Fig. 3-5). However, only sulfation of the first tyrosine of the motif seems to be functionally important,[132] contributing crucially to the binding affinity without interfering with specificity. The functional role of this posttranslational modification of the TSH receptor has been confirmed by demonstration of profound hypothyroidism due to resistance to TSH in mice with inactivation of Tpst2, one of the enzymes responsible for tyrosine sulfation.[134,135]

Activation of the Serpentine Portion of the TSH Receptor

Because it belongs to the rhodopsin-like GPCR family and displays many of the cognate signatures in primary structure, the serpentine portion of the TSH receptor is likely to share with rhodopsin common mechanisms of activation.[136,137] However, sequence signatures characteristic of the serpentine portion of the glycoprotein hormone receptors suggest the existence of idiosyncrasies associated with specific mechanisms of activation (see Fig. 3-5). In addition, the TSHR has been found to be activated by a wide spectrum of gain-of-function mutations.[138-140] Compilations of available data identify more than 30 residues, the mutation of which cause constitutive activation. Since many somatic mutations affecting a given residue have been found repeatedly, it is likely that we are close to a saturation map for spontaneous gain-of-function mutations. Attempts to translate this map into mechanisms of transition between inactive and active conformations of the receptor have been made, in the light of rhodopsin structural data. Three sequence patterns affected by gain-of-function mutations deserve special mention and may help in understanding how the TSH receptor is activated.

The first is centered on an aspartate in position 6.44 (Asp633) at the cytoplasmic side of transmembrane helix VI (TM-VI). When mutated to a variety of amino acids, the result is constitutive activation.[138,141,142] This suggested that the gain of function resulted from the breakage of (a) bond(s) rather than the creation of novel interaction(s) by the mutated residue, and the main partner of Asp6.44 was identified as Asn7.49 in transmembrane helix VII. From a series of site-directed mutagenesis studies,[141,143] it was tentatively concluded that in the inactive conformation of the TSH receptor, the side chain of Asp7.49 is normally "sequestered" by both Thr6.43 and Asp6.44, and that the active

conformation(s) require(s) establishment of novel interaction(s) of N7.49 involving most probably Asp in position 2.50.

The second: Glutamate 3.49 and arginine 3.50 of the highly conserved "D/ERY/W" motif at the bottom of TM-III form an ionic lock with aspartate 6.30 at the cytoplasmic end of TM-VI. Disruption of this ionic lock (e.g., by mutations affecting Asp6.30) leads to constitutively active mutant receptors.[143] Thus the movements of TM-III and TM-VI at the cytoplasmic side of the membrane (i.e., presumably an opening of the receptor) is necessary for receptor activation.[144] The existence of this ionic lock has, however, been questioned recently, since it is not found in the determined structure of the β₂-adrenergic receptor.[136]

The third: Serine 281 belongs to a GPHR-specific "YPSHC-CAF" sequence signature located at the carboxyl-terminal end of the LRR portion in the ectodomain of the receptors (see Fig. 3-5). After mutation of this serine residue had been shown to activate the TSH receptor constitutively,[145] this segment, sometimes referred to as the *hinge motif*, was shown to play an important role in activation of all three glycoprotein hormone receptors.[146] The functional effect of substitutions of S281 in the TSHR likely results in a "loss of structure" locally, since the more destructuring the substitutions, the stronger the activation.[146,147] This observation, together with results showing that mutation of specific residues in the extracellular loops of the TSHR cause constitutive activation,[148] and the previous demonstration of activation of TSH receptor by extracellular trypsinization,[149,150] led to the hypothesis that activation of the receptor could involve the rupture of an inhibitory interaction between the ectodomain and the serpentine domain (see later).[145]

Interaction Between the Ectodomain and the Serpentine Domain

Mutant TSHR constructs devoid of the ectodomain displayed a phenotype compatible with partial activation, thus confirming the inhibitory effect of the ectodomain on the serpentine portion already suggested by the partial activation of the receptor by a trypsin treatment. However, activation of cAMP production in cells transfected with truncated constructs was much lower than after full stimulation of the wild-type receptor by TSH or by mutation of Ser281.[151] These observations led to the following model for activation of the TSHR (Fig. 3-6).[151,152] In the resting state, the ectodomain would exert an inhibitory effect on the activity of an inherently noisy rhodopsin-like serpentine, qualifying pharmacologically as an inverse agonist of the serpentine. Upon activation, by binding of the hormone or secondary to mutation of S281 in the hinge region, the ectodomain would switch from inverse agonist to full agonist of the serpentine portion. The ability of the strongest S281 mutants to fully activate the receptor in the absence of hormone suggests that the ultimate agonist of the serpentine domain would be the "activated" ectodomain, with no need for an interaction between the hormone and the serpentine domain. This model in which the "real" agonist of the serpentine domain would be the activated

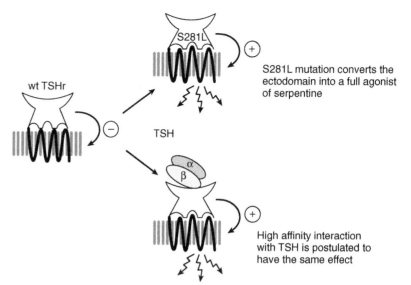

FIGURE 3-6. Model for activation of the thyrotropin receptor. Interactions between the ectodomain and the serpentine domains are implicated in the activation mechanism and functional specificity. The TSH receptor is represented with its ectodomain containing a concave, hormone-binding structure facing upwards, and a transmembrane serpentine portion. The basal state of the receptor is characterized by an inhibitory interaction between the ectodomain and the serpentine domain (indicated by the (−) sign). The ectodomain would function as a tethered inverse agonist of the serpentine portion. Mutation of Ser281 in the ectodomain into leucine switches the ectodomain from an inverse agonist into a full agonist of the serpentine domain (indicated by the (+) sign). Binding of TSH (indicated by $\alpha\beta$ dimeric structure) to the ectodomain is proposed to have a similar effect, converting it into a full agonist of the serpentine portion. The serpentine portion in the basal state is represented as a compact, black structure. The fully activated serpentine portion is depicted as a relaxed gray structure with arrows indicating activation of $G_{\alpha s}$.

ectodomain is confirmed by the identification of a monoclonal antibody recognizing the ectodomain and endowed with inverse agonistic activity.[153,154] Recent data suggest that the activation step might be achieved by interaction of charged residues of the α subunit of the hormone with acidic residues of the hinge region.[155]

Activation by Chorionic Gonadotropin

As indicated above, the sequence similarity between TSH and hCG, and between their receptors, allows for some degree of promiscuous stimulation of the TSH receptor by hCG during the first trimester of pregnancy, when hCG levels reach peak values. The inverse relation between TSH and hCG observed in most pregnant women is clear indication that their thyroid is subjected to the thyrotropic activity of hCG.[15] Whereas this situation is usually associated with euthyroidism, thyrotoxicosis may develop in cases of excessive hCG production (as it occurs in twin pregnancies or hydatidiform moles), or in rare patients harboring a mutant TSH receptor with increased sensitivity to hCG.[156]

Of note, the bioactivity of human TSH (and of all glycoprotein hormones, including hCG) is lower than that of bovine TSH and of other nonprimate mammals. This is due to positive selection in higher primates of α subunits in which several key basic amino acids have been substituted.[157] The observation that this phenomenon parallels the evolution of chorionic gonadotropin suggests that it may be related to protection against promiscuous stimulation of the TSH receptor by hCG during pregnancy.

Activation by Autoantibodies

Autoantibodies found in Graves' disease and some types of idiopathic myxedema can stimulate (TSAb) or block (TSBAb) TSH receptor, respectively. Epitopes recognized by TSAbs are being identified from precise mapping of binding sites of murine or human monoclonal antibodies endowed with TSAb activity on the partial crystal structure of the ectodomain[129] or models thereof.[158] However, the actual mechanisms implicated in activation of the receptor by TSAbs (and by TSH) are still unknown. Although most TSAbs do compete with TSH for binding to the receptor,[110,159] and despite similarity in interaction surfaces,[129] the precise targets of the hormone and autoantibodies are likely to be different, at least in part. It has indeed been shown that sulfated tyrosine residues, which are important for TSH binding,

are not implicated in recognition of TSH receptor by TSAbs.[160] Also, contrary to TSH, most TSAbs from Graves' patients display a delay in their ability to stimulate cAMP accumulation in transfected cells.[46] The availability of TSAb preparations purified from individual patients should allow exploration of these issues in a direct fashion.[161]

Activation by Thyrostimulin

Thyrostimulin has been identified as a novel agonist of the TSH receptor. A glycoprotein hormone, it is composed of two subunits, coined $\alpha2$ and $\beta5$, and activates the receptor with a lower EC50 than human TSH. It is produced by the pituitary in corticotrophs, but its physiologic significance remains mysterious.[2,162-164]

Down-Regulation of the TSH Receptor

Desensitization of some G protein–coupled receptors has been shown to involve phosphorylation of specific residues by G protein–receptor kinases (homologous desensitization) or PKA (heterologous desensitization) enzymes.[165] When compared with other G protein–coupled receptors, the TSH receptor contains few phosphorylatable serine or threonine residues in its intracellular loops and C-terminal tail, which probably accounts for the limited desensitization observed after stimulation by TSH. Acute desensitization of the receptor in the presence of TSH, presumably by phosphorylation, is weak and delayed.[166] Its internalization is rapidly followed by recycling to the cell surfaces, while the hormone is degraded in lysosomes.[167] Similarly, a weak down-regulation, confounded by the long life of both TSHR mRNA and protein, takes place but has little functional role.[123] On the other hand, in the presence of constant stimulation, cAMP accumulation is down-regulated mostly as a consequence of phosphodiesterase induction.[168] The persistence of hyperthyroidism in patients submitted to constant TSH stimulations in TSH-secreting pituitary adenomas or TSAb stimulation in Graves' disease testifies to the weakness of these negative regulations.

Dimerization

As do most rhodopsin-like GPCRs, the glycoprotein hormone receptors have been demonstrated to dimerize/oligomerize by a variety of experimental approaches, including FRET, BRET, and functional complementation of mutants.[169-171] The physiologic significance of this phenomenon remains unknown, but it has been shown to be associated with allosteric properties of the dimers/oligomers. TSH binding to the TSHR displays strong negative cooperativity,[169] which is classically considered to account for a shallow concentration action curve extending over more than two orders of magnitude.

Control of Thyroid Function

THYROID HORMONE SYNTHESIS

Thyroid hormone synthesis requires the uptake of iodide by active transport, thyroglobulin biosynthesis, oxidation and binding of iodide to thyroglobulin, and within the matrix of this protein, oxidative coupling of two iodotyrosines into iodothyronines. All these steps are regulated by the cascades just described.

Iodide Transport

Iodide is actively transported by the iodide Na^+/I^- symporter (NIS) against an electrical gradient at the basal membrane of the thyrocyte and diffuses by a specialized channel (pendrin or another channel)[172,173] from the cell to the lumen at the apical membrane. The opposite fluxes of iodide, from the lumen to the cell and from the cell to the outside, are generally considered to be passive and nonspecific. At least five types of control have been demonstrated.[90,91,172]

1. Rapid and transient stimulation of iodide efflux by TSH in vivo, which might reflect a general increase in membrane permeability. The cascade involved is not known.
2. Rapid activation of iodide apical efflux from the cell to the lumen by TSH. This effect, which contributes to the concentration of iodide at the site of its oxidation, is mediated—depending on the species—by Ca^{2+} and/or cAMP.[172,174] In human cells, it is mainly controlled by Ca^{2+} and therefore by the TSH effect on phospholipase C.
3. Delayed increase in the capacity (V_{max}) of the active iodide transport NIS in response to TSH. This effect is inhibited by inhibitors of RNA and protein synthesis and is due to activation of iodide transporter gene expression. This effect of TSH is reproduced by cAMP analogs in vitro and is therefore mediated by the cAMP cascade.[6] Expression of mRNA is enhanced by TSH and cAMP and decreased by iodide.[101,175] TSH enhancement of thyroid blood flow, more or less delayed depending on the species, also contributes to increase in the uptake of iodide.[6] Blood flow is inversely related to iodine levels in the thyroid.[176]
4. Rapid inhibition by iodide of its own transport in vivo and in vitro. This inhibitory effect requires an intact transport and oxidation function—that is, it fulfills the criteria of an XI effect. After several hours, the capacity of the active transport mechanism is greatly impaired (adaptation to the Wolff-Chaikoff effect).[91] The mechanism of the first effect is unknown but probably initially involves direct inhibition of the transport system itself (akin to the desensitization of a receptor), followed later by inhibition of NIS gene expression and NIS synthesis (akin to the down-regulation of a receptor).[101]
5. Inhibition by iodide of the thyroid blood flow. This effect does not fit the XI paradigm, since it takes place in patients treated with thyroperoxidase inhibitors.

Iodide Binding to Protein and Iodotyrosine Coupling

Iodide oxidation and binding to thyroglobulin and iodotyrosine coupling in iodothyronines are catalyzed by the same enzyme, thyroperoxidase, with H_2O_2 used as a substrate.[177] The same regulations therefore apply to the two steps. H_2O_2 is generated by an NADPH-oxidase system constituted by two DUOX proteins.[178,179] The system is very efficient in the basal state inasmuch as little of the iodide trapped can be chased by perchlorate in vivo. Also, in vitro the amount of iodine bound to proteins mainly depends on the iodide supply. Nevertheless, in human thyroid in vitro, stimulation of the iodination process takes place even at low concentrations of the anion, thus indicating that iodination is a second limiting step. Such stimulation is caused in all species by intracellular Ca^{2+} and is therefore a consequence of activation of the Ca^{2+}-PIP$_2$ cascade. In many species, phorbol esters and diacylglycerol, presumably through protein kinase C, also enhance iodination.[180] It is striking that in a species such as the human, in which TSH activates the PIP$_2$ cascade, cAMP inhibits H_2O_2 generation and iodination, whereas in a species (dog) in which TSH activates only the cAMP cascade, cAMP enhances iodination. Obviously, in the latter species, a supplementary cAMP control was necessary.[180,181]

Thyroperoxidase does not contain any obvious phosphorylation site in its intracellular tail. On the other hand, all the agents that activate iodination also activate H_2O_2 generation, and inhibition of H_2O_2 generation decreases iodination, which suggests that iodination is a substrate–driven process and that it is mainly controlled by iodide supply and H_2O_2 generation.[180,182] Congruent with the relatively high K_m of thyroperoxidase for H_2O_2, H_2O_2 is generated in disproportionate amounts with regard to the quantity of iodide oxidized. Negative control of iodination by iodide (the Wolff-Chaikoff effect) is accompanied and mostly explained by the inhibition of H_2O_2 generation. This effect of I^- is relieved by perchlorate and methimazole and thus pertains to the XI paradigm.[95,180]

Iodotyrosine coupling to iodotyrosines is catalyzed by the same system and is therefore subject to the same regulations as iodination. However, coupling requires that suitable tyrosyl groups in thyroglobulin be iodinated (i.e., that the level of iodination of the protein be sufficient). In the case of severe iodine deficiency or when thyroglobulin exceeds the iodine available, insufficient iodination of each thyroglobulin molecule will preclude iodothyronine formation, whatever the activity of the H_2O_2 generating system and thyroperoxidase. On the other hand, when the iodotyrosines involved in the coupling are present, coupling is controlled by the H_2O_2 concentration but independent of iodide.[177] In this case, H_2O_2 control has significance even at very low iodide concentrations.

Generation of H_2O_2 requires the reduced form of nicotinamide adenine dinucleotide phosphate (NADPH) as a coenzyme and is thus accompanied by NADPH oxidation. Limitation of the activity of the pentose phosphate pathway by NADP$^+$ insures that NADPH oxidation for H_2O_2 generation causes stimulation of this pathway. Also, excess H_2O_2 leaking back into the thyrocyte is reduced mainly by catalase but also by glutathione (GSH) peroxidase, and the oxidized GSH (GSSG) produced is reduced by NADPH-linked GSH reductase. Thus both the generation of H_2O_2 and to some extent the disposal of excess H_2O_2 by pulling NADP reduction and the pentose pathway lead to activation of this pathway—historically one of the earliest and unexplained effects of TSH.[6,180]

In the long term, in vivo or in vitro, the activity of the whole iodination system obviously also depends on the level of its constitutive enzymes. It is therefore not surprising that activation of thyrocytes by the cAMP cascade increases the thyroperoxidase gene expression, whereas dedifferentiating treatments with EGF and phorbol esters inhibit this expression and thus reduce the capacity and activity of the system. Apparent discrepancies in the literature about the effects of phorbol esters on iodination are mostly explained by the kinetics of these effects (acute stimulation of the system, delayed inhibition of expression of the involved genes).

THYROID HORMONE SECRETION

Secretion of thyroid hormone requires endocytosis of human thyroglobulin, its hydrolysis, and the release of thyroid hormones from the cell. Thyroglobulin can be ingested by the thyrocyte by three mechanisms.[6,183-185]

In *macropinocytosis*, which is the first, pseudopods engulf clumps of thyroglobulin. In all species this process is triggered by acute activation of the camp/PKA cascade and therefore by TSH.[186] Inactivation of the Rho small G proteins, resulting in microfilament depolarization and stress-fiber disruption, is probably involved in the process.[62] Stimulation of macropinocytosis is preceded and accompanied by an enhancement of thyroglobulin exocytosis and thus of membrane to the apical surface.[182,187,188] By *micropinocytosis*, the second process, small amounts of colloid fluid are ingested. This process does not appear to be greatly influenced by acute modulation of the regulatory cascades. It is enhanced in chronically stimulated thyroids and thyroid cells with induction of vesicle transport proteins Rab 5 and 7.[189,190] It probably accounts for most of basal secretion. A third (hypothesized) process is *receptor-mediated endocytosis*; it would be enhanced in chronically stimulated thyroid cells.[191-193] The protein involved could be megalin[194] and/or asialoglycoprotein. This process probably accounts for transcytosis of thyroglobulin.[195]

Contrary to the last named, the first two processes are not specific for the protein. They can be distinguished by the fact that macropinocytosis is inhibited by microfilament and microtubule poisons and by lowering of the temperature (below 23° C). Whatever its mechanism, endocytosis is followed by lysosomal digestion, with complete hydrolysis of thyroglobulin. The main iodothyronine in thyroglobulin is thyroxine. However, during its secretion, a small fraction is deiodinated by type I 5-deiodinases (DIO1 and DIO2) to triiodothyronine (T_3), thus increasing relative T_3 (the active hormone) secretion.[196]

The free thyroid hormones are released by an unknown mechanism, which may be transport or exocytosis. The iodotyrosines are deiodinated by specific deiodinases and their iodide recirculated in the thyroid iodide compartments. Under acute stimulation, a release (spillover) of amino acids and iodide from the thyroid is observed. A mechanism for lysosome uptake of poorly iodinated thyroglobulin on N-acetylglucosamine receptors and recirculation to the lumen has been proposed. Under normal physiologic conditions, endocytosis is the limiting step of secretion, but after acute stimulation, hydrolysis might become limiting with the accumulation of colloid droplets. Secretion by macropinocytosis is triggered by activation of the cAMP cascade and inhibited by Ca^{2+} at two levels: cAMP accumulation and cAMP action. It is also inhibited in some thyroids by protein kinase C downstream from cAMP. Thus the PIP_2 cascade negatively controls macropinocytosis.[81]

The thyroid also releases thyroglobulin. Inasmuch as this thyroglobulin was first demonstrated by its iodine, at least part of this thyroglobulin is iodinated; thus it must originate from the colloid lumen. Release is inhibited in vitro by various metabolic inhibitors and therefore corresponds to active secretion.[187,197] The most plausible mechanism is transcytosis from the lumen to the thyrocyte lateral membranes.[188] As for thyroid hormone, this secretion is enhanced by activation of the cAMP cascade and TSH and inhibited by Ca^{2+} and protein kinase C activation. Because thyroglobulin secretion does not require its iodination, it reflects the activation state of the gland regardless of the efficiency of thyroid hormone synthesis. Thyroglobulin serum levels and their increase after TSH stimulation constitute a very useful index of the functional state of the gland when thyroid hormone synthesis is impaired, as in iodine deficiency, congenital defects in iodine metabolism, treatment with antithyroid drugs, and the like.[198] Regulated thyroglobulin secretion should not be confused with the release of this protein from thyroid tumors, which corresponds in large part to exocytosis of newly synthesized thyroglobulin in the extracellular space rather than in the nonexistent or disrupted follicular lumen. In inflammation or after even mild trauma, opening of the follicles can cause unregulated leakage of lumen thyroglobulin. Transcytosis or leakage from the lumen yields iodinated thyroglobulin, whereas newly synthesized exocytotic thyroglobulin is not iodinated.

Control of Thyroid-Specific Gene Expression

The so-called thyroid-specific genes encode proteins that are either found in the thyroid exclusively, like thyroglobulin and thyroperoxidase, or that, although being also found in a few additional tissues, are primarily involved in thyroid function, like TSH receptor and sodium/iodide symporter. The transcription of these genes in the thyroid appears to rely on the coordinated action of a master set of transcription factors that includes at least the homeodomain protein TTF-1 (also known as *Nkx 2.1*, or *T/ebp*), the paired-domain protein Pax 8, and perhaps also the forkhead-domain protein TTF-2 (also known as *FoxE1*).[199,200] Loss-of-function mutant mice for TTF-1, Pax 8, or TTF-2 have been generated and allowed to identify a crucial role for these transcription factors in the development of the thyroid also. However, because none of these animals develop a normal mature thyroid, they could not be used to investigate the exact role of these key factors in the control of gene expression in the mature thyroid. Partial conditional inactivation of the *TITF1* gene that encodes the TTF-1 protein was also achieved in the mouse,[201] but since inactivation remains only partial in this model, its use is limited in the detailed investigation of the consequences of the absence of TTF-1 on differentiated thyroid cell function. Most of the work concerning this last aspect has thus been conducted either in primary cultures of thyrocytes[202] or in immortalized thyroid cell lines like FRTL-5 and PCCl3.[203] Although the data gathered to date agree on most basic aspects, significant differences have sometimes been observed between primary versus immortalized cell models.[204] Part of these discrepancies may result from the existence of occasional species-specific differences.[205]

The main regulator of thyroid function, the TSH signal, which is predominantly conveyed inside the cell by cAMP and PKA, up-regulates the expression of transcription factor Pax 8, both in primary cells[206] and established cell lines.[207] However, mice genetically deprived of TSH or of functional TSH receptor do not show reduced amounts of Pax 8 in their thyroids as compared to wild-type animals,[8] suggesting that compensatory mechanisms may ensure an adequate production of this factor when thyroid development takes place in the absence of the normal physiologic stimulus. Besides this control on the amount of Pax 8 protein, there is no firm evidence that TSH or cAMP exert any other control at the level of the master thyroid transcription factors identified presently.[204,208,209] The expression of several other transcription factors was shown to be up-regulated, often at least transiently, in response to TSH/cAMP in the thyroid, namely c-myc,[210] c-fos,[210] fos B, jun B, jun D,[211] CREM,[212] NGFI-B,[213] and CHOP.[214] A hypothetical role in the control exerted by TSH/cAMP on the expression of the thyroid-specific genes has been proposed for some of these factors,[212,214] but no final link has yet been established.[215] A recent report indicates that the dopamine and cAMP-regulated neuronal phosphoprotein DARPP-32 could play an essential role in this control.[216]

It is noteworthy that in addition to its control on the transcription of the individual thyroid-specific genes, which is detailed in a following discussion, TSH also regulates gene expression by acting at some posttranscriptional steps, as shown in the case of thyroglobulin.[217] Finally, many effects of TSH and cAMP on gene expression (including on thyroid-specific genes such as thyroglobulin) might be rather indirect and depend in part on the profound modifications of cell morphology and cytoskeleton that result from PKA activation.[31,62]

TGF-β has been shown to down-regulate the expression of thyroid-specific genes.[218,219] It seems to involve a reduction in the level of Pax 8 activity that is mediated by Smad proteins.[219,220] In human thyroid primary cultures, TGF-β inhibits most effects of cAMP on gene expression.[38] As above, this might be related in part to an inhibition of morphologic effects of TSH/cAMP. In all the species tested so far, EGF strongly represses thyroglobulin

and thyroperoxidase gene expression as well as iodide transport.[31,123,221-223] FGF has a similar action in some species including bovine.[17] The mechanisms have not been explored. As recently quantified by SAGE analysis in the thyroid cell line PCCl3,[224] exposure to a high dose of iodide also decreases the expression of most of the thyroid-specific genes within the thyrocyte.

THYROGLOBULIN

The regulatory DNA elements of the thyroglobulin gene have been characterized in several species.[199,205,225] The proximal promoter, as defined in transfection experiments, extends over 200 base pairs and contains binding sites for transcription factors TTF-1, TTF-2, and Pax 8 (Fig. 3-7). An upstream enhancer element containing binding sites for TTF-1 has been identified in beef and man.[226] In the latter, the enhancer region is longer and harbors additional binding sites for TTF-1 and cAMP responsive element–binding (CREB) protein.[227] Both TTF-1 and Pax 8 proteins were individually shown to exert a major control on thyroglobulin gene transcription.[228,229] By contrast, TTF-2 activity appears to be dispensable, because the thyroglobulin gene is expressed in cells devoid of TTF-2 protein.[228] Synergism in the transcriptional activation of the gene by TTF-1 and Pax 8 appears to rely on a direct interaction between these two factors[230] and on their coordinated action involving both the enhancer and proximal promoter sequences.[231] It has also been proposed recently that the transcriptional coactivators p300[232] and (or ?) TAZ, the transcriptional coactivator with PDZ-binding motif,[233] are involved in this activation. The known thyroglobulin gene regulatory elements were shown to be sufficient to drive the thyroid-restricted expression of a linked gene in living mice.[234] This thyroid-restricted expression likely results from the requirement for the simultaneous presence of both TTF-1 and Pax 8,

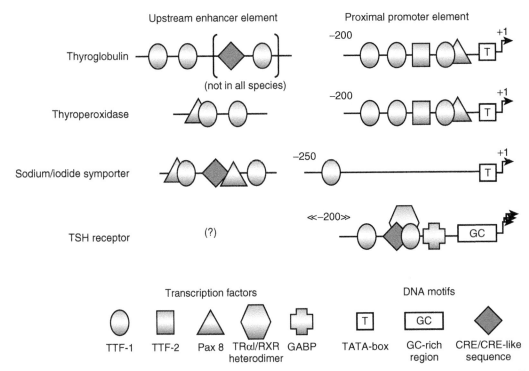

FIGURE 3-7. Schematic of the known regulatory elements of thyroglobulin, thyroperoxidase, sodium/iodide symporter, and TSH receptor genes. The organization of the proximal promoter and upstream enhancer elements of the different genes is depicted as determined in the species studied so far. Coordinates of the proximal promoters are in base pairs and refer to the transcription start site as +1. The positions of the upstream enhancer elements relative to the transcription start site are not indicated, since they vary extensively among the different species.

which occurs in thyroid only. It is associated with the tissue-specific demethylation of thyroglobulin gene sequences.[235] Demethylation of the DNA is supposed to relieve the constitutive silencing of the gene.[236]

Thyroglobulin gene transcription has been shown to require the presence of circulating TSH in the adult rat[237] and to be highly dependent on an elevated cAMP level in dog thyroid tissue slices,[238] in primary cultured cells,[222] and to a much lower extent in immortalized thyroid cell lines like FRTL-5.[239] Although they are devoid of classical cAMP-responsive element (CRE), the proximal promoter sequences are essentially involved in this control, as indicated by the observation of TSH/cAMP-induced changes in their chromatin structure[240] and their TSH/cAMP-dependent activity in transfection experiments.[241] It has, however, been demonstrated recently that the onset of thyroglobulin gene expression during thyroid development takes place normally in mouse strains deprived of either circulating TSH or functional TSH receptors.[7,8] This may be consistent with the observation that the thyroglobulin gene displays a low level of cAMP-independent transcription in primary cultured thyrocytes,[222] which might depend on insulin, as observed in different culture models.[242-244] In primary cultures of dog thyrocytes, the transcriptional activation of the thyroglobulin gene by cAMP after transient TSH withdrawal is also delayed as compared to that of the thyroperoxidase gene,[222] and unlike thyroperoxidase transcription, it requires an active protein synthesis for sustained transcription.[222] The increase in Pax 8 concentration consecutive to TSH/cAMP stimulation of the thyrocyte is not sufficient to account for the observed control on thyroglobulin gene transcription; TSH is still required for transcriptional activation even in cells expressing high levels of Pax 8 protein.[207] Thus, besides TTF-1 and Pax 8, at least one additional, still unidentified, factor is likely to play a key role in the control of thyroglobulin gene expression, as also suggested by the observation that in the course of thyroid development, both TTF-1 and Pax 8 are present well before a thyroglobulin gene is expressed.

In addition to the full-length thyroglobulin mRNA, a shorter transcript accumulates in the rat thyroid in response to TSH stimulation.[245] This transcript results from differential splicing and polyadenylation of the primary transcript and encodes a protein limited to the very N-terminal part of thyroglobulin. Because this truncated protein still contains a major hormonogenic site,[246] it could suggest that in conditions in which the balance of thyroid metabolism would favor hormone synthesis over iodine storage (e.g., shortage of iodine), the rat thyrocyte would manufacture a shorter thyroglobulin with a preserved hormonogenic ability but lacking many of the nonhormonogenic tyrosines.

THYROPEROXIDASE

In the species studied so far, the architecture of the proximal promoter region of the thyroperoxidase gene strikingly resembles that of the corresponding region of the thyroglobulin gene[247,248] (see Fig. 3-7). The upstream enhancer element also encompasses a pair of TTF-1 binding sites and contains an additional binding site for Pax 8, as compared to its counterpart in the thyroglobulin gene.[249,250] Here again, the combination of the upstream enhancer and proximal promoter supports the synergistic action of TTF-1 and Pax 8 on gene transcription.[231] The transcriptional coactivator p300 has also been reported to be involved in the activation of this promoter.[251]

Despite the existence of this high similarity, thyroperoxidase gene transcription is more tightly and more rapidly controlled

by TSH and cAMP than that of the thyroglobulin gene in primary cultured thyrocytes and does not require a concomitant protein synthesis.[222,252] Contrary to the thyroglobulin gene, the thyroperoxidase gene is not expressed in the absence of circulating TSH or functional TSH receptors in intact animals.[8] On the other hand, the constitutive hyperactivation of the cAMP cascade leads to an increased expression of the gene as compared to the normal situation.[253] In spite of their lack of a classical CRE, the proximal promoter sequences have been shown to mediate this TSH/cAMP control on transcription in transfection experiments.[247] Exposure to a high dose of iodide reduces thyroperoxidase gene expression, as well as that of thyroglobulin, sodium/iodide symporter, and thyrotropin receptor genes in PCCl3 thyroid cells.[224] Low doses of iodide also decrease thyroperoxidase gene expression in vivo, while the expression of thyroglobulin remains unaffected.[101] Thus, apart from their basic dependence on the presence of the transcription factors TTF-1 and Pax 8, which insures their shared thyroid-restricted expression, the thyroperoxidase and thyroglobulin genes distinguish themselves significantly regarding the control of their transcription. It is worth mentioning in this context that a synergistic action of Pax8 and pRb, the retinoblastoma protein, appears to be required for thyroperoxidase promoter activation, whereas this is not the case for thyroglobulin promoter activation.[254] It has also been postulated recently that the hormone-induced developmental activation of the thyroperoxidase gene involves the concerted action of TTF-2 and NF-1, both of which bind neighboring sequences in the gene promoter (see Fig. 3-7), resulting in the initial opening of the chromatin structure of the promoter.[255]

The existence of a major thyroperoxidase mRNA isoform has been detected in man.[256] It appears to encode a protein devoid of its normal enzymatic activity.

SODIUM/IODIDE SYMPORTER

Although the sodium/iodide symporter plays a key role in thyroid hormonogenesis, the expression of the corresponding gene is not restricted to the thyroid. Accordingly, the proximal promoter sequences identified so far do not exhibit a thyroid-specific activity in vitro,[257,258] even if this activity may be marginally increased in the presence of TTF-1.[259] The robust and appropriately controlled expression of this gene in the thyroid seems to be mediated essentially by the upstream enhancer element, which contains binding sites for both TTF-1 and Pax 8, and a cAMP-responsive element (CRE)-like DNA motif, which is involved in the control by TSH/cAMP[173,260] (see Fig. 3-7). The cAMP-response element modulator (CREM) has recently been proposed to be involved in this control.[261] As for the thyroperoxidase gene, TSH signaling is indispensable for sodium/iodide symporter gene transcriptional activation in vivo,[7,8] and iodide down-regulates the expression of the gene.[101,224] In addition, synergy between Pax8 and pRb appears to be required for the activation of both thyroperoxidase and sodium/iodide symporter promoters.[254] A very similar control is thus exerted on the expression of both of these genes in the thyroid, despite the fact that their known regulatory regions bear only limited resemblances.

THYROTROPIN RECEPTOR

The TSH receptor gene is also expressed in tissues other than the thyroid. Again, the promoter elements identified presently, which include binding sites for thyroid hormone receptor (TR)-α1/retinoid-X receptor (RXR) heterodimer,[262] GA-binding protein (GABP),[263] CREB protein,[264] and TTF-1[265] (see Fig. 3-7), do not display a clear thyroid-specific activity in transfection experiments, as could be expected. Contrary to the promoters described so far, the promoter of the TSH receptor gene does not contain a TATA-box motif but encompasses a GC-rich region preceding the multiple neighboring transcription start sites. Consistent with the presence of TTF-1 binding sites in the promoter region, the TSH receptor gene exhibits decreased activity in animals expressing reduced levels of TTF-1.[266] No other regulatory DNA element specifically involved in the thyroid-specific expression of this gene has been identified as yet. On the other hand, DNA demethylation events in the promoter region have been observed in thyroid cells expressing the TSH receptor gene, as compared to nonexpressing cells.[263]

Control of TSH receptor gene expression has been studied in the FRTL5 cell line,[267-269] the canine thyrocyte in primary culture,[123] cultured human thyrocytes,[270,271] and human thyroid cancer.[272,273] The general conclusion emerging from these studies is the extreme robustness of TSH receptor gene expression as compared with the other markers of thyroid cell differentiation (thyroglobulin and thyroperoxidase). In the dog, levels of TSH receptor mRNA remain virtually unchanged in animals subjected for 28 days to hyperstimulation by TSH secondary to treatment with methimazole or to TSH withdrawal achieved by administration of thyroxine.[123] In the same study, the effect of TSH or forskolin has been investigated in dog thyrocytes in primary culture. This experimental system has the advantage that the differentiation state of the cells can be manipulated at will: cAMP agonists maintain expression of the differentiated phenotype, whereas agents such as EGF, tetradecanoyl phorbol acetate (TPA), and serum lead to "dedifferentiation."[274] The results demonstrate that the dedifferentiating agents reduce accumulation of the receptor mRNA. However, contrary to what is observed with thyroglobulin and thyroperoxidase mRNA, the inhibition is never complete. TSH or forskolin are capable of promoting reaccumulation of the receptor mRNA, a maximum being reached after 20 hours. As with thyroglobulin but at variance with the thyroperoxidase gene, this stimulation requires ongoing protein synthesis.[123] Chronic stimulation of cultured dog thyrocytes by TSH for several days does not lead to any important down-regulation in mRNA. Similar data have been obtained with human thyrocytes in primary culture.[123,271] By contrast, negative regulation of receptor mRNA accumulation has been observed in immortal FRTL5 cells after treatment with TSH or TSAB.[267,269] This difference from human and canine cells must probably be interpreted in the general framework of the other known differences in phenotype and regulatory behavior of this cell line as compared with primary cultured thyrocytes (see later).[85] The presence in the promoter region of a CRE-like DNA motif which appears to be able to bind the CREB protein,[264] a transcriptional activator directly activated by cAMP, as well as the CREM isoform ICER,[212] a transcriptional repressor induced by cAMP, could explain both reported increase and decrease in gene expression following TSH stimulation, depending on the relative amounts of these factors (and likely of other CRE-binding proteins also) preexisting in the studied cells and the kinetics of the individual observations. Moreover, the binding site of the TRα1/RXR heterodimer identified in this promoter encompasses the CRE-like motif (see Fig. 3-7), which may add a further level of complexity depending on the availability of thyroid hormone in the experimental system. Recently, thyrotropin receptor mRNA was shown to be decreased in PCCl3 cells exposed to a high iodide concentration.[224]

The effect of malignant transformation on the amounts of TSH receptor mRNA has been studied in spontaneous tumors in humans,[272,273] in a murine transgenic model of thyroid tumor promoted by expression of the simian virus-40 large T oncogene,[275] and in FRTL5 cells transformed with v-ras.[268] In the last two models, expression of the TSH receptor gene was suppressed: the tumor or cell growth became TSH independent. In the transgenic animal model, loss of TSH receptor mRNA seemed to take place gradually, with early tumors still displaying some TSH dependence for growth. In the human tumors, a spectrum of phenotypes was observed. As expected, anaplastic tumors had completely lost the receptor mRNA, as well as other markers of thyrocyte differentiation (thyroglobulin and thyroperoxidase). In papillary carcinoma, variable amounts of TSH receptor mRNA were invariably found,[272] even in the tumors that had lost the capacity to express the thyroglobulin or thyroperoxidase genes.[272] These data agree well with the observations of thyrocytes in primary culture: expression of the TSH receptor gene is robust, and it persists in the presence of agents (or after several steps in tumor progression) that promote extinction of the other markers of thyroid cell differentiation. This evidence leads to the conclusion that the basic marker of the thyroid phenotype is probably the TSH receptor itself, which makes sense: the gene encoding the sensor of TSH—the major regulator of thyroid function, growth, and differentiated phenotype—is virtually constitutive in thyrocytes. From a pragmatic viewpoint, these data provide a rationale for the common therapeutic practice of suppressing TSH secretion in patients with a differentiated thyroid tumor.[276]

THYROID OXIDASES

Two distinct genes, *ThOX1* and *ThOX2* (also known as *DUOX-1* and *DUOX-2*), both significantly related to the gene encoding the phagocyte NADPH oxidase gp91[Phox], are expressed essentially in the thyroid, but not exclusively, at least for *ThOX2*.[179,277] In the dog, *ThOX* mRNAs accumulate in response to TSH/cAMP stimulation.[179] This effect is much less apparent in man,[179] and in the rat, conflicting results were obtained in vivo and in the established FRTL-5 cell line, respectively.[277] The proximal promoter sequences of both human *THOX1* and *THOX2* genes have been delineated using a functional assay.[278] These promoters do not exhibit a thyroid cell-restricted activity in vitro and are not controlled positively by TSH/cAMP, as could be expected. No known regulatory DNA motif could be identified within these promoter sequences. Notably, like the promoter of the TSH receptor gene, both of these promoters are devoid of a TATA-box motif. A recent report identified the ThOX-2 promoter as a target for either Pax8 or TTF-1,[279] but another study indicated that this control is likely to involve regulatory sequences other than the ones identified and cloned so far.[280]

Recently, genes encoding proteins required for the functional maturation of the thyroid oxidases were identified in the close vicinity of both *ThOX* genes, and named *DUOXA1* and *DUOXA2*, respectively.[281] Within each *ThOX-DUOXA* pair, the two genes are arranged in a head-to-head configuration, the distance separating the putative transcription starts being in the range of only 100 bp. This raises the question as to whether the ThOX promoter sequences identified previously[278] may also control transcription in the other direction.

Control of Growth and Differentiation

THYROID CELL TURNOVER

The thyroid is composed of thyrocytes (70%), endothelial cells (20%), and fibroblasts (10%) (proportions measured in dog thyroid). In a normal adult, the weight and composition of the tissue remain relatively constant. Because a low but significant proliferation is demonstrated in all types of cells, it must be assumed that the generation of new cells is balanced by a corresponding rate of cell death.[3,282,283] The resulting turnover is on the order of 1 per 5 to 10 years for human thyrocytes (i.e., 6 to 8 renewals in adult life, as in other species).[283] Normal cell population can therefore be modulated mainly at the level of proliferation and only secondarily by cell death. In growth situations—that is, either in normal development or after stimulation—the different cell types grow more or less in parallel, which implies a coordination between them.[16,34,284,285] Because TSH receptors and iodine metabolism and signaling coexist only in the thyrocyte in thyroid, this cell, sole receiver of the physiologic information, must presumably control the other types of cells by paracrine factors such as VEGF, FGF, IGF-1, NO, and the like.[16] The successful isolation of human thyroid endothelial cells will allow a more detailed study of these interactions.[286] TSH has been demonstrated to up-regulate the production of vascular endothelial cell growth factor (VEGF) by human thyrocytes.[287] It is interesting in this regard that the vascular support of the follicles reflects their activity, suggesting the concept of angiofollicular units.[288,289]

THE MITOGENIC CASCADES

In the thyroid, at least three families of distinct mitogenic pathways have been well defined (Fig. 3-8): (1) the hormone receptor–adenylyl cyclase–cAMP-dependent protein kinase system, (2) the hormone receptor–tyrosine protein kinase pathways, and (3) the hormone receptor–phospholipase C cascade.[3,290] The receptor–tyrosine kinase pathway may be subdivided into two branches; some growth factors, such as EGF, induce proliferation and repress differentiation expression, whereas others, such as FGF in dog cells or IGF-1 and insulin, are either mitogenic or are necessary for the proliferation effect of other factors without being mitogenic by themselves, but they do not inhibit differentiation expression.[28,242] In human thyroid cells, IGF-1 is required for the mitogenic action of TSH or EGF, but by itself it only weakly stimulates proliferation.[78] In dog and human thyrocytes in primary cultures, after induction of insulin receptors by TSH, physiologic concentrations of insulin permit the proliferative action of TSH.[20,21] In FRTL5 and rat cells, and in mouse thyroid in vivo,[291] IGF-1 is weakly mitogenic per se,[292] whereas in pig thyroid cells, it produces a strong effect.[293] Expression of both human IGF-1 and IGF-1R in mouse thyroid induces a mild goiter and a decrease in serum TSH level—that is, an increase in non-TSH-activated thyroid function.[291] Similarly, relatively high serum IGF-1 levels in a human population are associated with higher goiter frequency.[294]

It should be noted that TSH directly stimulates proliferation while maintaining the expression of differentiation. Differentiation expression, as evaluated by NIS or by thyroperoxidase and thyroglobulin mRNA content or nuclear transcription, is induced by TSH, forskolin, cholera toxin, and cAMP analogs.[3] These effects are obtained in all the cells of a culture, as shown by in situ hybridization experiments.[242] They are reversible; they can be obtained either after the arrest of proliferation or during the cell-division cycle.[223,242] Moreover, the expression of differentiation, as measured by iodide transport, is stimulated by concentrations of TSH lower than those required for proliferation.[78]

All the proliferation effects of TSH are mimicked by nonspecific modulators of the cAMP cascade (e.g., cholera toxin and forskolin, which stimulate adenylate cyclase), cAMP analogs (which activate the cAMP-dependent protein kinases), and even

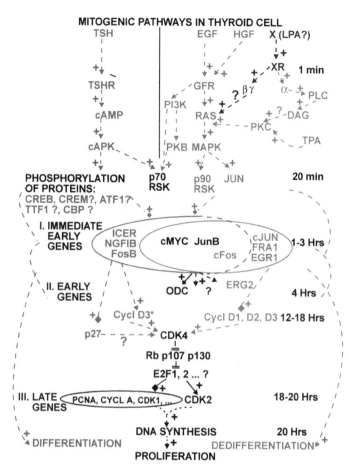

FIGURE 3-8. Mitogenic pathways in the thyroid. Data from the thyroid cell systems are integrated into the present general scheme of cell proliferation cascades. In the first line, known activators of various cascades in dog and human thyroid cells are shown. Various levels indicate a time sequence and postulated causal relationships from initial interaction of extracellular signal with its receptor to endpoints: proliferation and differentiation expression. In dog but not in human thyroid cells, acetylcholine through muscarinic receptors activates the phospholipase C cascade. *cAPK,* Cyclic adenosine monophosphate-dependent kinase; *CDK,* cyclin-dependent kinase; *DAG,* diacylglycerol; $------\rightarrow+$, stimulation; $------|+$, inhibition; $------ \blacklozenge +$, induction; *GFR,* growth factor receptor; *ODC,* ornithine decarboxylase; *PI3K,* phosphatidylinositol 3-kinase; *PKB,* protein kinase B; *PLC,* phospholipase C; *RSK,* ribosomal S6 kinase.

synergistic pairs of cAMP analogs acting on the different sites of these two kinases.[78,295,296] They are reproduced in vitro and in vivo by expression of the adenosine A$_2$ receptor, which is constitutively activated by endogenous adenosine,[253] and by constitutively active G$_{s\alpha}$[297] and cholera toxin.[298] They are inhibited by antibodies blocking G$_s$.[299] Inhibition of cAMP-dependent protein kinases (PKA) inhibits the proliferation and differentiation effects of cAMP.[300,301] Stimulation of PKA by selective cAMP analogs that do not activate EPAC proteins is sufficient to fully mimic mitogenic effects of TSH and forskolin in dog thyrocytes.[61] There is, therefore, no doubt that the mitogenic and differentiating effects of TSH are mainly and probably entirely mediated by cAMP-dependent protein kinases. A complementary role of the Rap guanyl nucleotide exchange factor EPAC and of Rap1 has been proposed in cell lines and in mice,[302-304] but it is not observed in canine thyroid primary cultures.[61] Permanent abolition of G$_q$ expression in mouse thyroid leads as expected to an inhibition of iodide oxidation and thyroid hormone synthesis but also to hypotrophy of the gland.[305] This suggests at least a necessary chronic permissive role of the G$_q$ phospholipase C cascade. In dog thyroid cells, carbamylcholine acting through the G$_q$ cascade has the same permissive effects on TSH mitogenic action as IGF-1, perhaps through activation of PKB.[88,306]

EGF also induces proliferation of thyroid cells from various species.[3,16,78] However, the action of EGF is accompanied by a general and reversible loss of differentiation expression, assessed as described earlier.[274] The effects of EGF on differentiation can be dissociated from its proliferative action. Indeed, they are obtained in cells that do not proliferate in the absence of insulin and in human cells, in which the proliferative effects are weaker, or in pig cells at concentrations lower than the mitogenic concentrations.[3]

Finally, the tumor-promoting phorbol esters, the pharmacologic probes of the protein kinase C system, and analogs of diacylglycerol also enhance the proliferation and inhibit the differentiation of thyroid cells. These effects are transient because of desensitization of the system by protein kinase C inactivation.[3,78,307,308] Activation of the G_q/phospholipase C (PLC)/PKC cascade by a more physiologic agent, such as carbamylcholine, in dog thyroid cells does not reproduce all the effects of phorbol esters. In particular, prolonged stimulation of this cascade by carbamyl choline permits the cAMP-dependent mitogenesis of dog thyrocytes,[306] but unlike phorbol esters, it does not induce proliferation in the presence of insulin.[309] The *Ras* protooncogene is strongly activated by phorbol esters but very weakly by carbachol.[88] Thus we cannot necessarily equate the effects of phorbol esters and prolonged stimulation of the PLC cascade. The dedifferentiating effects of phorbol esters do not require their mitogenic action either. Thus the effects of TSH, EGF, and phorbol esters on differentiation expression are largely independent of their mitogenic action.[3]

In several thyroid cell models, very high insulin concentrations are necessary for growth even in the presence of EGF. We now know that this prerequisite mainly reflects a requirement for IGF-1 receptor.[3,76,292,310] It is interesting that in FRTL5 cells, as in cells from thyroid nodules, this requirement may disappear, perhaps because the cells secrete their own somatomedins and thus become autonomous with regard to these growth factors.[76,311] By contrast, in primary cultures of normal dog and human thyrocytes, very low concentrations of insulin, acting on insulin receptors, are sufficient to support the mitogenic effects of TSH and cAMP when insulin receptors have been induced to high levels by TSH.[20,21] This puzzling regulation, which is reminiscent of the induction of insulin receptors during the differentiation of adipocytes, suggests that thyroid might well be revealed as a more specific target of circulating insulin than hitherto recognized.

In the action of growth factors on receptor protein tyrosine kinase pathways, the effects on differentiation expression vary with the species and the factor involved: from stimulation (e.g., insulin, as well as IGF-2 in dog and FRTL5 cells),[243] to an absence of effect,[312] to transitory inhibition of differentiation during growth (FGF and HGF in dog cells),[28,313] to full but reversible dedifferentiation effects (EGF in dog and human cells).[77,274] *Ret/PTC* rearrangements, activating mutations of *Ras*, as well as oncogenic mutation of *B-Raf*, which are responsible for most differentiated carcinoma, constitutively activate the signaling cascades of growth factors.[314-316]

The kinetics of the induction of thymidine incorporation into nuclear DNA of dog thyroid cells is similar for TSH, forskolin, EGF, and TPA. Whatever the stimulant, a minimal delay of about 16 to 20 hours takes place before the beginning of labeling—that is, the beginning of DNA synthesis.[317] This is the minimal amount of time required to prepare the necessary machinery. For the cAMP and EGF pathways, the stimulatory agent has to be present during this whole prereplicative period; any interruption in activation (e.g., by washing out the stimulatory forskolin) greatly delays the start of DNA synthesis.[318] This limitation explains why norepinephrine and prostaglandin E, which also activate the cAMP cascade, do not induce growth and differentiation: the rapid desensitization of their receptors does not allow a sustained rise in cAMP levels.

The three main types of mitogenic cascade, specifically the growth factor–protein tyrosine kinase, phorbol ester–protein kinase C, and TSH-cAMP cascades, are fully distinct at the level of their primary intracellular signal and/or the first signal-activated protein kinase.[3]

Iodide actually inhibits the cAMP and the Ca^{2+}-phosphatidylinositol cascades and in a more delayed and chronic effect decreases the sensitivity of the thyroid to the TSH growth response. These effects are relieved, according to the general paradigm of Van Sande, by perchlorate and methimazole[95,319] in that they are mediated by a postulated organified derivative of iodide, iodohexadecanal.[97]

Steps in the Mitogenic Cascades

The phenomenology of EGF, TPA, and TSH proliferative action cells has been partially elucidated using dog thyroid primary cultures.[3,85] The mechanisms of TSH/cAMP mitogenic effects have also been investigated using immortal rat thyroid cell lines (FRTL-5, WRT, and PC Cl3 cells).[86] Whereas the signaling cascades involved in the action of growth factors and IGF-1 are likely to be well conserved in the different thyroid systems, as generally observed in the other cell types, the mechanistic logistics of cell-cycle regulation by cAMP has disappointingly turned out to strongly diverge in the various thyroid in vitro models.[85] These divergences do not only reflect species differences.[3] Among the apparently similar rat thyroid cell lines, or even among different subclones of FRTL-5 cells, major differences have been observed.[85] For instance, the PI3 kinase/PKB cascade is activated by cAMP in WRT cells[320] but inhibited by cAMP in PC Cl3 cells.[321] The induction of c-Jun by TSH/cAMP in FRTL-5 cells and its repression by cAMP in WRT cells,[322] as in dog[323] and human thyrocytes, likely reflect major differences in upstream signaling cascades and should result in divergent expression of downstream target genes, such as cyclin D1. Cyclin D1 synthesis, an accepted endpoint of mitogenic cascades, is indeed induced by cAMP in FRTL-5 and PC Cl3 cells, but repressed by cAMP in dog and human thyroid primary cultures.[85,324] The reasons for such discrepancies are unclear. Some signaling features, when they lead to selective proliferative advantages, might have been acquired during the establishment and continuous cultures of the cell lines and stabilized by subcloning. Many mechanisms demonstrated in the dog thyroid primary culture system so far apply to normal human thyrocytes, but much remains to be defined.[85] In the following lines, we thus rely mostly on these systems.

Three biochemical aspects of the proliferative response occurring at different times of the prereplicative phase have been considered. The pattern of protein phosphorylation induced within minutes by TSH is reproduced by forskolin and cAMP analogs. It totally diverges from the phosphorylations induced by EGF and phorbol esters.[325] EGF, HGF, and phorbol ester actions rapidly converge on the activation of Ras[88] and the resulting activation of p42/p44 MAP kinases and p90[RSK].[74,75,87] PI-3-kinase and its effector enzyme PKB are activated for several hours only by insulin and IGF-1, the effect of EGF being short lived.[74]

This activity is therefore the one specific feature of insulin action and presumably the mechanism of the facilitating effect on mitogenesis. In dog thyrocytes, only HGF can trigger cell proliferation in the absence of insulin/IGF-1; this is explained by the fact that only this factor strongly activates both PI3 kinase and MAP kinase cascades.[74] Only insulin, IGF-1 and HGF also markedly enhance general protein synthesis and induce cell hypertrophy.[211] By contrast, TSH and cAMP are very unique as mitogens, since they do not activate Ras, the PI3kinase/PKB pathway, or any of different classes of MAP kinases in dog thyrocytes.[74,75,87,88] TSH and cAMP also do not activate MAP kinases in human thyrocytes.[75] The phosphorylation and activation of p70[S6K] and thus likely the mTOR cascade constitutes the only early convergence point of growth factor and cAMP-dependent mitogenic cascades.[74,326] A recent study has demonstrated the crucial role of this cascade for TSH-elicited thyroid follicular hyperplasia in vivo in mice.[327] Indeed, as found in dog thyroid primary cultures[74] and PCCl3 cells (Blancquaert and Roger, unpublished), TSH stimulates in mice the mTOR/p70[S6K] axis without activating PKB, and a rapamycin derivative abrogates the hyperplastic (but interestingly, not the hypertrophic) responses to TSH.[327] The cAMP-dependent mitogenesis and gene expression appears to require the phosphorylation by PKA and activity of CREB/CREM transcription factors.[328,329]

As in other types of cells, EGF and TPA first enhance c-fos and c-myc mRNA and protein concentrations in dog thyrocytes. On the other hand, TSH and forskolin strongly, but for a short period, enhance the c-myc mRNA concentration and with the same kinetics as the enhancement of the c-fos mRNA concentration by EGF/TPA. In fact, cAMP first enhances and then decreases c-myc expression. This second phenomenon is akin to what has been observed in the fibroblast, in which cAMP negatively regulates growth. As in fibroblasts, EGF and TPA enhance c-Jun, junB, junD, and egr1 expression. However, as in fibroblasts, activators of the cAMP cascade decrease c-Jun and egr1 expression. Therefore, c-Jun is not, as has been claimed, a gene whose expression is universally necessary for growth.[211,323]

The investigation of the pattern of proteins synthesized in response to the various proliferation stimuli has suggested very early that the proliferation of dog thyroid cells is controlled during G1 phase by at least two largely distinct cAMP-dependent or cAMP-independent pathways.[330] Recent microarray analyses have confirmed and extended this concept in human thyrocytes.[63,331] Nevertheless, the different mitogenic cascades are expected to finally modulate the level and activity of proteins that are the primary regulators of the cell-cycle machinery. As generally considered, mitogenic signals regulate the mammalian cell cycle by stimulating the accumulation of D-type cyclins and their assembly through an ill-defined mechanism, with their partners the cyclin-dependent kinases (CDKs) 4 and 6. These complexes operate in mid- to late G1 phase to promote progression through the restriction point and thus commit cells to replicate their genome.[332] In the current model, this key decision depends on the initiation by cyclin D-CDK complexes of the phosphorylation of the growth/tumor suppressor protein pRb, which triggers the activation of transcription factors, including those of the E2F family, the synthesis of cyclin E and then cyclin A, and CDK2 activation by these cyclins. Activated CDK2 in turn further phosphorylates pRb and other substrates and initiates and organizes the progression through the DNA synthesis phase.[332] The down-regulation of CDK inhibitors of the CIP/KIP family, including p27[kip1], by mitogenic factors and/or their sequestration by cyclin D-CDK complexes participate to CDK2

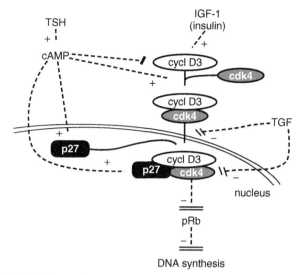

FIGURE 3-9. Targets of cell-cycle regulatory effects of TSH, insulin/IGF-1 and TGF-β, as demonstrated in the dog thyroid primary culture system. *Diamond/rectangle arrowheads* represent inductions/repressions; the other *dashed arrows* are activations (+) and inhibitions (−). TSH (cAMP) does not induce D cyclins, but it assembles and then activates the cyclin D3-CDK4-p27 holoenzyme by inducing the activating Thr172-phosphorylation of CDK4. IGF-1 and insulin allow the accumulation of the required cyclin D3. TGF-β inhibits the nuclear translocation of the cyclin D3-CDK4 complex, its association to p27, and its activation by TSH(cAMP). See text for full explanation.

activation, but their proposed role of adaptor and/or nuclear anchor for cyclin D-CDK complexes suggests positive influences on cell-cycle progression as well.[333] These mechanisms have been well studied in dog thyroid cells[324] (Fig. 3-9). As expected, the different mitogenic stimulations (TSH, cAMP, growth factors) require the activity of CDK4[334] and converge on the inactivating phosphorylation of pRb and related proteins p107 and p130[335] on the phosphorylation and nuclear translocation of CDK2, and on the induction of cyclin A and cdc2.[336] These effects are dependent on insulin.[335,337] What is strikingly different between the cascades is the mechanism of D-type cyclin-CDK4 activation. TSH, unlike all the other known mitogenic factors, does not induce the accumulation of D cyclins,[338] but it paradoxically stimulates the expression of the CDK "inhibitor" p27[kip1].[339] However, the predominant cyclin, D3, is required for the proliferation stimulated by TSH but not in the proliferation of dog thyrocytes stimulated by EGF or HGF that induce cyclins D1 and D2, in addition to increasing cyclin D3 levels.[338] The formation and the nuclear translocation of essential cyclin D3-CDK4 complexes depend on the synergistic interaction of TSH and insulin.[337,338] These complexes are absent from cells stimulated by TSH or insulin alone. Paradoxically, in the absence of insulin, TSH inhibits the basal accumulation of cyclin D3.[337] Conversely, insulin alone stimulates the required cyclin D3 accumulation, and it overcomes in large part the inhibition by TSH,[337] but it is unable to assemble cyclin D3-CDK4 complexes in the absence of TSH. In the presence of insulin, TSH (cAMP) unmasks some epitopes of cyclin D3 and induces the assembly of cyclin D3-CDK4 complexes and their import into nuclei,[337,338] where these complexes are anchored by their association with p27[kip1].[340,341] This also sequesters p27 away from CDK2 complexes,[340] thus contributing to CDK2 activation. Moreover, cAMP exerts an additional crucial function in very late G1 phase to stimulate the enzymatic activity of cyclin D3-cdk4-p27 complexes, which involves the stimulation of the activating Thr172-

phosphorylation of CDK4.[324,342] TGF-β selectively inhibits the cAMP-dependent proliferation of dog thyrocytes by preventing the association of the cyclin D3-CDK4 complex with nuclear p27[kip1] and the activating phosphorylation of CDK4.[340,341]

The investigation of cell-cycle regulatory proteins has thus clearly established that both CDK4 activation and pRb phosphorylation result from distinct but complementary actions of TSH and insulin, rather than from their interaction at an earlier step of the signaling cascades[306,337] (see Fig. 3-9). Together with the fact that the necessary increase of cell mass before division depends on insulin/IGF-1 but not TSH,[211] these observations provide a molecular basis for the well-established physiologic concept that in the regulation of normal thyroid cell proliferation, TSH is the "decisional" mitotic trigger, while locally produced IGF-1 and/or circulating insulin are supporting "permissive" factors.[3] Of note, in all these experiments, the facilitative action of insulin can be replaced by activation of the G_q/PLC cascade by carbamylcholine.[306]

Studies of protein phosphorylation, proto-oncogene expression, and cell-cycle regulatory proteins in dog thyrocytes allow discrimination between two models of cAMP action on proliferation in this system: a direct effect on the thyrocyte or an indirect effect through the secretion and autocrine action of another growth factor. If the effect of TSH through cAMP involved such an autocrine loop, one would expect to find faster kinetics of action of the growth factor and at least some common parts in the patterns of protein phosphorylation and protein synthesis induced by cAMP and the growth factor. The results do not support such a hypothesis, at least for the growth factors tested[3] (see Fig. 3-8). Nor do the data on cAMP action in the dog and human thyrocyte systems support a major role for various mechanisms involving cross-signaling of cAMP with growth factor pathways, as claimed in rat thyroid cell line studies (reviewed and discussed in[85]). Indeed, in primary cultures of normal human thyrocytes, EGF+serum increases cyclin D1 and p21 accumulation, and it stimulates the assembly and activity of cyclin D1-CDK4-p21. By contrast, TSH (cAMP) represses cyclin D1 and p21, but it stimulates the activating phosphorylation of CDK4 and the pRb-kinase activity of preexisting cyclin D3-CDK4 complexes.[343] Cyclin D1 and cyclin D3 are thus differentially used in the distinct mitogenic stimulations by growth factors and TSH and potentially in hyperproliferative diseases generated by the overactivation of their respective signaling pathways.

The validity of these concepts in vivo has been established by using transgenic mice models. The expression in thyroid of oncogene E7 of HPV16, which sequestrates pRb protein, leads to thyroid growth and euthyroid goiter. Expression in the thyroid of the adenosine A_2 receptor, which behaves as a constitutive activator of adenylyl cyclase, induces thyroid growth, goitrogenesis, and hyperthyroidism.[253] Similar, albeit weaker, phenotypes are obtained in mice expressing constitutive G_s (the G protein activating adenylyl cyclase)[297] or cholera toxin.[298] On the contrary, the expression in thyroid of a dominant negative CREB provokes a marked thyroid hypotrophy, suggesting the crucial role of CREB and its activating phosphorylation by PKA.[329] By contrast, transgenic mice overexpressing both human IGF-1 and IGF-1 receptor in their thyroid (TgIGF-1–TgIGF-IR) develop only a mild thyroid hyperplasia and respond to a goitrogenic effect of antithyroid drugs while maintaining a comparatively low serum TSH level. This indicates some autonomy of these thyroids, as in acromegalic patients, and a much greater sensitivity to endogenous TSH.[291] Recently, thyrocyte-specific deficiency of G_q/G_{11} (the G proteins activating PLCb) in mice was shown to

impair not only the TSH-stimulated iodine-organification and thyroid hormone synthesis, but also TSH-dependent development of goiter.[305] It remains to be defined whether this impaired follicular cell hyperplasia could result in part from the lack of induction of VEGF and angiogenesis[305] which normally accompany goitrogenesis. Nevertheless, the phenotype of these mice underscores the role in TSH-dependent goitrogenesis of PLC, which is activated by TSH but even more strongly by neurotransmitters. Noteworthy, section of inferior laryngeal nerve in rats was similarly found to impair both thyroid function and growth stimulated by TSH.[344] Moreover, activation of G_q/PLC by carbamylcholine can facilitate cAMP-dependent mitogenesis in dog thyrocytes cultured without insulin or IGF-1.[306] On the other hand, expression of Ret (which is a constitutive growth factor receptor) in papillary thyroid carcinoma (PTC) leads to growth, cancer, and hypothyroidism.[345,346]

PROLIFERATION AN DIFFERENTIATION
(Fig. 3-10)

The incompatibility at the cell level of a proliferation and differentiation program is commonly accepted in biology. In general, cells with a high proliferative capacity are poorly differentiated, and during development, such cells lose this capacity as they progressively differentiate. Some cells even lose all potential to divide when reaching their full differentiation, a phenomenon called *terminal differentiation*. Conversely, in tumor cells, proliferation and differentiation expression are inversely related. Activation of Ras and p42/p44 MAP kinases, induction of c-Jun, sustained expression of c-myc, induction of cyclin D1 and downregulation of p27[kip1] all have been shown to be causatively associated not only with proliferation but also with loss of differentiation in a large variety of systems, sometimes independently of proliferation effects. It is therefore not surprising that in thyroid cells, the general mitogenic agents and pathways, phorbol esters and the protein kinase C pathway, EGF, and in calf and porcine cells, FGF and the protein tyrosine kinase pathway, induce both proliferation and the loss of differentiation expression. The effects of the cAMP cascade are in striking contrast with this general concept. Indeed, TSH and cAMP induce proliferation of dog thyrocytes while maintaining differentiation expression; both

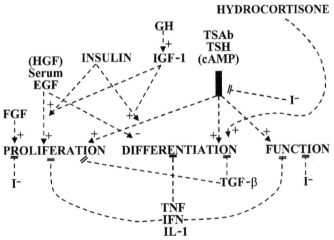

FIGURE 3-10. Main controls of the principal biological variables of the human thyrocyte. *EGF*, Epidermal growth factor; *FGF*, fibroblast growth factor; *GH*, growth hormone; *HGF*, hepatocyte growth factor; *I⁻*, iodide; *IGF-1*, insulin-like growth factor; *IFN*, interferon; *IL-1*, interleukin-1; *TGF-β*, transforming growth factor β; *TNF*, tumor necrosis factor; *TSAb*, thyroid-stimulating immunoglobulins; +, positive control (stimulation); −, negative control (inhibition).

proliferation and differentiation programs can be triggered by TSH in the same cells at the same time.[242] This situation is by no means unique, because neuroblasts in the cell cycle may simultaneously differentiate. It is tempting to relate this apparent paradox to the unique characteristics of the cAMP-dependent mitogenic pathway, such as the lack of activation (or even the inhibition) of the Ras/MAP kinase/c-Jun/cyclin D1 cascade, as demonstrated in dog and human thyrocytes. For instance, if one generalization could be made about proto-oncogenes, it is the dedifferentiating role of *c-myc*. A rapid and dramatic decrease in c-myc mRNA by antisense myc sequences induces differentiation of a variety of cell types. It is therefore striking that in the case of the thyrocyte, in which activation of the cAMP cascade leads to both proliferation and differentiation, the kinetics of the *c-myc* gene appears to be tightly controlled. After a first phase of 1 hour of higher levels of *c-myc* mRNA, *c-myc* expression is decreased below control levels. In this second phase, cAMP decreases *c-myc* mRNA levels, as it does in proliferation-inhibited fibroblasts. It even depresses EGF-induced expression. The first phase could be necessary for proliferation, whereas the second phase could reflect stimulation of differentiation by TSH.[210,347] The specific involvement of cyclin D3 in the cAMP-dependent mitogenic stimulation of dog and human thyrocytes is also interesting in this context.[343] We have recently shown that the differential utilization of cyclin D1 or cyclin D3 affects the site specificity of the pRb-kinase of CDK4, including in dog and human thyrocytes.[343,348] In addition to inhibiting E2F-dependent gene transcription related to cell-cycle progression, pRb plays positive roles in the induction of tissue-specific gene expression by directly interacting with a variety of transcription factors, including Pax8 in thyroid cells.[254] Whether the selective utilization of cyclin D3 in the TSH cascade, associated with a more restricted pRb-kinase activity, could allow the preservation of some differentiation-related functions of pRb thus remains to be examined. Indeed, unlike cyclins D1 and D2, cyclin D3 is highly expressed in several quiescent tissues in vivo, and its expression is not only stimulated by mitogenic factors but also induced during several differentiation processes associated with a repression of cyclin D1.[349]

We now consider the distinct cAMP-dependent mitogenic pathway, which appears to be adjuncted to the more general mechanisms used by growth factors, as pertaining to the specialized differentiation program of thyroid cells.[82] In dog thyrocytes, the proliferation in response to serum or growth factors specifically extinguishes their capacity to respond to TSH/cAMP as a mitogenic stimulus.[350] Similarly, in less differentiated thyroid cancers generated by the subversion of growth factor mechanisms, the TSH dependence of growth is generally found to be lost, and in various cell lines derived from thyroid carcinomas, cAMP and PKA activation even inhibit CDK4 activity and cell-cycle progression.[351]

Because the cell renewal rate is very low in the thyroid (once every 8 years in adults), the role of apoptosis is also very low. However, under different circumstances, the apoptotic role can greatly increase, such as after the arrest of an important stimulation in vitro[352] and in vivo.[353-355]

REFERENCES

1. Moeller LC, Alonso M, Liao X, et al: Pituitary-thyroid setpoint and thyrotropin receptor expression in consomic rats, Endocrinology 148:4727–4733, 2007.
2. Nakabayashi K, Matsumi H, Bhalla A, et al: Thyrostimulin, a heterodimer of two new human glycoprotein hormone subunits, activates the thyroid-stimulating hormone receptor, J Clin Invest 109:1445–1452, 2002.
3. Dumont JE, Lamy F, Roger PP, et al: Physiological and pathological regulation of thyroid cell proliferation and differentiation by thyrotropin and other factors, Physiol Rev 72:667–697, 1992.
4. Vassart G, Dumont JE: The thyrotropin receptor and the regulation of thyrocyte function and growth, Endocr Rev 13:596–611, 1992.
5. Brabant G, Bergmann P, Kirsch CM, et al: Early adaptation of thyrotropin and thyroglobulin secretion to experimentally decreased iodine supply in man, Metabolism 41:1093–1096, 1992.
6. Dumont JE: The action of thyrotropin on thyroid metabolism, Vitam Horm 29:287–412, 1971.
7. Marians RC, Ng L, Blair HC, et al: Defining thyrotropin-dependent and -independent steps of thyroid hormone synthesis by using thyrotropin receptor-null mice, Proc Natl Acad Sci U S A 99:15776–15781, 2002.
8. Postiglione MP, Parlato R, Rodriguez-Mallon A, et al: Role of the thyroid-stimulating hormone receptor signaling in development and differentiation of the thyroid gland, Proc Natl Acad Sci U S A 99:15462–15467, 2002.
9. Abramowicz MJ, Duprez L, Parma J, et al: Familial congenital hypothyroidism due to inactivating mutation of the thyrotropin receptor causing profound hypoplasia of the thyroid gland, J Clin Invest 99:3018–3024, 1997.
10. Toyoda N, Nishikawa M, Horimoto M: Synergistic effect of thyroid hormone and thyrotropin on iodothyronine 5'-adenosinase in FRTL-5 rat thyroid cells, Endocrinology 127:1199–1205, 1990.
11. Paire A, Bernier-Valentin F, Rabilloud R, et al: Expression of alpha- and beta-subunits and activity of Na+ K+ ATPase in pig thyroid cells in primary culture: modula-

tion by thyrotropin and thyroid hormones, Mol Cell Endocrinol 146:93–101, 1998.
12. Ying H, Suzuki H, Zhao L, et al: Mutant thyroid hormone receptor beta represses the expression and transcriptional activity of peroxisome proliferator-activated receptor gamma during thyroid carcinogenesis, Cancer Res 63:5274–5280, 2003.
13. Glinoer D, de Nayer P, Bourdoux P, et al: Regulation of maternal thyroid during pregnancy, J Clin Endocrinol Metab 71:276–287, 1990.
14. Hershman JM, Lee HY, Sugawara M, et al: Human chorionic gonadotropin stimulates iodide uptake, adenylate cyclase, and deoxyribonucleic acid synthesis in cultured rat thyroid cells, J Clin Endocrinol Metab 67:74–79, 1988.
15. Glinoer D: The regulation of thyroid function in pregnancy: pathways of endocrine adaptation from physiology to pathology, Endocr Rev 18:404–433, 1997.
16. Dumont JE, Maenhaut C, Pirson I, et al: Growth factors controlling the thyroid gland, Baillieres Clin Endocrinol Metab 5:727–754, 1991.
17. Gerard CM, Roger PP, Dumont JE: Thyroglobulin gene expression as a differentiation marker in primary cultures of calf thyroid cells, Mol Cell Endocrinol 61:23–35, 1989.
18. Cheung NW, Lou JC, Boyages SC: Growth hormone does not increase thyroid size in the absence of thyrotropin: a study in adults with hypopituitarism, J Clin Endocrinol Metab 81:1179–1183, 1996.
19. Dormitzer PR, Ellison PT, Bode HH: Anomalously low endemic goiter prevalence among Efe pygmies, Am J Phys Anthropol 78:527–531, 1989.
20. Burikhanov R, Coulonval K, Pirson I, et al: Thyrotropin via cyclic AMP induces insulin receptor expression and insulin co-stimulation of growth and amplifies insulin and insulin-like growth factor signaling pathways in dog thyroid epithelial cells, J Biol Chem 271:29400–29406, 1996.
21. Van Keymeulen A, Dumont JE, Roger PP: TSH induces insulin receptors that mediate insulin costimulation of growth in normal human thyroid cells, Biochem Biophys Res Commun 279:202–207, 2000.

22. Ahrén B: Regulatory peptides in the thyroid gland—a review on their localization and function, Acta Endocrinol (Copenh) 124:225–232, 1991.
23. Raspé E, Laurent E, Andry G, et al: ATP, bradykinine, TRH and TSH activate the Ca2+ inositol cascade of human thyrocytes in primary culture, Mol Cell Endocrinol 81:175–183, 1991.
24. Raspé E, Andry G, Dumont JE: Adenosine triphosphate, bradykinin, and thyrotropin-releasing hormone regulate the intracellular Ca2+ concentration and the 45Ca2+ efflux of human thyrocytes in primary culture, J Cell Physiol 140:608–614, 1989.
25. Ozawa S, Spaulding SW: Epidermal growth factor inhibits radioiodine uptake but stimulates deoxyribonucleic acid synthesis in newborn rat thyroids grown in nude mice, Endocrinology 127:604–612, 1990.
26. Paschke R, Eck T, Herfurth J, et al: Stimulation of proliferation and inhibition of function of xenotransplanted human thyroid tissue by epidermal growth factor, J Endocrinol Invest 18:359–363, 1995.
27. De Vito WJ, Chanoine JP, Alex S, et al: Effect of in vivo administration of recombinant acidic fibroblast growth factor on thyroid function in the rat: induction of colloid goiter, Endocrinology 131:729–735, 1992.
28. Roger PP, Dumont JE: Factors controlling proliferation and differentiation of canine thyroid cells cultured in reduced serum conditions: effects of thyrotropin, cyclic AMP and growth factors, Mol Cell Endocrinol 36:79–93, 1984.
29. Westermark K, Karlsson FA, Westermark B: Epidermal growth factor modulates thyroid growth and function in culture, Endocrinology 112:1680–1686, 1983.
30. Eggo MC, King WJ, Black EG, et al: Functional human thyroid cells and their insulin-like growth factor-binding proteins: regulation by thyrotropin, cyclic 3',5' adenosine monophosphate, and growth factors, J Clin Endocrinol Metab 81:3056–3062, 1996.
31. Lamy F, Taton M, Dumont JE: Control of protein synthesis by thyrotropin and epidermal growth factor in human thyrocytes: role of morphological changes, Mol Cell Endocrinol 73:195, 1990.
32. Kraiem Z, Sadeh O, Yosef M, et al: Mutual antagonistic interactions between the thyrotropin (adenosine

3′,5′-monophosphate) and protein kinase C/epidermal growth factor (tyrosine kinase) pathways in cell proliferation and differentiation of cultured human thyroid follicles, Endocrinology 136:585–590, 1995.
33. Becks GP, Logan A, Phillips ID, et al: Increase of basic fibroblast growth factor (FGF) and FGF receptor messenger RNA during rat thyroid hyperplasia: temporal changes and cellular distribution, J Endocrinol 142:325–338, 1994.
34. Bidey SP, Hill DJ, Eggo MC: Growth factors and goitrogenesis, J Endocrinol 160:321–332, 1999.
35. Derwahl M, Broecker M, Kraiem Z: Clinical review 101: thyrotropin may not be the dominant growth factor in benign and malignant thyroid tumors, J Clin Endocrinol Metab 84:829–834, 1999.
36. Roger PP: Thyrotropin-dependent transforming growth factor beta expression in thyroid gland [comment], Eur J Endocrinol 134:269–271, 1996.
37. Grubeck-Loebenstein B, Buchan G, Sadeghi R, et al: Transforming growth factor beta regulates thyroid growth, J Clin Invest 83:764–770, 1989.
38. Taton M, Lamy F, Roger PP, et al: General inhibition by transforming growth factor beta1 of thyrotropin and cAMP responses in human thyroid cells in primary culture, Mol Cell Endocrinol 95:13–21, 1993.
39. Logan A, Smith C, Becks GP, et al: Enhanced expression of transforming growth factor-beta 1 during thyroid hyperplasia in rats, J Endocrinol 141:45–57, 1994.
40. Franzen A, Piek E, Westermark B, et al: Expression of transforming growth factor-beta1, activin A, and their receptors in thyroid follicle cells: negative regulation of thyrocyte growth and function, Endocrinology 140:4300–4310, 1999.
41. Helmbrecht K, Kispert A, von Wasielewski R, et al: Identification of a Wnt/beta-catenin signaling pathway in human thyroid cells, Endocrinology 142:5261–5266, 2001.
42. Lyons J, Landis CA, Harsh G, et al: Two G protein oncogenes in human endocrine tumors, Science 249:655–659, 1990.
43. Parma J, Duprez L, Vansande J, et al: Somatic mutations in the thyrotropin receptor gene cause hyperfunctioning thyroid adenomas, Nature 365:649–651, 1993.
44. Vasseur C, Rodien P, Beau I, et al: A chorionic gonadotropin-sensitive mutation in the follicle-stimulating hormone receptor as a cause of familial gestational spontaneous ovarian hyperstimulation syndrome, N Engl J Med 349:753–759, 2003.
45. Smits G, Campillo M, Govaerts C, et al: Glycoprotein hormone receptors: determinants in leucine-rich repeats responsible for ligand specificity, EMBO J 22:2692–2703, 2003.
46. Van Sande J, Costa MJ, Massart C, et al: Kinetics of thyrotropin-stimulating hormone (TSH) and thyroid-stimulating antibody binding and action on the TSH receptor in intact TSH receptor-expressing CHO cells, J Clin Endocrinol Metab 88:5366–5374, 2003.
47. Dumont JE, Roger PP, Ludgate M: Assays for thyroid growth immunoglobulins and their clinical implications: methods, concepts and misconceptions, Endocr Rev 8:448–452, 1987.
48. Zakarija M, Jin S, McKenzie JM: Evidence supporting the identity in Graves' disease of thyroid-stimulating antibody and thyroid growth-promoting immunoglobulin G as assayed in FRTL-5 cells, J Clin Invest 81:879–884, 1988.
49. Zakarija M, McKenzie JM: Do thyroid growth-promoting immunoglobulins exist? J Clin Endocrinol Metab 70:308–310, 1990.
50. Contempré B, Le Moine O, Dumont JE, et al: Selenium deficiency and thyroid fibrosis. A key role for macrophages and transforming growth factor beta (TGF-beta), Mol Cell Endocrinol 124:7–15, 1996.
51. Thompson SD, Franklyn JA, Watkinson JC, et al: Fibroblast growth factors 1 and 2 and fibroblast growth factor receptor 1 are elevated in thyroid hyperplasia, J Clin Endocrinol Metab 83:1336–1341, 1998.
52. Fusco A, Santoro M, Grieco M, et al: RET/PTC activation in human thyroid carcinomas, J Endocrinol Invest 18:127–129, 1995.
53. Pierotti MA, Bongarzone I, Borrello MG, et al: Rearrangements of TRK proto-oncogene in papillary thyroid carcinomas, J Endocrinol Invest 18:130–133, 1995.
54. Trovato M, Villari D, Bartolone L, et al: Expression of the hepatocyte growth factor and c-met in normal thyroid, non-neoplastic, and neoplastic nodules, Thyroid 8:125–131, 1998.
55. Aasland R, Akslen LA, Varhaug JE, et al: Co-expression of the genes encoding transforming growth factor-alpha and its receptor in papillary carcinomas of the thyroid, Int J Cancer 46:382–387, 1990.
56. Vella V, Pandini G, Sciacca L, et al: A novel autocrine loop involving IGF-II and the insulin receptor isoform-A stimulates growth of thyroid cancer, J Clin Endocrinol Metab 87:245–254, 2002.
57. Blaydes JP, Schlumberger M, Wynford-Thomas D, et al: Interaction between p53 and TGF beta 1 in control of epithelial cell proliferation, Oncogene 10:307–317, 1995.
58. Vanvooren V, Allgeier A, Cosson E, et al: Expression of multiple adenylyl cyclase isoforms in human and dog thyroid, Mol Cell Endocrinol 170:185–196, 2000.
59. Van Sande J, Mockel J, Boeynaems JM, et al: Regulation of cyclic nucleotide and prostaglandin formation in human thyroid tissues and in autonomous nodules, J Clin Endocrinol Metab 50:776–785, 1980.
60. de Rooij J, Zwartkruis FJT, Verheijen MHG, et al: Epac is a Rap1 guanine-nucleotide-exchange factor directly activated by cyclic AMP, Nature 396:474–477, 1998.
61. Dremier S, Milenkovic M, Blancquaert S, et al: Cyclic adenosine 3′,5′-monophosphate (cAMP)-dependent protein kinases, but not exchange proteins directly activated by cAMP (Epac), mediate thyrotropin/cAMP-dependent regulation of thyroid cells, Endocrinology 148:4612–4622, 2007.
62. Fortemaison N, Blancquaert S, Dumont JE, et al: Differential involvement of the actin cytoskeleton in differentiation and mitogenesis of thyroid cells: inactivation of Rho proteins contributes to cyclic adenosine monophosphate-dependent gene expression but prevents mitogenesis, Endocrinology 146:5485–5495, 2005.
63. van Staveren WC, Solis DW, Delys L, et al: Gene expression in human thyrocytes and autonomous adenomas reveals suppression of negative feedbacks in tumorigenesis, Proc Natl Acad Sci U S A 103:413–418, 2006.
64. Ketelbant-Balasse P, Van Sande J, Neve P, et al: Time sequence of 3′,5′-cyclic AMP accumulation and ultrastructural changes in dog thyroid slices after acute stimulation by TSH, Horm Metab Res 8:212–215, 1976.
65. Cleator JH, Ravenell R, Kurtz DT, et al: A dominant negative Galphas mutant that prevents thyroid-stimulating hormone receptor activation of cAMP production and inositol 1,4,5-trisphosphate turnover: competition by different G proteins for activation by a common receptor, J Biol Chem 279:36601–36607, 2004.
66. Van Sande J, Dequanter D, Lothaire P, et al: Thyrotropin stimulates the generation of inositol 1,4,5-trisphosphate in human thyroid cells, J Clin Endocrinol Metab 91:1099–1107, 2006.
67. Esteves R, Van Sande J, Dumont JE: Nitric oxide as a signal in thyroid, Mol Cell Endocrinol 90:R1–R3, 1992.
68. Munari-Silem Y, Audebet C, Rousset B: Protein kinase C in pig thyroid cells: activation, translocation and endogenous substrate phosphorylating activity in response to phorbol esters, Mol Cell Endocrinol 54:81–90, 1987.
69. Van Sande J, Raspe E, Perret J, et al: Thyrotropin activates both the cyclic AMP and the PIP_2 cascades in CHO cells expressing the human cDNA of TSH receptor, Mol Cell Endocrinol 74:R1–R6, 1990.
70. Laurent E, Mockel J, Van Sande J, et al: Dual activation by thyrotropin of the phospholipase C and cAMP cascades in human thyroid, Mol Cell Endocrinol 52:273–278, 1987.
71. Mockel J, Laurent E, Lejeune C, et al: Thyrotropin does not activate the phosphatidylinositol bisphosphate hydrolyzing phospholipase C in the dog thyroid, Mol Cell Biol 82:221–227, 1991.
72. Mockel J, Lejeune C, Dumont JE: Relative contribution of phosphoinositides and phosphatidylcholine hydrolysis to the actions of carbamylcholine, thyrotropin, and phorbol esters on dog thyroid slices: regulation of cytidine monophosphate-phosphatidic acid accumulation and phospholipase-D activity. II. Actions of phorbol esters, Endocrinology 135:2497–2503, 1994.
73. Lejeune C, Mockel J, Dumont JE: Relative contribution of phosphoinositides and phosphatidylcholine hydrolysis to the actions of carbamylcholine, thyrotropin (TSH), and phorbol esters on dog thyroid slices: regulation of cytidine monophosphate-phosphatidic acid accumulation and phospholipase-D activity. I. Actions of carbamylcholine, calcium ionophores, and TSH, Endocrinology 135:2488–2496, 1994.
74. Coulonval K, Vandeput F, Stein RC, et al: Phosphatidylinositol 3-kinase, protein kinase B and ribosomal S6 kinases in the stimulation of thyroid epithelial cell proliferation by cAMP and growth factors in the presence of insulin, Biochem J 348:351–358, 2000.
75. Vandeput F, Perpete S, Coulonval K, et al: Role of the different mitogen-activated protein kinase subfamilies in the stimulation of dog and human thyroid epithelial cell proliferation by cyclic adenosine 5′-monophosphate and growth factors, Endocrinology 144:1341–1349, 2003.
76. Williams DW, Williams ED, Wynford-Thomas D: Evidence for autocrine production of IGF-1 in human thyroid adenomas, Mol Cell Endocrinol 61:139–147, 1989.
77. Errick JE, Ing KW, Eggo MC, et al: Growth and differentiation in cultured human thyroid cells: effects of epidermal growth factor and thyrotropin, In Vitro Cell Dev Biol 22:28–36, 1986.
78. Roger PP, Taton M, Van Sande J, et al: Mitogenic effects of thyrotropin and adenosine 3′,5′-monophosphate in differentiated normal human thyroid cells in vitro, J Clin Endocrinol Metab 66:1158–1165, 1988.
79. Heldin NE, Bergström D, Hermansson A, et al: Lack of responsiveness to TGF-β_1 in a thyroid carcinoma cell line with functional type I and type II TGF-β receptors and Smad proteins, suggests a novel mechanism for TGF-β insensitivity in carcinoma cells, Mol Cell Endocrinol 153:79–90, 1999.
80. Dumont JE, Miot F, Erneux C, et al: Negative regulation of cyclic AMP levels by activation of cyclic nucleotide phosphodiesterases: the example of the dog thyroid, Adv Cyclic Nucleotide Res 16:325–336, 1984.
81. Mockel J, Van Sande J, Decoster C, et al: Tumor promoters as probes of protein kinase C in dog thyroid cell: inhibition of the primary effects of carbamylcholine and reproduction of some distal effects, Metabolism 36:137–143, 1987.
82. Roger PP, Reuse S, Maenhaut C, et al: Multiple facets of the modulation of growth by cAMP, Vitam Horm 51:59–191, 1995.
83. Stork PJ, Schmitt JM: Crosstalk between cAMP and MAP kinase signaling in the regulation of cell proliferation, Trends Cell Biol 12:258–266, 2002.
84. Richards JS: New signaling pathways for hormones and cyclic adenosine 3′,5′-monophosphate action in endocrine cells, Mol Endocrinol 15:209–218, 2001.
85. Kimura T, Van Keymeulen A, Golstein J, et al: Regulation of thyroid cell proliferation by TSH and other factors: a critical evaluation of in vitro models, Endocr Rev 22:631–656, 2001.
86. Rivas M, Santisteban P: TSH-activated signaling pathways in thyroid tumorigenesis, Mol Cell Endocrinol 213:31–45, 2003.
87. Lamy F, Wilkin F, Baptist M, et al: Phosphorylation of mitogen-activated protein kinases is involved in the epidermal growth factor and phorbol ester, but not in the thyrotropin/cAMP, thyroid mitogenic pathways, J Biol Chem 268:8398–8401, 1993.
88. Van Keymeulen A, Roger PP, Dumont JE, et al: TSH and cAMP do not signal mitogenesis through Ras activation, Biochem Biophys Res Commun 273:154–158, 2000.
89. Bray GA: Increased sensitivity of the thyroid in iodine-depleted rats to the goitrogenic effects of thyrotropin, J Clin Invest 47:1640–1647, 1968.
90. Wolff J: Congenital goiter with defective iodide transport, Endocr Rev 4:240, 1983.
91. Wolff J: Iodide goiter and the pharmacologic effects of excess iodide, Am J Med 47:101–124, 1969.
92. Cochaux P, Van Sande J, Swillens S, et al: Iodide-induced inhibition of adenylate cyclase activity in horse and dog thyroid, Eur J Biochem 170:435–442, 1987.
93. Laurent E, Mockel J, Takazawa K, et al: Stimulation of generation of inositol phosphates by carbamylcholine and its inhibition by phorbol esters and iodide in dog thyroid cells, Biochem J 263:795–801, 1989.

94. Corvilain B, Laurent E, Lecomte M, et al: Role of the cyclic adenosine 3′,5′-monophosphate and the phosphatidylinositol-Ca²⁺ cascades in mediating the effects of thyrotropin and iodide on hormone synthesis and secretion in human thyroid slices, J Clin Endocrinol Metab 79:152, 1994.

95. Van Sande J, Grenier G, Willems C, et al: Inhibition by iodide of the activation of the thyroid cyclic 3′,5′-AMP system, Endocrinology 96:781–786, 1975.

96. Dugrillon A, Bechtner G, Uedelhoven WM, et al: Evidence that an iodolactone mediates the inhibitory effect of iodine on thyroid cell proliferation but not on adenosine 3′,5′-monophosphate formation, Endocrinology 127:337–343, 1990.

97. Panneels V, Macours P, Van den BH, et al: Biosynthesis and metabolism of 2-iodohexadecanal in cultured dog thyroid cells, J Biol Chem 271:23006–23014, 1996.

98. Panneels V, Van Sande J, Van den BH, et al: Inhibition of human thyroid adenylyl cyclase by 2-iodoaldehydes, Mol Cell Endocrinol 106:41–50, 1994.

99. Panneels V, Van den BH, Jacoby C, et al: Inhibition of H₂O₂ production by iodoaldehydes in cultured dog thyroid cells, Mol Cell Endocrinol 102:167–176, 1994.

100. Many MC, Mestdagh C, Van Den Hove MF, et al: In vitro study of acute toxic effects of high iodide doses in human thyroid follicles, Endocrinology 131:621–630, 1992.

101. Uyttersprot N, Pelgrims N, Carrasco N, et al: Moderate doses of iodide in vivo inhibit cell proliferation and the expression of thyroperoxidase and Na⁺/I⁻ symporter mRNAs in dog thyroid, Mol Cell Endocrinol 131:195–203, 1997.

102. Dias JA, Van Roey P: Structural biology of human follitropin and its receptor, Arch Med Res 32:510–519, 2001.

103. Ascoli M, Fanelli F, Segaloff DL: The lutropin/chorionic gonadotropin receptor, a 2002 perspective, Endocr Rev 23:141–174, 2002.

104. Szkudlinski MW, Fremont V, Ronin C, et al: Thyroid-stimulating hormone and thyroid-stimulating hormone receptor structure-function relationships, Physiol Rev 82:473–502, 2002.

105. Cornelis S, Uttenweiler-Joseph S, Panneels V, et al: Purification and characterization of a soluble bioactive amino-terminal extracellular domain of the human thyrotropin receptor, Biochemistry 40:9860–9869, 2001.

106. Rapoport B, Chazenbalk GD, Jaume JC, et al: The thyrotropin (TSH) receptor: interaction with TSH and autoantibodies, Endocr Rev 19:673–716, 1998.

107. de Bernard S, Misrahi M, Huet JC, et al: Sequential cleavage and excision of a segment of the thyrotropin receptor ectodomain, J Biol Chem 274:101–107, 1999.

108. Couet J, Sar S, Jolivet A, et al: Shedding of human thyrotropin receptor ectodomain: involvement of a matrix metalloprotease, J Biol Chem 271:4545–4552, 1996.

109. Mizutori Y, Chen CR, Latrofa F, et al: Evidence that shed thyrotropin receptor A subunits drive affinity maturation of autoantibodies causing Graves' disease, J Clin Endocrinol Metab 94:927–935, 2009.

110. Rapoport B, McLachlan SM: The thyrotropin receptor in Graves' disease, Thyroid 17:911–922, 2007.

111. Beau I, Misrahi M, Gross B, et al: Basolateral localization and transcytosis of gonadotropin and thyrotropin receptors expressed in Madin-Darby canine kidney cells, J Biol Chem 272:5241–5248, 1997.

112. Angers S, Salahpour A, Bouvier M: Dimerization: An emerging concept for G protein-coupled receptor ontogeny and function, Annu Rev Pharmacol Toxicol 42:409–435, 2002.

113. Libert F, Passage E, Lefort A, et al: Localization of human thyrotropin receptor gene to chromosome region 14q3 by in situ hybridization, Cytogenet Cell Genet 54:82–83, 1990.

114. Rousseau-Merck MF, Misrahi M, Loosfelt H, et al: Assignment of the human thyroid stimulating hormone receptor (TSHR) gene to chromosome 14q31, Genomics 8:233–236, 1990.

115. Gross B, Misrahi M, Sar S, et al: Composite structure of the human thyrotropin receptor gene, Biochem Biophys Res Commun 177:679–687, 1991.

116. Ikuyama S, Niller HH, Shimura H, et al: Characterization of the 5′-flanking region of the rat thyrotropin receptor gene, Mol Endocrinol 6:793–804, 1992.

117. Roselli-Rehfuss L, Robbins LS, Cone RD: Thyrotropin receptor messenger ribonucleic acid is expressed in most brown and white adipose tissues in the guinea pig, Endocrinology 130:1857–1861, 1992.

118. Bell A, Gagnon A, Grunder L, et al: Functional TSH receptor in human abdominal preadipocytes and orbital fibroblasts, Am J Physiol Cell Physiol 279:C335–C340, 2000.

119. Crisp MS, Lane C, Halliwell M, et al: Thyrotropin receptor transcripts in human adipose tissue, J Clin Endocrinol Metab 82:2003–2005, 1997.

120. Bassett JH, Williams AJ, Murphy E, et al: A lack of thyroid hormones rather than excess thyrotropin causes abnormal skeletal development in hypothyroidism, Mol Endocrinol 22:501–512, 2008.

121. Nakao N, Ono H, Yamamura T, et al: Thyrotrophin in the pars tuberalis triggers photoperiodic response, Nature 452:317–322, 2008.

122. Ono H, Hoshino Y, Yasuo S, et al: Involvement of thyrotropin in photoperiodic signal transduction in mice, Proc Natl Acad Sci U S A 105:18238–18242, 2008.

123. Maenhaut C, Brabant G, Vassart G, et al: In vitro and in vivo regulation of thyrotropin receptor mRNA levels in dog and human thyroid cells, J Biol Chem 267:3000–3007, 1992.

124. Lapthorn AJ, Harris DC, Littlejohn A, et al: Crystal structure of human chorionic gonadotropin, Nature 369:455–461, 1994.

125. Wu H, Lustbader JW, Liu Y, et al: Structure of human chorionic gonadotropin at 2.6-angstrom resolution from MAD analysis of the selenomethionyl protein, Structure 2:545–558, 1994.

126. Fox KM, Dias JA, Van Roey P: Three-dimensional structure of human follicle-stimulating hormone, Mol Endocrinol 15:378–389, 2001.

127. Fan QR, Hendrickson WA: Structure of human follicle-stimulating hormone in complex with its receptor, Nature 433:269–277, 2005.

128. Kajava AV, Vassart G, Wodak SJ: Modeling of the 3-dimensional structure of proteins with the typical leucine-rich repeats, Structure 3:867–877, 1995.

129. Sanders J, Chirgadze DY, Sanders P, et al: Crystal structure of the TSH receptor in complex with a thyroid-stimulating autoantibody, Thyroid 17:395–410, 2007.

130. Smits G, Govaerts C, Nubourgh I, et al: Lysine 183 and glutamic acid 157 of the TSH receptor: two interacting residues with a key role in determining specificity toward TSH and human CG, Mol Endocrinol 16:722–735, 2002.

131. Caltabiano G, Campillo M, De Leener A, et al: The specificity of binding of glycoprotein hormones to their receptors, Cell Mol Life Sci 65:2484–2492, 2008.

132. Costagliola S, Panneels V, Bonomi M, et al: Tyrosine sulfation is required for agonist recognition by glycoprotein hormone receptors, EMBO J 21:504–513, 2002.

133. Bonomi M, Busnelli M, Persani L, et al: Structural differences in the hinge region of the glycoprotein hormone receptors: evidence from the sulfated tyrosine residues, Mol Endocrinol 20:3351–3363, 2006.

134. Westmuckett AD, Hoffhines AJ, Borghei A, et al: Early postnatal pulmonary failure and primary hypothyroidism in mice with combined TPST-1 and TPST-2 deficiency, Gen Comp Endocrinol 156:145–153, 2008.

135. Sasaki N, Hosoda Y, Nagata A, et al: A mutation in Tpst2 encoding tyrosylprotein sulfotransferase causes dwarfism associated with hypothyroidism, Mol Endocrinol 21:1713–1721, 2007.

136. Palczewski K, Kumasaka T, Hori T, et al: Crystal structure of rhodopsin: a G protein–coupled receptor, Science 289:739–745, 2000.

137. Ridge KD, Abdulaev NG, Sousa M, et al: Phototransduction: crystal clear, Trends Biochem Sci 28:479–487, 2003.

138. Parma J, Duprez L, Van Sande J, et al: Diversity and prevalence of somatic mutations in the thyrotropin receptor and Gs alpha genes as a cause of toxic thyroid adenomas, J Clin Endocrinol Metab 82:2695–2701, 1997.

139. Refetoff S, Dumont JE, Vassart G: Thyroid disorders. In Scriver CR, Sly WS, Childs B, et al, editors: The Metabolic and Molecular Bases of Inherited Diseases, New York, 2001, McGraw-Hill, pp 4029–4076.

140. Duprez L, Parma J, Van Sande J, et al: Germline mutations in the thyrotropin receptor gene cause non-autoimmune autosomal dominant hyperthyroidism, Nat Genet 7:396–401, 1994.

141. Govaerts C, Lefort A, Costagliola S, et al: A conserved Asn in transmembrane helix 7 is an on/off switch in the activation of the thyrotropin receptor, J Biol Chem 276:22991–22999, 2001.

142. Neumann S, Krause G, Chey S, et al: A free carboxylate oxygen in the side chain of position 674 in transmembrane domain 7 is necessary for TSH receptor activation, Mol Endocrinol 15:1294–1305, 2001.

143. Claeysen S, Govaerts C, Lefort A, et al: A conserved Asn in TM7 of the thyrotropin receptor is a common requirement for activation by both mutations and its natural agonist, FEBS Lett 517:195–200, 2002.

144. Ballesteros JA, Jensen AD, Liapakis G, et al: Activation of the beta(2)-adrenergic receptor involves disruption of an ionic lock between the cytoplasmic ends of transmembrane segments 3 and 6, J Biol Chem 276:29171–29177, 2001.

145. Duprez L, Parma J, Costagliola S, et al: Constitutive activation of the TSH receptor by spontaneous mutations affecting the N-terminal extracellular domain, FEBS Lett 409:469–474, 1997.

146. Nakabayashi K, Kudo M, Kobilka B, et al: Activation of the luteinizing hormone receptor following substitution of Ser-277 with selective hydrophobic residues in the ectodomain hinge region, J Biol Chem 275:30264–30271, 2000.

147. Ho SC, Van Sande J, Lefort A, et al: Effects of mutations involving the highly conserved S281HCC motif in the extracellular domain of the thyrotropin (TSH) receptor on TSH binding and constitutive activity, Endocrinology 142:2760–2767, 2001.

148. Parma J, Van Sande J, Swillens S, et al: Somatic mutations causing constitutive activity of the thyrotropin receptor are the major cause of hyperfunctioning thyroid adenomas: identification of additional mutations activating both the cyclic adenosine 3′,5′-monophosphate and inositol phosphate-Ca²⁺ cascades, Mol Endocrinol 9:725–733, 1995.

149. Van Sande J, Massart C, Costagliola S, et al: Specific activation of the thyrotropin receptor by trypsin, Mol Cell Endocrinol 119:161–168, 1996.

150. Chen CR, Chazenbalk GD, McLachlan SM, et al: Evidence that the C terminus of the A subunit suppresses thyrotropin receptor constitutive activity, Endocrinology 144:3821–3827, 2003.

151. Vlaeminck-Guillem V, Ho SC, Rodien P, et al: Activation of the cAMP pathway by the TSH receptor involves switching of the ectodomain from a tethered inverse agonist to an agonist, Mol Endocrinol 16:736–746, 2002.

152. Vassart G, Pardo L, Costagliola S: A molecular dissection of the glycoprotein hormone receptors, Trends Biochem Sci 29(3):119–126, 2004.

153. Chen CR, McLachlan SM, Rapoport B: Suppression of thyrotropin receptor constitutive activity by a monoclonal antibody with inverse agonist activity, Endocrinology 148:2375–2382, 2007.

154. Chen CR, McLachlan SM, Rapoport B: Identification of key amino acid residues in a thyrotropin receptor monoclonal antibody epitope provides insight into its inverse agonist and antagonist properties, Endocrinology 149:3427–3434, 2008.

155. Kleinau G, Krause G: Thyrotropin and homologous glycoprotein hormone receptors: structural and functional aspects of extracellular signaling mechanisms, Endocr Rev. 2009.

156. Rodien P, Bremont C, Samson ML, et al: Familial gestational hyperthyroidism caused by a mutant thyrotropin receptor hypersensitive to human chorionic gonadotropin, N Engl J Med 339:1823–1826, 1998.

157. Szkudlinski MW, Teh NG, Grossmann M, et al: Engineering human glycoprotein hormone superactive analogues, Nat Biotechnol 14:1257–1263, 1996.

158. Costagliola S, Bonomi M, Morgenthaler NG, et al: Delineation of the discontinuous-conformational epitope of a monoclonal antibody displaying full in vitro and in vivo thyrotropin activity, Mol Endocrinol 18:3020–3034, 2004.

159. Costagliola S, Morgenthaler NG, Hoermann R, et al: Second generation assay for thyrotropin receptor antibodies has superior diagnostic sensitivity for Graves' disease, J Clin Endocrinol Metab 84:90–97, 1999.

160. Costagliola S, Franssen JDF, Bonomi M, et al: Generation of a mouse monoclonal TSH receptor antibody with stimulating activity, Biochem Biophys Res Commun 299:891–896, 2002.

161. Morgenthaler NG, Minich WB, Willnich M, et al: Affinity purification and diagnostic use of TSH receptor autoantibodies from human serum, Mol Cell Endocrinol 212:73–79, 2003.
162. Okada SL, Ellsworth JL, Durnam DM, et al: A glycoprotein hormone expressed in corticotrophs exhibits unique binding properties on thyroid-stimulating hormone receptor, Mol Endocrinol 20:414–425, 2006.
163. Nagasaki H, Wang Z, Jackson VR, et al: Differential expression of the thyrostimulin subunits, glycoprotein alpha$_2$ and beta$_5$ in the rat pituitary, J Mol Endocrinol 37:39–50, 2006.
164. Dos SS, Bardet C, Bertrand S, et al: Distinct expression patterns of glycoprotein hormone-α_2 (GPA2) and -β_5 (GPB5) in a basal chordate suggest independent developmental functions, Endocrinology. 2009.
165. Raymond JR, Hnatowich M, Lefkowitz RJ, et al: Adrenergic receptors. Models for regulation of signal transduction processes, Hypertension 15:119–131, 1990.
166. Delbeke D, Van Sande J, Swillens S, et al: Cooling enhances adenosine 3′,5′ monophosphate accumulation in thyrotropin stimulated dog thyroid slices, Metabolism 31:797–804, 1982.
167. Baratti-Elbaz C, Ghinea N, Lahuna O, et al: Internalization and recycling pathways of the thyrotropin receptor, Mol Endocrinol 13:1751–1765, 1999.
168. Persani L, Lania A, Alberti L, et al: Induction of specific phosphodiesterase isoforms by constitutive activation of the cAMP pathway in autonomous thyroid adenomas, J Clin Endocrinol Metab 85:2872–2878, 2000.
169. Urizar E, Montanelli L, Loy T, et al: Glycoprotein hormone receptors: link between receptor homodimerization and negative cooperativity, EMBO J 24:1954–1964, 2005.
170. Tao YX, Johnson NB, Segaloff DL: Constitutive and agonist-dependent self-association of the cell surface human lutropin receptor, J Biol Chem 279:5904–5914, 2004.
171. Latif R, Graves P, Davies TF: Ligand-dependent inhibition of oligomerization at the human thyrotropin receptor, J Biol Chem 277:45059–45067, 2002.
172. Nilsson M, Björkman U, Ekholm R, et al: Polarized efflux of iodide in porcine thyrocytes occurs via a cAMP-regulated iodide channel in the apical plasma membrane, Acta Endocrinol (Copenh) 126:67–74, 1992.
173. Rodriguez AM, Perron B, Lacroix L, et al: Identification and characterization of a putative human iodide transporter located at the apical membrane of thyrocytes, J Clin Endocrinol Metab 87:3500–3503, 2002.
174. Raspé E, Dumont JE: Control of the dog thyrocyte plasma membrane iodide permeability by the Ca2+-phosphatidylinositol and adenosine 3′,5′-monophosphate cascades, Endocrinology 135:986–995, 1994.
175. Saito T, Endo T, Kawaguchi A, et al: Increased expression of the Na^+/I^- symporter in cultured human thyroid cells exposed to thyrotropin and in Graves' thyroid tissue, J Clin Endocrinol Metab 82:3331–3336, 1997.
176. Arntzenius AB, Smit LJ, Schipper J: Inverse relation between iodine intake and thyroid blood flow: color Doppler flow imaging in euthyroid humans, J Clin Endocrinol Metab 73:1051–1055, 1991.
177. Nunez J, Pommier J: Formation of thyroid hormones, Vitam Horm 39:175–229, 1982.
178. Dupuy C, Ohayon R, Valent A, et al: Purification of a novel flavoprotein involved in the thyroid NADPH oxidase. Cloning of the porcine and human cDNAs, J Biol Chem 274:37265–37269, 1999.
179. De Deken X, Wang D, Many MC, et al: Cloning of two human thyroid cDNAs encoding new members of the NADPH oxidase family, J Biol Chem 275:23227–23233, 2000.
180. Corvilain B, Van Sande J, Laurent E, et al: The H_2O_2-generating system modulates protein iodination and the activity of the pentose phosphate pathway in dog thyroid, Endocrinology 128:779–785, 1991.
181. Björkman U, Ekholm R: Hydrogen peroxide generation and its regulation in FRTL-5 and porcine thyroid cells, Endocrinology 130:393–399, 1992.
182. Björkman U, Ekholm R: Accelerated exocytosis and H_2O_2 generation in isolated thyroid follicles enhance protein iodination, Endocrinology 122:488–494, 1988.
183. Dumont JE, Boeynaems JM, de Coster C, et al: Biochemical mechanisms in the control of thyroid function and growth, Adv Cyclic Nucleotide Res 9:723, 1978.
184. Bernier-Valentin F, Kostrouch Z, Rabilloud R, et al: Analysis of the thyroglobulin internationalization process using in vitro reconstituted thyroid follicles: evidence for a coated vesicle-dependent endocytic pathway, Endocrinology 129:2194–2201, 1991.
185. Deshpande V, Venkatesh SG: Thyroglobulin, the prothyroid hormone: chemistry, synthesis and degradation, Biochim Biophys Acta 1430:157–178, 1999.
186. Deery WJ, Heath JP: Phagocytosis induced by thyrotropin in cultured thyroid cells is associated with myosin light chain dephosphorylation and stress fiber disruption, J Cell Biol 122:21–37, 1993.
187. Chambard M, Depetris D, Gruffat D, et al: Thyrotropin regulation of apical and basal exocytosis of thyroglobulin by porcine thyroid monolayers, J Mol Endocrinol 4:193–199, 1990.
188. Herzog V: Pathways of endocytosis in thyroid follicle cells, Int Rev Cytol 91:107–139, 1984.
189. Croizet-Berger K, Daumerie C, Couvreur M, et al: The endocytic catalysts, Rab5a and Rab7, are tandem regulators of thyroid hormone production, Proc Natl Acad Sci U S A 99:8277–8282, 2002.
190. Rocmans PA, Ketelbant-Balasse P, Dumont JE, et al: Hormonal secretion by hyperactive thyroid cells is not secondary to apical phagocytosis, Endocrinology 103:1834–1848, 1978.
191. Van Den Hove MF, Couvreur M, De Visscher M: A new mechanism for the reabsorption of thyroid iodoproteins: selective fluid pinocytosis, Eur J Biochem 122:415–422, 1982.
192. Lemansky P, Herzog V: Endocytosis of thyroglobulin is not mediated by mannose-6-phosphate receptors in thyrocytes. Evidence for low-affinity-binding sites operating in the uptake of thyroglobulin, Eur J Biochem 209:111–119, 1992.
193. Marino M, McCluskey RT: Role of thyroglobulin endocytic pathways in the control of thyroid hormone release, Am J Physiol Cell Physiol 279:C1295–C1306, 2000.
194. Marino M, Zheng G, McCluskey RT: Megalin (gp330) is an endocytic receptor for thyroglobulin on cultured fisher rat thyroid cells, J Biol Chem 274:12898–12904, 1999.
195. Lisi S, Chiovato L, Pinchera A, et al: Impaired thyroglobulin (Tg) secretion by FRTL-5 cells transfected with soluble receptor associated protein (RAP): evidence for a role of RAP in the Tg biosynthetic pathway, J Endocrinol Invest 26:1105–1110, 2003.
196. Laurberg P: Mechanisms governing the relative proportions of thyroxine and 3,5,3′-triiodothyronine in thyroid secretion, Metabolism 33:379–392, 1984.
197. Unger J, Boeynaems JM, Van Herle A, et al: In vitro nonbutanol-extractable iodine release in dog thyroid, Endocrinology 105:225–231, 1979.
198. Van Herle AJ, Vassart G, Dumont JE: Control of thyroglobulin synthesis and secretion. (First of two parts), N Engl J Med 301:239–249, 1979.
199. Damante G, Tell G, Di Lauro R: A unique combination of transcription factors controls differentiation of thyroid cells, Prog Nucleic Acid Res Mol Biol 66:307–356, 2001.
200. Damante G, DiLauro R: Thyroid-specific gene-expression, Biochim Biophys Acta 1218:255–266, 1994.
201. Kusakabe T, Kawaguchi A, Hoshi N, et al: Thyroid-specific enhancer-binding protein/NKX2.1 is required for the maintenance of ordered architecture and function of the differentiated thyroid, Mol Endocrinol 20:1796–1809, 2006.
202. Roger PP, Christophe D, Dumont JE, et al: The dog thyroid primary culture system: a model of the regulation of function, growth and differentiation expression by cAMP and other well-defined signaling cascades, European J Endocrinol 137:579–598, 1997.
203. Medina DL, Suzuki K, Pietrarelli M, et al: Role of insulin and serum on thyrotropin regulation of thyroid transcription factor-1 and *Pax-8* genes expression in FRTL-5 thyroid cells, Thyroid 10:295–303, 2000.
204. Pouillon V, Pichon B, Donda A, et al: TTF-2 does not appear to be a key mediator of the effect of cyclic AMP on thyroglobulin gene transcription in primary cultured dog thyrocytes, Biochem Biophys Res Commun 242:327–331, 1998.
205. Donda A, Javaux F, Van Renterghem P, et al: Human, bovine, canine and rat thyroglobulin promoter sequences display species-specific differences in an in vitro study, Mol Cell Endocrinol 90:R23–R26, 1993.
206. Van Renterghem P, Vassart G, Christophe D: Pax 8 expression in primary cultured dog thyrocyte is increased by cyclic AMP, Biochim Biophys Acta 1307:97–103, 1996.
207. Mascia A, Nitsch L, Di Lauro R, et al: Hormonal control of the transcription factor Pax8 and its role in the regulation of thyroglobulin gene expression in thyroid cells, J Endocrinol 172:163–176, 2002.
208. Van Renterghem P, Dremier S, Vassart G, et al: Study of *TTF-1* gene expression in dog thyrocytes in primary culture, Mol Cell Endocrinol 112:83–93, 1995.
209. Zannini M, Acebron A, DeFelice M, et al: Mapping and functional role of phosphorylation sites in the thyroid transcription factor-1 (TTF-1), J Biol Chem 271:2249–2254, 1996.
210. Reuse S, Maenhaut C, Dumont JE: Regulation of protooncogenes c-fos and c-myc expressions by protein tyrosine kinase, protein kinase C, and cyclic AMP mitogenic pathways in dog primary thyrocytes: a positive and negative control by cyclic AMP on c-myc expression, Exp Cell Res 189:33–40, 1990.
211. Deleu S, Pirson I, Coulonval K, et al: IGF-1 or insulin, and the TSH cyclic AMP cascade separately control dog and human thyroid cell growth and DNA synthesis, and complement each other in inducing mitogenesis, Mol Cell Endocrinol 149:41–51, 1999.
212. Lalli E, Sassonecorsi P: Thyroid-stimulating hormone (TSH)-directed induction of the *Crem* gene in the thyroid gland participates in the long-term desensitization of the TSH receptor, Proc Natl Acad Sci U S A 92:9633–9637, 1995.
213. Pichon B, Jimenez-Cervantes C, Pirson I, et al: Induction of nerve growth factor-induced gene-B (NGFI-B) as an early event in the cyclic adenosine monophosphate response of dog thyrocytes in primary culture, Endocrinology 137:4691–4698, 1996.
214. Pomerance M, Carapau D, Chantoux F, et al: CCAAT/enhancer-binding protein-homologous protein expression and transcriptional activity are regulated by 3′,5′-cyclic adenosine monophosphate in thyroid cells, Mol Endocrinol 17:2283–2294, 2003.
215. Pichon B, Vassart G, Christophe D: A canonical nerve growth factor-induced gene-B response element appears not to be involved in the cyclic adenosine monophosphate-dependent expression of differentiation in thyrocytes, Mol Cell Endocrinol 154:21–27, 1999.
216. Garcia-Jimenez C, Zaballos MA, Santisteban P: DARPP-32 (dopamine and 3′,5′-cyclic adenosine monophosphate-regulated neuronal phosphoprotein) is essential for the maintenance of thyroid differentiation, Mol Endocrinol 19:3060–3072, 2005.
217. Davies E, Dumont JE, Vassart G: Thyrotropin-stimulated recruitment of free monoribosomes on to membrane-bound thyroglobulin synthesizing polyribosomes, Biochem J 172:227–231, 1978.
218. Colletta G, Cirafici AM, Dicarlo A: Dual effect of transforming growth factor-beta on rat thyroid cells: inhibition of thyrotropin-induced proliferation and reduction of thyroid-specific differentiation markers, Cancer Res 49:3457–3462, 1989.
219. Nicolussi A, D'Inzeo S, Santulli M, et al: TGF-beta control of rat thyroid follicular cells differentiation, Mol Cell Endocrinol 207:1–11, 2003.
220. Costamagna E, Garcia B, Santisteban P: The functional interaction between the paired domain transcription factor Pax8 and Smad3 is involved in transforming growth factor-beta repression of the sodium/iodide symporter gene, J Biol Chem 279:3439–3446, 2004.
221. Roger PP, Van Heuverswyn B, Lambert C, et al: Antagonistic effects of thyrotropin and epidermal growth factor on thyroglobulin mRNA level in cultured thyroid cells, Eur J Biochem 152:239–245, 1985.
222. Gerard CM, Lefort A, Christophe D, et al: Control of thyroperoxidase and thyroglobulin transcription by cAMP: evidence for distinct regulatory mechanisms, Mol Endocrinol 3:2110–2118, 1989.
223. Pohl V, Abramowicz M, Vassart G, et al: Thyroperoxidase mRNA in quiescent and proliferating thyroid epithelial cells: expression and subcellular localization studied by in situ hybridization, Eur J Cell Biol 62:94–104, 1993.
224. Leoni SG, Galante PA, Ricarte-Filho JC, et al: Differential gene expression analysis of iodide-treated rat thyroid follicular cell line PCCl3, Genomics 91:356–366, 2008.

225. Blackwood L, Onions DE, Argyle DJ: Characterization of the feline thyroglobulin promoter, Domest Anim Endocrinol 20:185–201, 2001.

226. Christophe-Hobertus C, Christophe D: Two binding sites for thyroid transcription factor 1 (TTF-1) determine the activity of the bovine thyroglobulin gene upstream enhancer element, Mol Cell Endocrinol 149:79–84, 1999.

227. Berg V, Vassart G, Christophe D: A zinc-dependent DNA-binding activity co-operates with cAMP-responsive-element-binding protein to activate the human thyroglobulin enhancer, Biochem J 323:349–357, 1997.

228. Mascia A, DeFelice M, Lipardi C, et al: Transfection of TTF-1 gene induces thyroglobulin gene expression in undifferentiated FRT cells, Biochim Biophys Acta 1354:171–181, 1997.

229. di Magliano MP, Di Lauro R, Zannini M: Pax8 has a key role in thyroid cell differentiation, Proc Natl Acad Sci U S A 97:13144–13149, 2000.

230. Di Palma T, Nitsch R, Mascia A, et al: The paired domain-containing factor Pax8 and the homeodomain-containing factor TTF-1 directly interact and synergistically activate transcription, J Biol Chem 278:3395–3402, 2003.

231. Miccadei S, De Leo R, Zammarchi E, et al: The synergistic activity of thyroid transcription factor 1 and Pax8 relies on the promoter/enhancer interplay, Mol Endocrinol 16:837–846, 2002.

232. Grasberger H, Ringkananont U, Lefrancois P, et al: Thyroid transcription factor 1 rescues PAX8/p300 synergism impaired by a natural PAX8 paired domain mutation with dominant negative activity, Mol Endocrinol 19:1779–1791, 2005.

233. Di Palma T, D'Andrea B, Liguori GL, et al: TAZ is a coactivator for Pax8 and TTF-1, two transcription factors involved in thyroid differentiation, Exp Cell Res 315:162–175, 2009.

234. Ledent C, Parmentier M, Vassart G: Tissue-specific expression and methylation of a thyroglobulin-chloramphenicol acetyltransferase fusion gene in transgenic mice, Proc Natl Acad Sci U S A 87:6176–6180, 1990.

235. Libert F, Vassart G, Christophe D: Methylation and expression of the human thyroglobulin gene, Biochim Biophys Acta 134:1109–1113, 1986.

236. Pichon B, Christophe-Hobertus C, Vassart G, et al: Unmethylated thyroglobulin promoter may be repressed by methylation of flanking DNA sequences, Biochem J 298:537–541, 1994.

237. Van Heuverswyn B, Streydio C, Brocas H, et al: Thyrotropin controls transcription of the thyroglobulin gene, Proc Natl Acad Sci U S A 81:5941–5945, 1984.

238. Van Heuverswyn B, Leriche A, Van Sande J, et al: Transcriptional control of thyroglobulin gene expression by cyclic AMP, FEBS Lett 188:192–196, 1985.

239. Avvedimento VE, Tramontano D, Ursini MV: The level of thyroglobulin mRNA is regulated by TSH both in vitro and in vivo, Biochem Biophys Res Commun 122:472–477, 1984.

240. Hansen C, Gerard C, Vassart G, et al: Thyroid-specific and cAMP-dependent hypersensitive regions in thyroglobulin gene chromatin, Eur J Biochem 178:387–393, 1988.

241. Christophe D, Gérard C, Juvenal G, et al: Identification of a cAMP-responsive region in thyroglobulin gene promoter, Mol Cell Endocrinol 64:5–18, 1989.

242. Pohl V, Roger PP, Christophe D, et al: Differentiation expression during proliferative activity induced through different pathways: in situ hybridization study of thyroglobulin gene expression in thyroid epithelial cells, J Cell Biol 111:663–672, 1990.

243. Ortiz L, Zannini M, Di Lauro R, et al: Transcriptional control of the forkhead thyroid transcription factor TTF-2 by thyrotropin, insulin, and insulin-like growth factor I, J Biol Chem 272:23334–23339, 1997.

244. Fayet G, Hovsepian S: Isolation of a normal human thyroid cell line: hormonal requirement for thyroglobulin regulation, Thyroid 12:539–546, 2002.

245. Graves PN, Davies TF: A second thyroglobulin messenger RNA species (rTg-2) in rat thyrocytes, Mol Endocrinol 4:155–161, 1990.

246. Mercken L, Simons MJ, Vassart G: The 5′-end of bovine thyroglobulin mRNA encodes a hormonogenic peptides, FEBS Lett 149:285–287, 1982.

247. Abramowicz MJ, Vassart G, Christophe D: Functional study of the human thyroid peroxidase gene promoter, Eur J Biochem 203:467–473, 1992.

248. Francis-Lang H, Price M, Polycarpou-Schwarz M, et al: Cell-type-specific expression of the rat thyroperoxidase promoter indicates common mechanism for thyroid-specific gene expression, Mol Cell Biol 12:576–588, 1992.

249. Mizuno K, Gonzalez FJ, Kimura S: Thyroid-specific enhancer-binding protein (T/EBP): cDNA cloning, functional characterization, and structural identity with thyroid transcription factor TTF-1, Mol Cell Biol 11:4927–4933, 1991.

250. Esposito C, Miccadei S, Saiardi A, et al: PAX 8 activates the enhancer of the human thyroperoxidase gene, Biochem J 331:37–40, 1998.

251. De Leo R, Miccadei S, Zammarchi E, et al: Role for p300 in Pax 8 induction of thyroperoxidase gene expression, J Biol Chem 275:34100–34105, 2000.

252. Gérard C, Lefort A, Libert F, et al: Transcriptional regulation of the thyroperoxidase gene by thyrotropin and forskolin, Mol Cell Endocrinol 60:239–242, 1988.

253. Ledent C, Dumont JE, Vassart G, et al: Thyroid expression of an A2 adenosine receptor transgene induces thyroid hyperplasia and hyperthyroidism, EMBO J 11:537–542, 1992.

254. Miccadei S, Provenzano C, Mojzisek M, et al: Retinoblastoma protein acts as Pax 8 transcriptional coactivator, Oncogene 24:6993–7001, 2005.

255. Cuesta I, Zaret KS, Santisteban P: The forkhead factor FoxE1 binds to the thyroperoxidase promoter during thyroid cell differentiation and modifies compacted chromatin structure, Mol Cell Biol 27:7302–7314, 2007.

256. Niccoli P, Fayadat L, Panneels V, et al: Human thyroperoxidase in its alternatively spliced form (TPO2) is enzymatically inactive and exhibits changes in intracellular processing and trafficking, J Biol Chem 272:29487–29492, 1997.

257. Tong Q, Ryu KY, Jhiang SM: Promoter characterization of the rat Na⁺/I⁻ symporter gene, Biochem Biophys Res Commun 239:34–41, 1997.

258. Behr M, Schmitt TL, Espinoza CR, et al: Cloning of a functional promoter of the human sodium/iodide-symporter gene, Biochem J 331:359–363, 1998.

259. Endo T, Kaneshige M, Nakazato M, et al: Thyroid transcription factor-1 activates the promoter activity of rat thyroid Na⁺/I⁻ symporter gene, Mol Endocrinol 11:1747–1755, 1997.

260. Taki K, Kogai T, Kanamoto Y, et al: A thyroid-specific far-upstream enhancer in the human sodium/iodide symporter gene requires Pax-8 binding and cyclic adenosine 3′,5′-monophosphate response element-like sequence binding proteins for full activity and is differentially regulated in normal and thyroid cancer cells, Mol Endocrinol 16:2266–2282, 2002.

261. Fenton MS, Marion KM, Hershman JM: Identification of cyclic adenosine 3′,5′-monophosphate response element modulator as an activator of the human sodium/iodide symporter upstream enhancer, Endocrinology 149:2592–2606, 2008.

262. Saiardi A, Falasca P, Civitareale D: The thyroid-hormone inhibits the thyrotropin receptor promoter activity: evidence for a short loop regulation, Biochem Biophys Res Commun 205:230–237, 1994.

263. Yokomori N, Tawata M, Saito T, et al: Regulation of the rat thyrotropin receptor gene by the methylation-sensitive transcription factor GA binding protein, Mol Endocrinol 12:1241–1249, 1998.

264. Saiardi A, Falasca P, Civitareale D: Synergistic transcriptional activation of the thyrotropin receptor promoter by cyclic AMP-responsive-element-binding protein and thyroid transcription factor-1, Biochem J 310:491–496, 1995.

265. Civitareale D, Castelli MP, Falasca P, et al: Thyroid transcription factor-1 activates the promoter of the thyrotropin receptor gene, Mol Endocrinol 7:1589–1595, 1993.

266. Moeller LC, Kimura S, Kusakabe T, et al: Hypothyroidism in thyroid transcription factor 1 haploinsufficiency is caused by reduced expression of the thyroid-stimulating hormone receptor, Mol Endocrinol 17:2295–2302, 2003.

267. Saji M, Akamizu T, Sanchez M: Regulation of thyrotropin receptor gene expression in rat FRTL-5 thyroid cells, Endocrinology 130:520–533, 1992.

268. Berlingieri MT, Akamizu T, Fusco A: Thyrotropin receptor gene expression in oncogene-transfected rat thyroid cells: correlation between transformation, loss of thyrotropin-dependent growth, and loss of thyrotropin receptor gene expression, Biochem Biophys Res Commun 173:172–178, 1990.

269. Akamizu T, Ikuyama S, Saji M, et al: Cloning, chromosomal assignment, and regulation of the rat thyrotropin receptor: expression of the gene is regulated by thyrotropin, agents that increase cAMP levels, and thyroid autoantibodies, Proc Natl Acad Sci U S A 87:5677–5681, 1990.

270. Kung AW, Collison K, Banga JP, et al: Effect of Graves' IgG on gene transcription in human thyroid cell cultures. Thyroglobulin gene activation, FEBS Lett 232:12–16, 1988.

271. Huber GK, Weinstein SP, Graves PN, et al: The positive regulation of human thyrotropin (TSH) receptor messenger ribonucleic acid by recombinant human TSH is at the intranuclear level, Endocrinology 130:2858–2864, 1992.

272. Brabant G, Maenhaut C, Kohrle J, et al: Human thyrotropin receptor gene: expression in thyroid tumors and correlation to markers of thyroid differentiation and dedifferentiation, Mol Cell Endocrinol 82:R7–R12, 1991.

273. Ohta K, Endo T, Onaya T: The mRNA levels of thyrotropin receptor, thyroglobulin and thyroid peroxidase in neoplastic human thyroid tissues, Biochem Biophys Res Commun 174:1148–1153, 1991.

274. Roger PP, Van Heuverswyn B, Lambert C, et al: Antagonistic effects of thyrotropin and epidermal growth factor on thyroglobulin mRNA level in cultured thyroid cells, Eur J Biochem 152:239–245, 1985.

275. Ledent C, Dumont JE, Vassart G, et al: Thyroid adenocarcinomas secondary to tissue-specific expression of Simian virus-40 large T-antigen in transgenic mice, Endocrinology 129:1391–1401, 1991.

276. Mazzaferri EL: Papillary and follicular thyroid cancer: a selective approach to diagnosis and treatment, Annu Rev Med 32:73–91, 1981.

277. Dupuy C, Pomerance M, Ohayon R, et al: Thyroid oxidase (THOX2) gene expression in the rat thyroid cell line FRTL-5, Biochem Biophys Res Commun 277:287–292, 2000.

278. Pachucki J, Wang D, Christophe D, et al: Structural and functional characterization of the two human ThOX/Duox genes and their 5′-flanking regions, Mol Cell Endocrinol 214:53–62, 2004.

279. D'Andrea B, Iacone R, Di Palma T, et al: Functional inactivation of the transcription factor Pax8 through oligomerization chain reaction, Mol Endocrinol 20:1810–1824, 2006.

280. Christophe-Hobertus C, Christophe D: Human thyroid oxidases genes promoter activity in thyrocytes does not appear to be functionally dependent on thyroid transcription factor-1 or Pax8, Mol Cell Endocrinol 264:157–163, 2007.

281. Grasberger H, Refetoff S: Identification of the maturation factor for dual oxidase. Evolution of an eukaryotic operon equivalent, J Biol Chem 281:18269–18272, 2006.

282. Christov K: Cell population kinetics and DNA content during thyroid carcinogenesis, Cell Tissue Kinet 18:119–131, 1985.

283. Coclet J, Foureau F, Ketelbant P, et al: Cell population kinetics in dog and human adult thyroid, Clin Endocrinol (Oxf) 31:655–665, 1989.

284. Smeds S, Wollman SH: 3H-thymidine labeling of endothelial cells in thyroid arteries, veins, and lymphatics during thyroid stimulation, Lab Invest 48:285–291, 1983.

285. Many MC, Denef JF, Haumont S: Precocity of the endothelial proliferation during a course of rapid goitrogenesis, Acta Endocrinol (Copenh) 105:487–491, 1984.

286. Patel VA, Logan A, Watkinson JC, et al: Isolation and characterization of human thyroid endothelial cells, Am J Physiol Endocrinol Metab 284:E168–E176, 2003.

287. Sato K, Yamazaki K, Shizume K, et al: Stimulation by thyroid-stimulating hormone and Grave's immunoglobulin G of vascular endothelial growth factor mRNA expression in human thyroid follicles in vitro and flt mRNA expression in the rat thyroid in vivo, J Clin Invest 96:1295–1302, 1995.

288. Gerard CM, Many MC, Daumerie C, et al: Structural changes in the angiofollicular units between active and

hypofunctioning follicles align with differences in the epithelial expression of newly discovered proteins involved in iodine transport and organification, J Clin Endocrinol Metab 87:1291–1299, 2002.
289. Gerard AC, Xhenseval V, Colin IM, et al: Evidence for coordinated changes between vascular endothelial growth factor and nitric oxide synthase III immunoreactivity, the functional status of the thyroid follicles, and the microvascular bed during chronic stimulation by low iodine and propylthiouracil in old mice, Eur J Endocrinol 142:651–660, 2000.
290. Takasu N, Komiya I, Nagasawa Y, et al: Stimulation of porcine thyroid cell alkalinization and growth by EGF, phorbol ester, and diacylglycerol, Am J Physiol 258:E445–E450, 1990.
291. Clement S, Refetoff S, Robaye B, et al: Low TSH requirement and goiter in transgenic mice overexpressing IGF-I and IGF-I receptor in the thyroid gland, Endocrinology 142:5131–5139, 2001.
292. Tramontano D, Cushing GW, Moses AC, et al: Insulin-like growth factor-I stimulates the growth of rat thyroid cells in culture and synergizes the stimulation of DNA synthesis induced by TSH and Graves' IgG, Endocrinology 119:940–942, 1986.
293. Saji M, Tsushima T, Isozaki O, et al: Interaction of insulin-like growth factor I with porcine thyroid cells cultured in monolayer, Endocrinology 121:749–756, 1987.
294. Volzke H, Friedrich N, Schipf S, et al: Association between serum insulin-like growth factor-I levels and thyroid disorders in a population-based study, J Clin Endocrinol Metab 92:4039–4045, 2007.
295. Roger PP, Servais P, Dumont JE: Stimulation by thyrotropin and cyclic AMP of the proliferation of quiescent canine thyroid cells cultured in a defined medium containing insulin, FEBS Lett 157:323–329, 1983.
296. Van Sande J, Lefort A, Beebe S, et al: Pairs of cyclic AMP analogs, that are specifically synergistic for type I and type II cAMP-dependent protein kinases, mimic thyrotropin effects on the function, differentiation expression and mitogenesis of dog thyroid cells, Eur J Biochem 183:699–708, 1989.
297. Michiels FM, Caillou B, Talbot M, et al: Oncogenic potential of guanine nucleotide stimulatory factor alpha subunit in thyroid glands of transgenic mice, Proc Natl Acad Sci U S A 91:10488–10492, 1994.
298. Zeiger MA, Saji M, Gusev Y, et al: Thyroid-specific expression of cholera toxin A1 subunit causes thyroid hyperplasia and hyperthyroidism in transgenic mice, Endocrinology 138:3133–3140, 1997.
299. Meinkoth JL, Goldsmith PK, Spiegel AM, et al: Inhibition of thyrotropin-induced DNA synthesis in thyroid follicular cells by microinjection of an antibody to the stimulatory G protein of adenylate cyclase, Gs, J Biol Chem 267:13239–13245, 1992.
300. Kupperman E, Wen W, Meinkoth JL: Inhibition of thyrotropin-stimulated DNA synthesis by microinjection of inhibitors of cellular Ras and cyclic AMP-dependent protein kinase, Mol Cell Biol 13:4477–4484, 1993.
301. Dremier S, Pohl V, Poteet-Smith C, et al: Activation of cyclic AMP-dependent kinase is required but may not be sufficient to mimic cyclic AMP-dependent DNA synthesis and thyroglobulin expression in dog thyroid cells, Mol Cell Biol 17:6717–6726, 1997.
302. Saavedra AP, Tsygankova OM, Prendergast GV, et al: Role of cAMP, PKA and Rap1A in thyroid follicular cell survival, Oncogene 21:778–788, 2002.
303. Ribeiro-Neto F, Urbani J, Lemee N, et al: On the mitogenic properties of Rap1b: cAMP-induced G(1)/S entry requires activated and phosphorylated Rap1b, Proc Natl Acad Sci U S A 99:5418–5423, 2002.
304. Hochbaum D, Hong K, Barila G, et al: Epac, in synergy with cAMP-dependent protein kinase (PKA), is required for cAMP-mediated mitogenesis, J Biol Chem 283:4464–4468, 2008.
305. Kero J, Ahmed K, Wettschureck N, et al: Thyrocyte-specific Gq/G11 deficiency impairs thyroid function and prevents goiter development, J Clin Invest 117:2399–2407, 2007.
306. Van Keymeulen A, Deleu S, Bartek J, et al: Respective roles of carbamylcholine and cyclic adenosine monophosphate in their synergistic regulation of cell cycle in thyroid primary cultures, Endocrinology 142:1251–1259, 2001.
307. Bacharach LK, Eggo MC, Mak WW, et al: Phorbol esters stimulate growth and inhibit differentiation in cultured thyroid cells, Endocrinology 116:1603–1609, 1985.
308. Roger PP, Reuse S, Servais P, et al: Stimulation of cell proliferation and inhibition of differentiated expression by tumor-promoting phorbol esters in dog thyroid cells in primary culture, Cancer Res 46:898, 1986.
309. Raspe E, Reuse S, Roger PP, et al: Lack of correlation between the activation of the Ca^{2+}-phosphatidylinositol cascade and the regulation of DNA synthesis in the dog thyrocyte, Exp Cell Res 198:17–26, 1992.
310. Ollis CA, Hill DJ, Munro DS: A role for insulin-like growth factor-I in the regulation of human thyroid cell growth by thyrotropin, J Endocrinol 123:495–500, 1989.
311. Maciel RMB, Mores AC, Villone G, et al: Demonstration of the production and physiological role of insulin-like growth factor II in rat thyroid follicular cells in culture, J Clin Invest 82:1546–1553, 1988.
312. De Vita G, Berlingieri MT, Visconti R, et al: Akt/protein kinase B promotes survival and hormone-independent proliferation of thyroid cells in the absence of dedifferentiating and transforming effects, Cancer Res 60:3916–3920, 2000.
313. Dremier S, Taton M, Coulonval K, et al: Mitogenic, dedifferentiating, and scattering effects of hepatocyte growth factor on dog thyroid cells, Endocrinology 135:135–140, 1994.
314. Gire V, Marshall CJ, Wynford-Thomas D: Activation of mitogen-activated protein kinase is necessary but not sufficient for proliferation of human thyroid epithelial cells induced by mutant Ras, Oncogene 18:4819–4832, 1999.
315. Melillo RM, Santoro M, Ong SH, et al: Docking protein FRS2 links the protein tyrosine kinase RET and its oncogenic forms with the mitogen-activated protein kinase signaling cascade, Mol Cell Biol 21:4177–4187, 2001.
316. Kimura ET, Nikiforova MN, Zhu Z, et al: High prevalence of BRAF mutations in thyroid cancer: genetic evidence for constitutive activation of the RET/PTC-RAS-BRAF signaling pathway in papillary thyroid carcinoma, Cancer Res 63:1454–1457, 2003.
317. Roger PP, Servais P, Dumont JE: Induction of DNA synthesis in dog thyrocytes in primary culture: synergistic effects of thyrotropin and cyclic AMP with epidermal growth factor and insulin, J Cell Physiol 130:58–67, 1987.
318. Roger PP, Servais P, Dumont JE: Regulation of dog thyroid epithelial cell cycle by forskolin, an adenylate cyclase activator, Exp Cell Res 172:282–292, 1987.
319. Becks GP, Eggo MC, Burrow GN: Organic iodide inhibits deoxyribonucleic acid synthesis and growth in FRTL5 cells, Endocrinology 123:545–550, 1988.
320. Tsygankova OM, Saavedra A, Rebhun JF, et al: Coordinated regulation of Rap1 and thyroid differentiation by cyclic AMP and protein kinase A, Mol Cell Biol 21:1921–1929, 2001.
321. Lou LG, Urbani J, Ribeiro-Neto F, et al: cAMP inhibition of Akt is mediated by activated and phosphorylated Rap1b, J Biol Chem 277:32799–32806, 2002.
322. Tominaga T, Dela Cruz J, Burrow GN, et al: Divergent patterns of immediate early gene expression in response to thyroid-stimulating hormone and insulin-like growth factor I in Wistar rat thyrocytes, Endocrinology 135:1212–1219, 1994.
323. Reuse S, Pirson I, Dumont JE: Differential regulation of protooncogenes c-Jun and Jun D expressions by protein tyrosine kinase, protein kinase C, and cyclic-AMP mitogenic pathways in dog primary thyrocytes: TSH and cyclic-AMP induce proliferation but down-regulate c-Jun expression, Exp Cell Res 196:210–215, 1991.
324. Bockstaele L, Kooken H, Libert F, et al: Regulated activating Thr172 phosphorylation of cyclin-dependent kinase 4(CDK4): its relationship with cyclins and CDK "inhibitors," Mol Cell Biol 26:5070–5085, 2006.
325. Contor L, Lamy F, Lecocq R, et al: Differential protein phosphorylation in induction of thyroid cell proliferation by thyrotropin, epidermal growth factor, or phorbol ester, Mol Cell Biol 8:2494–2503, 1988.
326. Cass LA, Meinkoth JL: Differential effects of cyclic adenosine 3′,5′-monophosphate on p70 ribosomal S6 kinase, Endocrinology 139:1991–1998, 1998.
327. Brewer C, Yeager N, Di Cristofano A: Thyroid-stimulating hormone initiated proliferative signals converge in vivo on the mTOR kinase without activating AKT, Cancer Res 67:8002–8006, 2007.
328. Uyttersprot N, Costagliola S, Dumont JE, et al: Requirement for cAMP-response element (CRE) binding protein/CRE modulator transcription factors in thyrotropin-induced proliferation of dog thyroid cells in primary culture, Eur J Biochem 259:370–378, 1999.
329. Nguyen LQ, Kopp P, Martinson F, et al: A dominant negative CREB (cAMP response element-binding protein) isoform inhibits thyrocyte growth, thyroid-specific gene expression, differentiation, and function, Mol Endocrinol 14:1448–1461, 2000.
330. Lamy F, Roger PP, Lecocq R, et al: Protein synthesis during induction of DNA replication in thyroid epithelial cells: evidence for late markers of distinct mitogenic pathways, J Cell Physiol 138:568–578, 1989.
331. Hebrant A, van Staveren WC, Delys L, et al: Long-term EGF/serum-treated human thyrocytes mimic papillary thyroid carcinomas with regard to gene expression, Exp Cell Res 313:3276–3284, 2007.
332. Bartek J, Bartkova J, Lukas J: The retinoblastoma protein pathway and the restriction point, Curr Opin Cell Biol 8:805–814, 1996.
333. Sherr CJ, Roberts JM: CDK inhibitors: positive and negative regulators of G1-phase progression, Genes Dev 13:1501–1512, 1999.
334. Lukas J, Bartkova J, Bartek J: Convergence of mitogenic signalling cascades from diverse classes of receptors at the cyclin D-cyclin-dependent kinase-pRb-controlled G(1) checkpoint, Mol Cell Biol 16:6917–6925, 1996.
335. Coulonval K, Maenhaut C, Dumont JE, et al: Phosphorylation of the three Rb protein family members is a common step of the cAMP-, the growth factor, and the phorbol ester-mitogenic cascades but is not necessary for the hypertrophy induced by insulin, Exp Cell Res 233:395–398, 1997.
336. Baptist M, Lamy F, Gannon J, et al: Expression and subcellular localization of CDK2 and cdc2 kinases and their common partner cyclin A in thyroid epithelial cells: comparison of cyclic AMP-dependent and -independent cell cycles, J Cell Physiol 166:256–273, 1996.
337. Van Keymeulen A, Bartek J, Dumont JE, et al: Cyclin D3 accumulation and activity integrate and rank the comitogenic pathways of thyrotropin and insulin in thyrocytes in primary culture, Oncogene 18:7351–7359, 1999.
338. Depoortere F, Van Keymeulen A, Lukas J, et al: A requirement for cyclin D3-cyclin-dependent kinase (CDK)-4 assembly in the cyclic adenosine monophosphate-dependent proliferation of thyrocytes, J Cell Biol 140:1427–1439, 1998.
339. Depoortere F, Dumont JE, Roger PP: Paradoxical accumulation of the cyclin-dependent kinase inhibitor p27kip1 during the cAMP-dependent mitogenic stimulation of thyroid epithelial cells, J Cell Sci 109:1759–1764, 1996.
340. Depoortere F, Pirson I, Bartek J, et al: Transforming growth factor beta(1) selectively inhibits the cyclic AMP-dependent proliferation of primary thyroid epithelial cells by preventing the association of cyclin D3-CDK4 with nuclear p27(kip1), Mol Biol Cell 11:1061–1076, 2000.
341. Coulonval K, Bockstaele L, Paternot S, et al: The cyclin D3-CDK4-p27(kip1) holoenzyme in thyroid epithelial cells: activation by TSH, inhibition by TGFbeta, and phosphorylations of its subunits demonstrated by two-dimensional gel electrophoresis, Exp Cell Res 291:135–149, 2003.
342. Paternot S, Coulonval K, Dumont JE, et al: Cyclic AMP-dependent phosphorylation of cyclin D3-bound CDK4 determines the passage through the cell cycle restriction point in thyroid epithelial cells, J Biol Chem 278:26533–26540, 2003.
343. Paternot S, Dumont JE, Roger PP: Differential utilization of cyclin D1 and cyclin D3 in the distinct mitogenic stimulations by growth factors and TSH of human thyrocytes in primary culture, Mol Endocrinol 20:3279–3292, 2006.
344. Romeo HE, Diaz MC, Ceppi J, et al: Effect of inferior laryngeal nerve section on thyroid function in rats, Endocrinology 122:2527–2532, 1988.
345. Jhiang SM, Sagartz JE, Tong Q, et al: Targeted expression of the ret/PTC1 oncogene induces papillary

thyroid carcinomas, Endocrinology 137:375–378, 1996.

346. Powell DJ Jr, Russell J, Nibu K, et al: The RET/PTC3 oncogene: metastatic solid-type papillary carcinomas in murine thyroids, Cancer Res 58:5523–5528, 1998.

347. Pirson I, Coulonval K, Lamy F, et al: c-myc expression is controlled by the mitogenic cAMP-cascade in thyrocytes, J Cell Physiol 168:59–70, 1996.

348. Paternot S, Arsenijevic T, Coulonval K, et al: Distinct specificities of pRb phosphorylation by CDK4 activated by cyclin D1 or cyclin D3: differential involvement in the distinct mitogenic modes of thyroid epithelial cells, Cell Cycle 5:61–70, 2006.

349. Bartkova J, Lukas J, Strauss M, et al: Cyclin D3: requirement for G1/S transition and high abundance in quiescent tissues suggest a dual role in proliferation and differentiation, Oncogene 17:1027–1037, 1998.

350. Roger PP, Baptist M, Dumont JE: A mechanism generating heterogeneity in thyroid epithelial cells: suppression of the thyrotropin/cAMP-dependent mitogenic pathway after cell division induced by cAMP-independent factors, J Cell Biol 117:383–393, 1992.

351. Rocha AS, Paternot S, Coulonval K, et al: Cyclic AMP inhibits the proliferation of thyroid carcinoma cell lines through regulation of CDK4 phosphorylation, Mol Biol Cell 19:4814–4825, 2008.

352. Dremier S, Golstein J, Mosselmans R, et al: Apoptosis in dog thyroid cells, Biochem Biophys Res Commun 200:52–58, 1994.

353. Rognoni JB, Penel C, Golstein J, et al: Cell kinetics of thyroid epithelial cells during hyperplastic goiter involution, J Endocrinol 114:483–490, 1987.

354. Riesco JM, Juanes JA, Carretero J, et al: Cell proliferation and apoptosis of thyroid follicular cells are involved in the involution of experimental non-tumoral hyperplastic goiter, Anat Embryol (Berl) 198:439–450, 1998.

355. Tamura M, Kimura H, Koji T, et al: Role of apoptosis of thyrocytes in a rat model of goiter. A possible involvement of Fas system, Endocrinology 139:3643–3646, 1998.

356. Rasmussen SG, Choi HJ, Rosenbaum DM, et al: Crystal structure of the human beta$_2$ adrenergic G protein–coupled receptor, Nature 450:383–387, 2007.

Chapter 4

THYROID HORMONE METABOLISM

DONALD L. ST. GERMAIN

Secretion of thyroxine (T_4) and triiodothyronine (T_3) from the thyroid gland provides an overall "set point" for the activity of this hormonal axis. However, as in the case of other hormones, in particular, those from the adrenal cortex and gonads, mechanisms governing the cellular uptake and metabolism of thyroid hormones have an important influence on their plasma concentrations. These "prereceptor" processes are also critical determinants of the cellular level of T_3 available for binding to nuclear thyroid hormone receptors. The metabolic fate of thyroid hormones in peripheral tissues thus serves as an important control mechanism of thyroid hormone action.

The principal secretory product of the thyroid gland, T_4, undergoes a complex series of intracellular metabolic alterations in peripheral tissues, as shown in Fig. 4-1. Some of these reactions, such as 5'-deiodination of T_4 to form T_3 or decarboxylation and deamination of T_3 to form the acetic acid analogue termed Triac, result in compounds with considerably greater intrinsic biopotency because of their increased affinity for thyroid hormone receptors.[1,2] Other reactions result in the formation of apparently inactive compounds, such as reverse T_3 (rT_3) formed by 5'-deiodination of T_4 or the sulfated and glucuronidated forms of T_4 and T_3 formed by conjugation of the phenolic ring hydroxyl group.[3,4] Progressive deiodination of T_4, T_3, and rT_3 results in the formation of various diiodinated and monoiodinated thyronines and eventually thyronine (T_0) itself.[5] Most of these compounds are believed to have little or no biological activity. Exceptions to this generalization may be the compounds 3,5-diiodothyronine (3,5-T_2) and 3,3'-T_2, which have been demonstrated to have effects on mitochondrial function[6] and to increase metabolic rate.[7-9] In addition, the monoiodinated compound 3-iodothyronamine, formed in vivo by sequential deiodination and decarboxylation, produces bradycardia and dramatic decreases in body temperature and metabolic rate when administered to experimental animals.[10,11] This effect, opposite to that expected of a thyroid hormone, is believed to result from a nongenomic mechanism via a G protein–coupled trace amine receptor.[10]

The enzymatic processes shown in Fig. 4-1 are not mutually exclusive. Indeed, modification of an iodothyronine molecule at one site may markedly alter its susceptibility to other metabolic reactions. For example, Tetrac and Triac are much better substrates for glucuronidation than are T_4 and T_3.[12] The acetic acid analogues and sulfated conjugates also are markedly better substrates for deiodination in the liver and kidney than are the native compounds.[13,14] In contrast, sulfation of iodothyronines in certain organs may effectively block further metabolism because these conjugates are poorly reactive with the deiodinase isoforms expressed in other tissues.[15,16]

HORMONE KINETICS AND PRODUCTION

Deiodination at the 5' or 5 position accounts for approximately 80% of the daily disposal of T_4, with the other processes shown in Fig. 4-1 responsible for the remaining metabolism of this compound.[5] Such approximations may underestimate the role of both deiodinative and nondeiodinative pathways, however. Many of the products of these reactions, including T_3 and rT_3, are present primarily in the intracellular compartment and may undergo degradation before they have a chance to exchange with

ALTERNATE ROUTES

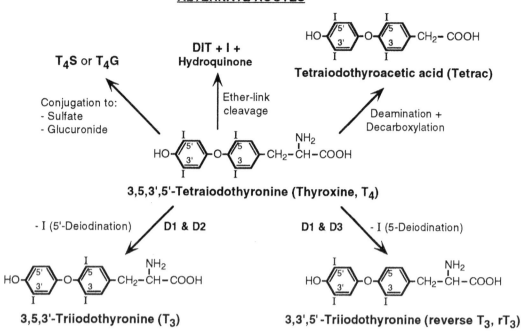

DEIODINATION

FIGURE 4-1. Graphic representation of the pathways of iodothyronine metabolism. The types 1 and 2 deiodinases (D1, D2) catalyze removal of the 5' (or chemically equivalent 3') iodine from T_4 and other iodothyronine substrates. Types 1 and 3 enzymes catalyze 5 (or chemically equivalent 3) deiodination. A variety of less common reactions occur via alternative enzymatic pathways. The metabolites shown are subject to further deiodination to form diiodothyronines, monoiodothyronines, and tyrosine. (From St. Germain DL, Galton VA: The deiodinase family of selenoproteins. Thyroid 7:655–658, 1997.)

the plasma pool. It thus is difficult in human kinetic studies that use plasma sampling techniques alone to assess the contribution of these processes to overall thyroid hormone metabolism. For example, it has been demonstrated that most of the thyronine (T_0) excreted in the urine is in the form of its acetic acid analogue,[17] thus suggesting that deamination plays a more prominent role in thyroid hormone metabolism than is apparent from the very low circulating levels of Tetrac and Triac. Such concerns have led to the concept that "hidden pools" of thyroid hormone metabolites may be present in tissues.[18]

Table 4-1[19-21] provides estimates of various kinetic parameters of thyroid hormone production and metabolism in humans.[5,22,23] The high affinity of T_4 for plasma binding proteins, along with its greater production rate, accounts for its relatively high concentration in serum, as well as its long serum half-life. In contrast, T_3 and rT_3 are present at much lower serum concentrations because of their lower production rates, greater metabolic clearance rates, and lower affinity for thyroxine-binding globulin (TBG). In addition, these two triiodothyronines appear to reside primarily within the intracellular compartment; thus their volumes of distribution are significantly greater than that of T_4.

The rate of T_4 production remains remarkably constant in healthy adults, with alterations noted only during pregnancy and in the aged. Although not well documented, increased T_4 secretion probably occurs during pregnancy in response to several factors, including thyroidal stimulation by human chorionic gonadotropin, an increase in the size of the extrathyroidal T_4 pool resulting from increased TBG levels, and an increase in the rate of T_4 and T_3 degradation because of high levels of 5-deiodinase activity in the pregnant uterus and placenta.[24,25] One clinical consequence is the need to increase the replacement dose of T_4 by 25% to 50% in hypothyroid women during preg-

nancy.[26] Thyroid function appears to be well preserved through age 80 in healthy individuals, although a slight decrease in T_4 production and clearance is noted after the age of 60 years, and free T_3 levels are lower in centenarians.[27,28] That being the case, the decreased T_4 requirements of elderly hypothyroid patients probably result more from the presence of chronic illness and the use of concurrent medications than from the aging process per se.[29,30]

DEIODINATION AND THE IODOTHYRONINE DEIODINASES

The potential importance of deiodination to thyroid hormone action was first recognized nearly 50 years ago when Gross and Pitt-Rivers demonstrated that although T_3 was considerably more potent than T_4,[31] it was present in the thyroid in much lower amounts.[32] This observation suggested that T_3 was derived largely from T_4 by metabolism in extrathyroidal tissues. This thesis was later proved by Braverman et al., who demonstrated the presence of T_3 in the serum of athyreotic subjects injected with T_4.[33]

Table 4-1. Normal Thyroid Hormone Kinetics in Humans

Property	T_4*	T_3*	rT_3*
Total serum concentration, µg/dL	8.1	0.11	0.012
Free serum concentration, ng/dL	1.2	0.29	0.04
Distribution volume, L	10	35	90
Metabolic clearance rate, L/day/70 kg	1.2	24	111
Serum half-life, day	7	1	0.2
Production or disposal rate, mg/day/70 kg	100	31	39

Data from Chopra[19,20] and Faber et al.[21]

T_4, Thyroxine; T_3, 3,5,3'-triiodothyronine; rT_3, reverse triiodothyronine.

*Conversion factors: T_4, 1 mg = 1.3 nmol; T_3 and rT_3, 1 mg = 1.5 nmol.

Research over the past three decades has confirmed the physiologic importance of the 5′- and 5-deiodination processes, has defined the biochemical parameters of these enzymatic reactions, has determined important regulatory factors that influence deiodinase activities, and has identified key structural determinants of the proteins that catalyze these reactions.[34,35]

Three deiodinase isoforms, termed D1, D2, and D3, are present in vertebrate species. These differ in their catalytic properties, patterns of tissue expression, and mechanisms of regulation.[34,36,37] The 5′- and 5-deiodination reactions catalyzed by these enzymes can be considered broadly as activating and inactivating processes, respectively.

BIOCHEMICAL CHARACTERISTICS

The biochemical properties of the deiodinases are outlined in Table 4-2.[38-45] They are in essence oxidoreductases in that they catalyze the substitution of hydrogen for iodine on the iodothyronine substrate. No other catalytic properties of these enzymes have yet been identified, nor do other known enzymes possess deiodinase activity. The enzymes are remarkable in terms of their substrate specificity and the precise location of the iodine removed.[16] D1 is unique in that it can catalyze either 5′- or 5-deiodination, depending on the reacting substrate. Thus rT_3 is efficiently deiodinated only at the 5′ position by D1. In contrast, T_4 and T_3 are poor substrates for this enzyme unless they are first sulfated. This reaction markedly enhances their rate of 5-deiodination and further reduces their susceptibility to 5′-deiodination.[46] That D1 is relatively inefficient in converting T_4 to T_3 presents a considerable paradox, given that a significant proportion of T_3 production has traditionally been believed to occur in the liver and other D1-expressing tissues (vide infra).

D2 catalyzes only 5′-deiodination and very efficiently converts T_4 to T_3.[16] The T_3 thus formed is a poor substrate for 5′-deiodination and is not further metabolized by this enzyme. In contrast, rT_3 is a good substrate for D2 as well as D1 and frequently is used in research assays to quantitate 5′-deiodinase activity. D3 exclusively catalyzes 5-deiodination[16] and thus serves to convert T_4 and T_3 to rT_3 and $3,3'-T_2$, respectively—metabolites with little affinity for the nuclear thyroid hormone receptors.

The deiodinases all require the availability of reduced thiol cofactors for efficient catalytic cycling.[39] These cofactors presumably function to displace iodine from an enzyme intermediate formed during the reaction and thus to regenerate the active deiodinase.[47] In in vitro assay systems using tissue homogenates or cellular subfractions, dithiothreitol typically is added as a cofactor. This small, nonnative four-carbon dithiol efficiently supports deiodination of all three enzymes. Kinetic data derived from broken cell preparations using dithiothreitol as cofactor have demonstrated a Michaelis-Menten constant (K_m) value for D1 of approximately 2.3 µmol/L (for T_4 5′-deiodination), whereas D2 and D3 manifest much lower K_m values in the nanomolar range (see Table 4-2).[39] Based on this analysis, D1 sometimes is referred to as a "high K_m" enzyme, whereas D2 is said to catalyze a "low K_m" 5′-deiodination process. This distinction is somewhat spurious, however, because the kinetic properties of the deiodinases are clearly dependent on the thiol cofactors used in the assay system.[48] Thus, when the native thiol cofactor glutathione or thioredoxin is used, K_m values for D1 in the nanomolar range are obtained. Unfortunately, the cofactor system supporting deiodination in intact cells remains unknown,[49] and evidence suggests that glutathione and thioredoxin may not serve this role.[50] Thus the physiologic significance of the kinetic parameters derived in vitro remains uncertain.

INHIBITORS

In addition to differences in their catalytic properties, the deiodinases show differential susceptibilities to certain inhibitors[39] (see Table 4-2). Most notable is the marked sensitivity of D1 to the antithyroid drug propylthiouracil (PTU). This agent forms an inactive complex with D1 by binding covalently to its active site. Notably, D2 and D3 show little or no susceptibility to inhibition by PTU. The related thioureylene drugs carbimazole and methimazole have no inhibitory effect on deiodination.[47]

Gold compounds such as aurothioglucose are known to react with the active site selenocysteine residue in glutathione peroxidase and impair its activity.[51] This compound also inhibits all three deiodinase isoforms, with D1 again showing a significantly greater sensitivity to this effect.[52-54] Other drugs that affect thyroid

Table 4-2. Characteristics of Iodothyronine Deiodinases

Characteristic	D1	D2	D3
Reaction catalyzed	5 or 5′	5′	5
Substrate preference	5: $T_4S > T_3S \gg T_3, T_4$ 5′: $rT_3, rT_3S > T_2S \gg T_4$	$T_4 > rT_3$	$T_3 > T_4$
K_m (DTT as cofactor)	T_4S (5): 0.3 µmol/L rT_3 (5′): 0.06 µmol/L T_4 (5′): 2.3 µmol/L	T_4 (5′): 1 nmol/L	T_3 (5): 6 nmol/L T_4 (5): 37 nmol/L
Molecular mass, kDa	29	30	32
Selenocysteine	Present	Present	Present
Homodimer	Yes	Yes	Yes
Chromosomal location (human)	1p32-p33	14q24.3	14q32
Location	Liver, kidney, thyroid, pituitary	Pituitary, brain, brown fat, thyroid,* heart,* skeletal muscle*	Brain, skin, uterus, placenta, fetus
Activity in hypothyroidism	↓ (Liver, kidney) ↑ (Thyroid)	↑ (All tissues)	↓ (Brain)
Activity in hyperthyroidism	↑ (Liver, kidney) ↑ (Thyroid)	↓ (Most tissues) ↑ (Thyroid)*	↑ (Brain)
Inhibitors			
PTU	++++	+	+/−
Aurothioglucose	++++	++	++
Iopanoic acid	+++	++++	+++

Data from St. Germain and Galton,[38] Leonard and Visser,[39] Jakobs et al.,[40] Celi et al.,[41] Hernández et al.,[42] Leonard et al.,[43,45] and Curcio-Morelli et al.[44]

DTT, Dithiothreitol; *PTU*, propylthiouracil; T_4, thyroxine; T_4S, thyroxine sulfate; T_3, 3,5,3′-triiodothyronine; rT_3, reverse triiodothyronine; T_2S, 3,3′-diiodothyronine sulfate.
*Human only.

hormone metabolism include the iodinated radiographic contrast agents iopanoic acid (Telepaque) and sodium ipodate (Oragrafin). These small phenolic compounds act as substrate analogues and inhibit all three deiodinases in a competitive manner. To date, no selective inhibitors of D2 or D3 have been described—a situation that has significantly limited experimental investigations into their physiologic roles.

TISSUE PATTERNS OF EXPRESSION

An intriguing feature of the deiodinases is their pattern of tissue expression (see Table 4-2). The liver, kidney, thyroid gland, and pituitary gland express high levels of D1, with lesser amounts found in the brain.[16,55,56] In contrast, D2 is most abundant in the pituitary gland and brown adipose tissue (in rodents), with significant amounts also noted in the central nervous system.[16] Studies using in situ hybridization and immunocytochemistry have demonstrated that D2 expression in the brain appears to be confined to certain subpopulations of astroglial cells, such as the tanycytes lining the third ventricle of the hypothalamus, which suggests that they serve as the principal site of T_3 production in this tissue.[57-59] In humans, D2 expression appears more widespread; the mRNA for this enzyme has been noted in the heart, skeletal muscle, and thyroid gland,[54,60] as well as in coronary artery smooth muscle cells.[61]

In adult mammals, D3 expression occurs primarily in the brain, with significant amounts also present in the skin.[62,63] The brain is thus the only tissue that expresses all three deiodinases, although these are generally found in different subregions of this tissue and in different cell types. Thus, as opposed to the expression of D2 by glial cells, D3 is expressed primarily in neurons.[64,65]

Finally, as detailed below, deiodinase expression patterns during pregnancy and development are of critical importance, with high levels of D3 activity present in the uterus, the placenta, and several fetal tissues.[66,67]

STRUCTURAL CHARACTERISTICS

Important structural features of the deiodinases have been deduced from the results of molecular cloning experiments.[37] All the enzymes have a molecular mass of approximately 29 to 32 kDa, function as homodimers,[43-45] and are selenoproteins in that they contain the uncommon amino acid selenocysteine as the reactive residue in the catalytic cleft (Fig. 4-2).[68] The importance of this amino acid to enzymatic activity is demonstrated by experiments in which selenocysteine has been replaced by cysteine. Such a substitution decreases the catalytic efficiency of the mutant protein to less than 1% of that of the native enzyme.[69] In the case of D3, the cysteine mutant also demonstrates an altered substrate preference.[70] It is remarkable that substitution of selenocysteine for a serine residue in a monoclonal antibody

raised against T_4 confers on the protein deiodinase activity with catalytic properties similar to the D1, including sensitivity to PTU inhibition.[71]

The importance of selenocysteine to deiodination likely derives from its being ionized at physiologic pH, thus serving as a much more potent nucleophile than cysteine.[72] Incorporation of selenocysteine into the deiodinases and other selenoproteins occurs at the time of translation and is directed by a specific stem-loop structure in the 3′-untranslated region of the mRNA termed a selenocysteine insertion sequence.[73] A unique tRNA (Sec-tRNA[Sec]), a specific RNA binding protein, and a specialized elongation factor also are required for efficient synthesis of selenoproteins.[74,75]

In earlier studies, it was suggested that a 29 kDa (p29) nonselenoprotein, almost identical in sequence to a member of the Dickkopf protein family (Dkk3), was a substrate binding subunit of the D2.[76] However, Montero-Pedrazuela et al. have demonstrated a marked difference in spatial expression patterns in the brain of the p29 and the D2 selenodeiodinase,[77] and as recently reported, mice deficient in the Dkk3 protein do not have any consistent alterations in thyroid hormone status or D2 activity in their tissues.[78] These findings strongly suggest that the p29 protein is not relevant to D2 activity or to thyroid hormone homeostasis.

The overall amino acid identity of the three deiodinase isoforms is less than 30%. However, a high degree of homology is present in the regions of the selenocysteine and a conserved histidine residue (Fig. 4-3A). These areas show significant structural similarities to the thioredoxin-fold family of proteins and to α-L-iduronidase, respectively.[79] Based on these structural homologies, Callebaut et al.[79] and others have reported mutagenesis studies that define further the structure-function correlates of the deiodinase isoforms, including the identification of a key serine residue in the D1 active catalytic site that appears to confer sensitivity to PTU.[80]

In addition, all deiodinases contain a hydrophobic region near the N-terminus,[81] and subcellular fractionation studies have confirmed that these enzymes are integral membrane proteins.[82,83] Such studies, along with fluorescent microscopy of epitope-tagged enzymes, have demonstrated that the D2 is located in the endoplasmic reticulum,[82,84] whereas a significant fraction of the D3 has been reported to be in the plasma membrane.[85] The location of the D1 may vary in different tissues; in renal epithelial cells, the D1 has been localized to the basolateral plasma membranes,[86] whereas in the liver, it appears to reside in the endoplasmic reticulum (Pallud, Croteau, and St. Germain, unpublished observations). Studies by Friesema et al.[87] demonstrate that the catalytic effectiveness of all three deiodinases is markedly increased when specific thyroid hormone transporters are coexpressed with the deiodinases in cultured cells. This finding indicates that the active catalytic sites of these enzymes are located in the intracellular compartment.

GENETIC CONSIDERATIONS AND KNOCKOUT MOUSE MODELS

The three deiodinase isoforms are coded in mammals by three different genes located in humans on chromosomes 1 (D1) and 14 (D2 and D3), as indicated in Table 4-2.[40-42] Although their genetic structure appears relatively simple in that they contain only four, three, and a single exon, respectively (Fig. 4-3B),[40,88,89] surprising complexities that may influence expression patterns have been identified.[90,91] For example, the *DIO3* gene locus also expresses antisense transcripts from the *DIO3os* gene coded on

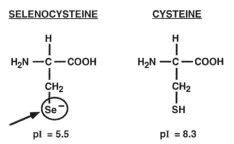

FIGURE 4-2. Comparison of the structures of selenocysteine and cysteine. Selenocysteine is ionized at physiologic pH, which likely contributes to the catalytic efficiencies of the deiodinases.

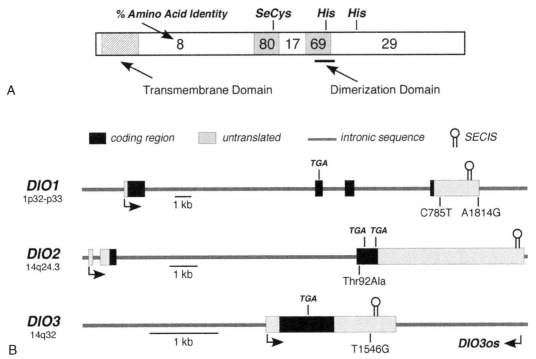

FIGURE 4-3. Structural features of the deiodinase proteins and genes. **A,** The proteins are composed of 257 to 278 amino acids with predicted molecular masses of 29 to 32 kDa. The hydrophobic transmembrane domain near the amino terminus, the selenocysteine residue (SeC), and two histidines (His) essential for catalytic activity are conserved in all three isoforms. The percentage of amino acid identity between the three isoforms in different portions of the molecule is given. A high degree of homology is noted in the regions surrounding the selenocysteine and one of the histidines. The dimerization domain as defined in the D1 is also shown. **B,** The structures of the genes, including the locations of the selenocysteine-encoding TGA codons and the regions coding for the selenocysteine insertion sequences (SECIS) located in the 3′-untranslated regions, are shown. Polymorphisms identified in each of the genes are also shown. *DIO3os* refers to the gene that encodes transcripts from the opposite DNA strand in the *DIO3* locus and that remains incompletely characterized.

the opposite DNA strand, and in the mouse fetus, the D3 is imprinted; transcription preferentially occurs from the paternal allele.[91] In humans the *DIO3* is also located within an imprinted region of chromosome 14.[91] This pattern of organization and expression of the D3 often is observed for genes important in development.[92]

To enhance our understanding of the physiologic roles of the deiodinases, genetic knockout models of each of the isoforms have been developed and partially characterized (Table 4-3).[93-100] D1-deficient mice show no general phenotypic abnormalities, although serum T_4 and rT_3 levels are modestly elevated, and the excretion patterns of iodothyronines in the feces and of iodine in the urine are significantly altered.[93] D2-deficient mice are viable and fertile in a protected laboratory setting. However, observed impairments in hearing,[96] thermogenesis,[95] and neurocognition[97] in these mutants would likely result in lethality in the wild. These animals also manifest elevated T_4 and thyroid-stimulating hormone (TSH) levels and show a marked selective resistance to the feedback effects of T_4, demonstrating the importance of D2 in pituitary thyrotroph regulation.[94] This contrasts with D1-deficient mice, in which TSH levels are normal.[93] This implies that the D1 expressed in the pituitary is not involved in TSH regulation.

A striking finding in the D1- and D2-deficent mouse models is that serum T_3 levels are normal.[93,94] Indeed, in mice cross-bred to yield a combined D1 and D2 deficiency, the serum T_3 level is only minimally decreased (V. A. Galton, unpublished observations).[101] This finding is both unexpected and difficult to explain, given that 5′-deiodination in peripheral tissues is supposed to contribute 80% of the T_3 production in humans and 45% in rats,

with the remainder secreted directly from the thyroid.[34,102] Given that the combined D1/D2 knockout mouse has been unequivocally shown to lack all 5′-deiodinating capacity, it is clear that at least in the rodent, thyroidal production and secretion of T_3, perhaps combined with a decreased rate of T_3 clearance from D1 deficiency, can compensate and maintain serum T_3 levels that are essentially normal in the face of an inability to convert T_4 to T_3 in all tissues. A surprising corollary to this observation is that a D1 deficiency does not appear to significantly compromise T_3 secretion from the rodent thyroid, a tissue in which this enzyme is highly expressed and previously was thought to be essential for T_3 production.[102,103] This suggests that under physiologic conditions, D1 acts primarily as a "scavenger" enzyme that prevents the buildup of lesser iodothyronines (rT_3, T_2s, T_1) and sulfated derivatives in the thyroid gland, blood, and tissues.

The extent to which humans may be able to compensate for at least a partial impairment in 5′-deiodinating capacity has recently been reported. Although to date no mutations in the deiodinase genes in humans have been described, Dumitrescu et al.[104] have described two families with partially inactivating mutations in the selenocysteine insertion sequence-binding protein2 (SBP2), which is essential for the synthesis of selenoproteins, including the deiodinases.[74] Affected individuals demonstrate short stature and delayed bone age along with modest abnormalities in serum thyroid hormone levels, including increases in total T_4 and rT_3.[104] Notably, total serum T_3 levels were only minimally reduced, whereas TSH levels were at the upper part of the reference range and proved relatively resistant to suppression by administered T_4, but not T_3. These findings are very similar to those observed in knockout mice with a com-

Table 4-3. Phenotypic Features of Deiodinase
Knockout Mice

___

D1-Deficient Mouse[93]

Viable
Normal growth
Normal fertility
Elevated serum T_4 and rT_3, normal serum T_3 and TSH in adults
Enhanced fecal excretion endogenous iodothyronines

D2-Deficient Mouse

Viable[94]
Mild growth delay in males[94]
Normal fertility[94]
Elevated serum T_4 and TSH, normal serum T_3[94]
Pituitary resistance to T_4[94]
Impaired thermogenesis[95,98]
Impaired hearing[96]
Mild impairment neurocognition[231]

D3-Deficient Mouse[99,100]

Increased perinatal mortality
Marked growth retardation
Impaired fertility in females and males
Hyperthyroidism in the perinatal period
Moderate hypothyroidism in adulthood
Impaired responsiveness of the thyroid gland, pituitary, and hypothalamus

___

bined deficiency in D1 and D2, as noted previously. Indeed, a deficiency in D2 activity was demonstrated in cultured skin fibroblasts from affected patients.[104]

Mice deficient in D3 present the most severe phenotype, likely as a result of the importance of this enzyme during the developmental period. Observed abnormalities include significant perinatal mortality, growth retardation, impaired fertility, and altered systemic thyroid hormone levels during the perinatal period (transient hyperthyroidism) and in adulthood (moderate hypothyroidism).[99,100] Multiple abnormalities, including impaired response of the thyroid gland to TSH and of the pituitary to TRH, have been observed at all levels of the thyroid axis in the D3-deficient adult mouse. The response to hypothyroidism of TRH mRNA production in the hypothalamus and of pituitary TSH production is also markedly impaired. Many of these abnormalities are similar to those observed in human infants born to mothers with poorly controlled hyperthyroidism during pregnancy[105,106] or to rodents treated with large doses of thyroid hormone during the perinatal period.[107,108] These findings demonstrate that strict control of thyroid hormone levels during development by D3 is critical for proper development of the thyroid axis.

REGULATION

The deiodinases are regulated by multiple hormones, growth factors, and environmental and nutritional factors.[34] Foremost among these are the thyroid hormones themselves; alterations in thyroid status induce profound changes in enzyme activity (see Table 4-2). Hypothyroidism is associated with a marked decrease in D1 and D3 levels, whereas D2 activity increases severalfold. Opposite changes occur in hyperthyroidism. These changes result from both pretranslational and posttranslational mechanisms.[34] For example, D1 and D3 mRNA levels are increased in the hyperthyroid state,[53,109] and D2 mRNA is decreased.[54] Hyperthyroidism also results in rapid downregulation of D2 activity by ubiquitination of the D2 protein.[110,111] This induces a reversible conformational change in the enzyme's dimerization structure, which results in reversible loss of activity and eventually may

target the enzyme for proteasomal degradation.[112] Considerable progress has been made in defining the molecular mechanisms involved in transcriptional control of the deiodinases; this topic has been reviewed recently by Gereben et al.[37] Of particular interest has been the observation by Simonides et al.[113] that hypoxia induces D3 expression in several cell culture systems, as well as in ischemic myocardium.

Other important regulatory effects on deiodinase activity are noted in the thyroid gland, where TSH and thyroid-stimulating immunoglobulins stimulate both D1 and D2 activity[60]; in brown adipose tissue, where cold exposure,[114] bile acids,[115] or intracerebroventricular administration of leptin[116] markedly stimulates D2 activity; and in the liver, where nutritional deprivation, diabetes, tumor necrosis factor, and other cytokines decrease D1 activity (see also below).[109,117,118] In addition, D2 activity in the brain displays a significant diurnal variation.[119] Although the physiologic significance of this remains to be determined, in some seasonal breeding species, rhythmic alterations in D2 and D3 activity in the central nervous system, perhaps mediated by melatonin,[120] appear to be integral responses to changes in the photoperiod.[121,122]

Alternative Routes of Iodothyronine Metabolism

In addition to deiodination, iodothyronines are metabolized by multiple other mechanisms.[123] In this regard, conjugation of the phenolic ring hydroxyl group to sulfate or glucuronide probably represents the second most prevalent mechanism of thyroid hormone metabolism.[16] Sulfation and glucuronidation are inactivating reactions because the compounds formed are devoid of thyromimetic activity, do not bind to nuclear thyroid hormone receptors, and are rapidly metabolized by D1 or excreted in bile.[4,16] However, sulfation is a reversible process that occurs through the action of tissue sulfatases or bacterial sulfatases in the intestine.[124] Thus T_3 sulfate (T_3S) injected into hypothyroid rats demonstrates approximately 20% of the thyromimetic activity of native T_3 because of liberation of this active hormone.[125]

Sulfotransferases in the cytoplasm of many tissues serve to catalyze the formation of iodothyronine sulfate conjugates. In rat tissue homogenates, $3,3'$-T_2 and T_3 appear to be the best substrates for sulfation.[46] Although the exact enzymes mediating iodothyronine sulfation are uncertain, the phenol sulfotransferases found in human liver and kidney have been demonstrated in vitro to possess this activity.[126] Sensitive and specific radioimmunoassays for various iodothyronine sulfates have been developed and used to demonstrate detectable but very low levels of T_3S, rT_3S, and T_4S in normal adult human serum.[46] These low circulating levels probably reflect the rapid metabolism of these compounds by D1. Evidence for this thesis comes from experiments in animals and humans, in which treatment with inhibitors of D1 activity, such as PTU or iopanoic acid, results in marked increases in iodothyronine sulfoconjugate levels in both serum and bile.[127,128] In other circumstances where D1 activity is low or impaired, such as during fetal life, in hypothyroidism, or in nonthyroidal illness, serum levels of these compounds also are elevated, either in absolute terms or relative to the native, unconjugated iodothyronines.[16] To date, the physiologic role of sulfation in thyroid hormone economy has not been clearly defined, although it appears to represent an important component of the degradative process.

Glucuronidation of iodothyronines followed by their secretion into bile represents another pathway of iodothyronine clearance. Studies in humans, however, suggest that this pathway accounts for less than 1% of the total clearance of T_4 by the liver, and only minute amounts of these conjugates are present in plasma.[5,129]

Two enzymes, L-amino acid oxidase and thyroid hormone aminotransferase, have been implicated in catalyzing the deamination of T_4 and T_3 to their acetic acid analogues Tetrac and Triac, respectively.[130] Current evidence suggests, however, that these reactions occur to only a limited extent in normal humans. Triac has intrinsic biological activity equivalent to that of T_3 when tested in in vitro assay systems,[130] and it binds with greater avidity than T_3 to the β isoform of the thyroid hormone receptor.[1] Injection of Triac into humans or animals results in significant physiologic effects; however, relatively large doses are required because of its apparent rapid clearance and degradation via deiodination and glucuronidation.[131] Despite its short half-life, Triac has been used successfully in the treatment of thyroid hormone resistance states.[1] As in the case of sulfated conjugates, levels of Triac and its conjugates increase in circumstances in which D1 activity is low or impaired, such as during fasting or treatment with PTU or iopanoic acid.[130] The physiologic relevance of these observations is uncertain but could be important, given Triac's significant intrinsic activity. As noted earlier, the novel compound 3-iodothyronamine, formed by sequential deiodination and decarboxylation of thyroid hormones, may have important physiologic effects in some species, although its role in humans has not yet been defined.[10,11]

A final mechanism of thyroid hormone metabolism involves oxidative cleavage of the ether link of T_4 and T_3 by phagocytosing leukocytes.[132] Current evidence suggests that this pathway is a minor one for iodothyronine degradation, except in the special circumstances of severe bacterial infection.

Thyroid Hormone Uptake Into Cells

Although some nongenomic effects of thyroid hormones may be triggered directly by hormones residing within the extracellular space via binding to cell surface receptors,[133] the effects of these compounds on gene transcription, as well as on other cellular events, require their uptake into the cellular compartment. Similarly, the metabolic processes described above likely take place in various intracellular locations.[87] Thus, the uptake of thyroid hormones into cells is a prerequisite for their affecting physiologic functions and for their metabolism.

Several membrane proteins capable of transporting thyroid hormones into and perhaps out of cells have been identified recently.[134] Members of the organic anion-transporting polypeptide (OATP) family[135] and the monocarboxylate transporter (MCT) family[136] have been best characterized with regard to their capacity to affect cellular uptake and facilitate metabolism of various thyroid hormones. OATP1C1 has a relatively high affinity for T_4 and rT_3 and is highly expressed in capillaries in the rodent brain, suggesting a role in the transport of T_4 across the blood-brain barrier. It also is widely expressed in the human brain.[137] The MCT8 transporter facilitates cellular uptake of T_3 and T_4 when expressed in *Xenopus laevis* oocytes and cultured COS1 cells, and results in marked enhancement in the rate of iodothyronine metabolism by the deiodinases.[87,138] The transporter is expressed in the choroid plexus and neuronal cells in the brain, as well as in the liver, kidney, heart, and placenta.[134] It also appears to facilitate thyroid hormone exit from cells, which is likely important for overall cellular homeostasis.[134]

Recently, knockout mouse models of MCT8 deficiency have been described that verify the importance of this transporter in thyroid hormone homeostasis.[139,140] Key features of these mice include elevations in serum T_3 level, decreases in serum T_4 and rT_3 levels, and decreased brain content of T_3. Deiodinase activities are also altered in several tissues secondary to tissue-specific patterns of thyroid hormone uptake. Thus, D1 expression is increased in the liver as the result of thyrotoxicosis in that organ (despite MCT8 deficiency) from high serum T_3 levels, whereas the relative brain hypothyroidism results in elevated D2 activity and decreased D3 activity in that tissue. It is surprising to note that the neurologic phenotype of MCT8-deficient mice appears to be mild. This contrasts sharply with the severe phenotype of humans bearing mutations in MCT8, which results in the Allan-Herndon-Dudley syndrome.[141] Male patients with this disorder (the *MCT8* gene is located on the X chromosome) display poor muscle tone, an inability to speak, and severe mental retardation. Serum thyroid hormone parameters in these patients are analogous to those observed in MCT8-deficient mice. The striking differences in neurological phenotype between the two species is as yet unexplained.

An Integrated View of Thyroid Hormone Metabolism

The preceding discussion has served to highlight the extraordinary complexity of thyroid hormone metabolism. Two critical features of this intricate system are apparent. First, the uptake and metabolic fate of iodothyronines vary significantly in different organs and even in different cell types within an organ, thus providing multiple mechanisms whereby thyroid hormone content and action can regulate differential metabolic control over physiologic processes. Second, these metabolic processes and in particular the rates of deiodination are regulated by several factors, which suggests that alterations in thyroid hormone metabolism may be important in adapting to internal and external homeostatic challenges.

ALTERED THYROID STATES

Several examples of these principles can be cited, starting first with the response to alterations in thyroid hormone status. Experimental studies, as well as clinical experience, indicate that serum T_3 levels tend to be maintained within the normal range in patients with moderate degrees of hypothyroidism despite the attendant hypothyroxinemia.[142,143] Several factors, including an increase in the relative proportion of T_3 secreted from the thyroid gland and an increase in the proportion of T_4 converted to T_3 in extrathyroidal tissue, appear to be responsible for this finding[144] (Fig. 4-4). Both of these effects result from increased rates of 5′-deiodination. Thus in the thyroid gland, D1 and D2 activities are stimulated by the increase in TSH that accompanies hypothyroidism.[60] In peripheral tissues, T_4 to T_3 conversion mediated by D2, which recently has been postulated to be the major source of plasma T_3 in euthyroid humans,[145] is also relatively enhanced by increased D2 activity.[54] As a result, T_4 is used more efficiently for T_3 production. In addition, the rate of T_3 clearance in extrathyroidal tissues is decreased. This decrease probably results in

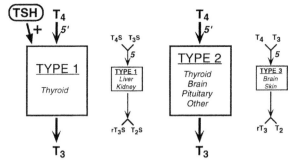

FIGURE 4-4. Autoregulation of thyroid hormone metabolism that accompanies the hypothyroid state, as might occur in iodine deficiency. D1 activity in the thyroid is stimulated by thyroid-stimulating hormone (TSH). Although this enzyme is relatively inefficient in converting T_4 to T_3, in the high T_4 environment of the thyroid gland, this may serve to increase the proportion of T_3 formed and secreted by this organ. Concurrently, D1 activity in extrathyroidal tissues is reduced, thereby decreasing the degradation of T_4 and T_3 by the 5-deiodination of their sulfated analogues. D2 activity is increased in all tissues that express this enzyme, which increases the proportion of T_4 to T_3 conversion in both the thyroid and peripheral tissues. Finally, D3 activity is decreased, again serving to diminish T_4 and T_3 degradation by 5-deiodinase processes. The net effect of these changes is to increase the relative rate of T_3 production and decrease T_3 degradation, thereby preserving the circulating and tissue levels of this active hormone in the presence of a diminished supply of T_4.

part from diminished 5-deiodination caused by the decreases in D1 and D3 activity that have been observed in the hypothyroid state. The physiologic importance of these extrathyroidal mechanisms, which in essence act as a form of peripheral autoregulation to help maintain T_3 levels, is easily demonstrated by the administration of varying doses of T_4 to athyreotic individuals. Under such circumstances, the circulating T_3/T_4 ratio is highest when low doses of T_4 are given, and the ratio progressively declines as full replacement and then supraphysiologic doses are provided.[142,143] Alterations in the rates of nondeiodinative pathways may contribute to this response. The net effect of these metabolic adaptations is to minimize the decrease in circulating T_3 levels in the face of impaired secretion from the thyroid gland.

In the hyperthyroid state that occurs with Graves' disease, D1 activity is markedly increased both in peripheral tissues (as a result of the thyrotoxic state) and in the thyroid gland (because of thyroid-stimulating immunoglobulins that mimic the D1-stimulating effects of TSH).[34] Although relatively inefficient in converting T_4 to T_3, this enhanced D1 activity has been shown recently to be the major source of circulating T_3 in this condition, as well as in toxic multinodular goiter, with much of the D1-mediated T_3 production occurring in the hyperactive thyroid gland itself.[103] However, given the marked increase in thyroidal T_4 and T_3 production in the hyperthyroid state, the increase in D1 expression in extrathyroidal tissues appears to be paradoxical in that it would serve to further increase serum T_3 levels. But such may not be the case; the administration of high doses of T_3 to D1-deficient mice results in both higher serum T_3 levels and a greater degree of tissue thyrotoxicosis as compared with thyrotoxic wild-type animals.[93] Thus, enhanced expression of D1 in the liver and kidney of hyperthyroid animals may serve to actually mitigate the increase in serum T_3, and thus the degree of thyrotoxicosis, presumably as a result of the inactivating 5-deiodinating capability of this enzyme.

The changes in D2 and D3 activity observed in hypothyroidism and hyperthyroidism have important additional effects. In organs that express these enzymes, alterations in activity provide a local mechanism for the maintenance of T_3 concentrations at the cellular level. Thus in the hypothyroid rat infused with increasing doses of T_4, normalization of the T_3 content of D2-expressing tissues, such as the cerebral cortex, cerebellum, and brown adipose tissue, is attained at much lower infusion rates than are required by other tissues.[146] This presumably reflects an enhanced rate of T_4 to T_3 conversion in these tissues by the elevated D2 activity. In contrast, the increased level of D3 expression in the brain that accompanies hyperthyroidism may explain why nuclear T_3 levels are observed to be normal in most regions of this organ under this abnormal condition.[147] The deiodinases thus appear to provide an additional level of autoregulation in tissues where thyroid hormone effects are especially critical.

DEVELOPMENT

Thyroid hormones are of unquestioned importance to the developing fetus and during the neonatal period; hypothyroidism at this time can result in the clinical syndrome of cretinism characterized by severe neurologic impairment.[148] However, exposure during development to excessive levels of thyroid hormones promotes premature differentiation of fetal tissues and thus is also detrimental.[149,150] Throughout most of gestation, circulating levels of total T_4 and total T_3 in the mammalian fetus are extremely low,[151] although significant amounts of free hormone have been demonstrated in amniotic fluid and fetal serum.[152] Thus a key role of the uteroplacental unit is to limit access of the large pool of maternal thyroid hormones to the fetus while at the same time allowing small, but appropriate amounts of hormone to reach the developing embryo.[153] This is accomplished by expression in the pregnant uterus[25,154] and in the placenta[67] of exceedingly high levels of D3 activity. (D2 is also expressed in these tissues, although its role remains undefined.[66,155]) Uterine D3 and D2 activities are regulated in a complex fashion by estrogens, progesterone, and probably other factors.[156,157] However, the marked rise in uterine D3 expression observed during pregnancy is induced immediately and directly by implantation and represents an integral aspect of the uterine decidualization reaction.[156] As implied above, high levels of D3 in the pregnant uterus and subsequently in the placenta do not result in a complete barrier to the transfer of maternal thyroid hormones to the fetus, as evidenced by the finding of significant levels of T_4 and T_3 at term in the serum of athyreotic infants.[158] Transporter proteins such as MCT8 likely also play an important role in thyroid hormone homeostasis in the fetal-placental unit.[159]

Most mammalian fetal tissues, including the human fetal brain,[160,161] also express deiodinases, with D3 activity largely predominating in the early and mid stages of development.[66] During the later stages of gestation and in the neonatal period, after fetal thyroid function has been initiated, expression of 5'-deiodinases becomes more prevalent. In this regard, expression of D2 in the fetal and neonatal brain appears to be critically important for supplying T_3 for the normal development of this tissue.[162] This concept has been verified directly with regard to cochlear development; failure of the normal induction of D2 expression in the rodent cochlea shortly after birth results in marked hearing impairment.[96,163] However, D2 expression in the developing brain may not be essential, or even important, in all brain regions, as demonstrated by the observation that the neurologic phenotype of the D2KO mouse is relatively mild compared with the rodent with developmental hypothyroidism.[97] This observation points to an important role of T_3 derived from the serum, which is the sole source of brain T_3 in the developing D2KO mouse, in neurologic development.

The ordered and timely expression of the deiodinases during development is also critically important in lower species such as the metamorphosing tadpole.[164-167]

An important aspect of thyroid hormone metabolism during development relates to the very high levels of sulfated iodothyronines that circulate in the fetus, most likely as a result of the low D1 levels that occur during development and the fact that these metabolites are not efficiently degraded by D3.[168] This observation has led to speculation that fetal T_3S could serve as a reservoir of T_3 that becomes available later in pregnancy through the actions of tissue sulfatases.[169]

FASTING AND ILLNESS

Profound changes occur in thyroid hormone economy during states of fasting and severe systemic illness, as detailed elsewhere in this volume. In humans, as well as in various animal models, the hallmark features induced by these conditions consist of marked decreases in the serum levels of total and free T_3, accompanied by an inappropriately normal or reduced serum TSH level.[170,171] Serum T_4 levels are also reduced in fasted rodents and in critically ill humans. These alterations in circulating thyroid hormone levels are accompanied by reduced tissue levels of T_3,[172] and the severity of these changes in acute illness correlates closely with patient mortality rates.[173] This generalized suppression of the thyroid axis is hypothesized by some observers to be of adaptive benefit in that it is associated with a significant decline in basal metabolic rate (BMR) in both humans and rodents,[174,175] and it appears to lessen protein and fat catabolism.[176,177]

The triggering and homeostatic mechanisms that underlie this response of the thyroid axis are complex and remain poorly understood despite decades of experimental observations. Given the importance of the deiodinases in the maintenance of peripheral and tissue thyroid hormone levels, alterations in the expression and activity of these enzymes have been postulated to play important roles in the development of this syndrome.[171] In particular, decreases in serum and tissue T_3 levels observed in nutritional deprivation and illness have been attributed, at least in part, to the decreases in D1 activity and/or increases in D3 activity observed experimentally in the liver, muscle, heart, and other tissues of humans and experimental animals.[109,113,173,178-180] In fasted or ill rodents, increased activity of D2 and decreased activity of D3 locally in the hypothalamus have been postulated to result in increased T_3 levels in this tissue, thereby preventing or blunting the rise in TRH, and subsequently TSH, that otherwise would be expected to result from decreased serum T_3 and T_4 levels.[181-183]

However, it is important to note that these concepts are based entirely on indirect evidence. For example, the current concept that peripheral T_3 production rates are diminished in fasting and illness is derived largely from in vivo kinetic studies that attempt to define rates of T_4 and T_3 production and clearance from serum measurements alone.[184] Unfortunately, such studies are prone to misinterpretation. Thus, in the only two studies in which the in vivo rate of T_4 to T_3 conversion was measured directly in whole animals subjected to fasting, by injecting animals with $^{[125]}I$-T_4 and quantifying $^{[125]}I$-T_3 appearance, the fraction of T_4 converted to T_3 was approximately doubled, and total T_3 production was unchanged.[185,186] It thus appears that much of the T_3 produced during fasting remains in the tissues, where it may be metabolized via other pathways, and is not exchanged with the plasma T_3 pool.[186] Such results serve to highlight the methodologic

shortcomings inherent in kinetic studies of thyroid hormone metabolism in humans or rodents, where sampling is limited to the plasma compartment.

Caution should also be exercised in inferring causality between in vitro–determined deiodination rates in tissue homogenates and observed alterations in systemic thyroid hormone parameters.[173] Studies conducted in deiodinase-deficient animals call into question the validity of such correlations. Thus, the changes in serum T_4, T_3, and TSH observed in fasted D1/D2KO mice are virtually identical to those in fasted wild-type mice (Galton/St. Germain, unpublished observations), and D3KO mice subjected to bacterial infection develop a nonthyroidal illness–type syndrome to the same extent as do infected wild-type mice.[187] Notably, however, changes in deiodinase activities could affect T_3 availability in selected cells or tissues and therefore could be important in the *local* response to nutritional deprivation, hypoxia, or inflammation, as suggested by Simonides et al.[113]

THERMOGENESIS

T_3 and other thyroid hormone derivatives (e.g., 3,5-T_2, 3-iodothyronamine) have been implicated in the control of metabolic rate and thermogenesis by both genomic and nongenomic mechanisms[11,188] (vide supra). D2 has been demonstrated to be a key modulator of T_3 availability and thus thermogenesis in brown adipose tissue (BAT) and other organs.[95] The importance of D2 in energetic pathways has been highlighted recently by the report that in mice, the induction of D2 in BAT by bile acids, working through a unique G protein–coupled receptor (TGR5), protects against diet-induced obesity and insulin resistance.[115] This suggests that the selective induction of D2 in thermogenic tissues could have therapeutic value in the treatment of obesity and diabetes. In this regard, da Silva et al.[189] recently demonstrated that the small polyphenolic molecule kaempferol stimulates D2 activity and energy expenditure in cultured human skeletal muscle myoblasts.

EFFECTS OF SELENIUM

Nutritional selenium deprivation in experimental animals leads to characteristic changes in deiodinase activities and serum thyroid hormone levels.[68] The most profound changes are noted in the liver and kidney, where marked decreases in D1 activity are noted secondary to impaired translation of selenoproteins.[190] In tissues where selenium levels are better preserved, such as the thyroid gland and brain, deiodinase activities are altered to a lesser extent or not at all.[102,191,192] Thus changes in serum thyroid hormone levels in selenium deficiency resemble those observed in other model systems where D1 activity is impaired, namely, T_4 is increased and little change occurs in T_3 or TSH.[193] Similar observations in circulating hormone levels have been noted in human populations susceptible to selenium deficiency.[194,195] In these circumstances, dietary selenium supplementation results in small but significant decreases in serum T_4 levels and increases in the T_3/T_4 ratio, thus suggesting restoration of D1 activity. The clinical consequences of these changes have not been determined. It is notable that a recently reported randomized control trial of selenium supplementation in patients in an intensive care unit with severe sepsis found no direct effect of selenium on free and total serum thyroid hormone levels, although patient morbidity seemed to be lessened.[196]

Of note are reported cases of worsening hypothyroidism developing in individuals with combined selenium and iodine deficiency who were given selenium supplements alone.[197] It is postulated that under such circumstances, restoration of D1 activity enhances T_4 metabolism and thereby worsens the iodine-induced hypothyroxinemic state. Thus concurrent iodine and selenium supplementation is required to restore thyroid hormone economy in this situation.

DRUG EFFECTS

Numerous drugs are known to affect the metabolism of thyroid hormones by directly interfering with enzymatic mechanisms or by altering the regulation of these processes.[198] The effect of PTU in inhibiting D1 activity provides it with a theoretical advantage over methimazole for use in the treatment of hyperthyroidism. In this condition, the increased expression of D1, combined with elevations in T_4 levels, probably contributes to the overproduction of T_3 in the thyroid gland.[103] However, this effect of PTU is noted only with relatively high doses of the drug (>1000 mg/day). At the usual doses prescribed for treating hyperthyroidism, methimazole (10 mg three times daily) actually results in more rapid restoration of the euthyroid state than does PTU (100 mg three times daily).[199]

As noted previously, oral radiographic contrast dyes (e.g., iopanoic acid, sodium ipodate) are potent competitive inhibitors of all three deiodinase isoforms. Although they now are rarely used in clinical medicine as diagnostic agents, the rapidity with which they lower circulating T_3 levels makes them extremely useful in the treatment of severe hyperthyroidism. For example, treatment of patients with Graves' disease with sodium ipodate (1 g daily per os) has been noted to lower serum T_3 levels by 58% within 24 hours of initiation of therapy—a decrease that is much greater than that noted with PTU (200 mg three times daily)[200] or a saturated solution of potassium iodide (12 drops SSKI daily).[201] Of importance, these decreases in serum T_3 levels are associated with rapid improvement in cardiovascular complications, with beneficial effects on systemic resistance and cardiac output noted within 3 to 6 hours after treatment initiation.[202] However, because of the high iodine content of these drugs, escape from their T_3-lowering effects and exacerbation of hyperthyroidism may occur after several days of therapy.[201] It thus is important that PTU or methimazole be administered concurrently to impair thyroidal secretion, and that use of the contrast agent be discontinued when thyrotoxicosis has been adequately controlled. It is notable that iopanoic acid (1 g daily per os for 13 days) has been used successfully to rapidly control the hyperthyroid state prior to thyroidectomy in patients with severe amiodarone-induced thyrotoxicosis.[203] (Iopanoic acid is currently available only from compounding pharmacies.)

Propranolol, in relatively modest doses (80 mg/day), also blocks the conversion of T_4 to T_3 by acting as a competitive inhibitor of 5'-deiodinase activity.[204] This drug therefore results in a 20% to 30% decrease in serum T_3 levels and a slight elevation in serum T_4 in hyperthyroid patients. Other commonly used β-blockers do not have this effect. High doses of glucocorticoids (e.g., 2 mg of dexamethasone four times daily) have been demonstrated to lower T_3 levels within 24 hours in hyperthyroid patients with Graves' disease,[205] as well as in euthyroid individuals.[23] This activity provides part of the rationale for the use of these agents in severe thyrotoxicosis. Animal studies have demonstrated that this effect is due, at least in part, to diminished total body production of T_3, and indeed, decreased D1 activity has been observed in the liver of dexamethasone-treated rats.[206] In addition, D2 activity in the brain of experimental animals is altered by several neuropharmacologic agents.[207]

Finally, the antiarrhythmic agent amiodarone is another iodine-rich compound that competitively inhibits the conversion of T_4 to T_3 and thus frequently causes a rise in serum T_4 levels and a modest decrease in serum T_3.[208] Although most patients who take this drug remain euthyroid as judged by normal serum TSH levels, the large quantities of iodine liberated during the course of its metabolism can result in hypothyroid or hyperthyroid states, with the latter at times being extremely difficult to treat.[209]

Emerging Roles of the Deiodinases in Human Disease

Germline mutations in the deiodinase genes that significantly affect their function or levels of expression have not yet been identified in humans. However, in addition to the conditions noted above, several human disease states are associated with alterations in deiodinase activities. Thus, those rare individuals with inactivating mutations in the SBP2 RNA-binding protein manifest a significant decrease in D2 activity[104] (vide supra). As a second example, patients with the McCune-Albright syndrome, which stems from activating mutations of the α subunit of the G stimulatory protein, have recently been demonstrated to have increases in thyroidal D1 and D2 activities.[210] This provides an explanation for the increase in the serum T_3/T_4 ratio that is frequently encountered in these patients and the occurrence during childhood of frank T_3 toxicosis. The increase in these 5'-deiodinases is believed to be secondary to the elevation in thyroidal cyclic adenosine monophosphate (cAMP) levels that is known to stimulate D2 expression.[211]

High levels of D1 and/or D2 expression also have been observed in metastatic foci of thyroid follicular carcinoma, again resulting in an increased T_3/T_4 ratio in patients with this disease.[212,213] In cases of widely metastatic disease, T_3 toxicosis may develop, depending on the amount of thyroxine supplementation that is provided.[213,214] Thus, in patients with this condition, monitoring of the serum T_3 level, in addition to serum T_4 and TSH, is indicated to avoid a thyrotoxic state. Increased D2[215] and D1[216] activities also have been observed in toxic adenomas of the thyroid gland, and this likely contributes to the thyrotoxic state.

Perhaps the most dramatic example of deiodinase overexpression is the extraordinarily high level of D3 activity observed in some infantile hepatic hemangiomas.[217] The "ectopic" D3 expression in these typically large tumors results in markedly enhanced clearance rates of T_4 and T_3, which overwhelm the synthetic capability of the thyroid gland and lead to a state of "consumptive hypothyroidism." Very large doses of thyroid hormone supplements typically need to be administered if these patients are to be maintained in a euthyroid state. Recently, a 3-month-old infant with this condition was treated successfully with liver transplantation.[218] Two cases of adults with consumptive hypothyroidism—one with a vascular hepatic tumor[219] and another with a large fibrous abdominal tumor—have been described.[220] D3 expression has also been reported in TSH-secreting pituitary adenomas, which may contribute to the observed resistance of these tumors to feedback by thyroid hormones.[221]

Finally, polymorphisms in the three human deiodinase genes have been reported (Fig. 4-3B), and much interest has been focused on possible clinical associations with these genetic variations.[222] For example, Mentuccia et al.[223] identified a polymorphism in the coding region of the human *DIO2* gene that results in a nonconserved amino acid substitution of alanine for threonine at position 92 (Thr92Ala). Evidence has been presented that suggests that patients homozygous for the alanine variant exhibit decreased D2 activity in skeletal muscle.[224] In an initial study, the alanine variant was found to be common in Pima Indians and Mexican Americans (allele frequencies of 0.75 and 0.42, respectively), in whom it was strongly associated with insulin resistance, and in patients carrying a second polymorphism in the β_3-adrenergic receptor (Trp64Arg), with obesity.[223] In small studies that used a different population group, an association with insulin resistance was again noted. However, studies of larger unselected populations have found no association between the alanine variant and the risk for diabetes or obesity.[225,226] A similar lack of consistency between study results has been noted with regard to a possible association between this variant and hypertension.[227,228] In other studies, polymorphisms in the 3′-untranslated region of the human *DIO1* gene have been associated with small (3% to 7%) but significant differences in serum free T_4, total T_3, and free T_3 levels in older subjects, as well as with changes in body composition.[229,230]

Summary

The extrathyroidal systems that mediate thyroid hormone uptake and metabolism work in concert with the hypothalamic-pituitary-thyroid axis to regulate the availability and thus influence the action of thyroid hormones in peripheral tissues. The presence and activity of these metabolic pathways differ significantly between tissues and with developmental state, thus allowing T_3 content to vary from organ to organ, and even from cell type to cell type. These prereceptor processes represent critical adaptive mechanisms that help to maintain T_3 homeostasis in response to environmental and internal stresses. Knowledge of these pathways is important for understanding the changes in tissue and plasma thyroid hormone levels that accompany a variety of thyroidal and nonthyroidal diseases, as well as for optimizing therapy for hypothyroidism and hyperthyroidism. Further studies will likely provide additional insight into the biochemistry and physiologic roles of the enzymes and transporters that mediate these important homeostatic processes.

REFERENCES

1. Takeda T, Suzuki S, Liu RT, et al: Triiodothyroacetic acid has unique potential for therapy of resistance to thyroid hormone, J Clin Endocrinol Metab 80:2033–2040, 1995.
2. Yen PM, Ando S, Feng X, et al: Thyroid hormone action at the cellular, genomic and target gene levels, Mol Cell Endocrinol 246:121–127, 2006.
3. Pittman HA, Brown RW, Register HBJ: Biological activity of 3,3′,5′-triiodo-DL-thyronine, Endocrinology 70:79–83, 1962.
4. Spaulding SW, Smith TJ, Hinkle PM, et al: Studies on the biological activity of triiodothyronine sulfate, J Clin Endocrinol Metab 74:1062–1067, 1992.
5. Engler D, Burger AG: The deiodination of the iodothyronines and their derivatives in man, Endo Reviews 5:151–184, 1984.
6. Lombardi A, Lanni A, de Lange P, et al: Acute administration of 3,5-diiodo-L-thyronine to hypothyroid rats affects bioenergetic parameters in rat skeletal muscle mitochondria, FEBS Letters 581:5911–5916, 2007.
7. Moreno M, Lombardi A, Beneduce L, et al: Are the effects of T3 on resting metabolic rate in euthyroid rats entirely caused by T3 itself? Endocrinology 143:504–510, 2002.
8. Grasselli E, Canesi L, Voci A, et al: Effects of 3,5-diiodo-L-thyronine administration on the liver of high fat diet-fed rats, Exp Biol Med 233:549–557, 2008.
9. Lanni A, Moreno M, Lombardi A, et al: 3,5-diiodo-L-thyronine powerfully reduces adiposity in rats by increasing the burning of fats, FASEB J 19:1552–1554, 2005.
10. Scanlan TS, Suchland KL, Hart ME, et al: 3-Iodothyronamine is an endogenous and rapid-acting derivative of thyroid hormone, Nat Med 10:638–642, 2004.
11. Braulke LJ, Klingenspor M, DeBarber A, et al: 3-Iodothyronamine: a novel hormone controlling the balance between glucose and lipid utilization, J Comp Phys B, Biochem, System, Environ Physiol 178:167–177, 2008.
12. Moreno M, Kaptein E, Goglia F, et al: Rapid glucuronidation of tri- and tetraiodothyroacetic acid to ester glucuronides in human liver and to ether glucuronides in rat liver, Endocrinology 135:1004–1005, 1994.
13. Sorimachi K, Yasumura Y: High affinity of triiodothyronine (T3) for nonphenolic ring deiodinase and high affinity of tetraiodothyroacetic acid (TETRAC) for phenolic ring deiodinase in cultured monkey hepatocarcinoma cells and in rat liver homogenates, Endocrinol Jap 28:775–783, 1981.
14. Rutgers M, Heusdens FA, Visser TJ: Metabolism of triiodothyroacetic acid (TA₃) in rat liver. I. Deiodination of TA₃ and TA₃ sulfate by microsomes, Endocrinology 125:424–432, 1989.

15. Santini F, Hurd RE, Chopra IJ: A study of metabolism of deaminated and sulfoconjugated iodothyronines by rat placental iodothyronine 5-monodeiodinase, Endocrinology 131:1689–1694, 1992.
16. Visser TJ: Pathways of thyroid hormone metabolism, Acta Med Aust 23:10–16, 1996.
17. Chopra IJ, Boado RJ, Geffner DL, et al: A radioimmunoassay for measurement of thyronine and its acetic acid analog in urine, J Clin Endocrinol Metab 67:480–487, 1988.
18. LoPresti JS, Anderson KP, Nicoloff JT: Does a hidden pool of reverse triiodothyronine (rT3) production contribute to total thyroxine (T4) disposal in high T4 states in man? J Clin Endocrinol Metab 70:1479–1484, 1990.
19. Chopra IJ: Nature, sources, and relative biologic significance of circulating thyroid hormones. In Braverman LE, Utiger RD, editors: The Thyroid, ed 6. New York, 1991, Lippincott, 136–143.
20. Chopra IJ: Simultaneous measurement of free thyroxine and free 3,5,3′-triiodothyronine in undiluted serum by direct equilibrium dialysis/radioimmunoassay: evidence that free triiodothyronine and free thyroxine are normal in many patients with the low triiodothyronine syndrome, Thyroid 8:249–257, 1998.
21. Faber J, Rogowski P, Kirkegaard C, et al: Serum free T4, T3, rT3, 3,3′-diiodothyronine and 3′,5′-diiodothyronine measured by ultrafiltration, Acta Endocrinol 107:357–365, 1984.
22. Nicoloff JT, Low JC, Dussault JH, et al: Simultaneous measurements of thyroxine and triiodothyronine peripheral turnover kinetics in man, J Clin Invest 51:473–483, 1972.
23. LoPresti JS, Eigen A, Kaptein E, et al: Alterations in 3,3′,5′-triiodothyronine metabolism in response to propylthiouracil, dexamethasone, and thyroxine administration in man, J Clin Invest 84:1650–1656, 1989.
24. Glinoer D: The regulation of thyroid function in pregnancy: pathways of endocrine adaptation from physiology to pathology, Endo Reviews 18:404–433, 1997.
25. Huang SA, Dorfman DM, Genest DR, et al: Type 3 iodothyronine deiodinase is highly expressed in the human uteroplacental unit and in fetal epithelium, J Clin Endocrinol Metab 88:1384–1388, 2003.
26. Alexander EK, Marqusee E, Lawrence J, et al: Timing and magnitude of increases in levothyroxine requirements during pregnancy in women with hypothyroidism, N Engl J Med 351:241–249, 2004.
27. Mariotti S, Barbesino G, Caturegli P, et al: Complex alteration of thyroid function in healthy centenarians, J Clin Endocrinol Metab 77:1130–1134, 1993.
28. Gregerman RI, Gaffney GW, Shock NW: Thyroxine turnover in euthyroid man with special reference

to changes with age, J Clin Invest 41:2065–2074, 1962.
29. Kabadi UM: Variability of L-thyroxine replacement dose in elderly patients with primary hypothyroidism, J Fam Pract 24:473–477, 1987.
30. Peeters RP: Thyroid hormones and aging, Hormones 7:28–35, 2008.
31. Gross J, Pitt-Rivers R: 3:5:3′-triiodothyronine. 2. Physiological activity, Biochem J 53:652–656, 1953.
32. Gross J, Pitt-Rivers R: 3:5:3′-triiodothyronine. 1. Isolation from thyroid gland and synthesis, Biochem J 53:645–652, 1953.
33. Braverman LE, Ingbar SH, Sterling K: Conversion of thyroxine to triiodothyronine in athyreotic human subjects, J Clin Invest 49:855–864, 1970.
34. Bianco AC, Salvatore D, Gereben B, et al: Biochemistry, cellular and molecular biology, and physiological roles of the iodothyronine selenodeiodinases. Endo Reviews 23:38–89, 2002.
35. Köhrle J: Iodothyonine deiodinases, Meth Enzymol 347:125–167, 2002.
36. Kohrle J: Thyroid hormone transporters in health and disease: advances in thyroid hormone deiodination. Best Prac Res Clin Endocrinol Metab 21:173–191, 2007.
37. Gereben B, Zeold A, Dentice M, et al: Activation and inactivation of thyroid hormone by deiodinases: local action with general consequences, Cell Mol Life Sci 65:570–590, 2008.
38. St. Germain DL, Galton VA: The deiodinase family of selenoproteins, Thyroid 7:655–668, 1997.
39. Leonard JL, Visser TJ: Biochemistry of deiodination. In Hennemann G, editor: Thyroid Hormone Metabolism. New York, 1986, Marcel Dekker, 189–229.
40. Jakobs TC, Koehler MR, Schmutzler C, et al: Structure of the human type I iodothyronine 5′-deiodinase gene and location to chromosome 1p32–p33, Genomics 42:361–363, 1997.
41. Celi FS, Canettieri G, Yarnell DP, et al: Genomic characterization of the coding region of the human type II 5′-deiodinase, Mol Cell Endocrinol 141:49–52, 1998.
42. Hernández A, Park J, Lyon GJ, et al: Localization of the type 3 iodothyronine deiodinase (DIO3) gene to human chromosome 14q32 and mouse chromosome 12F1, Genomics 53:119–121, 1998.
43. Leonard JL, Visser TJ, Leonard DM: Characterization of the subunit structure of the catalytically active type I iodothyronine deiodinase, J Biol Chem 276:2600–2607, 2001.
44. Curcio-Morelli C, Gereben B, Zavacki AM, et al: In vivo dimerization of types 1, 2, and 3 iodothyronine selenodeiodinases, Endocrinology 144:937–946, 2003.

45. Leonard JL, Simpson G, Leonard DM: Characterization of the protein dimerization domain responsible for assembly of functional selenodeiodinases, J Biol Chem 280:11093–11100, 2005.
46. Visser TJ: Role of sulfation in thyroid hormone metabolism, Chem Biol Interact 92:293–303, 1994.
47. Visser TJ: Mechanism of inhibition of iodothyronine-5′-deiodinase by thioureylenes and sulfite, Biochim Biophys Acta 611:371–378, 1980.
48. Sharifi J, St. Germain DL: The cDNA for the type I iodothyronine 5′-deiodinase encodes an enzyme manifesting both high K_m and low K_m activity, J Biol Chem 267:12539–12544, 1992.
49. Sarma BK, Mugesh G: Thiol cofactors for selenoenzymes and their synthetic mimics, Organ Biomol Chem 6:965–974, 2008.
50. Croteau W, Bodwell JE, Richardson JM, et al: Conserved cysteines in the type 1 deiodinase selenoprotein are not essential for catalytic activity, J Biol Chem 237:25230–25236, 1998.
51. Chaudiere J, Tappel AL: Interaction of gold(I) with the active site of selenium-glutathione peroxidase, J Inorg Biochem 20:313–325, 1984.
52. Berry MJ, Kieffer JD, Harney JW, et al: Selenocysteine confers the biochemical properties characteristic of the type 1 iodothyronine deiodinase, J Biol Chem 266:14155–14158, 1991.
53. Croteau W, Whittemore SL, Schneider MJ, et al: Cloning and expression of a cDNA for a mammalian type III iodothyronine deiodinase, J Biol Chem 270:16569–16575, 1995.
54. Croteau W, Davey JC, Galton VA, et al: Cloning of the mammalian type II iodothyronine deiodinase: a selenoprotein differentially expressed and regulated in the human brain and other tissues, J Clin Invest 98:405–417, 1996.
55. Kohrle J, Schomburg L, Drescher S, et al: Rapid stimulation of type I 5′-deiodinase in rat pituitaries by 3,3′,5′-triiodo-L-thyronine, Mol Cell Endocrinol 108:17–21, 1995.
56. Visser TJ, Leonard JL, Kaplan MM, et al: Kinetic evidence suggesting two mechanisms for iodothyronine 5′-deiodination in rat cerebral cortex, Proc Natl Acad Sci USA 79:5080–5084, 1982.
57. Guadaño-Ferraz A, Obregón MJ, St. Germain DL, et al: The type 2 iodothyronine deiodinase is expressed primarily in glial cells in the neonatal rat brain, Proc Natl Acad Sci USA 94:10391–10396, 1997.
58. Tu HM, Kim SW, Salvatore D, et al: Regional distribution of type 2 thyroxine deiodinase messenger ribonucleic acid in rat hypothalamus and pituitary and its regulation by thyroid hormone, Endocrinology 138:3359–3368, 1997.
59. Diano S, Leonard JL, Meli R, et al: Hypothalamic type II iodothyronine deiodinase: a light and electron microscopic study, Brain Res 976:130–134, 2003.
60. Salvatore D, Tu H, Harney JW, et al: Type 2 iodothyronine deiodinase is highly expressed in human thyroid, J Clin Invest 98:962–968, 1996.
61. Kasahara T, Tsunekawa K, Seki K, et al: Regulation of iodothyronine deiodinase and roles of thyroid hormones in human coronary artery smooth muscle cells, Atherosclerosis 186:207–214, 2006.
62. Kaplan MM, Yaskoski KA: Phenolic and tyrosyl ring deiodination of iodothyronines in rat brain homogenates, J Clin Invest 66:551–562, 1980.
63. Huang T, Chopra IJ, Beredo A, et al: Skin is an active site of inner ring monodeiodination of thyroxine to 3,3′,5′-triiodothyronine, Endocrinology 117:2106–2113, 1985.
64. Heuer H, Maier MK, Iden S, et al: The monocarboxylate transporter 8 linked to human psychomotor retardation is highly expressed in thyroid hormone-sensitive neuron populations, Endocrinology 146:1701–1706, 2005.
65. Alkemade A, Friesema EC, Unmehopa UA, et al: Neuroanatomical pathways for thyroid hormone feedback in the human hypothalamus, J Clin Endocrinol Metab 90:4322–4334, 2005.
66. Bates JM, St. Germain DL, Galton VA: Expression profiles of the three iodothyronine deiodinases, D1, D2 and D3, in the developing rat, Endocrinology 140:844–851, 1999.
67. Roti E, Fang SL, Green K, et al: Human placenta is an active site of thyroxine and 3,3′,5-triiodothyronine tyrosyl ring deiodination, J Clin Endocrinol Metab 53:498–501, 1981.
68. St. Germain DL: Selenium, deiodinases, and endocrine function. In Hatfield DL, editor: Selenium: Its Molecular Biology and Role in Human Health. Boston, 2001, Kluwer Academic Publishers, 189–202.
69. Berry MJ, Maia AL, Kieffer JD, et al: Substitution of cysteine for selenocysteine in type I iodothyronine deiodinase reduces the catalytic efficiency of the protein but enhances its translation, Endocrinology 131:1848–1852, 1992.
70. Kuiper GG, Klootwijk W, Visser TJ: Substitution of cysteine for selenocysteine in the catalytic center of type II iodothyronine deiodinase reduces catalytic efficiency and alters substrate preference, Endocrinology 144:2505–2513, 2003.
71. Lian G, Ding L, Chen M, et al: A selenium-containing catalytic antibody with Type I deiodinase activity. [Erratum appears in Biochem Biophys Res Commun Jul 6;285(1):159], Biochem Biophys Res Comm 283:1007–1012, 2001.
72. Stadtman TC: Selenocysteine, Ann Rev Biochem 65:83–100, 1996.
73. Driscoll DM, Copeland PR: Mechanism and regulation of selenoprotein synthesis. Ann Rev Nutr 23:17–40, 2003.
74. Hoffmann PR, Berry MJ: Selenoprotein synthesis: a unique translational mechanism used by a diverse family of proteins, Thyroid 15:769–775, 2005.
75. Squires JE, Berry MJ: Eukaryotic selenoprotein synthesis: mechanistic insight incorporating new factors and new functions for old factors, IUBMB Life 60:232–235, 2008.
76. Leonard DM, Stachelek SJ, Safran M, et al: Cloning, expression and functional characterization of the substrate binding subunit of rat type II iodothyronine 5′-deiodinase, J Biol Chem 275:25195–25201, 2000.
77. Montero-Pedrazuela A, Bernal J, Guadano-Ferraz A: Divergent expression of type 2 deiodinase and the putative thyroxine-binding protein p29, in rat brain, suggests that they are functionally unrelated proteins, Endocrinology 144:1045–1052, 2003.
78. Barrantes IdB, Montero-Pedrazuela A, Guadano-Ferraz A, et al: Generation and characterization of dickkopf3 mutant mice, Mol Cell Biol 26:2317–2326, 2006.
79. Callebaut I, Curcio-Morelli C, Mornon J-P, et al: The iodothyronine selenodeiodinases are thioredoxin-fold family proteins containing a glycoside hydrolase clan GH-A-like structure, J Biol Chem 278:36887–36896, 2003.
80. Kuiper GGJM, Klootwijk W, Morvan Dubois G, et al: Characterization of recombinant Xenopus laevis type I iodothyronine deiodinase: substitution of a proline residue in the catalytic center by serine (Pro132Ser) restores sensitivity to 6-propyl-2-thiouracil, Endocrinology 147:3519–3529, 2006.
81. Toyoda N, Berry MJ, Harney JW, et al: Topological analysis of the integral membrane protein, type 1 iodothyronine deiodinase (D1), J Biol Chem 270:12310–12318, 1995.
82. Courtin F, Pelletier G, Walker P: Subcellular localization of thyroxine 5′-deiodinase activity in bovine anterior pituitary, Endocrinology 117:2527–2533, 1985.
83. Schoenmakers CH, Pigmans IG, Visser TJ: Investigation of type I and type III iodothyronine deiodinases in rat tissues using N-bromoacetyl-iodothyronine affinity labels, Mol Cell Endocrinol 107:173–180, 1995.
84. Baqui MMA, Gerebon B, Harney JW, et al: Distinct subcellular localization of transiently expressed types 1 and 2 deiodinases as determined by immunofluorescence confocal microscopy, Endocrinology 141:4309–4312, 2000.
85. Baqui M, Botero D, Gereben B, et al: Human type 3 iodothyronine selenodeiodinase is located in the plasma membrane and undergoes rapid internalization to endosomes, J Biol Chem 278:1206–1211, 2003.
86. Leonard JL, Ekenbarger DM, Frank SJ, et al: Localization of type I iodothyronine 5′-deiodinase to the basolateral plasma membrane in renal cortical epithelial cells, J Biol Chem 266:11262–11269, 1991.
87. Friesema ECH, Kuiper GGJM, Jansen J, et al: Thyroid hormone transport by the human monocarboxylate transporter 8 and its rate-limiting role in intracellular metabolism, Mol Endocrinol 20:2761–2772, 2006.
88. Celi FS, Canettieri G, Mentuccia D, et al: Structural organization and chromosomal localization of the human type II deiodinase gene, Eur J Endocrinol 143:267–271, 2000.
89. Hernández A, Lyon GJ, Schneider MJ, et al: Isolation and characterization of the mouse gene for the type 3 iodothyronine deiodinase, Endocrinology 140:124–130, 1999.
90. Gereben B, Kollar A, Harney JW, et al: The mRNA structure has potent regulatory effects on type 2 iodothyronine deiodinase expression, Mol Endocrinol 16:1667–1679, 2002.
91. Hernandez A, Fiering S, Martinez E, et al: The gene locus encoding iodothyronine deiodinase type 3 (Dio3) is imprinted in the fetus and expresses antisense transcripts, Endocrinology 143:4483–4486, 2002.
92. Reik W, Walter J: Genomic imprinting: parental influence on the genome. Nat Rev Genetics 2:21–32, 2001.
93. Schneider MJ, Fiering SN, Thai B, et al: Targeted disruption of the type 1 selenodeiodinase gene (Dio1) results in marked changes in thyroid hormone economy in mice, Endocrinology 147:580–589, 2006.
94. Schneider MJ, Fiering SN, Pallud SE, et al: Targeted disruption of the type 2 selenodeiodinase gene (Dio2) results in a phenotype of pituitary resistance to T4, Mol Endocrinol 15:2137–2148, 2001.
95. de Jesus LA, Carvalho SD, Ribeiro MO, et al: The type 2 iodothyronine deiodinase is essential for adaptive thermogenesis in brown adipose tissue, J Clin Invest 108:1379–1385, 2001.
96. Ng L, Goodyear RJ, Woods CA, et al: Hearing loss and retarded cochlear development in mice lacking type 2 iodothyronine deiodinase, Proc Natl Acad Sci USA 101:3473–3479, 2004.
97. Galton VA, Wood ET, St. Germain EA, et al: Thyroid hormone homeostasis and action in the type 2 deiodinase-deficient brain during development, Endocrinology 148:3080–3088, 2007.
98. Christoffolete MA, Linardi CC, de Jesus L, et al: Mice with targeted disruption of the Dio2 gene have cold-induced overexpression of the uncoupling protein 1 gene but fail to increase brown adipose tissue lipogenesis and adaptive thermogenesis, Diabetes 53:577–584, 2004.
99. Hernandez A, Martinez E, Fiering S, et al: Type 3 deiodinase is critical for the maturation and function of the thyroid axis, J Clin Invest 116:476–484, 2006.
100. Hernandez A, Martinez ME, Liao XH, et al: Type 3 deiodinase deficiency results in functional abnormalities at multiple levels of the thyroid axis, Endocrinology 148:5680–5687, 2007.
101. Christoffolete MA, Arrojo e Drigo R, Gazoni F, et al: Mice with impaired extrathyroidal thyroxine to 3,5,3′-triiodothyronine conversion maintain normal serum 3,5,3′-triiodothyronine concentrations, Endocrinology 148:954–960, 2007.
102. Chanoine J, Braverman LE, Farwell AP, et al: The thyroid gland is a major source of circulating T3 in the rat, J Clin Invest 91:2709–2713, 1993.
103. Laurberg P, Vestergaard H, Nielsen S, et al: Sources of circulating 3,5,3′-triiodothyronine in hyperthyroidism estimated after blocking of type 1 and type 2 iodothyronine deiodinases. [see comment], J Clin Endocrinol Metab 92:2149–2156, 2007.
104. Dumitrescu AM, Liao X-H, Abdullah MSY, et al: Mutations in SECISBP2 result in abnormal thyroid hormone metabolism. Nat Genetics 37:1247–1252, 2005.
105. Kempers MJE, van Trotsenburg ASP, van Tijn DA, et al: Disturbance of the fetal thyroid hormone state has long-term consequences for treatment of thyroidal and central congenital hypothyroidism, J Clin Endocrinol Metab 90:4094–4100, 2005.
106. Kempers MJE, van Trotsenburg ASP, van Rijn RR, et al: Loss of integrity of thyroid morphology and function in children born to mothers with inadequately treated Graves' disease, J Clin Endocrinol Metab 2006–2042, 2007.
107. Bakke JL, Lawrence NL, Bennett J, et al: The late effects of neonatal hyperthyroidism upon the feedback regulation of TSH secretion in rats, Endocrinology 97:659–664, 1975.
108. Dussault JH, Coulombe P, Walker P: Effects of neonatal hyperthyroidism on the development of the hypothalamic-pituitary-thyroid axis in the rat, Endocrinology 110:1037–1042, 1982.

109. O'Mara BA, Dittrich W, Lauterio TJ, et al: Pretranslational regulation of type I 5′-deiodinase by thyroid hormones and in fasted and diabetic rats, Endocrinology 133:1715–1723, 1993.
110. Gereben B, Goncalves C, Harney JW, et al: Selective proteolysis of human type 2 deiodinase: a novel ubiquitin-proteasomal mediated mechanism for regulation of hormone activation, Mol Endocrinol 14:1697–1708, 2000.
111. Curcio-Morelli C, Zavacki AM, Christofollete M, et al: Deubiquitination of type 2 iodothyronine deiodinase by von Hippel-Lindau protein-interacting deubiquitinating enzymes regulates thyroid hormone activation, J Clin Invest 112:189–196, 2003.
112. Sagar GDV, Gereben B, Callebaut I, et al: Ubiquitination-induced conformational change within the deiodinase dimer is a switch regulating enzyme activity, Mol Cell Biol 27:4774–4783, 2007.
113. Simonides WS, Mulcahey MA, Redout EM, et al: Hypoxia-inducible factor induces local thyroid hormone inactivation during hypoxic-ischemic disease in rats, J Clin Invest 118:975–983, 2008.
114. Silva JE, Larsen PR: Adrenergic activation of triiodothyronine production in brown adipose tissue, Nature 305:712–713, 1983.
115. Watanabe M, Houten SM, Mataki C, et al: Bile acids induce energy expenditure by promoting intracellular thyroid hormone activation. [see comment], Nature 439:484–489, 2006.
116. Cettour-Rose P, Burger AG, Meier CA, et al: Central stimulatory effect of leptin on T3 production is mediated by brown adipose tissue type II deiodinase, Am J Physiol 283:E980–987, 2002.
117. Nagaya T, Fujieda M, Otsuka G, et al: A potential role of activated NF-kappa B in the pathogenesis of euthyroid sick syndrome, J Clin Invest 106:393–402, 2000.
118. Yu J, Koenig RJ: Regulation of hepatocyte thyroxine 5′-deiodinase by T3 and nuclear receptor coactivators as a model of the sick euthyroid syndrome, J Biol Chem 275:38296–38301, 2000.
119. Campos-Barros A, Musa A, Flechner A, et al: Evidence for circadian variations of thyroid hormone concentrations and type II 5′-iodothyronine deiodinase activity in the rat central nervous system, J Neurochem 68:795–803, 1997.
120. Yasuo S, Yoshimura T, Ebihara S, et al: Temporal dynamics of type 2 deiodinase expression after melatonin injections in Syrian hamsters, Endocrinology 148:4385–4392, 2007.
121. Yasuo S, Watanabe M, Nakao N, et al: The reciprocal switching of two thyroid hormone-activating and -inactivating enzyme genes is involved in the photoperiodic gonadal response of Japanese quail, Endocrinology 146:2551–2554, 2005.
122. Nakao N, Ono H, Yamamura T, et al: Thyrotrophin in the pars tuberalis triggers photoperiodic response, Nature 452:317–322, 2008.
123. Wu S-Y, Green WL, Huang W-S, et al: Alternate pathways of thyroid hormone metabolism, Thyroid 15:943–958, 2005.
124. Kung MP, Spaulding SW, Roth JA: Desulfation of 3,5,3′-triiodothyronine sulfate by microsomes from human and rat tissues, Endocrinology 122:1195–1200, 1988.
125. Santini F, Hurd RE, Lee B, et al: Thyromimetic effects of 3,5,3′-triiodothyronine sulfate in hypothyroid rats, Endocrinology 133:105–110, 1993.
126. Kester MH, Kaptein E, Roest TJ, et al: Characterization of human iodothyronine sulfotransferases, J Clin Endocrinol Metab 84:1357–1364, 1999.
127. Chopra IJ, Wu SY, Teco GN, et al: A radioimmunoassay for measurement of 3,5,3′-triiodothyronine sulfate: studies in thyroidal and nonthyroidal diseases, pregnancy, and neonatal life, J Clin Endocrinol Metab 75:189–194, 1992.
128. Eelkman Rooda SJ, Kaptein E, Rutgers M, et al: Increased plasma 3,5,3′-triiodothyronine sulfate in rats with inhibited type I iodothyronine deiodinase activity, as measured by radioimmunoassay, Endocrinology 124:740–745, 1989.
129. Van Middlesworth L: Metabolism and excretion of thyroid hormones. In Greer M, Solomon DH, editors: Handbook of Physiology: Endocrinology. Washington, D.C., 1974, American Physiological Society, 215–231.
130. Siegrist-Kaiser CA, Burger AG: Modification of the side chain of thyroid hormones. In Wu S-Y, Visser TJ, editors: Thyroid Hormone Metabolism. Boca Raton, 1994, CRC Press, 175–198.
131. Liang H, Juge-Aubry CE, O'Connell M, et al: Organ-specific effects of 3,5,3′-triiodothyroacetic acid in rats, Eur J Endocrinol 137:537–544, 1997.
132. Green WL: Ether-link cleavage of iodothyronines. In Wu S-Y, Visser, TJ, editors: Thyroid hormone metabolism, Boca Raton, 1994, CRC Press, 199–221.
133. Davis PJ, Leonard JL, Davis FB: Mechanisms of nongenomic actions of thyroid hormone, Front Neuroendocrinol 29:211–218, 2008.
134. Visser WE, Friesema ECH, Jansen J, et al: Thyroid hormone transport in and out of cells, Trends Endocrinol Metab 19:50–56, 2008.
135. Hagenbuch B: Cellular entry of thyroid hormones by organic anion transporting polypeptides, Best Pract Res Clin Endocrin Metab 21:209–221, 2007.
136. Visser WE, Friesema ECH, Jansen J, et al: Thyroid hormone transport by monocarboxylate transporters, Best Pract Res Clin Endocrin Metab 21:223–236, 2007.
137. Pizzagalli F, Hagenbuch B, Stieger B, et al: Identification of a novel human organic anion transporting polypeptide as a high affinity thyroxine transporter, Mol Endocrinol 16:2283–2296, 2002.
138. Friesema EC, Ganguly S, Abdalla A, et al: Identification of monocarboxylate transporter 8 as a specific thyroid hormone transporter, J Biol Chem 278:40128–40135, 2003.
139. Dumitrescu AM, Liao XH, Weiss RE, et al: Tissue-specific thyroid hormone deprivation and excess in monocarboxylate transporter (mct) 8-deficient mice, Endocrinology 4036–4043, 2006.
140. Trajkovic M, Visser TJ, Mittag J, et al: Abnormal thyroid hormone metabolism in mice lacking the mom-carboxylate transporter 8, J Clin Invest 117:627–635, 2007.
141. Schwartz CE, Stevenson RE: The MCT8 thyroid hormone transporter and Allan-Herndon-Dudley syndrome, Best Pract Res Clin Endocrin Metab 21:307–321, 2007.
142. Lum SM, Nicoloff JT, Spencer CA, et al: Peripheral tissue mechanism for maintenance of serum triiodothyronine values in a thyroxine-deficient state in man, J Clin Invest 73:570–575, 1984.
143. Keck FS, Loos U, Duntas L, et al: Evidence for peripheral autoregulation of thyroxine conversion. In Medeiros-Neto G, Gaitan E, editors: New York, 1986, Plenum Medical Book Co., 525–530.
144. Nicoloff JT, LoPresti JS: Alternate pathways of thyroid hormone metabolism. In Wu S-Y, editor: Thyroid Hormone Metabolism. Boston, 1991, Blackwell Scientific Publications, 55–64.
145. Maia AL, Kim BW, Huang SA, et al: Type 2 deiodinase is the major source of plasma T3 in euthyroid humans, J Clin Invest 115:2524–2533, 2005.
146. Escobar-Morreale H, Obregón MJ, Escobar del Rey F, et al: Replacement therapy for hypothyroidism with thyroxine alone does not ensure euthyroidism in all tissues, as studied in thyroidectomized rats, J Clin Invest 96:2828–2838, 1995.
147. Broedel O, Eravci M, Fuxius S, et al: Effects of hyper- and hypothyroidism on thyroid hormone concentrations in regions of the rat brain, Am J Physiol 285:E470–480, 2003.
148. Porterfield SP, Hendrich CE: The role of thyroid hormones in prenatal and neonatal neurological development—current perspectives, Endo Reviews 14:94–106, 1993.
149. Daneman D, Howard NJ: Neonatal thyrotoxicosis: intellectual impairment and craniosynostosis in later years, J Pediatr 97:257–259, 1980.
150. Figueiredo BC, Almazan G, Ma Y, et al: Gene expression in the developing cerebellum during perinatal hypo- and hyperthyroidism, Mol Brain Res 17:258–268, 1993.
151. Burrow GN, Fisher DA, Larsen PR: Maternal and fetal thyroid function, N Engl J Med 331:1072–1078, 1994.
152. Calvo RM, Jauniaux E, Gulbis B, et al: Fetal tissues are exposed to biologically relevant free thyroxine concentrations during early phases of development, J Clin Endocrinol Metab 87:1768–1777, 2002.
153. Morreale de Escobar G, Obregon MJ, Escobar del Rey F: Is neuropsychological development related to maternal hypothyroidism or to maternal hypothyroxinemia? J Clin Endocrinol Metab 85:3975–3987, 2000.
154. Galton VA, Martinez E, Hernandez A, et al: Pregnant rat uterus expresses high levels of the type 3 iodothyronine deiodinase, J Clin Invest 103:979–987, 1999.
155. Galton VA, Martinez E, Hernandez A, et al: The type 2 iodothyronine deiodinase is expressed in the rat uterus and induced during pregnancy, Endocrinology 142:2123–2128, 2001.
156. Wasco EC, Martinez E, Grant KS, et al: Determinants of iodothyronine deiodinase activities in rodent uterus, Endocrinology 144:4253–4261, 2003.
157. Kester MHA, Kuiper GGJM, Versteeg R, et al: Regulation of type III iodothyronine deiodinase expression in human cell lines, Endocrinology 147:5845–5854, 2006.
158. Vulsma T, Gons MH, de Vijlder JJM: Maternal-fetal transfer of thyroxine in congenital hypothyroidism due to a total organification defect or thyroid agenesis, N Engl J Med 321:13–16, 1989.
159. James SR, Franklyn JA, Kilby MD: Placental transport of thyroid hormone, Best Pract Res Clin Endo Metab 21:253–264, 2007.
160. Chan S, Kachilele S, McCabe CJ, et al: Early expression of thyroid hormone deiodinases and receptors in human fetal cerebral cortex. Develop Brain Res 138:109–116, 2002.
161. Kester HA, Martinez de Mena R, Obregon MJ, et al: Iodothyronine levels in the human developing brain: major regulatory roles of iodothyronine deiodinases in different areas, J Clin Endocrinol Metab 89:3117–3128, 2004.
162. Calvo R, Obregón MJ, Ruiz de Ona C, et al: Congenital hypothyroidism, as studied in rats: crucial role of maternal thyroxine but not 3,5,3′-triiodothyronine in the protection of the fetal brain, J Clin Invest 86:889–899, 1990.
163. Campos-Barros A, Amma LL, Faris JS, et al: Type 2 iodothyronine deiodinase expression in the cochlea before the onset of hearing, Proc Natl Acad Sci USA 97:1287–1292, 2000.
164. Becker KB, Stephens KC, Davey JC, et al: The type 2 and type 3 iodothyronine deiodinases play important roles in coordinating development in Rana catesbeiana tadpoles, Endocrinology 138:2989–2997, 1997.
165. Marsh-Armstrong N, Huang H, Remo BF, et al: Asymmetric growth and development of the Xenopus laevis retina during metamorphosis is controlled by type III deiodinase, Neuron 24:871–878, 1999.
166. Huang H, Cai L, Remo BF, et al: Timing of metamorphosis and the onset of the negative feedback loop between the thyroid gland and the pituitary is controlled by type II iodothyronine deiodinase in Xenopus laevis, Proc Natl Acad Sci USA 98:7348–7353, 2001.
167. Cai L, Brown DD: Expression of type II iodothyronine deiodinase marks the time that a tissue responds to thyroid hormone-induced metamorphosis in Xenopus laevis, Devel Biol 266:87–95, 2004.
168. Fisher DA, Polk DH, Wu SY: Fetal thyroid hormone metabolism, Thyroid 4:367–371, 1994.
169. Santini F, Chopra IJ, Wu S-Y, et al: Metabolism of 3,5,3′-triiodothyronine sulfate by tissues of the fetal rat: a consideration of the role of desulfation of 3,5,3′-triiodothyronine sulfate as a source of T3, Pediatr Res 31:541–544, 1992.
170. Wartofsky L, Burman K: Alterations in thyroid function in patients with systemic illness: the "euthyroid sick syndrome." Endo Reviews 3:164–217, 1982.
171. Peeters RP, Debaveye Y, Fliers E, et al: Changes within the thyroid axis during critical illness. Crit Care Clinics 22:41–55, 2006.
172. Peeters RP, Van der Geyten S, Wouters PJ, et al: Tissue thyroid hormone levels in critical illness, J Clin Endocrinol Metab 90:6498–6507, 2005.
173. Peeters RP, Wouters PJ, van Toor H, et al: Serum 3,3′,5′-triiodothyronine (rT3) and 3,5,3′-triiodothyronine/rT3 are prognostic markers in critically ill patients and are associated with postmortem tissue deiodinase activities, J Clin Endocrinol Metab 90:4559–4565, 2005.
174. Wells S, Campbell R: Decrease in resting metabolic rate during rapid weight loss is reversed by low dose thyroid hormone treatment, Metabolism 35:289–291, 1986.

175. Forsum E, Hillman PE, Nesheim MC: Effect of energy restriction on total heat production, basal metabolic rate, and specific dynamic action of food in rats, J Nutr 111:1691–1697, 1981.

176. Carter WJ, Shakir KM, Hodges S, et al: Effect of thyroid hormone on metabolic adaptation to fasting, Metabolism 24:1177–1183, 1975.

177. Gardner DF, Kaplan MM, Stanley CA, et al: Effect of tri-iodothyronine replacement on the metabolic and pituitary responses to starvation, N Engl J Med 300:579–584, 1979.

178. Boelen A, Kwakkel J, Alkemade A, et al: Induction of type 3 deiodinase in inflammatory cells of mice with chronic local inflammation, Endocrinology 146:5128–5134, 2005.

179. Peeters RP, Wouters PJ, Kaptein E, et al: Reduced activation and increased inactivation of thyroid hormone in tissues of critically ill patients, J Clin Endocrinol Metab 88:3202–3211, 2003.

180. Olivares EL, Marassi MP, Fortunato RS, et al: Thyroid function disturbance and type 3 iodothyronine deiodinase induction after myocardial infarction in rats—a time course study, Endocrinology 148:4786–4792, 2007.

181. Chang M, Reddy CC: Active transcription of the selenium-dependent glutathione peroxidase gene in selenium-deficient rats, Biochem Biophys Res Comm 181:1431–1436, 1991.

182. Coppola A, Hughes J, Esposito E, et al: Suppression of hypothalamic deiodinase type II activity blunts TRH mRNA decline during fasting, FEBS Letters 579:4654–4658, 2005.

183. Sanchez E, Singru PS, Fekete C, et al: Induction of type 2 iodothyronine deiodinase in the mediobasal hypothalamus by bacterial lipopolysaccharide: role of corticosterone, Endocrinology 149:2484–2493, 2008.

184. Lankford SP, Cosson P, Bonifacino JS, et al: Transmembrane domain length affects charge-mediated retention and degradation of proteins within the endoplasmic reticulum, J Biol Chem 268:4814–4820, 1993.

185. Kinlaw WB, Schwartz HL, Oppenheimer JH: Decreased serum triiodothyronine in starving rats is due primarily to diminished thyroidal secretion of thyroxine, J Clin Invest 75:1238–1241, 1984.

186. Yen YM, DiStefano JJ III, Yamada H, et al: Direct measurement of whole body thyroid hormone pool sizes and interconversion rates in fasted rats: hormone regulation implications, Endocrinology 134:1700–1709, 1994.

187. Boelen A, Kwakkel J, Wieland CW, et al: Impaired bacterial clearance in type 3 deiodinase deficient mice infected with Streptococcal pneumoniae, Endocrinology 150:1984–1989, 2009.

188. Kim B: Thyroid hormone as a determinant of energy expenditure and the basal metabolic rate, Thyroid 18:141–144, 2008.

189. da Silva WS, Harney JW, Kim BW, et al: The small polyphenolic molecule kaempferol increases cellular energy expenditure and thyroid hormone activation, Diabetes 56:767–776, 2007.

190. DePalo D, Kinlaw WB, Zhao C, et al: Effect of selenium deficiency on type I 5′-deiodinase, J Biol Chem 269:16223–16228, 1994.

191. Meinhold H, Campos-Barros A, Walzog B, et al: Effects of selenium and iodine deficiency on type I, type II, and type III iodothyronine deiodinases and circulating thyroid hormones in the rat, Exp Clin Endocrinol 101:87–93, 1993.

192. Bates JM, Spate VL, Morris JS, et al: Effects of selenium deficiency on tissue selenium content, deiodinase activity, and thyroid hormone economy in the rat during development, Endocrinology 141:2490–2500, 2000.

193. Chanoine J, Safran M, Farwell AP, et al: Effects of selenium deficiency on thyroid hormone economy in rats, Endocrinology 131:1787–1792, 1992.

194. Olivieri O, Girelli D, Azzini M, et al: Low selenium status in the elderly influences thyroid hormones, Clin Sci 89:637–642, 1995.

195. Kauf E, Dawczynski H, Jahreis G, et al: Sodium selenite therapy and thyroid-hormone status in cystic fibrosis and congenital hypothyroidism, Biol Trace Elem Res 40:247–253, 1994.

196. Angstwurm MWA, Schopohl J, Gaertner R: Selenium substitution has no direct effect on thyroid hormone metabolism in critically ill patients, Eur J Endo 151:47–54, 2004.

197. Contempré B, Duale NL, Dumont JE, et al: Effect of selenium supplementation on thyroid hormone metabolism in an iodine and selenium deficient population, Clin Endocrinol 36:579–583, 1992.

198. Cavalieri RR: Effects of drugs on human thyroid hormone metabolism. In Hennemann G, editor: Thyroid Hormone Metabolism. New York, 1986, Marcel Dekker, Inc., 359–379.

199. Okamura K, Ikenoue H, Shiroozu A, et al: Reevaluation of the effects of methylmercaptoimidazole and propylthiouracil in patients with Graves' hyperthyroidism, J Clin Endocrinol Metab 65:719–723, 1987.

200. Wu S, Shyh T, Chopra IJ, et al: Comparison of sodium ipodate (Oragrafin) and propylthiouracil in early treatment of hyperthyroidism, J Clin Endocrinol Metab 54:630–634, 1982.

201. Roti E, Robuschi G, Manfredi A, et al: Comparative effects of sodium ipodate and iodide on serum thyroid hormone concentrations in patients with Graves' disease, Clin Endocrinol 22:489–496, 1985.

202. Seclen SN, Pretell EA, Tapia FA, et al: Rapid amelioration of severe cardiovascular complications of thyrotoxic patients with sodium ipodate. In Medeiros-Neto G, Gaitan E, editors: Frontiers in Thyroidology. New York, 1986, Plenum Medical Book Company, 1101–1105.

203. Bogazzi F, Miccoli P, Berti P, et al: Preparation with iopanoic acid rapidly controls thyrotoxicosis in patients with amiodarone-induced thyrotoxicosis before thyroidectomy, Surgery 132:1114–1117, 2002.

204. Wiersinga WM: Propranolol and thyroid hormone metabolism, Thyroid 1:273–277, 1991.

205. Chopra IJ, Williams DE, Orgiazzi J, et al: Opposite effects of dexamethasone on serum concentrations of 3,3′,5′-triiodothyronine (reverse T3) and 3,3′5-triiodothyronine (T3), J Clin Endocrinol Metab 41:911–920, 1975.

206. Cavaleri RH, Castle JN, McMahon FA: Effects of dexamethasone on kinetics and distribution of triiodothyronine in the rat, Endocrinology 114:215–221, 1984.

207. Eravci M, Pinna G, Meinhold H, et al: Effects of pharmacological and nonpharmacological treatments on thyroid hormone metabolism and concentrations in rat brain, Endocrinology 141:1027–1040, 2000.

208. Newman CM, Price A, Davies DW, et al: Amiodarone and the thyroid: a practical guide to the management of thyroid dysfunction induced by amiodarone therapy, Heart 79:121–127, 1998.

209. Ursella S, Testa A, Mazzone M, et al: Amiodarone-induced thyroid dysfunction in clinical practice, Eur Rev Med Pharm Sci 10:269–278, 2006.

210. Celi FS, Coppotelli G, Chidakel A, et al: The role of type 1 and type 2 5′-deiodinase in the pathophysiology of the 3,5,3′-triiodothyronine toxicosis of McCune-Albright syndrome, J Clin Endocrinol Metab 93:2383–2389, 2008.

211. Bartha T, Kim SW, Salvatore D, et al: Characterization of the 5′-flanking and 5′-untranslated regions of the cyclic adenosine 3′,5′-monophosphate-responsive human type 2 iodothyronine deiodinase gene, Endocrinology 141:229–237, 2000.

212. Kim BW, Daniels GH, Harrison BJ, et al: Overexpression of type 2 iodothyronine deiodinase in follicular carcinoma as a cause of low circulating free thyroxine levels, J Clin Endocrinol Metab 88:594–598, 2003.

213. Miyauchi A, Takamura Y, Ito Y, et al: 3,5,3′-Triiodothyronine thyrotoxicosis due to increased conversion of administered levothyroxine in patients with massive metastatic follicular thyroid carcinoma, J Clin Endocrinol Metab 93:2239–2242, 2008.

214. Takano T, Miyauchi A, Ito Y, et al: Thyroxine to triiodothyronine hyperconversion thyrotoxicosis in patients with large metastases of follicular thyroid carcinoma, Thyroid 16:615–618, 2006.

215. Murakami M, Araki O, Hosoi Y, et al: Expression and regulation of type II iodothyronine deiodinase in human thyroid gland, Endocrinology 142:2961–2967, 2001.

216. Brtko J, Bobalova J, Podoba J, et al: Thyroid hormone receptors and type I iodothyronine 5′-deiodinase activity of human thyroid toxic adenomas and benign cold nodules, Exp Clin Endo Diab 110:166–170, 2002.

217. Huang SA, Tu HM, Harney JW, et al: Severe hypothyroidism caused by type 3 iodothyronine deiodinase in infantile hemangiomas, N Engl J Med 343:185–189, 2000.

218. Balazs AE, Athanassaki I, Gunn SK, et al: Rapid resolution of consumptive hypothyroidism in a child with hepatic hemangioendothelioma following liver transplantation, Ann Clin Lab Sci 37:280–284, 2007.

219. Huang SA, Fish SA, Dorfman DM, et al: A 21-year-old woman with consumptive hypothyroidism due to a vascular tumor expressing type 3 iodothyronine deiodinase, J Clin Endocrinol Metab 87:4457–4461, 2002.

220. Ruppe MD, Huang SA, Jan de Beur SM: Consumptive hypothyroidism caused by paraneoplastic production of type 3 iodothyronine deiodinase, Thyroid 15:1369–1372, 2005.

221. Tannahill LA, Visser TJ, McCabe CJ, et al: Dysregulation of iodothyronine deiodinase enzyme expression and function in human pituitary tumours, Clin Endocrinol 56:735–743, 2002.

222. Peeters RP, van Toor H, Klootwijk W, et al: Polymorphisms in thyroid hormone pathway genes are associated with plasma TSH and iodothyronine levels in healthy subjects, J Clin Endocrinol Metab 88:2880–2888, 2003.

223. Mentuccia D, Proietti-Pannunzi L, Tanner K, et al: Association between a novel variant of the human type 2 deiodinase gene Thr92Ala and insulin resistance: evidence of interaction with the Trp64Arg variant of the beta-3-adrenergic receptor, Diabetes 51:880–883, 2002.

224. Canani LH, Capp C, Dora JM, et al: The type 2 deiodinase A/G (Thr92Ala) polymorphism is associated with decreased enzyme velocity and increased insulin resistance in patients with type 2 diabetes mellitus, J Clin Endocrinol Metab 90:3472–3478, 2005.

225. Maia AL, Dupuis J, Manning A, et al: The type 2 deiodinase (DIO2) A/G polymorphism is not associated with glycemic traits: the Framingham Heart Study, Thyroid 17:199–202, 2007.

226. Grarup N, Andersen MK, Andreasen CH, et al: Studies of the common DIO2 Thr92Ala polymorphism and metabolic phenotypes in 7342 Danish white subjects, J Clin Endocrinol Metab 92:363–366, 2007.

227. Gumieniak O, Perlstein TS, Williams JS, et al: Ala92 type 2 deiodinase allele increases risk for the development of hypertension. [see comment], Hypertension 49:461–466, 2007.

228. Maia AL, Hwang S-J, Levy D, et al: Lack of association between the type 2 deiodinase A/G polymorphism and hypertensive traits: the Framingham Heart Study, Hypertension 51:e22–23, 2008.

229. de Jong FJ, Peeters RP, den Heijer T, et al: The association of polymorphisms in the type 1 and 2 deiodinase genes with circulating thyroid hormone parameters and atrophy of the medial temporal lobe, J Clin Endocrinol Metab 92:636–640, 2007.

230. Peeters RP, van den Beld AW, van Toor H, et al: A polymorphism in type I deiodinase is associated with circulating free insulin-like growth factor I levels and body composition in humans, J Clin Endocrinol Metab 90:256–263, 2005.

231. Galton V, Wood E, St. Germain EA, et al: Thyroid hormone homeostasis and action in the type 2 deiodinase-deficient rodent brain during development. Endocrinology 148:3080–3088, 2007.

Chapter 5

MECHANISMS OF THYROID HORMONE ACTION

PAUL WEBB, KEVIN PHILLIPS, and JOHN D. BAXTER

The award of the 1909 Nobel Prize to Theodore Kocher for pioneering work on thyroid gland surgery lent timely recognition to the field of the thyroid gland and its actions, an area of study that was already several centuries in the making.[1] Several Renaissance scholars, including Leonardo da Vinci, contributed to the early description of the thyroid gland and the realization that its swelling led to goiter. Later investigators linked goiter and cretinism to dietary deficiency of iodine (a key component of thyroid hormone) and uncovered links between altered thyroid gland function and apparently unconnected symptoms of hyperthyroidism (thyrotoxicosis or Graves' disease) and hypothyroidism (or myxedema). Classic experiments of Murray in 1891 revealed that sheep thyroid gland extracts could be used to treat, and even cure, myxedema. Later searches for the active principle culminated in the isolation of thyroxine (T_4; 3,5,3′,5′-tetra-iodo-L-thyronine) in 1914 by Kendall (who later, with others, received the Nobel Prize for discovering the therapeutic effects of the adrenal steroid cortisone on rheumatoid arthritis), the description of thyroxine structure and chemical synthesis by Harrington in the 1920s and the discovery of the major active form of thyroid hormone, triiodothyronine (T_3; 3,5,3′-tri-iodo-L-thyronine), by Pitt-Rivers about 3 decades later. It is now known that thyroid hormones influence virtually every tissue and cell type; they play important roles in growth, development, and differentiation in fetal life and early childhood and act as master regulators of multiple metabolic processes in the adult. The past 50 years have witnessed great increases in our knowledge of thyroid hormone action, with the last 2 decades in particular producing very rapid advancements in understanding the functions of thyroid hormone receptors (TRs), members of the nuclear hormone receptor (NR) family. In this chapter, we review current knowledge of the mechanisms of thyroid hormone action.[2-5]

Synthesis and Control of Secretion of Thyroid Hormones

Synthesis and regulation of thyroid hormone production is discussed elsewhere in this book. Reiteration of some of these aspects is warranted, since it is the availability of the active hormone that determines receptor function, and many aspects of the mechanisms of thyroid hormone action are revealed by examining the mechanisms of this process. Thyroid hormone levels are generally maintained within defined concentration ranges (biological set-points) by several different regulatory mechanisms, including:

1. Spontaneous release of hormones from the hypothalamus and pituitary that stimulate thyroid hormone production
2. Feedback inhibition of production and release of these hypothalamic and pituitary hormones
3. Rates of intracellular conversion of T_4 to T_3
4. Metabolic destruction of both of these forms of the hormone[6]

Thyroid hormones are derivatives of tyrosine that are produced in the thyroid gland and secreted into the general circulation. Thyroid hormone synthesis occurs via iodination of tyrosine residues in a large protein called *thyroglobulin*, coupling of iodinated tyrosines, and enzymatic cleavage to liberate free thyroxine (T_4). Recent human genetic linkage studies suggest that regulation of thyroid hormone production is complex, with up to eight different loci influencing biological set-point.[7-9] Some of these probably correspond to known genes involved in synthesis of thyroid hormones and feedback inhibition of thyroid hormone production (see later discussion), but most of these loci are not identified.

T_4 is the major form of thyroid hormone secreted from the gland, and much of this T_4 is converted to T_3 in peripheral tissues. Since T_3 binds to TRs with higher affinity than T_4, it is thought T_3 is the major active form of thyroid hormone. Smaller amounts of alternate forms of thyroid hormone are also made in, and secreted by, the thyroid gland. These products are metabolites of thyroxine and include T_3, reverse T_3 (rT_3), and others. Overall amounts of secreted T_4 are much higher (more than 20-fold) than any of these alternate forms of thyroid hormone.

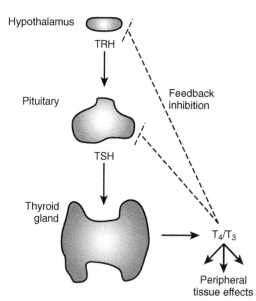

FIGURE 5-1. Regulation of thyroid hormone production in the hypothalamic-pituitary axis. Thyroid hormone is produced in the thyroid gland under control of thyroid-stimulating hormone (TSH). Circulating hormones exert multiple effects on different tissues in the periphery and also feed back to inhibit hypothalamic signals that stimulate TSH release and pituitary production of TSH, thereby maintaining thyroid hormone levels in defined limits.

The thyroid gland may also produce thyronamines (discussed in more detail later[10]), compounds that may constitute part of a completely distinct arm of the thyroid hormone signaling system; circulating levels of the most potent currently known thyronamine (3-iodothyronamine) appear higher than those of T_3.

The negative feedback loop that controls thyroid hormone levels works through the hypothalamus and pituitary (hypothalamic-pituitary-thyroid [HPT] axis (Fig. 5-1). Thyrotropin-releasing hormone (TRH) is released from the hypothalamus and stimulates the synthesis and release of thyroid-stimulating hormone (TSH) by thyrotrophic cells in the pituitary gland. TSH is released into the circulation, where it stimulates the synthesis and release of T_4 and to a lesser extent, T_3. The circulating thyroid hormones block release of both TRH and TSH through repression of the transcription of genes that encode the TRH pre-pro-hormone and the α and β subunits of TSH and also by down-regulating TRH receptors in the pituitary. Together, these actions result in repression of hormone synthesis and release in response to high circulating levels of T_4 and T_3. This process helps maintain thyroid hormone levels within defined limits.

Thyroid hormone production is also subject to additional influences. For example, rates of thyroid hormone synthesis and release often become depressed in conditions of inflammation and illness.

Thyroid Hormone Action in the Periphery

Plasma thyroid hormone constitutes the reservoir for distribution to target tissues. Higher hormone levels are generally correlated with increased TH response. However, there are differences in availability of hormone in peripheral tissues, which are conse-

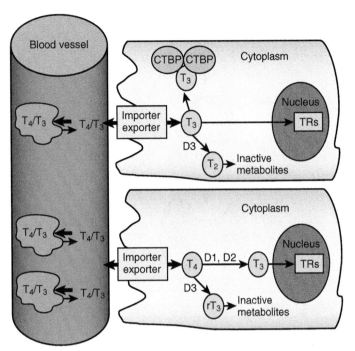

FIGURE 5-2. Peripheral actions of thyroid hormone. The figure summarizes possible fates of thyroid hormone in the periphery. Hormones are mostly transported as complexes with serum binding globulins with limited amounts of free T_4 and T_3. Hormones are actively taken up into cells by facilitated transport mechanisms, where they undergo several different fates. The *upper cell* represents possible intracellular fates of T_3; it can be sequestered in complexes with CTBP dimers, undergo conversion to inactive metabolites, or enter the nucleus to interact with TRs. The *lower cell* represents fates of T_4, which is either activated by metabolic modification to form T_3 or converted to inactive metabolites. It should be noted that expression of DI and D2 is under transcriptional control, making this step an important control point in thyroid hormone response.

quences of variations in transport processes and metabolic conversions that generate T_3 and degrade T_4 and T_3 to inactive forms. The activity of these pathways means that the correlation between plasma hormone levels and response is not absolute.

Both major forms of thyroid hormone (T_4 and T_3) are transported in the circulation in complex with plasma proteins (Fig. 5-2). The ratio of total T_4 to T_3 in plasma is about 60:1. This is higher than the 20-fold ratio of T_4 to T_3 that is initially secreted by the thyroid gland because of greater plasma binding of T_4 versus T_3, resulting in greater clearance rates of T_3. About 99.98% of total circulating T_4 and 99.7% of T_3 form noncovalent interactions with serum proteins, mostly to thyroxine-binding globulin but to a lesser extent to thyroxine-binding prealbumin, albumin and lipoproteins. The fact that less T_3 circulates in complex with plasma proteins means that the ratio of free T_4 to T_3 is around three- to sixfold, with typical circulating free hormone levels around 20 picomolar (pM) T_4 and 6 pM T_3, respectively. The free fraction is biologically active and can enter target tissues. Thus, interactions with plasma binding proteins help to ensure even hormone delivery throughout the body.

IMPORT AND EXPORT

Thyroid hormone entry into cells is mediated by specific transporters (see Fig. 5-2).[11-13] While early models suggested that lipophilic thyroid hormone molecules enter cells by diffusion across the plasma membrane, and this may occur to some extent, it is now clear that T_4 and T_3 entry mostly involves facilitated

transport, a form of passive diffusion that requires membrane transport proteins.

Several proteins involved in thyroid hormone import and efflux across the plasma membrane of target cells have been identified. However, the quantitative contributions of these and possibly other transporters to overall thyroid hormone entry and export have not been established, and concentrations of various transporters in different tissues may vary. Potential transporters include members of several different multigene families: monocarboxylate transporters (MCTs), organic anion transporters (OATP), L-amino acid transporters, multidrug resistance–associated proteins, fatty acid translocase, and Na⁺/taurocholate-cotransporting polypeptide.

Presently, the best-characterized thyroid hormone transporter is the X-linked MCT8 isoform, which is important for thyroid hormone import into the brain. Expression of the *MCT8* gene in cultured cells and frog oocytes enhances thyroid hormone transport into cells. Inactivating human *MCT8* mutations are associated with severe neurologic defects in affected males, suggesting that MCT8-dependent thyroid hormone transport into neurons is essential for proper brain development. There are also changes in circulating thyroid hormones (low T_4 and high T_3). Analysis of *MCT8* mutants in cultured cells reveals that the mutations abolish T_3 transport, likely explaining elevated circulating T_3 levels. Targeted deletion of the mouse *MCT8* gene leads to alterations in thyroid hormone levels that are similar to those of affected humans, although mice are devoid of the neurologic defects. Here, liver thyroid hormone levels are normal, suggesting that other transporters are more important in this tissue.

Of other transporters, recent observations show that a closely related protein, MCT10, can also mediate T_4 and T_3 import into cells. MCT10 is a more effective transporter than MCT8 and displays a preference for T_3. It is widely expressed and particularly abundant in the liver, intestine, kidney, and placenta. Finally, OATP1C1-expressing cells exhibit preferential import of T_4 and rT_3. The protein is distributed widely in the brain, with locations consistent with a specific role in thyroid hormone transport across the blood-brain barrier. It is not clear whether there are other high-affinity thyroid hormone transporters that are yet to be identified or whether apparently low-affinity transporters may play a physiologically important role in some tissues.

Less is known about mechanisms involved in thyroid hormone export from cells. It is clear that MCT8 and MCT10 enhance both thyroid hormone uptake and export, but it is not clear whether these proteins are physiologically relevant hormone exporters or whether other, undescribed, exporters may also play a role.

In some tissues—brown fat in the mouse is an example—hormone response is dependent on T_3 that is generated from intracellular T_4. The implication here is that free T_4 mostly penetrates these cells, where it constitutes a reservoir for T_3 generation, and that tissue uptake of T_3 is much lower. Regulated conversion of T_4 to T_3 provides an important control point; induction of the type 2 deiodinase via induction of second messenger pathways regulates T_3 levels and therefore the extent of the thyroid hormone response (also discussed later).

ACCUMULATION OF THYROID HORMONE IN CELLS

While free thyroid hormones are present at low concentrations in the circulation, levels of hormone can be much higher in target tissues. Although the extent to which this pool of hormone is active is not known, this observation suggests that there are

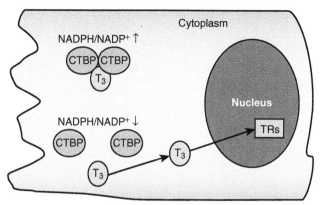

FIGURE 5-3. Thyroid hormone interactions with CTBP. Intracellular T_3 can bind CTBP dimers and become sequestered in the cytoplasm. CTBP dimer formation is sensitive to intracellular NADPH/NADP$^+$ concentrations such that free hormone will probably be released in response to reductions of NADPH levels.

mechanisms which permit thyroid hormone accumulation in target cells.

T_3 binds with nanomolar affinity to an intracellular protein that was originally called *cytoplasmic T_3-binding protein* (CTBP).[14] This protein is found at high abundance in the kidney and, to a lesser extent, in liver. Because CTBP was later found to be homologous to mu-crystallin, a protein abundant in the lens of the kangaroo eye, the gene is now often called *CRYM*. Overexpression of CRYM in stable cell lines increases maximal cellular T_3 binding capacity and decreases T_3 efflux rates. However, these effects are coupled to reduced transcriptional responses to T_3, suggesting that CRYM sequesters T_3 in an inactive cytoplasmic complex, away from nuclear TRs.

CRYM is important for thyroid hormone action in vivo. Mice with a targeted *CRYM* gene deletion appear normal but exhibit moderate decreases in circulating T_4 (25%) and T_3 (13%) levels and perhaps more importantly, also exhibit extremely rapid rates of T_3 entry into and escape from target tissues, presumably because there is no CRYM to sequester cytoplasmic hormone from export mechanisms. Human patients with a natural CRYM mutation that blocks its ability to bind T_3 (K314T) are deaf, a known consequence of defective thyroid hormone signaling during development. Interestingly, CRYM requires NADPH for dimerization and T_3 binding (Fig. 5-3). As NADPH levels are reflective of levels of cellular reducing power and anabolic capacity, it is conceivable that CRYM may sequester or release T_3 in response to alterations in cellular metabolic status. This notion is attractive but not proven.

There could be other T_3-binding proteins in addition to CRYM and the nuclear TRs (which are described later). Radioisotope-labeled T_3 interacts with proteins in the endoplasmic reticulum, mitochondrion, and nuclear envelope.[2] These putative T_3-binding proteins have not been identified, and the functional significance of these interactions is unknown.

DEIODINASES IN THYROID HORMONE ACTIVATION AND INACTIVATION

The thyroid gland produces mostly thyroxine. Limited amounts of T_3 and rT_3 are secreted by the gland, but more than 80% of both these forms of thyroid hormone are produced in the periphery via actions of specific deiodinases, D1, D2, and D3.[15,16] D1 and D2 remove the iodine group from the 5′ position of the outer thyronine ring. As T_3 binds to TRs with higher affinity than T_4,

the actions of D1 and D2 deiodinases serve to increase thyroid hormone activity through generation of T_3, and this represents a step-up in activity. Conversely, the action of D3 decreases hormone activity and represents a step down by removing the iodine group from the 5 position of the inner thyronine ring and converting T_4 and T_3 to rT_3 and 3,3′-T_2, respectively, neither of which interacts substantially with nuclear TRs at physiologic concentrations. Changes in deiodinase expression and activity are important control points in thyroid hormone signaling; they influence the production and availability of the biologically active form of thyroid hormone, T_3.

D2 activity generates most plasma T_3 in euthyroid (defined as levels of thyroid hormone within normal range) conditions via conversion of T_4 to T_3 in peripheral tissues. Comparisons of rates of T_3 production by D2 and D1 indicate that D2 is probably more important for T_4 to T_3 conversion at physiologic T_4 concentrations; it displays a higher K_m value for substrate than D1 and is likely to be sensitive to alterations in T_4 concentrations and more active than D1 at physiologic hormone concentrations. In addition, environmental stimuli regulate D2 activity catalyzing local T_3 production from T_4 in certain tissues. For example, signals such as cold exposure increase D2 expression in brown fat (discussed earlier), and the resulting increase in intracellular T_3 promotes induction of uncoupling protein with consequent heat generation. These lines of evidence suggest that D2 is important in generating T_3 that activates TRs. Accordingly, D2 is located in the perinuclear region where it can deliver T_3 efficiently to TRs.

D1 acts in a similar way to D2, but its functions are not as clear as with D2, because it displays a relatively high K_m value for T_4 to T_3 conversion (i.e., the enzyme binds the T_4 substrate with low affinity). D1 is highly expressed in liver and kidney, and its expression is induced by thyroid hormone. While previous models suggested that D1 is important for regulation of circulating T_3, more recent models suggest that D1 may only contribute substantially to plasma T_3 in conditions of thyroid hormone excess. D1 may also be involved in 5′ deiodination of other forms of thyroid hormone, including rT_3.

D3 is important for clearance of plasma T_3.[17] It is highly expressed in human placenta, where it is thought to be important for protection of the developing fetus from effects of maternal thyroid hormones. D3 is also highly expressed in the brain and skin. Increased D3 levels may account for reductions of circulating thyroid hormone levels that are often observed in critically ill patients and states of inflammation. Finally, D3 is often overexpressed in vascular tumors, and this in turn can result in marked reductions in circulating thyroid hormone levels.

ALTERNATE METABOLIC FATES OF THYROID HORMONE: INACTIVE AND ACTIVE DERIVATIVES

In addition to 5′ deiodination, T_4 undergoes other modifications which are generally believed to inactivate the hormone.[18] About 45% of circulating T_4 is converted to rT_3 and 35% to T_3. T_3 and rT_3 undergo further deiodinations to create T_4 derivatives with all possible combinations of iodinated and deiodinated inner and outer rings (3,3′-T_2, 3,5-T_2, 3′,5-T_2, 3′-T_1, 3-$T1$ and T_0), none of which bind significantly to nuclear TRs. T_4 and T_3 can also be inactivated by glucuronidation in liver, followed by secretion into the bile or by sulfation in liver and kidney and excretion in the urine.

The fact that most secreted T_4 is rapidly converted to apparently inactive forms of the hormone has led investigators to question whether some of these T_4 derivatives have unappreciated functions in activation of alternate receptors or as metabolic precursors of different active forms of the hormone. As mentioned earlier, one of the most prominent, rT$_3$, is a very weak thyroid hormone partial agonist that is unlikely to exert significant actions through the TRs. However, there are two cases in which alternate metabolic modification of T$_4$ does produce biologically active forms of hormone:

1. Deamination of the thyroid hormone alanine side group produces acetic acid derivatives of T$_4$ (tetraiodoacetic acid, Tetrac) and T$_3$ (triiodoacetic acid, Triac).[19] Both are exclusive products of extrathyroidal metabolism; they are undetectable in the thyroid gland. Although they comprise about 2% of total circulating thyroid hormone, they are present at high levels in liver, where Triac represents about 14% of total thyroid hormones. Tetrac and Triac are excreted in the urine, suggesting that deamination may promote thyroid hormone clearance from the body. However, Triac binds to TRs with high affinity and acts as a potent activator. It also exhibits TR isoform preference (it preferentially binds the beta form of TR) and interacts weakly with CTBP/CRYM, suggesting that it may evade cytoplasmic sequestration by this protein. While these observations raise the issue that Triac has a distinct function from T$_3$, this idea is not proven.

2. Decarboxylation of thyroid hormone alanine side group produces amine derivatives (thyronamines) that are directly analogous to different iodinated forms of thyroid hormone.[10] Thyronamines have been detected in the thyroid gland, central nervous system, fat, and other tissues. They are bound to transporter proteins in the circulation and, though completely quantitative analyses of circulating thyronamine levels have not been published, early estimates of their abundance suggest that they are present at concentrations that are at least similar to or greater than rT$_3$ or T$_3$.[10] At the time of writing, an endocrine role for thyronamines has not been formally proven, but there is clear evidence of biological activity. Each thyronamine has been chemically synthesized and tested in cell culture in animal models; one derivative with a single iodine substituent at the 3 position of the inner thyronine ring (T$_1$-amine) binds and activates a cell surface G-coupled protein receptor (trace amine–associated receptor 1; TAAR1) at physiologic concentrations (subnanomolar). T$_1$-amine induces profound hypothermia, bradycardia, and reduced cardiac output in mice and alters metabolism in several species; it reduces metabolic rate and increases lipid utilization in a pattern that is reminiscent of sleep or hibernation. T$_1$-amine may prove to be an important endocrine hormone, and it is interesting to suggest that T$_4$ derivatives such as rT$_3$ may be metabolic precursors of this compound.

Actions of Thyroid Hormone

Thyroid hormones exert profound influences on nearly all tissues (Fig. 5-4).[2] Receptors for thyroid hormones (TRs) are expressed fairly ubiquitously, although well-defined target tissues such as liver and heart express higher levels of TRs than others, and there are differences in distributions of particular TR isoforms[20] (described in more detail in a following discussion). Essentially, thyroid hormone is needed for proper growth and development

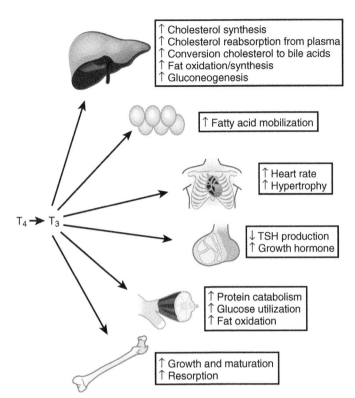

FIGURE 5-4. Tissue effects of thyroid hormones: summary of thyroid hormone effects on different tissues.

of the fetus and children and exerts widespread influences on multiple aspects of metabolism in adults.

Analysis of gene expression patterns in mouse knockout models has confirmed that TRs mediate nearly all thyroid hormone responses, and that many of these effects involve changes in gene expression. While actual influences of thyroid hormone on gene expression are complex, there are important underlying principles.[2] First, developmental defects that arise in cretinism and children born to hypothyroid mothers are not reversed by later hormone replacement, whereas adults with thyroid hormone imbalances exhibit metabolic disturbances that in most cases can be readily reversed by restoring TH levels to correct levels. This implies that hormone must trigger key developmental events in defined temporal windows, but thyroid hormone–regulated genes involved in metabolic regulation remain sensitive to alterations in hormone levels and continuously couple gene expression to thyroid status. Consideration of gene expression patterns, described in more detail later, reveals that some genes are induced in multiple tissues (D1 is an example), whereas other target genes are regulated in a manner that is highly tissue- and context-specific. Thus, thyroid hormone is a primary regulator of some genes, but hormone must cooperate with other factors to induce expression of other genes. Specific effects of thyroid hormone follow.

BASAL METABOLIC RATE

One of the most important effects of thyroid hormone involves changes in basal metabolic rate (BMR) in multiple tissues.[21-24] Thyroid hormones stimulate oxygen consumption (indicative of enhanced metabolism) in multiple locations, including skeletal muscle, liver, kidney, and intestine. Increases in BMR are probably partly related to increased mitochondrial activity and number. Importantly, thyroid hormones induce expression of uncoupling proteins (UCPs), mitochondrial membrane proteins that dissipate the proton gradient in the absence of ATP synthesis, thereby converting potential energy to heat. This effect is probably a contributor to thyroid hormone–dependent increases in BMR.

Thyroid hormone does not always enhance BMR. For example, BMR is not enhanced by thyroid hormone in most regions of the brain, and the hormone actually suppresses metabolic activity in the pituitary. The receptors in these tissues are functional, suggesting that key mediators of thyroid hormone regulation of BMR are blocked or absent.

TISSUE EFFECTS

Thyroid hormone exerts specific effects on growth, development, and metabolism in a variety of tissues. Some of these effects are summarized briefly here:

Liver

Thyroid hormones exert multiple effects on the liver.[2,25] They are potent mitogens in this tissue, especially in growing animals. Thyroid hormone also influences multiple metabolic processes. There is stimulation of fatty acid β-oxidation and gluconeogenesis, both key aspects of fasting response.[26] However, thyroid hormone can also stimulate expression of enzymes involved in lipogenesis and generation of NADPH-reducing equivalents that are required for fat synthesis and protection against reactive oxygen species. Since it is thought that fat oxidation and synthesis do not occur simultaneously, these processes are probably separated spatially or temporally, and thyroid hormone must cooperate with other signaling mechanisms to regulate these effects.

Thyroid hormone plays a major role in regulation of cholesterol metabolism in liver in rodents, and studies of patients with thyroid excess and deficiency states suggest that some of these pathways are also thyroid hormone regulated in humans. The hormone induces expression of enzymes involved in cholesterol synthesis but also increases levels of the low-density-lipoprotein (LDL) cholesterol receptor, which promotes cholesterol uptake from the circulation. Likewise, thyroid hormone increases expression of apolipoprotein A1, the key protein component of high-density lipoprotein (HDL) and increases expression of an HDL receptor (SR-B1). Consequently, thyroid hormone excess may promote increased cholesterol flux from the plasma to the liver through both the LDL and HDL pathways. Additionally, thyroid hormone stimulates cholesterol efflux and cholesterol to bile acid conversion. Collectively these mechanisms account for the net reductions of serum cholesterol levels that are observed with thyroid hormone and a net reverse cholesterol transport reflected by an increased flow of bile acids into the gut. Although not observed with T3, some thyroid hormone analogues promote a lowering of plasma triglycerides that may be due to net suppression of triglyceride synthesis through poorly defined mechanisms.

Adipose Tissue[27]

Thyroid hormones promote differentiation of precursors into white fat and induce lipogenic enzymes in pre-adipocytes from young rats and cell lines, but they also increase lipolysis in animals and humans. However, the lipolytic effects must predominate, because there is a net loss of fat in hyperthyroid states and a gain in hypothyroidism.

Thyroid hormone stimulates adaptive thermogenesis in brown adipose tissues. In cold or in response to overeating, there is increased local production of T3 via transcriptional induction of D2. This T3 cooperates with norepinephrine outputs from the sympathetic nervous system to induce uncoupling proteins that promote dissipation of the mitochondrial protein gradient as heat rather than ATP storage. Whereas previous reports suggested that adaptive thermogenesis was only important for temperature regulation in human newborns and in small mammals, recent studies have suggested that brown fat may also be important in adult humans. There are currently no reports of how thyroid hormones regulate development of this potentially important tissue.

Heart and Blood Vessels[28,29]

Thyroid hormones have multiple effects on the cardiovascular system. One influence is to increase cardiac output. Excess thyroid hormone is associated with increased heart rate, atrial arrhythmias, and development of heart failure. Conversely, reduced thyroid hormone is associated with reduced heart rate, lower vascular resistance, and increased blood volume. Thyroid hormone regulates genes involved in cardiac contractility. There is induction of the sarcoplasmic reticulum Ca^{2+} ATPase 2 (SERCA2), involved in calcium reuptake during the diastolic phase, and α myosin heavy chain (MHC), a fast ATPase required for heart contractility that is expressed in adult heart. Conversely, thyroid hormone inhibits expression of βMHC, a slow ATPase expressed in embryonic heart and up-regulated in stress conditions that diminish cardiac function. Thus, changes in thyroid hormone response in heart may be an important component of heart failure. Thyroid hormones also inhibit injury at sites of stroke, attenuate cardiac remodeling, and improve hemodynamics.

Pituitary[2]

Thyroid hormones repress production of pituitary TSH and hypothalamic TRH. This feedback loop is critical for maintenance of normal thyroid homeostasis and can be deranged in diseases. Thyroid hormones also stimulate expression of factors such as growth hormone, which influence growth and metabolism of many other tissues.

Muscle[2]

Thyroid hormones promote muscle catabolism and increase skeletal muscle energy expenditure in adults. Thyroid hormone induces the insulin-sensitive glucose transporter in muscle and also promotes fat burning.[30] These effects may help to sensitize muscle to insulin response. Accordingly, a human D2 gene polymorphism that reduces activity of the enzyme in muscle leads to a 20% reduction in insulin-dependent glucose disposal in humans and is correlated with insulin resistance in human populations that harbor this alteration.

Skeletal System[31]

Thyroid hormone is required for normal bone growth and maturation in children. Juvenile hypothyroidism causes delayed bone formation and short stature, whereas thyrotoxicosis leads to increased growth and advanced skeletal development. In adults, however, thyroid hormone excess promotes bone resorption. Thyroid hormone excess can lead to osteoporosis, especially in postmenopausal women.

Brain[32,33]

Thyroid hormone regulates brain development, and hypothyroidism results in mental retardation and multiple neurologic defects. Slow mentation and other CNS disturbances characterize hypothyroidism. In hyperthyroidism, there can be episodes of anxiety and even psychosis.

Intestine

Thyroid hormone is required for normal maturation of the small intestine. TRα1 is required for proliferation of intestinal epithelial progenitor cells via induction of the β-catenin proto-oncogene.[34]

Skin[35]

Thyroid hormone is important for skin function, and thyroid hormone imbalances are often first manifested in changes in appearance. Hypothyroidism leads to cold and dry, thickened skin. There is also increased hair loss. Conversely, hyperthyroidism leads to warm, moist, and smooth skin with fine soft hair. Hormone effects are a combination of inhibitory changes in keratin expression, sterol biosynthesis, diminished sebaceous gland secretion, and increased collagen breakdown.

SYSTEMATIC ANALYSIS OF THYROID HORMONE TARGET GENES

Many thyroid hormone–responsive genes involved in the responses described earlier are known.[2] For example, in liver, thyroid hormone induces carnitine palmitoyl transferase 1a (that mediates the rate-limiting step in fatty acid oxidation); glucose-6-phosphatase and phosphoenolpyruvate carboxykinase (rate-limiting steps in gluconeogenesis); the NR coregulator PGC-1α, which is an important transcriptional coregulator that stimulates genes important for mitochondrial biogenesis, gluconeogenesis, and fat oxidation; CYP-7a1 (cholesterol-to–bile acid conversion); fatty acid synthetase; acetyl-CoA carboxylase; malic enzyme (increases fat synthesis); and spot 14, which is required for fat synthesis in some tissues and up-regulated in contexts in which carbohydrates are converted to fat. Many other hormone-responsive genes are probably still unknown.

The earliest systematic attempt to define thyroid hormone response was performed in the late 1970s. Use of two-dimensional (2D) gels to analyze extracts from radiolabeled methionine–pulsed cells revealed that about 1% of 1000 rat liver proteins change in response to altered thyroid hormone.[36,37] There were inductions and repressions, and the studies began to define the "domain" of the thyroid hormone response. Recent advances in gene-profiling technology have permitted much more detailed descriptions of hormone-dependent alterations in gene profile. Presently there have been relatively few systematic genome-wide descriptions of thyroid hormone responses.[25,26,38,39] An early study of thyroid hormone action in mouse liver revealed that about 1% of mouse genes change in response to altered thyroid hormone (hypothyroid versus hyperthyroid),[25] confirming estimates from 2D gels. This study revealed target genes involved in carbohydrate, fat, and amino acid metabolism and unexpected thyroid hormone–regulated pathways; for example, genes involved in apoptosis are induced. The experiment also provided insights into patterns of thyroid hormone–responsive gene expression. Most regulated genes (>65%) in liver were repressed by thyroid hormone. This preponderance of negatively regulated genes is not seen in all tissues. Target genes are generally up-regulated by hormones in human muscle primary culture.

Later studies of thyroid hormone patterns of gene expression in TR knockout mice provided insights into TR-specific effects and subtle differences in thyroid hormone–responsive gene expression and are discussed in more detail later in the chapter. Systematic screening of thyroid hormone–responsive genes should provide detailed descriptions of novel target genes and pathways in different tissues.

THYROID HORMONE–REGULATED MICRORNAs

MicroRNAs (miRs) are small (18 to 25 nucleotides), noncoding RNAs that hybridize with coding mRNAs to inhibit translation and, in some cases, also promote mRNA degradation.[40] The enormous roles these miRs play in regulation is just beginning to be appreciated. MiRs are produced by cleavage and processing of large primary transcripts, which often code for proteins. Thus, many of the influences that regulate expression of parental primary transcripts also regulate expression of the associated miR. While effects of thyroid hormone on miR expression have not been studied extensively, one miR (miR-208) lies within a noncoding region of the thyroid hormone–responsive human αMHC transcript (and is therefore up-regulated by thyroid hormone itself). MiR-208 is implicated in up-regulation of stress-dependent cardiac responses. It is likely that other thyroid hormone–responsive miRs exist, and they may play important roles in hormone effects on protein translation.

History of the Mechanism of Action of Thyroid Hormones

As the physiologic effects of thyroid hormones became known, investigators focused on roles of these hormones on stimulating the basal metabolic rate and on the liver.[1,2] It was originally proposed that the hormones directly uncouple oxidative phosphorylation and that the primary site of action of thyroid hormones was at the mitochondria; here, investigators related actions of thyroid hormones to those of dinitrophenol. Later studies revealed other influences of thyroid hormones, including cholesterol reduction, that were hard to relate to mitochondrial actions. The notion that thyroid hormones directly uncouple mitochondrial oxidative phosphorylation did not provide a coherent unifying hypothesis to explain all actions of thyroid hormone.

In the late 1960s, Tata and colleagues conducted a number of measurements of the effects of thyroid hormones on the liver.[41] He found that thyroid hormone–dependent increases in metabolic rate were blocked by actinomycin D, an inhibitor of RNA and, secondarily, protein synthesis. Also, there was an increased uptake of radiolabeled uridine into trichloric acid (TCA) precipitable material following administration of TH to animals, as well as increased activity of RNA polymerase, suggesting that TH stimulates RNA synthesis. Similar studies were being conducted with NR ligands such as with glucocorticoids, estrogens, and progestins, and there was great controversy as to whether these ligands acted through (1) transcriptional control, (2) precursor uptake, or (3) posttranscriptional control. The experiments did not address high specificity of TH responses, and as a result, controversy remained as to which of the three mechanisms applied to thyroid hormone action. Nevertheless, this study represented the first fundamentally correct proposal for the mechanism of thyroid hormone action.

DISCOVERY OF THYROID HORMONE RECEPTORS AND THEIR MECHANISM OF ACTION

TRs were identified in the 1970s.[42,43] Following the discovery of several nuclear receptors, including the estrogen and glucocorticoid receptors, investigators in the thyroid hormone field utilized similar approaches to look for TRs. Specific binding of radiolabeled T_3 to liver cells was initially discovered by Oppenheimer and colleagues using intact cells and later characterized further by Samuels and colleagues, who found that the mechanism of TR actions differed mechanistically from the steroid receptors, which translocate into the nucleus on ligand binding. For TRs, hormone could bind directly to nuclei, and the location of receptors did not alter with T_3.

In the late 1970s and early 1980s, multiple aspects of the receptors were revealed.[36,44] Analysis of properties of TRs revealed a single class of high-affinity binding sites with K_d values for T_3 in the 0.1 nM range. Specific hormone-binding sites were observed in extracts of several responsive tissues, including liver, anterior pituitary, brain, and heart. Estimates of the number of binding sites per cell suggested that the proteins are rare; highly responsive tissues only contained about 10,000 specific hormone-binding sites per cell. Evidence that the receptor preparations correspond to physiologic hormone targets came from observations that affinities for different thyroid hormones parallel their biological potencies (Triac>T_3>T_4>rT_3). Partial TR purification and photo-affinity labeling revealed two major nuclear hormone-binding proteins with molecular weights of 46 and 57 kD, which were later found to correspond to products of distinct genes—the TR α and β isoforms—described later in the chapter. TRs were also found to be associated with chromatin, and preferentially with active chromatin, suggesting that they influence gene expression through interactions with DNA.[45-48]

DISCOVERY THAT THYROID HORMONES REGULATE SPECIFIC mRNAS AND GENE TRANSCRIPTION

As molecular biology techniques became available, it was possible to isolate specific mRNAs from tissues where they were abundant and to translate them. By the 1970s, regulation of specific mRNAs had been demonstrated for estrogens, progestins, and glucocorticoids. Growth hormone (GH) mRNA was abundant in rat pituitary cells, and Baxter and colleagues were able to demonstrate that thyroid hormones could specifically regulate GH mRNA, conclusively demonstrating for the first time that thyroid hormones alter the levels of specific mRNAs. The same group cloned rat GH gene sequences, and these permitted demonstrations that thyroid hormones increased mRNA hybridizable to a rat GH cDNA probe. The cloned GH sequences were also used in so-called "polymerase run-on experiments" that showed that hormones stimulate transcription rather than induce some posttranscriptional modification of the mRNA. These studies resolved the controversies prevalent at the time of experiments by Tata and colleagues, discussed previously. Thus the fundamental concept of thyroid hormone action whereby the receptor regulates the transcription of specific genes was established.

DISCOVERY THAT TRs BIND PREFERENTIALLY TO ACTIVE CHROMATIN AND SPECIFIC DNA SEQUENCES

Studies during the 1970s and 1980s also set the stage for understanding the nature of TR binding sites and their relationship to active chromatin. GH genomic DNA was used for interaction studies with partially purified TR preparations, demonstrating that TRs bound to specific DNA sequences. These experiments were forerunners of the now familiar concept that receptors act by binding to specific thyroid hormone response elements (TREs). That the receptors could affect DNA was further evidenced by the finding that they induce bending of rat or human TR DNA binding sites. Subcellular fractionation revealed that TRs were associated with chromatin, and preferentially with active chromatin, suggesting a relationship between the receptors and transcriptionally active chromatin.[45-48] These studies set the stage for definition of thyroid hormone response elements (TREs).

CLONING OF TRS

TRs were cloned in 1986.[49,50] They were identified as cellular homologs of a retroviral oncogene (cancer-causing gene), v-erbA,[51] which causes erythroblastoma in chickens. Isolation of these cDNAs occurred after those for other members of the NR family, the glucocorticoid and estrogen receptors, which led to the realization that v-erbA was derived from an NR. Both of the v-erbA homologs bound thyroid hormone with high affinity and appropriate specificity. The Vennstrom group clone was most closely related to v-erbA and was originally designated as c-erbA, but it is now called *thyroid hormone receptor α* (TRα). As compared to TRα, v-erbA contains 17 different amino acid substitutions and a C-terminal truncation, which are now known to prevent the viral oncogene from binding hormone.[49] The Evans group clone encoded a highly homologous but distinct 57-kD protein that was closely related to TRα and v-erbA but was the product of the *THRB* gene.[50] The characterization of TR genes (*THRA* and *THRB*), which encode the two major TR isoforms (TRα1 and TRβ1) and several variants that arise from differential splicing (described later), helped to reveal that TRs belong to the NR family, which includes receptors for the steroid hormones, vitamins A and D, and other small lipophilic molecules.[4]

Identification of these receptor cDNAs paved the way for many studies of receptor structure and function. Although it was known at the time that NRs were composed of modular domains, the receptor structures provided the primary sequences in these domains and the abilities to express them and study their functions. In addition, the availability of TR cDNAs paved the way for functional studies, analog development, and improvements in understanding TR mechanisms. While these studies are not described in historical context, there have been rapid advancements in understanding of TR action, including the definition that unliganded TRs are transcriptionally active, leading to a new paradigm for thyroid hormone action; definition of TRE sequences; identification of retinoid X receptor (RXR) heterodimer partners and coregulators; x-ray structural analysis of DBDs and LBDs, which demonstrated a new and unexpected concept that the receptor folds around the ligands; improved understanding of TR function through generation of TR gene knockout animals; and development of new thyroid hormone analogs with selective actions.

Thyroid Hormone Receptors: Mechanism

TRs work by altering gene expression in response to changes in thyroid hormone concentrations (mostly T_3).[2,38] This alteration in gene transcription profile is believed to account for most of the observed physiologic effects of thyroid hormones, although there are also actions of thyroid hormones that do not involve transcription (discussed later). Unlike the case with steroid receptors, TRs are active in the absence of hormone.

HORMONE BINDING AND OCCUPANCY

Measurements of thyroid hormone affinity for its receptors reveal that T_3 binds to purified and recombinant TRs with high affinity. T_3 binds with about 10- to 15-fold greater affinity than T_4 (K_d values are around 2 nM for T_4 and 0.2 nM for T_3). These values appear higher than measured concentrations of circulating free hormones (0.02 nmol for T_4 and 0.06 nmol with T_3), implying that receptor occupancy could be minor in normal conditions. However, based on direct estimates of occupancy of nuclear TRs in different tissues after radiolabeled T_3 and T_4 injection into hypothyroid rats, about 25% to 35% of liver and kidney TRs and 58% of pituitary TRs become occupied with thyroid hormones in euthyroid conditions. Thus, there appear to be mechanisms to bring the hormone into the correct range to bind and activate receptors. One possibility was described earlier: intracellular generation of T_3 from T_4 leads to increased T_3 production in target cells. Facilitated transport alone would not be enough to concentrate T_3, but combinations of transport and cytoplasmic sequestration by CTBP/CRYM or similar proteins could play a role. Finally, TR complexes with stabilizing coactivators could display higher affinities for target hormones than isolated TRs tested in vitro or partially purified from cell extracts. In any case, it is clear that thyroid hormone concentrations are in the correct range to achieve reasonable receptor occupancy in target tissues under euthyroid conditions.

TR ACTION

Unlike classic models of hormone action in which unliganded receptor is inactive and hormone binding triggers its activity, TRs are transcriptionally active in the absence and in the presence of hormone (Fig. 5-5).[52] Rather than activating the receptor, hormone binding alters the spectrum of its actions.

TRs bind constitutively to specific DNA sequences termed *thyroid hormone response elements* (TREs) in the proximal promoter of positively regulated target genes. As noted earlier, TRs function mostly via heterodimerization with another NR, RXR,

which is a partner for many members of the NR family. RXR binds vitamin A derivatives and unsaturated fatty acids but is thought in many cases to be silent and unoccupied by ligands, when it forms complexes with TRs. Unliganded TRs repress transcription of positively regulated genes by recruiting corepressors such as the NR corepressor (N-CoR), silencing mediator of retinoid and thyroid hormone–responsive transcription (SMRT) and alien. Corepressors actively silence gene transcription by binding histone de-acetylases (mainly HDAC3) which condense local chromatin to prevent access of RNA polymerase II to target promoters.[53] Hormone reverses these inhibitory effects and further stimulates gene expression by promoting corepressor release and subsequent recruitment of several different coactivator complexes which enhance transcription in different ways: ATP-dependent remodeling of local chromatin, catalysis of specific histone modifications that mark the genes for transcriptional activity, and enhancement of recruitment and processivity of the basal transcription machinery.

The converse process can also occur.[54] Unliganded TRs stimulate gene transcription, and binding of T_3 overcomes this process, resulting in repression of gene transcription. Generally, hormone also suppresses transcription below levels stimulated by the unliganded TRs. One model to explain this phenomenon is that coactivators and corepressors exert opposite actions at this type of gene, and there are several examples where so-called NR coactivators repress gene transcription, and corepressors act as coactivators that bind to the "corepressor binding site" (Fig. 5-6). However, several mechanisms of NR repression have been described, so there are other possibilities. For example, ligand-dependent activation of peroxisome proliferator–activated receptors (PPARs) and liver X receptors permits covalent attachment of lysine residue in the LBD to a large 100-amino-acid protein called *small ubiquitin-like modifier* (SUMO), which arrests corepressor complexes at target promoters (Fig. 5-7).[54] This effect counters proinflammatory stimuli that promote corepressor release and gene induction and therefore acts as a repressive mechanism. Negative gene regulation may not involve direct receptor/DNA contacts.[55] Although promoters of some genes that are repressed in response to ligand contain variant TREs, negative regulation may also involve TR interactions with heterolo-

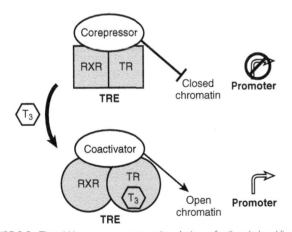

FIGURE 5-5. Thyroid hormone receptor action. Actions of unliganded and liganded TRs at positively regulated genes. The receptor binds DNA as a heterodimer with RXR in the absence and presence of the hormone. Unliganded TRs recruit corepressors, which repress gene transcription by condensing local chromatin structure and blocking coactivator binding. Hormone binding promotes a conformational change, which leads to exchange of corepressor for coactivators, which reverses effects of coactivators.

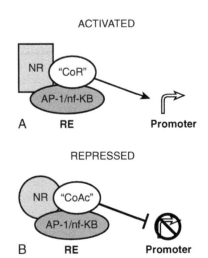

FIGURE 5-6. Transcriptional repression mechanisms. Transcriptional activation can occur by recruitment of a coactivator that binds to the corepressor binding surface. Transcriptional activation is mediated by a corepressor that binds the coactivator surface. In some cases, these proteins may be the same as coactivators and corepressors that mediate TR actions at classical TREs, with reversed functions.

REPRESSED-BASAL STATE

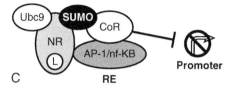

A   RE

ACTIVATED/PRO-INFLAMMATORY
SIGNALS

B   RE   Promoter

REPRESSED + PRO-INFLAMMATORY
STIMULI

C   RE

FIGURE 5-7. Repression by corepressor arrest. An alternative mode of transcriptional repression demonstrated for NRs at proinflammatory genes. **A,** Genes are constitutively repressed and **B,** activated by dismissal of corepressor complexes in response to proinflammatory signals. **C,** Liganded NRs repress transcription in the face of these proinflammatory stimuli by recruiting enzymes (including ubc9) which SUMOlate the liganded receptor LBD. SUMO modification, in turn, arrests the corepressor complex at the promoter.

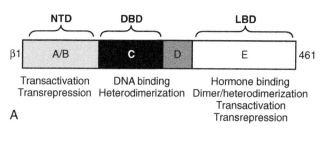

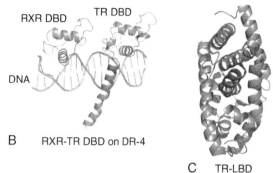

FIGURE 5-8. TR secondary and tertiary structure. Schematic representation of TR structures. **A,** The upper diagram represents TRβ secondary structure with domain positions marked. **B,** X-ray structures of the TR DBD on DNA in complex with RXR and the **C,** TR LBD. The two TR domain structures overlap in the "hinge" D-domain region.

gous DNA-bound transcription factors (such as AP-1 and CREB) instead of promoter DNA itself, as has been demonstrated for other NRs. Further investigation will be needed to clarify mechanisms of transcriptional repression at individual genes.

Models of thyroid hormone response emphasize differences in TR complex formation in the absence of hormone and the presence of saturating levels of hormone. As discussed previously, physiologic levels of hormone do not saturate all receptors under these conditions,[39] so thyroid hormone–responsive genes will probably be occupied by a mix of liganded and unliganded TRs, with different associated factors. The consequences of partial occupancy of DNA-bound receptors with hormone are far from clear; there could be active competition between liganded and unliganded TRs for the same sites in the same cells, stochastic choices between formation of liganded and unliganded TR-associated complexes in different cells, or other differences.

Receptor Structure and Function

SECONDARY STRUCTURE

TRs and other NRs are single polypeptide chains that adopt a common modular domain structure. Particular functions can be assigned to specific receptor domains (Fig. 5-8).[2,4] Use of basic recombinant DNA technology to create short cDNA fragments corresponding to each domain and targeted mutagenesis coupled with expression and functional analysis revealed the role of each domain.

The central DNA-binding domain (DBD) is highly conserved throughout the NR family. The DBD mediates receptor-DNA contact, contains a surface that mediates DNA-dependent heterodimer formation with RXR, and possibly has binding sites for other proteins with regulatory functions.

The amino acid sequences of the C-terminal ligand-binding domain (LBD) are relatively well conserved within the NR family, and the domain has a highly conserved common fold. The LBD is multifunctional and contains a ligand-binding cavity, a

hormone-dependent transcription function (AF-2) that binds coactivators, an overlapping corepressor binding surface exposed in the absence of ligands, and a major surface that mediates homodimer formation and heterodimer formation (with RXRs). The LBD may also harbor surfaces that mediate formation of alternate oligomers (trimers, heterotrimers, and tetramers) and interactions with heat shock proteins.

The amino-terminal domain (NTD) is poorly conserved among NRs, suggesting that it is primarily responsible for many of the unique activities of particular receptor subtypes. Transfection analysis reveals that the NTD contains a complex transactivation function (AF-1) that binds coactivators and corepressors, complements AF-2 in some contexts, and acts independently in others. TR AF-1 is required for optimal hormone response at certain promoters and in certain cell types. Accordingly, this domain also harbors binding sites for corepressors and coactivators.

DBD STRUCTURE

The DBD contains two zinc "fingers," protein domains of approximately 30 amino acids in length that require zinc ions for protein folding and stability. The zinc ion is coordinated by tetrahedral contacts with the side chains of four well conserved cysteine residues. Together, the two zinc finger motifs form a single functional DNA-binding domain.

The TR DBD x-ray structure was solved in complex with that of its heterodimer partner RXR on a thyroid hormone receptor response element (TRE), a direct repeat of the consensus sequence AGGTCA spaced by four bases (DR-4 element, see Fig. 5-8).[56,57] DNA contacts are mediated by a large α-helix in the first zinc finger, which docks into the major groove of DNA. This conserved region of the receptor contains the P-box, which dictates NR DNA element recognition specificity. Both the second zinc finger and a long carboxyl-terminal α-helix termed the *C-terminal extension* (CTE) also make DNA contacts. The second zinc finger interacts with the major groove, and the CTE interacts with the DNA minor groove and phosphate backbone. The organization of the CTE is unique to the TR, and these additional CTE-dependent DNA contacts may explain why TRs, unlike many other NRs, exhibit the capacity to bind to DNA as monomers (developed in following discussions).

RXR and TR DBDs interact with the DR-4 element in a head-to-tail manner, with RXR upstream. This polarity is dictated by the specific heterodimer contact surfaces, which involve multiple interactions between zinc finger regions of both receptors and between the outer face of the TR CTE and RXR. The 5′ location of RXR was already inferred by biochemical analysis[58]; introduction of the glucocorticoid receptor P-box sequence into TR permitted the RXR-TR complex to recognize a hybrid response element composed of one classic TR half-site (AGGTCA) and an equivalent glucocorticoid receptor response element half-site (TCTTGT) but only when the GR binding half-site is placed downstream in the 3′ position. This reflects that the TR preferentially associates with the downstream position.

RXR/TR pairs bind preferentially to DR-4 elements, whereas other RXR/NR pairs recognize direct AGGTCA repeats with different spacings.[58] Comparison of RXR/TR structures with other RXR/nuclear receptor pairs reveals that the CTE sets this spacing preference.[57] All NR CTEs fold across the core of the DBD, but different CTEs adopt different trajectories and occlude receptor binding to the wrong element. For RXR-TRs, spacings of less than 4 bp would not be permitted because of steric clashes between the CTE and the RXR DBD. Conversely, introduction of extra bases between the half-sites will impose geometric constraints that prevent proper engagement of the RXR-TR DBD heterodimer surface.

LBD STRUCTURE

Although there are now many publicly available NR LBD x-ray structures, TR (rat TRα) was the first structure solved in complex with native hormone (it was reported simultaneously with the structure of the liganded retinoic acid receptor, RAR).[59-61] Strikingly, the ligand was buried in the core of the LBD; this was contrary to contemporary models which assumed that ligand would interact with an allosteric site on the receptor surface. The ligand-binding pocket is small and well tailored to cognate agonists such as T_3 and Triac. This organization implies that admission of hormone into the core of the domain promotes its folding into an active conformation.

TR LBD structure strongly resembles other NRs.[4,62] The domain is almost entirely helical, composed of 12 α-helices. The α-helices fold into three layers: two outer layers comprise three distinct helices, the central layer comprises two helices, with the additional space occupied by hormone. Several short helical loops and β sheets link the individual α-helices. N-terminal LBD helix (H1) constitutes a backbone that links helical layers. C-terminal helix (H12) adopts different positions in the presence and absence of hormone and dictates cofactor interactions that influence receptor activity.

All NR LBDs possess the same fold, despite having only weak primary sequence similarity. TR LBDs share only 15% primary sequence identity with the progesterone receptor LBD, yet the two receptors exhibit a very similar structure, with only slight variations in the length of α-helices. Most structural variability occurs in the loops between conserved helices and in the extensions to C-terminal H12 (sometimes called the *F-domain*) that are present in other NRs but not the TRs. The overall conformation similarities of TRs and other NRs suggest that findings that apply to TRs will be general for other NRs and vice versa. Much has been learned about the function and interactions of NR homo-heterodimer surfaces, coregulator binding surfaces, and hormone effects on receptor structure with a combination of x-ray crystallography, approaches to assess LBD dynamics, and mutational analysis, to be discussed later.

HINGE STRUCTURE

The hinge domain (or D-domain) was first identified as a poorly conserved region that links the DBD and LBD. Original models suggested that it would behave as an unstructured peptide that facilitates rotation between the LBD and DBD in different contexts. However, TRβ LBD and DBD x-ray structures contain overlapping amino acids, and these reveal that residues that were originally assigned to the hinge actually comprise extensions of H1 of the LBD and the C-terminal portion of the DBD CTE.[60,63] The true unstructured hinge is only 3 to 6 amino acids long. Presently it is not clear whether this short region is sufficient for true rotational flexibility between domains. Interestingly, the C-terminal helix of the DBD CTE region appears as a completely unstructured peptide in some LBD crystals but not others, and it has been suggested that this region of the receptor could either fold into a functional helix or unfold to improve rotational flexibility in different contexts.[63]

NTD STRUCTURE

There are no published studies of TR NTD structure. NR N-terminal domains (NTDs) are important for transcriptional response and integration of NR ligand signals with second messenger pathways, but this region is poorly conserved throughout the receptor family and not at all defined at the level of tertiary structure.[64] Current models indicate that NR NTDs are composed of intrinsically unfolded domains; these types of proteins consist of multiple and potentially overlapping subregions that acquire active conformation on interaction with target cofactors.[64]

FULL-LENGTH RECEPTORS

No high-resolution structures of TRs or RXR-TR fragments that make up more than one domain have yet been resolved. There are published low-resolution solution x-ray structures of liganded TR DBD-LBD dimers, and an unusual tetrameric form of unliganded TR DBD-LBD.[65] However, these data provide sufficient resolution to determine likely shapes of the molecules, but not enough to define the trace of the protein backbone. Use of these low-resolution structures to dock high-resolution x-ray structural models of DBDs and LBDs suggests that in the dimer in solution, LBDs and DBDs are in close proximity to their counterparts in the neighboring subunit and that the DBDs are relatively distant from the LBDs, implying that the hinge is extended. In the solution tetramer, LBD pairs dock against each other with DBDs protruding in an X shape. Here, however, the DBDs are closer to the LBDs than they appear in the dimer, implying that there may be rearrangements in the hinge that are dependent on the oligomeric state of the LBD.

A recent structure of full-length liganded PPARγ in complex with liganded RXRα on a DNA element provides a guide to expected principles of organization of the full-length RXR-TR complex.[66] The PPARγ-RXRα heterodimer binds to a DR-1 element, with PPARγ in the 5′ position, unlike the TR which occupies the 3′ position (Fig. 5-9). LBDs and DBDs adopt the expected conformation and engage in the expected heterodimer contacts predicted from LBD and DBD structures and mutational

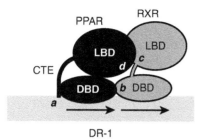

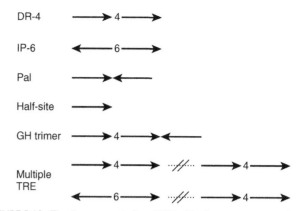

FIGURE 5-9. Schematic of full-length PPAR and RXR on a DR-1 element. Shown are expected and unexpected interaction points. The PPAR DBD CTE makes additional DNA contacts (**a**) outside of the consensus half-site. DBDs and LBDs are in predicted heterodimer contacts (**b, c**). Additionally, the PPAR LBD binds the RXR DBD (**d**). NTDs are unstructured and are not shown.

FIGURE 5-10. The diverse organization of TREs. The figure represents a schematic of orientations (*arrows*) and spacings (*numbers between arrows*) of AGGTCA half-sites observed in natural TREs. With multiple TREs, the orientations can differ between elements.

analysis, described more fully for the TRs later. However, the PPAR CTE portion of the hinge makes unexpected DNA contacts 5′ to the AGGTCA motif. Moreover, the complex is nonsymmetrical, the PPARγ LBD is close to the RXR DBD, and this facilitates unexpected heterodimer contacts which involve LBD surfaces around helix 3 and the β-sheet region and the surface of the RXR DBD on the opposite side of the molecule from the DNA-binding surface. The RXRα hinge appears unstructured and flexible. This permits the RXR LBD to adopt a more distant position from the DBD than the PPAR LBD and raises the possibility that the RXR hinge is a potential source of rotational flexibility in response-element recognition. Finally, NTDs of both receptors are disordered, in keeping with the prediction that these domains can only adopt appropriate conformation on contact with partners. It will be interesting to determine the structures of full-length TR/RXR to learn how TRs adapt to different elements and whether there are unexpected heterodimer contacts between LBDs and DBDs of these receptors.

VARIABLE TRE SEQUENCE AND CONFORMATIONAL ADAPTATION TO DNA

Published liganded TR LBD x-ray structures are monomers.[67] However, many NR LBDs have been crystallized as homodimers and heterodimers; there is a surface that binds both homo- and heterodimer partners which is large and comprises residues from helices 9, 10, 11, 7, and 8.[68] Targeted mutagenesis of TRs and RXRs confirms that dimer and heterodimer formation is similar to this common interface, with a hotspot of particularly hydrophobic residues at the junction of H10 and H11 playing very important roles in binding.[68]

Most TREs are composed of DR-4 elements, but there is significant variation in sequence and arrangement of TREs (Fig. 5-10) which results in TR isoform and oligomer-specific differences in DNA recognition. TRs and RXR-TRs bind to direct repeats with different spacing, inverted palindromes (IP), and palindromes (pal).[58,69] TRα- and TRβ-RXR heterodimers bind preferentially to DR-4 but also bind to IP-6 elements (where the DNA binding sites are in an inverted position with respect to each other, with a 6-nucleotide spacer) and palindromic (Pal) elements (where the DNA binding sites are arranged in a head-to-tail position with respect to each other, without spacer DNA). In contrast, TRβ homodimers bind strongly to IPs, weakly to consensus DR-4 elements, and not at all to Pal elements. TRα homodimers bind very weakly, if at all, to these TREs. In addition, TRβ homodimers bind strongly to a subset of variant DR-4 elements,[70] implying that additional sequence differences can facilitate homodimer interactions. RXR-TRs are the major TR

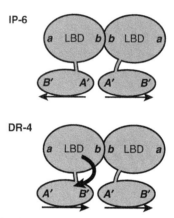

FIGURE 5-11. Predicted orientations of TR DBD and LBD on IP-6 and DR-4 elements. A need for swivel between domains at DR-4 elements? At an inverted palindrome, the LBDs and DBDs can bind in the same orientation, back to back, as indicated by positions of surfaces on DBDs (A′B″) and LBDs (a, b). At a direct repeat, the DBDs are in head-to-tail orientation, but the LBDs interact through the same surface that is utilized at the IP-6 element. Thus the LBD of the 5′ partner must rotate with respect to the 3′ partner. The source of this rotational flexibility is not clear, but the fact that RXR occupies this site in RXR-TR heterodimers suggests that the RXR hinge is one likely source.

species in living cells, but TRβ homodimers can clearly modulate transcription from some TREs in cell culture and yeast.[69] Moreover, blockade of RXR expression only inhibits T3 response at a subset of target genes.[71] Both observations suggest that alternate oligomeric forms of TR can mediate thyroid hormone responses. The precise contributions of RXR-TRs versus other TR oligomers to T3 signals at different genes in physiologic conditions are not yet clear.

TRs and RXR-TRs must undergo significant conformational adaptation to bind different TREs.[58] RXR-TR heterodimer and TR-TR homodimer formation involves the same interface at the junction of H10-H11, irrespective of TRE organization. Consideration of relative orientations of LBD and DBD required for binding to each TRE indicates that with DR-4 elements, the upstream LBD must rotate with respect to the DBD to form the heterodimer surface in a head-to-head fashion (Fig. 5-11). Since RXR-TRs preferetially bind DR-4 elements, it is likely that this rotation is provided by the upstream RXR. The TR DBD and LBD do not need to rotate for inverted palindromes, where TR-TR homodimer formation is strongest. Thus, RXR is probably responsible for flexible response-element recognition, and this may contribute to its function as a near-universal heterodimer partner for NRs. The unstructured appearance of the RXR hinge domain observed in the PPAR-RXR full-length structure mentioned earlier suggests that this could be one candidate for the source of flexibility.

ALTERNATE TREs

There are examples where TRs may interact with DNA in other ways.[58] Several response elements are composed of TRE half-sites that bind TR monomers. TRα and TRβ are unusual in the nuclear receptor family, with their high capacity to bind as monomers to AGGTCA half-sites in addition to more conventional interactions with DNA elements as dimers and heterodimers. In these cases, the recognition site is extended to include the core half-site and additional 5′ flanking sequences.

Natural TREs often contain multiple copies of half-sites. The spot 14 promoter contains two DR-4 elements, and the SERCa2 promoter contains a DR-4 element and two IP elements. In most cases, it is not known whether TRs recognize these elements as separate RXR-TR heterodimers or TR-TR homodimers or as larger assemblies, such as tetramers or heterotetramers. There is one clear example of the latter possibility. The rat growth-hormone promoter contains an unusual trimeric TRE that consists of a classic DR-4 element and a downstream half-site that forms a palindrome, the 3′ DR-4 half-site[72] (Fig. 5-12). TRβ, but not TRα, forms homotrimers and heterotrimers with RXR that bind this element with high efficiency and cooperativity. Thus TRβ must contain additional subunit interaction surfaces, if it simultaneously engages in typical homo/heterodimer contacts and also binds another TRβ subunit in the 3′ position. TRβ0, a TR splice variant that lacks the NTD and is abundantly expressed in frogs, birds, and reptiles, binds this element with high affinity, suggesting that all surfaces are in the DBD-LBD region.

There is significant variation in TRE half-site spacing and sequence in naturally occurring TREs that likely has consequences for TR activity.[4,58] TRs preferentially recognize DR-4 and IP-6 elements but also bind similar elements with different spacings, including DR-3, DR-7, and IP-4. Actual half-site sequences diverge considerably from the classic AGGTCA half-site. In fact, negatively regulated genes sometimes contain weak TR binding sites that instead conform to the consensus TGGTTT-GGGGTCCA.[55] These influences will affect the affinity of the receptor for the element but may also influence receptor activity in other ways. DNA contact alters DBD structure, and a small subset of glucocorticoid-receptor DBD mutations that mimic allosteric switches which occur on DNA binding affect activity of AF-1 and AF-2 and change the response element–specific

behavior of the receptor. One of these, a lysine residue at the base of the first zinc finger domain that contacts DNA, alters the activity of all NRs (including TR); it changes NRs from ligand-mediated repressors to ligand-mediated activators at promoters with AP-1 sites, where the receptor acts in the absence of direct DNA contact. Thus the nature of the DNA sequence element could alter both TR conformation and activity.

Hormone Effects on Receptor Structure

Presently there are few true unliganded NR LBD structures that permit direct comparison of liganded and unliganded states, and it is not clear how well such unliganded structures reflect the actual organization of unliganded receptors in the cell, where they are found in complexes with stabilizing protein partners.[61] However, x-ray structural analysis, nuclear magnetic resonance, and hydrogen-deuterium exchange studies, which can reveal different aspects of receptor dynamics, and results of structure-directed mutagenesis approaches have revealed many interesting facts about the nature of these hormone-dependent alterations.

LBD H12 POSITION AND COREGULATOR INTERACTIONS

The major known effect of hormone binding is stabilization of H12 in an active position in which it packs against the body of the LBD to form a surface called *activation function 2* (AF-2)[52,61] (Fig. 5-13). Comparisons of liganded TR and other liganded NR structures reveal that H12 is docked against the LBD in a similar position in all "active" liganded structures. Conversely, examination of unliganded structures and structures of NRs in complex with antagonists or partial agonists reveal that H12 can adopt various "inactive" or "partly active" conformations, all highly distinct from the active position of H12. This suggests that H12 may be unstable in the absence of an activating ligand. The idea that ligand binding stabilizes H12 has been confirmed by dynamics studies in which PPARγ H12 mobility was measured directly.[73]

H12 position influences coregulator interactions.[52] In the active position, H12 docks against the body of the LBD to form a surface-exposed hydrophobic cleft composed of residues from

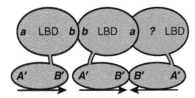

Growth hormone TRE

FIGURE 5-12. Predicted TR interactions with a complex TRE in the growth hormone promoter. The growth hormone TRE comprises three TRE half-sites arranged as a classic DR-4 element and a downstream half-site. The fact that there is cooperative binding suggests that the TR in the 3′ position in the DR-4 element must interact with both its upstream and downstream partner, although the mechanism for the latter interaction is not known.

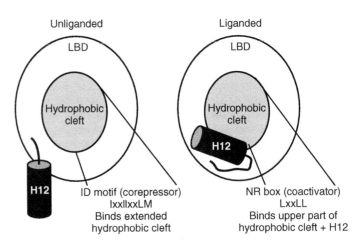

FIGURE 5-13. Helix 12 position and coregulator binding. TR C-terminal helix 12 is displaced away from the hydrophobic cleft without bound hormone, exposing a large hydrophobic cleft composed of residues form helices 3, 4, 5, and 6. This serves as interaction site for three-turn α-helical motifs from corepressors (IDs). With hormone, H12 packs over the lower part of the corepressor binding surface, blocking corepressor binding and creating a new binding site for coactivator NR boxes (LxxLL).

helices (H) 3, 4, 5, and 12. Saturation mutagenesis reveals that this surface corresponds to the hormone-dependent activation function, AF-2. Mutations in the AF-2 surface abolish LBD hormone-dependent transcriptional activity and interactions with coactivator proteins. AF-2 is not needed for heterodimer formation or for hormone binding, implying that these mutations in the AF-2 surface do not generally disrupt NR structure. Targeted mutation of LBD surface residues and examination of activities of the receptors in the unliganded state reveals that the corepressor binding surface overlaps with the upper part of AF-2 but also extends outside AF-2 and includes the region of the body of the LBD over which H12 is positioned in the active state. Thus, H12 is probably displaced in the absence of hormone, exposing an extended hydrophobic surface capable of corepressor binding, while hormone promotes H12 packing over the lower part of this surface, simultaneously inhibiting corepressor binding and completing the AF-2 surface.

Identification of NR recognition motifs in coactivators and corepressors and their subsequent co-crystallization with receptor LBDs helped to confirm the basic formulation for hormone-dependent coregulator exchange, outlined previously. TR and NR coactivators contain a common recognition motif, short α-helical sequences of the consensus sequence Leu-X-X-Leu-Leu (NR boxes). Co-crystallization of TR and other NRs with representative NR box peptides (12 to 15 amino acids) confirmed that they bind to the AF-2 cleft defined by mutation studies. Corepressors contain a common NR recognition motif composed of consensus sequence Ile-X-X-Ile-Ile-X-X-Leu-Met (these are variously referred to as *interaction domains* [IDs] or *corepressor NR boxes* [CoRNR boxes]). These peptides make up a three-turn α-helix, longer than coactivator NR boxes. A co-crystal of the PPARα LBD with an antagonist and a representative ID motif confirm that the corepressor ID interacts with the extended surface defined by targeted mutagenesis.

TR ANTAGONISTS: THE EXTENSION HYPOTHESIS

It has been possible to create TR antagonists based on x-ray structural analysis and knowledge of TR activation functions and interacting partners, outlined earlier.[61] The "extension hypothesis" proposes that the design of agonist-like compounds with appropriately placed bulky extensions will prevent H12 from folding into the active conformation, thereby blocking coactivator binding (Fig. 5-14). Several competitive TR antagonists have been produced using the principles of this hypothesis. Moreover,

later crystallization of estrogen-receptor LBDs in complex with the known antagonists tamoxifen and raloxifene revealed that both of these ligands possess extensions that displace H12.

Further chemical analysis of TR ligands with extensions revealed surprises; ligands with large extensions often behave as agonists or partial agonists. Chemical analysis revealed that the position of the extension is important, that the extension requires an inflexible linker for a bridge to the hormone-like moiety, and that the chemical nature of the extension is also important. Thus, more needs to be learned about rules of TR antagonism. The fact that some compounds with bulky extensions act as agonists suggests that the TR must adapt to bind large ligands and form a partially active conformation. The structural basis for this surprising effect is discussed later with two compounds, T_4 and GC-24.

OTHER INFLUENCES OF H12 REARRANGEMENT

Repositioning of NR H12 may influence NR function in other ways. The possibility that H12 position regulates hormone binding is discussed in the section on hormone binding and release. In addition, NR H12 may also play roles in LBD-LBD interactions. Unliganded RXR LBDs form tetramers which consist of pairs of LBD dimers linked by a large interface that overlaps lower parts of H3 and H11. In addition, H12 of one LBD subunit docks in the H3-H5 region (part of the AF-2 surface) of an LBD in the neighboring pair, enhancing tetramer interactions. Ligand promotes dissociation of LBD tetramers to form dimers and monomers, and this is probably initiated by hormone-dependent repositioning of H12, an event which would weaken the tetramer interaction.

LIGAND STABILIZES LBD STRUCTURE

Hormone effects on TR LBD are probably more extensive than simple repositioning of H12.[74-77] NR LBDs are somewhat mobile and unstable without ligand or association with cofactors, forming a so-called molten globular organization; hormone promotes widespread stabilization of domain structure.

The overall rearrangements that stabilize the domain may be functionally important. For TRs, homodimer interactions are inhibited by hormone in vitro, whereas RXR-TR LBD interactions are not. This implies that the homodimer and heterodimer interaction surfaces, though overlapping, are not identical, and that hormone promotes rearrangements in regions of the LBD surface that are specific for homodimer contact. Targeted mutagenesis suggests that conserved surface salt-bridge clusters within the TR H7-H8 region and H11 play a role in this effect.[77] For other NRs, ligand binding leads to rearrangements in the same region of the LBD surface that expose a short peptide sequence that is a target for covalent attachment of SUMO peptides,[54] an important event in some mechanisms of ligand-dependent repression, as described earlier. Finally, T_3 promotes increased packing of H1 against the remaining LBD core (H2-H12 region). Remarkably, this can even be recapitulated in cis, using separate fragments for the H2-H12 and H1 region. Since H1 links the LBD to DBD, this event could conceivably communicate information about hormone binding to the DBD.

MECHANISMS OF LIGAND BINDING AND RELEASE

The ways ligand enters and leaves the buried TR hormone-binding pocket remain unknown.[78,79] Hormone is completely enclosed within the domain, and entry/exit routes are not obvious from consideration of the structure alone. One possibility is that

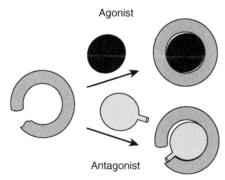

Agonist

Antagonist

FIGURE 5-14. The extension hypothesis. Agonist binding promotes folding of the TR LBD around the ligand, thereby completing the coactivator binding surface shown in Fig. 5-13. Antagonists should comprise a hormone-like moiety that recognizes the hormone-binding pocket but would contain a bulky extension group that would prevent complete closing of the LBD and disturb the AF-2 surface.

the major ligand entry and exit route lies under H12. In this model, referred to as the *mousetrap model*, H12 displacement in the absence of hormone opens the ligand entry route. Here, hormone-induced folding of H12 over the entry site traps ligand until H12 is displaced and the ligand is released. Interestingly, T_4 displays a very high dissociation rate from TR LBDs, likely explaining low affinity for receptor. A crystal structure of the TR-LBD with T_4 revealed that subtle rearrangements in side chains in the hormone-binding pocket create extra space to permit the receptor to accommodate the bulky 5′ iodine group, but that H12 packing is relatively inefficient. Inefficient H12 packing could increase T_4 dissociation because it opens an exit route from the LBD.

There are other possible sites for hormone entry and exit. The H1-H3 loop is highly mobile and disordered in crystal structures and was proposed to be a distinct ligand entry route in the report of the first TR crystal structure. Use of molecular dynamics computer simulations, where information from x-ray structures is used to simulate molecular motions in macromolecules, revealed three possible exit routes. (These were under H12, through the H1-H3 loop, and via opening of the H8-H11 region near the dimer surface.) Further analysis indicated that ligand exit through H1-H3 appears most energetically favorable in aqueous solution. Accordingly, mutations which affect the degree of disorder within the H1-H3 loop region enhance ligand dissociation rates. Thus TRs may harbor more than one ligand entry/exit route.

CONFORMATIONAL FLEXIBILITY IN THE HORMONE-BINDING POCKET

A major surprise derived from recent x-ray and functional studies of TRs is that the TRβ LBD can adapt to bind a ligand that is much larger than classical thyroid hormones and still fold into an active conformation.[76] A structure of TRβ with a synthetic agonist (GC-24) that contains a bulky 3′ phenyl extension reveals a different mechanism for adaptation from that described for T_4 (Fig. 5-15). Here, helices 3 and 11 part to form an extension to the pocket.[76] This phenomenon may be useful for drug design; GC-24 is highly TRβ selective, suggesting that it is possible to capitalize on TR isoform-specific differences in flexibility. The surprising implications of this finding are that TRs could bind and be activated by larger ligands than expected, although it is not clear whether natural ligands with appropriately placed extensions exist.

The reasons that the H3-H11 opens to extend the conventional hormone-binding pocket is not clear; one hypothesis is that the GC-24 extension is accommodated within a region of

receptor that can open up to allow ligand exit under H12.[76] There may be other regions of TR open to extend the pocket, as described earlier; some compounds with bulky 5′ extensions different from the GC-24 3′ extension can also act as agonists.

TR Interacting Proteins

Multiple TR interacting coactivators or corepressors have been identified (Fig. 5-16). The organization of these proteins is summarized briefly here. As already described, the liganded LBD recognizes coactivator NR box peptides (LxxLL), and the unliganded LBD binds IDs (CoRNR boxes, IxxIIxxLM). These motifs are often reiterated multiple times in the coregulator molecules. TRs exhibit clear preferences for certain coactivator and corepressor motifs (including the second NR box of the coactivator SRC2 [SRC2-2] and the first ID motif of N-CoR [ID3]).[39,80,81] The structural basis for this preference is not clear but must involve sequences outside the box. The significance of the latter interaction was confirmed in a mouse knockout model in which the N-CoR exon overlapping ID3 was eliminated in liver; unliganded TR-dependent suppression of TR target genes was strongly affected.

TRs may also interact with coactivators and corepressors via surfaces other than well-established NR and CoRNR boxes; TR AF-1 (NTD) is implicated in interactions with coactivator and corepressors, and the TR hinge domain is implicated in contacts with the coregulator PGC-1. The structural underpinnings of these interactions are not clear.

In addition to NR contact surfaces, coactivators and corepressors contain effector domains which mediate transcriptional activation or silencing. Both classes of coregulator protein exist as large complexes, and the effector domains often comprise docking sites for other components of the complex. Alternatively, some coactivators act as chromatin-modifying enzymes; for example, some coactivators act as histone acetyl transferases (HATs) and arginine methyltransferases, and effector domains may correspond to active enzymes.

TRs and other NRs recruit multiple coactivators with different functions.[82] Estrogen receptors recruit more than 60 different coactivators to target promoters, and it is likely that TRs will

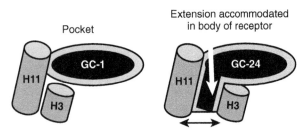

FIGURE 5-15. Plasticity of the TR hormone-binding pocket. Compounds such as T_3, Triac, and GC-1 (an agonist that is the parental molecule for GC-24) are buried in the hormone-binding pocket, defined in the first TR x-ray structure. In this structure, H3 and H11 are linked. GC-24 resembles GC-1 but also contains an additional bulky 3′ hydrophobic group that should not be accommodated in the buried pocket. Here, an x-ray structure reveals that H3 and H11 part to form a hitherto unsuspected extension to the buried pocket. In spite of this significant rearrangement, the overall conformation of the LBD surface is mostly similar, and the AF-2 surface is active.

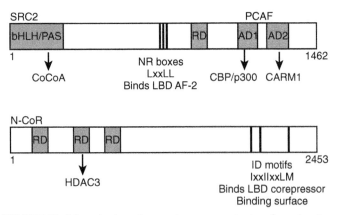

FIGURE 5-16. Schematic of coactivator and corepressor structure. Secondary structure of a representative coactivator (SRC2) and a corepressor (N-CoR) are shown. The positions of the NR interaction domains (inputs—NR boxes that bind TR AF-2 and IDs that bind the TR corepressor binding surface, respectively) are marked by *thin black lines*. The positions of independent domains that modulate gene expression (outputs) are also marked by *gray boxes*. These generally comprise binding sites for other factors, which are named beneath the diagram.

prove to bind a similar complement of proteins. The best known TR cofactors are the steroid-receptor coactivators (SRCs); these are implicated in chromatin modification, owing to their ability to recruit HATs such as p300 and pCAF and arginine methyltransferases such as CARM1. Other TR cofactors include the TRAP220/med1 subunit of the mediator complex, which contacts the basal transcription machinery, the metabolic coregulator PGC-1α, and many others. Some coactivators target TRs to protein degradation complexes, implying that TR turnover is an important component of transcriptional activation. Other coactivator complexes are implicated in modification of the basal transcription machinery that binds RNA polymerase, changes in RNA polymerase processivity, enzymatic modification of transcription factors, and alterations in RNA processing. Generally, individual coactivator complexes are recruited to target promoters sequentially with defined order and kinetics, implying that they must play different roles and function at different stages in transcriptional response.

As mentioned earlier, unliganded TRs interact with three known corepressors, N-CoR, SMRT, and alien.[83] Like coactivators, these proteins form large complexes with auxiliary proteins; however, they serve to silence transcription. These auxiliary factors include HDACs, which condense local chromatin, enzymes which methylate DNA, a repressive promoter modification, and factors that target corepressors and associated factors to protein degradation complexes. The extent to which the three TR corepressors fulfill analogous functions is not clear. Targeted deletion of the *N-CoR* and *SMRT* genes leads to an embryonic-lethal phenotype, implying that one corepressor cannot compensate for the other.

There are examples of coactivators and corepressors that co-opt the classical binding mode of the other type of protein. Receptor-interacting protein 140 (RIP140) is a repressor with LxxLL motifs that binds to liganded nuclear receptors, including the TRs, and dampens their activity.[84] This action is thought to repress NR activity in fat. RIP140 knockout mice are hypermetabolic and resistant to development of diet-induced obesity. Conversely, the adenoviral E1 protein is a coactivator that contains an ID/CoRnR box motif and binds unliganded TRs,[85] and truncated versions of N-CoR that lack repression domains may fulfill a similar function.

Structure and Function of TR Isoforms

TRα AND TRβ

TRα1 and TRβ1 are similar in primary sequence (Fig. 5-17), structure, and mechanism of action, but they are not completely identical in function.[2,86-88] Phenotypes of human patients with TRβ mutations that cause resistance to thyroid hormone syndrome (RTH) and mouse TR knockout models reveal that TRα and TRβ play distinct roles in T_3 effects on different responses, genes, and tissues. These differential actions are often ascribed to differences in the receptor tissue distribution,[20] but this is not proven. That TRα and TRβ may act differently to regulate some genes, which is also likely, also needs to be considered. In this regard, TRβ displays stronger activity at alternate inverted palindromic TREs than TRα, and this correlates with the extent of TR-TR homodimer binding to these elements. Moreover, TRs display different ligand preferences with TRβ binding to Triac, with about two- to threefold higher affinity than TRα. It is not clear whether these differences are functionally important, but the findings are suggestive of different mechanisms.

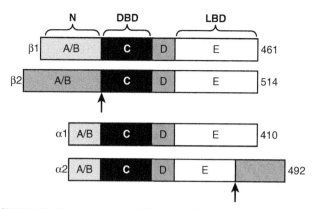

FIGURE 5-17. Schematic of major TR isoforms. Secondary structural diagram of TRβ and TRα isoforms showing locations of differential splicing events that alter receptor secondary structure. Differential splice junctions are indicated by *arrows*.

ALTERNATE TR SPLICE PRODUCTS

Both TR genes produce alternate protein products by combinations of differential exon splicing and promoter usage (see Fig. 5-17). The major differentially spliced THRA product is called *TRα2*. Here, the first 370 amino acids are identical to TRα, but an alternate C-terminus alters LBD sequences encoding H11 and H12, resulting in a TR that does not bind hormone. It is proposed that TRα2 can associate with wild-type TRs and block their actions in response to ligand (referred to as *dominant inhibitor activity*), especially in tissues where it is present in large amounts (e.g., brain, testis, kidney, and brown fat). TRα2 dampens T_3 responses in transfection assays, and knockout mice that lack TRα2 display heightened thyroid hormone sensitivity in vivo. The mechanism of this dominant negative effect is unclear; many models of dominant negative activity require functional homodimer or heterodimer formation, but TRα2 appears to display reduced dimer formation through the altered LBD H10-H11 region that is reflected in reduced DNA binding of TRα2 relative to wild-type TRα.

There are minor TRα variants. TRα3 lacks the first 39 amino acids found in the unique α2 region. Its function is obscure. Two further isoforms, TRΔα1 and TRΔα2, are expressed in the intestine. These contain portions of the TR C-terminus and may act as dominant inhibitors of TRα1. Interestingly, the antisense strand of the THRA locus encodes another NR, called *rev-erbA* (from reverse ERBA), which plays important roles in diurnal rhythm. For some species, rev-erbA has been demonstrated to bind heme and respond to differences in heme redox state. There is no evidence that rev-erbA has any functional relationship with TRs.

TRβ1 splice variants are created by differential splicing of the *THRB* gene NTD exon. The major alternate hormone-binding form is called *TRβ2* and is created as a result of transcriptional initiation at an isoform-specific promoter and alternative exon splicing, which creates a completely unique isoform-specific NTD. TRβ2 is predominantly expressed in pituitary and hypothalamus, although low levels of expression are detectable in liver, and this form of TRβ2 is believed to play an important role in negative regulation of thyroid hormone production through the hypothalamic-pituitary axis. TRβ2 is also expressed in the cochlea and retinal photoreceptor cells and is needed for appropriate development of color vision.

The distinct N-terminus of TRβ2 possesses a unique transactivation function. At positively regulated genes and reporters,

TRβ2 fails to suppress basal transcriptional activity in the absence of hormone and instead activates gene transcription in the absence of exogenous ligand. The TRβ2 NTD is thought to mediate the recruitment of coactivators independently of the LBD and may also exert antirepressive activities by blocking actions of corepressor gene-silencing functions.

There are other TRβ1 splice variants with obscure function. TRβ0 (present in reptiles and birds) lacks the NTD, and TRβ3 contains a unique short 24-amino-acid NTD. In addition, there is a truncated C-terminal TRβ receptor, TRΔβ3, which lacks part of the LBD and does not bind to T_3.

RESISTANCE TO THYROID HORMONE

Inherited human TR mutations cause resistance to thyroid hormone syndrome (RTH).[89] Symptoms of RTH, coupled with genetic analysis of TR mutations, yielded some of the first insights into differential actions of TRβ and TRα isoforms.

Patients with RTH exhibit reduced sensitivity to thyroid hormone.[89] In most cases, circulating thyroid hormone levels are elevated to variable extents, but TSH levels (which should be suppressed by elevated hormone levels) are elevated (sometimes resulting in goiter) or normal. This is caused by failure of feedback inhibition of hormone synthesis through the hypothalamic-pituitary axis due to the reduced sensitivity of TRβ to thyroid hormone (see Fig. 5-1). Overall, the elevated thyroid hormone levels overcome the resistance and produce a mostly euthyroid state. (In some cases, a variant of the syndrome results in central but not peripheral resistance to thyroid hormone, where TSH levels are high, and there can be symptoms of frank hyperthyroidism.) However, there can also be a mix of hypo- and hyperthyroid phenotypes of variable clinical penetrance. Commonly there is tachycardia (hyperthyroid symptom) and attention deficit. To a lesser extent, there can be some mild mental retardation, skeletal malformations, and hearing abnormalities (hypothyroid manifestations). Most (>80%) RTH is caused by mutations in the LBD coding regions of the *TRβ* gene. Mutations in *TRα* have never been detected. The fact that there is elevated heart rate therefore suggested that normal TRα is responsible for this hyperthyroid effect and provided the first evidence for TR isoform–specific activities, later confirmed by gene knockout studies.

RTH can also be caused by mutations in other genes involved that play roles in thyroid hormone response. Cases have been described in which the target genes identified involve a thyroid hormone membrane transporter and enzymes required for transfer of an essential cofactor, selenium, to the active site of deiodinases.[90]

ANALYSIS OF TR ISOFORM ACTION IN MICE

Functions of TR isoforms have been investigated in mouse models by targeted deletion of TR genes and knock-in of TR alleles with dominant negative activities.[18,88,91,92]

TR KNOCKOUTS

Several mouse TR knockout strains are available. For TRα, mice with deletions that eliminate all TRα isoforms (TRα$^{0/0}$), TRα1, and TRα2 (TRα$^{-/-}$; this strain preserves expression of minor TRα isoforms), TRα1$^{-/-}$ and TRα2$^{-/-}$ are reported. For TRβ, strains that lack all TRβ isoforms (TRβ$^{-/-}$) or TRβ2 (TRβ2$^{-/-}$) are available. Finally, strains that lack both TR isoforms have been created by crossing of TRα$^{0/0}$ and TRβ$^{-/-}$ strains (for example, TRα$^{0/0}$β$^{-/-}$). All TR knockout mice are viable and fertile. There are some complications in interpretation of the phenotypes of the mice.

Targeted deletions often affect more than one TR splice variant, and in some cases, deletion of one TR isoform leads to compensatory biological responses in TR isoform expression. Additionally, different mouse genetic backgrounds influence the presentation of the phenotype. In spite of these qualifications, several clear lessons about TR activity and TR isoform-specific actions can be drawn from these studies:

1. Mice that lack TRs (TRα$^{0/0}$β$^{-/-}$) fail to mount known thyroid hormone responses. This is interpreted as strong evidence that nuclear TRs mediate many known effects of thyroid hormones.

2. The mice exhibit clear developmental defects (such as dwarfism) and very high circulating thyroid hormone levels. Nevertheless, the overall phenotype is relatively mild compared to hypothyroid mice. This suggests that most harmful effects of hypothyroidism stem from unbalanced actions of unliganded TR isoforms, rather than lack of receptors per se, and emphasize the potent actions of unliganded TRs.

3. Deletions that target TRα or TRβ yield different phenotypes. TRα sets heart rate, in agreement with observed phenotypes of humans with RTH mutations. TRα is also involved in growth and development of the skeleton, muscle, and small intestine and plays an important role in body temperature regulation and setting metabolic rate. Conversely, TRβ plays major roles in regulation of serum cholesterol levels and feedback inhibition of thyroid hormone production and significant roles in regulating metabolic rate by directly inducing mitochondrial uncoupling proteins. Some genes respond selectively to particular TR isoforms. TRβ1 is needed for induction of spot 14, CYP7A1, Dio1, malic enzyme, and other liver-specific genes. Conversely, TRα1, but not TRβ1, is needed for induction of SERCa1 in muscle. Conceivably, differential actions could either reflect differences in TR tissue distributions or fundamental differences in mechanism of TRα1 and TRβ1. Evidence in favor of the latter possibility is that TRβ$^{-/-}$TRα2$^{-/-}$ mice exhibit elevated expression of TRα1 in liver such that total liver T_3-binding activity approaches wild-type levels, but this is not sufficient to rescue defects in T_3 induction of CYP7A1.

4. Alternate spliced TR isoforms play specific roles. As expected from the tissue distribution of TRβ2, this form of TR mediates feedback inhibition of thyroid hormone production through the hypothalamic-pituitary axis. TRα2$^{-/-}$ mice exhibit features of hyperthyroidism, including elevated heart rate, weight loss, and elevated body temperature. Consideration of phenotypic differences of TRα$^{0/0}$ (no TRα isoforms expressed) and TRα$^{-/-}$ mice (TRΔα1 and TRΔα2 expressed) reveal that some thyroid hormone responses are preserved in the intestine of the latter strain of mice.

KNOCK-INS

TR function has been probed with targeted (knock-in) mutagenesis. These experiments were first performed in order to create mouse models of RTH. These experiments were successful; a PV knock-in mutant (a highly dominant negative TR with altered H12 sequence) displayed several features of RTH, including elevated thyroid hormone with normal TSH, goiter, short stature, and tachycardia.

Mice strains that express analogous TRα mutants have also been created. The goal of these studies was to probe natural function of TRα with dominant negative versions of the protein. However, mouse strains bearing different mutations exhibit a range of phenotypes from lean and hypermetabolic to obese and insulin resistant. This suggests that TRα plays an important role in metabolic rate, but that different mutations affect these processes in different ways.

TR Mutations in Disease: Structure-Function

Studies of effects of TR mutations that arise in RTH and cancer on TR action have yielded important clues about the roles of TRs in these diseases and fundamental processes of receptor activation.

RTH

Analysis of RTH patient families revealed an autosomal dominant inheritance pattern which was explained by analysis of the effects of TRβ mutations on receptor function. RTH mutant TRs continue to bind corepressor at hormone concentrations in which it would normally be released. Projection of positions of RTH mutations onto the x-ray structural models of TR LBDs reveals that many map to the ligand-binding pocket, explaining why the mutations decrease T_3-binding affinity. Other mutations uncouple hormone binding from corepressor release. These tend to affect residues close to H12. The net result of increased corepressor binding is dominant negative activity; the mutant TR inhibits activity of the wild-type counterpart encoded by the other allele. This dominant negative activity explains the autosomal dominance of the inheritance pattern.

It is clear that dominant negative activity requires integrity of the dimer/heterodimer surface. Nevertheless, the molecular basis of this effect is not totally understood. Most TRs form heterodimers with RXRs, so there may be competition between heterodimers of wild-type RXR/mutant TRs and wild-type RXR/TRs for DNA binding sites. Alternatively, direct homodimer interactions between wild-type and mutant TRs may explain these effects.

A small number of RTH mutations in the LBD affect residues that appear far from the functional elements of this domain. These were studied to gain insights into coupling of hormone binding to response. Most mutations affect residues that are essential for TR LBD stability. Structural analysis reveals that these residues often participate in polar side-chain interactions that link helices. The mutations appear to destabilize the H1-H3 loop, a possible ligand escape route, and reduce ligand affinity by increasing dissociation rates.

While most patients exhibit generalized resistance that is manifested in the pituitary and periphery, others display so-called pituitary resistance—normal peripheral responses with a specific failure of feedback inhibition. The molecular basis for differences between pituitary and generalized resistance is not known. One possibility is that there are differential effects of mutations on activities of TRβ1 (widely expressed) versus TRβ2 (limited distribution, including the pituitary) whereby the TRβ1 is normal or near normal, and the TRβ2 is impaired, leading to decreased suppression of TSH release. Alternatively, since TR actions in the hypothalamic-pituitary axis often involve transcriptional repression, it is possible that pituitary resistance mutations preferentially affect ligand-dependent TR repression mechanisms.

CANCER

Cancer genome sequencing analysis has revealed that TR mutations occur frequently in cancer (including liver, kidney, thyroid gland, and breast).[93] Presently, the significance of these mutations in cancer etiology is not completely clear, but it is well established that mutated TRs can cause cancer; as described earlier, v-erbA is a non-hormone-binding form of TRα that actively represses transcription and causes erythroblastoma.[51] Moreover, mouse models which contain a targeted mutation of TRβ (knock-in) that resembles the human PV RTH mutant develop thyroid cancer at increased rates.

TR mutants that emerge in cancer often resemble RTH mutants; the mutations preserve repression at the expense of hormone binding and transcriptional activation. This led to the suggestion that localized RTH may contribute to some forms of cancer. However, other TR cancer mutants appear to lack dominant negative activity, such as those that disrupt DNA binding, presumably eliminating TR activity at target genes. There is also a correlation in other cases with loss of nuclear localization; unlike TRα, which is predominantly nuclear, v-erbA displays nuclear and cytoplasmic localization. Moreover, TRα partly relocalizes to the cytoplasm in cancers. The connections between TR structure-function and oncogenesis require further investigation.

Gene and Context-Specific Variations in TR Actions

There are variations in the mechanism of thyroid hormone response at different target genes.[2,38] Comparisons of gene expression patterns in livers of wild-type thyroidectomized and thyroid hormone–treated mice with similar $TR^{-/-}$ knockout mice reveals that most positively regulated genes adhere to the classic model of thyroid hormone action; transcription is suppressed by unliganded TRs and activated beyond basal levels with hormone. However, many genes deviate from this pattern (Fig. 5-18). Some are not suppressed by unliganded TRs but continue to be activated by the hormone, whereas others are suppressed by unliganded TRs, with hormone only partly relieving basal suppression. Similar variations are observed with negatively regulated genes.[38] Some genes are activated by unliganded TRs with hormone-suppressing transcription below basal levels, while others are not activated by unliganded TRs but continue to be repressed by hormone. It is tempting to suggest that these variations in transcriptional response must reflect promoter-specific differences in corepressor/coactivator function or recruitment patterns, but this is not proven.

The reasons that TRs exhibit different actions at different genes are less clear. One possibility is that different mechanisms are consequences of promoter organization. Different TREs could preferentially recruit different TR oligomeric forms with unique activities (RXR-TRs, TR-TRs, monomers) or induce different TR conformations with unique activities. Alternatively, variations in mechanism could reflect differential interactions with auxiliary transcription factors or cofactors that bind to subsets of TR-regulated target promoters. This issue will require better knowledge of TRE sequence and TR target gene–promoter architecture. Other possible reasons that TRs could display context-selective activities relate to differences in expression of TR isoforms, availability of TR cofactors, or differential auxiliary modifications

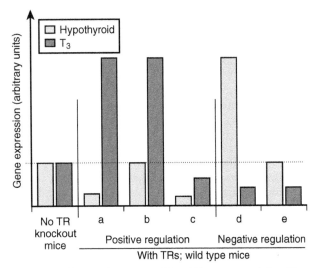

FIGURE 5-18. Differences in patterns of thyroid hormone regulation. Observed patterns of TR-responsive gene expression in knockout mice. Most positively regulated genes conform to pattern **a**; they are suppressed without ligand via corepressor recruitment and activated with ligand via coactivator recruitment. Other positively regulated genes differ and conform to patterns **b** and **c**; some lack basal repression, others are not activated beyond basal levels in response to hormone binding. Negatively regulated genes show similar variations. It is likely that different patterns correspond to variations in the mechanism of TR action at different genes.

(including phosphorylation, ubiquitination, SUMOlation, and the like).

Alternative Modes of TH Action

While most effects of thyroid hormone are mediated by nuclear TRs, there are some cases in which the hormones can exert rapid effects on cells that are unlikely to involve nuclear TRs.[94,95] There are two possible mechanisms of these effects. It is now known that conventional nuclear TRs circulate in and out of the nucleus, and cytoplasmic TRs could mediate rapid effects of thyroid hormones. Alternatively, there may be alternate proteins that bind thyroid hormones and transduce thyroid hormone signals. Both mechanisms appear to be at play for thyroid hormones.

Like other NRs, cytoplasmic TRs associate with the p85 subunit of phospho-inositol kinase (PI3K). This event triggers PI3K activity, which increases second messenger signaling events such as phosphorylation of important signaling molecules such as AKT, mTOR, and p70rsk. This effect on the TR triggers increased insertion of Na^+K^+-ATPase into membranes, increasing the activity of this pump protein. These effects are also implicated in protective effects of thyroid hormones in models of stroke. Interestingly, one RTH mutant (PV) exhibits increased activity through this pathway, which may contribute to its oncogenic actions in mice.

There is also evidence for alternate thyroid hormone–binding proteins in the membrane. T_4 and Tetrac interact with integrin $\alpha V\beta 3$ to trigger activation of MAP/ERK kinase cascades, alter intracellular protein trafficking, and increase activity of membrane pumps, including the Na^+ protein antiporter. Use of Tetrac as a molecular probe for activities of this pathway reveals functions in angiogenesis and stem cell proliferation.

Since membrane and cytoplasmic signaling pathways can target transcription factors, it is conceivable that these actions of thyroid hormone could also affect transcription. Cytoplasmic and nuclear signaling pathways can also intersect at the level of increased receptor phosphorylation.

Selective Modulation

Excess TH production by the thyroid gland can produce beneficial effects, including reductions in serum LDL cholesterol and body fat.[96] However, hyperthyroid patients also exhibit tachycardia (elevated heart rate) with atrial arrhythmias and can develop congestive heart failure. TH excess also causes muscle wasting, osteoporosis in postmenopausal women, and other symptoms, including fatigue, shortness of breath, and temperature sensitivity.[97]

Scientists have often suggested that TH derivatives could separate beneficial effects of TH from deleterious effects. Early human trials with dextrothyroxine (D-T_4, the D-enantiomer of T_4 that was contaminated also by small amounts of L-T_4 that may have contributed to both beneficial and harmful effects) were performed as part of the coronary drug project (CDP) in the late 1960s to determine whether different compounds improved survival in men who had suffered one heart attack.[98] This arm of the study was curtailed because of increased mortality, even though serum cholesterol was reduced. Other human trials involved Triac, which exhibited a small therapeutic window where beneficial effects on serum cholesterol are seen without increases in heart rate. Other groups identified synthetic TH analogs that reduce cholesterol without effects on heart, but these were not pursued for human use. In the last 10 to 15 years, improved understanding of TR structure and function and TH analog chemistry has led to creation of new, potent thyromimetics with clearer selective activities. Since analysis of RTH and mouse gene knockout models described previously revealed that TRα mediates tachycardia, several groups set out to create analogs that would selectively activate TRβ and promote the beneficial effects of TH, such as the lowering of serum cholesterol, while sparing the heart.[96,99-101] Tests in animal models revealed that they also display liver uptake selectivity and vary in their abilities to accumulate in extrahepatic tissues, complicating interpretations of their profile of actions and side effects. Nevertheless, several compounds have shown promising effects on serum lipids and obesity in preclinical animal models and on serum lipids in early human clinical trials[15] without obvious harmful effects on heart, muscle, or bone. In addition, some of the drugs cause rapid loss in body weight and white fat and potentially beneficial reductions in blood glucose. These compounds, and future derivatives, will improve treatments of thyroid hormone imbalances and could represent novel treatments for metabolic disease in euthyroid subjects.

Consideration of mechanisms of TR action outlined in this chapter suggests other ways to generate selective TR modulators. These include TR ligands that accumulate selectively in some tissues but not others, ligands that selectively affect some mechanisms of gene regulation but not others, and ligands that differentially affect classical nuclear and cytoplasmic/membrane pathways of thyroid hormone action or combinations thereof. It is likely that better understanding of TR function will lead to much better pharmaceuticals to modulate this important hormone-signaling pathway.

REFERENCES

1. Sawin CT: The heritage of the thyroid: A brief history. In Braverman LE, Utiger RD, Ingbar SH, Werner SC, editors: Werner and Ingbar's The Thyroid: A Fundamental and Clinical Text, ed 9, Philadelphia, 2000, Lippincott Williams & Wilkins, pp 3–7.
2. Yen PM: Physiological and molecular basis of thyroid hormone action, Physiol Rev 81:1097–1142, 2001.
3. Zhang J, Lazar MA: The mechanism of action of thyroid hormones, Annu Rev Physiol 62:439–466, 2000.
4. Laudet V, Gronemeyer H: The Nuclear Receptor Facts Book, London, 2002, Academic Press.
5. Flamant F, et al: International Union of Pharmacology. LIX. The pharmacology and classification of the nuclear receptor superfamily: thyroid hormone receptors, Pharmacol Rev 58:705–711, 2006.
6. Leonard JL, Koehrle J: Intracellular pathways of iodothyronine metabolism. In Braverman LE, Utiger RD, Ingbar SH, et al, editors: Werner and Ingbar's the thyroid: a fundamental and clinical text, ed 9, Philadelphia, 2000, Lippincott Williams & Wilkins, pp 136–173.
7. Panicker V, et al: A common variation in deiodinase 1 gene DIO1 is associated with the relative levels of free thyroxine and triiodothyronine, J Clin Endocrinol Metab 93:3075–3081, 2008.
8. Panicker V, et al: Genetic loci linked to pituitary-thyroid axis set points: a genome-wide scan of a large twin cohort, J Clin Endocrinol Metab 93:3519–3523, 2008.
9. Sorensen HG, et al: Identification and consequences of polymorphisms in the thyroid hormone receptor alpha and beta genes, Thyroid 18:1087–1094, 2008.
10. Scanlan TS, et al: 3-Iodothyronamine is an endogenous and rapid-acting derivative of thyroid hormone, Nat Med 10:638–642, 2004.
11. Visser WE, Friesema EC, Jansen J, et al: Thyroid hormone transport in and out of cells, Trends Endocrinol Metab 19:50–56, 2008.
12. Friesema EC, et al: Effective cellular uptake and efflux of thyroid hormone by human monocarboxylate transporter 10, Mol Endocrinol 22:1357–1369, 2008.
13. Dumitrescu AM, Refetoff S: Novel biological and clinical aspects of thyroid hormone metabolism, Endocr Dev 10:127–139, 2007.
14. Suzuki S, Mori J, Hashizume K: mu-crystallin, a NADPH-dependent T(3)-binding protein in cytosol, Trends Endocrinol Metab 18:286–289, 2007.
15. Berkenstam A, et al: The thyroid hormone mimetic compound KB2115 lowers plasma LDL cholesterol and stimulates bile acid synthesis without cardiac effects in humans, Proc Natl Acad Sci U S A 105:663–667, 2008.
16. Gereben B, et al: Cellular and Molecular Basis of Deiodinase-Regulated Thyroid Hormone Signaling, Endocr Rev, 2008.
17. Huang SA, Bianco AC: Reawakened interest in type III iodothyronine deiodinase in critical illness and injury, Nat Clin Pract Endocrinol Metab 4:148–155, 2008.
18. Moreno M, et al: Metabolic effects of thyroid hormone derivatives, Thyroid 18:239–253, 2008.
19. Sherman SI, et al: Augmented hepatic and skeletal thyromimetic effects of tiratricol in comparison with levothyroxine, J Clin Endocrinol Metab 82:2153–2158, 1997.
20. Bookout AL, et al: Anatomical profiling of nuclear receptor expression reveals a hierarchical transcriptional network, Cell 126:789–799, 2006.
21. Silva JE: Thermogenic mechanisms and their hormonal regulation, Physiol Rev 86:435–464, 2006.
22. Silva JE, Bianco SD: Thyroid-adrenergic interactions: physiological and clinical implications, Thyroid 18:157–165, 2008.
23. Videla LA, Fernandez V, Tapia G, et al: Thyroid hormone calorigenesis and mitochondrial redox signaling: upregulation of gene expression, Front Biosci 12:1220–1228, 2007.
24. Kim, B: Thyroid hormone as a determinant of energy expenditure and the basal metabolic rate, Thyroid 18:141–144, 2008.
25. Feng X, Jiang Y, Meltzer P, et al: Thyroid hormone regulation of hepatic genes in vivo detected by complementary DNA microarray, Mol Endocrinol 14:947–955, 2000.
26. Weitzel JM, et al: Hepatic gene expression patterns in thyroid hormone-treated hypothyroid rats, J Mol Endocrinol 31:291–303, 2003.

27. Obregon MJ: Thyroid hormone and adipocyte differentiation, Thyroid 18:185–195, 2008.
28. Klein I, Danzi S: Thyroid disease and the heart, Circulation 116:1725–1735, 2007.
29. Wiersinga WM: The role of thyroid hormone nuclear receptors in the heart: evidence from pharmacological approaches, Heart Fail Rev 2008 Dec 19 [Epub ahead of print].
30. Crunkhorn S, Patti ME: Links between thyroid hormone action, oxidative metabolism, and diabetes risk? Thyroid 18:227–237, 2008.
31. Bassett JH, Williams GR: Critical role of the hypothalamic-pituitary-thyroid axis in bone, Bone 43:418–426, 2008.
32. Samuels MH: Cognitive function in untreated hypothyroidism and hyperthyroidism, Curr Opin Endocrinol Diabetes Obes 15:429–433, 2008.
33. Williams GR: Neurodevelopmental and neurophysiological actions of thyroid hormone, J Neuroendocrinol 20:784–794, 2008.
34. Plateroti M, Kress E, Mori JI, et al: Thyroid hormone receptor alpha1 directly controls transcription of the beta-catenin gene in intestinal epithelial cells, Mol Cell Biol 26:3204–3214, 2006.
35. Doshi DN, Blyumin ML, Kimball AB: Cutaneous manifestations of thyroid disease, Clin Dermatol 26:283–287, 2008.
36. Baxter JD, et al: Thyroid hormone receptors and responses, Recent Prog Horm Res 35:97–153, 1979.
37. Ivarie RD, Baxter JD, Morris JA: Interaction of thyroid and glucocorticoid hormones in rat pituitary tumor cells. Specificity and diversity of the responses analyzed by two-dimensional gel electrophoresis, J Biol Chem 256:4520–4528, 1981.
38. Yen PM, Feng X, Flamant F, et al: Effects of ligand and thyroid hormone receptor isoforms on hepatic gene expression profiles of thyroid hormone receptor knockout mice, EMBO Rep 4:581–587, 2003.
39. Astapova I, et al: The nuclear corepressor, NCoR, regulates thyroid hormone action in vivo, Proc Natl Acad Sci U S A 105:19544–19549, 2008.
40. van Rooij E, et al: Control of stress-dependent cardiac growth and gene expression by a microRNA, Science 316:575–579, 2007.
41. Tata JR, et al: The action of thyroid hormones at the cell level, Biochem J 86:408–428, 1963.
42. Oppenheimer JH, Schwartz HL, Surks MI: Tissue differences in the concentration of triiodothyronine nuclear binding sites in the rat: liver, kidney, pituitary, heart, brain, spleen, and testis, Endocrinology 95:897–903, 1974.
43. Surks MI, Koerner DH, Oppenheimer JH: In vitro binding of L-triiodothyronine to receptors in rat liver nuclei. Kinetics of binding, extraction properties, and lack of requirement for cytosol proteins, J Clin Invest 55:50–60, 1975.
44. Nelson C, et al: Discrete cis-active genomic sequences dictate the pituitary cell type-specific expression of rat prolactin and growth hormone genes, Nature 322:557–562, 1986.
45. MacLeod KN, Baxter JD: DNA binding of thyroid hormone receptors, Biochem Biophys Res Commun 62:577–583, 1975.
46. Spindler BJ, MacLeod KM, Ring J, et al: Thyroid hormone receptors. Binding characteristics and lack of hormonal dependency for nuclear localization, J Biol Chem 250:4113–4119, 1975.
47. Latham KR, Ring JC, Baxter JD: Solubilized nuclear "receptors" for thyroid hormones. Physical characteristics and binding properties, evidence for multiple forms, J Biol Chem 251:7388–7397, 1976.
48. MacLeod KM, Baxter JD: Chromatin receptors for thyroid hormones. Interactions of the solubilized proteins with DNA, J Biol Chem 251:7380–7387, 1976.
49. Sap J, et al: The c-erb-A protein is a high-affinity receptor for thyroid hormone, Nature 324:635–640, 1986.
50. Weinberger C, et al: The c-erb-A gene encodes a thyroid hormone receptor, Nature 324:641–646, 1986.
51. Privalsky ML: v-erb A, nuclear hormone receptors, and oncogenesis, Biochim Biophys Acta 1114:51–62, 1992.
52. Glass CK, Rosenfeld MG: The coregulator exchange in transcriptional functions of nuclear receptors, Genes Dev 14:121–141, 2000.

53. Lazar MA: Nuclear receptor corepressors, Nucl Recept Signal 1:e001, 2003.
54. Ricote M, Glass CK: PPARs and molecular mechanisms of transrepression, Biochim Biophys Acta 1771:926–935, 2007.
55. Shibusawa N, Hollenberg AN, Wondisford FE: Thyroid hormone receptor DNA binding is required for both positive and negative gene regulation, J Biol Chem 278:732–738, 2003.
56. Rastinejad F, Perlmann T, Evans RM, et al: Structural determinants of nuclear receptor assembly on DNA direct repeats, Nature 375:203–211, 1995.
57. Khorasanizadeh S, Rastinejad F: Nuclear-receptor interactions on DNA-response elements, Trends Biochem Sci 26:384–390, 2001.
58. Desvergne B: How do thyroid hormone receptors bind to structurally diverse response elements? Mol Cell Endocrinol 100:125–131, 1994.
59. Wagner RL, et al: A structural role for hormone in the thyroid hormone receptor, Nature 378:690–697, 1995.
60. Wagner RL, et al: Hormone selectivity in thyroid hormone receptors, Mol Endocrinol 15:398–410, 2001.
61. Webb P, et al: Design of thyroid hormone receptor antagonists from first principles, J Steroid Biochem Mol Biol 83:59–73, 2002.
62. Weatherman RV, Fletterick RJ, Scanlan TS: Nuclear-receptor ligands and ligand-binding domains, Annu Rev Biochem 68:559–581, 1999.
63. Nascimento AS, et al: Structural rearrangements in the thyroid hormone receptor hinge domain and their putative role in the receptor function, J Mol Biol 360:586–598, 2006.
64. Kumar R, Thompson EB: Transactivation functions of the N-terminal domains of nuclear hormone receptors: protein folding and coactivator interactions, Mol Endocrinol 17:1–10, 2003.
65. Figueira AC, et al: Low-resolution structures of thyroid hormone receptor dimers and tetramers in solution, Biochemistry 46:1273–1283, 2007.
66. Chandra V, et al: Structure of the intact PPAR-gamma-RXR-nuclear receptor complex on DNA, Nature 456:350–356, 2008.
67. Ribeiro RC, et al: X-ray crystallographic and functional studies of thyroid hormone receptor, J Steroid Biochem Mol Biol 65:133–141, 1998.
68. Ribeiro RC, et al: Definition of the surface in the thyroid hormone receptor ligand binding domain for association as homodimers and heterodimers with retinoid X receptor, J Biol Chem 276:14987–14995, 2001.
69. Velasco LF, et al: Thyroid hormone response element organization dictates the composition of active receptor, J Biol Chem 282:12458–12466, 2007.
70. Wu Y, Xu B, Koenig RJ: Thyroid hormone response element sequence and the recruitment of retinoid X receptors for thyroid hormone responsiveness, J Biol Chem 276:3929–3936, 2001.
71. Diallo EM, Wilhelm KG Jr, Thompson DL, et al: Variable RXR requirements for thyroid hormone responsiveness of endogenous genes, Mol Cell Endocrinol 264:149–156, 2007.
72. Mengeling BJ, Lee S, Privalsky ML: Coactivator recruitment is enhanced by thyroid hormone receptor trimers, Mol Cell Endocrinol 280:47–62, 2008.
73. Kallenberger BC, Love JD, Chatterjee VK, et al: A dynamic mechanism of nuclear receptor activation and its perturbation in a human disease, Nat Struct Biol 10:136–140, 2003.
74. Pissios P, Tzameli I, Kushner P, et al: Dynamic stabilization of nuclear receptor ligand binding domains by hormone or corepressor binding, Mol Cell 6:245–253, 2000.
75. Pissios P, Tzameli I, Moore DD: New insights into receptor ligand binding domains from a novel assembly assay, J Steroid Biochem Mol Biol 76:3–7, 2001.
76. Togashi M, et al: Conformational adaptation of nuclear receptor ligand binding domains to agonists: potential for novel approaches to ligand design, J Steroid Biochem Mol Biol 93:127–137, 2005.
77. Togashi M, Nguyen P, Fletterick R, et al: Rearrangements in thyroid hormone receptor charge clusters that stabilize bound 3,5',5-triiodo-L-thyronine and inhibit

homodimer formation, J Biol Chem 280:25665–25673, 2005.

78. Martinez L, et al: Molecular dynamics simulations reveal multiple pathways of ligand dissociation from thyroid hormone receptors, Biophys J 89:2011–2023, 2005.

79. Martinez L, Webb P, Polikarpov I, et al: Molecular dynamics simulations of ligand dissociation from thyroid hormone receptors: evidence of the likeliest escape pathway and its implications for the design of novel ligands, J Med Chem 49:23–26, 2006.

80. Moore JM, et al: Quantitative proteomics of the thyroid hormone receptor-coregulator interactions, J Biol Chem 279:27584–27590, 2004.

81. Webb P, et al: The nuclear receptor corepressor (N-CoR) contains three isoleucine motifs (I/LXXII) that serve as receptor interaction domains (IDs), Mol Endocrinol 14:1976–1985, 2000.

82. Lonard DM, O'Malley BW: Nuclear receptor coregulators: judges, juries, and executioners of cellular regulation, Mol Cell 27:691–700, 2007.

83. Privalsky ML: The role of corepressors in transcriptional regulation by nuclear hormone receptors, Annu Rev Physiol 66:315–360, 2004.

84. White R, et al: Role of RIP140 in metabolic tissues: connections to disease, FEBS Lett 582:39–45, 2008.

85. Meng X, et al: E1A and a nuclear receptor corepressor splice variant (N-CoRI) are thyroid hormone receptor

coactivators that bind in the corepressor mode, Proc Natl Acad Sci U S A 102:6267–6272, 2005.

86. Lazar MA: Thyroid hormone receptors: multiple forms, multiple possibilities, Endocr Rev 14:184–193, 1993.

87. O'Shea PJ, Williams GR: Insight into the physiological actions of thyroid hormone receptors from genetically modified mice, J Endocrinol 175:553–570, 2002.

88. Forrest D, Vennstrom B: Functions of thyroid hormone receptors in mice, Thyroid 10:41–52, 2000.

89. Yen PM: Molecular basis of resistance to thyroid hormone, Trends Endocrinol Metab 14:327–333, 2003.

90. Refetoff S, Dumitrescu AM: Syndromes of reduced sensitivity to thyroid hormone: genetic defects in hormone receptors, cell transporters and deiodination, Best Pract Res Clin Endocrinol Metab 21:277–305, 2007.

91. Liu YY, et al: A mutant thyroid hormone receptor alpha antagonizes peroxisome proliferator-activated receptor alpha signaling in vivo and impairs fatty acid oxidation, Endocrinology 148:1206–1217, 2007.

92. Sjogren M, et al: Hypermetabolism in mice caused by the central action of an unliganded thyroid hormone receptor alpha1, EMBO J 26:4535–4545, 2007.

93. Yen PM, Cheng SY: Germline and somatic thyroid hormone receptor mutations in man, J Endocrinol Invest 26:780–787, 2003.

94. Davis PJ, Leonard JL, Davis FB: Mechanisms of nongenomic actions of thyroid hormone, Front Neuroendocrinol 29:211–218, 2008.

95. Furuya F, Lu C, Guigon CJ, et al: Nongenomic activation of phosphatidylinositol 3-kinase signaling by thyroid hormone receptors, Steroids 74:628–634, 2009.

96. Webb P: Selective activators of thyroid hormone receptors, Expert Opin Investig Drugs 13:489–500, 2004.

97. Biondi B, Cooper DS: The clinical significance of subclinical thyroid dysfunction, Endocr Rev 29:76–131, 2008.

98. The coronary drug project. Findings leading to further modifications of its protocol with respect to dextrothyroxine. The coronary drug project research group, JAMA 220:996–1008, 1972.

99. Baxter JD, et al: Selective modulation of thyroid hormone receptor action, J Steroid Biochem Mol Biol 76:31–42, 2001.

100. Baxter JD, Webb P, Grover G, et al: Selective activation of thyroid hormone signaling pathways by GC-1: a new approach to controlling cholesterol and body weight, Trends Endocrinol Metab 15:154–157, 2004.

101. Scanlan TS: Sobetirome: a case history of bench-to-clinic drug discovery and development, Heart Fail Rev 2008 Nov 11 [Epub ahead of print].

Chapter 6

THYROID FUNCTION TESTING

ROY E. WEISS and SAMUEL REFETOFF

The physician considers the possible presence of thyroid disease when certain signs and symptoms are elicited on history and physical examination. Only an accurate diagnosis can lead to effective treatment, and, occasionally, that might include recognition of the boundary between physiology and pathology. Accurate diagnosis of thyroid disease requires an understanding of thyroid physiology and pathophysiology of thyroid disorders. Precise diagnosis based solely on history and physical examination is not possible owing to the many nonspecific findings that can be associated with thyroid dysfunction. Therefore, in most instances, the diagnosis ultimately depends on the accurate interpretation of thyroid function tests. Often, interpretation of these tests can be difficult because of previous therapy, effects of medications, and concurrent nonthyroidal illnesses. The aim of this chapter is to provide the reader with the necessary information about the execution, use, and interpretation of thyroid function tests and their application in the diagnosis and treatment of patients with thyroid disorders. As we learn more about the normal physiology of the thyroid gland and thyroid hormone action, it is becoming clear that variation in thyroid physiology within and among populations has blurred the boundary between physiology and pathology.

During the past 5 decades, clinical thyroidology has witnessed the introduction of a multitude of diagnostic tests and procedures. These laboratory tests provide greater sensitivity and specificity that enhance the likelihood of early detection of occult thyroid disease with only minimal clinical findings or obscured by coincidental nonthyroid disease. These tests also assist in the exclusion of thyroid dysfunction when symptoms and signs closely mimic thyroid pathology. On the other hand, the wide choice of complementary and overlapping tests indicates that each has its limitations and that no single test is reliable in all circumstances. In addition, genetic analyses can be useful in diagnosing several of the inherited thyroid disorders.

Thyroid tests can be classified into broad categories according to the information they provide at the functional, etiologic, or anatomic level:

1. Tests that directly assess the level of thyroid gland activity and the integrity of hormone biosynthesis, such as thyroidal radioactive iodide uptake (RAIU) and perchlorate discharge, and the salivary-to-blood ratio of radioactive iodine are carried out in vivo.
2. Tests that measure the concentrations of thyroid hormones and their transport in blood are performed in vitro and provide indirect assessment of the level of thyroid hormone–dependent metabolic activity.
3. Tests that attempt to directly measure the impact of thyroid hormone on peripheral tissues are nonspecific because they often are altered by a variety of nonthyroidal processes.
4. Tests that detect substances, such as thyroid autoantibodies, that are generally absent in healthy individuals are useful in establishing the cause of some thyroid illnesses.
5. Invasive tests for histologic examination or enzymatic studies, such as biopsy, occasionally are required to establish a definite diagnosis. Gross abnormalities of the thyroid gland, detected by palpation, can be assessed by scintiscanning, by ultrasonography and by computerized tomography.
6. Tests to evaluate the integrity of the hypothalamic-pituitary-thyroid axis at the level of (a) the response of the pituitary gland to thyroid hormone excess or deficiency, (b) the ability of the thyroid gland to respond to thyrotropin (thyroid-stimulating hormone [TSH]), and (c) pituitary responsiveness to thyrotropin-releasing hormone (TRH) are intended to identify the primary organ affected by the disease process that is manifested as thyroid dysfunction—in other words, primary (thyroid), secondary (pituitary), or tertiary (hypothalamic) malfunction.
7. Analysis of the genes that are known to be involved in thyroid hormone transport into the cell (monocarboxylase transporter 8 [MCT8]) as well as thyroid hormone transport in the blood (albumin, prealbumin, and thyroxine-binding globulin), in thyroid hormone synthesis (sodium/iodine symporter [NIS] and thyroid peroxidase, dual oxidases, pendrin and thyroglobulin), in thyroid hormone action (thyroid hormone receptor β gene), or in thyroid gland formation and responsiveness (TSH receptor, PAX8, thyroid transcription factor [TTF]-1 and TTF-2) can be a useful molecular tool for the diagnosis of inherited thyroid disease.
8. Finally, several special tests will be briefly described. Some are valuable in the elucidation of rare inborn errors of hormone biosynthesis; others are used mainly as research tools.

Each test has inherent limitations, and no single procedure is diagnostically adequate for the entire spectrum of possible thyroid abnormalities. The choice, execution, application, and interpretation of each test require an understanding of the thyroid physiology and biochemistry. Thyroid tests not only assist in the diagnosis and management of thyroid illnesses, they also allow one to better understand the pathophysiology underlying a specific disease.

In Vivo Tests of Thyroid Gland Activity and Integrity of Hormone Synthesis and Secretion

In contrast to all other tests, these procedures provide a means to directly evaluate thyroid gland function. Common to these investigations is the administration of radioisotopes to the patient that cannot be distinguished by the body from the naturally occurring stable iodine isotope (^{127}I). Formerly, these tests were used to diagnose hypothyroidism and thyrotoxicosis, but this application has been supplanted by measurement of serum TSH and thyroid hormone concentrations in blood. Also, alterations in thyroid gland activity and the uptake and metabolism of iodine are not necessarily coupled to the amount of hormone that is produced and secreted. These tests are time consuming and relatively expensive, and they expose the patient to radiation. Nevertheless, they still have some specific applications, including evaluation of congenital hypothyroidism and the diagnosis of inborn errors of thyroid hormonogenesis. Administration of radioisotopes can also be used to demonstrate ectopic thyroid tissue and to establish the cause of some forms of thyrotoxicosis. Finally, measurement of tissue uptake of radioiodide is used as a means of estimating the dose of radioiodide to be delivered to the thyroid gland or to metastatic tissue in the treatment of thyrotoxicosis and thyroid carcinoma, respectively.

The principle of radioisotope thyroid scanning is based on the fact that iodine is an integral part of thyroid hormone molecules,

Table 6-1. Commonly Used Isotopes for in Vivo Studies and Radiation Dose Delivered

| Nuclide | Principal Photon Energy, keV | Physical Decay | | Estimated Radiation Dose (mrad/μCi) Administered | | Average Dose Given for Scanning Purposes, μCi |
		Mode	Half-Life, Days	Thyroid*	Total Body	
$^{131}I^-$	364	β (0.606 MeV)	8.1	1340	0.08	50
$^{125}I^-$	28	Electron capture	60	825	0.06	50
$^{123}I^-$	159	Electron capture	0.55	13	0.03	200
$^{132}I^-$	670	β (2.12 MeV)	0.10	15	0.1	50†
$^{99m}TcO_4^-$	141	Isometric transition	0.25	0.2	0.01	2500

*Calculations take into account the rate of maximal uptake and the residence time of the isotope, as well as gland size. For the iodine isotopes, average data for adult euthyroid people used were a $t_{1/2}$ uptake of 5 hours, a biological $t_{1/2}$ of 50 days, maximal uptake of 20%, and gland size of 15 g (see also Quimby et al.[4] and MIRD[2,3]).
†Dose used for early thyroid uptake studies.

and although several other tissues (salivary glands, mammary glands, lacrimal glands, the choroid plexus, and the parietal cells of the stomach) can extract iodide from blood, only the thyroid gland stores iodine for an appreciable period. Because the kidneys continually filter blood iodide, the final fate of most iodine atoms is to be trapped by the thyroid gland or to be excreted in urine. When a tracer of iodide is administered to the patient, it rapidly becomes mixed with the stable extrathyroidal iodide pool and thereafter is handled in an identical manner to the stable isotope. Thus, the thyroidal content of radioiodine gradually increases and that in the extrathyroidal body pool gradually declines until virtually no free iodide is left. This end point normally is reached between 24 and 72 hours after administration of the iodide isotope.

A number of important physiologic parameters can be derived from measurement of RAIU by the thyroid gland, measurement of urinary excretion, and/or determination of the stable iodide concentration in plasma and urine: (1) the rate of thyroidal iodine uptake (thyroid iodide clearance), (2) fractional thyroid RAIU, (3) absolute iodide uptake by the thyroid gland, and (4) urinary excretion of radioiodide, or iodide clearance. After complete removal of the administered radioiodide from the circulation, depletion of the radioisotope from the thyroid gland can be monitored by direct counting over the gland. Radioiodine that reappears in the circulation in protein-bound form can be measured, and this value can be used to estimate the intrathyroidal turnover of iodine and the secretory activity of the thyroid gland. In the absence of availability of whole-body gamma counters, determination of iodine transport can be estimated by measurement of the radioactivity ratio of saliva to blood following ingestion of ^{123}I.

Further useful information can be generated by combining the administration of radioisotopes with agents that are known to normally stimulate or inhibit thyroid gland activity, thus providing information on the control of thyroid gland activity. Administration of radioiodide followed by scanning allows examination of the anatomy of functional thyroid tissue. The latter two applications of in vivo tests using radioiodide will be discussed under their respective headings.

A number of radioisotopes are now available for investigative procedures, and the provision of more sophisticated and sensitive detection devices has substantially decreased the dose and radiation exposure required for these studies. The potential hazard of irradiation resulting from the administration of radioisotopes should always be kept in mind, however. Children are particularly vulnerable, and doses of x-rays as small as 20 rad to the thyroid gland are associated with an increased risk of thyroid malignancy.[1] However, no danger from isotopes used for the diagnosis of thyroid diseases has been substantiated. Administration of radioisotopes during pregnancy and breast-feeding is absolutely contraindicated because of placental transport of the isotopes and excretion into breast milk, respectively.

Table 6-1[2-4] lists the isotopes most commonly used for in vivo studies of thyroid function. Isotopes with slower physical decay, such as ^{125}I and ^{131}I, are particularly suitable for long-term studies. Conversely, isotopes with faster decay, such as ^{123}I and ^{132}I, usually deliver a lower radiation dose and are advantageous in short-term and repeated studies. Because the peak photon energy γ-emission differs among isotopes, simultaneous studies can be performed with two different isotopes.

THYROIDAL RADIOIODIDE UPTAKE

The iodide radioisotope usually is given orally in a capsule or in liquid form, and the quantity that is accumulated by the thyroid gland at various intervals is measured with a gamma scintillation counter. It is important to correct for the background activity of isotope circulating in the blood of the neck region (particularly during the early periods after administration). Background correction is achieved by subtracting counts obtained over the region of the thigh. A dose of the same radioisotope, usually 10%, placed in a neck "phantom" is also counted as a "standard." The percentage of RAIU is calculated from the counts accumulated per constant time unit.

The percentage of RAIU 24 hours after the administration of radioiodide is most useful because in most instances, the thyroid gland has reached the plateau of isotope accumulation, and the best separation between high, normal, and low uptake is obtained at this time. Normal values for 24 hour RAIU in most parts of North America are 5% to 30%. In many other parts of the world, normal values range from 15% to 50%. Lower normal values are due to the increase in dietary iodine intake after the enrichment of foods, particularly mass-produced bread (150 μg of iodine per slice) containing this element. Over the past 3 decades, the mean ingestion of dietary iodine in the United States, although still within the recommended minimum for adults of 125 μg/day, has dramatically declined to approximately 240 to 300 μg/day for men and 190 to 210 μg/day for women.[5] The inverse relationship between the daily dietary intake of iodine and the RAIU test is clearly illustrated in Fig. 6-1. Therefore, normal values of RAIU uptake will depend on the iodine content in a geographic region and also are related to age (with children having a higher iodine

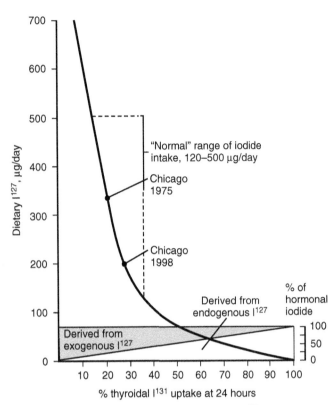

FIGURE 6-1. Relationship of 24-hour thyroidal radioiodide (^{131}I) uptake (RAIU) to dietary content of stable iodine (^{127}I). Uptake increases with decreasing dietary iodine. If iodine intake is below the amount provided from thyroid hormone degradation, the latter contributes a larger proportion of the total iodine taken up by the thyroid. With dietary habits in the United States, the average 24 hour thyroidal RAIU is below 20%. (Data from DeGroot LJ, Reed Larsen P, Hennemann G, et al: The Thyroid and Its Diseases. New York, John Wiley & Sons, 1984.)

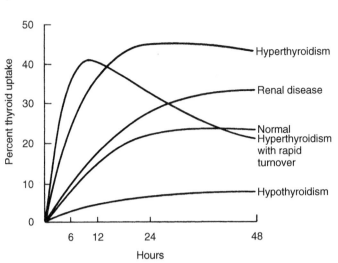

FIGURE 6-2. Examples of thyroidal radioiodide uptake curves under various pathologic conditions. Note the prolonged uptake in renal disease caused by decreased urinary excretion of the isotope and the early decline in thyroidal radioiodine content in some patients with thyrotoxicosis associated with a small but rapidly turning over intrathyroidal iodine pool. (Data from DeGroot LJ, Reed Larsen P, Hennemann G, et al: The Thyroid and Its Diseases. New York, John Wiley & Sons, 1984.)

intake than adults). In Japan, the mean dietary iodine is six times higher than in the United States.

The intake of large amounts of iodide (>5 mg/day), mainly from the use of iodine-containing radiologic contrast media, antiseptics, vitamins, and drugs such as amiodarone, suppresses RAIU values to a level that is hardly detectable with the usual equipment and doses of isotope. Depending on the type of iodine preparation and the period of exposure, depression of RAIU can last for weeks, months, or even years. Even external application of iodide can suppress RAIU. It therefore is important to inquire about individual dietary habits and sources of excess iodide intake. Because dietary assessment of iodine ingestion can be somewhat inaccurate owing to the variable content of iodine added to various foods, measurement of iodine excretion is a more accurate assessment of the iodine balance. Spot urine iodine measurements were compiled from 1971 to 1974 and from 1988 to 1994 in the National Health and Nutrition Examination Surveys I and III, respectively, and have been found to be decreasing, in accordance with what was stated.[6] Clinically, if one suspects that the patient had a large iodine load prior to an RAIU, a urine iodine measurement can be obtained. Urine iodine concentrations greater than 100 µg/day usually are associated with RAIU of 20% or less. Therefore, urine iodine can be useful in determining the feasibility of using RAIU.

RAIU is a measure of the avidity of the thyroid gland for iodide and its rate of clearance relative to the kidney, but results of this test do not equate with hormone production or release. Disease states resulting in excessive production of thyroid hormone most often are associated with increased thyroidal RAIU, and those causing hormone underproduction generally are associated with decreased thyroidal RAIU (Fig. 6-2). Some important exceptions to these rules include the high uptake values that are seen in certain hypothyroid patients and the low values noted in some hyperthyroid patients. Increased thyroidal RAIU with hormonal insufficiency can be caused by severe iodide deficiency and by most inborn errors of hormonogenesis. Lack of substrate in the former and specific enzymatic block of hormone synthesis in the latter cause hypothyroidism that is poorly compensated by TSH-induced thyroid gland overactivity. The increase in serum TSH, in response to the low circulating level of thyroid hormone, stimulates thyroidal iodine uptake by the NIS and hence increases RAIU. This can be a point of confusion for the clinician who is confronted with an increased RAIU in a patient who is suspected to have thyroiditis on the basis of blood tests. Alternatively, decreased thyroidal RAIU with hormonal excess typically is encountered in the syndrome of transient thyrotoxicosis (both deQuervain's and painless thyroiditis) after the ingestion of exogenous hormone (thyrotoxicosis factitia), with iodide-induced thyrotoxicosis (Jod-Basedow disease), rarely in patients with metastatic functioning thyroid carcinoma or struma ovarii, and in patients with thyrotoxicosis who have a moderately high intake of iodide. High or low thyroidal RAIU as a result of low or high dietary iodine intake, respectively, might not be associated with significant changes in thyroid hormone secretion.

Various factors, including diseases that affect the value of the 24 hour thyroidal RAIU, are listed in Table 6-2. Several variations of the RAIU test have been devised that have particular value under special circumstances. Some of these variations are briefly described.

EARLY THYROID RADIOIODIDE UPTAKE AND ^{99M}TC UPTAKE MEASUREMENTS

The combination of severe thyrotoxicosis and a low intrathyroidal iodine concentration may result in an accelerated turnover rate of iodine in some patients. This produces a rapid initial

Table 6-2. Diseases and Other Factors That Affect 24 Hour Thyroidal RAIU

Increased RAIU

Hyperthyroidism (Graves' disease, Plummer's disease, toxic adenoma, trophoblastic disease, resistance to thyroid hormone, TSH-producing pituitary adenoma)
Nontoxic goiter (endemic, inherited biosynthetic defects, generalized resistance to thyroid hormone, Hashimoto's thyroiditis)
Excessive hormonal loss (nephrosis, chronic diarrhea, hypolipidemic resins, diet high in soybean)
Decreased renal clearance of iodine (renal insufficiency, severe heart failure)
Recovery of the suppressed thyroid (withdrawal of thyroid hormone and antithyroid drug administration, subacute thyroiditis, iodine-induced myxedema)
Iodine deficiency (endemic or sporadic dietary deficiency, excessive iodine loss as in pregnancy or in the dehalogenase defect)
TSH administration

Decreased RAIU

Hypothyroidism (primary or secondary)
Syndromes of TSH resistance
Thyroid dysgenesis (hypoplasia, ectopy, or agenesis)
Na/I symporter defect
Defect in iodide concentration (inherited trapping defect, early phase of subacute thyroiditis, transient hyperthyroidism)
Suppressed thyroid gland caused by thyroid hormone (hormone replacement, thyrotoxicosis factitia, struma ovarii)
Iodine excess (dietary, drugs, and other iodine contaminants)
Miscellaneous drugs and chemicals (see Tables 6-10 and 6-13)

RAIU, Radioactive iodine uptake; *TSH,* thyroid-stimulating hormone.

uptake of radioiodide, which reaches a plateau before 6 hours, followed by a decline through release of the isotope in hormonal or other forms (see Fig. 6-2). Although this phenomenon is rare, some laboratories choose to routinely measure early RAIU, usually at 2, 4, or 6 hours. As was mentioned above, early measurements require accurate determination of the background activity contributed by circulating isotope. Radioisotopes with a shorter half-life, such as ^{123}I and ^{132}I, are more suitable in this context.

Because thyroidal uptake in the very early period after administration of radioiodide reflects mainly iodide trapping activity, ^{99m}Tc as the pertechnetate ion (^{99m}TcO$_4^-$) may be used. In euthyroid patients, thyroid trapping is maximal at about 20 minutes and is approximately 1% of the administered dose. This test, when coupled with the administration of triiodothyronine (T$_3$), has been used to evaluate thyroid gland suppressibility in thyrotoxic patients who are treated with antithyroid drugs.

PERCHLORATE DISCHARGE TEST

The perchlorate discharge test is used to detect defects in intrathyroidal iodide organification. It is based on the following physiologic principle. Iodide is "trapped" in the thyroid gland by an active transport mechanism that is mediated by NIS.[7] Once in the gland, iodine is rapidly bound to thyroglobulin (Tg), and retention no longer requires active transport. Several ions, such as thiocyanate (SCN$^-$) and perchlorate (ClO$_4^-$), inhibit NIS-mediated iodide transport and cause release of the intrathyroidal iodide that is not bound to thyroid protein. Thus, intrathyroidal radioiodine loss after the administration of an inhibitor of iodide trapping measures intrathyroidal iodide that is not protein bound and indicates the presence of an iodide-binding defect.

In the standard test, epithyroid counts are obtained every 10 or 15 minutes after the administration of radioiodide. Two hours

later, 1 g of KClO$_4$ is administered orally, and repeated epithyroid counts continue to be obtained for an additional 2 hours. We generally give this dose to patients 6 years or older and give 500 mg to children between the ages of 2 and 6 years. In normal individuals, radioiodide accumulation in the thyroid gland ceases after administration of the iodide transport inhibitor, and little or no loss of the accumulated thyroidal radioactivity occurs after induction of the "trapping" block. An organification defect is indicated if a loss of 5% or more is noted. The severity of the defect is proportional to the extent of radioiodide discharged from the gland and is complete when virtually all the activity accumulated by the gland is lost. The test is positive in the inborn defect of iodide organification caused by thyroid peroxidase (TPO) defects or by mutations in the chloride/iodide transport protein (pendrin) when associated with sensorineural deafness known as Pendred's syndrome and in defects of the H$_2$O$_2$-generating enzyme, dual oxidase 2 (DUOX2), or its maturation factor, DUOXA2. The test may also be positive during the administration of iodide organification–blocking agents or after treatment with radioactive iodine.

IODINE SALIVA-TO-PLASMA RATIO TEST

An abnormal iodine (I$^-$) saliva-to-plasma (S/P) ratio is pathognomonic of the iodine-trapping defect. The test can be carried out without interruption of thyroid hormone treatment. Furthermore, the measurement of I$^-$ S/P can distinguish between a trapping defect and thyroid agenesis, which cannot be determined by RAIU. The I$^-$ S/P ratio can be measured in a medical center without access to a gamma camera. The test is based on the observation that all tissues that normally concentrate iodide are affected by the trapping defect.[8] The presence of an I$^-$ transport defect in the parietal cells of the stomach and the choroid plexus of these patients has been used diagnostically by measurement of the gastric fluid-to-plasma and cerebrospinal fluid (CSF)-to-plasma ratios of radioiodide, following the administration of isotope.

One hour after the oral administration of 5 μCi of Na^{125}I, saliva is collected without stimulation over a period of 5 to 10 minutes. At the same time, a venous blood sample is obtained. After defrothing of the saliva and removal of cell debris by centrifugation (approximately 10 minutes at 500 × g) and separation of the serum, the S/P ratio of radioiodide is determined by counting equal volumes of these fluids in a gamma scintillation counter. A normal I$^-$ S/P is 25. Affected individuals who are not able to concentrate iodide and therefore cannot secrete it into their saliva have a very low S/P. An I$^-$ S/P of approximately 1 is diagnostic of a complete trapping defect, and a value between 1 and 20 is consistent with a partial defect.

Measurement of Hormone Concentration and Other Iodinated Compounds and Their Transport in Blood

The tests most commonly used for evaluating thyroid hormone–dependent metabolic status consist of measurements of free thyroid hormone concentrations. This approach is used because of the development of simple, sensitive, and specific methods for measuring these iodothyronines, and because of the lack of specific tests for direct measurement of the metabolic effects of these hormones on target tissues. Other advantages are the requirement of only a small blood sample and the large number of determinations that can be completed by a laboratory during a regular workday. In fact, although a clinician may entertain a diagnosis of thyroid dysfunction, the certainty of the diagnosis is confirmed only after measurement of the thyroid hormone concentrations and thyrotropin (TSH, see later).

The principal source of all hormonal iodine-containing compounds or their precursors is the thyroid gland, whereas peripheral tissues are the source of the products of their degradation. Their chemical structures and normal concentrations in serum are given in Fig. 6-3. It is important to note that the concentration of each substance is dependent not only on the amount synthesized and secreted by the thyroid gland, but also on its affinity for carrier serum proteins, distribution in tissues, rate of degradation, and, finally, clearance.

Quantitatively, the major secretory product of the thyroid gland is thyroxine (T_4), with T_3 being next in relative abundance. They are synthesized and stored in the thyroid gland as part of a larger molecule, Tg, which is degraded to release the two iodothyronines in a ratio favoring T_4 by 10- to 20-fold. Under normal circumstances, only minute amounts of Tg escape into the circulation. On a molar basis, it is the least abundant iodine-containing compound in blood. With the exception of T_4, Tg, and small amounts of diiodotyrosine (DIT) and monoiodotyrosine (MIT), all other iodine-containing compounds that are found in normal human serum are produced mainly in extrathyroidal tissues by a stepwise process of deiodination of T_4. An alternative pathway of T_4 metabolism that involves deamination and decarboxylation but retention of the iodine residues gives rise to tetraiodothyroacetic acid (TETRAC) and triiodothyroacetic acid (TRIAC).[9,10] Conjugation to form sulfated iodoproteins also occurs. Sulfoconjugates of T_4, T_3, and reverse T_3 (rT_3) have been identified in human biological fluids. Additionally, maternal serum levels of 3,3'-diiothyronine sulfate (T_2S) may reflect on the status of fetal thyroid function. Circulating iodalbumin is generated by intrathyroidal iodination of serum albumin. Small amounts of iodoproteins may be formed in peripheral tissues or in serum by covalent linkage of T_4 and T_3 to soluble proteins. The physiologic function of circulating iodine compounds other than T_4 and T_3 remains unknown, with the exception of rT_3. rT_3 levels are elevated during fasting and during significant nonthyroidal illness. In such instances, measurement of rT_3 can help the clinician to distinguish between these conditions and central hypothyroidism.

NAME	Abbre-viation	Molec-ular Weight	FORMULA	NORMAL CONCENTRATION[a] (range)	
				ng / dL	pmol / L
3,5,3',5'-tetraiodothyronine (Thyroxine)	T_4	777	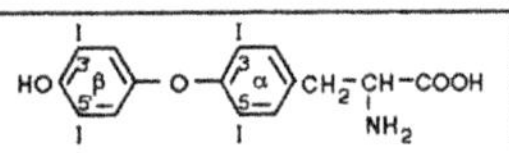	5,000 - 12,000	64,000 - 154,000
3,5,3'-triiodothyronine (Liothyronine)	T_3	651	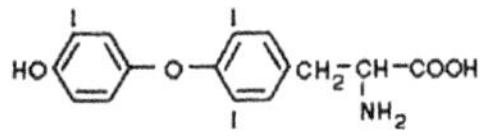	80 - 190[b]	1,200 - 2,900
3,3',5'-triiodothyronine (Reverse T_3)	rT_3	651	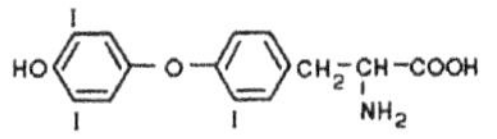	14 - 30	220 - 480
3.5-diiodothyronine	3,5-T_2	525	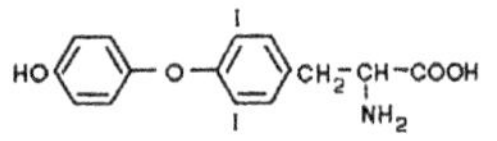	0.20 - 0.75[b]	3.8 - 14
3,3'-diiodothyronine	3,3'-T_2	525	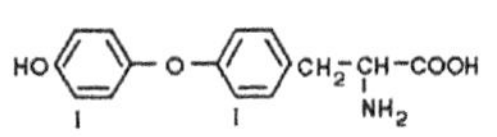	1 - 8[b]	19 - 150
3'5'-diiodothyronine	3'5'-T_2	525	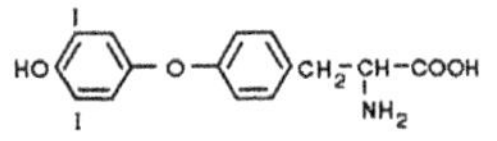	1.5 - 9.0[b]	30 - 170
3'-monoiodothyronine	3'-T_1	399	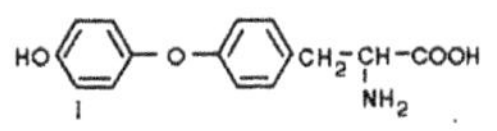	0.6 - 4	15 - 100
3-monoiodothyronine	3-T_1	399	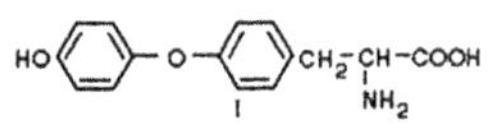	< 0.5 - 7.5	< 13 - 190
3,5,3',5'-tetraiodothyroacetic acid (TETRAC)	T_4A	748	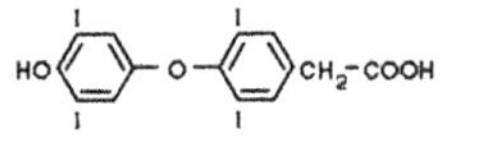	< 8 - 60	< 105 - 800
3,5,3'-triiodothyroacetic acid (TRIAC)	T_3A	622	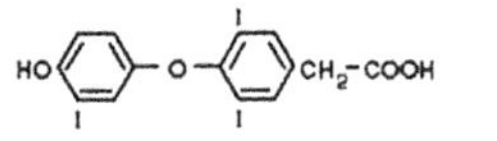	1.6 - 3	26 - 48
3,5-diiodotyrosine	DIT	433	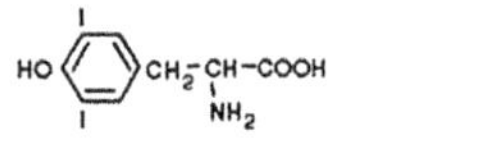	1 - 23	23 - 530
3-monoiodotyrosine	MIT	307	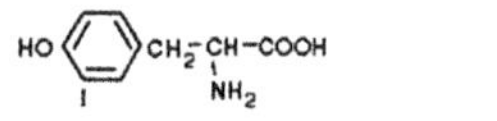	90 - 390[c]	2,900 - 12,700
thyroglobulin	Tg	660,000	glycoprotein made of two identical subunits	< 100 - 2,500	1.5 - 38

FIGURE 6-3. Iodine-containing compounds in the serum of healthy adults. a, Iodothyronine concentrations in the euthyroid population are not normally distributed. Therefore, calculation of the normal range on the basis of 95% confidence limits for a Gaussian distribution is accurate. b, Significant decline with old age. c, Probably an overestimation because of cross-reactivity by related substances.

MEASUREMENT OF TOTAL THYROID HORMONE CONCENTRATION IN SERUM

Iodometry

Because iodine is an integral part of the thyroid hormone molecule, it is not surprising that determination of the iodine content in serum was the first method used over 6 decades ago for the identification and quantitation of thyroid hormone.[11] Measurement of protein-bound iodine was the earliest method used routinely for the estimation of thyroid hormone concentration in serum. This test measured the total quantity of iodine precipitable with serum proteins, 90% of which is T_4. The normal range was 4 to 8 mg of iodine per deciliter of serum.

Efforts to measure serum thyroid hormone levels with greater specificity and with lesser interference from nonhormonal iodinated compounds led to the development of measurement of butanol-extractable iodine and T_4 iodine by column techniques. All such chemical methods for the measurement of thyroid hormone in serum have been replaced by ligand assays, which are devoid of interference by even large quantities of nonhormonal iodine-containing substances.

Radioimmunoassays

Concentrations of thyroid hormones in serum can be measured by radioimmunoassays (RIAs). The principle of these assays relies on competition between the hormone being measured with the same isotopically labeled compound for binding to a specific class of immunoglobulin G (IgG) molecule present in the antiserum. In assays for thyroid hormones, the hormone needs to be liberated from serum hormone–binding proteins, mainly thyroxine-binding globulin (TBG). Methods used to achieve such liberation include extraction, competitive displacement of the hormone being measured, and inactivation of TBG.[12-14] Rarely, circulating antibodies against thyronines develop in some patients and interfere with RIAs carried out on unextracted serum samples. Depending on the method used for the separation of bound from free ligand, the values that are obtained may be spuriously low or spuriously high in the presence of such antibodies.

The wide choice of commercial kits available for most RIA procedures makes these assays accessible to all medical centers. RIAs have been adapted for the measurement of T_4 in small samples of dried blood spots on filter paper and are used in screening for neonatal hypothyroidism.

Despite the ready availability of these kits, the specificity of the various antibodies can result in a twofold difference in hormone measurement when assessed by the College of American Pathologists Proficiency Testing Program.[15]

Nonradioactive Methods

Serum concentrations of T_4 and T_3 have been measured by radioimmunoassay since the early 1970s and more recently have been measured by nonisotopic methods. Assays for total T_4 and T_3 in unextracted serum include a reagent such as 8-anilinonaphthalene sulfonic acid that blocks T_4 and T_3 binding to serum proteins, so that total hormone is available for competition with the assay antibody. Assays were then developed that were based on the principle of the radioligand assay but do not use radioactive material. These assays, which use ligand conjugated to an enzyme, have largely replaced RIAs. The enzyme-linked ligand competes with the ligand being measured for the same binding sites on the antibody. Quantitation is carried out by spectrophotometry of the color reaction developed after addition of the enzyme substrate. Both homogeneous (enzyme-multiplied immunoassay technique) and heterogeneous (enzyme-linked immunosorbent) assays for T_4 have been developed. In the homogeneous assays, no separation step is required, thus providing easy automation. In one such assay, T_4 is linked to malate dehydrogenase to inhibit enzyme activity. The enzyme is activated when the T_4-enzyme conjugate is bound to T_4-specific antibody. Active T_4 conjugates to other enzymes such as peroxidase and alkaline phosphatase have also been developed. This assay has also been adapted for the measurement of T_4 in dried blood samples used in mass screening programs for neonatal hypothyroidism. Other nonradioisotopic immunoassays use fluorescence excitation for detection of the labeled ligand, a technique that is finding increasing application. Such assay methods use a variety of chemiluminescent molecules, such as 1,2-dioxetanes, luminol and derivatives, acridinium esters, oxalate esters, and firefly luciferins, as well as many sensitizers and fluorescent enhancers. One such assay that uses T_4 conjugated to β-galactosidase and fluorescence measurements of the hydrolytic product of 4-methylumbelliferyl-β-D-galactopyranoside has been adapted for use in a microanalytic system requiring only 10 μL of serum. One commercial electrochemiluminescence immunoassay by Roche Elecsys Systems (Mannheim, Germany) uses a competitive test principle with antibodies specifically derived against T_4 or T_3. Endogenous T_4 or T_3 released by the action of 8-anilino-1-naphthalene sulfonic acid competes with the added biotinylated T_4 derivative for the binding sites on the antibodies labeled with the ruthenium complex. Only 15 μL of sample is required. Application of the voltage to the reaction mixture induces chemiluminescent emission, which is measured by a photomultiplier.

Additionally, quantitative measurement of T_4 and T_3 can be done by high-performance liquid chromatography,[16] gas chromatography, and mass spectrometry.[17-20]

Serum Total T_4

The usual concentration of total T_4 (TT$_4$) in adults ranges from 5 to 12 μg/dL (64 to 154 nmol/L). When concentrations are below or above this range in the absence of thyroid dysfunction, they are usually the result of an abnormal level of serum TBG. Such abnormalities are commonly seen during the hyperestrogenic state of pregnancy and during the administration of estrogen-containing compounds, which results in a significant elevation of serum TT$_4$ levels in euthyroid individuals. Similar elevations can be seen in subjects with different forms of hepatitis, and if not appreciated the patient can be misdiagnosed as having hyperthyroidism. Far less commonly, TBG excess is inherited.[21]

Serum TT$_4$ is virtually undetectable in the fetus until midgestation. Thereafter, it rapidly increases and reaches high normal adult levels during the last trimester. A further acute but transient rise occurs within hours after delivery. Values remain above the adult range until 6 years of age, but subsequent age-related changes are minimal, so in clinical practice, the same normal range of TT$_4$ applies to both sexes and all ages.

Small seasonal variations and changes related to high altitude, cold, and heat have been described. Rhythmic variations in serum TT$_4$ concentration are of two types: variations related to postural changes in serum protein concentration[22] and those resulting from true circadian variation. Postural changes in protein concentration do not alter the free T_4 (FT$_4$) concentration, however.

Although levels of serum TT$_4$ below the normal range are usually associated with hypothyroidism and above this range are

Table 6-3. Conditions Associated With Changes in Serum TT_4 Concentration and Relationship to Clinical Status

| Clinical Status | Serum TT_4 Concentration | | |
	High	Low	Normal
Thyrotoxic	Hyperthyroidism (all causes, including Graves' disease, Plummer's disease, toxic thyroid adenoma, early phase of subacute thyroiditis) Thyroid hormone leak (early stage of subacute thyroiditis, transient thyrotoxicosis) Excess of exogenous or ectopic T_4 (thyrotoxicosis factitia, struma ovarii) Predominantly pituitary resistance to thyroid hormone TSH-secreting pituitary tumor	Intake of excess amounts of T_3 (thyrotoxicosis factitia)	Low TBG (congenital or acquired) T_3 thyrotoxicosis (untreated or recurrent post-therapy); more common in iodine-deficient areas Drugs competing with T_4 binding to serum proteins (see also entry under euthyroid with low TT_4) Hypermetabolism of nonthyroidal origin (Luft's syndrome)
Euthyroid	High TBG (congenital or acquired) Familial dysalbuminemic hyperthyroxinemia Transthyretin abnormality Endogenous T_4 antibodies Replacement therapy with T_4 only Treatment with D-T_4 Generalized resistance to thyroid hormone	Low TBG (congenital or acquired) Endogenous T_4 antibodies Mildly elevated or normal T_3 T_3 replacement therapy Iodine deficiency Treated thyrotoxicosis Chronic thyroiditis Congenital goiter Drugs competing with T_4 binding to serum proteins (see Table 6-4)	Normal state
Hypothyroid	Severe generalized resistance to thyroid hormone	Thyroid gland failure Primary (all causes, including gland destruction, severe iodine deficiency, inborn error of hormonogenesis) Secondary (pituitary failure) Tertiary (hypothalamic failure) Consumption hypothyroidism (hemangiomas)	High TBG (congenital or acquired) Deiodinase defect Thyroid transporter defect

T_3, Triiodothyronine; T_4, thyroxine; TBG, thyroxine-binding globulin; TSH, thyroid-stimulating hormone; TT_4, total T_4.

associated with thyrotoxicosis, it must be stressed that the TT_4 level does not always correspond to the FT_4 concentration, which represents the metabolically active fraction (see below). The TT_4 concentration in serum may be altered by independent mechanisms: (1) an increase or decrease in the supply of T_4, as is seen in most cases of thyrotoxicosis and hypothyroidism, respectively; (2) changes caused solely by alterations in T_4 binding to serum proteins; and (3) compensatory changes in the serum TT_4 concentration caused by high or low serum levels of T_3. Conditions associated with changes in serum TT_4 and their relationship to the metabolic status of the patient are listed in Table 6-3.

Serum TT_4 levels are low in conditions that are associated with decreased TBG concentrations, in the presence of abnormal TBGs with reduced binding affinity, and when the available T_4-binding sites on TBG are partially saturated by competing drugs present in blood in high concentration (Table 6-4). Conversely, TT_4 levels are high when the serum TBG concentration is high. In this situation, the person remains euthyroid provided that feedback regulation of the thyroid gland is intact.

Although changes in transthyretin (TTR) concentration rarely give rise to significant alterations in TT_4 concentration, the presence of a variant serum albumin with high affinity for T_4 or antibodies against T_4 produce apparent elevations in the measured TT_4 concentration, whereas the metabolic status remains normal. The variant albumin is inherited as an autosomal dominant trait termed familial dysalbuminemic hyperthyroxinemia (FDH).

Another possible cause of discrepancy between the observed serum TT_4 concentration and the metabolic status of the patient is divergent changes in serum total T_3 (TT_3) and TT_4 concentrations with alterations in the serum T_3/T_4 ratio. The most common situation is that of an elevated TT_3 concentration. The source of T_3 may be endogenous, as in T_3 thyrotoxicosis, or exogenous, as

during ingestion of T_3. In the former situation, contrary to the common variety of thyrotoxicosis, elevation in the serum TT_3 concentration is not accompanied by an increase in the TT_4 level. In fact, the serum TT_4 level is normal and occasionally low. This finding indicates that the pathogenesis of T_3 thyrotoxicosis is the direct secretion of T_3 from the thyroid gland rather than the peripheral conversion of T_4 to T_3. Ingestion of pharmacologic doses of T_3 results in thyrotoxicosis associated with severe depression of the serum TT_4 concentration. Moderate hypersecretion of T_3 can be associated with euthyroidism and a low serum TT_4 concentration. This situation, occasionally referred to as T_3 euthyroidism, may be more prevalent than T_3 thyrotoxicosis. It is believed to constitute a state of compensatory T_3 secretion as a physiologic adaptation of the failing thyroid gland, such as after treatment of thyrotoxicosis, in some cases of chronic thyroiditis, or during iodine deprivation. The serum TT_4 concentration is also low in normal persons receiving replacement doses of T_3. Conversely, serum TT_4 levels are above the upper limit of normal in 15% to 50% patients treated with exogenous T_4 and having normal serum TSH. Because of the relatively slow rate of metabolism and the large extrathyroidal T_4 pool, the serum concentration of the hormone varies little with the time of sampling in relation to ingestion of the daily dose.

Serum Total T_3

Triiodothyronine is principally responsible for the effects of thyroid hormones on the target organs. T_3 is formed extrathyroidally via 5′ deiodination of T_4. Thus, serum T_3 concentration reflects the functional state of the peripheral tissue rather than the secretory performance of the thyroid gland. Like T_4, 99% of T_3 is present in protein-bound form. However, the affinity of T_3 to TBG is 10-fold lower than that of T_4.

Table 6-4. Compounds That Affect Thyroid Hormone Serum Transport Proteins

Substance	Common Use
Increase TBG Concentration	
Estrogens[22,396,397]	Ovulation suppressants and anticancer
Heroin and methadone[398]	Opiates (in addicts)
Clofibrate[399]	Hypolipidemic
5-Fluorouracil[400]	Anticancer
Perphenazine[401]	Tranquilizer
Tamoxifen[402,403]	Chemotherapy
Raloxifene[403-405]	Osteoporosis
Decrease TBG Concentration	
Androgens and anabolic steroids[406,407]	Virilizing, anticancer, and anabolic
Glucocorticoids[408] intracranial pressure	Antiinflammatory and anti-immunosuppressive; decrease
L-Asparaginase[409]	Antileukemic
Nicotinic acid[410,411]	Hypolipidemic
Interfere With Thyroid Hormone Binding to TBG and/or TTR	
Salicylates and salsalate[387,412]	Antiinflammatory, analgesic, and antipyretic
Carbamazepine[387,412]	
Diphenylhydantoin and analogues[413,414]	Anticonvulsive and antiarrhythmic
Diazepam[415]	Antianxiety
Furosemide[416]	Diuretic
Sulfonylureas[417]	Hypoglycemic
Dinitrophenol[411]	Uncouples oxidative phosphorylation
Free fatty acids[417]	
o,p'-DDD[418]	Antiadrenal
Phenylbutazone[419]	Antiinflammatory
Halofenate[420]	Hypolipidemic
Fenclofenac[392,421]	NSAID
Mefenamic	NSAID
Diclofenac	NSAID
Heparin (IV)[422]	Anticoagulant
Enoxaparin[422]	
Orphenadrine[423]	Spasmolytic
Monovalent anions (SCN⁻, ClO_4^-)[424]	Antithyroid
Thyroid hormone analogues, including dextroisomers[425]	Cholesterol reducing

NSAID, Nonsteroidal antiinflammatory drug; *o,p'-DDD,* 2,4'-dichlorodiphenyldichloroethane (mitotane); *TBG,* thyroxine-binding globulin; *TTR,* transthyretin.

Normal serum TT_3 concentrations in the adult range from 80 to 190 ng/dL (1.2 to 2.9 nmol/L). Sex differences are small, but age differences are more dramatic. In contrast to serum TT_4, the TT_3 concentration at birth is low, about half the normal adult level. It rises rapidly within 24 hours to about double the normal adult value, followed by a decrease over the subsequent 24 hours to a level in the upper adult range, which persists for the first year of life. A decline in the mean TT_3 level has been observed in old age, although not in healthy subjects,[23,24] which suggests that a fall in TT_3 might reflect the prevalence of nonthyroidal illness rather than an effect of age alone. Although a positive correlation between serum TT_3 level and body weight has been observed, this might be related to overeating.[25] Rapid and profound reductions in serum TT_3 can be produced within 24 to 48 hours of total calorie or carbohydrate-only deprivation.

Most conditions that cause serum TT_4 levels to increase are associated with high TT_3 concentrations. Thus, serum TT_3 levels are usually elevated in thyrotoxicosis and reduced in hypothyroidism. However, in both conditions, the TT_3/TT_4 ratio is elevated relative to normal euthyroid persons. This elevation is due to the disproportionate increase in serum TT_3 concentration in thyrotoxicosis and a lesser diminution in hypothyroidism relative to the TT_4 concentration. Accordingly, measurement of the serum TT_3 level is a more sensitive test for the diagnosis of hyperthyroidism, and measurement of TT_4 is more useful in the diagnosis of hypothyroidism.

Under certain conditions, changes in the serum TT_3 and TT_4 concentrations are disproportionate or occur in the opposite direction (Table 6-5). Such conditions include the syndrome of thyrotoxicosis with normal TT_4 and FT_4 levels (T_3 thyrotoxicosis). In some patients, treatment of thyrotoxicosis with antithyroid drugs normalizes the serum TT_4 but not the TT_3 level and produces a high TT_3/TT_4 ratio. In areas of limited iodine supply and in patients with limited thyroidal ability to process iodide, euthyroidism can be maintained at low serum TT_4 and FT_4 levels by increased direct thyroidal secretion of T_3. Although these changes have a rational physiologic explanation, the significance of discordant serum TT_4 and TT_3 levels under other circumstances is less well understood.

The most common cause of discordant serum concentrations of TT_3 and TT_4 is a selective decrease in serum TT_3 caused by decreased conversion of T_4 to T_3 in peripheral tissues. This reduction is an integral part of the pathophysiology of a number of nonthyroidal acute and chronic illnesses and calorie deprivation. In these conditions, the serum TT_3 level is often lower than that commonly found in patients with frank primary hypothyroidism. However, no clear clinical evidence of hypometabolism is found in this situation. In some individuals, decreased T_4-to-T_3 conversion is an inherited condition.[26] A combination of high TT_3 and low TT_4 is typical in subjects with loss-of-function mutations in the iodothyronine cell membrane transporter, MCT8.[27]

A variety of drugs are responsible for producing changes in the serum TT_3 concentration without apparent metabolic consequences. Drugs that compete with hormone binding to serum proteins decrease serum TT_3 levels, generally without affecting the free T_3 (FT_3) concentration (see Table 6-4). Some drugs such as glucocorticoids[28] depress the serum TT_3 concentration by interfering with the peripheral conversion of T_4 to T_3. Others, such as phenobarbital,[29] depress the serum TT_3 concentration by stimulating the rate of intracellular hormone degradation and clearance. Most have multiple effects. These effects are combinations of those described above, as well as inhibition of the hypothalamic-pituitary axis or thyroidal hormonogenesis.

Changes in serum TBG concentration have an effect on the serum TT_3 concentration similar to that on TT_4. The presence of endogenous antibodies to T_3 can also result in apparent elevation of serum TT_3, but as in the case of high TBG, it does not cause hypermetabolism.

Administration of commonly used replacement doses of T_3, usually on the order of 75 μg/day or 1 μg/kg body weight per day,[30] results in serum TT_3 levels in the thyrotoxic range. Furthermore, because of rapid gastrointestinal absorption and a relatively fast degradation rate, the serum level varies considerably according to the time of sampling in relation to hormone ingestion.

MEASUREMENT OF TOTAL AND UNSATURATED THYROID HORMONE–BINDING CAPACITY IN SERUM

The concentration of thyroid hormone in serum is dependent on its supply, as well as on the abundance of hormone-binding sites on serum proteins; therefore, estimation of the latter has proved useful in the correct interpretation of values obtained from mea-

Table 6-5. Conditions That May Be Associated With Discrepancies Between the Concentration of Serum TT_3 and TT_4

Serum			Metabolic Status		
TT_3/TT_4 Ratio	TT_3	TT_4	Thyrotoxic	Euthyroid	Hypothyroid
↑	↑	N	T_3 thyrotoxicosis (endogenous)	Endemic iodine deficiency (T_3 autoantibodies)*	—
↑	N	↓	—	Treated thyrotoxicosis (T_4 autoantibodies)*	Endemic cretins (severe iodine deficiency)
↑	↑	↓	Pharmacologic doses of T_3 (exogenous T_3 toxicosis) Partially treated thyrotoxicosis	T_3 replacement (especially 1 to 3 hours after ingestion) Endemic iodine deficiency	T_3 autoantibodies*
↓	↓	N	—	Most conditions associated with reduced conversion of T_4 to T_3 Chronic or severe acute illness† Trauma (surgical, burns) Fasting and malnutrition Drugs‡ (T_3 autoantibodies)	—
↓	N	↑	Severe nonthyroidal illness associated with thyrotoxicosis	Neonates (first 3 weeks of life) T_4 replacement Familial hyperthyroxinemia resulting from T_4 binding albumin–like variant (T_4 autoantibodies)*	—
↓	↓	↑	—	At birth Acute nonthyroidal illness with transient hyperthyroxinemia	T_4 autoantibodies*
↑	↑	↓	—	Large hemangiomas	Type 3 deiodinase excess[426] MCT8 defect[27]

TT_3, Total triiodothyronine; TT_4, total thyroxine.
*Artifactual values depend on the method of hormone determination in serum.
†Hepatic and renal failure, diabetic ketoacidosis, myocardial infarction, infectious and febrile illness, cancers.
‡Glucocorticoids, iodinated contrast agents, amiodarone, propranolol, propylthiouracil.

surement of the total hormone concentration. These results have been used to provide an estimate of the free hormone concentration, which is important in differentiating changes in serum total hormone concentrations caused by alterations in binding proteins in euthyroid patients from those caused by abnormalities in thyroid gland activity that give rise to hypermetabolism or hypometabolism.

In Vitro Uptake Tests

In vitro uptake tests measure the unoccupied thyroid hormone–binding sites on TBG. They use labeled T_3 or T_4 and some form of synthetic absorbent to measure the proportion of radiolabeled hormone that is not tightly bound to serum proteins. Because ion exchange resins often are used as absorbents, the test became known as the resin T_3 or T_4 uptake test, which describes the technique rather than the entity measured.

The test is usually carried out by incubating a sample of the patient's serum with a trace amount of labeled T_3 or T_4. The labeled hormone, not bound to available binding sites on TBG present in the serum sample, is absorbed onto an anion exchange resin and measured as resin-bound radioactivity. Values correlate inversely with the concentration of unsaturated TBG. Various methods use different absorbing materials to remove the hormone that is not tightly bound to TBG. Labeled T_3 generally is used because of its less firm, yet preferential, binding to TBG. Depending on the method, typical normal results for T_3 uptake are 25% to 35% or 45% to 55%. Thus, it is more valuable to express results of the uptake tests as a ratio of the result obtained in a normal control serum run in the same assay as the test samples. Normal values will then range on either side of 1.0, usually from 0.85 to 1.15.

Uptake of tracer by the absorbent is inversely proportional to the number of unsaturated binding sites (unoccupied by endogenous thyroid hormone) in serum TBG. Thus, uptake is increased when the amount of unsaturated TBG is reduced as a result of

excess endogenous thyroid hormone or a decrease in the concentration of TBG. In contrast, uptake is decreased when the amount of unsaturated TBG is increased as a result of a low serum thyroid hormone concentration or an increase in the concentration of TBG. Because the test can be affected by either or both independent variables—serum total thyroid hormone and TBG concentrations—the results cannot be interpreted without knowledge of the hormone concentration. As a rule, parallel increases or decreases in serum TT_4 concentration and the T_3 uptake test indicate hyperthyroidism and hypothyroidism, respectively, whereas discrepant changes in serum TT_4 and T_3 uptake suggest abnormalities in TBG binding. However, abnormalities in hormone and TBG concentrations can coexist in the same patient. For example, a hypothyroid patient with a low TBG level will typically show a low TT_4 level and normal T_3 uptake results (Fig. 6-4). Several nonhormonal compounds, because of structural similarities, compete with thyroid hormone for its binding site on TBG. Some are used as pharmacologic agents and thus may alter the in vitro uptake test, as well as the total thyroid hormone concentration in serum. A list is provided in Table 6-4.

TBG and TTR Measurements

The concentrations of TBG and TTR in serum can be estimated by measurement of their total T_4-binding capacity at saturation or measured directly by immunologic techniques.[31,32]

The TBG concentration in serum can be determined by RIA,[32] and both TBG and TTR can be measured by Laurell's rocket immunoelectrophoresis, by radial immunodiffusion, or by enzyme immunoassay; commercial methods are available. The true mean value for TBG is 1.6 mg/dL (260 nmol/L), with a range of 1.1 to 2.2 mg/dL (180 to 350 nmol/L) in serum. In adults, the normal range for TTR is 16 to 30 mg/dL (2.7 to 5.0 mmol/L). Concentrations of TBG and TTR in serum vary with age, gender, pregnancy, and posture. Determination of the concentration of

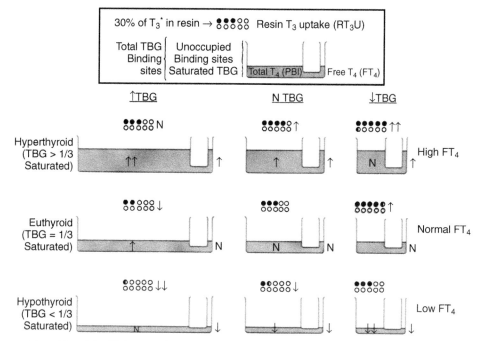

FIGURE 6-4. Graphic representation of the relationship between the serum total thyroxine (T_4) concentration, the resin triiodothyronine uptake (rT_3U) test, and the free T_4 (FT_4) concentration in various metabolic states and in association with changes in thyroxine-binding globulin (TBG). The principle of communicating vessels is used as an illustration. The height of fluid in the small vessel represents the level of FT_4; the total amount of fluid in the large vessel, the total T_4 concentration; and the total volume of the large vessel, the TBG capacity. *Dots* represent resin beads; *black dots* represent those carrying the radioactive T_3 tracer (T_3^*). The rT_3U test result *(black dots)* is inversely proportional to the unoccupied TBG-binding sites represented by the unfilled capacity of the large vessel.

these proteins in serum is particularly helpful for evaluation of extreme deviations from normal, as in congenital abnormalities of TBG. In most instances, however, the in vitro uptake test, in conjunction with the serum TT_4 level, gives an approximate estimation of the TBG concentration.

ESTIMATION OF FREE THYROID HORMONE CONCENTRATION

Most thyroid hormones in the blood are bound to serum protein carriers, thus leaving only a minute fraction of free hormone in the circulation that is capable of mediating biological activities. A reversible equilibrium exists between bound and unbound hormone, and it is the latter that represents the fraction of the hormone capable of traversing cellular membranes to exert its effects on body tissues. Although changes in serum hormone-binding proteins affect both the total hormone concentration and the corresponding circulating free fraction, in a euthyroid person, the absolute concentration of free hormone remains constant and correlates with the tissue hormone level and its biological effect. Information concerning this value is probably the most important parameter in the evaluation of thyroid function because it relates to the patient's metabolic status, although other mechanisms exist for the cell to control the active amount of thyroid hormone via autoregulation of receptors[33] and regulation of deiodinase activity.[34,35] Rarely, a defect in thyroid hormone transport into cells would abolish the free hormone and the metabolic effect correlation.[27]

With few exceptions, the free hormone concentration is high in thyrotoxicosis, low in hypothyroidism, and normal in euthyroidism, even in the presence of profound changes in TBG concentration, provided that the patient is in a steady state. Notably, the FT_4 concentration may be normal or even low in patients with T_3 thyrotoxicosis and in those ingesting pharmacologic doses of T_3. The concentration of FT_4 may be outside the normal range in the absence of an apparent abnormality in thyroid hormone–dependent metabolic status. This situation is frequently observed in severe nonthyroidal illness, during which both high and low values have been reported. As expected, when a euthyroid state is maintained by the administration of T_3 or by predominant thyroidal secretion of T_3, the FT_4 level is also depressed. More consistently, patients with a variety of nonthyroidal illnesses have low FT_3 levels. This decrease is characteristic of all conditions associated with depressed serum TT_3 concentrations caused by diminished conversion of T_4 to T_3 in peripheral tissues by deiodinase enzymes. Both FT_4 and FT_3 values may be out of line in patients receiving a variety of drugs (see below). Marked elevations in both FT_4 and FT_3 concentrations in the absence of hypermetabolism are typical of patients with the inherited condition of resistance to thyroid hormone. The FT_3 concentration is usually normal or even high in hypothyroid individuals living in areas of severe endemic iodine deficiency. Their FT_4 levels are, however, normal or low. Free hormone concentrations also do not reflect the metabolic status of the patient with inherited defects in hormone transport into cells of hormone metabolism.[36]

Direct Measurement of Free T_4 and Free T_3

Direct measurement of absolute FT_4 and FT_3 concentrations is technically difficult and until recently has been limited to research assays. To minimize perturbations of the relationship between free and bound hormone, these hormones must be separated by ultrafiltration or by dialysis involving minimal dilution and little alteration in pH or electrolyte composition. The separated free hormone is then measured directly by RIA or chromatography.[37] These assays are probably the most accurate available, but small, weakly bound, dialyzable substances or drugs may be removed from the binding proteins, and the free hormone concentration measured in their presence might not fully reflect the free concentration in vivo. Direct immunometric assays adapted to automation, although not reliable under specific conditions, have replaced more labor intensive methods (see below).

Isotopic Equilibrium Dialysis

This method has been the gold standard for the estimation of FT_4 or FT_3 for more than 40 years. It is based on a determination of the proportion of T_4 or T_3 that is unbound, or free, and thus is able to diffuse through a dialysis membrane (i.e., the dialyzable fraction). To carry out the test, a sample of serum is incubated with a trace amount of labeled T_4 or T_3. The labeled tracer rapidly equilibrates with the respective bound and free endogenous hormones. The sample is then dialyzed against buffer at a constant temperature until the concentration of free hormone on either side of the dialysis membrane has reached equilibrium. The dialyzable fraction is calculated from the proportion of labeled hormone in the dialysate. The contribution from radioiodide present as contaminant in the labeled tracer hormone should be eliminated by purification[38] and by various techniques of precipitation of the dialyzed hormone.[39] FT_4 and FT_3 levels can be measured simultaneously by addition to the sample of T_4 and T_3 labeled with two different radioiodine isotopes. Ultrafiltration is a modification of the dialysis technique. Results are expressed as the fraction (dialyzable fraction of T_4 or T_3) or percentage (%FT_4 or %FT_3) of the respective hormones that dialyzed, and the absolute concentrations of FT_4 and FT_3 are calculated from the product of the total concentration of the hormone in serum and its respective dialyzable fraction. Typical normal values for FT_4 in adults range from 1.0 to 3.0 ng/dL (13 to 39 pmol/L), and those for FT_3 range from 0.25 to 0.65 ng/dL (3.8 to 10 nmol/L).

Results achieved by these techniques generally are comparable to those determined by direct one-step methods (see below) but are more likely to differ with extremely low or extremely high TBG concentrations or in the presence of circulating inhibitors of protein binding, especially in situations of nonthyroidal illness. The measured dialyzable fraction may be altered by the temperature at which the assay is run, the degree of dilution, the time allowed for equilibrium to be reached, and the composition of the diluting fluid. The calculated value is dependent on an accurate measurement of TT_4 or TT_3 and may be incorrect in patients with T_4 or T_3 autoantibodies. Some of these problems, particularly those arising from dilution, can be surmounted by using commercially available dialysis methods or ultrafiltration methods of free from bound hormone that do not necessitate serum dilution. In addition, the antibody that is used on the ultrafiltrate must be of high affinity to achieve acceptable precision.

Index Methods

Because determination of free hormone by equilibrium dialysis is cumbersome and technically demanding, many clinical laboratories have used a method by which an FT_4 index (FT_4I) or an FT_3 index (FT_3I) is derived from the product of the TT_4 or TT_3 (determined by immunoassay) and the value of an in vitro uptake test (see above). Although the results are not always in agreement with the values obtained by dialysis, these techniques are rapid and simple. They are more likely to fail at extremely low or extremely high TBG concentrations, in the presence of abnormal binding proteins, in patients with nonthyroidal illness, or in the presence of circulating inhibitors of protein binding.

The theoretical contention that the FT_4I is an accurate estimate of the absolute FT_4 concentration can be confirmed by the linear correlation between these two parameters. This statement is true provided that results of the in vitro uptake test (T_3 or T_4 uptake) are expressed as the thyroid hormone–binding ratio, which is determined by dividing the tracer counts bound to the solid matrix by counts bound to serum proteins. Values are corrected for assay variations by using appropriate serum standards and are expressed as the ratio of a normal reference pool. The normal range is slightly narrower than the corresponding TT_4 in healthy euthyroid patients with a normal TBG concentration. It is 6.0 to 10.5 mg/dL (77 to 135 nmol/L) when calculated from TT_4 values. The FT_4I is high in thyrotoxicosis and low in hypothyroidism, irrespective of the TBG concentration. Euthyroid patients with TT_4 values outside the normal range as a result of TBG abnormalities have a normal FT_4I. Lack of correlation between the FT_4I and the metabolic status of the patient has been observed in the same circumstances as those described for similar discrepancies when the FT_4 concentration was measured by dialysis.

Methods for estimation of the FT_3I are also available but are rarely used in routine clinical evaluation of thyroid function. Like the FT_4I, it correlates well with the absolute FT_3 concentration. The test corrects for changes in TT_3 concentration resulting from variations in TBG concentration.

Estimation of Free T_4 and Free T_3 Based on TBG Measurements

Because most T_4 and T_3 in serum are bound to TBG, their free concentrations can be calculated from their binding affinity constants to TBG and molar concentrations of hormones and TBG. A simpler calculation of the T_4/TBG and T_3/TBG ratios yields values that are similar to but less accurate than the FT_4I and FT_3I, respectively.

Two-Step Immunoassays

In these assays, the free hormone is first immunoextracted by a specific bound antibody (first step), frequently fixed to the tube (coated tube).[40] After washing, labeled tracer is added and is allowed to equilibrate between the unoccupied sites on the antibody and those of serum thyroid hormone–binding proteins. The free hormone concentration will be inversely related to the antibody-bound tracer, and values are determined by comparison to a standard curve. Values that are obtained with this technique are generally comparable to those determined by direct methods. They are more likely to differ in the presence of circulating inhibitors of protein binding and in sera from patients with nonthyroidal illness.

Analogue (One-Step) Immunoassays

In these assays, a labeled analogue of T_4 or T_3 directly competes with the endogenous free hormone for binding to antibodies.[41] In theory, these analogues are not bound by the thyroid hormone–binding proteins in serum. However, various studies have found significant protein binding to the variant albumin-like protein, to TTR, and to iodothyronine autoantibodies. Such binding results in discrepant values in other assays in a number of conditions, including nonthyroidal illness, pregnancy, and familial dysalbuminemic hyperthyroxinemia (FDH).[42] A growing number of commercial kits are available, some of which have been modified to minimize these problems.[43,44] Nonetheless, their accuracy remains controversial, although such commercial methods are increasingly being adopted in the routine clinical chemistry laboratory. Commercially available kits for measurement of free T_4 values are compared in Table 6-6.

Table 6-6. Commercial Free T$_4$ Methods

Name	Methodology	Manufacturer
Amberlite MAB	Serum free T$_4$ inhibits binding of peroxidase anti-T$_4$ monoclonal antibody T$_3$-coated solid phase.	Amersham, UK
Chiron ACS:180	Serum free T$_4$ competes with acridinium ester labeled T$_4$. Anti-T$_4$ antibody linked to magnetic particles.	Chiron Diagnostics, MA, USA
AxSYM	Anti-T$_4$ coated microparticles. T$_3$-alkaline phosphatase binds to the unoccupied sites.	Abbott Labs, IL, USA
Elecsys	Anti-T$_4$ antibody labeled with ruthenium. Unoccupied antibody binds to biotinylated T$_4$, which is linked to streptavidin-coated microparticles. Magnetic separation.	Boehringer Manheim, IN, USA
Diagnostic Product Immulite	T$_4$ analogue tracer (does not bind TBG or TTR) competes with serum free T$_4$ for a limited number of T$_4$ antibody binding sites. Alkaline phosphatase–labeled antianalogue binds to solid phase, and generated signal is inversely proportional to free T$_4$.	Diag Prod, CA, USA
Corning Nichols Dialysis	Dialysis against 12-fold buffer volume, followed by radioimmunoassay of T$_4$ in the dialysate.	Nichols Institute, CA, USA

Automated Measurement of Free T$_4$ and Free T$_3$

During the 1990s, through the introduction of random access immunoassay analyzers that operate with chemiluminescent or fluorescent labels, measurements of free thyroid hormones became automated and therefore allowed rapid processing of multiple samples. Although the initial financial burden of such equipment is considerable, they reduce labor costs, demand few handling skills on behalf of the operator, and provide random access so that samples can be tested on demand. Precision studies have shown highly reproducible data with this approach.[45,46] Comparison of results between different automated analyzers and with manual free thyroid hormone assays, including the gold standard of equilibrium dialysis, has revealed good correlation over a broad range of free thyroid hormone concentrations.[47,48]

Considerations in Selection of Methods for the Estimation of Free Thyroid Hormone Concentration

No single method for the estimation of free hormone concentration in serum is infallible in the evaluation of thyroid hormone–dependent metabolic status. Each test has inherent advantages and disadvantages depending on specific physiologic and pathologic circumstances. For example, methods based on measurement of total thyroid hormone and TBG cannot be used in patients with absent TBG secondary to inherited TBG deficiency. Under such circumstances, the concentration of free thyroid hormone is dependent on interaction of the hormone with serum proteins that normally play a negligible role (TTR and albumin). When alterations in thyroid hormone binding do not affect T$_4$ and T$_3$ equally, discrepant results of FT$_4$I are obtained when labeled T$_4$ or T$_3$ is used in the in vitro uptake test. For example, euthyroid patients with FDH and those who have endogenous antibodies with greater affinity for T$_4$ will have high TT$_4$ but a

normal T$_3$ uptake test, which will result in an overestimation of the calculated FT$_4$I. In such instances, calculation of the FT$_4$I from a T$_4$ uptake test may provide more accurate results. Conversely, reduced overall binding affinity for T$_4$, which affects T$_3$ to a lesser extent, will underestimate the FT$_4$I derived from a T$_3$ uptake test. Similarly, use of T$_4$ and T$_3$ uptake for estimation of the free hormone concentration is satisfactory in the presence of alterations in TBG concentration but not with alterations of the affinity of TBG for the hormone.

Methods based on equilibrium dialysis are most appropriate for estimation of the free thyroid hormone level in patients with all varieties of abnormal binding to serum proteins, provided that the true concentration of total hormone has been accurately determined. All methods for the estimation of FT$_4$ may give high or low values in patients with severe nonthyroidal illness who are believed to be euthyroid. This finding has been attributed, at least in part, to the presence of inhibitors of thyroid hormone binding to serum proteins, as well as to the various adsorbents that are used in the test procedures. Some of these inhibitors have been postulated to leak from tissues of the diseased patient. Such discrepancies are even more pronounced during transient states of hyperthyroxinemia or hypothyroxinemia associated with acute illness, after withdrawal of treatment with thyroid hormone, and in patients with acute changes in TBG concentration.

The contribution of various drugs that interfere with binding of thyroid hormone to serum proteins or with the in vitro tests should also be taken into account in the choice and interpretation of tests (see Table 6-4). Although the free thyroid hormone concentration in serum would appear to determine the amount of hormone that is available to body tissues, factors that govern their cell membrane uptake, transport to the nucleus, and functional interactions with nuclear receptors and cofactors ultimately determine their biological effects.

MEASUREMENTS OF IODINE-CONTAINING HORMONE PRECURSORS AND PRODUCTS OF DEGRADATION

The last 4 decades have witnessed the development of RIAs for the measurement of a number of naturally occurring, iodine-containing substances that have little, if any, thyromimetic activity. Some of these substances are products of T$_4$ and T$_3$ degradation in peripheral tissues. Others are predominantly, if not exclusively, of thyroidal origin. Because they are devoid of significant metabolic activity, with the exception of rT$_3$, measurement of their concentration is of value only in the research setting for detecting abnormalities in the metabolism of thyroid hormone in peripheral tissues, as well as defects of hormone synthesis and secretion. The application of tandem mass spectrometry in the measurement of these substances undoubtedly will result in a better understanding of their changes and their pathophysiologic implications.

3,3′,5′-Triiodothyronine or Reverse T$_3$

rT$_3$ is principally a product of T$_4$ degradation in peripheral tissues, namely, liver and kidney. It is also secreted by the thyroid gland, but the amounts are practically insignificant.[49] rT$_3$ is an inactive product of T$_4$ degradation. Thus, measurement of the rT$_3$ concentration in serum reflects both tissue supply and metabolism of T$_4$ and identifies conditions that favor this particular pathway of T$_4$ degradation.

When total rT$_3$ (TrT$_3$) is measured in unextracted serum, a competitor of rT$_3$ binding to serum proteins must be added.

Several chemically related compounds may cross-react with the antibodies. The strongest cross-reactivity is observed with 3,3'-diiodothyronine (3,3'-T_2), but such cross-reactivity does not present a serious methodologic problem because of its relatively low level in human serum. Although cross-reactivity with T_3 and T_4 is less likely, these compounds are more often the cause of rT_3 overestimation because of their relative abundance, particularly in thyrotoxicosis. Free fatty acids interfere with the measurement of rT_3 by RIA.[50] The normal range in adult serum for TrT_3 is 14 to 30 ng/dL (0.22 to 0.46 nmol/L), although varying values have been reported. It is elevated in subjects with high TBG and in some individuals with FDH.[51] Serum TrT_3 levels are normal in hypothyroid patients who are treated with T_4, which indicates that peripheral T_4 metabolism is an important source of circulating rT_3. Values are high in thyrotoxicosis and low in untreated hypothyroidism. High values are normally found in cord blood and in newborns.

With only a few exceptions, notably uremia and human immunodeficiency virus (HIV) infection and acquired immunodeficiency syndrome (AIDS), serum TrT_3 concentrations are elevated in all circumstances that cause low serum T_3 levels in the absence of obvious clinical signs of hypothyroidism. These conditions include, in addition to the newborn period, a variety of acute and chronic nonthyroidal illnesses, calorie deprivation, and the influence of a growing list of clinical agents and drugs (Table 6-7).

The current clinical application of TrT_3 measurement in serum is in the differential diagnosis of conditions associated with alterations in serum T_3 and T_4 concentrations when thyroid gland and metabolic abnormalities are not readily apparent.

Table 6-7. Agents That Alter the Extrathyroidal Metabolism of Thyroid Hormone

Substance	Common Use
Inhibit Conversion of T_4 to T_3	
PTU[427-429]	Antithyroid
Glucocorticoids (hydrocortisone, prednisone dexamethasone)[214]	Antiinflammatory and immunosuppressive; decrease intracranial pressure
Propranolol[430,431]	Adrenergic blocker (antiarrhythmic, antihypertensive)
Interleukin-6[432]	Cancer therapy
Iodinated contrast agents: ipodate (Oragrafin), iopanoic acid (Telepaque)[433,434]	Radiologic contrast media
Amiodarone[435-437]	Antianginal and antiarrhythmic
Clomipramine[438]	Tricyclic antidepressant
Stimulate Hormone Degradation	
Diphenylhydantoin[243,439]	Anticonvulsive and antiarrhythmic
Carbamazepine[440]	Anticonvulsant
Phenobarbital[440]	Hypnotic, tranquilizing, and anticonvulsive
Rifampin[441]	Antituberculosis drug
Ritonavir	Antiviral
Sertraline[442]	Depression
Decrease Absorption/Increase Fecal Excretion of Thyroid Hormone	
Cholestyramine[443] Colestipol	Hypolipidemic resins
Soybeans[444]	Diet
Calcium carbonate[445]	
Ferrous sulfate[355]	Anemia
Sucralfate[446]	Antiulcer
Aluminum hydroxide[353,447]	Antacid

PTU, Propylthiouracil; T_3, triiodothyronine; T_4, thyroxine.

The dialyzable fraction of rT_3 in normal adult serum is 0.2% to 0.32%, or approximately the same as that of T_3. The corresponding serum free rT_3 (FrT_3) concentration is 50 to 100 pg/dL (0.77 to 1.5 pmol/L). In the absence of gross TBG abnormalities, variations in serum FrT_3 concentration closely follow those of TrT_3. Reverse T_3 is measured by RIA in serum, plasma, or amniotic fluid samples. Antigen from patient samples competes with radioactive tracer (^{125}I-rT_3) for binding sites on an antibody. After incubation, the amount of tracer that is bound to antibody will be inversely proportional to the amount of antigen in the sample. The radioactivity of the tracer bound to antibody is counted, and the amount of antigen or rT_3 from the patient's serum is determined from this. Typically, 0.1 mL of undiluted sample is required.

3,5-Diiodothyronine

The normal adult range for total 3,5-diiodothyronine (3,5-T_2) in serum measured by direct RIAs is 0.20 to 0.75 ng/dL (3.8 to 14 pmol/L). That 3,5-T_2 is derived from T_3 is supported by the observations that conditions associated with high and low serum T_3 levels have elevated and reduced serum concentrations of 3,5-T_2, respectively. Thus, high serum 3,5-T_2 levels have been reported in hyperthyroidism, and low levels have been reported in the serum of hypothyroid patients, in newborns, during fasting, and in patients with liver cirrhosis.

3,3'-Diiodothyronine

Normal concentrations in adults probably range from 1 to 8 ng/dL (19 to 150 pmol/L). Levels are clearly elevated in hyperthyroidism and in the newborn. Values have been found to be normal or depressed in nonthyroidal illnesses, in agreement with the demonstration of reduced monodeiodination of rT_3 to 3,3'-T_2. In vivo turnover kinetic studies and measurement of 3,3'-T_2 in serum after the administration of T_3 and rT_3 have clearly shown that 3,3'-T_2 is the principal metabolic product of these two triiodothyronines.

3',5'-Diiodothyronine

Reported concentrations of 3',5'-diiodothyronine (3',5'-T_2) in the serum of normal adults have a mean overall range of 1.5 to 9.0 ng/dL (30 to 170 pmol/L).[52,53] Values are high in hyperthyroidism and in the newborn. Being the derivative of rT_3 monodeiodination, 3',5'-T_2 levels are elevated in serum during fasting and in chronic illness, in which the level of the rT_3 precursor is also high. Administration of dexamethasone also produces an increase in the serum 3',5'-T_2 level.

3'-Monoiodothyronine

The concentration of 3'-monoiodothyronine (3'-T_1) in the serum of normal adults, as measured by RIA, has been reported to range from 0.6 to 2.3 ng/dL (15 to 58 pmol/L) and from less than 0.9 to 6.8 ng/dL (<20 to 170 pmol/L). Its two immediate precursors, 3,3'-T_2 and 3',5'-T_2, are the main cross-reactants in the RIA. Serum levels are very high in hyperthyroidism and low in hypothyroidism. The concentration of 3'-T_1 in serum is elevated in all conditions associated with high rT_3 levels, including the newborn period, nonthyroidal illness, and fasting. This finding is not surprising because the immediate precursor of 3'-T_1 is 3',5'-T_2, a product of rT_3 deiodination, which is also present in serum in high concentration under the same circumstances. Elevated serum levels of 3'-T_1 in renal failure are attributed to decreased clearance inasmuch as the concentrations of its precursors are not increased.

3-Monoiodothyronine

Experience with the measurement of $3\text{-}T_1$ in serum is limited. Normal values in the serum of adult humans determined by ^{3}H-labeled $3\text{-}T_1$ in a specific RIA ranged from less than 0.5 to 7.5 ng/dL (<13 to 190 pmol/L). The mean concentration of $3\text{-}T_1$ in the serum of thyrotoxic patients and in cord blood was significantly higher; $3\text{-}T_1$ appears to be a product of in vivo deiodination of $3,3'\text{-}T_2$.

Tetraiodothyroacetic Acid and Triiodothyroacetic Acid

The iodoamino acids TETRAC (T_4A) and TRIAC (T_3A), products of deamination and oxidative decarboxylation of T_4 and T_3, respectively, have been detected in serum by direct RIA measurements. Reported mean concentrations in the serum of healthy adults have been 8.7 ng/dL[54] and 2.6 ng/dL (range, 1.6 to 3.0 ng/dL or 26 to 48 pmol/L)[25] for T_3A, and 28 ng/dL (range, <8 to 60 mg/dL or <105 to 800 pmol/L) for T_4A. Serum T_4A levels are reduced during fasting and in patients with severe illness, although the percentage of conversion of T_4 to T_4A is increased.[55,56] The concentration of serum T_3A remains unchanged during the administration of replacement doses of T_4 and T_3.[25] It has been suggested that intracellular rerouting of T_3 to T_3A during fasting is responsible for the maintenance of normal serum TSH levels in the presence of low T_3 concentrations.

3,5,3'-Triiodothyronine Sulfate and 3,3'-Diiodothyronine Sulfate

Sulfation of iodothyronines results in the inactivation of thyroid hormones and enhances their excretion in urine and bile. An RIA procedure is available to measure 3,5,3'-triiodothyronine sulfate (T_3S) in ethanol extracted serum samples. Concentrations of T_3S in normal adults range from 4 to 10 ng/dL (50 to 125 pmol/L). Although the principal source of T_3S is T_3 and the former binds to TBG, values are high in the newborn period and low in pregnancy. This observation suggests different rates of T_3S generation or metabolism in the mother and fetus. T_3S values are high in thyrotoxicosis (including patients taking suppressive doses of thyroxine), in patients receiving amiodarone therapy,[57] and in patients with nonthyroidal illness.

The mean serum concentration of T_2S in normal subjects is 0.86 ± 0.59 nmol/L, with a detection threshold between 0.17 and 0.5 nmol/L, depending on the assay. The values of T_2S were higher in hyperthyroid patients (2.2 ± 0.06) and in subjects with nonthyroidal illness (6.0 ± 1.5). It was also detectable in normal urine and amniotic fluid.[9]

Diiodotyrosine and Monoiodotyrosine

Although RIA methods have been developed for the measurement of DIT and MIT, because of limited experience, their value in clinical practice remains unknown. Early reports gave a normal mean value for DIT in the serum of normal adults of 156 ng/dL (3.6 nmol/L),[58] with a progressive decline caused by refinement of techniques to values as low as 7 ng/dL with a range of 1 to 23 ng/dL (0.02 to 0.5 nmol/L). Thus, the normal range of 90 to 390 ng/dL (2.9 to 12.7 nmol/L) for MIT is undoubtedly an overestimation. Iodotyrosine that has escaped enzymatic deiodination in the thyroid gland appears to be the principal source of DIT in serum. Iodothyronine degradation in peripheral tissues is probably a minor source of iodotyrosines because the administration of large doses of T_4 to normal subjects produces a decline rather than an increase in the serum DIT level. DIT is metabolized to MIT in peripheral tissues. Serum levels of DIT are low during pregnancy and high in cord blood. Recently, high-performance liquid chromatography (HPLC) tandem mass spectrometry was used for the measurement of iodotyrosines in urine in patients with defects in iodotyrosine deiodinase.[59]

Thyronamine and 3-Iodothyronamine

Thyronamines are a novel class of endogenous signaling molecules that differ from T_4 and other T_4 derivatives owing to the absence of the carboxylate group of the β alanine side chain. Measurement of these compounds can be done by liquid chromatography and tandem mass spectrometry.[60] Only two compounds in this class, thronamine (T_0AM) and 3-tiodothyronamine ($3\text{-}T_1AM$), have been detected in tissues and are believed to function physiologically as thyroid hormone antagonists.[61,62] Thyronamines are isozyme-specific substrates of deiodinases.[60]

Thyroglobulin

RIA methods were the methods first used routinely for measurement of Tg in serum, although other methods using immunoradiometric assay, immunochemiluminescent assay, and enzyme-linked immunosorbent assay technology have been reported and are gaining increasing popularity. They are specific and, depending on the sensitivity of the assay, capable of detecting Tg in the serum of approximately 90% of euthyroid healthy adults. When antisera are used in high dilutions, virtually no cross-reactivity with iodothyronines or iodotyrosines occurs. Results obtained from analysis of sera containing Tg autoantibodies may be inaccurate depending on the antiserum that is used.[63] Because of the importance of Tg measurement in the management of thyroid cancer, methods for its determination in the presence of antibodies have been devised. The simplest, and probably the most accurate, is the estimation of Tg recovery after its addition to the sample being tested.[64,65] The presence of TPO antibodies does not interfere with the Tg RIA. Despite the reliability of measurements of serum Tg, it is clear that different assay methods may result in values that are discrepant by up to 30%, even though reference preparations are available. Typically, immunochemiluminometric assay (ICMA) methods underestimate the serum Tg value, whereas RIA methods overestimate it, so it is essential that clinical decisions be based on serial measurements using the same assay.

Tg concentrations in the serum of normal adults range from less than 1 to 25 ng/mL (<1.5 to 38 pmol/L), with mean levels of 5 to 10 ng/mL.[66] On a molar basis, these concentrations of Tg are minute relative to the circulating iodothyronines: 5000-fold lower than the corresponding concentration of T_4 in serum. Values tend to be slightly higher in women than in men. In the neonatal period and during the third trimester of pregnancy, mean values are approximately fourfold and twofold higher.[67,68] They gradually decline throughout infancy, childhood, and adolescence.[69] The positive correlation between the levels of serum Tg and TSH indicates that pituitary TSH regulates the secretion of Tg.

Elevated serum Tg levels reflect increased secretory activity by stimulation of the thyroid gland or damage to thyroid tissue, whereas values below or at the level of detectability indicate a paucity of thyroid tissue or suppressed activity. Patients with acromegaly have elevated serum Tg levels, but it is unclear whether this is a direct effect of growth hormone. Tg levels in a variety of conditions affecting the thyroid gland have been reviewed[70,71] and are listed in Table 6-8.

Interpretation of a serum Tg value should take into account the fact that Tg concentrations may be high under normal physiologic conditions or may be altered by drugs. Administration of

Table 6-8. Conditions Associated With Changes in Serum Tg Concentration Listed According to the Presumed Mechanism

Increased

TSH Mediated
Acute and transient (TSH and TRH administration, neonatal period)
Chronic stimulation
    Iodine deficiency, endemic goiter, goitrogens
    Reduced thyroidal reserve (lingual thyroid)
    TSH-producing pituitary adenoma
    Resistance to thyroid hormone
    TBG deficiency

Non–TSH Mediated
Thyroid stimulators
    IgG (Graves' disease)
    hCG (trophoblastic disease)
Trauma to the thyroid (needle aspiration and surgery of the thyroid gland, ^{131}I therapy)
Destructive thyroid pathology
    Subacute thyroiditis
    Painless thyroiditis
    Postpartum thyroiditis
Abnormal release
    Thyroid nodules (toxic, nontoxic, multinodular goiter)
    Differentiated nonmedullary thyroid carcinoma
Abnormal clearance (renal failure)
Amiodarone-induced hyperthyroidism
Acromegaly
Cord blood

Decreased

TSH Suppression
Administration of thyroid hormone

Decreased Synthesis
Athyrosis (postoperative, congenital)
Tg synthesis defect

hCG, Human chorionic gonadotropin; *IgG,* immunoglobulin G; *TBG,* thyroxine-binding globulin; *Tg,* thyroglobulin; *TRH,* thyrotropin-releasing hormone; *TSH,* thyroid-stimulating hormone.

iodine and antithyroid drugs increases the serum Tg level, as do states associated with hyperstimulation of the thyroid gland by TSH or other substances with thyroid-stimulating activity. This increase in serum Tg concentration is due to increased thyroidal release of Tg rather than to changes in its clearance.[72] Administration of TRH and TSH also transiently increases the serum level of Tg.[73] Trauma to the thyroid gland, such as that occurring during diagnostic and therapeutic procedures, including percutaneous needle biopsy, surgery, or ^{131}I therapy, can produce a striking although short-lived elevation in the Tg level in serum.[73,74] Pathologic processes with destructive effects on the thyroid gland also produce transient although more prolonged increases.[75] Tg is undetectable in serum after total ablation of the thyroid gland, as well as in normal people receiving suppressive doses of thyroid hormone. It is thus a useful test in the differential diagnosis of thyrotoxicosis factitia,[76] especially when transient thyrotoxicosis with low RAIU or suppression of thyroidal RAIU by iodine is an alternative possibility.

Reverse transcriptase polymerase chain reaction is a sensitive technique to measure the presence of mRNA of different genes in peripheral blood. Initial results were promising that this highly sensitive method would be useful in the management of patients with thyroid cancer[77]; however, subsequent studies have demonstrated that this measurement is of limited clinical value.[78,79]

The most striking elevations in serum Tg concentrations have been observed in patients with metastatic differentiated nonmedullary thyroid carcinoma, even after total surgical and radioio-dide ablation of all normal thyroid tissue. It usually persists despite full thyroid hormone suppressive therapy, suggesting excessive autonomous release of Tg by the neoplastic cells. The determination is thus of particular value in the follow-up and management of thyroid cancer metastases, particularly when they fail to concentrate radioiodide. Follow-up of such patients with sequential serum Tg determinations helps in the early detection of tumor recurrence or growth and in assessment of the efficacy of treatment. Measurement of serum Tg is also useful in patients with metastases, particularly to bone, in whom no evidence of a primary site is noted and thyroid malignancy is being considered in the differential diagnosis. On the other hand, serum Tg levels are of no value in the differential diagnosis of primary thyroid cancer because levels may be within the normal range in the presence of differentiated thyroid cancer and high in a variety of benign thyroid diseases. In fact, levels of Tg greater than 100 mg/dL can often be seen in subjects with multinodular goiters and can raise the possibility of metastatic disease. Whether early detection of recurrent thyroid cancer after initial ablative therapy could be achieved by serum Tg measurement without cessation of hormone replacement therapy is debatable because Tg secretion by the tumor is modulated by TSH and could be suppressed by the administration of thyroid hormone. Although the presence of an elevated Tg level with suppressed TSH is an indicator of probable recurrence, suppressed Tg with suppressed TSH is not a reliable indicator of the absence of recurrence. The introduction of recombinant human TSH allows stimulation of thyroid tissue for the measurement of Tg without cessation of replacement treatment.

In the early phase of subacute thyroiditis, Tg levels are high. Declining serum Tg levels during the course of antithyroid drug treatment of patients with Graves' disease may indicate the onset of a remission.[80] Tg may be undetectable in the serum of neonates with dyshormonogenetic goiters caused by defects in Tg synthesis,[81] but levels are very high in some hypothyroid infants with thyromegaly or ectopy.[82] Measurement of serum Tg in hypothyroid neonates is useful in differentiating infants with complete thyroid agenesis from those with hypothyroidism resulting from other causes and thus in most cases obviates the need for diagnostic administration of radioiodide.

Measurement of Thyroid Hormone and Its Metabolites in Other Body Fluids and in Tissues

Clinical experience with measurement of thyroid hormone and its metabolites in body fluids other than serum and in tissues is limited for several reasons. Analyses carried out in urine and saliva do not appear to give information additional to that determined from measurements carried out in serum. Amniotic fluid, CSF, and tissues are less readily accessible for sampling. Their likely application in the future will depend on information that they could provide beyond that obtained from similar analyses in serum.

URINE

Because thyroid hormone is filtered in the urine predominantly in free form, measurement of the total amount excreted over 24 hours offers an indirect method for estimation of the free hormone concentration in serum. The 24 hour excretion of T_4 in normal adults ranges from 4 to 13 μg and from 1.8 to 3.7 μg, depending on whether total or only conjugated T_4 is measured. Corresponding normal ranges for T_3 are 2.0 to 4.0 μg and 0.4 to 1.9 μg.[83-86] Striking seasonal variations have been shown for the urinary excretion of both hormones, with a nadir during the hot summer months in the absence of significant changes in serum TT_4 and TT_3. As expected, values are normal in pregnancy and in nonthyroidal illnesses and are high in thyrotoxicosis and low in hypothyroidism. The test might not be valid in the presence of gross proteinuria and impairment in renal function.

AMNIOTIC FLUID

From week 12 of gestation onward, fetal serum concentrations of T_4 and TSH steadily rise that correlate with concentrations in the amniotic fluid[87] and are independent of maternal concentrations.[87,88] Determination of fetal thyroid status is a clinical challenge, and although percutaneous umbilical blood sampling is technically possible, it is a demanding procedure that poses a risk for fetal bradycardia and hemorrhage. Amniocentesis, in contrast, is easier, safer, and more readily available. All iodothyronines measured in blood have also been detected in amniotic fluid. With the exception of T_3, $3,3'-T_2$, and $3'-T_2$, the concentration at term is lower than that in cord serum.[89] This fact cannot be fully explained by the low TBG concentration in amniotic fluid.

The TT_4 concentration in amniotic fluid averages 0.5 μg/dL (65 nmol/L) with a range of 0.15 to 1.0 μg/dL and thus is very low when compared with values in maternal and cord serum. The FT_4 concentration is, however, twice as high in amniotic fluid relative to serum. The TT_3 concentration is also low relative to maternal serum, being on average 30 ng/dL (0.46 nmol/L) in both amniotic fluid and cord serum. rT_3, on the other hand, is very high in amniotic fluid, on average 330 ng/dL (5.1 nmol/L) during the first half of gestation and declining precipitously at about the 30th week of gestation to an average of 85 ng/dL (1.3 nmol/L), which is also found at term.

A recent study sought to establish normal amniotic fluid reference intervals for TSH, total T_4, and free T_4 using automated immunoassays.[90] Results showed TSH from less than 0.1 to 0.5 mU/L, with a median of 0.1 mU/L; total T_4 from 2.3 to 3.9 μg/dL (30 to 50 nmol/L), with a median of 3.3 μg/dL (4 nmol/L); and free T_4 from less than 0.4 to 0.7 ng/dL (5 to 9 pmol/L), with a median of 0.4 ng/dL (5 pmol/L).

CEREBROSPINAL FLUID

T_4, T_3, and rT_3 concentrations have been measured in human CSF.[91-93] The concentrations of both TT_4 and TT_3 are approximately 50-fold lower than those found in serum. However, the concentrations of these iodothyronines in free form are similar to those in serum. In contrast, the level of TrT_3 in CSF is only 2.5-fold lower than that of serum, whereas that of FrT_3 is 25-fold higher. This difference is probably due to the presence in CSF of a larger proportion of TTR, which has high affinity for rT_3. All the thyroid hormone–binding proteins that are present in serum are also found in CSF, although in lower concentrations. The concentrations of TT_4 and FT_4 are increased in thyrotoxicosis and depressed in hypothyroidism. Severe nonthyroidal illness gives rise to increased TrT_3 and FrT_3 levels.

MILK

The TT_4 concentration in human milk is on the order of 0.03 to 0.5 μg/dL.[94] Analytic artifacts were responsible for the much higher values formerly reported.[95] TT_3 concentrations range from 10 to 200 ng/dL (0.15 to 3.1 nmol/L).[96] The concentration of TrT_3 ranges from 1 to 30 ng/dL (15 to 460 pmol/L). Thus, it is

unlikely that milk would provide a sufficient quantity of thyroid hormone to alleviate hypothyroidism in an infant. The serum levels of thyrotropin, T_4, free T_4, and T_3 are not significantly different between breastfed and bottle-fed babies.[97]

SALIVA

It has been suggested that only the free fraction of small nonpeptide hormones that circulate predominantly bound to serum proteins would be transferred to saliva and that their measurement, in this easily accessible body fluid, would provide a simple and direct means to determine their free concentration in blood. This hypothesis was confirmed for steroid hormones that are not tightly bound to serum proteins.[98] Levels of T_4 in saliva range from 4.2 to 35 ng/dL (54 to 450 pmol/L) and do not correlate with the concentration of FT_4 in serum.[99] This finding is, in part, due to the transfer of T_4 bound to small but variable amounts of serum proteins that reach the saliva.

EFFUSIONS

TT_4 measured in fluid obtained from serous cavities bears a direct relationship to the protein content and the serum concentration of T_4. Limited experience with Tg measurement in pleural effusions from patients with thyroid cancer metastatic to the lungs suggests that it might be of diagnostic value. Thyroglobulin levels are expectedly very high in fluid from thyroid nodules or cysts.

TISSUES

Because the response to thyroid hormone is expressed at the cellular level via nuclear receptors, it is logical to assume that hormone concentrations in tissues should correlate best with their action. Methods for extraction, recovery, and measurement of iodothyronines from tissues have been developed, but for obvious reasons, data from thyroid hormone measurements in human tissues are limited. Preliminary work has shown that under several circumstances, hormonal levels in tissues such as liver, kidney, and muscle usually correlate with those found in serum.[100]

Measurements of T_3 in cells most accessible for sampling in humans, namely, red blood cells, gave values of 20 to 45 ng/dL (0.31 to 0.69 nmol/L), or one-fourth those found in serum.[101] They are higher in thyrotoxicosis and lower in hypothyroidism.

The concentrations of all iodothyronines have been measured in thyroid gland hydrolysates. In normal glands, the molar ratios relative to the concentration of T_4 are on average as follows: $T_4/T_3 = 10$, $T_4/rT_3 = 80$, $T_4/3,5'-T_2 = 1400$, $T_4/3,3'-T_2 = 350$, $T_4/3',5'-T_2 = 1100$, and $T_4/3'-T_1 = 4400$. Information about the content of iodothyronines in hydrolysates of abnormal thyroid tissue is limited, and the diagnostic value of such measurements has not been established.

Measurement of Tg in metastatic tissue obtained by needle biopsy may be of value in the differential diagnosis, especially when the primary site is unknown and the histologic diagnosis is not conclusive.

Tests Assessing the Effects of Thyroid Hormone on Body Tissues

Because of the ubiquitous expression of thyroid hormone receptors, thyroid hormone regulates a variety of biochemical reactions in virtually all tissues. Thus, ideally, the adequacy of hormonal supply should be assessed by tissue responses rather than by parameters of thyroid gland activity or serum hormone concentrations, which are several steps removed from the site of thyroid hormone action. Unfortunately, tissue responses (metabolic indices) are nonspecific because they are altered by a variety of physiologic and pathologic mechanisms unrelated to thyroid hormone deprivation or excess. This would indicate that thyroid function tests might not be a reliable measure of thyroid hormone action at the cellular level. These conditions include, but are not limited to, nonthyroidal illness or euthyroid sick syndrome, alterations in T_4 binding by changes in transport proteins, resistance to thyroid hormone or TSH, subclinical hypothyroidism and hyperthyroidism, central causes of hypothyroidism, and use of medications such as lithium, amiodarone, and other iodine-containing medications, and centrally acting medications. The following review of biochemical and physiologic changes mediated by thyroid hormone has a dual purpose: (1) to outline some of the changes that can be used as clinical tests in the evaluation of metabolic status, and (2) to point out the changes in various determinations commonly used in the diagnosis of a variety of nonthyroidal illnesses that might be affected by the concomitant presence of thyroid hormone deficiency or excess.

CLINICAL SYMPTOM SCALES

Clinical symptom scales have been developed and used in the past to aid in the diagnosis of thyrotoxicosis and hypothyroidism. A weighted score involving 19 different signs and symptoms was able to discriminate between thyrotoxic and euthyroid patients with a relatively high degree of sensitivity.[102] The limitation of this scale is its basis on the presence or absence of symptoms and signs rather than on a range of degrees of their severity. A hyperthyroid scale was developed that looks at the following characteristics: nervousness, sweating, heat tolerance, hyperactivity, tremor, weakness, hyperdynamic precordium, diarrhea, appetite, and impairment of daily function.[103] Each of the symptoms or signs was graded on a scale of 0 to 4, 4 being the most severe. Newly diagnosed, untreated Graves' disease patients had significantly higher scores compared with the same patients after treatment and euthyroid patients. Although no correlation was found between the rating scale and serum levels of T_4, total T_3, and free T_4 index, a direct relationship was found between goiter size and the rating scale, and an inverse relationship was demonstrated with age.

Clinical evaluation of hypothyroidism, in contrast, is more difficult. In 1969, Billewicz and coworkers described a diagnostic index that scores the presence or absence of various symptoms and signs of hypothyroidism for the purpose of establishing a diagnosis.[104] Reevaluation found that only three signs—ankle reflex, puffiness, and slow movements—had a positive predictive value greater than 90%; the rest had positive and negative predictive values of around 70% or less.[105] The original index was revised to exclude cold intolerance and pulse rate because these findings had a positive predictive and a negative predictive value of less than 70% in combination with an age-correcting factor, resulting in a more sensitive scale. The new scale demonstrated 62% of all overt hypothyroid and 24% of subclinical hypothyroid patients as clinically hypothyroid, compared with 42% and 6% using Billewicz's index.

METABOLISM

Basal Metabolic Rate

The basal metabolic rate (BMR) has a long history in the evaluation of thyroid function. It measures oxygen consumption under basal conditions of overnight fast and rest from mental and physical exertion. Because standard equipment for the measurement of BMR might not be readily available, the BMR can be estimated from the oxygen consumed over a timed interval by analysis of samples of expired air. The test indirectly measures metabolic energy expenditure or heat production.

Results are expressed as the percentage of deviation from normal after appropriate corrections have been made for age, gender, and body surface area. Low values are suggestive of hypothyroidism, and high values reflect thyrotoxicosis. Normal BMR ranges from negative 15% to positive 5%, most hyperthyroid patients having a BMR of positive 20% or better and hypothyroid patients commonly having a BMR of negative 20% or lower. Different clinical states are known to alter BMR. Fever, pregnancy, pheochromocytoma, adrenergic agonist drugs, cancer, congestive heart failure, acromegaly, polycythemia, and Paget's disease of the bone are known to increase the BMR. Obesity, starvation or anorexia, hypogonadism, adrenal insufficiency, Cushing's syndrome, immobilization, and sedative drugs are known to decrease the BMR.

Metabolic Markers

Plasma homocysteine concentrations have been shown to increase in hypothyroidism and decrease in hyperthyroidism, indicating that free T_4 is an independent determinant of total homocysteine concentrations.[106-108] A longitudinal study of hyperthyroid and hypothyroid patients over 12 months of treatment showed that serum homocysteine levels started at higher levels in hypothyroid patients and at lower levels in hyperthyroid patients; with treatment, the values of both patient groups approached the same values. Lower folate levels and a lower creatinine clearance in hypothyroidism and a higher creatinine clearance in hyperthyroidism only partially explain these changes in homocysteine. The association of elevated homocysteine levels in subclinical hypothyroidism is less clear.[109] Free fatty acids in serum are higher in hyperthyroid patients than in controls or in hypothyroid patients and might be a marker of lipolysis.[110,111] Serum glycerol levels are significantly increased in hyperthyroid patients and are lower in hypothyroid patients versus controls. Ketone bodies are increased in hyperthyroidism.[112]

DEEP TENDON REFLEX RELAXATION TIME (PHOTOMOTOGRAM)

A delay in the relaxation time of the deep tendon reflexes, visible to the experienced eye, occurs in hypothyroidism. Several instruments have been devised to quantitate various phases of the Achilles tendon reflex. Although normal values vary according to the phase of the tendon reflex measured, the apparatus used, and individual laboratory standards, the approximate adult normal range for the half-relaxation time is 230 to 390 msec. Diurnal variation, differences with gender, and changes with age, cold exposure, fever, exercise, obesity, and pregnancy have been reported. However, the main reason for failure of this test as a diagnostic measure of thyroid dysfunction is the large overlap with values obtained in euthyroid individuals and alterations caused by nonthyroidal illnesses.[113]

TESTS RELATED TO CARDIOVASCULAR FUNCTION

Thyroid hormone affects the heart through regulation of cardiac gene expression as well as through nongenomic means. Evidence of thyroid hormone–regulated cardiac gene expression comes from in vivo studies of transcription of the cardiac myocyte gene α-myosin heavy chain (α-MHC). Myocyte genes that are positively regulated by thyroid hormones include α-MHC, sarcoplasmic reticulum Ca^{2+}-adenosine phosphatase (ATPase SERCA), and the voltage-gated potassium channels Kv1.4, Kv4.2, and Kv4.3.[114,115] These are all critical determinants of contractile activity and are downregulated in hypothyroidism. Genes that are negatively regulated by thyroid hormone include the β-myosin heavy chain (β-MHC) and phospholamban, which regulates contractile function through modulation of calcium cycling. These genes are upregulated in hypothyroidism.

Thyroid hormone can also affect the myocardium through nongenomic actions. Changes primarily involve membrane ion channels and ion pumps, but other possible extranuclear changes involving cell-surface proteins, signal transduction, and intracellular protein trafficking, myocardial contractility and metabolism, vascular smooth muscle, and myocardial mitochondria have been described.[116] Nongenomic actions of thyroid hormone, primarily T_3, on the plasma membrane of myocytes include (1) stimulation of the Na^+/H^+ antiporter through effects on the activity of protein kinase C,[117] (2) stimulation of Ca^{2+}-adenosine triphosphatase (ATPase) activity through activation of phospholipase C (PLC)[118] and presence of calmodulin, (3) prolonged activation of the Na^+ current through effects on protein kinase C activity, and (4) an increase in the inward rectifying K^+ current, which may be mediated via G protein–coupled receptors.[119] These extranuclear nontranscriptional effects of thyroid hormones on the performance characteristics of the ion channels in the heart result in changes in intracellular levels of calcium and potassium, which can increase inotropy and chronotropy. Noninvasive measures of cardiovascular hemodynamics using electrocardiogram, echocardiogram, and Doppler parameters have been found to be a sensitive measure of T_3 action on the cardiac and vascular smooth muscle cells.[120] Standardized measures of cardiac systolic function include (1) the pre-ejection period (PEP), which is the time from the QRS complex onset to the opening of the aortic valve, and (2) left ventricular ejection time, or the time from the opening of the aortic valve to the end of ventricular systole. Two other highly reproducible measures that are obtained via two-dimensional echocardiogram are the isovolumetric contraction time (ICT) and the isovolumetric relaxation time (IVRT), which are measures of early systole and of diastolic function, respectively. In hyperthyroidism secondary to Graves' disease and multinodular goiter, increased systolic function with shortened PEP, left ventricular ejection time (LVET), and ICT; reduced systemic vascular resistance; and supranormal diastolic dysfunction with shortened left ventricular relative thickness (LVRT) and rate of blood flow across the mitral valve have been demonstrated. In hypothyroidism, all measures of cardiac contractile performance are impaired. Cardiac function improved as soon as 24 hours after treatment and returned to normal levels by 1 week in a study using intravenous T_3 for 1 week in hypothyroid patients.[121] The geometry, cardiac function, and oxidative metabolism have also been assessed in hypothyroid patients by positron emission tomography (PET) and magnetic resonance imaging (MRI). Ejection fraction and myocardial efficiency were derived from the imaging measurements and were found to be decreased in hypothyroidism and improved with thyroid hormone treatment.[122] In hyperthyroidism, heart rate and cardiac output are expectedly higher. Peripheral vascular resistance is reduced. Differences in blood pressure, stroke volume, and ventricular mass are not observed.

NEUROBEHAVIORAL MARKERS OF THYROID HORMONE ACTION

A variety of neuropsychiatric scales have also been used to evaluate hyperthyroid and hypothyroid patients and their response to treatment,[123] including a specific thyroid symptom scale for hypothyroid patients.[124] A study of hyperthyroid patients found them to have abnormal scores on neuropsychological tests (IQ, memory, and attention span) that improved somewhat with propranolol therapy and more with antithyroid drug therapy. Disturbances in cognition in hypothyroidism include inattentiveness, inability to concentrate, slowing of thought processes and speech, inability to calculate and to understand complex questions, and alterations in perception.[125] In addition, memory deficits, particularly for recent events, have been found to occur in hypothyroidism. Furthermore, hypothyroidism in nondemented older adults is associated with impairments in learning, word fluency, visual-spatial abilities, attention, visual scanning, and psychomotor function. Several studies evaluating the effects of T_4 and T_3 treatment on neurocognitive function and psychiatric symptoms with varying outcomes, however, demonstrate that the underlying pathophysiologic mechanisms of thyroid hormone in the brain still need further elucidation.[126,127] The metabolic consequences of hypothyroidism have been studied with the use of imaging techniques such as ^{31}P nuclear magnetic spectroscopy, which demonstrated an increase in the phosphocreatinine/inorganic phosphate ratio after treatment for acute hypothyroidism.[128] A more recent study used PET to correlate the regional cerebral blood flow and cerebral glucose metabolism with the mental state in patients. Investigators demonstrated a generalized decrease in regional cerebral blood flow by 23.4% and in cerebral glucose metabolism by 12.1% and no specific local defects.[129]

MISCELLANEOUS BIOCHEMICAL AND PHYSIOLOGIC CHANGES RELATED TO THE ACTION OF THYROID HORMONE ON PERIPHERAL TISSUES

Thyroid hormone affects the function of a variety of peripheral tissues. Thus, hormone deficiency or excess can alter a number of the determinations that are used in the diagnosis of illnesses unrelated to thyroid hormone dysfunction. Knowledge of the determinations that may be affected by thyroid hormone is important in the interpretation of laboratory data.

Measurement of Substances Absent in Normal Serum

Tests that measure substances present in the circulation only under pathologic circumstances do not provide information on the level of thyroid gland function. They are of value in establishing the cause of the hormonal dysfunction or thyroid gland pathology.

THYROID AUTOANTIBODIES

In clinical practice, the antibodies that are most commonly measured are directed against Tg or thyroid cell microsomal proteins. The latter is principally represented by thyroperoxidase (TPO). Immunoassays have been developed with the use of purified and recombinant TPO.[130-132] Other circulating immunoglobulins, which are used less frequently as diagnostic markers, are those directed against a colloid antigen, T_4, and T_3. Immunoglobulins that have the property of stimulating the thyroid gland will be discussed in the next section.

A variety of techniques have been developed for the measurement of Tg and microsomal antibodies. These procedures include a competitive binding radioassay, complement fixation reaction, tanned red cell agglutination assay, Coon's immunofluorescent technique, and enzyme-linked immunosorbent assay. Although the competitive binding radioassay is a sensitive test, agglutination methods combine sensitivity and simplicity and have now largely superseded other methods. Current commercial kits use synthetic gelatin beads rather than red cells.

In the assay of Tg and TPO antibodies by hemagglutination, particulate material is coated with human Tg or solubilized thyroid microsomal proteins and is exposed to serial dilutions of the patient's serum. Agglutination of the coated particulate material occurs in the presence of antibodies that are specific to the antigen attached to their surface. To detect false-positive reactions, it is important to include a blank for each sample consisting of uncoated particles. Because of the common occurrence of a prozone or blocking phenomenon, it is necessary to screen all serum samples through at least six consecutive twofold dilutions. Results are expressed in terms of the highest serum dilution, or titer, that shows persistent agglutination. The presence of immune complexes, particularly in patients with high serum Tg levels, may mask the presence of Tg antibodies. Assays have been developed for the measurement of such Tg–anti-Tg immune complexes.[133]

Normally, the test response is negative, but results may be positive in up to 10% of the adult population. The frequency of positive test results is higher in women and with advancing age. The presence of thyroid autoantibodies in the apparently healthy population is thought to represent subclinical autoimmune thyroid disease rather than false-positive reactions. Nonetheless, it is difficult to compare results from such studies because some laboratories that use agglutination methods report low titers (1/10 to 1/40) as positive. It is important in reporting values that a method-specific normal range be used, and that assays be calibrated against internationally available reference preparations. The availability of such preparations allows the reporting of results in international units. The importance of using internationally available reference ranges is confirmed by preliminary evidence that suggests that TPO and Tg antibody testing might be less reliable in certain ethnic groups. TPO antibodies are detectable in approximately 95% of patients with Hashimoto's thyroiditis and 85% of those with Graves' disease, irrespective of the functional state of the thyroid gland. Similarly, Tg antibodies are positive in about 60% and 30% of adult patients with Hashimoto's thyroiditis and Graves' disease, respectively. Tg antibodies are less frequently detected in children with autoimmune thyroid disease. Although higher titers are more common in Hashimoto's thyroiditis, quantitation of the antibody titer carries little diagnostic implication. The tests are of particular value in the evaluation of patients with atypical or selected manifestations of autoimmune thyroid disease (ophthalmopathy and dermopathy). Positive antibody titers are predictive of postpartum thyroiditis.[134] Low antibody titers occur transiently in some patients after an episode of subacute thyroiditis,[135] presumably caused by antigen exposure. No increased incidence of thyroid autoantibodies is seen in patients with multinodular goiter, thyroid adenomas, or secondary hypothyroidism. In some patients with Hashimoto's thyroiditis and undetectable thyroid autoantibodies in their serum, intrathyroidal lymphocytes have been demonstrated to produce TPO antibodies.

The development of sensitive radioassays and quantitative enzyme-linked immunoassays has allowed measurement of the concentration of antibodies to TPO and Tg in absolute terms. Such methods provide sensitive, precise, and antigen-specific

means of revealing quantitative fluctuations in autoantibody concentrations.

Other antibodies that are directed against thyroid components (such as NIS) or other tissues have been detected in the serum of some patients with autoimmune thyroid disease. They do not exert a blocking effect on NIS,[136] and their diagnostic value has not been fully evaluated. Circulating antibodies that are capable of binding T_4 and T_3 have also been demonstrated in patients with autoimmune thyroid disease and might interfere with the measurement of T_4 and T_3 by immunometric techniques. Antibodies reacting with nuclear components, which are not tissue specific, and with cellular components of parietal cells and adrenal, ovarian, and testicular tissue are more commonly encountered in patients with autoimmune thyroid disease.[137] Their presence reflects the frequency of coexistence of several autoimmune disease processes in the same patient.

THYROID-STIMULATING IMMUNOGLOBULINS

A large number of names have been given to tests that measure abnormal gamma globulins present in the serum of some patients with autoimmune thyroid disease, in particular Graves' disease.[138] The interaction of these unfractionated immunoglobulins with thyroid follicular cells usually results in global stimulation of thyroid gland activity and only rarely causes inhibition. It has been recommended that these assays all be called TSH receptor antibodies with the phrase "measured by ... assay" to identify the type of method that was used for their determination. The tests will be described under three general categories: (1) those measuring thyroid-stimulating activity by using in vivo or in vitro bioassays, (2) tests based on competition of the abnormal immunoglobulin with binding of TSH to its receptor, and (3) measurement of the thyroid growth–promoting activity of immunoglobulins. Tests use both human and animal tissue material or cell lines.

Thyroid Stimulation Assays

The earliest assays used various modifications of the McKenzie mouse bioassay.[139,140] The abnormal gamma globulin with TSH-like biological properties has relatively longer in vivo activity, hence its name, long-acting thyroid stimulator (LATS). The assay measures the LATS-induced release of thyroid hormone from the mouse thyroid gland prelabeled with radioiodide. The presence of LATS in serum is pathognomonic of Graves' disease. However, depending on assay sensitivity, a variable percentage of untreated patients will show a positive LATS response. LATS activity may be found in the serum of patients with Graves' disease even in the absence of thyrotoxicosis. Although it is more commonly present in patients with ophthalmopathy, especially when accompanied by pretibial myxedema,[141] LATS activity does not appear to correlate with the presence of Graves' disease, its severity, or the course of complications. LATS crosses the placenta and may be found transiently in newborns of mothers possessing the abnormal gamma globulin.[142]

Attempts to improve the ability to detect thyroid-stimulating antibodies (TSAbs) in autoimmune thyroid disease led to the development of several in vitro assays using animal as well as human thyroid tissue. The ability of the patient's serum to stimulate endocytosis in fresh human thyroid tissue is measured by direct count of the intracellular colloid droplets formed. When such a technique is used, human thyroid stimulator activity has been demonstrated in serum samples from patients with Graves' disease that were devoid of LATS activity measured by the standard mouse bioassay.[143] TSAbs can be detected by measuring the accumulation of cyclic adenosine monophosphate (cAMP) or the stimulation of adenylate cyclase activity in human thyroid cell cultures and thyroid plasma membranes, respectively. Accumulation of cAMP in the cultured rat thyroid cell line FRTL5 has also been used as an assay for TSAb.[144] Stimulation of release of T_3 from human and porcine thyroid slices is another form of in vitro assay for TSAb. An in vitro bioassay using a cytochemical technique depends on the ability of thyroid-stimulating material to increase lysosomal membrane permeability to a chromogenic substrate, leucyl-β-naphthylamide, which then reacts with the enzyme naphthylamidase. Quantitation is by scanning and integrated microdensitometry.[145]

Cloning of the TSH receptor led to the development of an in vitro assay for TSAb in cell lines that express the recombinant TSH receptor.[146-148] This assay, based on the generation of cAMP, is specific for the measurement of human TSH receptor antibodies that have thyroid-stimulating activity and thus contrasts with assays based on binding to the TSH receptor (see below), which cannot distinguish between antibodies with thyroid-stimulating and TSH-blocking activity. Accordingly, the recombinant human TSH receptor assay measures antibodies that are relevant to the pathogenesis of autoimmune thyrotoxicosis and is more sensitive than the formerly used TSAb assays.[149] For example, 94% of serum samples were positive for TSAb compared with 74% when the same samples were assayed by using FRTL5 cells.[150]

One of the major drawbacks with the bioassays mentioned above is that they are unsuitable for use as routine laboratory tools. This problem has been largely circumvented, however, with the advent of a luminescence-linked bioassay for TSAbs. This assay uses Chinese hamster ovary cells stably transfected with the human TSH receptor and a cAMP-dependent luciferase reporter. With the use of an international TSAb standard, the assay responded in a dose-dependent manner, with 10 mIU/mL of standard generating a relative light unit score of greater than 10. The authors also reported that the assay was modified to allow use in a 96-well plate format, thereby permitting automated measurement of relative luminosity in a large number of samples.

Thyrotropin-Binding Inhibition Assays

The principle of binding inhibition assays dates to the discovery of another class of abnormal immunoglobulins in patients with Graves' disease: those that neutralize the bioactivity of LATS tested in the mouse.[151] This material, known as the LATS protector, is species specific; it has no biological effect on the mouse thyroid gland but is capable of stimulating the human thyroid.[152] The original assay was cumbersome, which limited its clinical application.

Techniques that are used currently, which may be collectively termed radioreceptor assays, are based on competition of the abnormal immunoglobulins and TSH for a common receptor-binding site on thyroid cells. The test is akin in principle to the radioligand assays, in which a natural membrane receptor takes the place of the binding proteins or antibodies. Various sources of TSH receptor are used, including human thyroid cells, their particulate or solubilized membrane, and cell membranes from porcine thyroids or guinea pig fat cells or recombinant human TSH receptor expressed in mammalian cells. Because the assays do not directly measure thyroid-stimulating activity, the abnormal immunoglobulins determined have been given a variety of names, such as thyroid-binding inhibitory immunoglobulins or antibodies and thyrotropin-displacing immunoglobulins. This type of assay has indicated that not all the antibodies that are detected stimulate the thyroid, and some are inhibitory. Even with modern techniques, the presence of inhibitory antibody is less sensitive and specific for Graves' disease than is the presence of stimulatory antibody activity.[153] The stimulatory and inhibitory effects can be differentiated only by functional assays, which typically measure the production of cAMP.

Thyroid Growth–Promoting Assays

Assays have also been developed that measure the growth-promoting activity of abnormal immunoglobulins. One such assay is based on the staining of nuclei from guinea pig thyroid cells in S phase by the Feulgen reaction.[154] Another assay measures the incorporation of ^{3}H-thymidine into DNA in FRTL cells.[155] Whether the thyroid growth–stimulating immunoglobulins that are measured by these assays represent a population of immunoglobulins distinct from those with stimulatory functional activity remains a subject of active debate.

Clinical Applications

Measurement of abnormal immunoglobulins that interact with thyroid tissue by any of the methods described above is not indicated as a routine diagnostic test for Graves' disease. It is useful, however, in a few selected clinical conditions: (1) in the differential diagnosis of exophthalmos, particularly unilateral exophthalmos, when the origin of this condition is otherwise not apparent; the presence of thyroid-stimulating immunoglobulins would obviate the necessity to undertake more complex diagnostic procedures described elsewhere[156]; (2) in the differential diagnosis of pretibial myxedema and other forms of dermopathy when the cause is unclear and it is imperative that the cause of the skin lesion be ascertained; (3) in the differentiation of Graves' disease from toxic nodular goiter when both are being considered as the possible cause of thyrotoxicosis, when other tests such as thyroid scanning and thyroid autoantibody tests have been inconclusive, and particularly when such a distinction would play a role in determining the course of therapy; (4) when nonautoimmune thyrotoxicosis is suspected in a patient with hyperthyroidism and diffuse or nodular goiter; (5) in Graves' disease during pregnancy, when high maternal levels of TSAb are a warning for the possible occurrence of neonatal thyrotoxicosis; and (6) in neonatal thyrotoxicosis, where serial TSAb determinations showing a gradual decrease may be helpful in distinguishing between intrinsic Graves' disease in an infant and transient thyrotoxicosis resulting from passive transfer of maternal TSAb. Some investigators have found the persistence of TSAbs to be predictive of relapse of Graves' thyrotoxicosis after a course of antithyroid drug therapy.[157]

OTHER SUBSTANCES WITH THYROID-STIMULATING ACTIVITY

Hyperthyroidism develops in some patients with trophoblastic disease as a result of the production and release of a thyroid stimulator that has been termed molar or trophoblastic thyrotropin or big placental TSH.[158] It is likely that the thyroid-stimulating activity in patients with trophoblastic disease is entirely due to the presence of high levels of human chorionic gonadotropin (hCG).[159] Thus, an RIA for hCG can be useful in the differential diagnosis of thyroid dysfunction, although the clinical status of the patient is likely to suggest this cause.

The thyroid-stimulating activity of hCG can be enhanced by mutations in the TSH receptor that increase its affinity for this placental hormone. The consequence is thyrotoxicosis limited to pregnancy and associated with hyperemesis gravidarum in women.[160]

EXOPHTHALMOS-PRODUCING SUBSTANCE

A variety of tests have been developed for measuring exophthalmogenic activity in serum. Although great uncertainty still exists regarding the pathogenesis of thyroid-associated eye disease, the role of the immune system appears to be central. Exophthalmogenic activity has also been detected in IgG fractions of some patients with Graves' ophthalmopathy. Autoantibodies directed toward a 64 kilodalton eye muscle protein have been identified in 73% of patients with active thyroid-associated ophthalmopathy,[161-163] although the role of these antibodies in the diagnosis and management of the ophthalmopathy is at present unclear.

TESTS OF CELL-MEDIATED IMMUNITY

Delayed hypersensitivity reactions to thyroid antigens are present in autoimmune thyroid diseases. Cell-mediated immunity can be measured in several ways: (1) the migration inhibition test, which measures the inhibition of migration of sensitized leukocytes when exposed to the sensitizing antigen; (2) the lymphotoxic assay, which measures the ability of sensitized lymphocytes to kill target cells when exposed to the antigen; (3) the blastogenesis assay, which scores the formation of blast cells after exposure of lymphocytes to a thyroid antigen; and (4) thymus-dependent (T) lymphocyte subset quantitation using monoclonal antibodies.

Anatomic and Tissue Diagnoses

The purpose of the procedures described in this section is to evaluate the anatomic features of the thyroid gland, to localize and determine the nature of abnormal areas, and eventually to provide a pathologic or tissue diagnosis.

THYROID SCINTISCANNING

Normal and abnormal thyroid tissue can be externally imaged by three scintiscanning methods: (1) with radionuclides that are concentrated by normal thyroid tissues, such as iodide isotopes and ^{99m}Tc given as the pertechnetate ion; (2) by administration of radiopharmaceutical agents that are preferentially concentrated by abnormal thyroid tissues; and (3) by fluorescent scanning, which uses an external source of ^{241}Am and does not require the administration of radioactive material. Each has specific indications, advantages, and disadvantages.

The physical properties, dosages, and radiation delivered by the most commonly used radioisotopes are listed in Table 6-1. The choice of scanning agent depends on the purpose of the scan, the age of the patient, and the equipment available. Radioiodide scans cannot be performed in patients who have recently ingested iodine-containing compounds. ^{123}I and ^{99m}TcO$_4^-$ are the radionuclides of choice because of the low radiation exposure. The radioisotope ^{131}I is still used for the detection of functioning metastatic thyroid carcinoma by total body scanning.

Radioiodide and ^{99m}Tc Scans

^{99m}TcO$_4^-$ is concentrated, and all iodide isotopes are concentrated and bound by thyroid tissue. Depending on the isotope that is used, scans are carried out at different times after administration: 20 minutes for ^{99m}TcO$_4^-$; 4 or 24 hours for ^{123}I; 24 hours for ^{125}I and ^{131}I; and 48, 72, and 96 hours when ^{131}I is used in the search for metastatic thyroid carcinoma. The appearance of the normal thyroid gland on scan may be best described as a narrow-winged butterfly. Each "wing" represents a thyroid lobe, which in the adult measures 5 ± 1 cm in length and 2.3 ± 0.5 cm in width. Common variants include the absence of a connecting isthmus, a large isthmus, asymmetry between the two lobes, and trailing activity extending to the cricoid cartilage (pyramidal lobe). The latter is more commonly found in conditions associated with diffuse thyroid hyperplasia. Occasionally, collection of saliva in the esophagus during ^{99m}TcO$_4^-$ scanning may simulate a pyramidal lobe, but this artifact can be eliminated by drinking water.

Indications for scanning are listed in Table 6-9. In clinical practice, scans most often are requested for evaluation of the functional activity of solitary nodules. However, owing to the widespread use of fine-needle aspiration in the initial evaluation of thyroid nodules, this indication has been less used, and scans generally are obtained to search for abnormal uptake of iodine outside the thyroid bed in patients with thyroid cancer and congenital hypothyroidism. Normally, the isotope is homogeneously distributed throughout both lobes of the thyroid gland. This diffuse distribution occurs in the enlarged gland of Graves' disease and may be seen in Hashimoto's thyroiditis. A mottled appearance may be noted in Hashimoto's thyroiditis and can occasionally be seen in Graves' disease, especially after therapy with radioactive iodide. Irregular areas of relatively diminished and occasionally increased uptake are characteristic of large multinodular goiters. The traditional nuclear medicine jargon classifies nodules as "hot," "warm," and "cold," according to their isotope-concentrating ability relative to the surrounding normal parenchyma. Hot, or hyperfunctioning, nodules are typically benign, although the presence of malignancy has been reported.[164,165] In a large series of patients in whom thyroid scans were undertaken and subsequent surgery was performed irrespective of the scan result, 84% were cold nodules, 11% were warm nodules, and 6% were hot nodules. A histopathologic diagnosis of thyroid cancer was made in 16% of cold, 9% of warm, and 4% of hot nodules.[166,167] These data demonstrate that cold nodules are most likely to harbor malignancy but that most cold nodules are benign and, furthermore, the finding of a hot nodule on thyroid isotope scanning does not exclude the presence of malignancy. Occasionally, a nodule that is functional on a ^{99m}TcO$_4^-$ scan will be found to be cold on an iodine scan; this pattern is found with both benign and malignant nodules.

Thyroid isotope scans are of particular value in identifying autonomous thyroid nodules because the remainder of the activity in the gland is suppressed. This can have important therapeutic implications in that hyperthyroid subjects with a hot thyroid nodule would more appropriately be treated with ^{131}I than with long-term use of antithyroid medications.

Table 6-9. Indications for Radionuclide Scanning

Detection of anatomic variants and search for ectopic thyroid tissue (thyroid hemiagenesis, lingual thyroid, struma ovarii)
Diagnosis of congenital athyrosis
Determination of the nature of abnormal neck or chest (mediastinal) masses
Evaluation of solitary thyroid nodules (functioning or nonfunctioning)
Evaluation of thyroid remnants after surgery
Detection of functioning thyroid metastases
Evaluation of focal functional thyroid abnormalities (suppressed or nonsuppressible tissue)

A search for functioning thyroid metastases is best accomplished by using 2 to 4 mCi of ^{131}I after ablation of normal thyroid tissue and cessation or reduction of the amount of hormone to allow TSH to increase above the upper limit of normal. In general, two methods are used for total body scanning of thyroid cancer patients following surgery and initial radioactive iodine ablation. In one instance, the patient is made hypothyroid by discontinuing the regular dose of levothyroxine (L-T_4) and taking 25 μg liothyronine (L-T_3) twice daily for 2 weeks followed by no exogenous thyroid hormone treatment. When the TSH is 20 mU/L or greater, then a 72-hour total body scan is done with 2 mCi [131]I. Alternatively, the patient can be made moderately hypothyroid by taking the routine dose of L-T_4 every other day.[168] This will result in an elevated TSH of 20 mU/L or greater without the severe symptoms of hypothyroidism experienced in the previous method. Recombinant human TSH (r-hTSH, Thyrogen) can be used as an alternative to thyroid hormone withdrawal with approximately the same overall sensitivity and specificity for detection of thyroid metastasis. According to the Thyrogen protocol for scanning, 0.9 mg of r-hTSH is given via intramuscular injections on day 1 and day 2. On day 3, 4 mCi of ^{131}I is given, and a total body scan is performed on day 5, 48 hours after isotope ingestion. Blood is obtained for TSH and Tg measurements on day 1 and day 5.[169,170]

Uptake is also found outside the thyroid gland in patients with lingual thyroids and in the rare ovarian dermoid tumor containing functioning thyroid tissue.

The scan can be used as an adjunct during TSH stimulation and T_3 suppression tests to localize suppressed normal thyroid tissue and autonomously functioning areas, respectively (see below). Applications other than those listed in Table 6-9 are of doubtful benefit and are rarely justified in view of the radiation exposure, expense, and inconvenience. [123]I single-photon emission computed tomography (CT) may also be useful in the evaluation of thyroid abnormalities.

[18]Fluorodeoxyglucose Positron Emission Tomography Scanning

Some patients with thyroid cancer metastases do not concentrate ^{131}I, even when it is given in therapeutic doses.[171] Although other imaging modalities such as ultrasound, CT scanning, and nuclear magnetic resonance imaging can be used to detect the locations of the metastases, none are 100% specific or sensitive (see below). Several studies have shown that in differentiated thyroid carcinoma, fluorodeoxyglucose (FDG) PET can be used to detect recurrence or metastases with a high degree of sensitivity (80% to 90%).[172-174] In addition, the combination of FDG PET and CT scanning can increase the yield of either modality alone.[174]

Other Isotope Scans

Because most test procedures, short of direct microscopic examination of thyroid tissue, fail to detect thyroid malignancy with any degree of certainty, efforts have been made to find other radioactive materials that would possibly be of diagnostic use. Several such agents that are concentrated by metabolically active tissues, irrespective of whether they have iodide-concentrating ability, have been tried. However, despite claims to the contrary, either they have had only limited value or their diagnostic usefulness has not been fully evaluated. These agents include ^{75}Se-methionine, [125]Ce, ^{67}Ga-citrate, ^{32}P-pyrophosphate, ^{99m}Tc, and [201]Th.[175]

Scanning with ^{131}I-labeled anti-Tg for the detection of occult metastatic thyroid malignancy that fails to concentrate ^{131}I showed early promising results.[176] However, the procedure has not proved clinically useful.

ULTRASONOGRAPHY

Ultrasonography is used to outline the thyroid gland and to characterize lesions differing in density from the surrounding tissue. The technique differentiates interphases of different acoustic densities by using sound frequencies in the megahertz range that are above the audible range. A transducer fitted with a piezoelectric crystal produces and transmits the signal and receives echo reflections. Interfaces of different acoustic densities reflect dense echoes, liquid transmits sound without reflections, and air-filled spaces do not transmit the ultrasound.[177]

One of the most useful applications of the ultrasonogram is in the differentiation of solid from cystic lesions. Purely cystic lesions are entirely sonolucent, whereas solid lesions produce multiple echoes as a result of multiple sonic interphases. Many lesions, however, are mixed (solid and cystic) and are termed complex lesions. Some tumors can have the same acoustic characteristics as the surrounding normal tissue, thus escaping echographic detection. True cystic lesions are usually benign, although most large thyroid nodules contain cystic areas. Carcinomas may also undergo infarction, which causes degenerative cystic change within their substance. In one large series of thyroid nodules, 69% were found to be solid, and 21% of these were subsequently shown to be malignant. Similarly, of the 19% of cystic lesions, 7% were malignant, and malignancy was also detected in 12% of the mixed lesions.[166,167] Thus, solid nodules, as determined by ultrasound scanning, were most likely to be malignant, but most were benign, and a similar proportion of cystic nodules were also malignant. Ultrasound scanning of thyroid nodules is poorly sensitive and specific as an indicator of the presence of malignancy in a thyroid mass.

Although high-resolution ultrasonography can detect thyroid nodules on the order of a few millimeters, lesions must be larger than 0.5 cm to allow differentiation between solid and cystic structures. A sonolucent pattern is frequently noted in glands with Hashimoto's thyroiditis, but this pattern has also been described in multinodular glands and in patients with Graves' disease.

Because sonography localizes the position and the depth of lesions, the procedure has been used to successfully guide the needle during aspiration biopsy. In complex lesions, sonographic guiding ensures sampling from the solid portion of the nodule. With experience and proper calibration, sonography can be used for estimation of thyroid gland size. Several recent reports have described treatment for toxic nodules provided by the injection of alcohol under sonographic guidance. Although ultrasonography has found virtually the same applications as scintiscanning, claims that the former may differentiate benign from malignant lesions are unfounded. Also, ultrasonography cannot be used for the assessment of substernal goiters because of interference from overlying bone.

The procedure is simple and painless and, at the frequencies of sound that are used, does not produce tissue damage. Because it does not require the administration of isotopes, it can be safely used in children and during pregnancy. Also, because the procedure is independent of iodine-concentrating mechanisms, it is valuable in the study of suppressed glands.

X-RAY PROCEDURES

A simple x-ray film of the neck and upper part of the mediastinum can provide valuable information regarding the location, size, and effect of a goiter on surrounding structures. Radiographs may show an asymmetrical goiter, an intrathoracic extension of the gland, and displacement or narrowing of the trachea. If any suggestion of posterior extension of the mass is seen, it is useful to take films during the swallow of x-ray contrast material. The soft tissue x-ray technique may disclose calcium deposits. Large deposits in flakes or rings are typical of an old multinodular goiter, whereas foci of finely stippled flecks of calcium are suggestive of papillary adenocarcinoma.

Information not related to anatomic abnormalities of the thyroid gland may be obtained from x-ray studies. In children with a history of hypothyroidism, an x-ray film of the hand to determine bone age could aid in estimating the onset and duration of thyroid dysfunction. Hypothyroidism leads to retardation in bone age and in infants produces dense calcification of epiphyseal plates most easily seen at the distal end of the radius. Longstanding myxedema produces pituitary hypertrophy, which especially in children, but also in adults, causes enlargement of the sella turcica on imaging of the pituitary region.

CT and MRI provide useful information on the location and architecture of the thyroid gland, as well as its relationship to surrounding tissues. An important application of CT is the assessment and delineation of obscure mediastinal masses and large substernal goiters.[178] The necessity to infuse iodine-containing contrast agents limits the application of CT in patients who are being considered for radioiodide therapy. CT and MRI have found firm application in another area of thyroid diseases: the evaluation of ophthalmopathy and mediastinal masses.

OTHER PROCEDURES

A barium swallow may be useful in evaluating impingement of a goiter on the esophagus, whereas a flow-volume loop[179] may be useful in allowing quantitative documentation of functional impingement on the upper part of the airway.

BIOPSY OF THE THYROID GLAND

Histologic examination of thyroid tissue for diagnostic purposes requires some form of an invasive procedure. The biopsy procedure depends on the intended type of microscopic examination. Core biopsy for histologic examination of tissue with preservation of architecture is obtained by closed needle or open surgical procedures; aspiration biopsy is performed to obtain material for cytologic examination.

Core Biopsy

Closed core biopsy is an office procedure that is carried out with the patient under local anesthesia. A large (about 15 gauge) cutting needle of the Vim-Silverman type is most commonly used. The needle is introduced under local anesthesia through a small skin nick, and firm pressure is applied over the puncture site for 5 to 10 minutes after withdrawal of the needle. In experienced hands, complications are rare, but they may be serious and can include transient damage to the laryngeal nerve, puncture of the trachea, laryngospasm, jugular vein phlebitis, and bleeding. With the improvement in cytology based on fine-needle aspiration (see below), the use of core and open biopsy has been virtually abandoned.

Percutaneous Fine-Needle Aspiration

The development of more sophisticated staining techniques for cytologic examination, the realization that fear of tumor dissemination along the needle track was not well founded, and especially the high diagnostic accuracy of the technique are responsible for the increasing popularity of percutaneous fine-needle aspiration (FNA).

The procedure is exceedingly simple and safe. The patient lies supine, with the neck hyperextended by placing a small pillow under the shoulders. Local anesthesia is not usually required. The skin is prepared with an antiseptic solution. The lesion, fixed between two gloved fingers, is penetrated with a fine (22 to 27 gauge) needle attached to a syringe. Suction is then applied while the needle is moved within the nodule. A nonsuction technique using capillary action has also been developed. The small amount of aspirated material, usually contained within the needle or its hub, is applied to glass slides and is spread. Some slides are air-dried and others are fixed before staining. Because biopsy of small nodules may be technically more difficult, the use of ultrasound to guide the needle is recommended. It is important that the slides be properly prepared, stained, and read by a cytologist who is experienced in the interpretation of material from thyroid gland aspirates. Newer molecular approaches have been used to analyze FNA material to help distinguish benign from malignant pathologies, although these techniques are currently in development stages.

The yield of false-positive and false-negative results is variable from one center to another, but both are acceptably low. Various centers have reported that the accuracy of this technique in distinguishing benign from malignant lesions may be as high as 95%. The false-positive rate is about 2%, and the false-negative rate is about 1% to 6%, cystic papillary carcinoma being the most common cause of false negative. Patients with an initial FNA that demonstrates frankly malignant or suspicious cytologic findings (including follicular neoplasms; see below) on first examination are immediately referred for surgery. Some clinicians recommend that repeat FNA be performed 6 to 12 months after the initial biopsy to reduce the risk of false-negative results. In one study, the second FNA changed the diagnosis in 7% of patients, and an additional four carcinomas were detected.

In one clinic in which the procedure is used routinely, the number of patients operated on decreased by one third, whereas the percentage of thyroid carcinomas among the patients who underwent surgery doubled.[180] When the results are suggestive of follicular neoplasia, surgery is required because follicular adenoma cannot be differentiated from follicular cancer by cytologic analysis alone. Because the sample obtained is not always representative of the lesion, surgical treatment is indicated for lesions that are highly suspicious for being malignant on clinical grounds. Other uses of aspiration biopsy include presumed lymphoma or invasive anaplastic carcinoma when biopsy might spare the patient an unnecessary neck exploration. Another application of needle aspiration is in the confirmation and treatment of thyroid cysts and autonomous thyroid nodules.[181] The latter are best diagnosed by the identification of a mutation in the TSH receptor in material obtained by FNA.[182,183]

Evaluation of the Hypothalamic-Pituitary-Thyroid Axis

The development of an RIA for the routine measurement of TSH in serum and the availability of synthetic TRH have placed increased reliance on tests that assess the hypothalamic-pituitary control of thyroid function. These tests allow the diagnosis of mild and subclinical forms of thyroid dysfunction and provide a means of differentiating between primary, pituitary (secondary), and hypothalamic (tertiary) thyroid gland failure.

THYROTROPIN

In recent years, dramatic improvements have been made in assays for TSH. The routine measurement of TSH in clinical practice initially used RIA techniques. These first-generation assays had a sensitivity level of 1 mU/L, which did not allow the separation of normal from reduced values. A major problem with early TSH RIAs was cross-reactivity with gonadotropins (luteinizing hormone, follicle-stimulating hormone, and hCG) that share with TSH a common α subunit.[184] Nevertheless, even older RIA methods for measurement of pituitary TSH correlated well with values obtained by bioassay techniques.[31] Another uncommon source of error is the presence in the serum sample of heterophilic antibodies induced by vaccination with materials contaminated with animal serum or the presence of endogenous TSH antibodies.[185] RIA techniques for the measurement of TSH in dry blood spots on filter paper are used in screening for neonatal hypothyroidism.

Newer techniques have been developed that use multiple antibodies to produce a "sandwich"-type assay in which one antibody (usually directed against the α subunit) serves to anchor the TSH molecule and another (usually monoclonal antibodies directed against the β subunit) is radioiodinated (immunoradiometric assay) or is conjugated with an enzyme (immunoenzymometric) or a chemiluminescent compound (chemiluminescent assay). In these assays, the signal should be directly related to the amount of the ligand present rather than being inversely related as in RIAs that measure the bound tracer. This technique results in decreased background "noise" and greater sensitivity, decreased interference from related compounds, and an expanded useful range. Initial improvements in the TSH assay resulted in assays with a sensitivity limit of 0.1 mU/L, a normal range of approximately 0.5 to 4.5 mU/L, and the ability to distinguish between low and normal TSH values.[186,187] Recently, commercial assays have been developed with an even higher sensitivity limit of 0.005 to 0.01 mU/L and a similar normal range but an expanded range between the lower limit of normal and the lower limit of sensitivity.[188,189]

The nomenclature for differentiating these various assays has not been standardized, with manufacturers applying various combinations of "high(ly)," "ultra," and "sensitive." It has been recommended that the sensitivity limit be used in defining the assays, with the early RIAs that detect values of 1 mU/L or greater being designated first-generation assays, those with a lower sensitivity limit of 0.1 mU/L being designated as second-generation assays, and those with a lower sensitivity limit of 0.01 mU/L or less being designated as third-generation assays. Determination of the appropriate sensitivity level has also been controversial. Some base the definition on the level with a coefficient of variation less than 20%; others define it as the lowest level that can be reliably differentiated from the zero TSH standard. At a minimum, for a TSH assay to be considered "sensitive," the overlap of TSH values in sera from clinically hyperthyroid and euthyroid individuals should be less than 5% and preferably less than 1%.

In a number of these third-generation assays, TSH that was detected in clinically toxic patients and elevated values that were found in euthyroid subjects were not confirmed when the samples were measured in other assays. In some cases, these discrepant results have been attributed to the presence of antibodies directed against the animal immunoglobulins used in the assay. These immunoglobulins act to bind the anchoring and detecting antibodies and lead to an overestimation of TSH. In some cases, this effect can be blocked by the addition of an excess of nonspecific immunoglobulin of the same species.[190]

The availability of random access immunoassay analyzers has revolutionized TSH measurements. These assays are highly reproducible and provide convenience and rapid throughput of large volumes of serum samples.

TSH appears abruptly in the pituitary and serum of the fetus at midgestation and can also be detected in amniotic fluid.[191,192] The mean TSH level is higher in cord blood than in maternal blood. A substantial increase, to levels several-fold above the upper range in adults, is observed during the first half-hour of life. Levels decline to near normal adult range by the third day of life. Minimal changes that are reported to occur during adult life and in early adolescence have no significant effect on the overall range of normal. In the absence of pregnancy, no significant gender differences have been observed. Although early studies failed to show diurnal TSH variation, significantly higher values have been recorded during the late evening and early night and are partially inhibited by sleep.[193] This diurnal rhythm of TSH is superimposed on continuous high-frequency, low-amplitude variations. The nocturnal TSH surge persists in patients with mild primary hypothyroidism[194,195] and is abolished in hypothalamic hypothyroidism[195,196] and in some patients during fasting and with nonthyroidal illness. It is enhanced by oral contraceptives[197] and is abolished by high levels of glucocorticoids.[193] The presence of seasonal variation has not been a uniform finding, but it is unlikely to affect the clinical interpretation of serum values. Various types of stressful stimuli have no significant effect on the basal serum TSH level, except for a rise during surgical hypothermia in infants but not in adults.[198] Various stimuli that elicit in normal humans a secretory response of some pituitary hormones, such as the administration of insulin, vasopressin, glucagon, bacterial pyrogens, arginine, prostaglandins, and chlorpromazine, have no effect on serum TSH. However, administration of any of a growing list of drugs has been found to alter the basal concentration of serum TSH and/or its response to exogenous TRH (Table 6-10). In the presence of a normally functioning hypothalamic-pituitary system, an inverse correlation is found between the serum concentration of FT_4 and TSH. Changes in the serum concentration of TT_4 as a result of TBG abnormalities or drugs competing with T_4 binding to TBG have no effect on the level of serum TSH. The pituitary is exquisitely sensitive to both minimal decreases and increases in thyroid hormone concentration, with a logarithmic change in TSH levels in response to changes in T_4 (Fig. 6-5). Thus, serum TSH levels should be elevated in patients with primary hypothyroidism and low or undetectable in those with thyrotoxicosis. Indeed, in the absence of hypothalamic pituitary disease, illness, or drugs, TSH is an accurate indicator of thyroid hormone status and the adequacy of thyroid hormone replacement.

In patients with primary hypothyroidism of whatever cause, levels may reach 1000 mU/L or higher. The magnitude of serum TSH elevation grossly correlates with the severity and, in part, with the duration of thyroid hormone deficiency. TSH concentrations above the upper limit of normal have been observed in the absence of clinical symptoms and signs of hypothyroidism and in the presence of serum T_4 and T_3 levels well within the normal range. This condition is most commonly encountered in patients with incipient hypothyroidism from Hashimoto's thyroiditis or with limited ability to synthesize thyroid hormone

Table 6-10. Agents That May Affect TSH Secretion

Substance	Common Use
Increase Serum TSH Concentration and/or Its Response to TRH	
Iodine (iodide and iodine-containing compounds)[434,448,449]	Radiologic contrast media, antiseptic, expectorant, antiarrhythmic, and antianginal
Lithium[450]	Treatment of bipolar psychoses
Dopamine antagonists	
Dopamine receptor blockers (metoclopramide,[451,452] domperidone[453])	Antiemetic
Dopamine-blocking agent (sulpiride[454])	Tranquilizer
Decarboxylase inhibitor (benserazide[455])	—
Dopamine-depleting agent (monoiodotyrosine[451])	—
L-Dopa inhibitors[456] (chlorpromazine, biperiden, haloperidol)	Neuroleptic
Cimetidine (histamine receptor blocker)[457]	Treatment of peptic ulcers
Clomiphene (antiestrogen)[247]	Induction of ovulation
Spironolactone[458]	Antihypertensive
Amphetamines[459]	Anticongestants and antiappetite
IL-2[338,339]	Immune system modulation
Decrease Serum TSH Concentration and/or Its Response to TRH	
Thyroid hormones (T_4 and T_3)	Replacement therapy, antigoitrogenic, and anticancer
Thyroid hormone analogues (DT₄,[460] 3′,3′,5-TRIAC,[461] etiroxate-HCl,[462] dimethyl-3 isopropyl-L-thyronine[463])	Cholesterol lowering and weight reducing
Dopaminergic agents (agonists) Dopamine[453,464]	Antihypotensive
L-Dopa[465] (dopamine precursor)	Diagnostic agent and antiparkinsonian
Cabergoline[466]	Antilactation and pituitary tumor suppression
Bromocriptine[466]	
Fusaric acid (inhibitor of dopamine hydroxylase)[465]	—
Pyridoxine (coenzyme of dopamine synthesis)	Vitamin and antineuropathic
Other dopaminergic agents[453,467] (pirbedil, apomorphine, lisuride)	Treatment for cerebrovascular diseases and migraine
Dopamine antagonist (pimozide)[244]	Neuroleptic
α-Noradrenergic blockers[468,469] (phentolamine, thioridazine)	Neuroleptic
Serotonin antagonists (metergoline,[470] cyproheptadine,[471] methysergide[472])	Antimigraine and appetite stimulators
Serotonin agonist (5-hydroxytryptophan)[452]	—
Glucocorticoids[473,474]	Antiinflammatory, antiimmunosuppressive, and anticancer; reduction of intracranial pressure
Acetylsalicylic acid[161]	Antiinflammatory, antipyretic, and analgesic
Growth hormone[162*]	Growth promoting
Somatostatin[163]	Antineoplastic
Octreotide[475]	
Opiates (morphine,[476] leuenkephalin,[477] heroin[398])	Analgesic
Clofibrate[478]	Hypolipidemic
Fenclofenac[392,421]	Nonsteroidal antiinflammatory drug
Bexarotene[479]	T cell lymphoma
IL-6[432]	Immune modulating

DT₄, Dextrothyroxine; IL, interleukin; T_3, triiodothyronine; T_4, thyroxine; TRH, thyrotropin-releasing hormone; TRIAC, triiodothyroacetic acid; TSH, thyroid-stimulating hormone.

*In hyposomatotrophic dwarfs.

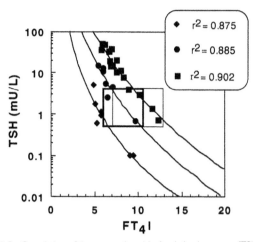

FIGURE 6-5. Correlation of the serum thyroid-stimulating hormone (TSH) concentration and the free thyroxine index (FT₄I) in three persons given increasing doses of levothyroxine. Note the logarithmic correlation between TSH and FT₄I and the variable individual requirement of T_4 to normalize the TSH level. Normal ranges are included in the heavily lined box, and those for subjects treated by levothyroxine replacement are in the lightly lined box.

because of prior thyroid surgery, radioiodide treatment, or severe iodine deficiency. No agreement has been reached on whether such patients have subclinical hypothyroidism or a "compensated state" in which euthyroidism is maintained by chronic stimulation of a reduced amount of functioning thyroid tissue through hypersecretion of TSH. Transient hypothyroidism occurs in some infants during the early neonatal period. In two circumstances, the usual inverse relationship between the serum level of TSH and T_4 is not maintained in patients with proven primary hypothyroidism. Treatment with replacement doses of T_4 may normalize or even produce serum levels of thyroid hormone above the normal range before high TSH levels have reached the normal range. This finding is particularly true in patients with severe neonatal or long-standing primary hypothyroidism, who might require 3 to 6 months of hormone replacement before TSH levels are fully suppressed. Conversely, serum TSH concentrations may remain low or normal for up to 5 weeks after withdrawal of thyroid hormone replacement when serum levels of T_4 and T_3 have already declined to values well below the lower range of normal. Causes of discrepancies between TSH and FT₄ and FT₃ levels are listed in Table 6-11.

At this time, it is uncertain what TSH level is appropriate for suppressive thyroid hormone therapy. The frequency with which patients have subnormal but detectable TSH values depends on both the population studied and the sensitivity of the assay (Fig. 6-6). When an assay is used with a sensitivity limit of 0.1 mU/L, 3% to 4% of hospitalized patients have been noted to have subnormal TSH. When patients with undetectable TSH in such an assay were reevaluated in an assay with a sensitivity limit of 0.005 mU/L, 3 of 77 (4%) with thyrotoxicosis and 32 of 37 (86%) with nonthyroidal illness or taking drugs were found to have a subnormal, but detectable, TSH level.[189] Thus, the more sensitive the assay, the more likely it is that patients with clinical thyrotoxicosis will have undetectable serum TSH, whereas those with illness will have a subnormal but detectable level. However, with progressively more sensitive assays, the likelihood that a clinically toxic patient will have detectable TSH will increase, and if patients who are receiving suppressive therapy are treated until the TSH is undetectable, they are more likely to have symptoms of thyrotoxicosis.

Persistent absence of a reverse correlation between the serum thyroid hormone and the TSH concentration has a very different connotation. A low serum level of thyroid hormone without clear elevation in the serum TSH concentration is suggestive of trophoprivic hypothyroidism (central or secondary hypothyroidism), especially when associated with obvious clinical stigmata of hypothyroidism.

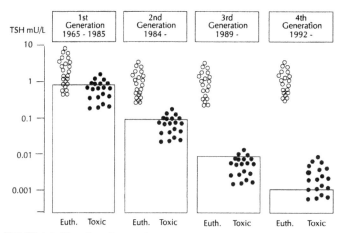

FIGURE 6-6. The effect of serum thyroid-stimulating hormone (TSH) assay sensitivity on the discrimination of euthyroid subjects (Euth) from those with thyrotoxicosis (Toxic). (Data from Spencer C: Clinical Diagnostics. Rochester, NY, Eastman Kodak, 1992.)

Table 6-11. Discrepancies Between TSH and Free Thyroid Hormone Levels

Elevated Serum TSH Value Without Low FT₄ or FT₃ Values

Subclinical hypothyroidism (inadequate replacement therapy, mild thyroid gland failure)
Recent increase in thyroid hormone dosage
Drugs
Inappropriate TSH secretion syndromes
Laboratory artifact

Subnormal Serum TSH Value Without Elevated FT₄ or FT₃ Values

Subclinical hyperthyroidism (excessive replacement therapy, mild thyroid gland hyperfunction, autonomous nodule)
Recent decrease in suppressive thyroid hormone dosage
Recent treatment for thyrotoxicosis (Graves' disease, toxic multinodular goiter, toxic nodule)
Resolution of thyrotoxic phase of thyroiditis
Nonthyroidal illness
Drugs
Central hypothyroidism

FT₃, Free triiodothyronine; *FT₄,* free thyroxine; *TSH,* thyroid-stimulating hormone.

Resistance to TSH is an inherited syndrome of variable thyroid sensitivity to a biologically active TSH molecule. The clinical features of this condition are (1) elevated serum TSH values with normal biological activity when tested in vitro, (2) absence of goiter but the presence of a normal or hypoplastic gland, and (3) normal ("compensated") or low ("not compensated") TSH levels depending on the degree of TSH insensitivity. Therefore, subjects with resistance to TSH can present as euthyroid hyperthyrotropinemia or with severe primary hypothyroidism. The index case of the first reported family with resistance to TSH due to a mutation in the thyroid-stimulating hormone receptor (TSHR) presented with a blood TSH on neonatal screening of 103 mU/L (normal, <20). Repeat measurement on the sixteenth day of life was 47 mU/L with a normal T₄; a radioiodide scan reveals a thyroid gland in the normal location and of normal size. The mother was found to be heterozygous for an abnormal TSHR, P162A, and the father was found to be heterozygous for another abnormal TSHR, I167N. All the children were compound heterozygous for the P162A and I167N and therefore had significant elevations of serum TSH.[199] In other cases of resistance to TSH, the TSH receptor gene had a normal sequence, and the molecular basis for the phenotype remains unknown.

In some cases, a mild elevation in the serum TSH level measured by RIA is probably due to the presence of immunoreactive TSH with reduced biological activity. Distinction between pituitary and hypothalamic hypothyroidism may be made on the basis of the TSH response to the administration of TRH, although the responses can be very variable (Table 6-12, and see below).

In another group of pathologic conditions, serum TSH levels might not be suppressed despite a clear elevation of serum free thyroid hormone levels. Because such a finding is incompatible with a normal thyroregulatory control mechanism of the pituitary, which is preserved in the more common forms of thyrotoxicosis, it has been termed inappropriate secretion of TSH. It implicitly suggests defective feedback regulation of TSH. When associated with the clinical and metabolic changes of thyrotoxicosis, it is usually due to TSH-secreting pituitary adenoma and rarely to partial resistance to thyroid hormone. The existence of hypothalamic hyperthyroidism can be questioned. Precise diagnosis requires additional studies, including radiologic examination of the pituitary gland and a TRH test. In addition, the presence of high circulating levels of the common α subunit (α-SU) of the pituitary glycoprotein hormones, with a subsequent disproportionately high α-SU/TSH molar ratio in serum, is characteristic, if not pathognomonic, of TSH-secreting pituitary tumors. Normal and occasionally high serum TSH levels associated with a clear elevation in serum FT₄ and FT₃ but no clear clinical evidence of hypothyroidism or symptoms and signs

Table 6-12. Differential Diagnosis of Euthyroid Hyperthyrotropinemia

Condition	Clinical State	History	THs	Diagnostic Test
Mouse heterophile antibody	Euthyroid	Not helpful	Normal	Measure antibody directly
Subclinical hypothyroidism	Euthyroid	inc Chol?	Normal	Repeat TSH; TRH stimulation test
AITD (early Hashimoto's)	Hypo-/euthyroid	Helpful	Low/normal	Measure antibodies
Recovering thyroiditis	Euthyroid	Helpful	Low/normal	¹²³I uptake; repeat tests
Central hypothyroidism	Hypothyroid	Helpful	Low/normal	TRH stimulation test
Nonthyroidal illness	Hypo-/?euthyroid	Helpful	Low	High rT₃
Deiodinase abnormality	Euthyroid	Not helpful	Low T₃, high T₄	Unknown
Mutation in TSHR-RTSH	Hypo-/euthyroid	Not helpful	Normal or low	Sequence TSHR family history

AITD, Autoimmune thyroid disease; *Chol,* cholesterol; *THs,* thyroid hormones T₄ and T₃; *RTSH,* resistance to TSH; *TRH,* thyrotropin-releasing hormone; *TSH,* thyroid-stimulating hormone; *TSHR,* thyroid-stimulating hormone receptor.

suggestive of both thyroid hormone deficiency and excess are typical of resistance to thyroid hormone.

Although TSH has been implicated in the pathogenesis of simple, nontoxic goiter, unless hypothyroidism supervenes or iodide deficiency is very severe, TSH levels are characteristically normal. Elevated TSH levels may occur in the presence of normal thyroid hormone levels and apparent euthyroidism in nonthyroidal diseases and with primary adrenal failure. A more common occurrence in severe acute and chronic illnesses is a normal or low serum TSH concentration despite low levels of T_3 and even low T_4 levels. TSH values may be transiently elevated during the recovery phase. Various hypotheses to explain these anomalous findings have been proposed, but a satisfactory explanation is not at hand.

A specific RIA for the β subunits of human TSH is also available but has not found clinical application. Measurement of TSH usually consists of the quantitation of the immunoreactive moiety. However, under certain physiologic and pathologic states, there can be a change in the ratio of immunoreactive and bioreactive TSH. For example, the nocturnal rise in TSH is due to less bioreactive TSH because of different glycosylation. In addition, in states of hypothalamic dysfunction, there is also a decrease in the bioreactive-to-immunoreactive ratio of TSH, usually due to an alteration in the degree of glycosylation of the TSH molecule. Bioassay of TSH is performed by using JP26$_{26}$ cells. This is a subclone of JP26, a line of Chinese hamster ovary cells that are stably transfected with a human TSH receptor cDNA. Standard bovine TSH or samples for TSH measurement are added with Rolipram, a cyclic adenosine monophosphate (cAMP) phosphodiesterase inhibitor. cAMP is measured in the dried cell extract by RIA.

THYROTROPIN-RELEASING HORMONE

The hypothalamic tripeptide TRH (protirelin) plays a central role in the regulation of pituitary TSH secretion. Several methods have been used for quantitation of TRH, but for many reasons measurement in humans has failed to provide information of diagnostic value. These reasons include high dilution of TRH by the time that it reaches the systemic circulation, rapid enzymatic degradation, and ubiquitous tissue distribution. Mean serum TSH levels of 5 and 6 pg/mL have been reported. It is uncertain whether measurements carried out in urine truly represent TRH.[200]

The TRH test measures the increase in pituitary TSH in serum in response to the administration of synthetic TRH. The magnitude of the TSH response to TRH is modulated by the thyrotroph response to active thyroid hormone and is thus almost always proportional to the concentration of free thyroid hormone in serum. The response is exquisitely sensitive to minor changes in the level of circulating thyroid hormones, which might not be detected by direct measurement. A direct correlation between basal serum TSH values and the maximal response to TRH has been observed even in the absence of thyroid hormone abnormalities, which suggests that the euthyroid state might be associated with a fine modulation of pituitary sensitivity to TRH.[200]

TRH normally stimulates pituitary prolactin secretion, and under certain pathologic conditions, the release of growth hormone and adrenocorticotropic hormone. Accordingly, the test has been used for the assessment of a variety of endocrine functions, some unrelated to the thyroid. In clinical practice, the TRH test is used mainly (1) to assess the functional integrity of pituitary thyrotrophs and thus to aid in differentiating hypothyroidism caused by intrinsic pituitary disease from hypothalamic

dysfunction, (2) in the diagnosis of mild thyrotoxicosis when results of other tests are equivocal, and (3) in the differential diagnosis of inappropriate TSH secretion, in particular, when a TSH-secreting adenoma is suspected.

TRH is effective when given intravenously as a bolus or by infusion,[201] intramuscularly,[202] or orally in single or repeated doses. Doses as small as 6 μg can elicit a significant TSH response, and a linear correlation exists between the incremental changes in serum TSH concentration and the logarithm of the TRH dose administered. The standard test uses a single TRH dose of 200 or 400 μg/1.73 m^2 body surface area, given by rapid intravenous injection. Serum is collected before and at 15 minutes and then at 30 minute intervals over a period of 120 to 180 minutes, although many clinicians choose to obtain a single postinjection sample at 15, 20, or 30 minutes. Normal individuals have a prompt increase in serum TSH, with a peak level at 15 to 40 minutes that is on the average 16 mU/L, or fivefold the basal level. The decline is more gradual, with a return of serum TSH to the preinjection level by 3 to 4 hours. Results can be expressed in terms of the peak level of TSH achieved, the maximal increment above the basal level, the peak TSH value expressed as a percentage of the basal value, or the integrated area of the TSH response curve. Determination of TSH before and 30 minutes after injection of TRH provides information concerning the presence or absence of TSH responsiveness but cannot detect delayed or prolonged responses.

At the time of this writing, TRH was not available in the United States. It can, however, be obtained for use in the United States after submission of an Investigational New Drug application from the Food and Drug Administration (FDA). It is manufactured by Ferring Arzneimittel, GmbH (Wittland 11; 24109 Kiel, Germany; telephone number: 0049 431 58520; fax number: 0049 431 585235) or the distributor UNIPHARMA SA (Via Pian Scairolo, 6; 6917 Barbengo, Switzerland).

The stimulatory effect of TRH is specific for pituitary TSH, its free α and β subunits, and prolactin. Under normal circumstances, no significant changes are observed in the serum levels of other pituitary hormones[203] or potential thyroid stimulators.[204] Responsiveness is present at birth,[205] is greater in women than in men, particularly in the follicular phase of the menstrual cycle, and may be blunted in older men, but this finding is not consistent. On average, the magnitude of the response is greater at 11:00 PM than at 11:00 AM, in accordance with the diurnal pattern of the basal TSH level, which correlates with its response to TRH. Repetitive administration of TRH to the same subject at daily intervals causes gradual blunting of the TSH response, presumably because of the increase in thyroid hormone concentration and also in part because of TSH "exhaustion." However, more than 1 hour must elapse between the increase in thyroid hormone concentration and TRH administration for inhibition of the TSH response to occur. A number of drugs and nonendocrine diseases may affect the magnitude of the response to varying extent.

TRH-induced secretion of TSH is followed by the release of thyroid hormone that can be detected by direct measurement of serum TT$_4$ and TT$_3$ concentrations. Peak levels are normally reached approximately 4 hours after the administration of TRH and are accompanied by an increase in serum Tg concentration. The incremental rise in serum TT$_3$ is relatively greater, and the peak is on average 50% above the basal level. Measurement of changes in serum thyroid hormone concentration after the administration of TRH has been proposed as an adjunctive test and is useful for evaluation of the integrity of the thyroid gland or the bioactivity of endogenous TSH.[206] The increase in RAIU is minimal and occurs only with high doses of TRH given orally.

Side effects from the intravenous administration of TRH, in decreasing order of frequency, include nausea, flushing or a sensation of warmth, desire to micturate, peculiar taste, lightheadedness or headache, dry mouth, urge to defecate, and chest tightness. They are usually mild, begin within a minute after the injection of TRH, and last for a few seconds to several minutes. A transient rise in blood pressure has been observed on occasion, but no other changes are seen in vital signs, urine analysis, blood count, or routine blood chemistry tests.[207] The occurrence of circulatory collapse is exceedingly rare. There have been several case reports of pituitary apoplexy in patients who received TRH testing with or without gonadotropin-releasing hormone. In many of these cases, the patient had a large pituitary tumor, which might predispose to this complication.

The test provides a means to distinguish between secondary (pituitary) and tertiary (hypothalamic) hypothyroidism (Fig. 6-7). Although the diagnosis of primary hypothyroidism can be easily confirmed by the presence of elevated basal serum TSH levels, secondary and tertiary hypothyroidism are typically associated with TSH levels that are low or normal. On occasion, the serum TSH concentration might be slightly elevated because of the secretion of biologically less potent molecules, but it remains inappropriately low for the degree of thyroid hormone deficiency. Differentiation between secondary and tertiary hypothyroidism cannot be made with certainty without the TRH test. In a case report of a family with congenital hypothyroidism secondary to hemizygous mutations in the TSH receptor gene, response of TSH to TRH was normal.[208] A TSH response is suggestive of a hypothalamic disorder, and failure to respond is compatible with intrinsic pituitary dysfunction. Furthermore, the typical TSH response curve in hypothalamic hypothyroidism shows a delayed peak with a prolonged elevation in serum TSH before return to the basal value (see Fig. 6-7). The finding of a lack of

TSH response in association with normal prolactin stimulation may be due to isolated pituitary TSH deficiency. Caution should be exercised in the interpretation of test results after withdrawal of thyroid hormone replacement or after treatment of thyrotoxicosis because despite a low serum thyroid hormone concentration, TSH may remain low and may not respond to TRH for several weeks. In the most common forms of thyrotoxicosis, the mechanism of feedback regulation of TSH secretion is intact but is appropriately suppressed by the excessive amounts of thyroid hormone. Thus, both the basal TSH level and its response to TRH are suppressed unless thyrotoxicosis is TSH induced. With the development of more sensitive TSH assays, the TRH test generally is not needed in the evaluation of a thyrotoxic patient with undetectable TSH. The differential diagnosis of conditions leading to inappropriate secretion of TSH may be aided by the TRH test result. Elevated basal TSH values that do not respond to TRH by a further increase are typical of TSH-secreting pituitary adenomas. In contrast, patients with high thyroid hormone levels but detectable serum TSH resulting from resistance to thyroid hormone have a normal or exaggerated TSH response to TRH that in most instances is suppressed by supraphysiologic doses of thyroid hormone. Because of the exquisite sensitivity of the pituitary gland to feedback regulation by thyroid hormone, small changes in the latter profoundly affect the response of TSH to TRH. Thus, patients with non–TSH-induced thyrotoxicosis of the mildest degree have a reduced TSH response to TRH, whereas those with primary hypothyroidism exhibit an accentuated response that is prolonged (see Fig. 6-7). These changes can occur in the absence of clinical or other laboratory evidence of thyroid dysfunction.

The TSH response to TRH is subnormal or absent in one third of apparently euthyroid patients with autoimmune thyroid disease, and even members of their family might not respond to TRH. Most, but not all, patients with a reduced TSH response to TRH will also show thyroid activity that is nonsuppressible

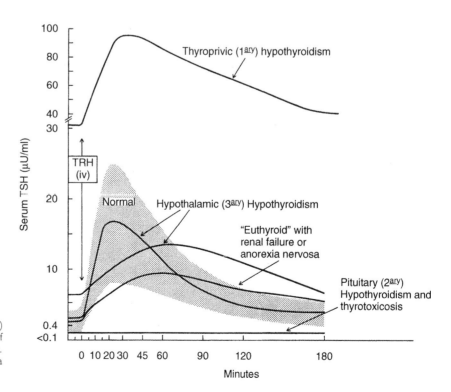

FIGURE 6-7. Typical serum thyroid-stimulating hormone (TSH) responses to the administration of a single intravenous bolus of thyrotropin-releasing hormone at time 0 in various conditions. The normal response is represented by the shaded area. Data used for this figure are the average of several studies.

by thyroid hormone. A common dissociation between these two tests is typified by a normal TSH response to TRH in a nonsuppressible patient. This finding is not surprising because patients with nonsuppressible thyroid glands often have limited capacity to synthesize and secrete thyroid hormone as a result of prior therapy or partial destruction of their glands by the disease process. Clinically, euthyroid patients who do not respond to TRH admittedly have a slight excess of thyroid hormone. It is less easy to reconcile the rare occurrence of TRH unresponsiveness in a patient whose TSH is suppressible by exogenous thyroid hormone. It should be remembered, however, that a suppressed pituitary can take a variable amount of time to recover, a phenomenon that might be the basis of such discrepancies. Despite discrepancies between the results of the TRH and T_3 suppression tests, use of the former is much preferred, particularly in elderly patients, in whom administration of T_3 can produce untoward effects.

OTHER TESTS OF TSH RESERVE

It has been reasoned that by virtue of different mechanisms of action, testing the TSH response by means other than TRH can provide information of diagnostic value that is not obtainable from stimulation and suppression of the pituitary by TRH and thyroid hormone, respectively. Trials using drugs such as metoclopramide and L-dopa have been carried out but so far have provided only limited additional information and so have not found a place in clinical practice. These tests have limited application in the study of patients with inappropriate secretion of TSH, in whom the distinction of autonomous secretion of TSH as compared with selective unresponsiveness to thyroid hormone inhibition is of diagnostic value.

Other tests indirectly measure pituitary TSH reserve during the rebound period after suppression of thyroid hormone synthesis or pituitary TSH secretion. Assessment of thyroid gland activity after withdrawal of antithyroid drugs or T_3 replacement has been proposed.[209,210]

THYROTROPIN STIMULATION TEST

The TSH stimulation test measures the ability of thyroid tissue to respond to exogenous TSH by an increase in iodide accumulation and hormone release and for the identification of residual thyroid cancer tissue. Formerly used to differentiate hypothyroidism caused by thyroid gland failure from that caused by TSH deficiency, the test was recently used in conjunction with a scintiscan to localize areas of suppressed thyroid tissue. Formerly, it required the intramuscular administration of one or three 5 to 10 U doses of bovine TSH. The test could cause discomfort, and even serious reactions to the heterologous TSH, and therefore is no longer used.

Recombinant human TSH (r-hTSH), Thyrogen (Genzyme Transgenics Corp., Cambridge, MA), was approved by the Food and Drug Administration over 6 years ago for the management of patients with thyroid cancer. Many studies have subsequently demonstrated the utility of r-hTSH to stimulate thyroid remnants, but few have evaluated its effect on intact thyroids. A single dose of 0.1 mg r-hTSH (compared with 0.9 mg given to thyroid cancer patients) was a potent stimulus for the release of T_4, T_3, and Tg in normal volunteers.[211] A very low dose of r-hTSH (0.01 mg) has been found to stimulate ^{131}I uptake in multinodular goiters, but no data are available on whether this very low dose is capable of stimulating TSH or Tg release from the thyroid gland. It has also been suggested that dosing of r-hTSH should be based on body surface area (BSA) as an inverse relationship between BSA and serum peak TSH after r-hTSH administration has been reported.[212]

THYROID SUPPRESSION TEST

Maintenance of thyroid gland activity that is independent of TSH can be demonstrated by the thyroid suppression test. Under normal conditions, administration of thyroid hormone in quantities sufficient to satisfy the body requirement suppresses endogenous TSH and results in a reduction in thyroid hormone synthesis and secretion. Because thyrotoxicosis resulting from excessive secretion of hormone by the thyroid gland implies that the feedback control mechanism is not operative or has been perturbed, it is easy to understand why, under such circumstances, the supply of exogenous hormone would also be ineffective in suppressing thyroid gland activity. The test has very limited application today, although it might be of value in patients who are euthyroid or only mildly thyrotoxic but are suspected of having abnormal thyroid gland stimulation or autonomy, particularly for confirmation of the diagnosis of resistance to thyroid hormone.

Usually, the test is carried out with 100 μg of liothyronine (L-T_3) given daily in two divided doses over a period of 7 to 10 days. A 24 hour RAIU is determined before and during the last 2 days of T_3 administration.[213] Normal individuals show suppression of RAIU by at least 50% when compared with the value before liothyronine treatment. No change or a lesser reduction is typical of not only Graves' disease but also other forms of endogenous thyrotoxicosis, including toxic adenoma, functioning carcinoma, and thyrotoxicosis caused by trophoblastic disease. The presence of nonsuppressibility indicates thyroid gland activity independent of TSH but not necessarily thyrotoxicosis. Euthyroid patients with autonomous thyroid function have a normal TSH response to TRH before the administration of liothyronine. However, inhibition of TSH secretion by exogenous T_3 does not suppress the autonomous activity of the thyroid gland. This discrepancy is the most commonly encountered difference between the results of the two related tests. When the T_3 suppression test is used in conjunction with a scintiscan, localized areas of autonomous function can be identified. The test can be carried out without the administration of radioisotopes by measuring serum T_4 before and 2 weeks after the ingestion of liothyronine. Although total suppression of T_4 secretion never occurs, even after prolonged treatment with liothyronine, reduction by at least 50% is normal.[214]

Variants of the test have been proposed to reduce the potential risks of liothyronine administration in elderly patients and in those with angina pectoris or congestive heart failure. However, with the availability of sensitive TSH assays, thyroid suppression tests are no longer indicated.

Specialized Thyroid Tests

A number of specialized tests are available for the evaluation of specific aspects of thyroid hormone biosynthesis, secretion, turnover, distribution, and absorption. Their primary application is investigative. They are only briefly mentioned here for the sake of completeness.

IODOTYROSINE DEIODINASE ACTIVITY

The iodotyrosine deiodinase test involves the intravenous administration of tracer MIT or DIT labeled with radioiodide. Urine collected over a period of 4 hours is analyzed by chromatography or resin column separation. Normally, only 4% to 8% of the radioactivity is excreted as such; the remainder appears in the urine in the form of iodide.[215] Excretion of larger amounts of the administered compound indicates an inability to deiodinate iodotyrosine. The test is useful in the diagnosis of a dehalogenase defect. This test undoubtedly will be replaced by measurement of MIT and DIT by tandem mass spectroscopy.

TEST FOR DEFECTIVE HORMONOGENESIS

After the administration of radioiodide, the isotopically labeled compounds synthesized in the thyroid gland and those secreted into the circulation can be analyzed by immunologic, chromatographic, electrophoretic, and density gradient centrifugation techniques.[216] Such tests serve to evaluate the synthesis and release of thyroid hormone, as well as delineate the formation of abnormal iodoproteins.

IODINE KINETIC STUDIES

The iodine kinetic procedure is used to evaluate overall iodide metabolism and to elucidate the pathophysiology of thyroid disease. Analysis involves follow-up of the fate of administered radioiodide tracer by measurement of thyroidal accumulation, secretion into blood, and excretion in urine and feces.[217] Double-tracer techniques and programs for computer-assisted analysis of data are available.

ABSORPTION OF THYROID HORMONE

Failure to achieve a normal serum thyroid hormone concentration after the administration of replacement doses of thyroid hormone is usually due to poor compliance, occasionally due to the use of inactive preparations, and rarely, if ever, due to malabsorption. The last can be evaluated by simultaneous oral and intravenous administration of the hormone labeled with two different iodine isotope tracers. The ratio of the two isotopes in blood is proportional to the net absorbed fraction of the orally administered hormone.[218,219] Under normal circumstances, approximately 80% of the T_4 and 95% of the T_3 administered orally are absorbed. Hypothyroidism and a variety of other unrelated conditions have little effect on the intestinal absorption of thyroid hormones. Absorption may be diminished in patients with steatorrhea, in some cases of hepatic failure, during treatment with cholestyramine, and with diets that are rich in soybeans and their products. Absorption of thyroid hormone can also be evaluated by the administration of a single oral dose of 100 µg of L-T_3 or 1 mg of levothyroxine (L-T_4), followed by their measurement in blood sampled at various intervals.[220] Standard values for normal absorption of L-T_4 are given in Fig. 6-8.

TURNOVER KINETICS OF T_4 AND T_3

Turnover kinetic studies require the intravenous administration of isotope-labeled tracer levothyroxine or liothyronine. The half-time of disappearance of the hormone is calculated from the rate of decrease in serum trichloroacetic acid–precipitable, ethanol-extractable, or antibody-precipitable isotope counts. Compartmental analysis can be used for calculation of the turnover parameters.[221,222] The calculated daily degradation or production rate (PR) is the product of the fractional turnover rate (K), the extrathyroidal distribution space (DS), and the average concentration of the hormone in serum. Noncompartmental analysis may be used for the calculation of kinetic parameters. The metabolic clearance rate (MCR) is defined as the dose of the injected labeled tracer divided by the area under its curve of disappearance. The PR is then calculated from the product of the MCR

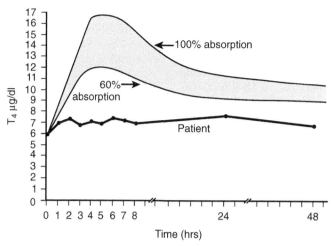

FIGURE 6-8. Absorption of oral L-T_4. Results of serum T_4 levels following ingestion of five 0.2 mg tablets of L-thyroxine. The pills were pulverized and suspended in water, and subjects ingested the thyroid hormone slurry with subsequent blood tests hourly for 8 hours, then again at 24 and 48 hours. An example of a subject with malabsorption of thyroid hormone is shown (*solid line*). Absorption in normal subjects is shown in the shaded area.

and the average concentration of the respective nonradioactive iodothyronine measured in serum over the period of the study. Simultaneous studies of T_4 and T_3 turnover kinetics can be carried out by injection of both hormones labeled with different iodine isotopes.

Average normal values in adults for T_4 and T_3, respectively, are as follows: = $T_{1/2}$ 7.0 and 0.8 days; K = 10% and 90% per day; DS = 11 and 30 L of serum equivalent; MCR = 1.1 and 25 L/day; and PR = 90 and 25 mg/day.

The hormonal PR is accelerated in thyrotoxicosis and diminished in hypothyroidism. In euthyroid patients with TBG abnormalities, the PR remains normal because changes in serum hormone concentration are accompanied by compensatory changes in the fractional turnover rate and the extrathyroidal hormonal pool. A variety of nonthyroidal illnesses can alter hormone kinetics.

METABOLIC KINETICS OF THYROID HORMONES AND THEIR METABOLITES

The kinetics of the production of various metabolites of T_4 and T_3 in peripheral tissues and their further metabolism can be studied. Most methods use radiolabeled iodothyronine tracers injected intravenously.[221,223,224] Their disappearance is monitored in serum samples obtained at various intervals after injection of the tracers by means of chromatographic and immunologic techniques of separation. Kinetic parameters can be calculated by noncompartmental analysis or by two- or multiple-compartment analysis. Estimates have been made by the differential measurement in urine of the isotopes derived from the precursor and its metabolite. They are in agreement with measurements carried out in serum.[225] Conversion rates of iodothyronines, principally generated in peripheral tissues, can be calculated from the ratio of their PR and that of their respective precursors. Some iodothyronines such as T_3 are secreted by the thyroid gland as well as generated in peripheral tissues. Studies to calculate the conversion rate require the administration of thyroid hormone to block thyroidal secretion.[226]

On average, 35% and 45% of T_4 are converted to T_3 and rT_3, respectively, in peripheral tissues. The conversion of T_4 to T_3 is greatly diminished in a variety of illnesses of nonthyroidal origin and in response to many drugs (see Table 6-7). Degradation and monodeiodination of iodothyronines can be estimated without the administration of isotopes. They are, however, less accurate. The conversion of T_4 to T_3 can be estimated semiquantitatively by the measurement of serum TT_3 after treatment with replacement doses of levothyroxine.

MEASUREMENT OF THE PRODUCTION RATE AND METABOLIC KINETICS OF OTHER COMPOUNDS

The metabolism and PRs of a variety of compounds related to thyroid physiology can be studied by using their radiolabeled congeners and by applying the general principles of turnover kinetics. Studies of TSH have demonstrated changes not only related to thyroid dysfunction but also associated with age and kidney and liver disease.[227,228] Studies of the turnover kinetics of TBG have shown that the slight increases and decreases in serum TBG associated with hypothyroidism and thyrotoxicosis, respectively, are due to changes in the degradation rate of TBG rather than synthesis.

TRANSFER OF THYROID HORMONE FROM BLOOD TO TISSUES

Transfer of hormone from blood to tissues can be estimated in vivo by two techniques. A direct method monitors accumulation of the administered labeled hormone tracer by surface counting over the organ of interest. An indirect method monitors the early disappearance from plasma of the simultaneously administered hormone and albumin, labeled with different radioisotope tracers.[229] The difference between the rates of disappearance of hormone and albumin represents the fraction of hormone that has left the vascular (albumin) space and presumably has entered tissues.

Molecular Diagnosis of Thyroid Disease

Molecular diagnosis of thyroid disease is useful when a specific genetic abnormality is suspected. Often, similar thyroid phenotypes can be the result of different causes. For example, hyperthyroxinemia with normal or elevated TSH can be the result of a binding protein disorder, resistance to thyroid hormone (RTH), or a TSH-secreting pituitary tumor. One of the first steps in determining the presence of a genetic defect is confirmation that the suspected phenotype is inherited, that is, that other family members have the same abnormality. The final diagnosis can then be aided by demonstration of an abnormal TBG in the case of an abnormal binding protein or a mutation in the thyroid hormone (TR) β gene in the case of RTH, whereas pituitary tumors are rarely inherited. A general approach to molecular diagnosis would be first extraction of genomic DNA from peripheral blood leukocytes. Identification of a specific mutation can be done by direct sequencing of the gene of interest or by the use of specific restriction endonucleases to digest an amplified fragment of the gene. The latter approach can be helpful in confirming common mutations but will not detect novel mutations. It is likely that genetic diagnosis of the common inherited diseases of the thyroid will become a cost-efficient method available in the clinical laboratory.

DYSALBUMINEMIAS

The most common form of inherited euthyroid hyperthyroxinemia is FDH. FDH is caused by a mutation in the albumin gene resulting in a protein with increased affinity for T_4 and T_3. The most common form is due to a missense mutation resulting in a change from arginine to histidine at codon 218 (R218H). Diagnosis can be made by demonstration of comigration of ^{125}I-thyroxine by nondenaturing electrophoresis or precipitation with antialbumin serum, or by molecular diagnosis. A variant albumin, L66P, has been described that has a 40-fold increased affinity for T_3 and only a 50% increased affinity for T_4. Subjects with this form of FDH, termed FDH-T_3, present with high levels of total T_3, normal or mildly elevated levels of T_4, and normal TSH.

Molecular diagnosis of the common form of FDH is made by polymerase chain reaction (PCR) amplification of exon 7 of the human serum albumin (HSA) gene using a mismatched oligonucleotide primers. The PCR product is cut by Dra III only in the presence of the mutant allele producing HSA R218H.[230] The other, less common mutation of albumin is diagnosed by sequencing exon 1 for L66P.[231]

PREALBUMIN-ASSOCIATED HYPERTHYROXINEMIA

Four mutations that are described in the transthyretin (TTR) gene result in increased (2.1- to 7.3-fold) affinity for T_4 in codons 6, 109, and 119.[232] Endonucleases that are useful in the identification of the TTR variants are $MspI^-$ for Gly6Ser in exon 2 and $BsoFI^-$ and $Fnu4H^+$ for Ala109Thr, $BsoFI^-$ for Ala109Val, and $NcoI^+$ for Thr119Met, all in exon 4.[233]

THYROXINE-BINDING GLOBULIN

Seventy-five to 80% of blood T_4 is bound to TBG; therefore, when there is an abnormality in the TBG, measurable changes in the serum total T_4 and T_3 levels are noted. Over 17 different mutant TBG molecules have been described. The TBG gene is located in the X-chromosome and results in more severe abnormalities in males than in females. Although direct measurement of TBG can be helpful as well as anodal or cathodal shift on isoelectric focusing, sequencing of the TBG gene usually leads to the molecular diagnosis.[234]

NA$^+$/I$^-$ SYMPORTER

The failure of the thyroid gland to actively accumulate I^- ("iodide trapping defect") in iodine-replete areas results in congenital hypothyroidism. Clinical diagnosis is suggested in hypothyroid subjects with elevated TSH and a goiter of variable size. Subjects have RAIUs of less than 2 and a saliva-to-plasma radioiodide ratio of less than 20% (see above). Definitive diagnosis is based on the identification of a mutation in the NIS gene.[235]

THYROID PEROXIDASE

TPO is a protein located in the apical plasma membrane of thyroid follicular cells with its catalytic domain facing the colloid space. It is responsible for iodine oxidation and trapping. When TPO is defective, administered radioiodide is partially or completely discharged after administration of perchlorate. Demonstration of linkage to the TPO gene, when several family members are suspected, or sequencing of the gene can be done to confirm the diagnosis.[236]

Other Mutations Causing Defects in Thyroid Hormone Synthesis (Dyshormonogenesis)

All steps in the pathway of hormone synthesis that involve protein catalysts can be defective and result in various degrees of hypothyroidism. In addition to NIS and TPO, described above, these include defects in Tg, the generation of H_2O_2 by the dual oxidase 2 (DUOX2) and its maturation factor (DUOXA2), and the dehalogenase enzyme (DEHAL or IYD) and the membrane protein, Pendrin, involved in iodide transport at the apical membrane of the thyrocyte (PDS or SLC26A4). The latter is associated with deafness caused by malformations of the vestibular system.[237]

TSH RECEPTOR

Loss of function of the TSH receptor is likely to cause the syndrome of resistance to TSH as described above. Molecular characterization of this syndrome requires sequencing of the TSH receptor.[238,239] In addition, somatic gain-of-function mutations of the TSH receptor are a common cause for autonomous toxic adenoma.

THYROID HORMONE RECEPTOR β

Patients with persistently elevated free thyroid hormone levels in the presence of a nonsuppressed TSH, goiter, and failure to respond to exogenous administration of L-T_3 are likely to have RTH. Most cases of RTH are due to mutations in the TRβ gene. More than 150 different mutations have been reported in association with this syndrome. In 10% to 15% of subjects with RTH, no mutation in the TRβ is seen.[240]

Genetic Defects Causing Thyroid Dysgenesis

Congenital hypothyroidism, the most common endocrine abnormality occurring at birth, is due in 80% of cases to developmental defects of the thyroid gland (dysgenesis). However, in only a small number of cases, it has been traced to a specific gene defect. In addition to mutations of the TSH receptor, which may cause thyroid hypoplasia, defects in the following transcription factors can cause dysgenesis: thyroid transcription factor 1 (TTF1), TTF2, and PAX8.[241]

Effects of Drugs on Thyroid Function

Many drugs can interfere with biochemical tests of thyroid function by interfering with the synthesis, transport, and metabolism of thyroid hormones or by altering the synthesis and secretion of thyrotropin (TSH). Only rarely, however, do these effects cause overt, clinically apparent thyroid disease. This section is not intended to provide exhaustive information on all drugs that can affect tests of thyroid function. Instead, the more commonly encountered agents, those with broad clinical applications, and those that are helpful in understanding the mechanisms of drug interactions are described.

MECHANISMS OF ACTION

Some drugs and hormones, such as estrogens and androgens, affect thyroid hormone transport in blood by altering the concentration of binding proteins in serum. Thyroid hormone transport may also be affected by substances that compete with the binding of thyroid hormone to its carrier proteins (see Table 6-4).

Some of the agents that can alter the extrathyroidal metabolism of thyroid hormone are listed in Table 6-7. Several drugs that are widely used in clinical practice (e.g., glucocorticoids, amiodarone, propranolol) inhibit the conversion of T_4 to T_3 in peripheral tissues. As expected, their most profound effect on thyroid function is a decrease in the serum concentration of T_3, usually with a concomitant increase in the rT_3 level. An increase in the serum T_4 concentration has been observed on occasion. When intrapituitary T_4-to-T_3 conversion is inhibited, the serum TSH concentration may rise. In the absence of inherent abnormalities in thyroid hormone synthesis or in its secretion, TSH levels should return to normal, and hypothyroidism should not ensue from the chronic administration of compounds that only partially interfere with T_4 monodeiodination. Other mechanisms by which some compounds affect the extrathyroidal metabolism of thyroid hormone involve acceleration of the overall rates of the deiodinative and nondeiodinative routes of hormone disposal. An example of a drug that acts principally through the former mechanism is phenobarbital,[242] and one that acts by way of the latter is diphenylhydantoin.[243] In such circumstances, thyroid hormone concentrations should remain unaltered. Furthermore, it has been anticipated, as well as observed, that hypothyroid patients who receive such drugs require higher doses of exogenous hormone to maintain a eumetabolic state. Some drugs have multiple effects.

A large array of drugs act on the hypothalamic-pituitary axis (see Table 6-10), although only a few have significant effects on thyroid function by way of this central mechanism. Furthermore, people undergoing drug treatment who have no thyroid disease seldom show important changes in the basal serum TSH concentration.

The most potent suppressors of pituitary TSH secretion are thyroid hormone and its analogues. Some of the TSH-inhibiting agents listed in Table 6-10—fenclofenac and salicylates—may act by increasing the free thyroid hormone level through interference with its binding to serum proteins. Other agents appear to have a direct inhibitory effect on the pituitary and possibly the hypothalamus. The most notable are dopamine and its agonists. They have been shown to suppress basal TSH levels in the euthyroid state and in patients with primary hypothyroidism. They also suppress the TSH response to TRH. As expected, dopamine antagonists amplify TSH secretion. A notable exception to this rule, which casts some doubt on the assumed mechanism of action of dopamine antagonists, is pimozide. This neuroleptic dopamine blocker has been shown to reduce elevated serum TSH levels in patients with primary hypothyroidism.[244]

Iodide and some iodine-containing organic compounds cause a rapid increase in the basal and TRH-stimulated levels of serum TSH. This effect is undoubtedly the result of a decrease in the serum thyroid hormone concentration caused by inhibition of hormone synthesis and secretion by the thyroid gland or by a selective decrease in the intrapituitary concentration of T_3 as with iopanoic acid and amiodarone. Indeed, a predominant block on the intrapituitary conversion of T_4 to T_3 has been demonstrated. It should be noted that iodide and iodine-containing compounds do not stimulate TSH secretion in patients in whom they induce excessive secretion of thyroid hormone.[245,246] A decrease in the free thyroid hormone concentration in serum, albeit minimal in magnitude, might also be responsible for the increase in TSH levels observed during treatment with clomiphene.[247] An increase in serum TSH concentration during lithium therapy is also believed to be caused by reduced thyroid hormone levels rather than by a direct effect of this ion on the pituitary.

It has been postulated that some agents might act by modifying the effect of TSH on its target tissue. For example, theophylline may potentiate the action of TSH through its inhibitory effect on phosphodiesterase, which may lead to an increase in the intracellular concentration of cAMP.[248] A handful of drugs appear to act by blocking some of the peripheral tissue effects of thyroid hormone. Others appear to mimic one or several manifestations of thyroid hormone effects on tissues. Guanethidine, which inhibits release of catecholamines from tissues, provides a beneficial effect in thyrotoxicosis by decreasing the BMR, pulse rate, and tremulousness.[249,250] This agent probably has no direct effect on the thyroid gland but might depress those manifestations of thyrotoxicosis that are mediated by sympathetic pathways. Among the multiple effects of the β-adrenergic blocker propranolol on thyroid hormone economy is a reduction in peripheral tissue responses to thyroid hormone.

SPECIFIC AGENTS

Hormones and Derivatives

Androgens

Androgens decrease the concentration of TBG in serum and thereby reduce levels of T_4 and T_3.[251,252] In addition, in hypothyroid patients who are taking levothyroxine, androgen administration was found to increase free T_4 levels and decrease TSH levels while causing the typical changes of reduction in TBG and total T_4; this clinical hyperthyroidism induced by androgen therapy necessitated a reduction in thyroid replacement doses.[253] The concentration of free hormone remains unaffected, and the degradation rate of T_4 is normal at the expense of an accelerated turnover rate. TSH levels are normal.[254] Anabolic steroids with weaker androgenic action have the same effect, although similar changes that are observed during danazol therapy have been attributed to its androgen-like properties.[255]

Estrogen and Selective Estrogen Receptor Modulators

Hyperestrogenism caused by pregnancy, hydatidiform moles, tumors, or treatment with estrogens is the most common cause of increased TBG, the major carrier of thyroid hormone in serum. Estrogens produce a dose-dependent increase in the complexity of oligosaccharide side chains, which proportionately increases the number of sialic acids in the TBG molecule, which in turn prolongs its survival in serum.[256] The concentrations of other serum proteins, ceruloplasmin, transferrin, and several that bind hormones (cortisol-binding globulin and testosterone-binding globulin) are also increased.[257] The consequences of increased TBG concentration in serum are higher serum levels of both T_4 and T_3 and, to a lesser extent, other metabolites of T_4 deiodination. At the usual doses of ethinyl estradiol (20 to 35 µg per day) and conjugated estrogen (0.625 mg per day), serum TBG concentrations increase by about 30% to 50%, and serum T_4 concentrations increase by 20% to 35%, starting at 2 weeks of therapy with attainment of steady state by 4 to 8 weeks.[258] Of note, in a study of transdermal versus oral estradiol in women with premature ovarian failure, serum levels of thyroid-binding globulin and T_4 were elevated only in the women using oral estradiol despite comparable serum estradiol levels in the two groups.[258]

Women with hypothyroidism that is being treated with thyroxine need on average 45% more thyroxine during pregnancy to maintain the euthyroid state. In Mandel's study of 12 pregnant women with primary hypothyroidism who were on thyroxine replacement, the mean serum TSH increased from 2.0 mU/L to 13.5 mU/L during pregnancy, the normal range being 0.5 to 5 mU/L.[259] Several reasons for this increased need include an increase in serum thyroxine-binding globulin from mother to fetus and increased maternal clearance of thyroxine. This increased need for thyroxine in pregnant women with hypothy-

roidism was further studied in postmenopausal women with hypothyroidism who were given estrogen replacement therapy. This study found small but potentially important decreases in serum free thyroxine and increases in serum thyrotropin that are thought to result from estrogen-induced increases in serum TBG concentration, which slows entry of thyroxine into cells, including those in the pituitary, resulting in reduced thyroid hormone action in tissue. From these studies, it can be concluded that in normal, euthyroid women, the estrogen-induced increase in TBG may result in at least a transient increase in T_4 secretion to compensate for and prevent mild hypothyroidism and an increase in TSH.

Tamoxifen blocks the estrogen-induced increase in TBG, whereas tamoxifen alone in postmenopausal women increases serum TBG, T_4, and T_3 levels.[260] Tamoxifen, a selective estrogen receptor modulator (SERM) used predominantly in the prevention and treatment of breast cancer, has been shown to elevate TBG levels with resultant increases in total T_4 and T_3 levels. In addition to causing significant elevations of TBG, tamoxifen has been shown to significantly suppress FT_3 and FT_4 levels after 6 months of treatment, accompanied by a significant increase in TSH after 1 year of treatment.

Some newer SERMs include raloxifene and droloxifene. These drugs also cause increases in TBG with mild to no increase in total thyroid hormone levels; the changes induced by these medications are less than those seen with estrogen use. Raloxifene, which was developed for treatment of osteoporosis, given at a dose of 60 mg orally per day, only mildly increased TBG levels with no significant change in TSH and free thyroid hormone levels in controls and in patients with subclinical hyperthyroidism. Droloxifene administered to postmenopausal women for 6 weeks resulted in an increase in TBG that was significant, but much less than that induced by 0.625 mg of estrogen/day for the same time period; this increase in TBG did not have any significant effect on thyroid hormone levels.

The consequences of increased TBG concentration in serum include higher serum levels of both T_4 and T_3 and, to a lesser extent, other metabolites of T_4 deiodination. The fractional turnover rate of T_4 is reduced principally because of an increase in the intravascular T_4 pool. On the other hand, the FT_4 and FT_3 concentrations and the absolute amount of hormone that was degraded each day remain normal.

Glucocorticoids

Physiologic amounts of glucocorticoids, as well as pharmacologic doses, influence thyroid function. The effects are variable and multiple, depending on the dose and the person's endocrine status. The type of glucocorticoid and the route of administration can also influence the magnitude of the effect.[261] Known effects include a decrease in the serum concentration of TBG and an increase in that of TTR,[42] inhibition of the outer-ring deiodination of T_4 and probably rT_3, suppression of TSH secretion, a possible decrease in hepatic binding of T_4, and an increase in the renal clearance of iodide.[262]

The decrease in serum concentration of TBG caused by the administration of pharmacologic doses of glucocorticoids results in a decrease in the serum TT_4 concentration and an increase in its free fraction. The absolute concentration of FT_4 and the FT_4I remain normal.

A more profound decrease is noted in the concentration of serum T_3 as opposed to T_4 in association with pharmacologic doses of glucocorticoids, and this difference cannot be ascribed to the reduced serum TBG level. It is caused by decreased conversion of T_4 to T_3 in peripheral tissues. A reduced T_3/T_4 ratio also occurs in hypothyroid patients receiving replacement doses of T_4. It is accompanied by an increase in the serum level of rT_3. This effect of the steroid is rapid and can be seen within 24 hours.

Earlier observations of cortisone-induced depression of uptake and clearance of iodide by the thyroid gland can now be attributed to the effect of this steroid on TSH secretion. Pharmacologic doses of glucocorticoids suppress the basal TSH level in euthyroid subjects and in patients with primary hypothyroidism and decrease their TSH response to TRH. Normal adrenocortical secretion appears to have a suppressive influence on pituitary TSH secretion inasmuch as patients with primary adrenal insufficiency have a significant elevation in serum TSH concentrations. Administration of moderate doses of hydrocortisone reduces the basal release of TSH and the T_3 and TSH response to TRH.[263]

No single change in thyroid function can be ascribed to a specific mode of action of glucocorticoids. For example, diminished thyroidal RAIU can be caused by the combined effects of TSH suppression and increased renal clearance of iodide. Similarly, a low serum TT_4 level is the result of suppressed thyroidal secretion caused by diminished TSH stimulation, as well as the decreased serum level of TBG. One of the common problems in clinical practice is to separate the effect of glucocorticoid action on pituitary function from that of other agents and those caused by acute and chronic illness. This situation arises often because steroids are commonly used in various autoimmune and allergic disorders as well as in the treatment of septic shock. The diagnosis of coexisting true hypothyroidism is difficult. Because of the suppressive effects of glucocorticoids on the hypothalamic-pituitary axis, low levels of serum T_4 and T_3 may not be accompanied by an increase in the serum TSH level, which would otherwise be diagnostic of primary hypothyroidism. In such circumstances, a depressed rather than an elevated serum rT_3 level may be helpful in the detection of coexistent primary thyroid failure.

Pharmacologic doses of glucocorticoids induce a prompt decline in serum T_4 and T_3 concentrations in thyrotoxic patients with autoimmune thyroid disease. Amelioration of the symptoms and signs in such patients may also be accompanied by a decrease in the elevated thyroidal RAIU and a diminution in TSH receptor antibody titer.[264] This effect of glucocorticoids might be caused in part by their immunosuppressive action, because it has been shown that administration of dexamethasone to hypothyroid patients with Hashimoto's thyroiditis causes an increase in the serum concentration of both T_4 and T_3.[265]

Growth Hormone

The effects of growth hormone (GH) replacement on the hypothalamic-pituitary-thyroid axis and thyroid function are controversial. Many of the differences between older studies and more recent studies may be related to different methods used for measurement of thyroid hormones, different study protocols, and different subjects studied. Furthermore, in studies that were performed years ago, the source of GH preparations from pituitary extracts had variable purity and possibly was contaminated with TSH. Most studies report changes in thyroid function, including a decrease in serum total T_4 and rT_3 with an elevation in T_3 levels caused by an increase in peripheral conversion of T_4 to T_3 and a decreased conversion of T_4 to rT_3. TSH responses to growth hormone have been more variable. Some researchers have suggested that GH inhibits TSH release, possibly via an

increase in somatostatinergic tone[266-268] or by negative feedback from increased T_3 levels. Others found no change in TSH levels on GH therapy. Controversy exists as to whether these changes in thyroid function tests truly represent the occurrence of central hypothyroidism with GH therapy, or whether they are only transient changes that do not need to be treated with T_4 supplementation. Wyatt and coworkers studied the acute effects of GH in euthyroid growth hormone–deficient children and found a decrease in T_4, FT_4I, and rT_3; increases in T_3 and T_3/T_4 ratio; and no change in baseline TSH or TRH-stimulated TSH. In addition, because patients remained clinically euthyroid without changes in cholesterol over the 1 year period of treatment, they concluded that these changes in thyroid function are transient and did not recommend thyroxine supplementation unless a persistent decline occurs in both T_3 and T_4.[269] A study by Porretti and coworkers of GH-deficient adults found significant and persistent decreases in rT_3 and free T_4 levels on low doses of recombinant human growth hormone (r-hGH) over a 6 month period, with 25.7% of free T_4 levels in the hypothyroid range. In addition, almost half of the initially euthyroid GH-deficient adults became clinically hypothyroid on r-hGH, despite no change in serum TSH. This group concluded that GH deficiency masks a state of central hypothyroidism that is manifested on GH replacement, and that subjects who demonstrate thyroid function abnormalities consistent with central hypothyroidism should be treated with T_4 supplementation.[270]

Neuropsychiatric Medications

Carbamazepine and Oxcarbazepine

Carbamazepine (CBZ) and oxcarbazepine (OCBZ), a newer antiepileptic drug that structurally resembles CBZ, have been shown to decrease thyroid hormone levels.[271] These drugs decrease total T_4 and free T_4, while T_3 and free T_3 may be slightly decreased to normal, with TSH remaining in the normal range.[272,273] Altered thyroid function from CBZ use has been attributed to induction of the hepatic P-450 enzyme system with consequent increases in thyroid hormone metabolism. More recently, however, in a study of 90 men with epilepsy, none of the observed changes in thyroid function tests correlated with the levels of a specific liver enzyme, GGT, or with serum drug levels of CBZ or OCBZ, suggesting that other mechanisms aside from liver enzyme induction may be involved. Immunologic mechanisms of the changes in thyroid hormone have also been evaluated. There is no association between concentrations of anti–TPO-ab or anti–Tg-ab with alterations in thyroid hormone concentrations.

OCBZ has a mechanism of action that does not appear to induce the hepatic P-450 system; in one study, replacement of CBZ with OCBZ resulted in deinduction of liver enzyme levels and short-term restoration of normal thyroid function in male epileptics.[274]

Despite decreased total and free T_4 levels, TSH levels in most studies remain in the normal range with no clinical evidence of hypothyroidism. These paradoxical findings of low free thyroid hormone levels with a normal TSH and euthyroid clinical picture are explained by measurement of free T_4 levels in undiluted human serum by ultrafiltration. In contrast to previous studies in which serum was diluted, free T_4 concentrations were normal by the ultrafiltration method of measurement in clinically euthyroid patients treated with phenytoin and CBZ; variations in free T_4 based on method of measurement indicate that TSH is the best indicator of thyroid function in these patients. Another proposed reason why TSH remains normal is the CBZ-induced increase in type 1 5′-deiodinase activity, which results in increased free T_3 and normalized TSH.[275]

Desipramine

A study of 28 severely depressed outpatients treated with desipramine, a tricyclic antidepressant, demonstrated a decrease in T_4 levels only in those whose depression responded to the medication without any change in other thyroid function tests.[276] In contrast, a study of another 39 outpatients with depression showed a nonsignificant reduction in TT_4 after 3 weeks of treatment with desipramine that rebounded by week 6.[277] Given that this change was nonsignificant and transient and that TSH levels were not changed, the authors concluded that there was no overall reduction in thyroid axis activity with desipramine, although a transient increase in type 1 5′-deiodinase activity might have occurred. Studies in vitro demonstrate that tricyclic antidepressants, namely, imipramine, desipramine, and clomipramine, have antithyroid effects and act by complexing with iodine and inactivating TPO.[278]

Diphenylhydantoin

Diphenylhydantoin (DPH) competes with thyroid hormone binding to TBG. This effect of DPH and diazepam, a related compound, has been exploited to study the conformational requirements for the interaction of thyroid hormone with its serum carrier protein. Although the affinity of DPH for TBG is far below that of T_4, when used in therapeutic doses the serum concentration that is achieved is high enough to cause significant occupancy of the hormone-binding sites on TBG. This effect of diphenylhydantoin is only partly responsible for the decrease in TT_4 and TT_3 concentrations in serum.

In addition to interference with serum protein binding, DPH induces and accelerates the conjugation and clearance of T_4 and T_3 by the liver and probably enhances the conversion of T_4 to T_3 via an increase in 5′ monodeiodinase activity.[279] The net result of DPH's effects on thyroid function is a decrease in the serum concentration of T_4 and rT_3 and less consistently T_3 because the enhanced conversion of T_4 to T_3 compensates for degradation of T_3.[275,279,280] Free thyroxine index is usually reduced, but the FT_4 measured by dialysis is normal. Basal and TRH-stimulated TSH values are usually in the normal range. A study of thyroid status assessed by peripheral parameters demonstrated that patients on long-term phenytoin as well as carbamazepine were eumetabolic.[281]

DPH reduces the intestinal absorption of T_4 and increases its nondeiodinative metabolism. At the usual therapeutic concentrations, this effect of the drug is probably more important than competition with T_4 for binding to TBG and is, by and large, responsible for the reduced concentration of T_4 in serum. Despite these observations, basal and TRH-stimulated TSH levels are within the normal range[282] or are only slightly elevated. This finding is partly the result of the increased generation of T_3 from T_4.

Both DPH and diazepam are commonly used in clinical practice, the former as an anticonvulsant and antiarrhythmic agent and the latter as an anxiolytic. Reduced serum levels of thyroid hormone in patients with therapeutic blood levels of DPH should not be viewed as indicative of thyroid dysfunction unless the TSH level is elevated. Treatment with T_4 in such patients does not alter parameters of cardiac function or symptoms that might be caused by hypothyroidism. DPH may slightly increase the dose required for thyroid hormone replacement in athyreotic subjects.[283]

Fluoxetine

Antidepressants with strong serotoninergic activity, such as clomipramine or fluoxetine, can induce decreases in T_3 levels. In Shelton and coworkers' study, fluoxetine was found to result in a reduction in T_3 levels after 6 weeks of treatment that was associated with decreased Hamilton Rating Scores for Depression.[277]

Lithium

Lithium is a commonly prescribed drug in bipolar affective disorders. It has long been known to cause significant abnormalities in thyroid status[284-289]; hence, thyroid function tests should be performed at 6 month intervals during lithium therapy. Overt hypothyroidism develops in up to 15% of patients, and as many as one third have evidence of subclinical hypothyroidism (elevated serum TSH with a normal free T_4 concentration).

Lithium-induced hypothyroidism that is clinically overt is frequently associated with the presence of autoimmune thyroiditis and high titers of thyroid autoantibodies in 24% of cases. These findings often predate commencement of lithium therapy[290] and occur more frequently in females.[291]

Possible mechanisms of lithium-induced thyroid dysfunction include direct inhibitory actions on thyroid function, including reduction in iodine-concentrating capacity and inhibition of iodotyrosine and iodothyronine biosynthesis.[292-294] Lithium also may inhibit the secretion of thyroid hormones by stabilizing the follicular cell microtubule system.[295] In vitro studies have suggested that lithium inhibits the peripheral conversion of T_4 to T_3, although this action has not been confirmed in vivo.[296] Despite the predilection of lithium-induced hypothyroidism in females and the high prevalence of thyroid autoantibodies, few data support a primary immunogenic role for lithium. It has been postulated that lithium alters the tertiary structure of macromolecules in thyroid membrane receptors or other membrane proteins, thus making these proteins more immunogenic,[297] although this activity is purely speculative. A central (pituitary or hypothalamic) mechanism of action of lithium has been proposed on the basis of its dopaminergic activity in the central nervous system. Although dopamine inhibits TSH secretion, serum prolactin levels are normal in patients treated with lithium, which argues against a central mode of action.

Hyperthyroidism associated with lithium has also been documented. Two retrospective studies demonstrated that the incidence of hyperthyroidism in patients treated with lithium was more than two to three times greater than the incidence of hyperthyroidism in the general population, with a prevalence of about 1.7% to 2.5% in patients taking lithium.[298] One study reported 14 cases of lithium-associated thyrotoxicosis, 8 of which resulted from toxic diffuse goiter, 2 from toxic multinodular goiter, 1 from toxic uninodular goiter, and 2 from painless thyroiditis. Most were treated initially with carbimazole; others required ^{131}I therapy. Another study of 300 patients with Graves' hyperthyroidism and 100 patients with painless thyroiditis found that the odds of lithium exposure were increased 4.7-fold in patients with silent thyroiditis compared with those of Graves' disease. Presumed mechanisms included lithium-induced or exacerbated autoimmune thyroiditis and a direct toxic effect of lithium on the thyroid. Carmaciu et al.[299] reported thyrotoxicosis occurring after complete or partial lithium withdrawal in two patients with bipolar affective disorder, suggesting either a glandular rebound phenomenon or a previous masking of latent hyperthyroidism by the lithium treatment. They postulated possible autoimmune thyroid disease triggered by lithium, disturbed iodine kinetics with overflow of iodine into thyroid hormone production after expansion of the intrathyroidal iodine pool, direct toxicity to thyroid follicular cells by lithium, and coincidental Graves' disease or other causes of hyperthyroidism.

Neuroleptics

Treatment with neuroleptics in schizophrenics has been shown to result in lower FT_4I values as well as higher basal TSH and TSH response to TRH, indicating development of hypothyroidism in these patients.[300] Phenothiazines (chlorpromazine, thioridazine, or trifluoperazine) have been found to result in low T_4 levels with normal or increased T_3 levels without other changes in thyroid indices. The cause of these changes may be secondary to decreased synthesis of thyroid hormone or modulation of deiodinase enzymes.[301,302] In vitro studies and in vivo animal studies demonstrated that chlorpromazine induced a decrease in RAIU.[303,304] However, in humans, an increase in RAIU and a decrease in renal clearance of iodide were observed after 6 weeks of treatment with chlorpromazine and procyclidine.[305]

A third mechanism that is suspected with phenothiazines is an immunogenic effect. Alimemazine, another phenothiazine drug, was found to induce class II MHC antigens on thyroid cells, especially Tg antigen expression. Chlorpromazine has also been shown to increase humoral autoimmunity and to block delayed-type hypersensitivity reactions.

Paroxetine

Konig et al.[306] showed a significant reduction of 11.2% in T_4 levels during treatment with 20 mg of paroxetine in 25 severely depressed patients.

Phenobarbital

Chronic administration of phenobarbital to animals induces increased binding of thyroid hormone to liver microsomes and enhanced deiodinating activity.[307] Phenobarbital administration reduces the biological effectiveness of the hormone by diverting it to microsomal degradative pathways. In humans, phenobarbital augments fecal T_4 clearance by nearly 100%, but serum T_4 levels and FT_4I remain near normal because of compensatory increases in T_4 secretion. Barbiturates therefore appear to have no important effect on thyroid-mediated metabolic action in normal humans who are not dependent on exogenous hormone supply. The augmented hepatic removal of T_4 induced by phenobarbital increases T_4 clearance and lowers T_4 levels and the FT_4I in patients with Graves' disease but has no effect on the clinical response.

Sertraline

Sertraline acts primarily by inhibiting serotonin reuptake and has minimal effects on norepinephrine and dopamine reuptake. It downregulates serotonin and norepinephrine receptors in the brain.

Elevated serum TSH concentrations and decreased serum FT_4I have been reported in nine L-T_4–treated patients with hypothyroidism after treatment with sertraline. The mechanism of these changes is uncertain. One reported case in which sertraline caused a low total serum T_4 concentration but normal concentrations of TSH and FT_4 in an adolescent patient suggested that sertraline only displaced the bound fraction of total T_4 and was not associated with true hypothyroidism.[308]

St. John's Wort

St. John's wort is an herbal product—*Hypericum perforatum*—that is used to treat depression. Its mechanism of action is unknown and is postulated to occur via serotonin. A small retrospective case control study found a probable association between St. John's wort and elevated TSH levels.[309]

Gypsywort

Lycopus europaeus extracts are traditionally used in patients with mild hyperthyroidism. In a prospective study, 62 patients with a serum TSH <1.0 mU/L demonstrated increased urinary T_4 in the treated group as well as heart rate and symptoms of hyperthyroidism.[310]

Valproic Acid

The changes in thyroid hormone levels are more controversial with valproic acid than with the above antiepileptics. Earlier studies found that valproic acid levels were associated with both normal and elevated serum levels of thyroid hormones and TSH.[47,311,312] More recently, however, valproic acid has not been shown to alter T_4 and FT_4I or TSH.

Dopaminergic Agents

Dopamine

It is now reasonably well established that endogenous brain dopamine plays a physiologic role in the regulation of TSH secretion through its effect on the hypothalamic-pituitary axis.[313] Dopamine exerts a suppressive effect on TSH secretion and can be regarded as antagonistic to the stimulatory action of TRH at the pituitary level. Much of the information about the role of dopamine in the control of TSH secretion in humans has been derived from observations made during the administration of agents with dopamine agonistic and antagonistic activity (see Table 6-10).

Dopamine infusion is commonly used in acutely ill hypotensive patients. It lowers the basal serum TSH level in both euthyroid and hypothyroid patients and blunts its response to the administration of TRH. Levodopa, the precursor of dopamine that is used in the treatment of Parkinson's disease and as a test agent in the diagnosis of pituitary disease, also suppresses the basal and TRH-stimulated serum TSH level in euthyroid subjects, as well as in patients with primary hypothyroidism. A similar effect has been observed during the administration of bromocriptine, a dopamine agonist that is used to treat some pituitary tumors and to suppress lactation during the puerperal period. Although the agent has been shown to diminish high serum TSH levels in patients with primary hypothyroidism, chronic administration does not produce a significant inhibitory effect on TRH-induced TSH secretion.[314] Metoclopramide, a dopamine antagonist that is used as a diagnostic agent and in the treatment of motility disorders, increases TSH secretion.[315]

Although some authors have cautioned that prolonged infusion of dopamine might induce secondary hypothyroidism and thus worsen the prognosis of severely ill patients, no evidence suggests that chronic treatment with dopaminergic drugs induces hypothyroidism in less critically ill patients. These drugs have been used in the treatment of pituitary-induced thyrotoxicosis. When measurements of basal or stimulated serum TSH levels are used in the differential diagnosis of primary and secondary hypothyroidism, the concomitant use of drugs with dopamine agonistic or antagonistic activity should be taken into account in the interpretation of results.

Cabergoline

A recent retrospective study of nine patients with prolactin-secreting pituitary tumors treated with cabergoline, a long-acting dopamine type 2 receptor agonist, demonstrated that a significant reduction in T_4 and T_3 levels did occur, with a slight but not significant decrease in TSH levels. Two of the nine patients required L-T_4 treatment based on symptoms and low T_4 levels.[312] This contrasts with a prior study of cabergoline in hyperprolactinemic patients, which was without effect on thyroid hormone levels or TRH-stimulated TSH levels.

Dobutamine

Dobutamine, another vasopressor that acts through β_1-adrenergic receptors on the heart and weakly on peripheral β_2 and α receptors, is used in the intensive care unit as well as in the outpatient management of congestive heart failure to increase cardiac output. Only two studies have looked at dobutamine's effects on thyroid function. Administration of dobutamine for 48 hours at a dose less than that typically used in clinical practice (4 ± 0.3 µg/kg/min) did not find a significant effect on TSH.[316] Dobutamine's effects on TSH were later studied by using incremental doses starting at 5 µg/kg/min and increasing every 3 minutes, reaching 50 µg/kg/min by 15 minutes in subjects undergoing outpatient dobutamine stress echocardiograms.[317] It was found that high-dose dobutamine treatment was associated with a small but significant decrease in TSH that can be detected within 15 minutes and was still present 15 minutes after discontinuation of the drug. The different findings in these two studies can be attributed to the very low dose that was used in Heinen and coworkers' study, which was much lower than the doses that are normally used for congestive heart failure or in the intensive care unit setting. In addition, the older study might have used a less sensitive TSH assay. The mechanism for the decrease in TSH in the latter study is unknown, but it is speculated to result from increased TSH clearance and/or central inhibitory effects on TRH and/or TSH production.

β-Adrenergic Receptor Blockers

Alprenolol

Alprenolol is an oral nonselective β-receptor blocker with intrinsic sympathomimetic activity. The effects of alprenolol on thyroid function were studied in a double-blind placebo-controlled trial in euthyroid subjects with a history of myocardial infarction.[318] The results indicated a direct effect of long-term alprenolol treatment on peripheral levels of serum T_4, T_3, and rT_3 in euthyroid subjects, resulting in significant elevation of rT_3. After withdrawal, increases were seen in total T_4, FT_4I, T_3, and FT_3I. These changes in thyroid hormones indicate alprenolol-induced inhibition of 5′ deiodinase in euthyroid subjects.[319]

Atenolol

Atenolol, unlike propranolol, does not cause significant decreases in T_3 levels in hyperthyroid patients. T_4 levels are unaffected by atenolol.[318,320]

Propranolol

Propranolol, a β-adrenergic blocker, is often used as an adjunct in the treatment of thyrotoxicosis. It is also used, in its own right, in the treatment of cardiac arrhythmias and hypertension. Propranolol does not affect the secretion or overall turnover rate of T_4 or TSH release or its regulatory mechanisms. A small to moderate lowering effect on serum T_4 has been reported in euthyroid subjects, as well as in patients with hyperthyroidism or in those with myxedema receiving L-T_3 replacement therapy. Such data,

combined with the findings of reciprocal increases in rT_3 and minimal increases in serum T_4 levels, suggest a mild blocking effect of this drug on the 5′-deiodination of iodothyronines in peripheral tissue. This effect does not appear to be related to the β-adrenergic blocking action of propranolol, because other β-blocking agents do not share the deiodinase-blocking property.[321,322]

Clearly, amelioration of the clinical manifestations of thyrotoxicosis is related to the β-adrenergic blocking action of propranolol rather than to its effect on thyronine metabolism. Whether in fact it alters the hypermetabolism of thyrotoxicosis is debatable.

Immune-Modulating Drugs

Interferons and interleukins have been associated with the development of both hypothyroidism and thyrotoxicosis.[323-327] They are used in the treatment of infectious diseases such as hepatitis, as well as in malignancies, including melanoma and renal cell carcinoma. Acute administration has been used as a model of illness because the effects are similar: interferon-α leads to a decrease in T_3, an increase in rT_3, and a fall in TSH.[324]

Cytokine-induced thyroid disease appears to be immune mediated. The incidence is much greater in females and in patients with positive TPO antibodies before the initiation of therapy.[323,325,326] During therapy, patients who were antibody positive can have a rise in titer, whereas antibody positivity can develop in previously negative patients. In patients who are treated with interferon, the incidence of thyroid disease is much higher in those with hepatitis C than in those with hepatitis B. Thyrotoxicosis often occurs as a manifestation of a destructive thyroiditis. In most patients, the thyroid disease resolves within several months after cessation of cytokine therapy.

Etanercept

Etanercept is a tumor necrosis factor (TNF) antagonist that works by binding to TNF-α and TNF-β, cytokines that are involved in the inflammatory response, blocking their interaction with the TNF receptor. It is used in rheumatoid arthritis, psoriatic arthritis, and ankylosing spondylitis. The development of transient hyperthyroidism in a patient with rheumatoid arthritis after 6 months of etanercept therapy has been reported.[328] No evidence of autoimmune thyroid disease was found, etanercept was continued, and after symptomatic control was achieved with propranolol, thyroid function normalized.

Interferon-α_2

Three types of thyroid dysfunction are associated with interferon-α_2 (IFN-α_2): autoimmune subclinical hypothyroidism, destructive thyroiditis, and Graves' hyperthyroidism,[329-331] all of which may occur at any time during the course of treatment, with a median date of onset of 17 weeks after initiation of treatment.[332] Several different mechanisms have been proposed for the effects of IFN-α_2 on thyroid function. IFN-α_{2b} has been shown to inhibit thyroid follicular cell proliferation and thyroglobulin release in vitro. Second, cell-surface expression of major histocompatibility class I and intercellular adhesion molecules has been found to be increased by IFN-α_{2b}, but not class II MHC molecules, implicating an autoimmune mechanism.[333] Risk factors for development of thyroid dysfunction with IFN-α_2, which might persist after discontinuation of the drug, include female gender, underlying malignancy, high doses used for a long duration, combination of immunotherapy especially with interleukin-2 (IL-2), and the presence of TPO antibodies before treatment is begun. The development of thyroid dysfunction does not seem to be related to IFN-α dosage or to the virologic response to treatment.[334]

Interferon-β_l

Interferon-β (IFN-β) is an approved treatment for multiple sclerosis, and antithyroid autoantibodies and thyroid dysfunction have been reported in such patients who are treated with IFN-β.[335,336] However, a recent longitudinal study of 156 patients with multiple sclerosis treated with IFN-β who were followed over a year did not demonstrate a significantly increased frequency of thyroid dysfunction over time. In addition, this study did not find any correlation of the thyroid dysfunction to antithyroid autoantibody positivity.[337]

In addition, the interferons (α, β, and γ), IL-1, and TNF-α are known to inhibit iodine organification and hormone release and to modulate Tg production and thyrocyte growth.

Interleukin-2 (Aldesleukin)

IL-2 causes thyroid impairment in 20% to 35% of patients. They present commonly with a painless thyroiditis with hyperthyroxinemia followed by primary hypothyroidism, which may last for months and possibly be irreversible. The mechanism of IL-2–induced autoimmune thyroid disease is unclear, although disruption of self-tolerance has been suggested.[338]

IL-2 has also been found to have a stimulatory effect in the hypothalamic-pituitary axis, resulting in an increase in TSH with a significant increase in T_4 and T_3 in vivo in HIV-positive patients without thyroid disease.[339] This finding was supported by an in vitro study of IL-2 on the anterior pituitary, which demonstrated IL-2 stimulation of TSH release.[340]

Interleukin-6

IL-6 is produced in response to inflammatory and noninflammatory stress and regulates the acute phase response. IL-6 is thought to be involved in the thyroid function abnormalities in nonthyroidal illness. Torpy and co-workers[340a] studied the effects of a single dose of IL-6 in healthy subjects and found a 27% decrease in TSH, elevation of FT_4, and elevation of rT_3. T_3/rT_3 levels are similar to levels seen in nonthyroidal illness and are thought to result from inhibition of type 1 5'-deiodinase. IL-6 also inhibits release of TSH.

Chemotherapy

Several combination chemotherapy regimens may result in an increased incidence of primary hypothyroidism. These include (1) cisplatin, bleomycin, vinblastine, etoposide, and dactinomycin, which resulted in primary hypothyroidism in 15% of testicular cancer patients who were treated with this combination compared with a control group[341]; (2) mechlorethamine, vinblastine, procarbazine, and prednisolone regimen in patients with Hodgkin's disease, which resulted in an elevated TSH in 44%,[342] although interpretation is difficult in the presence of concurrent radiation; and (3) brain irradiation, vincristine, carmustine, or lomustine, and procarbazine given to children with brain tumors not involving the hypothalamic-pituitary axis, which resulted in a 35% incidence of hypothyroidism, compared with a 10% incidence in those who received brain irradiation alone.[343]

5-Fluorouracil

5-Fluorourcil increases total T_4 and T_3 levels, but patients are clinically euthyroid with a normal FT_4I and a normal level of TSH, suggesting an effect on thyroid hormone–binding proteins.

Alklylating Agents (Cyclophosphamide and Ifosfamide)

Intravenous administration of cyclophosphamide and ifosfamide has been demonstrated to induce a transient increase in T_4 and FT_4 with a concomitant fall in TSH in the presence of normal Tg, T_3, and TBG concentrations. The changes are thought to be due to a release of thyroxine from extrathyroidal tissues such as the liver.[344]

Aminoglutethimide

Aminoglutethimide blocks several cytochrome P-450–mediated steroid hydroxylation steps, including those that are required for conversion of cholesterol to pregnenolone and for the aromatization of androgens to estrogens. Through these actions, it blocks adrenal steroidogenesis and the production of estrogens in extraglandular tissues and has been used in Cushing's syndrome and breast cancer as well as adrenal and prostate cancer.[345] In a study of breast cancer patients who were receiving only a low dose of 125 mg per day of aminoglutethimide, little effect on thyroid function was noted.[346] However, a dose of 1000 mg per day of aminoglutethimide in prostate cancer patients resulted in clinical and biochemical evidence of hypothyroidism in 31% with TSH above 10 mU/L.[347]

L-Asparaginase

L-Asparaginase affects serum thyroid hormone levels by inhibiting synthesis of TBG and albumin, resulting in low total but normal FT_4 values. It might also cause hypothalamic or pituitary hypothyroidism. This was suggested by a study of 14 children with acute leukemia who were being treated with L-asparaginase and prednisone, 9 of whom had low free T_4 levels with normal basal TSH and 6 of whom had blunted TSH response to TRH. The effects might be from the prednisone but might also be from the L-asparaginase.[348,349]

Sunitinib

Tyrosine kinase inhibitors target various growth factor receptors and are antitumorigenic and antiangiogenic. Sunitinib was approved by the Food and Drug Administration in 2006 for treatment of renal cell carcinoma and gastrointestinal stromal tumor and recently has been shown to be effective in advanced stages of metastatic thyroid cancer. Hypothyroidism has been reported by several investigators in patients taking sunitinib.[350-352] One proposed mechanism for the thyroid dysfunction is the blocking of iodine uptake.

Minerals and Resins

Aluminum Hydroxide

Reports of elevated TSH have been found in patients taking levothyroxine concurrently with aluminum hydroxide. This is presumably the result of decreased bioavailability of levothyroxine via a mechanism involving nonspecific adsorption, or complexing, of levothyroxine to the aluminum hydroxide.[353]

Calcium Carbonate

The coadministration of calcium carbonate and levothyroxine has been reported to decrease L-T_4 absorption and result in increased TSH levels and decreased serum T_4 levels.[354] Singh and coworkers[354] studied the effects of calcium carbonate administration on serum thyroid hormone levels and TSH in 20 patients with hypothyroidism on a stable regimen of L-T_4. With the use of calcium carbonate, levels of free and total T_4 were significantly reduced, and TSH concentrations were significantly increased, some levels being above the normal range. L-T$_4$ was found to adsorb to calcium carbonate in vitro in an acidic environment, which probably reduces its absorption and bioavailability.

Ferrous Sulfate

Ferrous sulfate has been reported to decrease thyroxine absorption via binding of L-T$_4$ to the ferrous sulfate when coadministered. This has been found to be clinically significant in some patients who manifested increased signs and symptoms of hypothyroidism as well as elevated TSH levels.[355]

High Fiber

Decreased T$_4$ bioavailability has also been reported with the use of dietary fiber through a mechanism involving nonspecific adsorption of T$_4$ to dietary fibers. The authors concluded that increased intake of dietary fiber might account for the need for larger than expected doses of L-T$_4$ in some hypothyroid patients.[353]

Soybeans

Interference of soy-based formulas with L-T$_4$ absorption was reported in infants with congenital hypothyroidism who were found to have increased L-T$_4$ requirements while taking soy formula and decreased requirements on discontinuation of the soy product.[356]

Sucralfate

Sucralfate also results in diminished levothyroxine absorption, presumably by intraluminal binding of the hormone. Separating dosing of sucralfate and levothyroxine by 8 hours prevented this effect.[357]

Iodide and Iodine-Containing Compounds

Iodine has complex effects on the thyroid gland and is recognized as causing both hypothyroidism and hyperthyroidism or inducing goiter formation. The effect of iodine on thyroid function is dependent on a number of variables: the total dose, the rate of administration, previous iodine status, and the presence or absence of underlying thyroid dysfunction.

Uptake and organification (the Wolff-Chaikoff effect) of iodine are inhibited in the presence of iodine excess. Under these circumstances, the stimulatory effect of TSH, via adenyl cyclase, is also reduced. Excess iodine may inhibit proteolytic enzymes that are responsible for cleaving T$_3$ and T$_4$ before release.[358] It has been recognized that iodine might also reduce the peripheral conversion of T$_4$ to T$_3$ by inhibition of 5'-monodeiodinase.[359] The net effect of excess iodine in some euthyroid individuals is hypothyroidism.

Some of the effects of iodine may have an immune basis. Correction of iodine deficiency in depleted areas results in an increased incidence of autoimmune thyroid disease.[360] One of the mechanisms proposed to explain this phenomenon involves increased iodination of Tg, which results in increased immunogenicity and subsequently leads to autoantibody formation. Indirect evidence for a primary immunogenic role has also been achieved through in vitro studies. Such experiments, which used cultured lymphocytes grown in the presence of iodine, revealed increased quantities of IgG production.[361] Patients with high titers of thyroid autoantibodies are also more likely to acquire hypothyroidism after iodine administration.[362]

Induction of hyperthyroidism by iodine is almost exclusively limited to patients who have underlying thyroid disease,[363] which often occurs secondary to iodine deficiency in the first place.

Administration of iodine to iodine-deficient subjects with nodular goiters can induce the autonomous secretion of excess thyroid hormone. Hyperthyroidism induced via these means is known as Jod-Basedow disease. Iodine-induced hyperthyroidism may also be seen in the absence of nodular goiter, especially in patients with autoantibodies to thyroid antigens.

Iodine can have profound and variable effects on thyroid function, although rarely in iodine-replete areas do these effects become clinically relevant. Only some drugs that contain very large doses of iodine can cause abnormalities in thyroid function in normal, healthy individuals. These drugs are discussed below.

Amiodarone

Amiodarone is a very potent and effective antiarrhythmic agent derived from benzofuran that contains large quantities of iodine (37% by weight). It bears some structural homology with thyroid hormones, and among its array of potential side effects,[364] abnormalities in thyroid function tests are common during its administration. These abnormalities are similar to those that are seen with iodine-containing contrast agents and include a marked decrease in serum T$_3$, an increase in rT$_3$, and a more modest elevation in the T$_4$ concentration. Basal and TRH-stimulated TSH levels are increased. All these changes can occur as early as 1 week after institution of amiodarone therapy. The principal mechanism of action is believed to be inhibition of T$_3$ generation from T$_4$ in peripheral tissues and in the pituitary gland.[365,366] Amiodarone also directly stimulates TSH secretion from cultured thyrotrophs. Metabolic studies in humans have shown clearance rates of T$_4$ and rT$_3$ to be reduced with a concomitant reduction in the rate of production of T$_3$.

Despite changes in thyroid function, clinically relevant thyroid dysfunction develops in only a minority of patients who take amiodarone. Hypothyroidism is reported to be more common in iodine-replete areas, whereas hyperthyroidism has a higher prevalence in iodine-deficient areas. The iodine dependence of both these diseases is confirmed by the improvement in both with the use of perchlorate to discharge iodine from the thyroid gland. A second form of thyrotoxicosis that is a destructive thyroiditis does not respond to antithyroid drugs or perchlorate but is responsive to steroid therapy.[367] The development of overt thyroid disease is also more common in subjects with a past history of thyroid disease and in those with goiter or evidence of autoimmune-related thyroid disease. Because most patients treated with amiodarone have abnormalities on thyroid function tests, clinical assessment of the patient is extremely important in the diagnosis of overt thyroid disease. Clinical assessment is complicated, however, by the α-adrenergic receptor and the β-adrenergic receptor blocking properties of the drug, which mask some of the symptoms and signs of hyperthyroidism. The clinical picture therefore might not be typical, and symptoms of tiredness and weight loss often predominate. Despite a paucity of symptoms, a number of serious and occasionally fatal cases of amiodarone-induced thyrotoxicosis have been reported.[368,369] Drug-induced thyroiditis can also cause thyrotoxicosis, which often is followed by transient hypothyroidism.

Amiodarone metabolites compete with thyroid hormone for its receptor, but it is uncertain to what extent this action is of physiologic relevance at the concentrations obtained at the tissue level. The bradycardia that almost invariably occurs when the drug is used in high doses might suggest the presence of hypothyroidism. Measurement of serum TSH, the most useful test in the differential diagnosis of this condition, may also give misleading results, however. If hypothyroidism is suspected, measurement of the serum rT_3 concentration could be helpful. Failure to show high serum levels of this iodothyronine in a patient receiving amiodarone can be considered indicative of hypothyroidism, and a suppressed serum TSH value with a normal serum T_3 concentration might indicate mild thyrotoxicosis. Overt hyperthyroidism should not be diagnosed on the basis of an elevated T_4 level alone; similarly, a modestly elevated TSH with a low T_3 concentration is not necessarily indicative of hypothyroidism.

Cellasene

Cellasene (from Rexall Sundown, Boca Raton, FL), a product containing ginkgo biloba, sweet clover, seaweed, grape seed oil, lecithin, and evening primrose oil, has been marketed all over the world as a miracle cure for cellulite. The seaweed in the product, similar to kelp, has 930 μg of iodine per recommended dose of three capsules, which could interfere with thyroid function.[370,371]

Iodinated Contrast Agents

Some radiographic contrast media contain large amounts of iodine; for example, a 3 g dose of ipodate (used in oral cholecystography) contains 1.8 g of iodine. The principal effect of this agent is to inhibit deiodination of T_4 to T_3 in peripheral tissues and in the pituitary,[372] which results in a profound decrease in the serum T_3 concentration and an increase in rT_3 and T_4 levels[373,374] in association with a rise in serum TSH. This effect occurs in all individuals and is not the consequence of released iodine. The serum T_4 concentration can reach values that are well within the thyrotoxic range. These changes are maximal 3 to 4 days after administration and disappear within 14 days.

Iodocontrast agents also decrease the hepatic uptake of T_4[375] and inhibit T_3 binding to its nuclear receptors. The antithyroidal effect of the iodine released from these agents is believed to be responsible for the falling T_4 level and amelioration of the symptoms and signs of thyrotoxicosis when they are administered to patients with Graves' thyrotoxicosis.

Miscellaneous

Antithyroid Drugs

Agents that act principally by inhibiting thyroid hormone synthesis are collectively called goitrogens or antithyroid drugs. A number of these compounds occur naturally in foodstuffs. Others are used in the treatment of thyrotoxicosis. A list of substances that inhibit thyroid hormone synthesis and secretion is provided in Table 6-13.

Highly Active Antiretroviral Therapy

D4T (stavudine) has been found to be associated with subclinical hypothyroidism. The incidence of thyroid dysfunction correlates with the cumulative dose and duration. The mechanism involved is uncertain, but D4T is thought to perhaps interfere directly with synthesis or catabolism of thyroid hormones.[376,377] In a study of 697 HIV-infected patients, treatment with stavudine and low CD4 cell count were associated with hypothyroidism.[378]

A regimen that includes D4T and lamivudine (3TC) and a protease inhibitor (indinavir or ritonavir) was found to be associated with immune restoration and thyroid-specific immunity resulting in Graves' disease in five patients.

Heparin

Serum FT_4 concentrations increase transiently after intravenous heparin administration.[379] This is caused by inhibition of protein

Table 6-13. Agents That Inhibit Thyroid Hormone Synthesis and Secretion

Substance	Common Use
Block Iodide Transport Into the Thyroid Gland	
Monovalent anions (SCN^-, ClO_4^-, NO_3^-)	Not in current use; ClO_4 test agent
Complex anions (monofluorosulfonate, difluorophosphate, fluoroborate)	—
Minerals	In diet
Lithium	Treatment of manic-depressive psychosis
Ethionamide	Antituberculosis drug
Impair Tg Iodination and Iodotyrosine Coupling	
Thionamides and thiourylenes (PTU, methimazole, carbimazole)	Antithyroid drugs
Sulfonamides (acetazolamide, sulfadiazine, sulfisoxazole)	Diuretic, bacteriostatic
Sulfonylureas (carbutamide, tolbutamide, metahexamide, ? chlorpropamide)	Hypoglycemic agents
Salicylamides (aminosalicylic acid)	Antituberculosis drugs
Ethionamide (p-aminobenzoic acid)	
Resorcinol	Cutaneous antiseptic
Amphenone and aminoglutethimide	Antiadrenal and anticonvulsive agents
Thiocyanate	No current use; in diet
Antipyrine (phenazone)	Antiasthmatic
Aminotriazole	Cranberry poison
Amphenidone	Tranquilizer
2,3-Dimercaptopropanol (BAL)	Chelating agent
Ketoconazole	Antifungal agent
Induction of Autoimmunity	
Interleukins	
Interferons α, β, γ	
Inhibitor of Deiodinase	
Alprenolol	
Inhibitors of Thyroid Hormone Secretion	
Iodide (in large doses)	Antiseptic, expectorant, and others
Lithium	
Mechanism Unknown	
p-Bromdylamine maleate	Antihistaminic
Phenylbutazone	Antiinflammatory agent
Minerals (calcium, rubidium, cobalt)	
Gabapentin	Psychoneurologic

BAL, Bronchoalveolar lavage; *PTU,* propylthiouracil; *Tg,* thyroglobulin.

binding of T_4 by free fatty acids generated by in vitro heparin-induced activation of lipoprotein lipase. This effect is seen not only with intravenous heparin, but also with subcutaneous enoxaparin.

Nitrophenols

2,4-Dinitrophenol elevates the BMR, lowers the serum T_4 concentration, accelerates the peripheral metabolism of T_4, and depresses thyroidal RAIU and secretion.[380,381] Its actions are probably complex. Like T_4, the drug stimulates metabolism by uncoupling oxidative phosphorylation in mitochondria. Part of the effect of dinitrophenol may be to mimic the action of thyroid hormone on hypothalamic or pituitary receptor control centers; this effect would account for the diminished thyroid activity. Dinitrophenol also displaces thyroid hormone from T_4-binding serum proteins; this action could lower the total hormone concentration in serum but should have no persistent effect on thyroid function. Dinitrophenol increases biliary and fecal excretion of T_4, and this action largely accounts for the rapid removal of hormone from the circulation. Deiodination of T_4 is also increased. 2,4-Dinitrophenol does not share some of the most important properties of T_4. It cannot initiate tadpole metamorphosis or provide substitution therapy in myxedema.

Rifampin

Rifampin, like phenobarbital and phenytoin, increases thyroid hormone metabolism by stimulating hepatic microsomal drug-metabolizing enzyme activity. In a study of healthy male volunteers who were given rifampin, hepatic microsomal enzyme activity assessed by antipyrine clearance demonstrated a significant increase, median thyroid volume increased, and FT_4 decreased.[382] The induced changes resolved after cessation of treatment, supporting the hypothesis that induced hepatic degradation of thyroid hormones results in a compensatory mechanism of increased thyroid volume, increased T_4 secretion, and maintenance of euthyroid status in normal volunteers. However, in patients who are on thyroid replacement, increased doses of L-T_4 might be necessary. Nolan and coworkers reported the case of a man, stable on levothyroxine, who exhibited significantly elevated TSH levels during rifampin therapy that returned to baseline 9 days after discontinuance of rifampin.[383]

Salicylates and Nonsteroidal Antiinflammatory Drug

Salicylate and its noncalorigenic congeners compete for thyroid hormone–binding sites on TTR and TBG in serum and thereby cause a decline in T_4 and T_3 concentrations and an increase in their free fractions. The turnover rate of T_4 is accelerated, but degradation rates remain normal.[384,385] Furthermore, they suppress thyroidal RAIU but do not retard iodine release from the thyroid gland.[386] Thus, the hypermetabolic effect of this drug was attributed to the increase in FT_4 and FT_3 fractions. If this proposed explanation were correct, hormonal release from the serum hormone–binding proteins should produce only temporary suppression of thyroidal RAIU and transient hypermetabolism. In fact, both effects have been observed during chronic administration of salicylates. In addition, this mechanism of action does not explain the lack of calorigenic effect of some salicylate congeners despite their ability to also displace thyroid hormone from its serum hormone–binding proteins. In vitro studies have demonstrated an inhibitory effect of salicylate on the outer-ring monodeiodination of both T_4 and rT_3, but lack of typical changes in the relative levels of serum iodothyronine suggests that this action is less important in vivo. Similar abnormalities in thyroid function tests have been noted in patients treated with salsalate.[387]

Acetylsalicylic acid mimics the action of thyroid hormone in several ways. For example, it lowers the serum cholesterol level,[388] but it does not provide a therapeutic effect in myxedema or lower TSH levels.[389] Administration of 8 g of aspirin daily raises the BMR and accelerates the circulation, suggesting that changes in blood flow in thyrotoxicosis and myxedema are secondary to heat production rather than to primary effects of the hormone on the circulation.

p-Aminosalicylic acid and p-aminobenzoic acid are closely related chemically to salicylate. They inhibit iodide binding in the thyroid gland and are goitrogenic.[390,391]

The proposed sequence of events based on studies of the effects of nonsteroidal antiinflammatory drugs (NSAIDs) and salicylates on thyroid function is an initial displacement of thyroid hormone from protein-binding sites, resulting in transient elevations of circulating free thyroid hormone levels, which temporarily suppress TSH and then cause a transient decrease in thyroid hormone concentrations. Salicylates at doses of more than 2.0 g per day and salsalate at doses of 1.5 to 3.0 g per day inhibit binding of T_4 and T_3 to TBG. In addition to aspirin and salsalates, other NSAIDs have been evaluated, the most common ones being fenclofenac and mefenamic acid, and have been found to displace thyroid hormones from protein-binding sites.[392] More recent studies have evaluated more commonly used NSAIDs, such as ibuprofen, naproxen, diclofenac, sulindac, and indomethacin, as compared with aspirin and salsalate.[393] One study of 25 healthy subjects who were given aspirin, salsalate, meclofenamate, ibuprofen, naproxen, or indomethacin at doses that patients usually choose for acute, limited, painful conditions showed that aspirin and salsalate induced decreases in mean total and free thyroid hormone measurements with associated changes in TSH after 1 week, confirming findings of older studies; it is interesting to note that meclofenamate induced acute increases in mean total T_4, T_3, and free T_3 levels at 2 hours after a single dose but did not affect mean levels of thyroid hormones over a period of 1 week.[394] Commonly used NSAIDs, such as ibuprofen, naproxen, and indomethacin, however, did not significantly affect thyroid hormone levels after a single dose or over 1 week of drug administration. Another study showed depression of T_3 with use of diclofenac sodium and naproxen but unchanged serum T_4 and T_3 in patients who were treated with diflunisal, ibuprofen, indomethacin, piroxicam, or sulindac. Aceclofenac, another NSAID, leads to significant redistribution of T_3 protein binding, displacement of T_3 from TBG, and increased binding to albumin.[395]

Acknowledgments

The authors would like to acknowledge the contributions of authors of past versions of this chapter, Drs. Sharon Wu, David Sarne, Neil J. L. Gittoes, Jayne A. Franklyn, Michael C. Sheppard. Supported in part by NIH Grants RR00055, DK15070, DK 58258, RR 18372, and DK07011 and The Seymour J. Abrams Center for Thyroid Research and Rabbi Morris Esformes Endowment.

REFERENCES

1. Modan B, Baidatz D, Mart H, et al: Radiation-induced head and neck tumours. Lancet 1:277–279, 1974.
2. Summary of current radiation dose estimates to humans from 123I, 124I, 125I, 126I, 130I, 131I, and 132I as sodium iodide, J Nucl Med 16:857–860, 1975.
3. MIRD/Dose Estimate Report No. 8. Summary of current radiation dose estimates to normal humans from 99mTc as sodium pertechnetate, J Nucl Med 17:74–77, 1976.
4. Quimby EH, Feitelberg S, Gross W: Radioactive Nuclides in Medicine and Biology, ed 3, Philadelphia, 1970, Lea & Febiger.
5. Iodine. In Dietary Reference Intakes for vitamin A, vitamin K, arsenic, boron, chromium, copper, iodine, iron, manganese, molybdenum, nickel, silicon, vanadium and zinc, Washington, D.C., 2001, National Academy Press, pp 258–289,
6. Hollowell JG, Staehling NW, Hannon WH, et al: Iodine nutrition in the United States. Trends and public health implications: iodine excretion data from National Health and Nutrition Examination Surveys I and III (1971–1974 and 1988–1994), J Clin Endocrinol Metab 83:3401–3408, 1998.
7. Dai G, Levy O, Carrasco N: Cloning and characterization of the thyroid iodide transporter, Nature 379:458–460, 1996.
8. Stanbury JB, Chapman EM: Congenital hypothyroidism with goitre: absence of an iodide-concentrating mechanism, Lancet 1:1162–1165, 1960.
9. Chopra IJ: A radioimmunoassay for measurement of 3,3'-diiodothyronine sulfate: Studies in thyroidal and nonthyroidal diseases, pregnancy, and fetal/neonatal life, Metabolism 53:538–543, 2004.
10. Gavin LA, Livermore BM, Cavalieri RR, et al: Serum concentration, metabolic clearance, and production rates of 3,5,3'-triiodothyroacetic acid in normal and athyreotic man, J Clin Endocrinol Metab 51:529–534, 1980.
11. Trevorrow V: Studies on the nature of the iodine in blood, J Biol Chem 127:737–750, 1939.

12. Fang VS, Refetoff S: Radioimmunoassay for serum triiodothyronine: evaluation of simple techniques to control interference from binding proteins, Clin Chem 20:1150–1154, 1974.
13. Larsen PR, Dockalova J, Sipula D, et al: Immunoassay of thyroxine in unextracted human serum, J Clin Endocrinol Metab 37:177–182, 1973.
14. Sterling K, Milch PO: Thermal inactivation of thyroxine-binding globulin for direct radioimmunoassay of triiodothyronine in serum, J Clin Endocrinol Metab 38:866–875, 1974.
15. Soukhova N, Soldin OP, Soldin SJ: Isotope dilution tandem mass spectrometric method for T4/T3, Clin Chim Acta 343:185–190, 2004.
16. Burman KD, Bongiovanni R, Garis RK, et al: Measurement of serum T4 concentration by high performance liquid chromatography, J Clin Endocrinol Metab 53:909–912, 1981.
17. Kahric-Janicic N, Soldin SJ, Soldin OP, et al: Tandem mass spectrometry improves the accuracy of free thyroxine measurements during pregnancy, Thyroid 17:303–311, 2007.
18. Tai SS, Sniegoski LT, Welch MJ: Candidate reference method for total thyroxine in human serum: use of isotope-dilution liquid chromatography-mass spectrometry with electrospray ionization, Clin Chem 48:637–642, 2002.
19. Thienpont LM, De Brabandere VI, Stockl D, et al: Development of a new method for the determination of thyroxine in serum based on isotope dilution gas chromatography mass spectrometry, Biol Mass Spectrom 23:475–482, 1994.
20. Yue B, Rockwood AL, Sandrock T, et al: Free thyroid hormones in serum by direct equilibrium dialysis and online solid-phase extraction—liquid chromatography/tandem mass spectrometry, Clin Chem 54:642–651, 2008.
21. Refetoff S: Inherited thyroxine-binding globulin abnormalities in man, Endocr Rev 10:275–293, 1989.
22. De Costre P, Buhler U, DeGroot LJ, et al: Diurnal rhythm in total serum thyroxine levels, Metabolism 20:782–791, 1971.
23. Franklyn JA, Ramsden DB, Sheppard MC: The influence of age and sex on tests of thyroid function, Ann Clin Biochem 22(Pt 5):502–505, 1985.
24. Westgren U, Burger A, Ingemansson S, et al: Blood levels of 3,5,3′-triiodothyronine and thyroxine: differences between children, adults, and elderly subjects, Acta Med Scand 200:493–495, 1976.
25. Welle S, O'Connell M, Danforth E Jr, et al: Decreased free fraction of serum thyroid hormones during carbohydrate overfeeding, Metabolism 33:837–839, 1984.
26. Dumitrescu AM, Liao XH, Abdullah MS, et al: Mutations in SECISBP2 result in abnormal thyroid hormone metabolism, Nat Genet 37:1247–1252, 2005.
27. Dumitrescu AM, Liao XH, Best TB, et al: A novel syndrome combining thyroid and neurological abnormalities is associated with mutations in a monocarboxylate transporter gene, Am J Hum Genet 74:168–175, 2004.
28. Chopra IJ, Williams DE, Orgiazzi J, et al: Opposite effects of dexamethasone on serum concentrations of 3,3′,5′-triiodothyronine (reverse T3) and 3,3′5-triiodothyronine (T3), J Clin Endocrinol Metab 41:911–920, 1975.
29. Davies PH, Franklyn JA: The effects of drugs on tests of thyroid function, Eur J Clin Pharmacol 40:439–451, 1991.
30. Busnardo B, Vagelista R, Girelli ME, et al: TSH levels and TSH response to TRH as a guide to the replacement treatment of patients with thyroid carcinoma, J Clin Endocrinol Metab 42:901–906, 1976.
31. Miyai K, Fukuchi M, Kumahara Y: Correlation between biological and immunological potencies of human serum and pituitary thyrotropin, J Clin Endocrinol Metab 29:1438–1442, 1969.
32. Refetoff S, Murata Y, Vassart G, et al: Radioimmunoassays specific for the tertiary and primary structures of thyroxine-binding globulin (TBG): measurement of denatured TBG in serum, J Clin Endocrinol Metab 59:269–277, 1984.
33. Sadow PM, Chassande O, Gauthier K, et al: Specificity of thyroid hormone receptor subtype and steroid receptor coactivator-1 on thyroid hormone action, Am J Physiol Endocrinol Metab 284:E36–46, 2003.
34. Hernandez A, St Germain DL: Thyroid hormone deiodinases: physiology and clinical disorders, Curr Opin Pediatr 15:416–420, 2003.
35. Koenig RJ: Ubiquitinated deiodinase: not dead yet, J Clin Invest 112:145–147, 2003.
36. Refetoff S, Dumitrescu AM: Syndromes of reduced sensitivity to thyroid hormone: genetic defects in hormone receptors, cell transporters and deiodination, Best Pract Res Clin Endocrinol Metab 21:277–305, 2007.
37. Nelson JC, Tomei RT: Direct determination of free thyroxin in undiluted serum by equilibrium dialysis/radioimmunoassay, Clin Chem 34:1737–1744, 1988.
38. Surks MI, DeFesi CR: Normal serum free thyroid hormone concentrations in patients treated with phenytoin or carbamazepine. A paradox resolved, JAMA 275:1495–1498, 1996.
39. Oppenheimer JH, Squef R, Surks MI, et al: Binding of thyroxine by serum proteins evaluated by equilibrum dialysis and electrophoretic techniques. Alterations in nonthyroidal illness, J Clin Invest 42:1769–1782, 1963.
40. Nuutila P, Koskinen P, Irjala K, et al: Two new two-step immunoassays for free thyroxin evaluated: solid-phase radioimmunoassay and time-resolved fluoroimmunoassay, Clin Chem 36:1355–1360, 1990.
41. Wilkins TA, Midgley JE, Barron N: Comprehensive study of a thyroxin-analog-based assay for free thyroxin ("Amerlex FT4"), Clin Chem 31:1644–1653, 1985.
42. Stockigt JR, Stevens V, White EL, et al: "Unbound analog" radioimmunoassays for free thyroxin measure the albumin-bound hormone fraction, Clin Chem 29:1408–1410, 1983.
43. Christofides ND, Sheehan CP: Enhanced chemiluminescence labeled-antibody immunoassay (Amerlite-MAB) for free thyroxine: design, development, and technical validation, Clin Chem 41:17–23, 1995.
44. Christofides ND, Sheehan CP: Multicenter evaluation of enhanced chemiluminescence labeled-antibody immunoassay ("Amerlite-MAB") for free thyroxine, Clin Chem 41:24–31, 1995.
45. Costongs GM, van Oers RJ, Leerkes B, et al: Evaluation of the DPC IMMULITE random access immunoassay analyser, Eur J Clin Chem Clin Biochem 33:887–892, 1995.
46. Letellier M, Levesque A, Daigle F, et al: Performance evaluation of automated immunoassays on the Technicon Immuno 1 system, Clin Chem 42:1695–1701, 1996.
47. Liewendahl K, Majuri H, Helenius T: Thyroid function tests in patients on long-term treatment with various anticonvulsant drugs, Clin Endocrinol (Oxf) 8:185–191, 1978.
48. Vogeser M, Jacob K: Measurement of free triiodothyronine in intensive care patients—comparison of two routine methods, Eur J Clin Chem Clin Biochem 35:873–875, 1997.
49. Chopra IJ: An assessment of daily production and significance of thyroidal secretion of 3,3′,5′-triiodothyronine (reverse T3) in man, J Clin Invest 58:32–40, 1976.
50. O'Connell M, Robbins DC, Bogardus C, et al: The interaction of free fatty acids in radioimmunoassays for reverse triiodothyronine, J Clin Endocrinol Metab 55:577–582, 1982.
51. Chopra IJ: A radioimmunoassay for measurement of 3,3′,5′-triiodothyronine (reverse T3), J Clin Invest 54:583–592, 1974.
52. Burman KD, Wright FD, Smallridge RC, et al: A radioimmunoassay for 3′,5′-diiodothyronine, J Clin Endocrinol Metab 47:1059–1064, 1978.
53. Chopra IJ, Geola F, Solomon DH, et al: 3′-5′-Diiodothyronine in health and disease: studies by a radioimmunoassay, J Clin Endocrinol Metab 47:1198–1207, 1978.
54. Nakamura Y, Chopra IJ, Solomon DH: An assessment of the concentration of acetic acid and propionic acid derivatives of 3,5,3′-triiodothyronine in human serum, J Clin Endocrinol Metab 46:91–97, 1978.
55. Pittman CS, Shimizu T, Burger A, et al: The nondeiodinative pathways of thyroxine metabolism: 3,5,3′,5-tetraiodothyroacetic acid turnover in normal and fasting human subjects, J Clin Endocrinol Metab 50:712–716, 1980.
56. Pittman CS, Suda AK, Chambers JB Jr, et al: Abnormalities of thyroid hormone turnover in patients with diabetes mellitus before and after insulin therapy, J Clin Endocrinol Metab 48:854–860, 1979.
57. Huang WS, Kuo SW, Chen WL, et al: Increased urinary excretion of sulfated 3,3′,5′-triiodothyronine in patients with nodular goiters receiving suppressive thyroxine therapy, Thyroid 6:91–96, 1996.
58. Nelson JD, Lewis JE: Radioimmunoassay of iodotyrosines. In: Abraham GE editor. Handbook of Radioimmunoassay, New York, 1979, Marcel Dekker.
59. Afink G, Kulik W, Overmars H, et al: Molecular characterization of iodotyrosine dehalogenase deficiency in patients with hypothyroidism, J Clin Endocrinol Metab 93:4894–4901, 2008.
60. Piehl S, Heberer T, Balizs G, et al: Thyronamines are isozyme-specific substrates of deiodinases, Endocrinology 149:3037–3045, 2008.
61. Chiellini G, Frascarelli S, Ghelardoni S, et al: Cardiac effects of 3-iodothyronamine: a new aminergic system modulating cardiac function, FASEB J 21:1597–1608, 2007.
62. Scanlan TS, Suchland KL, Hart ME, et al: 3-Iodothyronamine is an endogenous and rapid-acting derivative of thyroid hormone, Nat Med 10:638–642, 2004.
63. Spencer CA, Takeuchi M, Kazarosyan M, et al: Serum thyroglobulin autoantibodies: prevalence, influence on serum thyroglobulin measurement, and prognostic significance in patients with differentiated thyroid carcinoma, J Clin Endocrinol Metab 83:1121–1127, 1998.
64. Massart C, Maugendre D: Importance of the detection method for thyroglobulin antibodies for the validity of thyroglobulin measurements in sera from patients with Graves disease, Clin Chem 48:102–107, 2002.
65. Zophel K, Wunderlich G, Liepach U, et al: [Recovery test or immunoradiometric measurement of anti-thyroglobulin autoantibodies for interpretation of thyroglobulin determination in the follow-up of different thyroid carcinoma], Nuklearmedizin 40:155–163, 2001.
66. Van Herle AJ, Uller RP, Matthews NI, et al: Radioimmunoassay for measurement of thyroglobulin in human serum, J Clin Invest 52:1320–1327, 1973.
67. Pacini F, Pinchera A, Giani C, et al: Serum thyroglobulin in thyroid carcinoma and other thyroid disorders, J Endocrinol Invest 3:283–292, 1980.
68. Pezzino V, Filetti S, Belfiore A, et al: Serum thyroglobulin levels in the newborn, J Clin Endocrinol Metab 52:364–366, 1981.
69. Penny R, Spencer CA, Frasier SD, et al: Thyroid-stimulating hormone and thyroglobulin levels decrease with chronological age in children and adolescents, J Clin Endocrinol Metab 56:177–180, 1983.
70. Refetoff S, Lever EG: The value of serum thyroglobulin measurement in clinical practice, JAMA 250:2352–2357, 1983.
71. Torrens JI, Burch HB: Serum thyroglobulin measurement. Utility in clinical practice, Endocrinol Metab Clin North Am 30:429–467, 2001.
72. Izumi M, Kubo I, Taura M, et al: Kinetic study of immunoreactive human thyroglobulin, J Clin Endocrinol Metab 62:410–412, 1986.
73. Uller RP, Van Herle AJ: Effect of therapy on serum thyroglobulin levels in patients with Graves' disease, J Clin Endocrinol Metab 46:747–755, 1978.
74. Lever EG, Refetoff S, Scherberg NH, et al: The influence of percutaneous fine needle aspiration on serum thyroglobulin, J Clin Endocrinol Metab 56:26–29, 1983.
75. Smallridge RC, De Keyser FM, Van Herle AJ, et al: Thyroid iodine content and serum thyroglobulin: cues to the natural history of destruction-induced thyroiditis, J Clin Endocrinol Metab 62:1213–1219, 1986.
76. Mariotti S, Martino E, Cupini C, et al: Low serum thyroglobulin as a clue to the diagnosis of thyrotoxicosis factitia, N Engl J Med 307:410–412, 1982.
77. Ringel MD, Balducci-Silano PL, Anderson JS, et al: Quantitative reverse transcription-polymerase chain reaction of circulating thyroglobulin messenger ribonucleic acid for monitoring patients with thyroid carcinoma, J Clin Endocrinol Metab 84:4037–4042, 1999.
78. Grammatopoulos D, Elliott Y, Smith SC, et al: Measurement of thyroglobulin mRNA in peripheral blood as an adjunctive test for monitoring thyroid cancer, Molecular Pathology 56:162–166, 2003.
79. Span PN, Sleegers MJ, van den Broek WJ, et al: Quantitative detection of peripheral thyroglobulin mRNA has limited clinical value in the follow-up of thyroid cancer patients, Ann Clin Biochem 40:94–99, 2003.
80. Kawamura S, Kishino B, Tajima K, et al: Serum thyroglobulin changes in patients with Graves' disease

treated with long term antithyroid drug therapy, J Clin Endocrinol Metab 56:507–512, 1983.
81. Heinze HJ, Shulman DI, Diamond FB Jr, et al: Spectrum of serum thyroglobulin elevation in congenital thyroid disorders, Thyroid 3:37–40, 1993.
82. Czernichow P, Schlumberger M, Pomarede R, et al: Plasma thyroglobulin measurements help determine the type of thyroid defect in congenital hypothyroidism, J Clin Endocrinol Metab 56:242–245, 1983.
83. Burke CW, Shakespear RA, Fraser TR: Measurement of thyroxine and triiodothyronine in human urine, Lancet 2:1177–1179, 1972.
84. Chan V, Landon J: Urinary thyroxine excretion as index of thyroid function, Lancet 1:4–6, 1972.
85. Chan V, Landon J, Besser GM, et al: Urinary tri-iodothyronine excretion as index of thyroid function, Lancet 2:253–256, 1972.
86. Gaitan JE, Wahner HW, Gorman CA, et al: Measurement of triiodothyronine in unextracted urine, J Lab Clin Med 86:538–546, 1975.
87. Yoshida K, Sakurada T, Takahashi T, et al: Measurement of TSH in human amniotic fluid: diagnosis of fetal thyroid abnormality in utero, Clin Endocrinol (Oxf) 25:313–318, 1986.
88. Thorpe-Beeston JG, Nicolaides KH, McGregor AM: Fetal thyroid function, Thyroid 2:207–217, 1992.
89. Chopra IJ, Crandall BF: Thyroid hormones and thyrotropin in amniotic fluid, N Engl J Med 293:740–743, 1975.
90. Singh PK, Parvin CA, Gronowski AM: Establishment of reference intervals for markers of fetal thyroid status in amniotic fluid, J Clin Endocrinol Metab 88:4175–4179, 2003.
91. Hagen GA, Elliott WJ: Transport of thyroid hormones in serum and cerebrospinal fluid, J Clin Endocrinol Metab 37:415–422, 1973.
92. Nishikawa M, Inada M, Naito K, et al: 3,3′,5′-triiodothyronine (reverse T3) in human cerebrospinal fluid, J Clin Endocrinol Metab 53:1030–1035, 1981.
93. Siersbaek-Nielsen K, Hansen JM: Tyrosine and free thyroxine in cerebrospinal fluid in thyroid disease, Acta Endocrinol (Copenh) 64:126–132, 1970.
94. Mallol J, Obregon MJ, Morreale de Escobar G: Analytical artifacts in radioimmunoassay of L-thyroxin in human milk, Clin Chem 28:1277–1282, 1982.
95. Varma SK, Collins M, Row A, et al: Thyroxine, tri-iodothyronine, and reverse tri-iodothyronine concentrations in human milk, J Pediatr 93:803–806, 1978.
96. Jansson L, Ivarsson S, Larsson I, et al: Tri-iodothyronine and thyroxine in human milk, Acta Paediatr Scand 72:703–705, 1983.
97. Mizuta H, Amino N, Ichihara K, et al: Thyroid hormones in human milk and their influence on thyroid function of breast-fed babies, Pediatr Res 17:468–471, 1983.
98. Riad-Fahmy D, Read GF, Walker RF, et al: Steroids in saliva for assessing endocrine function, Endocr Rev 3:367–395, 1982.
99. Elson MK, Morley JE, Shafer RB: Salivary thyroxine as an estimate of free thyroxine: concise communication, J Nucl Med 24:700–702, 1983.
100. Reichlin S, Bollinger J, Nejad I, et al: Tissue thyroid hormone concentration of rat and man determined by radiommunoassay: biologic significance, Mt Sinai J Med 40:502–510, 1973.
101. Ochi Y, Hachiya T, Yoshimura M, et al: Determination of triiodothyronine in red blood cells by radioimmunoassay, Endocrinol Jpn 23:207–213, 1976.
102. Crooks J, Murray IP, Wayne EJ: Statistical methods applied to the clinical diagnosis of thyrotoxicosis, Q J Med 28:211–234, 1959.
103. Klein I, Trzepacz PT, Roberts M, et al: Symptom rating scale for assessing hyperthyroidism, Arch Intern Med 148:387–390, 1988.
104. Billewicz W, Chapman R, Crooks J, et al: Statistical methods applied to the diagnosis of hypothyroidism, Q J Med 38:255–266, 1969.
105. Zulewski H, Muller B, Exer P, et al: Estimation of tissue hypothyroidism by a new clinical score: evaluation of patients with various grades of hypothyroidism and controls, J Clin Endocrinol Metab 82:771–776, 1997.
106. Diekman MJ, van der Put NM, Blom HJ, et al: Determinants of changes in plasma homocysteine in hyperthyroidism and hypothyroidism, Clin Endocrinol (Oxf) 54:197–204, 2001.
107. Nedrebo BG, Ericsson UB, Nygard O, et al: Plasma total homocysteine levels in hyperthyroid and hypothyroid patients, Metabolism 47:89–93, 1998.
108. Nedrebo BG, Nygard O, Ueland PM, et al: Plasma total homocysteine in hyper- and hypothyroid patients before and during 12 months of treatment, Clin Chem 47:1738–1741, 2001.
109. Lindeman RD, Romero LJ, Schade DS, et al: Impact of subclinical hypothyroidism on serum total homocysteine concentrations, the prevalence of coronary heart disease (CHD), and CHD risk factors in the New Mexico Elder Health Survey, Thyroid 13:595–600, 2003.
110. Haluzik M, Nedvidkova J, Bartak V, et al: Effects of hypo- and hyperthyroidism on noradrenergic activity and glycerol concentrations in human subcutaneous abdominal adipose tissue assessed with microdialysis, J Clin Endocrinol Metab 88:5605–5608, 2003.
111. Riis AL, Gravholt CH, Djurhuus CB, et al: Elevated regional lipolysis in hyperthyroidism, J Clin Endocrinol Metab 87:4747–4753, 2002.
112. Beylot M, Riou JP, Bienvenu F, et al: Increased ketonaemia in hyperthyroidism. Evidence for a beta-adrenergic mechanism, Diabetologia 19:505–510, 1980.
113. Waal-Manning HJ: Effect of propranolol on the duration of the Achilles tendon reflex, Clin Pharmacol Ther 10:199–206, 1969.
114. Danzi S, Klein I: Thyroid hormone-regulated cardiac gene expression and cardiovascular disease, Thyroid 12:467–472, 2002.
115. Danzi S, Ojamaa K, Klein I: Triiodothyronine-mediated myosin heavy chain gene transcription in the heart, Am J Physiol Heart Circ Physiol 284:H2255–H2262, 2003.
116. Davis PJ, Davis FB: Nongenomic actions of thyroid hormone on the heart, Thyroid 12:459–466, 2002.
117. Incerpi S, Luly P, De Vito P, et al: Short-term effects of thyroid hormones on the Na/H antiport in L-6 myoblasts: high molecular specificity for 3,3′,5′triiodo-L-thyronine, Endocrinology 140:683–689, 1999.
118. Davis FB, Moffett MJ, Davis PJ, et al: Inositol phosphates modulate binding of thyroid hormone to human red cell membranes in vitro, J Clin Endocrinol Metab 77:1427–1430, 1993.
119. Kawano T, Chen L, Watanabe SY, et al: Importance of the G protein gamma subunit in activating G protein-coupled inward rectifier K(+) channels, FEBS Lett 463:355–359, 1999.
120. Mintz G, Pizzarello R, Klein I: Enhanced left ventricular diastolic function in hyperthyroidism: noninvasive assessment and response to treatment, J Clin Endocrinol Metab 73:146–150, 1991.
121. Ladenson PW, Goldenheim PD, Cooper DS, et al: Early peripheral responses to intravenous L-thyroxine in primary hypothyroidism, Am J Med 73:467–474, 1982.
122. Bengel FM, Nekolla SG, Ibrahim T, et al: Effect of thyroid hormones on cardiac function, geometry, and oxidative metabolism assessed noninvasively by positron emission tomography and magnetic resonance imaging, J Clin Endocrinol Metab 85:1822–1827, 2000.
123. Haggerty JJ Jr, Garbutt JC, Evans DL, et al: Subclinical hypothyroidism: a review of neuropsychiatric aspects, Int J Psychiatry Med 20:193–208, 1990.
124. Saravanan P, Chau WF, Roberts N, et al: Psychological well-being in patients on "adequate" doses of L-thyroxine: results of a large, controlled community-based questionnaire study, Clin Endocrinol (Oxf) 57:577–585, 2002.
125. Whybrow PC: Behavioral and psychiatric aspects of hypothyroidism. In Braverman L, Utiger R editors. Werner and Ingbar's The Thyroid, ed 8, Philadelphia, 2000, Lippincott Williams & Wilkins, pp 837–842,
126. Bunevicius R, Kazanavicius G, Zalinkevicius R, et al: Effects of thyroxine as compared with thyroxine plus triiodothyronine in patients with hypothyroidism, N Engl J Med 340:424–429, 1999.
127. Escobar-Morreale HF, Botella-Carretero JI, Gomez-Bueno M, et al: Thyroid hormone replacement therapy in primary hypothyroidism: a randomized trial comparing L-thyroxine plus liothyronine with L-thyroxine alone, Ann Intern Med 142:412–424, 2005.
128. Smith CD, Ain KB: Brain metabolism in hypothyroidism studied with 31P magnetic-resonance spectroscopy, Lancet 345:619–620, 1995.
129. Constant EL, de Volder AG, Ivanoiu A, et al: Cerebral blood flow and glucose metabolism in hypothyroidism: a positron emission tomography study, J Clin Endocrinol Metab 86:3864–3870, 2001.
130. Chang CC, Huang CN, Chuang LM: Autoantibodies to thyroid peroxidase in patients with type 1 diabetes in Taiwan, Eur J Endocrinol 139:44–48, 1998.
131. Kaufman KD, Filetti S, Seto P, et al: Recombinant human thyroid peroxidase generated in eukaryotic cells: a source of specific antigen for the immunological assay of antimicrosomal antibodies in the sera of patients with autoimmune thyroid disease, J Clin Endocrinol Metab 70:724–728, 1990.
132. Smyth PP, Shering SG, Kilbane MT, et al: Serum thyroid peroxidase autoantibodies, thyroid volume, and outcome in breast carcinoma, J Clin Endocrinol Metab 83:2711–2716, 1998.
133. Ohtaki S, Endo Y, Horinouchi K, et al: Circulating thyroglobulin-antithyroglobulin immune complex in thyroid diseases using enzyme-linked immunoassays, J Clin Endocrinol Metab 52:239–246, 1981.
134. Tamaki H, Katsumaru H, Amino N, et al: Usefulness of thyroglobulin antibody detected by ultrasensitive enzyme immunoassay: a good parameter for immune surveillance in healthy subjects and for prediction of post-partum thyroid dysfunction, Clin Endocrinol (Oxf) 37:266–273, 1992.
135. Volpe R, Row VV, Ezrin C: Circulating viral and thyroid antibodies in subacute thyroiditis, J Clin Endocrinol Metab 27:1275–1284, 1967.
136. Tonacchera M, Agretti P, Ceccarini G, et al: Autoantibodies from patients with autoimmune thyroid disease do not interfere with the activity of the human iodide symporter gene stably transfected in CHO cells, Eur J Endocrinol 144:611–618, 2001.
137. Bastenie PA, Bonnyns M, Vanhaelst L, et al: Diseases associated with autoimmune thyroiditis. In Bastenie PA, Ermans AM editors. Thyroiditis and Thyroid Function, Oxford, 1972, Pergamon.
138. Gupta MK: Thyrotropin receptor antibodies: advances and importance of detection techniques in thyroid diseases, Clin Biochem 25:193–199, 1992.
139. Furth ED, Rathbun M, Posillico J: A modified bioassay for the long-acting thyroid stimulator (LATS), Endocrinology 85:592–593, 1969.
140. McKenzie JM, Zakarija M: Fetal and neonatal hyperthyroidism and hypothyroidism due to maternal TSH receptor antibodies, Thyroid 2:155–159, 1992.
141. Kriss JP, Pleshakov V, Rosenblum AL, et al: Studies on the pathogenesis of the ophthalmopathy of Graves' disease, J Clin Endocrinol Metab 27:582–593, 1967.
142. Sunshine P, Kusumoto H, Kriss JP: Survival time of circulating long-acting thyroid stimulator in neonatal thyrotoxicosis: implications for diagnosis and therapy of the disorder, Pediatrics 36:869–876, 1965.
143. Onaya T, Kotani M, Yamada T, et al: New in vitro tests to detect the thyroid stimulator in sera from hyperthyroid patients by measuring colloid droplet formation and cyclic AMP in human thyroid slices, J Clin Endocrinol Metab 36:859–866, 1973.
144. Leedman PJ, Frauman AG, Colman PG, et al: Measurement of thyroid-stimulating immunoglobulins by incorporation of tritiated-adenine into intact FRTL-5 cells: a viable alternative to radioimmunoassay for the measurement of cAMP, Clin Endocrinol (Oxf) 37:493–499, 1992.
145. Petersen V, Hall R, Smith BF: A study of thyroid stimulating activity in human serum with the highly sensitive cytochemical bioassay, J Clin Endocrinol Metab 41:199–202, 1975.
146. Libert F, Lefort A, Gerard C, et al: Cloning, sequencing and expression of the human thyrotropin (TSH) receptor: evidence for binding of autoantibodies, Biochem Biophys Res Commun 165:1250–1255, 1989.
147. Ludgate M, Perret J, Parmentier M, et al: Use of the recombinant human thyrotropin receptor (TSH-R) expressed in mammalian cell lines to assay TSH-R autoantibodies, Mol Cell Endocrinol 73:R13–18, 1990.
148. Nagayama I, Yamamoto K, Saito K, et al: Subject-based reference values in thyroid function tests, Endocr J 40:557–562, 1993.
149. Botero D, Brown RS: Bioassay of thyrotropin receptor antibodies with Chinese hamster ovary cells transfected with recombinant human thyrotropin receptor: clinical utility in children and adolescents with Graves disease, J Pediatr 132:612–618, 1998.

150. Vitti P, Elisei R, Tonacchera M, et al: Detection of thyroid-stimulating antibody using Chinese hamster ovary cells transfected with cloned human thyrotropin receptor, J Clin Endocrinol Metab 76:499–503, 1993.
151. Adams DD, Kennedy TH: Occurrence in thyrotoxicosis of a gamma globulin which protects LATS from neutralization by an extract of thyroid gland, J Clin Endocrinol Metab 27:173–177, 1967.
152. Shishiba Y, Shimizu T, Yoshimura S, et al: Direct evidence for human thyroidal stimulation by LATS-protector, J Clin Endocrinol Metab 36:517–521, 1973.
153. Filetti S, Foti D, Costante G, et al: Recombinant human thyrotropin (TSH) receptor in a radioreceptor assay for the measurement of TSH receptor autoantibodies, J Clin Endocrinol Metab 72:1096–1101, 1991.
154. Drexhage HA, Bottazzo GF, Doniach D: Thyroid growth stimulating and blocking immunoglobulins. In Chayen J, Bitensky L editors. Cytochemical Bioassays, New York, 1983. Marcel Dekker.
155. Valente WA, Vitti P, Rotella CM, et al: Antibodies that promote thyroid growth. A distinct population of thyroid-stimulating autoantibodies, N Engl J Med 309:1028–1034, 1983.
156. Grove AS Jr: Evaluation of exophthalmos, N Engl J Med 292:1005–1013, 1975.
157. Cho BY, Shong MH, Yi KH, et al: Evaluation of serum basal thyrotrophin levels and thyrotrophin receptor antibody activities as prognostic markers for discontinuation of antithyroid drug treatment in patients with Graves' disease, Clin Endocrinol (Oxf) 36:585–590, 1992.
158. Hershman JM: Hyperthyroidism induced by trophoblastic thyrotropin, Mayo Clin Proc 47:913–918, 1972.
159. Nisula BC, Ketelslegers JM: Thyroid-stimulating activity and chorionic gonadotropin, J Clin Invest 54:494–499, 1974.
160. Rodien P, Bremont C, Sanson ML, et al: Familial gestational hyperthyroidism caused by a mutant thyrotropin receptor hypersensitive to human chorionic gonadotropin, N Engl J Med 339:1823–1826, 1998.
161. Dussault JH, Turcotte R, Guyda H: The effect of acetylsalicylic acid on TSH and PRL secretion after TRH stimulation in the human, J Clin Endocrinol Metab 43:232–235, 1976.
162. Porter BA, Refetoff S, Rosenfeld RL, et al: Abnormal thyroxine metabolism in hyposomatotrophic dwarfism and inhibition of responsiveness to TRH during GH therapy, Pediatrics 51:668–674, 1973.
163. Weeke J, Hansen AP, Lundaek K: Inhibition by somatostatin of basal levels of serum thyrotropin (TSH) in normal men, J Clin Endocrinol Metab 41:168–171, 1975.
164. Becker FO, Economou PG, Schwartz TB: The occurrence of carcinoma in "hot" thyroid nodules. Report of two cases, Ann Intern Med 58:877–882, 1963.
165. Mazzaferri EL: Management of a solitary thyroid nodule, N Engl J Med 328:553–559, 1993.
166. Ashcraft MW, Van Herle AJ: Management of thyroid nodules. I: History and physical examination, blood tests, x-ray tests, and ultrasonography, Head Neck Surg 3:216–230, 1981.
167. Ashcraft MW, Van Herle AJ: Management of thyroid nodules. II: Scanning techniques, thyroid suppressive therapy, and fine needle aspiration, Head Neck Surg 3:297–322, 1981.
168. Guimaraes V, DeGroot LJ: Moderate hypothyroidism in preparation for whole body 131I scintiscans and thyroglobulin testing, Thyroid 6:69–73, 1996.
169. Haugen BR, Pacini F, Reiners C, et al: A comparison of recombinant human thyrotropin and thyroid hormone withdrawal for the detection of thyroid remnant or cancer, J Clin Endocrinol Metab 84:3877–3885, 1999.
170. Ladenson PW, Braverman LE, Mazzaferri EL, et al: Comparison of administration of recombinant human thyrotropin with withdrawal of thyroid hormone for radioactive iodine scanning in patients with thyroid carcinoma, N Engl J Med 337:888–896, 1997.
171. Pineda JD, Lee T, Ain K, et al: Iodine-131 therapy for thyroid cancer patients with elevated thyroglobulin and negative diagnostic scan, J Clin Endocrinol Metab 80:1488–1492, 1995.
172. Dietlein M, Scheidhauer K, Voth E, et al: Fluorine-18 fluorodeoxyglucose positron emission tomography and iodine-131 whole-body scintigraphy in the follow-up of differentiated thyroid cancer, Eur J Nucl Med 24:1342–1348, 1997.
173. Feine U, Lietzenmayer R, Hanke JP, et al: Fluorine-18-FDG and iodine-131-iodide uptake in thyroid cancer, J Nucl Med 37:1468–1472, 1996.
174. Zimmer LA, McCook B, Meltzer C, et al: Combined positron emission tomography/computed tomography imaging of recurrent thyroid cancer, Otolaryngol Head Neck Surg 128:178–184, 2003.
175. Corstens F, Huysmans D, Kloppenborg P: Thallium-201 scintigraphy of the suppressed thyroid: an alternative for iodine-123 scanning after TSH stimulation, J Nucl Med 29:1360–1363, 1988.
176. Fairweather DS, Bradwell AR, Watson-James SF, et al: Detection of thyroid tumours using radio-labelled antithyroglobulin, Clin Endocrinol (Oxf) 18:563–570, 1983.
177. Barki Y: Ultrasonographic evaluation of neck masses—sonographic patterns in differential diagnosis, Isr J Med Sci 28:212–216, 1992.
178. Brown LR, Aughenbaugh GL: Masses of the anterior mediastinum: CT and MR imaging, AJR Am J Roentgenol 157:1171–1180, 1991.
179. Gittoes NJ, Miller MR, Daykin J, et al: Upper airways obstruction in 153 consecutive patients presenting with thyroid enlargement, BMJ 312:484, 1996.
180. Hamberger B, Gharib H, Melton LJ 3rd, et al: Fine-needle aspiration biopsy of thyroid nodules. Impact on thyroid practice and cost of care, Am J Med 73:381–384, 1982.
181. Bennedbaek FN, Karstrup S, Hegedus L: Percutaneous ethanol injection therapy in the treatment of thyroid and parathyroid diseases, Eur J Endocrinol 136:240–250, 1997.
182. Porcellini A, Ciullo I, Laviola L, et al: Novel mutations of thyrotropin receptor gene in thyroid hyperfunctioning adenomas. Rapid identification by fine needle aspiration biopsy, J Clin Endocrinol Metab 79:657–661, 1994.
183. Tassi V, Di Cerbo A, Porcellini A, et al: Screening of thyrotropin receptor mutations by fine-needle aspiration biopsy in autonomous functioning thyroid nodules in multinodular goiters, Thyroid 9:353–357, 1999.
184. Pierce JG: Eli Lilly lecture. The subunits of pituitary thyrotropin—their relationship to other glycoprotein hormones, Endocrinology 89:1331–1344, 1971.
185. Chaussain JL, Binet E, Job JC: Antibodies to human thyreotrophin in the serum of certain hypopituitary dwarfs, Rev Eur Etud Clin Biol 17:95–99, 1972.
186. Nicoloff JT, Spencer CA: Clinical review 12: The use and misuse of the sensitive thyrotropin assays, J Clin Endocrinol Metab 71:553–558, 1990.
187. Spencer CA, Schwarzbein D, Guttler RB, et al: Thyrotropin (TSH)-releasing hormone stimulation test responses employing third and fourth generation TSH assays, J Clin Endocrinol Metab 76:494–498, 1993.
188. Spencer CA, Takeuchi M, Kazarosyan M: Current status and performance goals for serum thyrotropin (TSH) assays, Clin Chem 42:140–145, 1996.
189. Spencer CA, Takeuchi M, Kazarosyan M, et al: Interlaboratory/intermethod differences in functional sensitivity of immunometric assays of thyrotropin (TSH) and impact on reliability of measurement of subnormal concentrations of TSH, Clin Chem 41:367–374, 1995.
190. Brennan MD, Klee GG, Preissner CM, et al: Heterophilic serum antibodies: a cause for falsely elevated serum thyrotropin levels, Mayo Clin Proc 62:894–898, 1987.
191. Fisher DA, Klein AH: Thyroid development and disorders of thyroid function in the newborn, N Engl J Med 304:702–712, 1981.
192. Kourides IA, Heath CV, Ginsberg-Fellner F: Measurement of thyroid-stimulating hormone in human amniotic fluid, J Clin Endocrinol Metab 54:635–637, 1982.
193. Brabant G, Brabant A, Ranft U, et al: Circadian and pulsatile thyrotropin secretion in euthyroid man under the influence of thyroid hormone and glucocorticoid administration, J Clin Endocrinol Metab 65:83–88, 1987.
194. Adriaanse R, Brabant G, Prank K, et al: Circadian changes in pulsatile TSH release in primary hypothyroidism, Clin Endocrinol (Oxf) 37:504–510, 1992.
195. Bartalena L, Martino E, Falcone M, et al: Evaluation of the nocturnal serum thyrotropin (TSH) surge, as assessed by TSH ultrasensitive assay, in patients receiving long term L-thyroxine suppression therapy and in patients with various thyroid disorders, J Clin Endocrinol Metab 65:1265–1271, 1987.
196. Brabant G, Prank K, Hoang-Vu C, et al: Hypothalamic regulation of pulsatile thyrotopin secretion, J Clin Endocrinol Metab 72:145–150, 1991.
197. Van Cauter E, Golstein J, Vanhaelst L, et al: Effects of oral contraceptive therapy on the circadian patterns of cortisol and thyrotropin (TSH), Eur J Clin Invest 5:115–121, 1975.
198. Wilber JF, Baum D: Elevation of plasma TSH during surgical hypothermia, J Clin Endocrinol Metab 31:372–375, 1970.
199. Sunthornthepvarakui T, Gottschalk ME, Hayashi Y, et al: Brief report: resistance to thyrotropin caused by mutations in the thyrotropin-receptor gene, N Engl J Med 332:155–160, 1995.
200. Emerson CH, Frohman LA, Szabo M, et al: TRH immunoreactivity in human urine: evidence for dissociation from TRH, J Clin Endocrinol Metab 45:392–399, 1977.
201. Haigler ED Jr, Hershman JM, Pittman JA Jr: Response to orally administered synthetic thyrotropin-releasing hormone in man, J Clin Endocrinol Metab 35:631–635, 1972.
202. Azizi F, Vagenakis AG, Portnay GI, et al: Pituitary-thyroid responsiveness to intramuscular thyrotropin-releasing hormone based on analyses of serum thyroxine, tri-iodothyronine and thyrotropin concentrations, N Engl J Med 292:273–277, 1975.
203. Ormston BJ, Kilborn JR, Garry R, et al: Further observations on the effect of synthetic thyrotropin-releasing hormone in man, Br Med J 2:199–202, 1971.
204. Hershman JM, Kojima A, Friesen HG: Effect of thyrotropin-releasing hormone on human pituitary thyrotropin, prolactin, placental lactogen, and chorionic thyrotropin, J Clin Endocrinol Metab 36:497–501, 1973.
205. Jacobsen BB, Andersen H, Dige-Petersen H, et al: Thyrotropin response to thyrotropin-releasing hormone in fullterm, euthyroid and hypothyroid newborns, Acta Paediatr Scand 65:433–438, 1976.
206. Shenkman L, Mitsuma T, Suphavai A, et al: Triiodothyronine and thyroid-stimulating hormone response to thyrotrophin-releasing hormone. A new test of thyroidal and pituitary reserve. Lancet 1:111–112, 1972.
207. Anderson MS, Bowers CY, Kastin AJ, et al: Synthetic thyrotropin-releasing hormone. A potent stimulator of thyrotropin secretion in man, N Engl J Med 285:1279–1283, 1971.
208. Park SM, Clifton-Bligh RJ, Betts P, et al: Congenital hypothyroidism and apparent athyreosis with compound heterozygosity or compensated hypothyroidism with probable hemizygosity for inactivating mutations of the TSH receptor, Clin Endocrinol (Oxf) 60:220–227, 2004.
209. Mornex R, Berthezene F: Comments on a proposed new way of measuring thyrotropin (TSH) reserve, J Clin Endocrinol Metab 31:587–589, 1970.
210. Stein RB, Nicoloff JT: Triiodothyronine withdrawal test–a test of thyroid-pituitary adequacy, J Clin Endocrinol Metab 32:127–129, 1971.
211. Ramirez L, Braverman LE, White B, et al: Recombinant human thyrotropin is a potent stimulator of thyroid function in normal subjects, J Clin Endocrinol Metab 82:2836–2839, 1997.
212. Vitale G, Lupoli GA, Ciccarelli A, et al: Influence of body surface area on serum peak thyrotropin (TSH) levels after recombinant human TSH administration, J Clin Endocrinol Metab 88:1319–1322, 2003.
213. Werner SC, Spooner M: A new and simple test for hyperthyroidism employing L-triiodothyronine and the twenty-four hour I-131 uptake method, Bull N Y Acad Med 31:137–145, 1955.
214. Duick DS, Stein RB, Warren DW, et al: The significance of partial suppressibility of serum thyroxine by triiodothyronine administration in euthyroid man, J Clin Endocrinol Metab 41:229–234, 1975.
215. Stanbury JB, Kassenaar AA, Meijer JW: The metabolism of iodotyrosines. I. The fate of mono- and di-iodotyrosine in normal subjects and in patients with various diseases, J Clin Endocrinol Metab 16:735–746, 1956.
216. Lissitzky S, Codaccioni JL, Bismuth J, et al: Congenital goiter with hypothyroidism and iodo-serum albumin replacing thyroglobulin, J Clin Endocrinol Metab 27:185–196, 1967.
217. DeGroot LJ: Kinetic analysis of iodine metabolism, J Clin Endocrinol Metab 26:149–173, 1966.

218. Hays MT: Absorption of oral thyroxine in man, J Clin Endocrinol Metab 28:749–756, 1968.
219. Hays MT: Absorption of triiodothyronine in man, J Clin Endocrinol Metab 30:675–676, 1970.
220. Ain KB, Refetoff S, Fein HG, et al: Pseudomalabsorption of levothyroxine, JAMA 266:2118–2120, 1991.
221. Curti GL, Fresco GF: A theoretical five-pool model to evaluate triiodothyronine distribution and metabolism in healthy subjects, Metabolism 41:3–10, 1992.
222. Oppenheimer JH, Schwartz HL, Surks MI: Determination of common parameters fo iodothyronine metabolism and distribution in man by noncompartmental analysis, J Clin Endocrinol Metab 41:319–324, 1975.
223. Bianchi R, Mariani G, Molea N, et al: Peripheral metabolism of thyroid hormones in man. I. Direct measurement of the conversion rate of thyroxine to 3,5,3′-triiodothyronine (T3) and determination of the peripheral and thyroidal production of T3, J Clin Endocrinol Metab 56:1152–1163, 1983.
224. Faber J, Heaf J, Kirkegaard C, et al: Simultaneous turnover studies of thyroxine, 3,5,3′ and 3,3′,5′-triiodothyronine, 3,5-, 3,3′-, and 3′,5′-diiodothyronine, and 3′-monoiodothyronine in chronic renal failure, J Clin Endocrinol Metab 56:211–217, 1983.
225. LoPresti JS, Fried JC, Spencer CA, et al: Unique alterations of thyroid hormone indices in the acquired immunodeficiency syndrome (AIDS), Ann Intern Med 110:970–975, 1989.
226. Lim VS, Fang VS, Katz AI, et al: Thyroid dysfunction in chronic renal failure. A study of the pituitary-thyroid axis and peripheral turnover kinetics of thyroxine and triiodothyronine, J Clin Invest 60:522–534, 1977.
227. Cavalieri RR, Searle GL: The kinetics of distribution between plasma and liver of 131-I-labeled L-thyroxine in man: observations of subjects with normal and decreased serum thyroxine-binding globulin, J Clin Invest 45:939–949, 1966.
228. Cuttelod S, Lemarchand-Beraud T, Magnenat P, et al: Effect of age and role of kidneys and liver on thyrotropin turnover in man. Metabolism 23:101–113, 1974.
229. Oppenheimer JH, Bernstein G, Hasen J: Estimation of rapidly exchangeable cellular thyroxine from the plasma disappearance curves of simultaneously administered thyroxine-131-I and albumin-125-I, J Clin Invest 46:762–777, 1967.
230. Sunthornthepvarakul T, Angkeow P, Weiss RE, et al: An identical missense mutation in the albumin gene results in familial dysalbuminemic hyperthyroxinemia in 8 unrelated families, Biochem Biophys Res Commun 202:781–787, 1994.
231. Sunthornthepvarakul T, Likitmaskul S, Ngowngarmratana S, et al: Familial dysalbuminemic hypertriiodothyroninemia: a new, dominantly inherited albumin defect, J Clin Endocrinol Metab 83:1448–1454, 1998.
232. Refetoff S, Dumont JE, Vassart G: Thyroid disorders. In Scriver CR, Beaudet AL, Sly WS, Valle D editors. The Metabolic and Molecular Basis of Inherited Disease, ed 8, New York, 2001, McGraw Hill, pp 4029–4075,
233. Saraiva MJ: Transthyretin mutations in health and disease, Hum Mutat 5:191–196, 1995.
234. Li P, Janssen OE, Takeda K, et al: Complete thyroxine-binding globulin (TBG) deficiency caused by a single nucleotide deletion in the TBG gene, Metabolism 40:1231–1234, 1991.
235. Pohlenz J, Rosenthal IM, Weiss RE, et al: Congenital hypothyroidism due to mutations in the sodium/iodide symporter. Identification of a nonsense mutation producing a downstream cryptic 3′ splice site, J Clin Invest 101:1028–1035, 1998.
236. Pannain S, Weiss RE, Jackson CE, et al: Two different mutations in the thyroid peroxidase gene of a large inbred Amish kindred: power and limits of homozygosity mapping, J Clin Endocrinol Metab 84:1061–1071, 1999.
237. Kopp P: Perspective: genetic defects in the etiology of congenital hypothyroidism, Endocrinology 143:2019–2024, 2002.
238. Fuhrer D, Lachmund P, Nebel IT, et al: The thyrotropin receptor mutation database: update 2003, Thyroid 13:1123–1126, 2003.
239. Wonerow P, Neumann S, Gudermann T, et al: Thyrotropin receptor mutations as a tool to understand thyrotropin receptor action, J Mol Med 79:707–721, 2001.
240. Pohlenz J, Weiss RE, Macchia PE, et al: Five new families with resistance to thyroid hormone not caused by mutations in the thyroid hormone receptor beta gene, J Clin Endocrinol Metab 84:3919–3928, 1999.
241. Van Vliet G: Development of the thyroid gland: lessons from congenitally hypothyroid mice and men, Clin Genet 63:445–455, 2003.
242. Cavlieri RR, Sung LC, Becker CE: Effects of phenobarbital on thyroxine and triiodothyronine kinetics in Graves' disease, J Clin Endocrinol Metab 37:308–316, 1973.
243. Faber J, Lumholtz IB, Kirkegaard C, et al: The effects of phenytoin (diphenylhydantoin) on the extrathyroidal turnover of thyroxine, 3,5,3′-triiodothyronine, 3,3′,5′-triiodothyronine, and 3′,5′-diiodothyronine in man, J Clin Endocrinol Metab 61:1093–1099, 1985.
244. Collu R, Jequier JC, Leboeuf G, et al: Endocrine effects of pimozide, a specific dopaminergic blocker, J Clin Endocrinol Metab 41:981–984, 1975.
245. Martino E, Safran M, Aghini-Lombardi F, et al: Environmental iodine intake and thyroid dysfunction during chronic amiodarone therapy, Ann Intern Med 101:28–34, 1984.
246. Vagenakis AG, Wang CA, Burger A, et al: Iodide-induced thyrotoxicosis in Boston, N Engl J Med 287:523–527, 1972.
247. Feldt-Rasmussen U, Lange AP, Date J, et al: Effect of clomifene on thyroid function in normal men, Acta Endocrinol (Copenh) 90:43–51, 1979.
248. Faglia G, Ambrosi B, Beck-Peccoz P, et al: The effect of theophylline on plasma thyrotropin (HTSH) response to thyrotropin releasing factor (TRF) in man, J Clin Endocrinol Metab 34:906–909, 1972.
249. Gaffney TE, Braunwald E, Kahler RL: Effects of guanethidine on tri-iodothyronine-induced hyperthyroidism in man, N Engl J Med 265:16–20, 1961.
250. Lee WY, Bronsky D, Waldstein SS: Studies of thyroid and sympathetic nervous system interrelationships. II. Effects of guanethidine on manifestations of hyperthyroidism, J Clin Endocrinol Metab 22:879–885, 1962.
251. Deyssig R, Weissel M: Ingestion of androgenic-anabolic steroids induces mild thyroidal impairment in male body builders, J Clin Endocrinol Metab 76:1069–1071, 1993.
252. Malarkey WB, Strauss RH, Leizman DJ, et al: Endocrine effects in female weight lifters who self-administer testosterone and anabolic steroids, Am J Obstet Gynecol 165:1385–1390, 1991.
253. Arafah BM: Decreased levothyroxine requirement in women with hypothyroidism during androgen therapy for breast cancer, Ann Intern Med 121:247–251, 1994.
254. Gross HA, Appleman MD Jr, Nicoloff JT: Effect of biologically active steroids on thyroid function in man, J Clin Endocrinol Metab 33:242–248, 1971.
255. Graham RL, Gambrell RD Jr: Changes in thyroid function tests during danazol therapy, Obstet Gynecol 55:395–397, 1980.
256. Ain KB, Mori Y, Refetoff S: Reduced clearance rate of thyroxine-binding globulin (TBG) with increased sialylation: a mechanism for estrogen-induced elevation of serum TBG concentration, J Clin Endocrinol Metab 65:689–696, 1987.
257. Doe RP, Mellinger GT, Swaim WR, et al: Estrogen dosage effects on serum proteins: a longitudinal study, J Clin Endocrinol 27:1081–1086, 1967.
258. Steingold KA, Matt DW, DeZiegler D, et al: Comparison of transdermal to oral estradiol administration on hormonal and hepatic parameters in women with premature ovarian failure, J Clin Endocrinol Metab 73:275–280, 1991.
259. Mandel SJ, Larsen PR, Seely EW, et al: Increased need for thyroxine during pregnancy in women with primary hypothyroidism, N Engl J Med 323:91–96, 1990.
260. Karami-Tehrani F, Salami S, Mokarram P: Competition of tamoxifen with thyroxine for TBG binding: ligand binding assay and computational data, Clin Biochem 34:603–606, 2001.
261. Gamstedt A, Jarnerot G, Kagedal B, et al: Corticosteroids and thyroid function. Different effects on plasma volume, thyroid hormones and thyroid hormone-binding proteins after oral and intravenous administration, Acta Med Scand 205:379–383, 1979.
262. Ingbar SH: The effect of cortisone on the thyroidal and renal metabolism of iodine, Endocrinology 53:171–181, 1953.
263. Samuels MH, McDaniel PA: Thyrotropin levels during hydrocortisone infusions that mimic fasting-induced cortisol elevations: a clinical research center study, J Clin Endocrinol Metab 82:3700–3704, 1997.
264. Benoit FL, Greenspan FS: Corticoid therapy for pretibial myxedema. Observations on the long-acting thyroid stimulator, Ann Intern Med 66:711–720, 1967.
265. Yamada T, Ikejiri K, Kotani M, et al: An increase of plasma triiodothyronine and thyroxine after administration of dexamethasone to hypothyroid patients with Hashimoto's thyroiditis, J Clin Endocrinol Metab 46:784–790, 1978.
266. Cobb WE, Reichlin S, Jackson IM: Growth hormone secretory status is a determinant of the thyrotropin response to thyrotropin-releasing hormone in euthyroid patients with hypothalamic-pituitary disease, J Clin Endocrinol Metab 52:324–329, 1981.
267. Eskildsen PC, Kruse A, Kirkegaard C: The pituitary-thyroid axis in acromegaly, Horm Metab Res 20:755–757, 1988.
268. Root AW, Snyder PJ, Rezvani I, et al: Inhibition of thyrotropin releasing hormone-mediated secretion of thyrotropin by human growth hormone, J Clin Endocrinol Metab 36:103–107, 1973.
269. Wyatt DT, Gesundheit N, Sherman B: Changes in thyroid hormone levels during growth hormone therapy in initially euthyroid patients: lack of need for thyroxine supplementation, J Clin Endocrinol Metab 83:3493–3497, 1998.
270. Porretti S, Giavoli C, Ronchi C, et al: Recombinant human GH replacement therapy and thyroid function in a large group of adult GH-deficient patients: when does L-T(4) therapy become mandatory? J Clin Endocrinol Metab 87:2042–2045, 2002.
271. Isojarvi JI, Turkka J, Pakarinen AJ, et al: Thyroid function in men taking carbamazepine, oxcarbazepine, or valproate for epilepsy, Epilepsia 42:930–934, 2001.
272. Caksen H, Dulger H, Cesur Y, et al: Evaluation of thyroid and parathyroid functions in children receiving long-term carbamazepine therapy, Int J Neurosci 113:1213–1217, 2003.
273. Haidukewych D, Rodin EA: Chronic antiepileptic drug therapy: classification by medication regimen and incidence of decreases in serum thyroxine and free thyroxine index, Ther Drug Monit 9:392–398, 1987.
274. Verrotti A, Scardapane A, Manco R, et al: Antiepileptic drugs and thyroid function, J Pediatr Endocrinol Metab 21:401–408, 2008.
275. Premachandra BN, Radparvar A, Burman K, et al: Apparent increase in type I 5′-deiodinase activity induced by antiepileptic medication in mentally retarded subjects, Horm Res 58:273–278, 2002.
276. Joffe RT, Singer W: Antidepressants and thyroid hormone levels, Acta Med Austriaca 19(Suppl 1):96–97, 1992.
277. Shelton RC, Winn S, Ekhatore N, et al: The effects of antidepressants on the thyroid axis in depression, Biol Psychiatry 33:120–126, 1993.
278. Rousseau A, Comby F, Buxeraud J, et al: Spectroscopic analysis of charge transfer complex formation and peroxidase inhibition with tricyclic antidepressant drugs: potential anti-thyroid action, Biol Pharm Bull 19:726–728, 1996.
279. Smith PJ, Surks MI: Multiple effects of 5,5′-diphenylhydantoin on the thyroid hormone system, Endocr Rev 5:514–524, 1984.
280. Curran PG, DeGroot LJ: The effect of hepatic enzyme-inducing drugs on thyroid hormones and the thyroid gland, Endocr Rev 12:135–150, 1991.
281. Tiihonen M, Liewendahl K, Waltimo O, et al: Thyroid status of patients receiving long-term anticonvulsant therapy assessed by peripheral parameters: a placebo-controlled thyroxine therapy trial, Epilepsia 36:1118–1125, 1995.
282. Cavalieri RR, Gavin LA, Wallace A, et al: Serum thyroxine, free T4, triiodothyronine, and reverse-T3 in diphenylhydantoin-treated patients, Metabolism 28:1161–1165, 1979.
283. Blackshear JL, Schultz AL, Napier JS, et al: Thyroxine replacement requirements in hypothyroid patients receiving phenytoin, Ann Intern Med 99:341–342, 1983.
284. Barclay ML, Brownlie BE, Turner JG, et al: Lithium associated thyrotoxicosis: a report of 14 cases, with statistical analysis of incidence, Clin Endocrinol (Oxf) 40:759–764, 1994.
285. Bschor T, Baethge C, Adli M, et al: Hypothalamic-pituitary-thyroid system activity during lithium aug-

mentation therapy in patients with unipolar major depression, J Psychiatry Neurosci 28:210–216, 2003.

286. Gyulai L, Bauer M, Bauer MS, et al: Thyroid hypofunction in patients with rapid-cycling bipolar disorder after lithium challenge, Biol Psychiatry 53:899–905, 2003.

287. Hullin R: The place of lithium in biological psychiatry. In Johnson F, Johnson S editors. Lithium in Medical Practice, Lancaster, 1978, MTP, p 433.

288. Pallisgaard G, Frederiksen K: Thyrotoxicosis in a patient treated with lithium carbonate for mental disease, Acta Med Scand 204:141–143, 1978.

289. Schou M, Amdisen A, Jensen S, et al: Occurrence of goitre during lithium treatment, BMJ 2:710–713, 1968.

290. Schorderet M: Lithium inhibition of cyclic AMP accumulation induced by dopamine in isolated retinae of the rabbit, Biochem Pharmacol 26:167–170, 1977.

291. Joffe RT, Kutcher S, MacDonald C: Thyroid function and bipolar affective disorder, Psychiatry Res 25:117–121, 1988.

292. Bagchi N, Brown TR, Mack RE: Studies on the mechanism of inhibition of thyroid function by lithium, Biochim Biophys Acta 542:163–169, 1978.

293. Lazarus JH, Muston HL: The effect of lithium on the iodide concentrating mechanism in mouse salivary gland, Acta Pharmacol Toxicol (Copenh) 43:55–58, 1978.

294. Leppaluoto J, Mannisto PT, Virkkunen P: On the mechanism of goitre formation during lithium treatment in the rat, Acta Endocrinol (Copenh) 74:296–306, 1973.

295. Bhattacharyya B, Wolff J: Stabilization of microtubules by lithium ion, Biochem Biophys Res Commun 73:383–390, 1976.

296. Blomqvist N, Lindstedt G, Lundberg PA, et al: No inhibition by Li+ of thyroxine monodeiodination to 3,5,3′-triiodothyronine and 3,3′,5′-triiodothyronine (reverse triiodothyronine), Clin Chim Acta 79:457–464, 1977.

297. Singer I, Rotenberg D: Mechanisms of lithium action, N Engl J Med 289:254–260, 1973.

298. Miller KK, Daniels GH: Association between lithium use and thyrotoxicosis caused by silent thyroiditis, Clin Endocrinol (Oxf) 55:501–508, 2001.

299. Carmaciu CD, Anderson CS, Lawton CA: Thyrotoxicosis after complete or partial lithium withdrawal in two patients with bipolar affective disorder, Bipolar Disord 5:381–384, 2003.

300. Martinos A, Rinieris P, Papachristou DN, et al: Effects of six weeks' neuroleptic treatment on the pituitary-thyroid axis in schizophrenic patients, Neuropsychobiology 16:72–77, 1986.

301. Gwinup G, Ogundipe O: Preliminary report: Decreased leukocyte alkaline phoshatase in hyperthyroidism, Metabolism 23:659–661, 1974.

302. Ramschak-Schwarzer S, Radkohl W, Stiegler C, et al: Interaction between psychotropic drugs and thyroid hormone metabolism—an overview, Acta Med Austriaca 27:8–10, 2000.

303. Mayer SW, Kelly FH, Morton ME: The direct antithyroid action of reserpine, chlorpromazine and other drugs, J Pharmacol Exp Ther 117:197–201, 1956.

304. Wiseman R Jr: The effect of acute and chronic administration of chlorpromazine on the I-131 distribution in normal rats, J Pharmacol Exp Ther 138:269–276, 1962.

305. Blumberg AG, Klein DF: Chlorpromazine-procyclidine and imipramine: effects on thyroid function in psychiatric patients, Clin Pharmacol Ther 10:350–354, 1969.

306. Konig F, Hauger B, von Hippel C, et al: Effect of paroxetine on thyroid hormone levels in severely depressed patients, Neuropsychobiology 42:135–138, 2000.

307. Schwartz HL, Kozyreff V, Surks MI, et al: Increased deiodination of L-thyroxine and L-triiodothyronine by liver microsomes from rats treated with phenobarbital, Nature 221:1262–1263, 1969.

308. Harel Z, Biro FM, Tedford WL: Effects of long term treatment with sertraline (Zoloft) simulating hypothyroidism in an adolescent, J Adolesc Health 16:232–234, 1995.

309. Ferko N, Levine MA: Evaluation of the association between St. John's wort and elevated thyroid-stimulating hormone, Pharmacotherapy 21:1574–1578, 2001.

310. Beer AM, Wiebelitz KR, Schmidt-Gayk H: Lycopus europaeus (Gypsywort): effects on the thyroidal param-

eters and symptoms associated with thyroid function, Phytomedicine 15:16–22, 2008.

311. Isojarvi JI, Pakarinen AJ, Myllyla VV: Thyroid function with antiepileptic drugs, Epilepsia 33:142–148, 1992.

312. Keogh MA, Wittert GA: Effect of cabergoline on thyroid function in hyperprolactinaemia, Clin Endocrinol (Oxf) 57:699, 2002.

313. Morley JE: Neuroendocrine control of thyrotropin secretion, Endocr Rev 2:396–436, 1981.

314. Kobberling J, Darragh A, Del Pozo E: Chronic dopamine receptor stimulation using bromocriptine: failure to modify thyroid function, Clin Endocrinol (Oxf) 11:367–370, 1979.

315. Samuels MH, Kramer P: Effects of metoclopramide on fasting-induced TSH suppression, Thyroid 6:85–89, 1996.

316. Heinen E, Herrmann J, Lippe J, et al: [Effect of dopamine and dobutamine on thyroid hormone concentration], Med Welt 34:696–699, 1983.

317. Lee E, Chen P, Rao H, et al: Effect of acute high dose dobutamine administration on serum thyrotrophin (TSH), Clin Endocrinol (Oxf) 50:487–492, 1999.

318. Jones MK, Birtwell J, Owens DR, et al: Beta-adrenoreceptor blocking drugs and thyroid hormones in hyperthyroid subjects, Postgrad Med J 57:207–209, 1981.

319. Perrild H, Pedersen F, Rasmussen SL, et al: Long-term alprenolol treatment affects serum T4, T3 and rT3 in euthyroid patients with ischaemic heart disease, Acta Endocrinol (Copenh) 105:190–193, 1984.

320. Rassu S, Masala A, Alagna S, et al: Acute effect of atenolol on serum thyroid hormones in hyperthyroid patients, J Endocrinol Invest 5:39–41, 1982.

321. Cutting CC, Tainter ML: Comparative effects of dinitrophenol and thyroxine on tadpole metamorphosis, Proc Soc Exp Biol Med 31:97–100, 1933.

322. How J, Khir AS, Bewsher PD: The effect of atenolol on serum thyroid hormones in hyperthyroid patients, Clin Endocrinol (Oxf) 13:299–302, 1980.

323. Amenomori M, Mori T, Fukuda Y, et al: Incidence and characteristics of thyroid dysfunction following interferon therapy in patients with chronic hepatitis C, Intern Med 37:246–252, 1998.

324. Corssmit EP, Heyligenberg R, Endert E, et al: Acute effects of interferon-alpha administration on thyroid hormone metabolism in healthy men, J Clin Endocrinol Metab 80:3140–3144, 1995.

325. Fernandez-Soto L, Gonzalez A, Escobar-Jimenez F, et al: Increased risk of autoimmune thyroid disease in hepatitis C vs hepatitis B before, during, and after discontinuing interferon therapy, Arch Intern Med 158:1445–1448, 1998.

326. Koh LK, Greenspan FS, Yeo PP: Interferon-alpha induced thyroid dysfunction: three clinical presentations and a review of the literature, Thyroid 7:891–896, 1997.

327. Schuppert F, Rambusch E, Kirchner H, et al: Patients treated with interferon-alpha, interferon-beta, and interleukin-2 have a different thyroid autoantibody pattern than patients suffering from endogenous autoimmune thyroid disease, Thyroid 7:837–842, 1997.

328. Allanore Y, Bremont C, Kahan A, et al: Transient hyperthyroidism in a patient with rheumatoid arthritis treated by etanercept, Clin Exp Rheumatol 19:356–357, 2001.

329. Prummel MF, Laurberg P: Interferon-alpha and autoimmune thyroid disease, Thyroid 13:547–551, 2003.

330. Wong V, Fu AX, George J, et al: Thyrotoxicosis induced by alpha-interferon therapy in chronic viral hepatitis, Clin Endocrinol (Oxf) 56:793–798, 2002.

331. Andrade LJ, Atta AM, D'Almeida Junior A, et al: Thyroid dysfunction in hepatitis C individuals treated with interferon-alpha and ribavirin—a review, Braz J Infect Dis 12:144–148, 2008.

332. Okanoue T, Sakamoto S, Itoh Y, et al: Side effects of high-dose interferon therapy for chronic hepatitis C, J Hepatol 25:283–291, 1996.

333. Selzer E, Wilfing A, Sexl V, et al: Effects of type I-interferons on human thyroid epithelial cells derived from normal and tumour tissue, Naunyn Schmiedebergs Arch Pharmacol 350:322–328, 1994.

334. Dalgard O, Bjoro K, Hellum K, et al: Thyroid dysfunction during treatment of chronic hepatitis C with interferon alpha: no association with either interferon dosage or efficacy of therapy, J Intern Med 251:400–406, 2002.

335. Monzani F, Caraccio N, Casolaro A, et al: Long-term interferon beta-1b therapy for MS: is routine thyroid assessment always useful? Neurology 55:549–552, 2000.

336. Olivieri A, Sorcini M, Battisti P, et al: Thyroid hypofunction related with the progression of human immunodeficiency virus infection, J Endocrinol Invest 16:407–413, 1993.

337. Durelli L, Ferrero B, Oggero A, et al: Thyroid function and autoimmunity during interferon beta-1b treatment: a multicenter prospective study, J Clin Endocrinol Metab 86:3525–3532, 2001.

338. Kroemer G, Francese C, Martinez C: The role of interleukin 2 in the development of autoimmune thyroiditis, Int Rev Immunol 9:107–123, 1992.

339. Witzke O, Winterhagen T, Saller B, et al: Transient stimulatory effects on pituitary-thyroid axis in patients treated with interleukin-2, Thyroid 11:665–670, 2001.

340. Karanth S, McCann SM: Anterior pituitary hormone control by interleukin 2, Proc Natl Acad Sci U S A 88:2961–2965, 1991.

340a. Torpy DJ, Tsigos C, Lotsikas AJ, et al: Acute and delayed effects of a single-dose injection of interleukin-6 on thyroid function in healthy humans, Metabolism 47:1289–1293, 1998.

341. Stuart NS, Woodroffe CM, et al: Long-term toxicity of chemotherapy for testicular cancer—the cost of cure, Br J Cancer 61:479–484, 1990.

342. Sutcliffe SB, Chapman R, Wrigley PF: Cyclical combination chemotherapy and thyroid function in patients with advanced Hodgkin's disease, Med Pediatr Oncol 9:439–448, 1981.

343. Ogilvy-Stuart AL, Shalet SM, Gattamaneni HR: Thyroid function after treatment of brain tumors in children, J Pediatr 119:733–737, 1991.

344. Reinhardt W, Sauter V, Jockenhovel F, et al: Unique alterations of thyroid function parameters after i.v. administration of alkylating drugs (cyclophosphamide and ifosfamide), Exp Clin Endocrinol Diabetes 107:177–182, 1999.

345. Santen RJ, Misbin RI: Aminoglutethimide: review of pharmacology and clinical use, Pharmacotherapy 1:95–120, 1981.

346. Dowsett M, Mehta A, Cantwell BM, et al: Low-dose aminoglutethimide in postmenopausal breast cancer: effects on adrenal and thyroid hormone secretion, Eur J Cancer 27:846–849, 1991.

347. Figg WD, Thibault A, Sartor AO, et al: Hypothyroidism associated with aminoglutethimide in patients with prostate cancer, Arch Intern Med 154:1023–1025, 1994.

348. Heidemann PH, Stubbe P, Beck W: Transient secondary hypothyroidism and thyroxine binding globulin deficiency in leukemic children during polychemotherapy: an effect of L-asparaginase, Eur J Pediatr 136:291–295, 1981.

349. Yeung SC, Chiu AC, Vassilopoulou-Sellin R, et al: The endocrine effects of nonhormonal antineoplastic therapy, Endocr Rev 19:144–172, 1998.

350. Desai J, Yassa L, Marqusee E, et al: Hypothyroidism after sunitinib treatment for patients with gastrointestinal stromal tumors, Ann Intern Med 145:660–664, 2006.

351. Wolter P, Stefan C, Decallonne B, et al: The clinical implications of sunitinib-induced hypothyroidism: a prospective evaluation, Br J Cancer 99:448–454, 2008.

352. Wong E, Rosen LS, Mulay M, et al: Sunitinib induces hypothyroidism in advanced cancer patients and may inhibit thyroid peroxidase activity, Thyroid 17:351–355, 2007.

353. Liel Y, Sperber AD, Shany S: Nonspecific intestinal adsorption of levothyroxine by aluminum hydroxide, Am J Med 97:363–365, 1994.

354. Singh N, Weisler SL, Hershman JM: The acute effect of calcium carbonate on the intestinal absorption of levothyroxine, Thyroid 11:967–971, 2001.

355. Campbell NR, Hasinoff BB, Stalts H, et al: Ferrous sulfate reduces thyroxine efficacy in patients with hypothyroidism, Ann Intern Med 117:1010–1013, 1992.

356. Jabbar MA, Larrea J, Shaw RA: Abnormal thyroid function tests in infants with congenital hypothyroidism: the influence of soy-based formula, J Am Coll Nutr 16:280–282, 1997.

357. Sherman SI, Tielens ET, Ladenson PW: Sucralfate causes malabsorption of L-thyroxine, Am J Med 96:531–535, 1994.

358. Wartofsky L, Ransil BJ, Ingbar SH: Inhibition by iodine of the release of thyroxine from the thyroid glands of patients with thyrotoxicosis, J Clin Invest 49:78–86, 1970.

359. Grubeck-Loebenstein B, Kleiber M: The influence of iodide upon thyroxine metabolism in euthyroid subjects (abstract), Acta Endocrinol 234(suppl):21, 1980.

360. McGregor A, Weetman A, Ratanachaiyavong S: Iodine: an influence on the development of autoimmune thyroid desease. In Hall R, Kobberling J, editors. Thyroid Disorder Associated with Iodine Deficiency, New York, 1985, Raven, p 209.

361. Sundick RS, Herdegen DM, Brown TR, et al: The incorporation of dietary iodine into thyroglobulin increases its immunogenicity, Endocrinology 120:2078–2084, 1987.

362. Braverman LE, Woeber KA, Ingbar SH: Induction of myxedema by iodide in patients euthyroid after radioiodine or surgical treatment of diffuse toxic goiter, N Engl J Med 281:816–821, 1969.

363. Fradkin JE, Wolff J: Iodide-induced thyrotoxicosis, Medicine (Baltimore) 62:1–20, 1983.

364. Vrobel TR, Miller PE, Mostow ND, et al: A general overview of amiodarone toxicity: its prevention, detection, and management, Prog Cardiovasc Dis 31:393–426, 1989.

365. Hershman JM, Nademanee K, Sugawara M, et al: Thyroxine and triiodothyronine kinetics in cardiac patients taking amiodarone, Acta Endocrinol (Copenh) 111:193–199, 1986.

366. Sogol PB, Hershman JM, Reed AW, et al: The effects of amiodarone on serum thyroid hormones and hepatic thyroxine 5′-monodeiodination in rats, Endocrinology 113:1464–1469, 1983.

367. Bartalena L, Brogioni S, Grasso L, et al: Treatment of amiodarone-induced thyrotoxicosis, a difficult challenge: results of a prospective study, J Clin Endocrinol Metab 81:2930–2933, 1996.

368. Georges JL, Normand JP, Lenormand ME, et al: Life-threatening thyrotoxicosis induced by amiodarone in patients with benign heart disease, Eur Heart J 13:129–132, 1992.

369. Hauptman PJ, Fyfe B, Mechanick J, et al: Fatal hyperthyroidism after amiodarone treatment and total lymphoid irradiation in a heart transplant recipient, J Heart Lung Transplant 12:513–516, 1993.

370. Dong BJ: How medications affect thyroid function, West J Med 172:102–106, 2000.

371. Lis-Balchin M: Parallel placebo-controlled clinical study of a mixture of herbs sold as a remedy for cellulite, Phytother Res 13:627–629, 1999.

372. Obregon MJ, Pascual A, Mallol J, et al: Marked decrease of the effectiveness of a T4 dose in iopanoic acid treated rats (abstract). Ann Endocrinol 40:72, 1979.

373. Beng CG, Wellby ML, Symons RG, et al: The effects of iopodate on the serum iodothyronine pattern in normal subjects, Acta Endocrinol (Copenh) 93:175–178, 1980.

374. Suzuki H, Kadena N, Takeuchi K, et al: Effects of three-day oral cholecystography on serum iodothyronines and TSH concentrations: comparison of the effects among some cholecystographic agents and the effects of iopanoic acid on the pituitary-thyroid axis, Acta Endocrinol (Copenh) 92:477–488, 1979.

375. Felicetta JV, Green WL, Nelp WB: Inhibition of hepatic binding of thyroxine by cholecystographic agents, J Clin Invest 65:1032–1040, 1980.

376. Calza L, Manfredi R, Chiodo F: Subclinical hypothyroidism in HIV-infected patients receiving highly active antiretroviral therapy, J Acquir Immune Defic Syndr 31:361–363, 2002.

377. Grappin M, Piroth L, Verges B, et al: Increased prevalence of subclinical hypothyroidism in HIV patients treated with highly active antiretroviral therapy, AIDS 14:1070–1072, 2000.

378. Beltran S, Lescure FX, Desailloud R, et al: Increased prevalence of hypothyroidism among human immunodeficiency virus-infected patients: a need for screening, Clin Infect Dis 37:579–583, 2003.

379. Jain R, Uy HL: Increase in serum free thyroxine levels related to intravenous heparin treatment, Ann Intern Med 124:74–75, 1996.

380. Cutting WC, Rytand DA, Tainter ML: Relationship between blood cholesterol and increased metabolism from dinitrophenol and thyroid, J Clin Invest 13:547–552, 1934.

381. Goldberg RC, Wolff J, Greep RO: The mechanism of depression of plasma protein bound iodine by 2,4 dinitrophenol, Endocrinology 56:560–566, 1955.

382. Christensen HR, Simonsen K, Hegedus L, et al: Influence of rifampicin on thyroid gland volume, thyroid hormones, and antipyrine metabolism, Acta Endocrinol (Copenh) 121:406–410, 1989.

383. Nolan SR, Self TH, Norwood JM: Interaction between rifampin and levothyroxine, South Med J 92:529–531, 1999.

384. Austen FK, Rubini ME, Meroney WH, et al: Salicylates and thyroid function. I. Depression of thyroid function, J Clin Invest 37:1131–1143, 1958.

385. Wolff J, Austen FK: Salicylates and thyroid function. II. The effect on the thyroid-pituitary interrelation, J Clin Invest 37:1144–1152, 1958.

386. Woeber KA, Barakat RM, Ingbar SH: Effects of salicylate and its noncalorigenic congeners on the thyroidal release of 131-I in patients with thyrotoxicosis, J Clin Endocrinol Metab 24:1163–1168, 1964.

387. McConnell RJ: Abnormal thyroid function test results in patients taking salsalate, JAMA 267:1242–1243, 1992.

388. Alexander WD, Johnson KW: A comparison of the effects of acetylsalicylic acid and DL-triiodothyronine in patients with myxoedema, Clin Sci (Lond) 15:593–601, 1956.

389. Yamamoto T, Woeber KA, Ingbar SH: The influence of salicylate on serum TSH concentration in patients with primary hypothyroidism, J Clin Endocrinol Metab 34:423–426, 1972.

390. Christensen LK: The metabolic effect of p-aminosalicylic acid, Acta Endocrinol (Copenh) 31:608–610, 1959.

391. Macgregor AG, Somner AR: The anti-thyroid action of para-aminosalicylic acid, Lancet 267:931–936, 1954.

392. Ratcliffe WA, Hazelton RA, Thomson JA, et al: The effect of fenclofenac on thyroid function tests in vivo and in vitro, Clin Endocrinol (Oxf) 13:569–575, 1980.

393. Bishnoi A, Carlson HE, Gruber BL, et al: Effects of commonly prescribed nonsteroidal anti-inflammatory drugs on thyroid hormone measurements, Am J Med 96:235–238, 1994.

394. Samuels MH, Pillote K, Asher D, et al: Variable effects of nonsteroidal antiinflammatory agents on thyroid test results, J Clin Endocrinol Metab 88:5710–5716, 2003.

395. Nadler K, Buchinger W, Semlitsch G, et al: [Effect of aceclofenac on thyroid hormone binding and thyroid function], Acta Med Austriaca 27:56–57, 2000.

396. Oppenheimer JH: Role of plasma proteins in the binding, distribution and metabolism of the thyroid hormones, N Engl J Med 278:1153–1162, 1968.

397. Snyder SM, Cavalieri RR, Ingbar SH: Simultaneous measurement of percentage free thyroxine and triiodothyronine: comparison of equilibrium dialysis and Sephadex chromatography, J Nucl Med 17:660–664, 1976.

398. Azizi F, Vagenakis AG, Portnay GI, et al: Thyroxine transport and metabolism in methadone and heroin addicts, Ann Intern Med 80:194–199, 1974.

399. McKerron CG, Scott RL, Asper SP, et al: Effects of clofibrate (Atromid S) on the thyroxine-binding capacity of thyroxine-binding globulin and free thyroxine, J Clin Endocrinol Metab 29:957–961, 1969.

400. Beex L, Ross A, Smals A, et al: 5-fluorouracil-induced increase of total serum thyroxine and triiodothyronine, Cancer Treat Rep 61:1291–1295, 1977.

401. Oltman JE, Friedman S: Protein-bound iodine in patients receiving perphenazine, JAMA 185:726–727, 1963.

402. Anker GB, Lonning PE, Aakvaag A, et al: Thyroid function in postmenopausal breast cancer patients treated with tamoxifen, Scand J Clin Lab Invest 58:103–107, 1998.

403. Draper MW, Flowers DE, Neild JA, et al: Antiestrogenic properties of raloxifene, Pharmacology 50:209–217, 1995.

404. Duntas LH, Mantzou E, Koutras DA: Lack of substantial effects of raloxifene on thyroxine-binding globulin in postmenopausal women: dependency on thyroid status, Thyroid 11:779–782, 2001.

405. Marqusee E, Braverman LE, Lawrence JE, et al: The effect of droloxifene and estrogen on thyroid function in postmenopausal women, J Clin Endocrinol Metab 85:4407–4410, 2000.

406. Barbosa J, Seal US, Doe RP: Effects of anabolic steroids on hormone-binding proteins, serum cortisol and serum nonprotein-bound cortisol, J Clin Endocrinol Metab 32:232–240, 1971.

407. Braverman LE, Ingbar SH: Effects of norethandrolone on the transport in serum and peripheral turnover of thyroxine, J Clin Endocrinol Metab 27:389–396, 1967.

408. Oppenheimer JH, Werner SC: Effect of prednisone on thyroxine-binding proteins, J Clin Endocrinol Metab 26:715–721, 1966.

409. Garnick MB, Larsen PR: Acute deficiency of thyroxine-binding globulin during L-asparaginase therapy, N Engl J Med 301:252–253, 1979.

410. O'Brien T, Silverberg JD, Nguyen TT: Nicotinic acid-induced toxicity associated with cytopenia and decreased levels of thyroxine-binding globulin, Mayo Clin Proc 67:465–468, 1992.

411. Shakir KM, Kroll S, Aprill BS, et al: Nicotinic acid decreases serum thyroid hormone levels while maintaining a euthyroid state, Mayo Clin Proc 70:556–558, 1995.

412. McConnell RJ: Changes in thyroid function tests during short-term salsalate use, Metabolism 48:501–503, 1999.

413. Surks MI, Sievert R: Drugs and thyroid function, N Engl J Med 333:1688–1694, 1995.

414. Tabachnick M, Hao YL, Korcek L: Effect of oleate, diphenylhydantoin and heparin on the binding of 125 I-thyroxine to purified thyroxine-binding globulin, J Clin Endocrinol Metab 36:392–394, 1973.

415. Schussler GC: Diazepam competes for thyroxine binding, J Pharmacol Exp Ther 178:204–209, 1971.

416. Stockigt JR, Lim CF, Barlow JW, et al: Interaction of furosemide with serum thyroxine-binding sites: in vivo and in vitro studies and comparison with other inhibitors, J Clin Endocrinol Metab 60:1025–1031, 1985.

417. Hershman JM, Craane TJ, Colwell JA: Effect of sulfonylurea drugs on the binding of triiodothyronine and thyroxine to thyroxine-binding globulin, J Clin Endocrinol Metab 28:1605–1610, 1968.

418. Marshall JS, Tompkins LS: Effect of o,p′-DDD and similar compounds on thyroxine binding globulin, J Clin Endocrinol Metab 28:386–392, 1968.

419. Abiodun MO, Bird R, Havard CW, et al: The effects of phenylbutazone on thyroid function, Acta Endocrinol (Copenh) 72:257–264, 1973.

420. Davis PJ, Hsu TH, Bianchine JR, et al: Effects of a new hypolipidemic agents, MK-185, on serum thyroxine-binding globulin (TBG) and dialyzable fraction thyroxine, J Clin Endocrinol Metab 34:200–208, 1972.

421. Taylor R, Clark F, Griffiths ID, et al: Prospective study of effect of fenclofenac on thyroid function tests, Br Med J 281:911–912, 1980.

422. Stevenson HP, Archbold GP, Johnston P, et al: Misleading serum free thyroxine results during low molecular weight heparin treatment, Clin Chem 44:1002–1007, 1998.

423. Wiersinga WM, Fabius AJ, Touber JL: Orphenadrine (Disipal), serum thyroxine and thyroid function, Acta Endocrinol (Copenh) 86:522–532, 1977.

424. Michajlovskij N, Langer P: Increase of serum free thyroxine following the administration of thiocyanate and other anions in vivo and in vitro, Acta Endocrinol (Copenh) 75:707–716, 1974.

425. Pages RA, Robbins J, Edelhoch H: Binding of thyroxine and thyroxine analogs to human serum prealbumin, Biochemistry 12:2773–2779, 1973.

426. Huang SA, Tu HM, Harney JW, et al: Severe hypothyroidism caused by type 3 iodothyronine deiodinase in infantile hemangiomas, N Engl J Med 343:185–189, 2000.

427. Escobar Del Rey F, Morreale De Escobar G: The effect of propylthiouracil, methylthiouracil and thiouracil on the peripheral metabolism of L-thyroxine in thyroidectomized, L-thyroxine maintained rats, Endocrinology 69:456–465, 1961.

428. Furth ED, Rives K, Becker DV: Nonthyroidal action of propylthiouracil in euthyroid, hypothyroid and hyperthyroid man, J Clin Endocrinol Metab 26:239–246, 1966.

429. Oppenheimer JH, Schwartz HL, Surks MI: Propylthiouracil inhibits the conversion of L-thyroxine to L-

triiodothyronine. An explanation of the antithyroxine effect of propylthiouracil and evidence supporting the concept that triiodothyronine is the active thyroid hormone, J Clin Invest 51:2493–2497, 1972.

430. Faber J, Friis T, Kirkegaard C, et al: Serum T4, T3 and reverse T3 during treatment with propranolol in hyperthyroidism, L-T4 treated myxedema and in normal man, Horm Metab Res 11:34–36, 1979.

431. Wiersinga WM, Touber JL: The influence of beta-adrenoceptor blocking agents on plasma thyroxine and triiodothyronine, J Clin Endocrinol Metab 45:293–298, 1977.

432. Torpy DJ, Tsigos C, Lotsikas AJ, et al: Acute and delayed effects of a single-dose injection of interleukin-6 on thyroid function in healthy humans, Metabolism 47:1289–1293, 1998.

433. Burgi H, Wimpfheimer C, Burger A, et al: Changes of circulating thyroxine, triiodothyronine and reverse triiodothyronine after radiographic contrast agents, J Clin Endocrinol Metab 43:1203–1210, 1976.

434. Wu SY, Chopra IJ, Solomon DH, et al: Changes in circulating iodothyronines in euthyroid and hyperthyroid subjects given ipodate (Oragrafin), an agent for oral cholecystography, J Clin Endocrinol Metab 46:691–697, 1978.

435. Burger A, Dinichert D, Nicod P, et al: Effect of amiodarone on serum triiodothyronine, reverse triiodothyronine, thyroxin, and thyrotropin. A drug influencing peripheral metabolism of thyroid hormones, J Clin Invest 58:255–259, 1976.

436. Franklyn JA, Davis JR, Gammage MD, et al: Amiodarone and thyroid hormone action, Clin Endocrinol (Oxf) 22:257–264, 1985.

437. Nademanee K, Piwonka RW, Singh BN, et al: Amiodarone and thyroid function, Prog Cardiovasc Dis 31:427–437, 1989.

438. Schlienger JL, Kapfer MT, Singer L, et al: The action of clomipramine on thyroid function, Horm Metab Res 12:481–482, 1980.

439. Larsen PR, Atkinson AJ Jr, Wellman HN, et al: The effect of diphenylhydantoin on thyroxine metabolism in man, J Clin Invest 49:1266–1279, 1970.

440. Rootwelt K, Ganes T, Johannessen SI: Effect of carbamazepine, phenytoin and phenobarbitone on serum levels of thyroid hormones and thyrotropin in humans, Scand J Clin Lab Invest 38:731–736, 1978.

441. Isley WL: Effect of rifampin therapy on thyroid function tests in a hypothyroid patient on replacement L-thyroxine, Ann Intern Med 107:517–518, 1987.

442. McCowen KC, Garber JR, Spark R: Elevated serum thyrotropin in thyroxine-treated patients with hypothyroidism given sertraline, N Engl J Med 337:1010–1011, 1997.

443. Northcutt RC, Stiel JN, Hollifield JW, et al: The influence of cholestyramine on thyroxine absorption, JAMA 208:1857–1861, 1969.

444. Van Wyk JJ, Arnold MB, Wynn J, et al: The effects of a soybean product on thyroid function in humans, Pediatrics 48:752–760, 1959.

445. Singh N, Singh PN, Hershman JM: Effect of calcium carbonate on the absorption of levothyroxine, JAMA 283:2822–2825, 2000.

446. Havrankova J, Lahaie R: Levothyroxine binding by sucralfate, Ann Intern Med 117:445–446, 1992.

447. Sperber AD, Liel Y: Evidence for interference with the intestinal absorption of levothyroxine sodium by aluminum hydroxide, Arch Intern Med 152:183–184, 1992.

448. Kleinmann RE, Vagenakis AG, Braverman LE: The effect of iopanoic acid on the regulation of thyrotropin secretion in euthyroid subjects, J Clin Endocrinol Metab 51:399–403, 1980.

449. Vagenakis AG, Rapoport B, Azizi F, et al: Hyperresponse to thyrotropin-releasing hormone accompanying small decreases in serum thyroid hormone concentrations, J Clin Invest 54:913–918, 1974.

450. Lazarus JH, John R, Bennie EH, et al: Lithium therapy and thyroid function: a long-term study, Psychol Med 11:85–92, 1981.

451. Delitala G, Devilla L, Lotti G: Domperidone, an extracerebral inhibitor of dopamine receptors, stimulates thyrotropin and prolactin release in man, J Clin Endocrinol Metab 50:1127–1130, 1980.

452. Kirkegaard C, Bjorum N, Cohn D, et al: Studies on the influence of biogenic amines and psychoactive drugs on the prognostic value of the TRH stimulation test in endogenous depression, Psychoneuroendocrinology 2:131–136, 1977.

453. Delitala G: Dopamine and T.S.H. secretion in man, Lancet 2:760–761, 1977.

454. Massara F, Camanni F, Belforte L, et al: Increased thyrotrophin secretion induced by sulpiride in man, Clin Endocrinol (Oxf) 9:419–428, 1978.

455. Delitala G, Devilla L, Lotti G: TSH and prolactin stimulation by the decarboxylase inhibitor benserazide in primary hypothyroidism, Clin Endocrinol (Oxf) 12:313–316, 1980.

456. Kirkegaard C, Bjorum N, Cohn D, et al: Thyrotrophin-releasing hormone (TRH) stimulation test in manic-depressive illness, Arch Gen Psychiatry 35:1017–1021, 1978.

457. Nelis GF, Van de Meene JG: The effect of oral cimetidine on the basal and stimulated values of prolactin, thyroid stimulating hormone, follicle stimulating hormone and luteinizing hormone, Postgrad Med J 56:26–29, 1980.

458. Smals AG, Kloppenborg PW, Hoefnagels WH, et al: Pituitary-thyroid function in spironolactone treated hypertensive women, Acta Endocrinol (Copenh) 90:577–584, 1979.

459. Morley JE, Shafer RB, Elson MK, et al: Amphetamine-induced hyperthyroxinemia, Ann Intern Med 93:707–709, 1980.

460. Gloebel B, Weinheimer B: TRH-test during D-T4 application, Nuc-Compact 8:44, 1977.

461. Medeiros-Neto G, Kallas WG, Knobel M, et al: Triac (3,5,3'-triiodothyroacetic acid) partially inhibits the thyrotropin response to synthetic thyrotropin-releasing hormone in normal and thyroidectomized hypothyroid patients, J Clin Endocrinol Metab 50:223–225, 1980.

462. Emrich D: [The influence of etiroxat-HCl on iodine metabolism in man (author's transl)], Arzneimittelforschung 27:422–426, 1977.

463. Tamagna EI, Hershman JM, Jorgensen EC: Thyrotropin suppression by 3,5-dimethyl-3'-isopropyl-L-thyronine in man, J Clin Endocrinol Metab 48:196–200, 1979.

464. Scanlon MF, Weightman DR, Shale DJ, et al: Dopamine is a physiological regulator of thyrotrophin (TSH) secretion in normal man, Clin Endocrinol (Oxf) 10:7–15, 1979.

465. Yoshimura M, Ochi Y, Miyazaki T, et al: Effect of intravenous and oral administration of L-dopa on HGH and TSH release, Endocrinol Jpn 19:543–548, 1972.

466. Giusti M, Lomeo A, Torre R, et al: Effect of subacute cabergoline treatment on prolactin, thyroid stimulating hormone and growth hormone response to simultaneous administration of thyrotrophin-releasing hormone and growth hormone-releasing hormone in hyperprolactinaemic women, Clin Endocrinol (Oxf) 30:315–321, 1989.

467. Miyal K, Onishi T, Hosokawa M, et al: Inhibition of thyrotropin and prolactin secretions in primary hypothyroidism by 2-Br-alpha-ergocryptine, J Clin Endocrinol Metab 39:391–394, 1974.

468. Lamberg BA, Linnoila M, Fogelholm R, et al: The effect of psychotropic drugs on the TSH-response to thyroliberin (TRH), Neuroendocrinology 24:90–97, 1977.

469. Nilsson KO, Thorell JI, Hokfelt B: The effect of thyrotrophin releasing hormone on the release of thyrotrophin and other pituitary hormones in man under basal conditions and following adrenergic blocking agents, Acta Endocrinol (Copenh) 76:24–34, 1974.

470. Delitala G, Rovasio PP, Masala A, et al: Metergoline inhibition of thyrotrophin and prolactin secretions in primary hypothyroidism, Clin Endocrinol (Oxf) 8:69–73, 1978.

471. Ferrari C, Paracchi A, Rondena M, et al: Effect of two serotonin antagonists on prolactin and thyrotrophin secretion in man, Clin Endocrinol (Oxf) 5:575–578, 1976.

472. Collu R: The effect of TRH on the release of TSH, PRL and GH in man under basal conditions and following methysergide, J Endocrinol Invest 1:121–124, 1978.

473. Dussault JH: The effect of dexamethasone on TSH and prolactin secretion after TRH stimulation, Can Med Assoc J 111:1195–1197, 1974.

474. Re RN, Kourides IA, Ridgway EC, et al: The effect of glucocorticoid administration on human pituitary secretion of thyrotropin and prolactin, J Clin Endocrinol Metab 43:338–346, 1976.

475. Bertherat J, Brue T, Enjalbert A, et al: Somatostatin receptors on thyrotropin-secreting pituitary adenomas: comparison with the inhibitory effects of octreotide upon in vivo and in vitro hormonal secretions, J Clin Endocrinol Metab 75:540–546, 1992.

476. Thomas JA, Shahid-Salles KS, Donovan MP: Effects of narcotics on the reproductive system, Adv Sex Horm Res 3:169–195, 1977.

477. May P, Mittler J, Manougian A, et al: TSH release-inhibiting activity of leucine-enkephalin, Horm Metab Res 11:30–33, 1979.

478. Kobayashi I, Shimomura Y, Maruta S, et al: Clofibrate and a related compound suppress TSH secretion in primary hypothyroidism, Acta Endocrinol (Copenh) 94:53–57, 1980.

479. Sherman SI, Gopal J, Haugen BR, et al: Central hypothyroidism associated with retinoid X receptor-selective ligands, N Engl J Med 340:1075–1079, 1999.

Chapter 7

THYROID IMAGING

MANFRED BLUM

More than half a century ago, imaging the thyroid gland was accomplished when the isotope I-131 and rectilinear scanning became available. Thyroid scintiscanning takes advantage of the thyroid gland's unique ability to concentrate the radioactive tracer of iodine and to organify it and produce thyroxine. Thus scintiscanning is a biomarker-imaging technique. Another biomarker is radiolabeled glucose to identify rapidly metabolizing tissue such as thyroid cancer, which is the basis of PET scanning. Unfortunately, neither of these techniques produce the precise anatomic localization offered by anatomic imaging methods such as ultrasonography, computed tomography (CT), and magnetic resonance imaging (MRI), which lack tissue specificity. Special computer software and advanced engineering permit bimodality scanning in which biomarker images from the positron emission tomography (PET) scan and anatomic CT or MRI images can be fused to produce excellent and precise correlation of metabolic activity and anatomic location. Although each type of imaging modality can answer specific diagnostic questions, any imaging procedure might be unnecessary and even misleading when used indiscriminately or inappropriately.

This chapter mainly discusses how the various thyroid imaging techniques can be integrated into patient management. Imaging in epidemiology or as an aid to teaching thyroidology will be mentioned briefly. As a basic principle in patient care, thyroid imaging should be used only when needed to arrive at a diagno-sis and to assist in planning therapy. Imaging procedures should not be used for the purpose of screening. Nor should they be done before the clinical history has been taken, a physical examination has been performed, and a differential diagnosis has been formulated. Imaging procedures should be used together with other laboratory data to answer specific diagnostic questions. Selection of the proper procedure is predicated on an understanding of the disease under consideration and an awareness of the known capabilities and limitations of the techniques. Imaging tests are not efficient in assessing the presence of cancer in a thyroid nodule. Furthermore, it is essential to precisely correlate the results of palpation with the image. Rarely is more than one imaging modality required to solve a problem. The exception is PET scanning, in which bimodality imaging that fuses PET and CT or MRI images is standard. As a guiding principle, when the information that is obtained from one imaging examination is inadequate and an additional type of imaging is required, the several images should be correlated to optimize their combined diagnostic value.

Radioiodine Uptake by the Thyroid

This subject will be summarized here briefly because scintigraphic images are dependent on proper accumulation of radioiodine by thyroid cells. Testing the extent to which the thyroid gland accumulates a tracer quantity of radioactive iodine is an application of thyroid iodine physiology that correlates with thyroid metabolic activity under normal circumstances. Inorganic iodide is cleared from the blood mainly by the thyroid gland and by the kidney. It is vitally important to keep in mind that the fetal thyroid and the lactating breast also concentrate iodide, so radioiodine must not be given to a pregnant or nursing woman. RAIU represents the fractional clearance of iodide (%) by the thyroid gland at a given time. There is a progression of iodine accumulation that peaks at about 24 hours after administration. Under physiologic conditions at this time, clearance by the thyroid is approximately 17 mL of blood per minute and by the kidneys 35 mL per minute. The net clearance is 52 mL per minute, and thyroid RAIU in a euthyroid person is about 30% $(17 \div [17 + 35] \times 100)$. Thyroid clearance is stimulated by thyrotropin, or thyroid-stimulating hormone (TSH), and is inversely proportional to dietary iodine intake. Renal clearance is independent of TSH or the iodide load and is reduced when the kidneys fail. Therefore, TSH excess, residence in an iodine-deprived geographic area, consuming a low-iodine (low-salt) diet, or severely decreased renal function will result in an elevated RAIU.

Conversely, a reduced RAIU will occur when TSH is deficient owing to pituitary failure, if excessive iodine is ingested, or if iodinated contrast radiographic dye or medications that are rich in iodine are administered. When these abnormalities are not present, hyperthyroidism or hypothyroidism cause increased or decreased RAIU, respectively. Faulty production of thyroid hormone, called *dyshormonogenesis*, has a variable effect on the progression of iodine accumulation and the RAIU, depending on where the enzyme defect is located in the metabolic sequence. Optimal interpretation of scintiscans of the thyroid requires a comprehension of this physiologic and pathophysiologic information.

Radioisotope Scintiscanning (Scintigraphy)

Scintigraphy provides information about the functional anatomy of an organ; it is a biomarker. When scintigraphy is applied to the thyroid gland, the resulting image, by showing the pattern of distribution of radioiodine or pertechnetate, reveals the location and volume of functioning thyroid tissue and answers the question of whether a particular nodule is functioning (how well it accumulates the reference tracer material). Thyroid scintiscanning is not to be confused with thyroid radioiodine uptake testing. The latter is a quantitative measure of the function of the entire gland in trapping and retaining iodine.

Common clinical indications for thyroid scintigraphy are listed in Table 7-1. In the assessment of a hyperthyroid patient with a single or multinodular goiter, scintigraphy provides information that no other imaging modality offers—namely, whether a nodule or nodules are the source of the hyperthyroidism.

RADIONUCLIDES USED IN THE DIAGNOSIS OF THYROID DISORDERS

Several radionuclides can be used for imaging the thyroid (Table 7-2). The choice depends in part on the clinical question to be addressed. Of the isotopes of iodine, ^{123}I is close to an ideal agent both for imaging and for determining thyroid uptake. [123]I exposes the gland to relatively low radiation doses.[1,2] The commonly administered activity (orally) of ^{123}I for imaging the thyroid ranges from 100 to 600 μCi (7.4 to 22 MBq). [123]I images of the gland may be obtained any time between 4 hours and 24 hours after administration.

Technetium-99m (^{99m}Tc) in the form of pertechnetate is trapped by the thyroid gland and other sites that concentrate iodide (salivary glands, gastric mucosa), but it is not organified in the thyroid and is therefore not a true tracer of iodine metabolism.[1] The radiation exposure to the thyroid from ^{99m}Tc is even lower than that from [123]I. [99m]Tc is readily available in nuclear medicine laboratories and is relatively inexpensive. ^{99m}Tc-pertechnetate is administered intravenously in amounts ranging from 2 to 10 mCi (74 to 370 MBq), and imaging of the thyroid is usually begun 15 to 30 minutes after injection.[2]

[123]I and ^{99m}Tc have largely replaced ^{131}I for thyroid scintigraphy. Radiation exposure to the thyroid from ^{131}I per microcurie administered is 100-fold higher than that from ^{123}I, and ^{131}I-labeled images of the gland are generally inferior in quality because of the high γ energy of [131]I.

The principal diagnostic use of ^{131}I is in whole-body scanning to search for functioning metastases that are potentially treatable with ^{131}I in patients who have had thyroid cancer surgery. The 8-day half-life of ^{131}I permits scanning over a period of several days, which facilitates proper identification of anatomic sites that accumulate inorganic iodine but do not produce or harbor thyroxine and also iodine excretory routes. In distinction to these transient foci of radioactivity, functioning metastases retain activity and slowly release their organic product. Thus the signal-to-noise ratio is enhanced greatly. The long half-life also allows for dosimetry in preparation for ^{131}I therapy. A high beta-particle radiation exposure to the thyroid gland (in contrast to all other organs and tissues) from ^{131}I, the long half-life, and selective concentration of the isotope by the thyroid together permit destruction of benign or malignant thyroid tissue.

SCINTISCANNING INSTRUMENTATION

In most nuclear medicine laboratories, the scintillation camera has largely replaced the rectilinear scanner for thyroid imaging. The camera is fitted with a pinhole collimator, which provides a

Table 7-1. Clinical Indications for Thyroid Scintigraphy

Clinical Setting	Purpose of Scintigraphy
1. Hyperthyroid patient with or without a goiter (diffuse or nodular)	To determine function of palpable nodule(s) To detect unsuspected cold nodule(s) in a diffusely hyperfunctioning gland To distinguish Graves' disease from toxic nodular goiter or other causes of thyrotoxicosis (e.g., destructive thyroiditides) To estimate volume of a functional gland before ^{131}I therapy
2. Euthyroid patient with a solitary nodule ("follicular neoplasm" on FNA) multinodular goiter	To determine whether the nodule is hyperfunctional To identify hypofunctional nodule(s) before FNA To estimate the volume and location of functional tissue in planning surgery or ^{131}I therapy
3. Patient suspected of having an ectopic thyroid	To identify a mass as functioning thyroid tissue (e.g., substernal goiter, lingual thyroid)
4. Patient who has had thyroid surgery for cancer	To define the amount of thyroid remnant (usually combined with whole-body scintigraphy)

Data from Cavalieri and McDougall[1] and Becker et al.[2]
FNA, Fine-needle aspiration.

Table 7-2. Radionuclides Used in Thyroid Scintigraphy

Radionuclide/ Chemical Form	Physical Half-Life	Type of Emission	Clinical Applications
[123]I-iodide	13 hours	Gamma	Thyroid scintigraphy (planar or SPECT)
[131]I-iodide	8 days	Gamma and beta	Whole-body scintigraphy (posttreatment for thyroid cancer) Radioiodine therapy
[99m]Tc-pertechnetate	6 hours	Gamma	Thyroid scintigraphy
[99m]Tc-sestamibi*	6 hours	Gamma	Localization of thyroid cancer metastases
[201]Tl-Cl⁻	77 hours	Gamma	Localization of thyroid cancer metastases
[18]F-fluorodeoxyglucose (FDG)	110 min	Positron	Localization of thyroid cancer metastases

SPECT, Single-photon emission computed tomography.
*Other radioactive agents that have been used for localizing metastases from thyroid cancer include ^{99m}Tc-tetrofosmin and ^{99m}Tc-labeled dimercaptosuccinic acid (DMSA) (V). Medullary thyroid carcinoma has been imaged with ^{99m}Tc-DMSA (V) and ^{111}In-octreotide (reviewed by Sisson[19]).

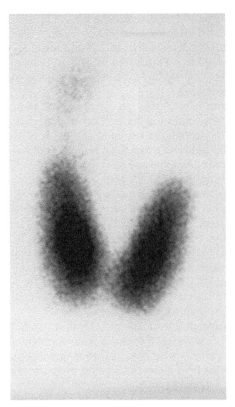

FIGURE 7-1. Scintiscan of the thyroid in a 72-year-old patient with Graves' hyperthyroidism. This image was obtained with a pinhole collimator 6 hours after oral administration of 200 μCi [123]I. Thyroid uptake was 24% at 6 hours. Note the diffuse pattern of ^{123}I distribution throughout the gland. The faint activity extending superiorly from the right lobe is a pyramidal lobe.

variable-size image of the gland and yields higher resolution than that obtained with a parallel-hole collimator or rectilinear scanner[3] (Fig. 7-1). The pinhole technique permits oblique views of the gland, which is an advantage in detecting posterior nodules, but accurate estimation of gland size is not possible. In dealing with thyroid nodules, it is important to correlate the image with the palpable lesion by placing radioactive spot markers on the skin overlying or adjacent to the nodule. Particular care must be taken in placing radioactive markers because parallax errors are possible with the pinhole method, and in the case of small nodules (<1 cm), skin markers may even be misleading. Furthermore, it is extremely difficult and undependable for a physician to palpate for thyroid pathology when a patient is "under" a gamma camera, which is necessary to correlate anatomy and image in the scanning position. The parallel-hole collimator technique is better at assessing size because it avoids parallax error, but standards of image contrast and intensity are arbitrary, and the assessment of thyroid dimensions is subjective and inconsistent. The resolution of nodules with this collimator is very poor.

Rectilinear scanners equipped with a focused collimator and a coaxial, narrow beam of light that is projected onto a palpated anatomic feature provide life-size images and allow accurate correlation of an image and the palpation. If desired, the pencil of light can be used to place markers over nodules and landmarks, or the scan film can be marked directly to localize a lesion or physical feature. The resolution of a rectilinear scanner image is not as high as that produced by a camera with a pinhole collimator.[3] These scanners are currently not commercially available.

Whole-body scintiscans, obtained by using either a scintillation camera or a rectilinear scanner and a special scanning table, are used in surveys for thyroid cancer metastases that involve the administration of ^{131}I or other radiolabeled agents. A scanning system that results in a composite image of the entire body provides more reliable anatomic orientation and is easier to interpret than multiple scans of isolated areas. However, spot-scans of a specific area such as the neck may offer superior anatomic detail.

Single-photon emission computed tomography (SPECT), which is widely used in nuclear medicine and requires more isotope than standard scintiscanning, provides three-dimensional images or tomographic slices through the organ of interest. When used with either ^{99m}Tc or ^{123}I, SPECT of the thyroid has an advantage over other methods of scintigraphy (including the pinhole technique) in defining the function of small nodules that may be obscured by overlying normal thyroid tissue.[4] SPECT is also useful for estimating the volume of functioning thyroid and for identifying thyroid tissue in ectopic sites such as the substernal area. [131]I SPECT whole-body scanning in thyroid cancer patients greatly enhances anatomic localization of metastases. Fusion of SPECT images with CT or MRI images provides the most impressive and precise anatomic localization.

Positron emission tomography (PET) requires special tomographic equipment that is capable of imaging the high-energy γ-rays produced by positron-emitting radionuclides (e.g., ^{18}F and ^{124}I).

As a caveat, with scanning in general and particularly with whole-body scanning, one must keep in mind that the scan image of a metastasis that accumulates abundant isotope might appear to be considerably larger than the mass. Especially in the neck, ultrasonography is the best way to estimate the volume of a metastasis.

PATIENT PREPARATION

For thyroid scanning, the patient need not be fasting on the morning of the study, but a heavy meal can retard absorption of iodide and reduce uptake values for the initial hours. Patients are asked about medications and dietary items that interfere with thyroid radioiodine uptake. When the uptake of radioiodine is low for any reason, the quality of the image is impaired. The most common interfering substances are radiographic contrast dyes, drugs that contain iodine (e.g., amiodarone), and iodine-containing food supplements such as kelp. Thyroid hormone in any form reduces thyroid radioiodine uptake except when autonomously functioning thyroid tissue is present or there is an abnormal thyroid stimulator. Because the administration of radioactive materials is contraindicated during pregnancy and breastfeeding, these aspects of the history must be included in the preliminary interview when appropriate.

DIAGNOSTIC APPLICATIONS OF THYROID SCINTIGRAPHY

The Thyroid Nodule

The terms *cold* and *hot* are commonly used to describe the functional activity of thyroid nodules as revealed by scintigraphy. These descriptors refer to the apparent amount of radionuclide in the lesion relative to that in surrounding normal thyroid tissue. Until recently, this distinction was diagnostically important to identify thyroid cancer. Nearly all malignant tumors in the thyroid concentrate less radioiodine or ^{99m}Tc than the normal gland and therefore appear cold (hypofunctional). However, since many benign tumors and nontumorous nodules are also

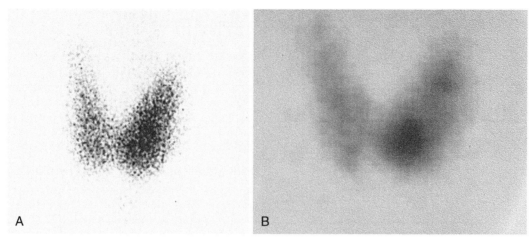

FIGURE 7-2. Thyroid scintiscans in a mildly hyperthyroid patient (suppressed serum thyroid-stimulating hormone, borderline-high free thyroxine and triiodothyronine levels) with a palpable 1.5-cm solitary nodule in the lower portion of the left thyroid lobe. **A,** Pinhole image showing that most of the ^{123}I uptake is in the lower pole of the left lobe, which corresponds to the palpable nodule. **B,** Single-photon emission computed tomographic (SPECT) image showing a more clearly delineated hyperfunctioning nodule in the lower pole and two smaller (nonpalpable) foci of uptake in the upper portion of the left lobe. Both pinhole and SPECT images were obtained 6 hours after administration of ^{123}I (200 µCi). The diagnosis was multiple autonomously functioning nodules.

cold, that characteristic is now of limited clinical use because of the advent of fine-needle biopsy (FNB). Now "hot versus cold" is important in the choice not to do an FNB in patients with a nodule when TSH is low and the nodule is hot; hot nodules are very rarely malignant, and the biopsy may be misleading by incorrectly suggesting malignancy (Fig. 7-2).

The term *warm nodule* is ambiguous and not helpful in assessing the risk of cancer. The term should not be used. A nodule that is not clearly delineated on a scintiscan may in fact be a cold nodule that is too small or too close to normal activity to be distinguishable from surrounding normal thyroid tissue. In general, a cold nodule must be almost 1 cm or larger in diameter to be detected by pinhole imaging.

Because the great majority of nodules are cold on radioisotope scintiscanning, and such cold nodules may be either benign or malignant, it is not cost effective to obtain a scintiscan as the initial diagnostic test in a euthyroid (normal TSH) patient with a nodule. A fine-needle aspiration (FNA) biopsy is usually performed first. However, when the FNA result indicates sheets of follicular cells that do not look malignant but could be a tumor, scintigraphy may be helpful to identify a hot nodule, thus avoiding surgery.

There are two kinds of hot nodules. The majority of them are reactive to elevated TSH in an otherwise failing thyroid gland and thus are compensatory. These are called *hyperplastic nodules*. The *hot* nodules associated with low TSH are autonomous nodules. They function autonomously because the TSH receptor of the thyroid cell has mutated and does not require TSH to stimulate cell activities such as the production of thyroxine or cell replication and nodule growth. The clone of the mutated cells is a benign tumor, which is the nodule, and may grow large enough over time to lead to hyperthyroidism ("toxic" nodule, TAN). When TAN-produced thyroid hormone levels increase, TSH falls, leading to suppression of the normal paranodular tissue in both thyroid lobes.[5] The chance of malignancy in a hot nodule is less than 1%.[1] Therefore, when TSH is undetectable in a patient with a thyroid nodule, a scintiscan may be the next appropriate test. In some cases, a hyperfunctioning nodule undergoes degeneration or hemorrhage, and therefore part of it, or uncommonly all of it, becomes hypofunctioning or cold. Some of the reported instances of cold areas in a hot nodule are in fact

cases of small, coexisting carcinomas in close proximity to a larger, benign hot nodule. Although documented cases have been reported in which the entire hot nodule is malignant, these cases are quite rare.

Occasionally, follicular neoplasms (including follicular adenomas and even some carcinomas) may appear hot on a ^{99m}Tc-pertechnetate image but cold on a radioiodine image, presumably because such tumors are able to trap but do not organify iodine. This type of discordance between ^{99m}Tc and radioiodine images occurs infrequently and must be recognized when ^{99m}Tc is used for thyroid scintiscanning.[5-7]

In the past, one spoke of a solitary thyroid nodule. We assumed incorrectly that if the rest of the thyroid gland was normal to palpation, it was free of nodules. Examination by ultrasound and correlation with pathology have disclosed that nonpalpable nodules occur commonly when a dominant nodule has been palpated.

Multinodular Goiter

Scintiscanning by itself does not reveal the etiology of a multinodular goiter. Scintiscanning has a role in the diagnostic assessment of multinodular goiter in some patients. When the nodules are discrete and larger than 1 cm in diameter, the scintiscan reveals the functional activity of a particular nodule relative to that of paranodular tissue (Fig. 7-3). When a nodule is clinically dominant—that is, a nodule that on palpation or by ultrasonography is different from the other nodules or is growing faster—the finding on scintiscan that this nodule contains all or most of the functional activity helps to guide management. Such a functioning nodule is unlikely to be malignant. When a multinodular goiter is large and causes symptoms and signs of compression of the trachea or esophagus, scintiscanning may complement other imaging modalities such as MRI or sonography. Either of the latter two methods depicts the extent of the goitrous mass, but only scintiscanning can reveal functioning tissue, information that is often helpful in making therapeutic decisions such as surgery or ^{131}I therapy.

In a hyperthyroid patient with a nodular goiter, there may be several different patterns on scintigraphy. The image may show many functioning, widely dispersed nodules, generally smaller than 0.5 cm, that have a salt-and-pepper appearance; a coarsely

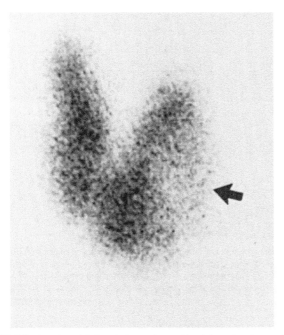

FIGURE 7-3. Anterior pinhole scintiscan of a multinodular goiter in a euthyroid patient. Physical examination revealed many firm nodules with the largest nodule (2 × 3 cm) in the left lobe. The image, obtained 24 hours after administration of 250 μCi [123]I (thyroid uptake, 23%), shows the left lobe nodule to be cold *(arrow)*. A functioning nodule is seen in the isthmus. Surgical excision of the gland showed all nodules to be mixed solid/cystic and benign.

patchy distribution may be evident, or a uniform pattern of uptake not unlike that of Graves' disease can be seen. In contrast, there may be a cold zone correlating with a nodule that should be evaluated by other means, such as sonography and aspiration biopsy.

In a hypothyroid patient with nodular goiter, the uptake is usually low (unless there is iodine deficiency or dyshormonogenesis), and thus the scintigraphic image shows a "patchy" distribution of radioisotope because of low "counts" that result in poor scan statistics. However, scintigraphy may be of clinical value to identify a reactive, hyperplastic, functional area that is rarely malignant.

Diffuse Goiter Including Graves' Disease

Assessing the thyroid uptake of radioiodine is diagnostically important to differentiate the low accumulation of the tracer in silent thyroiditis and its high accretion in hyperthyroid Graves' disease and for precise dosimetry of ^{131}I therapy. However, thyroid scintiscanning usually is not clinically useful in diffuse goiters. If assessing size is desired, an ultrasonogram offers superior results. Yet, some clinicians order scintiscans for patients with Graves' disease.

The pattern of isotope accumulation in Graves' disease usually is uniform, but irregular distribution may occur, especially in a geographic region where goiter is endemic. The heterogeneity should not be misconstrued as reflecting toxic nodular goiter when the clinical setting and serologic tests are more consistent with Graves' disease. At times, a patient with Graves' disease may have a palpable thyroid nodule or an unusually firm area, or a nonisotopic neck-imaging procedure might have disclosed an incidentaloma (discussed later) that leads to scintiscanning to assess whether it is cold, in which case sonography and aspiration biopsy might be appropriate. Similarly, a "routine" scintiscan might have revealed a cold area that should be investigated.

Substernal Goiter

A substernal goiter is suspected when chest radiographs or CT reveal an anterior mediastinal mass. A positive radioiodine scintigram definitively identifies such a mass as thyroid tissue. [123]I or ^{131}I is preferred over ^{99m}Tc in such cases because of interference by circulating ^{99m}Tc in the mediastinal blood vessels. SPECT (using ^{123}I) is of particular value in visualizing substernal thyroid tissue and SPECT/CT or MR can precisely localize it to an anatomical structure.

Scintigraphy in Patients With Thyroid Carcinoma

In general, thyroid carcinoma takes up and retains radioiodine much less efficiently than normal thyroid tissue does. Therefore, most thyroid cancers are cold nodules. However, after the thyroid gland has been removed surgically and under the stimulation of elevated TSH levels and iodine deprivation, the uptake in differentiated thyroid carcinoma is often sufficiently high to permit detection by scintigraphy and therapy with [131]I. Thus diagnostic imaging with radioiodine is indicated for patients who have recently undergone thyroid surgery for differentiated thyroid carcinoma. The rationale for imaging in such patients is to identify and quantify uptake in the thyroid remnant and to detect any functioning metastases in the neck or in distant sites. This information helps to determine the amount of ^{131}I that should be administered to ablate the normal remnant and treat functioning metastases.

To stimulate uptake of radioiodine by malignant thyroid tissue, it is necessary to raise serum TSH levels to 30 mU/L or higher.[7] In routine practice, levothyroxine therapy is discontinued for 5 to 6 weeks before administration of the diagnostic dose of radioiodine for imaging. To shorten the period of hypothyroidism, liothyronine (triiodothyronine [T_3]) is often given (25 to 50 μg/day in divided doses) for 3 weeks after discontinuation of levothyroxine therapy. T_3 therapy is discontinued 2 weeks before radioiodine administration. Alternatively, it is possible to prepare patients by giving their usual thyroxine dose every other day for 6 weeks, which induces mild hypothyroidism and raises the level of TSH to about 50 mIU/L.

Recently, recombinant human TSH (rhTSH, Thyrogen, Genzyme Corp., Cambridge, MA) has been developed and in clinical trials has been shown to stimulate uptake of ^{131}I by thyroid remnants and metastases and to raise serum thyroglobulin (Tg) levels in patients who remain euthyroid while taking thyroid hormone therapy.[8,9] The Food and Drug Administration has approved the use of rhTSH for radioiodine imaging and serum Tg testing in such patients and for the destruction (ablation) of thyroid tissue that remains after a total thyroidectomy has been performed because of thyroid cancer.

Patients who are scheduled to undergo diagnostic whole-body scintigraphy are advised to follow a low-iodine diet for at least 7 to 10 days before administration of the radioiodine. A simple low-iodine diet has been described.[10] It is even more important to avoid iodine-containing medications and radiographic contrast agents.

Diagnostic administration of ^{131}I may reduce the uptake of subsequent therapeutic ^{131}I by normal thyroid remnants or functioning metastases. This phenomenon, which has been termed *stunning*, seems to involve a sublethal, presumably temporary suppression of iodine uptake (reviewed elsewhere[11,12]). To avoid stunning, many authors recommend limiting the quantity of ^{131}I given for diagnostic imaging to 2 mCi (74 MBq)[11,13] or even less.[14] An alternative is to use ^{123}I for whole-body imaging,[15] but the present cost of this radionuclide in millicurie amounts is prohibitive for many centers. While ^{123}I offers superior imaging of deposits of thyroid tumor in the neck when compared to ^{131}I, its efficiency for deposits deep in the rest of the body remains to be established convincingly.

Physicians who interpret whole-body radioiodine scintigrams must be familiar with the distribution of inorganic iodine in the blood pool and extracellular fluid and its dynamics over time, the normal, nonthyroid sites that accumulate the radioactive iodine tracer, and the behavior of isotope-labeled thyroxine that has been produced in thyroid gland or metastases. The salivary glands, gastric mucosa, kidneys, and lactating breasts concentrate iodide but do not convert it to thyroxine. Nasal secretions, saliva, sweat, urine, stool, and milk may contain high concentrations of inorganic radioiodine and can cause artifacts, depending on the time after isotope administration. Skin and hair are easily contaminated with saliva, urine, or vomitus. Radioiodine-labeled thyroxine is observed later than inorganic iodide and has a different pattern of distribution, including the liver as part of the enterohepatic circulation of thyroxine. Nonthyroid tumors, inflammatory lesions, and cysts may occasionally contain radioiodine as part of their vasculature and result in a false-positive scintigram.[11,16]

In interpreting ^{131}I planar whole body scans, there may be atypical or cryptic findings. [131]I SPECT/CT is useful to characterize challenging foci more accurately, differentiate thyroid cancer from physiologic activity or nonthyroid pathology, and reduce false positives. By identifying nonthyroid cancer activity, SPECT/CT can reduce inappropriate treatment with [131]I.

[131]I scanning is not 100% sensitive for metastatic thyroid carcinoma. In some series, the rate of false-negative radioiodine scans approaches 35%.[17] When diagnostic ^{131}I scans are negative and metastases are suspected on the basis of elevated serum Tg levels, some advocate empirical treatment with [131]I. Scans that are done 1 week after ^{131}I therapy are frequently positive in these cases (reviewed by Clark and Hoelting[18]) (Fig. 7-4). Indeed, a routine pre-ablation scan after thyroidectomy for thyroid cancer may not be cost effective. Therefore, many centers employ a protocol of administering a standard therapeutic dose of ^{131}I without prescanning and perform the whole body scan a week later. This protocol is limited by an inability to do dosimetry for the treatment, which some authorities deem essential, and fails to assess for undetected metastases in the head or spine, which may swell after ^{131}I and cause neurologic complications.

It is useful in ^{131}I scan-negative, Tg-positive patients to search for metastases by performing sonography of the neck and, if negative, performing MRI of the neck and chest. Especially if ^{131}I therapy is anticipated, contrast CT studies are not employed, but noncontrast CT may suffice. The aim is to find metastases that either are surgically accessible or can be treated by external radiotherapy, if appropriate. When the above imaging techniques do not reveal a source of the elevated Tg, scintiscanning with other radiolabeled agents or fluoro-deoxyglucose (FDG)-PET scanning may succeed in localizing ^{131}I-negative metastases[19] (see Table 7-2).

Thallium (^{201}Tl) has been useful in localizing metastases in selected patients (reviewed by Cavalieri[12] and Sisson[19]). However, ^{201}Tl is concentrated by a variety of benign and malignant lesions other than thyroid carcinoma.

[99m]Tc-sestamibi (MIBI) is a cationic, lipophilic agent that concentrates in normal and neoplastic thyroid tissue and in a variety of other cancers. Experience indicates that like ^{201}Tl, ^{99m}Tc-MIBI can be useful in ^{131}I-negative patients in whom one has reason

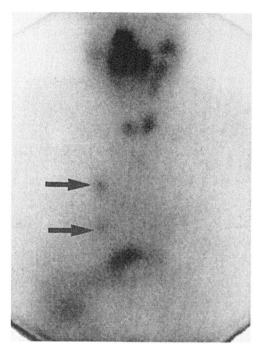

FIGURE 7-4. Anterior scintiscan of head, neck, chest, and upper part of the abdomen in a male patient who 72 hours previously had received 212 mCi ^{131}I as therapy for follicular thyroid carcinoma metastatic to the lung. The image shows intense activity in the nose, mouth, and salivary glands; small right and left thyroid lobe remnants; two discrete foci of uptake in the right side of the chest (arrows) corresponding to small lung nodules seen on computed tomography; and physiologic radioiodine in the stomach and bowel. The liver is faintly visualized, a common finding in post-therapy scintiscans with no pathologic significance.

to suspect persistent or recurrent tumor.[19,20] ^{99m}Tc-MIBI is the agent of choice for imaging Hürthle cell carcinoma, which typically takes up radioiodine poorly.[21]

Other agents that have been shown to concentrate in some metastatic differentiated thyroid tumors are ^{99m}Tc-tetrofosmin, which like MIBI is a myocardial perfusion imaging agent, and ^{99m}Tc-labeled dimercaptosuccinic acid in the pentavalent form (DMSA [V]) (reviewed by Sisson[19]). Clinical experience with these agents is still limited. Indium-111-labeled octreotide is used to localize metastatic medullary thyroid carcinoma.[22]

[18]Fluoro-2-Deoxyglucose Positron Emission Scanning

[18]F-fluoro-2-deoxyglucose ([18]FDG), a radiolabeled analogue of glucose, is actively concentrated in a variety of malignant tumors, including thyroid carcinoma.[23] [18]FDG uptake tends to be higher in thyroid tumors that are not well differentiated, in contrast to ^{131}I, which is accumulated by differentiated cancers. For this reason, ^{131}I-negative tumors are more often positive with [18]FDG, and [18]FDG-negative tumors tend to be positive with [131]I.[23] [18]FDG-PET scans show low background in the chest and liver, which gives this agent a relative advantage over ^{201}Tl and ^{99m}Tc-MIBI. Enhanced clinical value of PET images is obtained when they are fused with CT or MRI images. The last section of this chapter, Positron Emission Tomography and Bimodality CT or MRI Fusion Scanning, offers an in-depth discussion of the subject.

Nonisotopic Thyroid Imaging Tests

The nonisotopic thyroid-imaging tests consist of sonography, CT, and MRI. Sonography reveals how the tissue transmits and/

or reflects sound waves, CT is a computerized analysis of the relative density of tissues to x-rays, and MRI depicts the response of hydrogen atoms to a magnetic field. Both CT and MRI provide sectional images that can be electronically assembled in perpendicular planes. None of these techniques are a substitute for histopathology, and none differentiate benign and malignant lesions.

SONOGRAPHY (ECHOGRAPHY)

Sonography is efficiently used to (1) elucidate cryptic findings on physical examination, (2) identify nonpalpable nodules or the solid component of a complex nodule for guiding FNA, (3) determine the comparative size of nodules in patients who are under observation, (4) detect small nodules in patients who were exposed to therapeutic irradiation of the head or neck, (5) identify sonographic characteristics of a nodule that are associated with a greater than average risk of cancer, (6) improve the accuracy of needle placement in percutaneous biopsy, and (7) evaluate for recurrence of thyroid cancer after surgery, particularly in cervical lymph nodes.

Technical Aspects

Sonography uses high-frequency sound waves (ultrasound) in the megahertz range to produce a photographic image of the internal structure of the thyroid gland and its region.[24,25] No ionizing radiation is involved, nor is iodinated contrast material given. Sonography is safe; tissue damage has not been reported, and it is less costly than other imaging procedures. Preparation of the patient for the procedure is unnecessary, and it is performed without discontinuing TSH suppressive therapy. To image the thyroid gland and surrounding regions, the patient's neck is examined in the sagittal, transverse, and oblique planes with a probe called a *transducer* that both generates the sound energy and receives the reflected signal. The sound enters the body and is transmitted or reflected by interfaces within the tissues. Air does not transmit ultrasound, and calcified areas block its passage. The images are produced quickly and are assembled electronically in "real time." Each frame of the sonogram shows a static image, and sequential pictures depict motion. Swallowing is used to elevate the thyroid to examine the lower pole of an enlarged lobe, and this maneuver may facilitate identification of the esophagus. With the use of a signal having a frequency of 7.5 to 12 MHz, thyroid nodules and lymphadenopathy as small as 2 to 3 mm are identified in shades of gray. Dynamic information such as blood flow is added by using physics principles called the *Doppler effect.*[26] The signals are translated into colors to differentiate static fluid-filled cystic spaces and blood flowing through the vasculature. Thus the direction and velocity of flow and the degree of vascularity are revealed. Color is assigned to the signal by assuming that venous flow is parallel to, but in the opposite direction to, arterial flow. Arterial signals are made red, and the accompanying venous signals are made blue. The shade of a color is proportional to the direction of flow as it relates to the transducer and flow velocity.

Routine protocols for ultrasound scanning by a technologist are not satisfactory but unfortunately are used too often, degrading the value of the test. Rather, the ultrasound operator must be experienced and aware of the clinical question that has been posed to provide an appropriate answer. Close supervision by a sonographer-physician or endocrinologist who is expert in physical examination and ultrasonography is needed.

It is important to comprehend that the optimal clinical value of sonography depends on the quality of the ultrasound examination, including the maturity of the examiner and the characteristics of the equipment. Grossly misleading results are common with quick, incomplete studies and unsophisticated machines or readouts. Therefore, routine sonography in a medical or radiology office will require proper preparation of the professional and technical staff. Without study, training, and experience, there are likely to be unacceptable results and adverse outcomes.

Sonography of the Normal Thyroid Gland and Environs

With standard gray-scale technique, the normal thyroid gland has a homogeneous appearance like ground glass (Fig. 7-5). The surrounding muscles are of equal or lower echogenicity. Tissue planes are identified. The air-filled trachea, which does not transmit the ultrasound signal, is poorly imaged, and dense echoes represent its calcified tracheal ring anteriorly. The carotid artery and other blood vessels are echo-free unless calcified. Lateral and anterior to the carotid arteries is the jugular vein, which is frequently collapsed and can be identified when it is distended during a Valsalva maneuver. Small blood vessels on the surface of the thyroid and the inferior thyroid artery and vein can sometimes be seen. Color Doppler enhances the identification of blood vessels and flow. The esophagus is sometimes detected behind the thyroid and left of center, anteromedial to the longus colli muscle. It can be observed to distend after the patient swallows a sip of water. Lymph nodes can be seen normally as less than 1 × 3 mm, elliptical, uniform structures with an echo-dense central hilum. The parathyroid glands are not visualized unless they are enlarged. They are less dense to ultrasound than the thyroid gland because of the absence of iodine.

Generally, imaging procedures are not useful in patients whose thyroid gland is normal to palpation unless the patient has a history of exposure to therapeutic irradiation in youth or metastatic thyroid cancer has been discovered and a primary

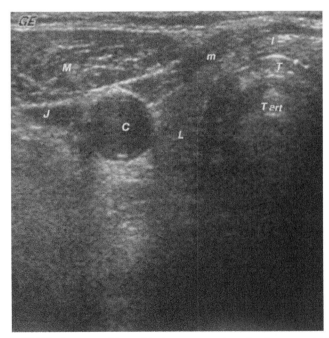

FIGURE 7-5. Sonogram of the neck in the transverse plane, showing a normal right thyroid lobe and isthmus. *C,* Carotid artery (note the enhanced echoes deep to the fluid-filled blood vessel); *I,* isthmus; *J,* jugular vein; *L,* thyroid lobe; *M,* sternocleidomastoid muscle; *m,* strap muscles; *T,* anterior portion of the tracheal ring (the dense white arc is calcification); *T art,* artifact in the trachea.

lesion in the gland is being sought. However, in selected circumstances, an ultrasound image may be used to supplement or confirm physical examination findings and identify the size and shape of regional structures accurately and relatively inexpensively. This test is useful when thyroid anatomy is in question but clinical perception is confused by obesity, great muscularity, distortion by abnormal adjacent structures, tortuous blood vessels, a prominent thyroid cartilage, metastatic tumor, lymphadenopathy, prior surgery, or examiner inexperience. On the other hand, the sonogram is so sensitive that many small, nonpalpable thyroid nodules may be detected. Management of these nodules, which are called *incidentalomas*, requires mature clinical judgment. Objective diagnostic evaluation of all of them is needless and impractical. Selective attention to those found in a patient with a high risk of cancer, those with special characteristics frequently seen in cancers, or those that grow is prudent. Neglecting all of them is inappropriate and occasionally dangerous.

Sonography When There Is Thyroid Enlargement (Goiter)

Enlargement of the thyroid gland is common. In general terms, enlargement may be diffuse and symmetrical, asymmetrical, smooth and uniform, or nodular. It is not generally necessary to obtain a sonogram to confirm thyroid enlargement unless a specific question has attracted clinical concern. Such questions may involve a dominant nodule, a tender spot, focal hardness, or substernal extension. At times, a physician may obtain a sonogram to explain a cryptic finding, such as differentiating goiter from fat or muscle, documenting a controversial observation, estimating the size of the thyroid gland for ^{131}I dosimetry, or assessing volume changes in response to suppressive therapy with thyroid hormone. Sonography has been used in population studies to objectively identify thyroid enlargement as a screen for iodine deprivation.

Sonography can show alterations of the echo pattern of the thyroid gland and its size. Cystic and/or hemorrhagic degeneration, which is depicted by an echo-free zone, is common (Fig. 7-6). These findings are not specific for any particular type of pathology. However, sonography can identify one region in a uniform goiter whose echo pattern is different from the rest of the goiter, which is suggestive of a focal lesion, especially if that focus is surrounded by a distinctive rim or halo.

Sonography in Patients With Thyroiditis and Graves' Disease

The greatest value of ultrasonography in patients with immune or inflammatory thyroid disease is to identify incidental focal lesions. However, because most focally distinct zones in these glands are not neoplastic, the need for their subsequent management requires judgment. In situations in which localized firm consistency, focal enlargement, or pain call attention to a part of Graves' or Hashimoto's goiter, or if a scintigram shows a cold area, a sonogram may demonstrate a region that has a distinctive appearance, which should be subjected to accurate aspiration biopsy (Fig. 7-7).

Sonography may demonstrate an image of the thyroid gland that correlates with subacute thyroiditis, Hashimoto's thyroiditis, and Graves' disease, but such correlation is of debatable practical diagnostic importance. Several types of thyroiditis show reduced echogenicity. During the active phase of subacute thyroiditis, the echogram is characterized by a severely reduced echo density of the thyroid gland that returns to a normal pattern with healing.[27]

Some patients with Hashimoto's thyroiditis have low echogenicity (see Fig. 7-7). Marcocci and co-workers reported that only 44 of 238 (18.5%) patients with autoimmune thyroiditis had diffuse hypoechogenicity, especially when they were hypothyroid.[28] The accuracy of a heterogeneous, hypoechoic sonographic pattern in diagnosing Hashimoto's thyroiditis was compared to that of anti-

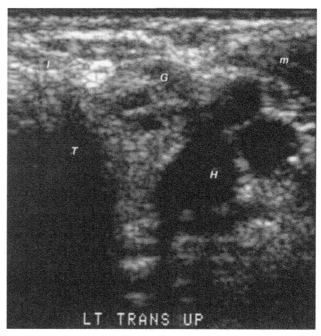

FIGURE 7-6. Sonogram of the left lobe of the thyroid gland in the transverse plane, showing a degenerated multinodular goiter. *G,* Heterogeneous goiter; *H,* hemorrhagic/cystic degenerated area; *I,* region of lobe adjacent to the enlarged isthmus; *m,* sternocleidomastoid muscle; *T,* trachea.

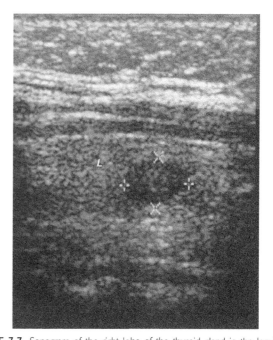

FIGURE 7-7. Sonogram of the right lobe of the thyroid gland in the longitudinal plane from a 33-year-old, 235-pound woman. The serum contained high titers of antithyroid antibodies. The thyroid gland was difficult to palpate, and examiners could not agree on the findings. Therefore, a sonogram was done. It shows a 7.7 × 10.0-mm nodule (× and + symbols) that is less echo-dense than the rest of the thyroid lobe. Fine-needle aspiration biopsy demonstrated and surgery confirmed papillary carcinoma. *L,* Thyroid lobe.

thyroid peroxidase antibody thyroid peroxidase antibody (TPOAb) concentration in 451 ambulatory patients with unknown thyroid status, excluding those with suspected hyperthyroidism or who were on drugs known to cause hypothyroidism. There was high intraobserver and interobserver agreement on the abnormal thyroid ultrasound patterns, which were judged highly indicative of autoimmune thyroiditis and allowed the detection of thyroid dysfunction with 96% probability.[29] Furthermore, in another investigation, patients with postpartum thyroiditis who had both high levels of antithyroid peroxidase antibody and a hypoechoic thyroid gland also had a high risk of long-term thyroid dysfunction.[30] Graves' disease goiters and a few goiters without thyroid autoantibodies have a similar appearance. In Graves' disease, color Doppler imaging can detect diffuse hyperemia in the thyroid gland,[31] a condition that has been called a "thyroid inferno."[32] Increased flow velocity in hyperthyroid patients has been demonstrated with duplex Doppler techniques.[33] However, neither the sensitivity nor the specificity of these observations is known.

Sonography of the Thyroid Nodule

Thyroid nodules are identified by sonography because they distort the uniform echo pattern or the shape of the gland. Most nodules have a less dense appearance than normal thyroid tissue does. Most of the remainder are more echogenic, and isoechogenicity is less common. Some nodules have a sonolucent rim called a *halo*. Nodules may contain regions of calcium (Fig. 7-8) that are extremely echo-dense. The echo texture within a small nodule tends to be uniform, but nodules larger than 2.5 cm usually have irregular zones that are free of echoes. These areas represent cystic and/or hemorrhagic degeneration that may occur in benign or malignant nodules (see Fig. 7-6). Such nodules are called *complex*. Careful examination of echo-free zones is necessary to discern internal echoes that represent septa or small solid regions that differentiate common, complex cystic nodules and

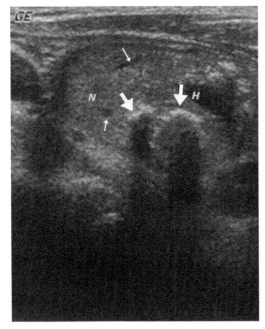

FIGURE 7-8. Sonogram of the neck in the longitudinal plane, showing a large nodule. The *small arrows* point to echo-free zones that Doppler examination identified as small blood vessels. The *thick straight arrows* point to calcifications. Note that passage of the ultrasound signal distal to the calcium is blocked in a linear fashion and creates an artifact. *H*, Hemorrhagic/cystic degenerated area; *N*, nodule.

a true thyroid cyst. A cyst is encountered once in approximately 500 to 1000 nodules and is globular shaped, smooth walled, and without internal echoes.

The prevalence of palpable thyroid nodules in members of the general population who are screened by palpation is 1.5% to 6.4%.[34] It is 10-fold greater when they have been screened by ultrasonography.[35] The prevalence of sonographically detectable nodules increases with age to around 50% in older adults. The risk of malignancy of palpable nodules is 5% to 15%; in ultrasonically detected nonpalpable nodules, the risk is smaller.[36] The major use of ultrasonography is to determine which of the many nodules are the relatively few malignancies. Sonography can help in this triage, but the ultrasonic appearance of a nodule cannot reliably differentiate benign lesions and cancer.[37] Table 7-3 lists the sonographic features of a nodule that are associated with high or low risk of thyroid cancer. Cancers may be minute or large, entirely solid or complex. Some features of a nodule can be helpful to select nodules that are likely malignant. The most reliable ultrasonic predictor of malignancy is vascular invasion, but this feature is observed uncommonly. Adenopathy associated with a nodule is also very good evidence, providing there is no other reason for enlarged nodes such as infection, as will be discussed later. It is important to realize that in children, adenopathy is a relatively nonspecific finding and must be interpreted with caution. The characteristics of nodules that studies have shown most useful for identifying carcinomas include the intensity of the echoes, the lack of sharpness and irregularity of the boundary of the nodule, the presence of an incomplete "halo" or calcifications, and internal structure, including vascularity.[38,39] However, there is considerable variation in the cancer-predictive value of these characteristics. The most optimistic data is a 97.2% positive predictive value for cytologically diagnosed cancer and 96.1% predictive value for benign disease among 1244 nodules in 900 patients who were stratified according to ultrasound characteristics on a scale of 1 to 5 assessing cancer-risk.[40] The author is considerably less confident. As a group, malignancies tend to be rather hypoechoic.[44,45] In one study, 62% of cancers were hypoechoic among 202 patients with nodules, and few were hyperechoic.[41] In another series, none of the 14 cancers were hyperechoic among 132 consecutive ultrasound-guided fine-needle aspiration biopsies.[42] However, most benign nodules are also of low echo density. Nevertheless, it can be said that hyperdense nodules are probably not cancerous and need not be biopsied unless there are other factors that indicate a high risk of cancer.[43] Internal cystic spaces in thyroid nodules are degenerative and have no cancer-predictive value. In distinction, cystic space in lymph adenopathy is important because it may be seen

Table 7-3. Ultrasonographic Features of a Thyroid Nodule and the Risk of Thyroid Cancer

Increased Risk of Thyroid Cancer	Decreased Risk of Thyroid Cancer
Hypoechoic	Hyperechoic
Microcalcifications	Large, coarse calcifications (except medullary cancer)
Central vascularity	Peripheral vascularity
Irregular margins	Looks like Napoleon or puff pastry
Incomplete halo	Comet-tail shadowing
Nodule is taller than wide	
Documented interval enlargement of a nodule	
Associated rounded adenopathy (especially with cystic spaces)	

more often with thyroid cancer than in inflammatory nodes. Deposits of calcium may be seen in benign or malignant nodules. Frequently, large irregular plaques or eggshell calcifications are found, and because benign nodules are more common than malignant ones, these concretions do not correlate with cancer. In distinction, punctate calcifications or microcalcifications are not common in nodules but have high specificity for thyroid cancer (95.2%), low sensitivity (59.3%), and a diagnostic accuracy of 83.8%.[36] They may represent psammoma bodies in papillary cancer. A halo around a nodule is thought to represent a boundary, capsule, or vasculature that may be seen in benign or malignant conditions.[44,45] Demonstrating in multiple images and in several planes that a halo is incomplete correlates with cancer, but the finding is of low specificity and sensitivity. Lack of distinctness of a nodule has little diagnostic value, but an ill-defined edge has been reported with infiltrating, poor-prognosis lesions.[46] In general, the shape of a nodule has limited diagnostic significance except that cancers tend to exhibit a tall and thin shape. The patterns of blood flow as depicted by Doppler examination offer insight into the potential for malignancy. An internal or central flow pattern in a hypofunctioning ("cold") nodule or lymph node should raise one's suspicion of malignancy. In one study of 125 nodules, 55 of 92 (60 percent) cold nodules had a peripheral flow pattern, 34 no internal flow, and only 3 had increased internal flow. All 3 cold nodules with an enhanced internal color flow pattern were carcinomas. However, among the 27 patients who had pathology correlation, there were a total of 7 cancers, only 3 of which had increased internal flow; the other 4 had either diffuse or no internal flow.[47] Another study of 203 patients, the addition of color flow Doppler imaging to conventional sonography only slightly increased the screening sensitivity and accuracy from 71.9% to 83.3% in identifying the 36 malignant thyroid nodules.[48]

Ultrasonic features of a nodule that specifically favor benign disease include hyperechogenicity and characteristics that suggest the presence of abundant colloid accumulation within the nodule. A "Napoleon" or puff-pastry, layered appearance of the nodule, or a bright spot with a trailing, fading comet tail have been reported with colloid nodules.

Thyroid palpation might not accurately predict the need for sonography in patients with a thyroid nodule. One suspects that routine sonography will be employed, especially when palpation is uncertain or skills are tentative.

Evidence is mounting in support of routine sonography for patients with palpable uninodular thyroid disease with or without a palpable goiter. Thyroid ultrasonography has been reported to show that among 114 patients who were referred because of a solitary thyroid nodule, ultrasonography detected additional nonpalpable thyroid nodules that were at least 1 cm in diameter in 27 patients and no nodules in 23. In this investigation, sonography provided information to the clinician that importantly altered management in 63% (109 of 173) of patients who were referred to a tertiary endocrine group. Sonography showed an indication for needle aspiration or demonstrated that the procedure was not necessary. Among 59 patients who were referred because of goiter, sonography revealed nonpalpable nodules that were at least 1 cm in diameter in 39 patients, requiring aspiration that was not anticipated.[49]

Sonography in Patients With a Dominant Palpable Nodule in a Goiter

Improved technology has permitted the detection of thyroid nodules as small as 2 mm, which can be the source of prob-

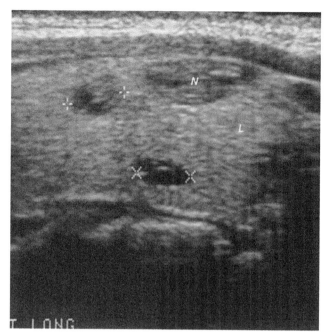

FIGURE 7-9. Sonogram of the right lobe of the thyroid gland in the longitudinal plane from a 44-year-old woman with one palpable nodule in the right thyroid lobe (N). The sonogram also shows two nonpalpable micronodules (+ +, 6.8 mm; × ×, 6.5 mm). L, Thyroid lobe; N, palpable nodule.

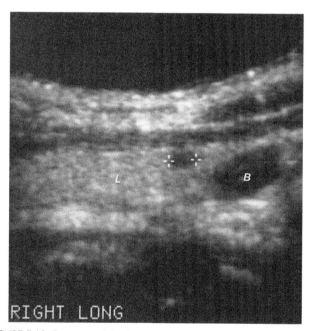

FIGURE 7-10. Sonogram of the right thyroid lobe in the longitudinal plane from a 51-year-old man with a history of radiation therapy in youth. A hypoechoic, 5.2-mm nodule (+ +) is located in the lower pole of the lobe just above the level of the thoracic inlet. B, Blood vessel demonstrated by Doppler examination; L, thyroid lobe.

lems.[36] Approximately 20% of all adults have nonpalpable micronodules that are of indeterminate significance, usually benign, and of no clinical consequence in most patients (Figs. 7-9, 7-10, and 7-11). Their discovery, usually by sonography of the neck but sometimes by CT or MRI during an investigation of cervical vascular or neurologic pathology or during thyroid sonography for a palpable thyroid nodule, may occasion needless expense, concern, and therapy. However, rarely one of these lesions represents occult thyroid cancer and could become a

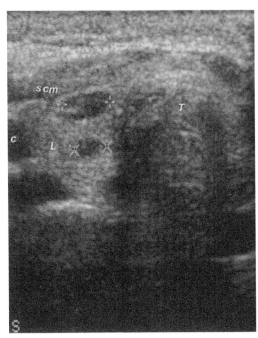

FIGURE 7-11. Sonogram of the left lobe of the thyroid gland in the longitudinal plane, showing two hypoechoic micronodules (+ +, 7.1 mm; × ×, 4.8 mm) that represent tumor in the contralateral thyroid lobe after partial thyroidectomy for papillary thyroid cancer. C, Carotid artery; L, thyroid lobe; scm, sternocleidomastoid muscle; T, artifact in the tracheal region.

clinically significant malignancy.[50] Therefore, a micronodule, or incidentaloma, should not be dismissed simply for reasons of cost-effectiveness, as some authorities have suggested. Overreaction and surgery are not suitable either. Rather, yearly reassessment seems appropriate. However, it remains for future investigation to determine the value of periodic sonography in examining for changes in the size or characteristics of a nodule, as well as the benefit if any of suppressive therapy with thyroid hormone.

It is common, when a solitary nodule is palpable, for sonography to demonstrate micronodules in the rest of the thyroid (see Fig. 7-9). This occurrence has the same pathologic significance as a dominant nodule in a patient with clinical multinodular goiter. FNA biopsy and cytology of the dominant nodule appear to be the most cost-effective approach.

Sonography of Lymphadenopathy

Ultrasonography may be useful to diagnose and monitor lymphadenopathy in patients, especially if they have thyroid cancer or a history of therapeutic irradiation in youth. However, one must be mindful that even in cancer patients, enlarged benign nodes are more common than malignant ones.

Consensus is growing that the shape of benign lymph nodes tends to be a thin oval, whereas malignant ones are plump and rounded (Fig. 7-12), but differences in size or homogeneity are not reliable indicators of pathology. Solbiati and co-workers evaluated 291 lymph nodes in 143 patients before thyroid cancer surgery and reported that the ultrasonic characteristics of lymph nodes correlated with the histologic findings.[51] A ratio of longitudinal diameter to transverse diameter of less than 1.5 was reported in 62% of metastatic nodes, and a ratio greater than 2 was reported in 79% of reactive nodes.[51] The absence of a nodal hilus was observed in 44% of malignant lesions but in only 8% of benign nodes.[52] Thus, ultrasound can detect head and neck

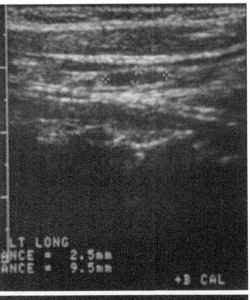

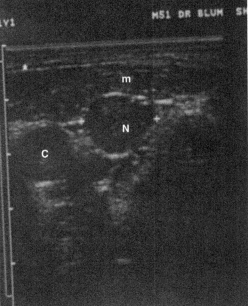

FIGURE 7-12. Sonograms showing lymphadenopathy. Upper panel, Sonogram in the longitudinal plane from a patient who had a thyroidectomy. A benign, thin elliptical, 2.5 × 9.5-mm lymph node (+ + and × ×) is present. Lower panel, Sonogram of the left side of the neck from a 51-year-old muscular man who had a thyroidectomy because of papillary thyroid carcinoma. The sonogram disclosed a nonpalpable, plump, 13-mm lymph node that was involved with metastatic cancer. The thyroid lobe is absent. C, Carotid artery; m, muscle; N, pathologic lymph node.

cancer metastases to cervical nodes with a sensitivity of 92.6%.[53] It has been reported that cystic degeneration of a pathologic node occurs with some frequency in papillary thyroid cancer but is uncommon with other head and neck cancers.[54] It is not clear whether additional information about lymphadenopathy may be offered by color and spectral Doppler studies.[55] Vascularity along the convexity of a node, remote from the hilus, may represent neovascularization of malignancy.[56] Distortion of adjacent soft tissue by a node signifies hardness that may be seen with cancer. Even when thyroid cells are not observed in an aspirate from a node, the biochemical detection of thyroglobulin (even in the presence of antithyroid antibodies in the serum) indicates a thyroid metastasis.[57]

Sonography in Patients With a History of Therapeutic Irradiation in Youth

Patients with a history of therapeutic irradiation in youth may have a risk of thyroid cancer that is as high as 30%. Therefore, some clinicians use sonography to screen irradiated people for tiny thyroid nodules before a mass becomes palpable. However, in the process, many more benign nodules are found than malignancies. The inefficiency of the selection process and the indolence of thyroid cancer have resulted in continuing controversy about the clinical relevance of sonographic identification of nodules and subsequent management. The approach to which the author subscribes is to obtain potentially useful baseline ultrasonic anatomic information but not act on it unless the sonogram strongly suggests malignancy (as discussed earlier), studies at intervals reveal changes, or other circumstances arise that heighten suspicion of malignancy.

Sonography to Monitor Changes in Thyroid Size

In a patient with thyroid disease, sonography can accurately and objectively assess the size of the thyroid gland or a nodule during the course of therapy or the emergence of a new nodule.[58] Because growth of a nodule can be difficult to perceive clinically, sonography may be useful in this context. Furthermore, inasmuch as most patients change doctors over the years, objective assessment of thyroid size greatly facilitates continuity of care. Comparison of serial records, even with different equipment, can demonstrate changes in the thyroid gland or in a nodule and lead to a change in treatment earlier than palpation alone would warrant.

Sonography in Patients With Known Thyroid Cancer

Sonography is useful in the management of a patient with thyroid carcinoma[59,60] and has become the most frequently used imaging procedure in patients who have had either a partial or a complete thyroidectomy. After a hemithyroidectomy, the procedure will detect even nonpalpable nodules in the contralateral lobe or lymphadenopathy that could represent tumor (see Fig. 7-11). In these patients and in those who have undergone a total (or near-total) thyroidectomy, sonography that is done without interrupting thyroid hormone therapy will detect recurrent carcinoma either in the thyroid bed or in lymph nodes before the mass has grown sufficiently large to be palpable[59,60] (see Fig. 7-12). Sonography is particularly useful in searching for a nonpalpable malignant lesion in a patient who has had a thyroidectomy when periodic assessment has disclosed an elevated Tg concentration. In contrast, one group of investigators have reported that even when Tg levels remain low or undetectable after stimulation with rhTSH, ultrasonography may identify lymph node metastases from thyroid cancer.[61]

Another circumstance in which sonography is useful is when thyroid cancer was diagnosed by detecting metastases of thyroid origin and the thyroid gland is normal by palpation. A sonogram may detect an occult primary thyroid tumor.

Intraoperative ultrasonography may enhance the ability to locate and surgically remove recurrent thyroid cancer that does not accumulate radioactive iodine. Experience in seven patients suggests that sonography was particularly helpful after external beam radiotherapy to identify tumor nodules of 20 mm or less and were invasive or adherent to the airway.[62]

Sonography in Conjunction With Needle Biopsy

In an attempt to enhance the utility of FNA biopsy, sonographic guidance has been used in selected circumstances to minimize

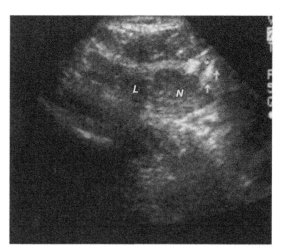

FIGURE 7-13. Sonogram of the right lobe of the thyroid gland in the transverse plane from a patient who is having fine-needle aspiration biopsy of an 8 × 11-mm nodule. The *arrows* point to the tip of the needle in the nodule. *L,* Thyroid lobe; *N,* nodule.

sampling errors[63] (Fig. 7-13). Ultrasound guidance for needle biopsy is generally reserved for (1) unusually deep nodules, particularly in an obese, muscular, or large-framed patient; (2) very small nodules; (3) nonpalpable nodules; (4) ultrasonically detected incidentalomas that are associated with cancer risk factors; (5) complex degenerated nodules if a prior aspiration has not been diagnostic; (6) suspicious nodules in a nodular goiter; and (7) nonpalpable adenopathy.[64,65] A special transducer to guide the needle is available but is cumbersome and not required. It is easier to explore the thyroid area of the neck with a hand-held transducer to locate the nodule and then insert the needle into the lesion under ultrasonic direct vision from another angle. The success rate is low for nodules that are smaller than 8 mm. Generally, correlation of the anatomy with the sonographic film without guided puncture is less costly and is adequate for nodules that are palpable unless a prior aspiration has been unsuccessful.

It has been reported from a goiter zone in Italy that as many as 52% of histologically malignant nodules in goiters were found only with the aid of ultrasound-guided FNAB. Therefore, the authors concluded that ultrasound-guided aspiration should be used in areas where multinodular goiter is endemic to assess nodules that are deemed suspicious by virtue of a hypoechoic pattern, a "blurred halo," microcalcifications, or intranodular color Doppler signal.[66]

Ultrasound-guided aspiration can facilitate biochemical analysis—for instance, calcitonin assay—or can lead to a nonneoplastic diagnosis such as tuberculosis[67] or amyloidosis.[68] It seems probable that soon cytologic material will be studied for subcellular components that are useful as tumor markers.

Sonography in Conjunction With Percutaneous Therapeutic Intervention

After an aspiration and cytologic examination have demonstrated that a nodule is benign, ultrasound-guided puncture of a nodule can have a therapeutic role to deliver medication precisely into the lesion and to spare the surrounding tissue.

Percutaneous injection of ethanol has been used to reduce the function of autonomous thyroid nodules.[69] One investigation has observed 34 patients for up to 3 years, who had percutaneous ethanol injection of autonomous thyroid nodules with a volume larger than 40 mL. The patients required 1 to 11 sessions of 3 to 14 mL of ethanol injection (total amount of ethanol per patient: 20 to 125 mL). The authors report recovery of extranodular uptake on isotope scan and normalization of TSH levels within 3 months from the end of the treatment in 30 of 34 patients and an average reduction in nodule volume of 62.9%. Four of 34 patients were refractory to the treatment, three of whom had had nodule volumes greater than 60 mL. There were no recurrences during 6 to 36 months of observation.[70] Another study examined 20 patients with autonomous thyroid nodules for 763 ± 452 days after ethanol injection. A mean of 2.85 ± 1.1 injections per patient and a mean volume of 4.63 mL of ethanol were required (nodule volume-dependent). After a mean time of 50 ± 23 days, TSH normalized and was maintained in 16 patients (80%), whose nodular volume reduced 60.8%. Four patients (20%) did not completely respond to the treatment.[71] Less impressive but clinically acceptable results have also been observed in a study that reported a "complete cure" in only 22 of 42 patients (52%), mainly in small nodules, and little or no hormonal response in four patients (9%). However, nodule volume decreased in all cases, and there were no recurrences or serious adverse effects.[72] In the reported series, "mild to moderate" local pain often occurred after the injections and lasted a day or two, and local hematomas were seen. Major complications such as permanent dysphonia or vascular thrombosis seem to be very uncommon. However, transient paralysis of the laryngeal nerve may occur. Thus, this technique may be an option for some, but not very large, autonomous nodules that cannot or should not be treated surgically or with ^{131}I.

Percutaneous injection of ethanol has also been used to treat toxic nodular goiter,[72,73] and thyroid masses that recur after nontoxic nodular goiters have been treated surgically,[73] with results that are similar to those described for autonomous nodules.

Recurrent cysts and cystic spaces in a degenerated solid lesion have been obliterated in this fashion.[74] Perhaps the procedure will have use in cosmetically unacceptable or very large structures.

Sonographically guided percutaneous ethanol injection may become a treatment option for patients with cervical nodal metastases from papillary thyroid cancer that are not amenable to further surgical or radioiodine therapy. In a study of 21 metastatic nodes in 14 patients, all treated lymph nodes decreased in volume, some impressively. No major complications have been reported.[75] It seems to the author that this option may be palliative when there are large nodes that threaten to impact on surrounding structures. However, since ethanol-treated nodes may increase in size owing to inflammation, caution is warranted, especially when there are bulky nodes in the thoracic inlet or if they are adjacent to vital structures.

Prospective studies will be required to ascertain whether precise, ultrasound-guided placement of medication will reduce the intensity or duration of pain after the injection and improve success over palpation-directed injection.

Sonography of the Fetal Thyroid

Ultrasonography in pregnancy is an interesting tool to assess thyroid status in utero. Gestational age-dependent and age-independent nomograms for fetal thyroid size have been developed by performing ultrasonograms in 200 fetuses between 16 and 37 weeks of gestation.[76] Fetal goiters and hypothyroidism have been studied, and successful treatment has been reported. It is thought that intrauterine recognition and treatment of con-

genital goitrous hypothyroidism can reduce obstetric complications and improve the prognosis for normal growth and mental development of affected fetuses. One report cited a fetal goiter that was diagnosed at 29 weeks of gestation during routine ultrasound examination. Fetal blood sampling performed at this time documented fetal hypothyroidism, and treatment was given using a series of intraamniotic injections of triiodothyronine and subsequently thyroxine. Following birth, neonatal serum TSH levels were within the normal range.[77] A case of fetal goitrous hypothyroidism associated with high-output cardiac failure was diagnosed at 32 weeks of gestation on the basis of ultrasound examination. The fetus's thyroid function was examined by amniocentesis and cordocentesis. The fetus was treated by injection of levothyroxine sodium into the amniotic fluid at 33 weeks of gestation. Thereafter, the goiter decreased in size, and the high-output cardiac failure improved.[78]

Sonography of the Newborn Thyroid

Normative data for thyroid length (cm), 1.94 (0.24) 0.9 to 2.5; breadth (cm), 0.88 (0.16) 0.5 to 1.4; depth (cm), 0.96 (0.17) 0.6 to 2.0; and volume (mL), 0.81 (0.24) 0.3 to 1.7 was investigated in 100 (49 male) healthy term Scottish neonates. There was considerable variation (−0.8 to +0.7 mL) between the two lobes in individual babies.[79]

Epidemiologic Use of Ultrasonography

Sonography has been used effectively even in the field in undeveloped areas to evaluate thyroid anatomy and size in iodine-deficient people or to search for cancer in radiation-exposed populations. Interobserver agreement on estimates of thyroid volume has been good in epidemiologic studies, but agreement on echogenicity has been poor.[80] One group correlated age, body size, and thyroid volume in an endemic goiter area.[81] Another such study concluded that systematic ultrasound screening was useful in Belarus for the early detection of thyroid carcinoma in children 4 to 14 years of age who were exposed to radioactive fallout because of the Chernobyl accident.[82]

The value of ultrasonographic mass screening to uncover thyroid carcinoma in a population with average cancer risk is controversial because of the presumed low benefit/cost of the screening. One group did thyroid sonograms on 1401 women who were scheduled to undergo a breast examination. Thyroid nodules were detected in 25.2% and thyroid cancer in 2.6% of all subjects. The size of the tumors was significantly smaller in the ultrasound-studied group than in a clinically detected cancer group (P < 0.05).[83]

SECTIONAL IMAGING: COMPUTED TOMOGRAPHY AND MAGNETIC RESONANCE IMAGING

CT and MRI are computer-assisted sectional imaging techniques that can be used to accurately define the regional anatomy of the neck and superior mediastinum, but they are expensive to perform.[84,85] Although these tests are not usually required in the diagnosis of a patient with a thyroid nodule or goiter, they can be useful in selected cases to answer specific clinical questions that cannot be addressed by sonography.

Computed Tomography

CT images are a reconstruction of a computer-assisted analysis of multiple x-rays of a region. Standard CT represents discontinuous thin slices through an anatomic region, and spiral CT provides a continuous assemblage of pictures.

In CT of the neck, the thyroid gland is distinctive in that it is relatively more radiopaque than the rest of the soft tissues of the neck because of its high iodine content. The thyroid is homogeneous except for regions of enhanced or reduced density that correspond to nodules, cysts, hemorrhage, and calcification. It is clear that sonography is far more sensitive than CT in detecting millimeter-sized nodules. To precisely define the gland for clinical purposes, the regional vasculature must be enhanced by the intravenous administration of iodinated contrast material, which is a major limitation to subsequent management when CT is used for thyroid diagnosis.[86,87]

Magnetic Resonance Imaging

MRI images are generated by computer-produced analysis of the interaction of electromagnetic waves of a specific frequency and the hydrogen atoms in a patient's body. To perform the test, the person must be housed within a magnetic field. Varying the magnetic field can selectively emphasize special properties of the hydrogen atoms. The two properties that are conventionally used in MRI are termed *T1* and *T2*. Because the hydrogen atoms of various tissues have specific T1 and T2 properties, differences between T1-weighted and T2-weighted images can be used to identify the thyroid gland, skeletal muscle, blood vessels, or lymph nodes.[88] The quality and diagnostic value of MRI are enhanced by the intravenous administration of noniodinated contrast agents such as gadolinium-labeled diethylenetriamine pentaacetic acid or by electronically repressing a relatively unique signal derived from fat (short τ inversion recovery). As with CT, MRI is not as sensitive as sonography in detecting small nodules.

In general, normal thyroid tissue tends to be slightly more intense than muscle on a T1-weighted image, and thyroid tumor usually appears even more intense, or brighter.[89] Although differences in the MRI characteristics of malignant and benign thyroid tissue have been suggested as a result of investigations in vitro,[89] the distinctions have rarely proved to be of clinical value.

Distinctions Between Computed Tomography and Magnetic Resonance Imaging

The relative clinical utility of CT and MRI in thyroid disease has not been examined critically and is controversial. However, the author is persuaded that when additional imaging is needed to supplement thyroid sonography, MRI is preferred, and CT should be used only when specifically needed. The major advantages of MRI are that ionizing radiation and iodinated contrast agents are not required. MRI seems to provide better spatial resolution, and reports have suggested superior differentiation of postoperative scar from recurrent tumor.[90,91] The use of MRI has been limited by discomfort for a claustrophobic patient, considerable noise, long test time, great demand for the equipment for other types of examinations, relatively high cost, and incompatibility with pacemakers or ferrous prostheses. "Open" MRI systems address some of these problems but currently provide inferior images. CT is more sensitive in detecting small metastases to lymph nodes[92] and the lungs.[93,94] The total examination time for CT is shorter than that for MRI, and access to CT scanners outside major centers is superior.

SECTIONAL IMAGING IN CLINICAL MANAGEMENT

Sectional imaging is too expensive and insufficiently specific to be useful in the initial diagnosis of the usual thyroid nodule or goiter. MRI or CT becomes necessary only when the results of physical examination and ultrasonography are inadequate to answer a clinical question about anatomy.

When CT is needed, alteration of thyroid function by iodine contrast material is a serious issue. If the patient has not had a thyroidectomy, the excessive iodide may cause hyperthyroidism, including cardiac arrhythmias, or may cause hypothyroidism, depending on the underlying thyroid condition. In patients with thyroid cancer who might need an ^{131}I whole-body scan or therapy, the excess iodine will delay diagnosis or therapy. Therefore, radioiodine studies should precede contrast-enhanced CT. In patients who are taking suppressive therapy and in whom contrast-enhanced CT is required, it is best to continue administration of thyroid hormone for several days after the contrast-enhanced CT to keep TSH suppressed while the dye is excreted. The radiologist and clinician must discuss these aspects before the performance of contrast-enhanced CT and consider a non-contrast-enhanced study, which may be adequate to answer the clinical question. Iodinated dye is not used for MRI examinations, which is a distinct advantage.

A preoperative sectional imaging examination is useful for a thyroid nodule or goiter only for special situations to supplement information from a sonogram. These situations include circumstances in which the clinical examination demonstrates a thyroid or extrathyroidal mass that is fixed to surrounding tissues, when an unusually large mass obstructs the thoracic inlet and impinges on other structures or extends substernally, when tracheal compression or invasion is noted, when evaluating substernal or retrotracheal extension for a possible transthoracic surgical approach, and as a surgical guide for palliation when the sonogram suggests that total excision is precluded.[95]

Although sonography is the primary imaging procedure for assessing patients after thyroid cancer surgery, sectional imaging is useful if recurrence has been demonstrated. The major uses in these patients are to confirm recurrent thyroid cancer when the sonogram is equivocal, detect lymphadenopathy in regions where sonography is technically unsatisfactory such as the mediastinum or near bone, investigate suspected invasion, and evaluate cryptic findings. For instance, after radical surgery, sectional imaging may be required to distinguish whether a palpable deep mass is tumor or part of a vertebra. It has been claimed that after postoperative edema, infection, or bleeding has resolved, recurrent thyroid carcinoma may be differentiated from scarring with MRI.[96]

At times, thyroid lesions are incidentally detected as part of CT or MRI examinations for cervical spine, vascular, or neurologic disease, as is also true of incidentalomas discovered by sonography. They provide no unique diagnostic problem but sometimes engender undue anxiety.

Positron Emission Tomography and Bimodality CT or MRI Fusion Scanning

OVERVIEW: PET WITH RESPECT TO THYROID CANCER

Sensitive and specific monitoring for recurrent or persistent thyroid cancer after total thyroidectomy or postsurgical radioactive iodine therapy is essential for optimal patient management. Surveillance can be accomplished with biomarker imaging (^{131}I whole-body scanning [WBS] or PET), anatomic imaging (ultrasonography [US], CT, or MRI), and a biochemical indicator, thyroglobulin.

Biomarker Imaging of Thyroid Cancer

Surveillance with ^{131}I WBS is the most specific imaging modality when thyroid cancer is iodine-avid. As discussed previously, this WBS offers a two-dimensional map of tissues that concentrate the radioactive iodine tracer and represents a biomarker of thyroid and other iodine-avid cells but only a general, imprecise indicator of anatomy. Its interpretation is highly objective and depends on an understanding of iodine metabolism, extrathyroid iodine-concentrating sites, thyroid physiology, and information about the physical structure of the body relative to the focus of radioactivity. Anatomic localization may be improved with SPECT, which may be employed after therapeutic doses of ^{131}I have been administered. This method produces cross-sectional image slices through the patient that are reformatted by computer software to provide 3-D pictures.

PET scanning provides a non-iodine biomarker for rapidly metabolizing thyroid cancer. PET depicts the accumulation of radioactive-tagged glucose by rapidly growing or dividing tissue or organs, aggressive neoplastic tissue, lymphoma, and also regions that are infected or otherwise inflamed and thus is not as specific for thyroid cancer as ^{131}I WBS. Indeed, benign thyroid adenomas, nodular hyperplasia, focal thyroiditis, Hashimoto's thyroiditis, Graves' disease, and thyroglossal duct cyst have been reported to accumulate excessive FDG.[97] Focal accumulation of FDG thought to be thyroid in origin on PET examination that is done to investigate nonthyroid malignancies has been reported in 1.2% to 4.3% of such studies.[98-102]

As a general rule, thyroid cancer that is well differentiated and concentrates ^{131}I utilizes relatively less glucose than poorly differentiated thyroid cancer that does not accumulate [131]I. Consequently, PET may reveal cancer in WBS-negative patients, especially when thyroglobulin is elevated.

Anatomic Imaging of Thyroid Cancer

There are several anatomic imaging methods for monitoring patients with thyroid cancer. Since most recurrence of thyroid cancer is in the neck, ultrasonography of the neck is the most frequently used method. US may reveal nodules down to the millimeter range, but it lacks specificity for the type of the tissue or its benign or malignant nature. CT and MRI of the neck or whole body may also offer anatomical information in selected circumstances, such as mediastinal, pulmonary, or bone metastases, but also lack specificity for thyroid cancer. In order to derive optimal information from CT, iodinated contrast medium is usually required, which may complicate further diagnosis and treatment of patients with thyroid cancer.

Bimodality Imaging of Thyroid Cancer

The utility of PET is enhanced greatly by precise fusion of its images and simultaneous CT or MRI. Simple visual correlation of PET images with ultrasound, CT, and MRI is time consuming, imperfect, and sometimes misleading. Technologic advances have permitted multimodality scanning so that the same instrument can perform a PET scan and CT or MRI (which is in the late stages of development) with the patient in exactly the same position. Software can then digitally fuse the two images to produce an accurate superimposition of function and anatomy. Thus a composite image is produced that shows a superimposition or co-registration of both glucose concentration and a nodule or anatomic structure in the proper physical context. Extraordinary anatomic localization of FDG-avid lesions can be achieved, but mismatch of the two modalities may be a source of confusion. Fusion of WBS and anatomic images has not been achieved, but assembling thyroid gland scintiscan images and US on a single computer screen has been described.[105]

A Biochemical Indicator of Thyroid Cancer

Assessment of the concentration of thyroglobulin in the serum when TSH is elevated is a very good marker for the presence of a postoperative thyroid remnant or recurrence of thyroid cancer only after a total thyroidectomy has been performed. Its presence in material aspirated from a metastatic lymph node is diagnostic of thyroid cancer.

PET SCANNING

To perform PET, radioactive-labeled glucose (FDG) is injected intravenously. The radiopharmaceutical "homes" to thyroid tumor in about an hour, and its residence in the tissue is transient. The isotope is a positron emitter, fluorine-18, which has a relatively short half-life of 110 minutes. A special scanner with pairs of detectors is required. The detectors in a PET scanner record gamma photons that are emitted at approximately 180 degrees to each other, which are coincidence events. Near-simultaneous detection of annihilation photons by a pair of detectors representing a line in space along which positron emission has occurred are captured and recorded. Thus one can localize their source along a straight line of coincidence. Current scanners consist of multiple rings of detectors that essentially constitute a cylinder of detectors around the patient. Computer-assisted statistical analysis of the pairs of data are constructed to identify points in space and are assembled to produce an image. The image is difficult to interpret because many organs actively concentrate and utilize glucose, so elucidation requires considerable education and experience with the technique to identify likely deposits of thyroid cancer.

Interpreting a PET scan is quite subjective and requires a detailed knowledge of the region and how specific anatomical structures and organs are likely to handle glucose. In many cases, the shape and location of the structure in question offers an "obvious" correlation between the image and its anatomic or pathologic basis. Nevertheless, occasionally conclusions drawn in this way may be incorrect. Good clinical judgment and appropriate skepticism are always in order.

Fusing the image obtained with the glucose bio-marker with CT and potentially with MRI has enhanced the accuracy, specificity, and utility of PET scanning and may alter clinical management, especially when thyroglobulin is elevated and ^{131}I WBS is negative.[106-111] For example, in the neck, PET scanning may reveal FDG activity in the region of the thyroid cartilage or low-level diffuse activity in extrathyroid regions that may be reported as abnormalities, suspicious findings, or nonspecific. The "philosophy" of the radiologist, the endocrinologist, or the surgeon, as well as clinical factors like "I know the thyroglobulin is positive and I must find a lesion" can contribute to image interpretation. In contrast, bimodality fusion scanning is more objective and has revealed that the activity in the region of the thyroid cartilage often represents the vocal cord muscles and can be differentiated from regional tumor.[106] These muscles are thin, linear in shape, oriented in the distribution of the vocal muscles, and the PET activity fuses to the muscles on an accurately co-registered CT examination. The diffuse glucose concentration elsewhere in the neck has now been attributed to the metabolism of brown fat, which has recently been identified in human adults as normal. Interestingly, it seems to be possible to reduce glucose activity in this brown fat by warming the person.

Does It Matter If TSH Is Suppressed or Elevated During FDG PET Scanning?

The studies to assess if TSH should be elevated during PET scanning have suffered from low power and debatable design. Firm conclusions cannot be drawn. The author's impression is that TSH elevation may improve sensitivity somewhat.

Some reports suggest that PET or PET/CT/MRI may be more sensitive to the presence of thyroid cancer when TSH is elevated rather than suppressed. In one study, 10 patients had FDG PET while TSH was suppressed and while it was elevated subsequent to the withdrawal of thyroid hormone. Although 17 lesions were found on both studies, the tumor-to-background ratio of activity increased in 15 of the patients when TSH was elevated compared to when it was suppressed. The change was attributable to increased uptake by the lesion and also to decrease in background activity.[112] A similarly designed examination of eight patients revealed more intense uptake of glucose by lesions in four patients and additional lesions in two of these four when TSH was elevated after the withdrawal of suppression.[113] Similarly, after the administration of human recombinant TSH (rhTSH), the number of "tumor-like lesions" increased from 22 when TSH was low to 78 to after rhTSH. Furthermore, the tumor-to-lesion ratio and standardized uptake value (SUV) also increased.[103] Among seven patients, rhTSH stimulation identified four lesions that were not seen during TSH suppression, and one patient had lesions after rhTSH not seen during suppression.[104]

Other studies have suggested that the two preparations are similarly effective. For instance, the relative efficacy of raising TSH by withdrawing L-thyroxine or administering rhTSH was studied in 15 patients who had elevated levels of thyroglobulin but negative WBS. The comparison consisted of seven patients whose TSH was elevated by withdrawing thyroxine and eight patients who had rhTSH. Abnormal FDG uptake was observed in four of the first and five of the second group.[105]

The Thyroid Incidentaloma in PET Scanning

Thyroid incidentalomas in FDG PET occur in 1.2% to 4.3% of patients undergoing PET because of nonthyroid malignancy,[98-104] as mentioned earlier. They are entirely similar to the incidentalomas that have been reported in thyroid ultrasonography. The majority of PET incidentalomas are benign but result in considerable anxiety, medical testing, and expense. There is considerable overlap in the SUV between benign and malignant incidentalomas.[103] One investigation disclosed that 70 of 1763 patients (4.0%) had excessive FDG accumulation in the thyroid region; 36.7% of the 70 lesions were malignant. The maximum SUV was significantly higher in the malignant lesions (10.7 verses 6.7). However, the overlap of maximum SUV was so great as to make the distinction meaningless (2.0 to 32.9 for malignant opposed to 2.3 to 33.1 for benign).[98] Therefore, lesions that are sufficiently large should be examined according to the criteria described for ultrasonography.

PET Scanning in the Initial Evaluation of Patients With Thyroid Nodules

Thyroid nodules are usually evaluated with fine-needle biopsy and cytology unless TSH is suppressed, in which case a ^{123}I scan is the appropriate next step. Ultrasonography is the cost-effective anatomic imaging study. PET scanning plays no role.

PET Scanning in the Initial Staging of Patients With Thyroid Cancer After Thyroidectomy

Ultrasonography (for the neck), TSH stimulated ^{131}I WBS, and TSH-stimulated, in vitro measurement of thyroglobulin play complementary and essential roles in the initial postoperative evaluation of patients with thyroid cancer. Uncontrolled clinical testing of patients with thyroid cancer and a few actual investigations have explored the feasibility, utility, and cost effectiveness of using PET scanning for initial screening. PET scanning can reveal some metastatic lesions but is not adequately useful clinically to routinely warrant this expensive, time-consuming, and isotope-requiring technique. However, PET scanning may be useful in the initial evaluation and staging of local cancer or metastases in patients with poorly differentiated or anaplastic thyroid cancer. The sensitivity of this application is unknown, but since anaplastic cancers usually do not adequately concentrate ^{131}I, and there may be extensive distant metastases, PET with CT or MRI are the appropriate imaging techniques in this setting rather than WBS. Similarly, with Hürthle cell thyroid cancer, where ^{131}I accumulation tends to be low, and medullary thyroid cancer, where there tends to be no uptake, PET scans are especially useful. Several studies have shown the value of PET scanning for Hürthle cell lesions[117-120] and for medullary tumors.[121-129]

PET Scanning in the Detection of Recurrence of Thyroid Cancer

As in the initial staging after surgery, ultrasonography of the neck, ^{131}I WBS, and measurement of thyroglobulin are the main tools to assess patients for recurrence of typical thyroid cancer. In selected cases, percutaneous fine-needle biopsy of suspicious nodules together with cytology and sometimes measurement of thyroglobulin in the aspirate complement these examinations. PET scanning seems to be cost effective when ^{131}I WBS is negative, but thyroglobulin is identified in either the blood or an aspirated specimen of tissue or fluid.

The role of FDG PET scanning (PET/CT or PET/MRI) in patients with thyroid cancer is the detection and localization of recurrence of the cancer when ^{131}I WBS is negative, but there is reason to believe that thyroid cancer deposits are present because thyroglobulin is elevated and/or ultrasonography shows a suspicious lesion.[130-136] This conclusion is based on observations that thyroid cancers that do not take up ^{131}I frequently concentrate FDG and are detectable on PET scanning. As an example, in one investigation among patients who were strongly suspected of persistent or recurrent cancer by traditional clinical criteria, FDG PET identified 17 of 18 sites that concentrated ^{131}I on WBS. Eleven additional sites that concentrated FDG but not ^{131}I were also disclosed. In contrast, there was normal FDG distribution in 19 of 27 patients who did not concentrate [131]I.[137]

Studies that evaluate the utility of PET scanning agree about a general value but vary as to specificity and sensitivity. False positives are uncommon. The result of PET alters clinical management in many of the patients.

PET Scanning in Patients With Hyperthyroidism and Lymphocytic Thyroiditis

PET scanning may be used in a variety of disorders to study the metabolism of glucose. For example, it has been found that there is enhanced uptake of glucose in hyperthyroid patients that correlates with increased levels of antithyroid antibodies, but it is unclear if the activity reflects thyroid cell or lymphocyte function.[138]

Novel Observations from PET Scanning

It is believed that thyroid cancers that are PET positive and ^{131}I WBS negative behave clinically in a more aggressive fashion than ^{131}I-positive lesions and are less differentiated histopathologically. A retrospective analysis demonstrated relatively reduced survival of patients older than 45 years, abnormal focal FDG uptake, and large volume of the FDG lesions. The variable that most strongly predicted survival was large FDG volume of lesions.[139] In contrast, a negative PET scan in a patient with known metastatic disease seems to confer a favorable survival advantage when compared with patients who are PET-positive.[140]

The expression of glucose transporters has been linked to abnormal PET FDG accumulation and to unfavorable prognosis in patients with thyroid cancer. This observation may offer insight into the mechanism of enhanced labeled-glucose accumulation by certain thyroid cancers. Studying the expression of types 1 to 5 glucose transporters in formalin-fixed, paraffin-embedded tissue samples from 45 patients with carcinoma, increased levels of glucose transporter type 1 (GLUT1) was found in the cancers of patients who had an unfavorable prognosis. Among these were anaplastic thyroid cancer and aggressively behaving follicular cancers. Low or no GLUT1 expression was observed in both normal thyroid tissue and well-differentiated tumors that had a good prognosis.[141]

Acknowledgment

The late Ralph R. Cavalieri, M.D., wrote the section on thyroid scintigraphy for the 4th edition of this textbook. I have reworked that section for the 5th and 6th editions.

REFERENCES

1. Cavalieri RR, McDougall IR: In vivo isotopic tests and imaging. In Braverman LE, Utiger RD, editors: The Thyroid: A Fundamental and Clinical Text, ed 7, Philadelphia, 1996, JB Lippincott, pp 352–376.
2. Becker DV, Charkes ND, Dworkin H, et al: Procedure guideline for thyroid scintigraphy: 1.0, J Nucl Med 37:1264–1266, 1996.
3. Sostre S, Ashare AB, Quinones JD, et al: Thyroid scintigraphy: pinhole images vs. rectilinear scans, Radiology 129:759–762, 1978.
4. Chen JJS, LaFrance ND, Allo MD, et al: Single-photon emission computed tomography of the thyroid, J Clin Endocrinol Metab 66:1240–1246, 1988.
5. Burch HB, Shakir F, Fitzsimmons TR, et al: Diagnosis and management of the autonomously functioning thyroid nodule: the Walter Reed Army Medical Center experience, 1975–1996, Thyroid 8:871–880, 1998.
6. Kusic Z, Becker DV, Saenger EL, et al: Comparison of Tc-99m and iodine-123 imaging of thyroid nodules: correlation with pathological findings, J Nucl Med 31:393–399, 1990.
7. Singer PA, Cooper DS, Daniels GH, et al: Treatment guidelines for patients with thyroid nodules and well-differentiated thyroid cancer, Arch Intern Med 156:2165–2172, 1996.
8. Meier CA, Braverman LE, Ebner SA, et al: Diagnostic use of recombinant human thyrotropin in patients with thyroid carcinoma (phase I/II study), J Clin Endocrinol Metab 78:188–196, 1994.
9. Ladenson P, Braverman L, Mazzaferri E, et al: Comparison of administration of recombinant human thyrotropin with withdrawal of thyroid hormone for radioactive iodine scanning in patients with thyroid carcinoma, N Engl J Med 337:888–896, 1997.
10. Lakshmanan M, Schaffer A, Robbins J, et al: A simplified low iodine diet in I-131 scanning and therapy of thyroid cancer, Clin Nucl Med 13:866–868, 1988.
11. Maxon HRI, Smith HS: Radioiodine I-131 in the diagnosis and treatment of metastatic well differentiated thyroid cancer, Endocrinol Metab Clin North Am 19:685–719, 1990.
12. Cavalieri RR: Nuclear imaging in the management of thyroid carcinoma, Thyroid 6:485–492, 1996.
13. McDougall IR: 74 MBq radioiodine ^{131}I does not prevent uptake of therapeutic doses of [131]I (i.e., does not cause stunning in differentiated thyroid cancer), Nucl Med Commun 18:505–512, 1997.
14. Muratet J-P, Daver A, Minier J-F, et al: Influence of scanning doses of iodine-131 on subsequent first ablative treatment outcome in patients operated on for differentiated thyroid carcinoma, J Nucl Med 39:1546–1550, 1998.
15. Park HM, Park YA, Zhou XH: Detection of thyroid remnants/metastases without stunning: an ongoing dilemma, Thyroid 7:277–280, 1997.
16. McDougall IR: Whole body scintigraphy with radioiodine-131: a comprehensive list of false-positives with some examples, Clin Nucl Med 20:869–875, 1995.
17. Schlumberger M, Parmentier C, de Vathaire F, et al: Iodine-131 and external radiation in the treatment of local and metastatic thyroid cancer. In Falk SA, editor: Thyroid Disease, ed 2, Philadelphia, 1997, Lippincott-Raven, pp 601–617.
18. Clark OH, Hoelting T: Management of patients with differentiated thyroid cancer who have positive serum thyroglobulin levels and negative radioiodine scans, Thyroid 4:501–505, 1994.
19. Sisson JC: Selection of the optimal scanning agent for thyroid cancer, Thyroid 7:295–302, 1997.
20. Dadparvar S, Chevres A, Tulchinsky M, et al: Clinical utility of technetium-99m methoxyisobutylisonitrile imaging in the treatment of differentiated thyroid carcinoma: comparison with thallium-201 and iodine-131 Na scintigraphy, and serum thyroglobulin quantitation, Eur J Nucl Med 22:1330–1338, 1995.
21. Yen T-C, Lin HD, Lee CH, et al: The role of technetium-99m sestamibi whole-body scans in diagnosis of metastatic Hürthle cell carcinoma of the thyroid gland after total thyroidectomy: a comparison with iodine-131 and thallium-201 whole-body scans, Eur J Nucl Med 21:980–983, 1994.
22. Baudin E, Lubroso J, Schlumberger M, et al: Comparison of octreotide scintigraphy and conventional imaging in medullary thyroid carcinoma, J Nucl Med 36:912–916, 1996.
23. Grunwald F, Schomburg A, Bender H, et al: Fluorine-18 fluorodeoxyglucose positron imaging tomography in the follow-up of differentiated thyroid cancer, Eur J Nucl Med 23:312–319, 1996.
24. Blum M, Goldman AB, Herskovic A, et al: Clinical applications of thyroid echography, N Engl J Med 287:1164–1169, 1972.
25. Butch RJ, Simeone JF, Mueller PR: Thyroid and parathyroid ultrasonography, Radiol Clin North Am 23:57, 1995.
26. Clarke DK, Cronan J, Scola F: Color Doppler sonography: anatomic and physiologic assessment of the thyroid, J Clin Ultrasound 23:215–223, 1995.
27. Blum M, Passalaqua AM, Sackler J, et al: Thyroid echography of subacute thyroiditis, Radiology 124:795–799, 1977.
28. Marcocci C, Vitti P, Cetani F, et al: Thyroid ultrasonography helps to identify patients with diffuse lymphocytic thyroiditis who are prone to develop hypothyroidism, J Clin Endocrinol Metab 72:209–213, 1991.
29. Raber W, Gessl A, Nowotny P, et al: Thyroid ultrasound versus antithyroid peroxidase antibody determination: a cohort study of four hundred fifty-one subjects, Thyroid 12:725–731, 2002.
30. Premawardhana LD, Parkes AB, Ammari F, et al: Postpartum thyroiditis and long-term thyroid status: prognostic influence of thyroid peroxidase antibodies and ultrasound echogenicity, J Clin Endocrinol Metab 85:71–75, 2000.
31. Fobbe F, Finke R, Reichenstein E, et al: Appearance of thyroid diseases using colour-coded duplex sonography, Eur J Radiol 9:29–31, 1989.
32. Ralls PW, Mayekawa DS, Lee K, et al: Color-flow Doppler sonography in Graves' disease: "thyroid inferno," Am J Roentgenol 150:781–784, 1988.
33. Hodgson KW, Lazarus JH, Wheeler MH, et al: Duplex scan-derived thyroid blood flow in euthyroid and hyperthyroid patients, World J Surg 12:470–475, 1988.
34. Vander JB, Gaston EA, Dawber TR: The significance of nontoxic thyroid nodules: final report of a 15-year study of the incidence of thyroid malignancy, Ann Intern Med 69:537–540, 1968.
35. Mazzaferri EL: Management of a solitary thyroid nodule, N Engl J Med 328:553–559, 1993.
36. Ridgway EC: Clinical review 30: clinician's evaluation of a solitary thyroid nodule, J Clin Endocrinol Metab 74:231–235, 1992.
37. Brander A, Viikinkoski P, Tuuhea LJ, et al: Clinical versus ultrasound examination of the thyroid gland in common clinical practice, J Clin Ultrasound 20:37–42, 1992.
38. James EM, Charboneau JW, Hay ID: The thyroid. In Rumack CM, Wilson SR, Charboneau JW, editors: Diagnostic Ultrasound, Vol 1, St Louis, 1991, Mosby-Year Book, p 507.
39. Simeone JF, Daniels GH, Hall DA, et al: Sonography in the follow-up of 100 patients with thyroid carcinoma, AJR Am J Roentgenol 148:45, 1987.
40. Ito Y, Amino N, Yokozawa T, et al: Ultrasonographic evaluation of thyroid nodules in 900 patients: comparison among ultrasonographic, cytological, and histological findings, Thyroid 2007 Nov 8 [Epub].
41. Solbiati L, Volterrani L, Rizzatto G, et al: The thyroid gland with low uptake lesions: evaluation by ultrasound, Radiology 155:187, 1985.
42. Cochand-Priollet B, Guillausseau PJ, Chagnon S, et al: The diagnostic value of fine-needle aspiration biopsy under ultrasonography in nonfunctional thyroid nodules: a prospective study comparing cytologic and histologic findings, Am J Med 97:152, 1994.
43. Solivetti FM, Bacaro D, Cecconi P, et al: Small hyperechogenic nodules in thyroiditis: usefulness of cytological characterization, J Exp Clin Cancer Res 23:433, 2004.
44. Solbiati L, Cioffi V, Ballarati E: Ultrasonography of the neck, Radiol Clin North Am 30:941–953, 1992.
45. Simeone JF, Daniels GH, Muller PR, et al: High-resolution real-time sonography of the thyroid, Radiology 145:431–435, 1982
46. Ito Y, Kobayashi K, Tomoda C, et al: Ill-defined edge on ultrasonographic examination can be a marker of aggressive characteristic of papillary thyroid microcarcinoma, World J Surg 29:1007, 2005.
47. Clark KJ, Cronan JJ, Scola FH: Color Doppler sonography: anatomic and physiologic assessment of the thyroid, J Clin Ultrasound 23:215, 1995.
48. Appetecchia M, Solivetti FM: The association of colour flow Doppler sonography and conventional ultrasonography improves the diagnosis of thyroid carcinoma, Horm Res 66:249–256, 2006.

49. Marqusee E, Benson CB, Frates MC, et al: Usefulness of ultrasonography in the management of nodular thyroid disease, Ann Intern Med 133:696–700, 2000.
50. Boehm TM, Rothose L, Wartofsky L: Occult follicular carcinoma of the thyroid with a solitary slowly growing metastasis, JAMA 235:2420, 1976.
51. Solbiati L, Rizzatto G, Bellotti E, et al: High resolution sonography of cervical lymph nodes in head and neck cancer: criteria for differentiation of reactive versus malignant nodes [abstract], Radiology 169:113, 1988.
52. Vassallo P, Wernecke K, Roos N, et al: Differentiation of benign from malignant superficial lymphadenopathy: The role of high-resolution US, Radiology 183:215–220, 1992.
53. Bruneton JN, Roux P, Caramella E, et al: Ear, nose, and throat cancer: ultrasound diagnosis of metastasis to cervical lymph nodes, Radiology 152:771–773, 1984.
54. Kessler A, Rappaport Y, Blank A, et al: Cystic appearance of cervical lymph nodes is characteristic of metastatic papillary thyroid carcinoma, J Clin Ultrasound 31:21–25, 2003.
55. Choi M, Lee JW, Jang KJ: Distinction between benign and malignant causes of cervical, axillary, and inguinal adenopathy: value of Doppler spectral waveform analysis, Am J Roentgenol 165:981–984, 1995.
56. Kuna SK, Bracic I, Tesic V, et al: Ultrasonographic differentiation of benign from malignant neck lymphadenopathy in thyroid cancer, J Ultrasound Med. 25:1531–1537, 2006.
57. Boi F, Baghino G, Atzeni F, et al: The diagnostic value for differentiated thyroid carcinoma metastases of thyroglobulin (Tg) measurement in washout fluid from fine-needle aspiration biopsy of neck lymph nodes is maintained in the presence of circulating anti-Tg antibodies, J Clin Endocrinol Metab 91:1364, 2006.
58. Blum M: Ultrasonography and computed tomography of the thyroid gland. In Ingbar SH, Braverman LE, editors: Werner's the Thyroid, ed 5, New York, 1986, JB Lippincott, pp 576–591.
59. Simeone JF, Daniels GH, Hall DA, et al: Sonography in the follow up of 100 patients with thyroid carcinoma, Am J Roentgenol 148:45–49, 1987.
60. Arora P, Blum M: Utility of ultrasonography in post surgical management of patients with thyroid carcinoma. Paper presented at the 74th Meeting of the American Thyroid Association, Nov 7–10, 2001, Washington, DC.
61. Torlontano M, Crocetti U, D'Aloiso L, et al: Serum thyroglobulin and ^{131}I whole body scan after recombinant human TSH stimulation in the follow-up of low-risk patients with differentiated thyroid cancer, Eur J Endocrinol 148:19–24, 2003.
62. Karwowski JK, Jeffrey RB, McDougall IR, et al: Intraoperative ultrasonography improves identification of recurrent thyroid cancer, Surgery 132:924–928, 2002.
63. Rizzatto G, Solbiati L, Croce F, et al: Aspiration biopsy of superficial lesions: ultrasonic guidance with a linear-array probe, Am J Roentgenol 148:623–625, 1987.
64. Takashima S, Yoshida J, Kishimoto H, et al: Nonpalpable lymph nodes of the neck: assessment with US and US-guided fine-needle aspiration biopsy [abstract], Radiology 197(Suppl):270, 1995.
65. Gharib H, Goellner JR, Johnson DA: FNA cytology of the thyroid: a 12-year experience with 11,000 biopsies, Clin Lab Med 13:699–710, 1995.
66. Deandrea M, Mormile A, Veglio M, et al: Fine-needle aspiration biopsy of the thyroid: Comparison between thyroid palpation and ultrasonography, Endocr Pract 8:282–286, 2002.
67. Chung SY, Oh KK, Chang HS: Sonographic findings of tuberculosis thyroiditis in a patient with Behcet's syndrome, J Clin Ultrasound 30:184–188, 2002.
68. Basaria S, Ayala AR, Westra WH, et al: Amyloidosis: role of fine-needle aspiration, Thyroid 13:313–314, 2003.
69. Ozdemir H, Ilgit ET, Yucel C, et al: Ultrasound guided percutaneous ethanol injection for the treatment of autonomous thyroid nodules, Am J Roentgenol 163:929–932, 1994.
70. Del Prete S, Russo D, Caraglia M, et al: Percutaneous ethanol injection of autonomous thyroid nodules with a volume larger than 40 ml: three years of follow-up, Clin Radiol 56:895–901, 2001.
71. Janowitz P, Ackmann S: Long-term results of ultrasound-guided ethanol injections in patients with autonomous thyroid nodules and hyperthyroidism, Med Klin 96:451–456, 2001.
72. Brkljacic B, Sucic M, Bozikov V, et al: Treatment of autonomous and toxic thyroid adenomas by percutaneous ultrasound-guided ethanol injection, Acta Radiol 42:477–481, 2001.
73. Solymosi T, Gal I: Treatment of recurrent nodular goiters with percutaneous ethanol injection: a clinical study of 12 patients, Thyroid 13:273–277, 2003.
74. Cho YS, Lee HK, Ahn IM, et al: Sonographically guided ethanol sclerotherapy for benign thyroid cysts: results in 22 patients, Am J Roentgenol 174:213–216, 2000.
75. Lewis BD, Hay ID, Charboneau JW, et al: Percutaneous ethanol injection for treatment of cervical lymph node metastases in patients with papillary thyroid carcinoma, Am J Roentgenol 178:699–704, 2002.
76. Ranzini AC, Ananth CV, Smulian JC, et al: Ultrasonography of the fetal thyroid: nomograms based on biparietal diameter and gestational age, J Ultrasound Med 20:613–617, 2001.
77. Agrawal P, Ogilvy-Stuart A, Lees C: Intrauterine diagnosis and management of congenital goitrous hypothyroidism, Ultrasound Obstet Gynecol 19:501–505, 2002.
78. Morine M, Takeda T, Minekawa R, et al: Antenatal diagnosis and treatment of a case of fetal goitrous hypothyroidism associated with high-output cardiac failure, Ultrasound Obstet Gynecol 19:506–509, 2002.
79. Perry RJ, Hollman AS, Wood AM, et al: Ultrasound of the thyroid gland in the newborn: normative data, Arch Dis Child Fetal Neonatal Ed 87:209–211, 2002.
80. Knudsen N, Bols B, Bulow I, et al: Validation of ultrasonography of the thyroid gland for epidemiological purposes, Thyroid 9:1069, 1999.
81. Semiz S, Senol U, Bircan O, et al: Correlation between age, body size and thyroid volume in an endemic area, J Endocrinol Invest 24:559–563, 2001.
82. Drozd V, Polyanskaya O, Ostapenko V, et al: Systematic ultrasound screening as a significant tool for early detection of thyroid carcinoma in Belarus, J Pediatr Endocrinol Metab 15:979–984, 2002.
83. Chung WY, Chang HS, Kim EK, et al: Ultrasonographic mass screening for thyroid carcinoma: a study in women scheduled to undergo a breast examination, Surg Today 31:763–767, 2001.
84. Blum M: Evaluation of thyroid function sonography, computed tomography and magnetic resonance imaging. In Becker KL, editor: Principles and Practice of Endocrinology and Metabolism, Philadelphia, 1990, JB Lippincott, pp 289–293.
85. Bahist B, Ellis K, Gold RP: Computed tomography of intrathoracic goiters, Am J Roentgenol 140:455–460, 1983.
86. Blum M, Reede DL, Seltzer TF, et al: Computerized axial tomography in the diagnosis and management of thyroid and parathyroid disorders, Am J Med Sci 287:34, 1984.
87. Blum M, Braverman LE, Holliday RA, et al: The thyroid: Diagnosis. In Wagner HN, Szabo Z, Buchanan JW, editors: principles of Nuclear Medicine, ed 2, Philadelphia, 1995, WB Saunders, pp 595–621.
88. Higgins CB, Auffermann W: MR imaging of thyroid and parathyroid glands: a review of current status, Am J Roentgenol 151:1095–1106, 1988.
89. Tennvall J, Biorklund A, Moller T, et al: Studies of MRI relaxation times in malignant and normal tissues of the human thyroid gland, Prog Nucl Med 8:142–148, 1984.
90. Glazer HS, Niemeyer JH, Balfe DM, et al: Neck neoplasms: MR imaging Part II. Posttreatment evaluation, Radiology 160:349–354, 1986.
91. Freeman M, Toriumi DM, Mafee MF: Diagnostic imaging techniques in thyroid cancer, Am J Surg 155:215–223, 1988.
92. Yousem DM, Som PM, Hackney DB, et al: Central nodal necrosis and extracapsular neoplastic spread in cervical lymph nodes: MR imaging versus CT, Radiology 182:753–759, 1992.
93. Webb WR, Sostman HD: MR imaging of thoracic disease: clinical uses, Radiology 182:621–630, 1992.
94. Davis SD: CT evaluation of pulmonary metastases in patients with extrathoracic malignancy, Radiology 180:1–12, 1991.
95. Auffernann W, Clark OH, Thurner S, et al: Recurrent thyroid carcinoma: characteristics on MR images, Radiology 168:753–757, 1988.
96. Takashima S, Morimoto S, Ikezoe J, et al: CT evaluation of anaplastic thyroid carcinoma, Am J Neuroradiol 11:361–367, 1990.
97. Schmid DT, Kneifel S, Stoeckli SJ, et al: Increased 18F-FDG uptake mimicking thyroid cancer in a patient with Hashimoto's thyroiditis, Eur Radiol 13(9):2119–2121, 2003.
98. Choi JY, Lee KS, Kim HJ, et al: Focal thyroid lesions incidentally identified by integrated 18F-FDG PET/CT: clinical significance and improved characterization, J Nucl Med 47(4):609–615, 2006.
99. Chen YK, Ding HJ, Chen KT, et al: Prevalence and risk of cancer of focal thyroid incidentaloma identified by 18F-fluorodeoxyglucose positron emission tomography for cancer screening in healthy subjects, Anticancer Res 25(2B):1421–1426, 2005.
100. Chu QD, Connor MS, Lilien DL, et al: Positron emission tomography (PET) positive thyroid incidentaloma: the risk of malignancy observed in a tertiary referral center, Am Surg 72(3):272–275, 2006.
101. Cohen MS, Arslan N, Dehdashti F, et al: Risk of malignancy in thyroid incidentalomas identified by fluorodeoxyglucose-positron emission tomography, Surgery 130(6):941–946, 2001.
102. Kang KW, Kim SK, Kang HS, et al: Prevalence and risk of cancer of focal thyroid incidentaloma identified by 18F-fluorodeoxyglucose positron emission tomography for metastasis evaluation and cancer screening in healthy subjects, J Clin Endocrinol Metab 88(9):4100–4104, 2003.
103. Kim TY, Kim WB, Ryu JS, et al: 18F-fluorodeoxyglucose uptake in thyroid from positron emission tomogram (PET) for evaluation in cancer patients: high prevalence of malignancy in thyroid PET incidentaloma, Laryngoscope 115(6):1074–1078, 2005.
104. Yi JG, Marom EM, Munden RF, et al: Focal uptake of fluorodeoxyglucose by the thyroid in patients undergoing initial disease staging with combined PET/CT for non-small cell lung cancer, Radiology 236(1):271–275, 2005.
105. Blum M, Noz M, Yee J, et al: Feasibility of simultaneous display of thyroid function & structure images: assemblage of scintiscanning and ultrasonography. American Thyroid Association: 77th Annual Meeting, Phoenix, Arizona October 11–15, 2006.
106. Chin BB, Patel P, Hammoud D: Combined positron emission tomography–computed tomography improves specificity for thyroid carcinoma by identifying vocal cord activity after laryngeal nerve paralysis, Thyroid 13(12):1183–1184, 2003.
107. Bockisch A, Brandt-Mainz K, Gorges R, et al: Diagnosis in medullary thyroid cancer with [18F]FDG-PET and improvement using a combined PET/CT scanner, Acta Med Austriaca 30(1):22–25, 2003.
108. Zimmer LA, McCook B, Meltzer C, et al: Combined positron emission tomography/computed tomography imaging of recurrent thyroid cancer, Otolaryngol Head Neck Surg 128(2):178–184, 2003.
109. Nahas Z, Goldenberg D, Fakhry C, et al: The role of positron emission tomography/computed tomography in the management of recurrent papillary thyroid carcinoma, Laryngoscope 115(2):237–243, 2005.
110. Palmedo H, Bucerius J, Joe A, et al: Integrated PET/CT in differentiated thyroid cancer: diagnostic accuracy and impact on patient management, J Nucl Med 47(4):616–624, 2006.
111. Zoller M, Kohlfuerst S, Igerc I, et al: Combined PET/CT in the follow-up of differentiated thyroid carcinoma: what is the impact of each modality? Eur J Nucl Med Mol Imaging 2006.
112. Moog F, Linke R, Manthey N, et al: Influence of thyroid-stimulating hormone levels on uptake of FDG in recurrent and metastatic differentiated thyroid carcinoma, J Nucl Med 41(12):1989–1995, 2000.
113. van Tol KM, Jager PL, Piers DA, et al: Better yield of (18)fluorodeoxyglucose-positron emission tomography in patients with metastatic differentiated thyroid carcinoma during thyrotropin stimulation, Thyroid 12(5):381–387, 2002.
114. Petrich T, Borner AR, Otto D, et al: Influence of rhTSH on [(18)F]fluorodeoxyglucose uptake by differentiated thyroid carcinoma, Eur J Nucl Med Mol Imaging 29(5):641–647, 2002.
115. Chin BB, Patel P, Cohade C, et al: Recombinant human thyrotropin stimulation of fluoro-D-glucose positron emission tomography uptake in well-differentiated

thyroid carcinoma, J Clin Endocrinol Metab 89(1):91–95, 2004.

116. Saab G, Driedger AA, Pavlosky W, et al: Thyroid-stimulating hormone-stimulated fused positron emission tomography/computed tomography in the evaluation of recurrence in ^{131}I-negative papillary thyroid carcinoma, Thyroid 16(3):267–272, 2006.

117. Plotkin M, Hautzel H, Krause BJ, et al: Implication of 2-18fluor-2-deoxyglucose positron emission tomography in the follow-up of Hurthle cell thyroid cancer, Thyroid 12(2):155, 2002.

118. Blount CL, Dworkin HJ: F-18 FDG uptake by recurrent Hürthle cell carcinoma of the thyroid using high-energy planar scintigraphy, Clin Nucl Med 21(11):831–833, 1996.

119. Lowe VJ, Mullan BP, Hay ID, et al: 18F-FDG PET of patients with Hürthle cell carcinoma, J Nucl Med 44(9):1402–1406, 2003.

120. Pryma DA, Schoder H, Gonen M, et al: Diagnostic accuracy and prognostic value of 18F-FDG PET in Hürthle cell thyroid cancer patients, J Nucl Med 47(8):1260–1266, 2006.

121. Gasparoni P, Rubello D, Ferlin G: Potential role of fluorine-18-deoxyglucose (FDG) positron emission tomography (PET) in the staging of primitive and recurrent medullary thyroid carcinoma, J Endocrinol Invest 20(9):527–530, 1997.

122. Musholt TJ, Musholt PB, Dehdashti F, et al: Evaluation of fluorodeoxyglucose-positron emission tomographic scanning and its association with glucose transporter expression in medullary thyroid carcinoma and pheochromocytoma: a clinical and molecular study, Surgery 122(6):1049–1060, 1997.

123. Brandt-Mainz K, Muller SP, Gorges R, et al: The value of fluorine-18 fluorodeoxyglucose PET in patients with medullary thyroid cancer, Eur J Nucl Med 27(5):490–496, 2000.

124. Adams S, Baum RP, Hertel A, et al: Metabolic (PET) and receptor (SPET) imaging of well- and less well-differentiated tumours: comparison with the expression of the Ki-67 antigen, Nucl Med Commun 19(7):641–647, 1998.

125. Diehl M, Risse JH, Brandt-Mainz K, et al: Fluorine-18 fluorodeoxyglucose positron emission tomography in medullary thyroid cancer: results of a multicentre study, Eur J Nucl Med 28(11):1671–1676, 2001.

126. Szakall S Jr, Bajzik G, Repa I, et al: [FDG PET scan of metastases in recurrent medullary carcinoma of the thyroid gland], Orv Hetil 143(21 Suppl 3):1280–1283, 2002.

127. Szakall S Jr, Esik O, Bajzik G, et al: 18F-FDG PET detection of lymph node metastases in medullary thyroid carcinoma, J Nucl Med 43(1):66–71, 2002.

128. de Groot JW, Links TP, Jager PL, et al: Impact of 18F-fluoro-2-deoxy-D-glucose positron emission tomography (FDG-PET) in patients with biochemical evidence of recurrent or residual medullary thyroid cancer, Ann Surg Oncol 11(8):786–794, 2004.

129. Gotthardt M, Battmann A, Hoffken H, et al: 18F-FDG PET, somatostatin receptor scintigraphy, and CT in metastatic medullary thyroid carcinoma: a clinical study and an analysis of the literature, Nucl Med Commun 25(5):439–443, 2004.

130. Khan N, Oriuchi N, Higuchi T, et al: PET in the follow-up of differentiated thyroid cancer, Br J Radiol 76(910):690–695, 2003.

131. Feine U, Lietzenmayer R, Hanke JP, et al: [18FDG whole-body PET in differentiated thyroid carcinoma. Flipflop in uptake patterns of 18FDG and ^{131}I], Nuklearmedizin 34(4):127–134, 1995.

132. Chung JK, So Y, Lee JS, et al: Value of FDG PET in papillary thyroid carcinoma with negative ^{131}I whole-body scan, J Nucl Med 40(6):986–992, 1999.

133. Alnafisi NS, Driedger AA, Coates G, et al: FDG PET of recurrent or metastatic ^{131}I-negative papillary thyroid carcinoma, J Nucl Med 41(6):1010–1015, 2000.

134. Helal BO, Merlet P, Toubert ME, et al: Clinical impact of (18)F-FDG PET in thyroid carcinoma patients with elevated thyroglobulin levels and negative ^{131}I scanning results after therapy, J Nucl Med 42(10):1464–1469, 2001.

135. Hung MC, Wu HS, Kao CH, et al: F18-fluorodeoxyglucose positron emission tomography in detecting metastatic papillary thyroid carcinoma with elevated human serum thyroglobulin levels but negative I-131 whole body scan, Endocr Res 29(2):169–175, 2003.

136. Caplan RH, Wickus GG, Manske BR: Long-term follow-up of a patient with papillary thyroid carcinoma, elevated thyroglobulin levels, and negative imaging studies, Endocr Pract 11(1):43–48, 2005.

137. Wang W, Macapinlac H, Larson SM, et al: [18F]-2-fluoro-2-deoxy-D-glucose positron emission tomography localizes residual thyroid cancer in patients with negative diagnostic ^{131}I whole body scans and elevated serum thyroglobulin levels, J Clin Endocrinol Metab 84:2291–2302, 1999.

138. Boerner AR, Voth E, Theissen P, et al: Glucose metabolism of the thyroid in Graves' disease measured by F-18-fluoro-deoxyglucose positron emission tomography, Thyroid 8(9):765–772, 1998.

139. Wang W, Larson SM, Fazzari M, et al: Prognostic value of [18F]fluorodeoxyglucose positron emission tomographic scanning in patients with thyroid cancer, J Clin Endocrinol Metab 85(3):1107–1113, 2000.

140. Robbins RJ, Wan Q, Grewal RK, et al: Real-time prognosis for metastatic thyroid carcinoma based on 2-[18F]fluoro-2-deoxy-D-glucose-positron emission tomography scanning, J Clin Endocrinol Metab 91(2):498–505, 2006.

141. Schonberger J, Ruschoff J, Grimm D, et al: Glucose transporter 1 gene expression is related to thyroid neoplasms with an unfavorable prognosis: an immunohistochemical study, Thyroid 12(9):747–754, 2002.

Chapter 8

AUTOIMMUNE THYROID DISEASE

ANTHONY P. WEETMAN

The Syndromes of Thyroid Autoimmunity

The concept of thyroid autoimmunity, the original exemplar of an organ-specific autoimmune disorder, arose from the seminal observations of Rose and Witebsky, who showed that thyroid autoantibodies and thyroiditis developed in rabbits that had been immunized with thyroid extract,[1] and from the observations of Roitt and colleagues, who first described thyroglobulin (TG) antibodies in the serum of patients with Hashimoto's thyroiditis.[2] Graves' disease became defined as an autoimmune disorder after the discovery of a long-acting thyroid stimulator in the serum of such patients[3] that subsequently was shown to be a specific immunoglobulin G (IgG) directed against the thyroid-stimulating hormone receptor (TSHR). Over the past 40 years, a huge volume of work founded on these discoveries has continued to improve our understanding of the origin and pathogenesis of these disorders. It is now appreciated that autoimmune hypothyroidism and Graves' disease share many features, with some patients progressing from one to the other, and that lesser degrees of thyroid autoimmunity (subclinical hypothyroidism, focal thyroiditis, postpartum thyroiditis) are remarkably common in the general population.

The main types of thyroid autoimmunity are summarized in Table 8-1. The prevalence of subclinical thyroid autoimmunity is difficult to define because the prevalence depends in part on the sensitivity of assays for thyroid autoantibodies, with sensitive assays detecting TG and thyroid peroxidase (TPO) antibodies in up to 20% of women. However, focal thyroiditis, which is closely associated with circulating thyroid autoantibodies, is present in up to 40% of white women and 20% of men at autopsy,[4] thus indicating that these figures do reflect the real prevalence of subclinical thyroid autoimmunity. Careful community studies have shown that such subclinical disease progresses only slowly and infrequently to overt thyroid dysfunction; the weighted prevalence of autoimmune hypothyroidism in the United States is 0.8 per 100 population, 95% of whom are women.[5]

Subclinical autoimmune thyroiditis may become clinically apparent in the postpartum period as the result of an exacerbation of the autoimmune process for reasons that are not yet clear. Typically, such women have TPO autoantibodies antepartum and experience transient thyroid dysfunction (thyrotoxicosis followed by hypothyroidism, or either phase alone) accompanied by a small painless goiter, with full recovery within a year after delivery.[6] It is now known that postpartum thyroiditis is a risk factor for future permanent hypothyroidism, which ensues in 20% to 30% of cases in the subsequent 5 years. Around 5% of pregnant white women have one or more episodes of postpartum thyroiditis.

Overt hypothyroidism caused by autoimmunity has two main forms: Hashimoto's (or goitrous) thyroiditis and primary myxedema, also known as atrophic thyroiditis. The former is characterized by a variably sized, firm goiter, often with an irregular surface; the goiter is typically painless, although a rare, painful variant occurs that, in contrast to subacute thyroiditis, might respond poorly to steroid treatment.[7] Such patients may have a goiter and normal thyroid function or subclinical or overt hypothyroidism, depending on the extent of the autoimmune

Table 8-1. Main Types of Thyroid Autoimmunity

Condition	Goiter	Thyroid Function	Features
Focal thyroiditis	No	Normal or subclinical hypothyroidism	May progress to overt hypothyroidism
Hashimoto's thyroiditis	Usually large	Normal or hypothyroid	Usually strongly positive for thyroglobulin and thyroid peroxidase autoantibodies
Atrophic thyroiditis	No	Hypothyroid	Probably end-stage disease
Silent thyroiditis; postpartum thyroiditis	Small	Transient thyrotoxicosis and/or hypothyroidism	May progress to permanent hypothyroidism
Graves'disease	Variable size	Hyperthyroid	Associated with ophthalmopathy and thyroid-stimulating antibodies

destructive process. However, in primary myxedema, the typical manifestation is clinically evident hypothyroidism, obviously without a goiter. Many attempts have been made to ascribe distinct genetic or pathogenic factors to these two disorders, but in most cases, a unique pathogenesis is not evident, and it seems most likely that they are simply at opposite ends of a spectrum of clinical features, with gradual diminution in the size of the goiter noted as disease progresses.

Similarly, Graves' disease shares many immunologic features with autoimmune hypothyroidism, and even the hallmark of Graves' disease, TSHR autoantibodies, can be found in some patients with autoimmune hypothyroidism, although their effects are masked by a more vigorous destructive autoimmune process (see below). Graves' disease is the most common autoimmune disorder in the United States, with an estimated weighted prevalence of 1.2 per 100, 88% of whom are women.[5] Many of these individuals progress to hypothyroidism, either spontaneously after successful treatment with antithyroid drugs or iatrogenically after radioiodine therapy or surgery.

This chapter provides an overview of the basic causative and pathologic factors involved in autoimmune thyroid disease.

Pathology

The typical appearance of Hashimoto's thyroiditis is termed *struma lymphomatosa* to indicate the extensive infiltration of the thyroid by lymphocytes, plasma cells, and macrophages.[7] As well as a diffuse infiltrate, germinal center formation may be particularly prominent, and giant (Langerhans) cells can occur. The thyroid follicular cells are destroyed to a variable extent, depending on the chronicity of the disease, and during this process, the remaining cells become hyperplastic and undergo oxyphil metaplasia, which gives rise to the so-called Askanazy or Hürthle cells. Variable fibrosis and, in rare cases, concurrent changes typical of Graves' disease appear—so-called hashitoxicosis.

Primary myxedema is characterized by extensive fibrosis, loss of normal lobular architecture, and gland atrophy; lymphocytic infiltration varies from minor to moderate. It remains to be established how frequently Hashimoto's thyroiditis progresses to primary myxedema. The extent of fibrosis in autoimmune hypothyroidism is directly correlated with the age of the patient,[8] compatible with the occurrence of such a progression, although little change in the pathologic appearance has been found in sequential biopsies over 10 to 20 years in those with Hashimoto's thyroiditis.[9] The histologic appearances of postpartum thyroiditis and silent thyroiditis resemble Hashimoto's thyroiditis, although oxyphil metaplasia and germinal centers are less frequent, whereas in focal thyroiditis, mild Hashimoto-like changes are

seen in localized areas of the thyroid, but most follicles are preserved.

The pathologic features of Graves' disease usually are obscured by prior treatment with antithyroid drugs, whose effects on the autoimmune process are considered later. Hypertrophy and hyperplasia of the thyroid follicles may be noted, the epithelium is columnar, and the colloid shrinks.[7] In addition, a variable degree of lymphocytic infiltration is present, sometimes with germinal center formation. Lymphoid hyperplasia also can be found in the thymus, lymph nodes, and spleen. Follicular involution and reversal of the lymphocytic infiltrate and hyperplasia occur with antithyroid drug treatment.

Thus, all forms of thyroid autoimmunity are associated with a lymphocytic infiltrate in the thyroid, and these lymphocytes are largely responsible for generating both T and B cell–mediated autoreactivity, although other sites such as thyroid-draining lymph nodes and bone marrow contain thyroid-autoreactive lymphocytes in autoimmune thyroid disease.[10] Many investigations have used peripheral blood lymphocytes from patients, but although these cells are readily accessible, they reflect the behavior of only a small proportion of autoreactive lymphocytes migrating in the blood compartment in what is essentially a localized disease.

The Basis of Autoimmune Disease

This section provides only an attenuated overview of the basic mechanisms underlying autoimmunity; the reader is referred elsewhere for a more comprehensive review.[11] For the purposes of this chapter, however, a brief summary of the normal immune response is followed by a description of how autoreactivity can arise.

THE NORMAL IMMUNE RESPONSE

The essence of the immune response is shown in Fig. 8-1. The initial step involves presentation of an antigen by an antigen-presenting cell (APC), such as a dendritic cell or macrophage, to a helper T cell, which recognizes the antigen by means of a specific T cell receptor (TCR).[12] Such T cells can be identified phenotypically by expression of the molecule CD4 (*CD* stands for cluster of differentiation and is used to define an array of surface molecules on lymphocytes and other cells). The antigen is first taken up by simple phagocytosis or by involvement of specific surface receptors, and it is processed by the APC so that fragments of 12 to 18 amino acids are generated. These fragments are the "epitopes" of the antigen, which binds to major histocompatibility complex (MHC) class II molecules expressed constitutively by the APC. The MHC (termed *HLA* in humans

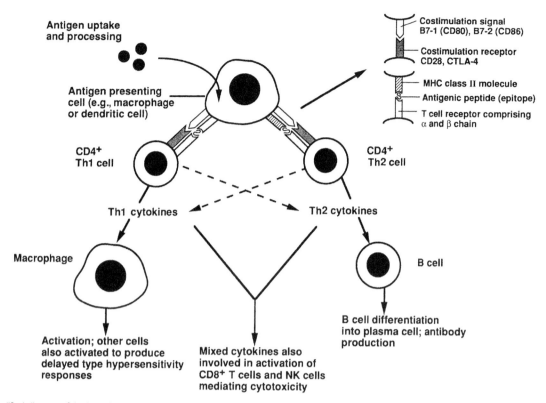

FIGURE 8-1. Simplified diagram of the key elements in a normal immune response, starting with antigen presentation. The type of immune response that is induced depends on the cytokine profile of the T helper cell that is stimulated. (From Weetman AP: Recent progress in thyroid autoimmunity: an overview for the clinician. Thyroid Today 19[2]:1–9, 1996.)

and *H-2* in mice) is a huge complex of genes that is of fundamental immunologic importance because class I (described below) and class II genes encode polymorphic molecules capable of binding a wide range of antigenic peptides.[13] The ability of an individual to mount an immune response to any given antigen depends in part on the inheritance of class I and II genes, which determine (1) whether appropriate T cells develop in the thymus, because MHC molecules can positively or negatively select T cells with particular antigenic specificities, as determined by their TCR and stage of development; and (2) whether an antigenic epitope can bind to an appropriate MHC molecule and therefore be presented to a mature T cell in adult life.

Formation of the trimolecular complex between the MHC class II molecule, antigenic epitope, and TCR is followed by activation of the CD4+ T cell, a process that involves expression of the interleukin-2 (IL-2) receptor and autocrine stimulation by IL-2 release and leads to T cell proliferation, secretion of other cytokines, and thus the development of effector function. However, many other molecules are involved in this interaction and act as stabilizers, signal transducers, or providers of so-called costimulatory or second signals (Fig. 8-2). In brief, interaction of a number of adhesion molecule ligands and receptors, such as intercellular adhesion molecule-1 (ICAM-1, CD54)/lymphocyte function-associated antigen-1 (LFA-1, CD11a/CD18) and LFA-3 (CD58)/CD2, allows initial binding of the T cell to an APC. CD4 interacts with a nonpolymorphic region on the MHC molecule to stabilize the trimolecular complex; this activity explains why helper T cells recognize antigen that is presented by class II rather than class I molecules. CD3 is composed of five peptides that are expressed uniquely by all T cells and serves to initiate the intercellular events after TCR ligation. Finally, a host of costimulatory signals can determine whether

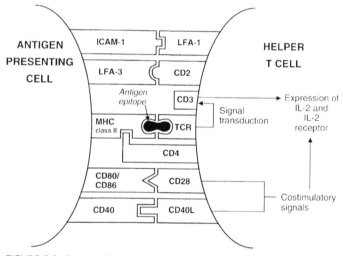

FIGURE 8-2. Diagram of the key molecular interactions in CD4+ T cell activation by an antigen-presenting cell (APC).

antigen recognition proceeds or is terminated because of the absence of an essential costimulator or the presence of an inhibitory signal.

The best defined costimulatory pathway involves the interaction of B7-1 (CD80) and B7-2 (CD86) on the APC with CD28, which transduces a stimulatory second signal, or cytotoxic T lymphocyte antigen type 4 (CTLA-4, now named CD152), which transduces an inhibitory second signal on the surface of the T cell.[14] Interaction of the TCR on naïve T cells with an MHC class II molecule plus epitope, in the absence of CD28 ligation, induces anergy (rather than stimulation) in the T cell; that is, the T cell is paralyzed and is unable to respond (Fig. 8-3). Similarly,

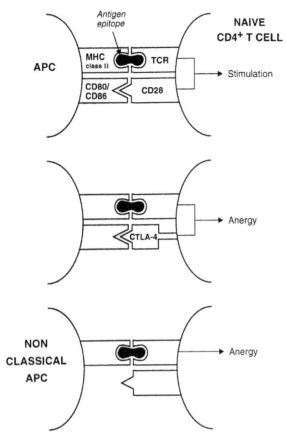

FIGURE 8-3. Mechanisms for anergy induction. The normal pathway for antigen presentation is shown in the *upper panel;* failure to provide an appropriate costimulatory signal *(lower panels)* results in anergy. Classic antigen-presenting cells (APCs) express costimulatory molecules, but class II–positive nonclassic APCs (e.g., thyroid cells) do not.

Table 8-2. Characteristics of Murine CD4$^+$ T Helper (Th) Cell Subsets; Similar but Not Identical Profiles Have Been Identified in Humans

Characteristic	Th1	Th2
Cytokine Profile		
IL-2	++	−
IL-3	++	++
IL-4	−	++
IL-5	−	++
IL-6	−	++
IL-10	−	++
Interferon-γ	++	−
Tumor necrosis factor	++	+
Lymphotoxin	++	+
Function		
Delayed-type hypersensitivity	++	−
B-cell help	+	++
Eosinophil/mast cell production	−	++

IL, Interleukin.

engagement of CTLA-4 results in T-cell anergy. As is discussed below, induction of anergy is an important mechanism in preventing autoimmune responses. Other important membrane-bound costimulatory signals exist, for instance, ICOS (inducible costimulator) ligand, which seems to be particularly important for eliciting responses from previously activated (or memory) T cells.[15] Thus, strikingly different outcomes are possible after

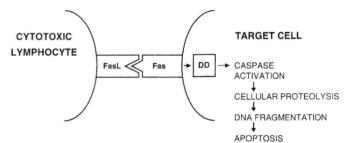

FIGURE 8-4. Interaction between Fas ligand (FasL) on cytotoxic lymphocytes and Fas on a target cell leads to signaling via the death domain (DD) proteins and apoptosis.

antigen presentation, depending on which costimulatory signals are delivered, and the signal that is delivered in turn depends on the maturity of the T cell and the type of APC involved.

Activated CD4$^+$ T cells can follow two broad pathways of function depending on their pattern of cytokine secretion (Table 8-2). Type 1 helper T (Th1) cells mediate delayed-type hypersensitivity responses, essentially the kind of destructive process that is seen in organ-specific endocrinopathies, whereas Th2 cells promote antibody production.[13] A number of factors, including TCR affinity and ligand density, the nature of the APC, and the presence of non–T-cell–derived IL-4 and IL-12, determine which pathway is followed.[16,17] Although this paradigm is undoubtedly useful, many helper T cells, particularly in humans, cannot be neatly classified according to the Th1/Th2 dichotomy. For example, a third subset, Th0 cells, produces a mix of Th1 and Th2 cytokines and is thought to be a precursor population; evidence suggests linear development of Th1 into Th2 cells via Th0 in humans.[18] Another recently identified subset, Th17, produces the cytokine IL-17 and is highly proinflammatory, with a potent role in causing autoimmunity.[17] Expanded clones of T cells arising from naïve T cells after ligation of the T cell receptor give rise to memory T cells, which help antibody production, promote inflammation, or regulate immune responses.[19]

CD8$^+$ T cells are typically cytotoxic but have in the past been assigned suppressor functions. Th1 and Th2 responses are mutually inhibitory; therefore, many suppressor phenomena may be due to a population of cells that are capable of secreting appropriate cytokines that can switch off an ongoing immune response (termed *immune deviation*). The best defined regulatory T cell subset is CD25$^+$ CD4$^+$, Foxp3$^+$ and is generated in the thymus; the emergence of autoimmune disease in animals when such thymic development is interfered with provides compelling evidence for the importance of these cells.[20,21] The cytotoxic function of activated CD8$^+$ T cells is directed against antigenic epitopes that are synthesized within the target cell and presented by MHC class I molecules; the two classic groups of antigens that are recognized by these cells are the products of viral infection or malignant transformation.[13] Destruction of target cells is mediated by two mechanisms: (1) the granule exocytosis pathway, which utilizes perforin and granzyme A and B; and (2) apoptosis, or programmed cell death. In the latter, engagement of Fas on the surface of the target cell with Fas ligand (FasL) on the T cell leads to activation of a chain of intracellular events that results in target cell apoptosis (Fig. 8-4). Fas expression is generalized, whereas FasL is restricted to cells of the immune system and to sites of immune privilege, as is described in the next section.

Mention should also be made of a further subdivision of T cells. Most T cells have a TCR that is a heterodimer composed of an α and a β chain. The genes for these chains are rearranged to ensure adequate diversity for antigen recognition. However, a small proportion of T cells have a TCR composed of a γ and a δ chain, and these receptors have a more restricted diversity.[22] The role of γδ T cells is unclear, but they may be important in mucosal immunity and protection against particular microorganisms.

Two other cell types are essential components of the immune response. B cells produce antibodies after differentiation into plasma cells, a process that is regulated by Th2 cytokines and CD40/CD40 ligand interaction with a helper T cell. Up to 10^7 different antibody specificities can be generated in humans by recombination and somatic mutation of the immunoglobulin genes.[23] During an immune response, these processes ensure selection of the most appropriate antibodies so that IgG molecules with the highest affinity for antigen are produced. Antibodies generally recognize specific determinants on an antigen that is intact rather than processed or fragmented, and these determinants are termed *epitopes*; however, unlike T cell epitopes, most B cell epitopes are conformational and are formed from discontinuous regions of the molecule.[24] As well as producing antibodies, B cells are important APCs in that they are able to take up antigen via this surface-bound immunoglobulin and enter into cognate recognition of appropriate T cells. This type of antigen presentation may be important in diversifying the T cell response because B cells present multiple epitopes of the antigen to T cells.

Killer and natural killer cells are CD3 negative and spontaneously destroy target cells with altered surface antigens (particularly reduced MHC class I), such as tumor cells.[13] Because killer and natural killer cells express receptors (CD16) for the constant (Fc) region of immunoglobulins, they also can bind to and kill antibody-coated targets, a process called antibody-dependent cell-mediated cytotoxicity (ADCC). This function also can be mediated by macrophages. Thus, although natural killer cells have little antigen specificity, they can be focused on a target via a specific antibody (Fig. 8-5).

SELF-TOLERANCE AND AUTOIMMUNITY

The immune system exists to eliminate foreign antigens but must remain tolerant of (i.e., must not respond to) autoantigens. We now know, particularly through experiments with transgenic mice, that individual mechanisms for ensuring self-tolerance (Table 8-3) are practically never completely successful; a few autoreactive T cells are present in all healthy individuals, although

in various states of nonreactivity. Failure of the control mechanisms for ensuring nonreactivity allows clonal expansion of these cells, with subsequent autoimmune disease if the response is sufficiently vigorous.

During development, the thymus is mainly responsible for eliminating autoreactive T cells (clonal deletion) and for positively selecting appropriate T cells to constitute the immune repertoire.[25,26] These processes depend on the interaction of endogenous peptides, presented by thymic APCs, with the naive TCR repertoire. Inevitably, a few T cells escape tolerance, which is particularly likely if specific endogenous antigens are unavailable for presentation in the thymus because of low abundance outside a developing organ, for example. For these antigens, peripheral tolerance, including both deletion and anergy (see Fig. 8-3), may be very important for regulation of self-reactivity.

As well as deletion and anergy, clonal ignorance provides effective protection against autoreactivity. Simply put, autoantigen-specific lymphocytes are harmless unless they become activated by autoantigen; therefore, autoimmune disease will not result from such cells if they do not come into contact with autoantigen, or if the necessary costimulatory signals are not provided. Autoreactive CD8$^+$ T cells and B cells remain harmless or "ignorant" of self-antigens unless activated by helper T cells; therefore, provided that the latter are controlled, autoimmune disease will not result. However, it should be noted that CD8$^+$ T cells and B cells are subject to central tolerance mechanisms in the fetal thymus or bone marrow and liver, respectively.[27] Another mechanism for conferring immunologic privilege at an anatomic site, whereby it becomes protected from

Table 8-3. Mechanisms for Maintaining Autoreactive T Cell Nonresponsiveness to Target Tissues

Mechanism	Reversibility
Thymic Presentation of Self-Antigens	
Deletion	No
Anergy	Yes
Peripheral Tolerance	
Deletion	No
Anergy	Yes
Clonal ignorance	Yes
Immunologic privilege at a target site	Yes
Active Suppression	
Cytokine network	Yes
Idiotype–anti-idiotype networks	Yes
Regulatory (Treg) cells	Yes

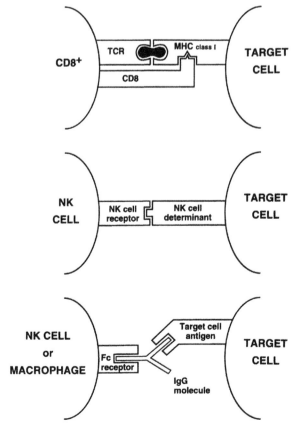

FIGURE 8-5. Recognition mechanisms involved in the interaction between cytotoxic effector cells and target cells in cell-mediated cytotoxicity. Various adhesion molecules are also involved in stabilizing these interactions.

recognition, is localized expression of FasL, which induces apoptosis in potentially autoaggressive lymphocytes entering the site; examples of such FasL expression are seen in Sertoli cells, corneal cells, and the placental trophoblast.

Subsidiary control over autoreactive T cells is provided by a number of suppressor mechanisms that often are now referred to as regulatory pathways and remain to be fully characterized. Inhibitory cytokines, such as those that produce reciprocal inhibition of Th1 and Th2 subset responses, provide one means of suppression of harmful autoimmune responses,[18] but antigen-specific suppressor phenomena have been defined in many situations, especially in animal cell transfer experiments.[20,28,29]

Tolerance to a self-antigen can be broken at one or more of the levels at which it operates (see Table 8-3) and may involve both genetic and environmental factors:

1. Autoreactive T cells might not be deleted or rendered anergic in the thymus (e.g., through inheritance of particular MHC genes or, in animals, after neonatal thymectomy).
2. T cells that escape thymic tolerance might fail to be deleted or rendered anergic in the periphery (e.g., because of abnormal provision of costimulatory signals; see Fig. 8-3).
3. Failure of immunologic tolerance might occur (e.g., because of altered FasL expression).
4. Cross-reactive exogenous antigens might induce a response against a normally "silent" autoantigen (e.g., myocarditis after streptococcal infection).
5. Suppressor mechanisms might fail to occur (e.g., provision of high concentrations of endogenous or exogenous cytokines).

Experimental Autoimmune Thyroiditis

The development of animal models of experimental autoimmune thyroiditis (EAT) (Table 8-4) has allowed profound insight into the development of thyroid autoimmunity, for example, Fig. 8-6 shows how autoimmune thyroid disease can arise in mice through modulation at the different stages of T cell tolerance, some of the principles of which were described in the preceding section. Several different types of EAT have been described,[30] and these types more or less resemble Hashimoto's thyroiditis, with lymphocytic infiltration of the thyroid, TG antibodies, and variable degrees of hypothyroidism.[30] Most recently, attempts to produce animal models of Graves' disease[31,32] have had some success, although they remain incompletely characterized. Key lessons from these animal models can be summarized as follows.

A strong genetic tendency is apparent in all models such that manipulations that readily induce EAT in one strain may induce no disease or a different autoimmune disease (such as oophoritis or gastritis) in a different strain. In both spontaneous and immunization-induced models, the MHC makes a contribution to genetic susceptibility, but it is clear that other non-MHC loci are also involved; in the OS chicken, for example, these loci control T cell responsiveness, glucocorticoid tonus, and intrinsic properties of the thyroid, which makes the OS chicken more susceptible to autoimmunity.[33] Perhaps the most elegant demonstration of susceptibility is the creation of HLA-DRB1*0301 (DR3) transgenic mice; HLA-DR3 is an MHC specificity that is known to confer susceptibility to autoimmune disease in humans (see below). Thyroiditis develops in HLA-DR3 but not HLA-DR2 transgenic mice after TG immunization, thereby confirming that this HLA-DRB1 polymorphism determines, at least in part, susceptibility to autoimmune thyroiditis.[34]

In addition, a number of environmental and endogenous factors contribute to susceptibility, and more must await discovery. Excess iodine exacerbates spontaneous thyroiditis, possibly through the generation of toxic metabolites that are formed with oxygen in the thyroid, but it is also known that a major T cell epitope on TG requires iodination for recognition by autoreactive T cells.[35] Antithyroid drugs suppress EAT with no reduction in thyroid hormone levels, which confirms the direct immunomodulatory effects of these drugs.[36]

The potential adverse effects of infection are illustrated by the absence of EAT in suitably thymectomized rats that are reared under germ-free conditions; transfer of normal gut microflora will induce disease.[37] It is possible that this result is due to the nonspecific effects of gut microflora, such as polyclonal lymphocytic activation or release of cytokines, or to some thyroid cross-reactive antigen. Environmental toxins, such as 3-methylcholanthrene, can induce EAT in genetically susceptible

Table 8-4. Summary of the Main Animal Models of Experimental Autoimmune Thyroiditis

Model	Antigen	Comments
Immunization usually with adjuvant (mouse, rat, rabbit, guinea pig)	TG, TPO, TSHR	Strain dependent, transient, and transferable via T cells; TSHR does not induce a Graves' disease–like model because the TSHR antibodies are without stimulatory action
Thymectomy induced (mouse, rat)	TG	Depends on time of thymectomy and strain, may require sublethal irradiation; transferable with T cells
T cell manipulations (mouse)	TG	Cyclosporine A and transfer of specific T cells to T cell–depleted animals induce thyroiditis
Spontaneous (chicken, dog, rat)	TG + other autoantigens	Thyroiditis occurs in OS chickens, beagles, NOD mice, and BB and Buffalo strain rats (NOD and BB animals also have autoimmune diabetes)
Virus induced (mouse)	TG + polyendocrine autoantigens	Reovirus infection of certain strains of mice
SCID mouse	TG, TPO, TSHR	SCID mice allow long-term study of transplanted thyroid tissue from patients with Graves' and Hashimoto's disease; disease does not develop in the mice themselves
cDNA Immunization (mouse)	TSHR	Allows production of monoclonal TSHR antibodies
Immunization with fibroblasts transfected with TSHR and MHC class II (mouse)	TSHR	Hyperthyroidism and histologic features of Graves' disease develop, but without lymphocytic infiltration

MHC, Major histocompatibility complex; *SCID*, severe combined immunodeficiency; *TG*, thyroglobulin; *TPO*, thyroid peroxidase; *TSHR*, thyroid-stimulating hormone receptor.

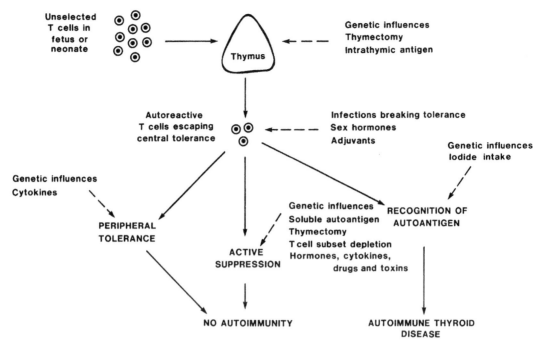

FIGURE 8-6. Control of autoreactive T cells in experimental autoimmune thyroiditis in mice. The sites at which genetic and other factors act are shown as *dashed lines;* the development of autoimmune thyroid disease depends on the balance between these multiple influences. (From Weetman AP, McGregor AM: Autoimmune thyroid disease: further developments in our understanding. Endocr Rev 15:788–830. © 1994, The Endocrine Society.)

strains of rats.[30] Similar to humans, female animals generally have more severe EAT than males do; this difference is dependent on sex hormones; estrogen administration worsens thyroiditis, whereas testosterone has the opposite effect.[38]

In all models, the role of T cells is paramount, as is illustrated by the effects of T cell manipulation on disease induction (see Table 8-4), and disease is transferred only poorly, if at all, by thyroid antibodies.[39] In general, transfer of both CD4+ and CD8+ autoreactive T cells from a donor with EAT is needed to induce EAT in a recipient. A key role for T regulatory cells in preventing EAT has been obvious for decades based on cell transfer experiments.[30] It is now established that naturally occurring CD4+, CD25+ T cells have a partial role in this regard, and additional contributions from antigen-activated T regulatory cells may occur.[40] Additional layers of regulation, including cytokine profiles, are likely to be involved, and it is clear from the multiple models of Graves' disease that a paradigm of TH1/Th2 balance is too simplistic to explain the type of autoimmune response involved.[41]

No correlation has been found between the level of TG antibodies and the severity of EAT,[30] further demonstrating the uncertain pathologic role for these autoantibodies in EAT. Indeed, in transgenic mice, it has been shown that tolerance is not induced in B cells by membrane-bound antigen expressed on thyroid cells, presumably because the preimmune B cells are sequestered from the antigen by basement membrane and endothelium.[42] Because tolerance is induced in T cells in this model, it appears that somehow thyroid surface antigens can affect the development of these cells, either by transport to the thymus or by some type of peripheral tolerance. This observation is important and implies that thyroid autoreactive B cells are frequent but remain ignorant; the frequent appearance of thyroid autoantibodies in otherwise healthy populations could be explained by the activation of these B cells if T cell tolerance breaks down or is bypassed.

Thyroid Autoantigens

THYROGLOBULIN

TG is a 660 kDa glycoprotein that is composed of two identical subunits and is secreted by thyroid follicular cells into the follicular lumen, where it is stored as colloid. Each TG molecule consists of around 100 tyrosine residues, a quarter of which are iodinated; at four to eight so-called hormonogenic sites, these residues couple to form the thyroid hormones triiodothyronine (T_3) and thyroxine (T_4). The sequence of human TG has been determined.[43] Despite considerable work, the exact location of T and B cell epitopes within TG is still uncertain, even in EAT, in which it is possible to immunize animals with defined peptides.[44] A key T cell epitope in the spontaneous thyroiditis of OS chickens contains iodine, and poorly iodinated TG is only weakly immunogenic.[35]

It has long been recognized that each 330 kDa TG subunit has two major B cell epitopes and a minor epitope.[45] However, as the titer of TG antibodies rises in Hashimoto's thyroiditis over time, other regions of the molecule become targets for autoantibodies—a process that is reflected in mice that are immunized with human TG, in which an array of epitopes subsequently develop.[46] The two major B cell epitopes on TG are conformational,[47] although linear epitopes have been identified that react with a small proportion of Hashimoto sera.[48]

THYROID PEROXIDASE

TPO, an apical 100 to 105 kDa protein that is responsible for tyrosine iodination and coupling, is the key enzyme in thyroid hormone synthesis. Many studies have confirmed the identity of the previously defined thyroid microsomal antigen as TPO.[49] Multiple T cell epitopes exist within the molecule, and individual patients respond to different sets of epitopes with no obvious clinical correlations.[50,51]

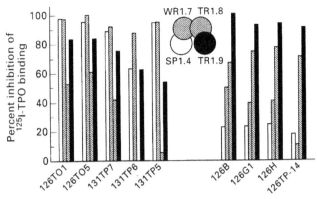

FIGURE 8-7. Epitopic domains on thyroid peroxidase (TPO). Domains A1, A2, B1, and B2 have been defined by the recombinant monoclonal TPO antibodies SP1.4, WR1.7, TR1.8, and TR1.9, respectively *(center of diagram)*, and the bars represent the inhibition of binding of these four monoclonal reagents *(shading of bars corresponds to the shading of the domains)* by a separate panel of TPO monoclonal antibodies. Those that bind predominantly to domain A are shown on the left, and those that bind predominantly to domain B are shown on the right. (From Guo J, McIntosh RS, Czarnocka B, et al: Relationship between autoantibody epitopic recognition and immunoglobulin gene usage. Clin Exp Immunol 111:408–414, 1998.)

It is also apparent that multiple B cell epitopes are present, some conformational and some linear, because TPO antibodies can recognize native, denatured, or denatured and reduced antigen.[52] As has been reviewed extensively elsewhere,[53] studies using human and murine monoclonal TPO antibodies have defined two neighboring major domains—A and B—that constitute the antibody reactivity of more than 80% of Hashimoto sera (Fig. 8-7). Some sera bind to epitopes overlapping the two domains. It is striking that the antibody response to TPO is restricted at the level of the germline heavy and light chain variable (V) regions.[53,54] Cocrystallization of TPO with monoclonal TPO antibody fragments is required for further elucidation of the epitopes within the main domains of this autoantigen.

THYROID-STIMULATING HORMONE RECEPTOR

TSHR is a member of the G protein–coupled receptor family; activation of TSHR by TSH or that subset of TSHR antibodies with stimulatory activity leads to intracellular signaling by the cyclic adenosine monophosphate (cAMP) pathway, although other signaling pathways operate at high ligand concentrations. TSHR has an extracellular domain, the A subunit, which is linked via a C peptide region to the B subunit, which comprises the transmembrane domain (organized in seven loops) and an intracellular domain.[55] Variants of TSHR have been described, in particular a form that does not include the transmembrane region and in which shed A subunits may induce or amplify the immune response to the receptor in Graves' disease.[56] The extrathyroidal expression of TSHR, particularly in the orbit, where it could serve as a cross-reactive autoantigen, may be crucial to the complications of Graves' disease.[57]

As with TPO, multiple T cell epitopes, including TSHR sequences that are recognized by 10% to 20% of healthy individuals, have been defined.[58,59] B cell epitopes are generally conformational, and it is clear that the response is heterogeneous both within and between patients because some antibodies can stimulate via the receptor in several ways, and other TSHR antibodies bind to the receptor without stimulating it, with a proportion of these antibodies interfering with TSH-mediated stimulation (Table 8-5).[60] Further characterization of these B cell epitopes has required the development of human TSHR monoclonal antibodies—a daunting task given the low frequency of TSHR antibody–secreting B cells and the difficulty of expressing the receptor in vitro in its native form.[61] Such reagents have shown far greater similarity of binding sites for blocking and stimulatory antibodies than had previously been suspected, and it is likely that these antibodies, together with TSH, bind to similar regions in the leucine-rich horseshoe portion of the TSHR ectodomain.[41,60]

OTHER AUTOANTIGENS

Cloning and sequencing of the Na^+/I^- symporter (NIS) have allowed confirmation of NIS as a fourth major thyroid autoantigen, first demonstrated with the use of cultured dog thyroid cells.[62] Up to a third of Graves' disease sera and 15% of Hashimoto sera contain antibodies that inhibit NIS-mediated iodide uptake in vitro.[63] Antibodies to thyroid hormones can be found in 10% to 25% of patients with autoimmune thyroid disease,[64] and nonspecific autoantibodies against DNA, tubulin, and other cytoskeletal proteins can be detected in a small proportion of patients.

Genetic Factors

The role of heredity in autoimmune thyroid disease has been illustrated by numerous studies showing a higher frequency of autoimmune thyroid disease or thyroid antibodies in family members of patients with autoimmune hypothyroidism and Graves' disease.[30] That both types of thyroid disease cluster together in families provides additional support for the notion that these conditions share causative and pathogenic features. A number of patterns of inheritance and candidate genes have been suggested, but ascertainment artifacts and the drawbacks of genetic association studies have produced many inconsistencies in results. Meticulous twin studies have shown a concordance rate of only 22% for Graves' disease—much lower than was previously thought.[65]

The most important susceptibility factor that has thus far been recognized is the association with particular HLA-DR alleles; the role that these MHC class II genes play in the immune response makes them excellent candidates.[66] HLA-DR3 is associated with Graves' disease and Hashimoto's thyroiditis in whites and gives a relative risk of between 2 and 6, whereas HLA-DR4

Table 8-5. Classification of Main Thyroid-Stimulating Hormone Receptor Antibodies

Antibody	Assay
TSAbs	Bioassay; usually measurement of cAMP production by primary cultures of thyroid cells, thyroid cell lines, (e.g., FRTL-5), or cells transfected with TSHR
Thyroid-blocking antibodies	Bioassay; measurement of inhibition of cAMP production after TSH-mediated stimulation of the TSHR; may operate at the level of TSH binding or receptor signaling
TSH binding-inhibiting immunoglobulins	Measurement of inhibition of radiolabeled TSH binding to TSHR by antibodies; unable to define functional activity
Long-acting thyroid stimulator	Original description of TSAb; used bioassay in whole mouse to assess effects of stimulator antibodies on radioiodine release

cAMP, Cyclic adenosine monophosphate; *FRTL-5,* Fischel rat thyroid line; *TSAb,* thyroid-stimulating antibodies; *TSH,* thyroid-stimulating hormone; *TSHR,* thyroid-stimulating hormone receptor.

and HLA-DR5 have been associated with goitrous but not atrophic thyroiditis in some white populations.[67] Postpartum thyroiditis has only a weak association with HLA-DR5. It should be noted that nonwhite populations have very different HLA associations.[68]

Detailed family studies have found only weak evidence of linkage between the HLA region and autoimmune thyroid disease.[69,70] These results imply the existence of other susceptibility loci. Of the candidates that have been tested, which include genes that encode immunoglobulins, TCR, and various cytokines, the most robust association has been seen with two linked polymorphisms of the CTLA-4 gene, which exists in both Graves' disease and autoimmune hypothyroidism and confers a relative risk of around 2.[67,68] The same polymorphism confers susceptibility for type 1 diabetes mellitus and therefore presumably reflects some generalized effect of a common functional variant of the CTLA-4 gene on autoreactive T cell regulation. A number of studies have employed genome-wide scans to identify new susceptibility genes, but their results indicate that no genes exert a major effect and, conversely, no upper limit is placed on the number of genes that have a small effect.[68a] The candidate gene approach has established that polymorphisms in PTPN22 and the IL-2 receptor (CD25), both integrally involved in T cell regulation, contribute to susceptibility, and a contribution to the Fc receptor–like-3 locus is likely.[69-72] The TSHR has been confirmed as a susceptiblity locus for Graves' disease but not Hashimoto's thyroiditis.[73]

Environmental Factors

Work in EAT has identified several environmental influences on thyroiditis (see earlier), and epidemiologic evidence supports a role for some of these environmental factors in humans; only these factors can explain the rapid changes in the prevalence of Hashimoto's thyroiditis recently described in Italy.[74] An excess of thyroid autoantibodies and thyroiditis occurs after iodination programs[75]; as in EAT, iodine might increase the immunogenicity of thyroid autoantigens or may have a role in the generation of toxic metabolites. Radioiodine given therapeutically can rarely induce autoimmune responses in patients with nodular goiters.[76] The mechanism is obscure but could relate to the release of thyroid autoantigens (possibly altered by radiation damage and therefore more immunogenic) or to the effect of ^{131}I on radiation-sensitive regulatory T cell subsets. Occupational exposure to ionizing radiation also may be a risk factor.[77]

No convincing evidence has indicated a role for infection in autoimmune hypothyroidism, except for the high frequency of this condition in patients with congenital rubella syndrome; however, an association has been proposed between *Yersinia* infection and Graves' disease, and *Yersinia* contains proteins that mimic TSHR immunologically.[78] The relative importance of this association has not been established but seems low, given the relative frequencies of Graves' disease and *Yersinia* infection. Autoimmune thyroid disease occurs only rarely, if at all, after subacute thyroiditis.[79] Epidemiologic studies suggest that inferior levels of prosperity and hygiene may actually protect against the development of thyroid autoimmunity.[80]

A number of retrospective surveys have identified stress during the year before the initial evaluation as an important risk factor for Graves' disease, but these surveys suffer from potential flaws in their dependence on recall and other sources of bias.[81] Any such effect presumably results from the neuroendocrine responses to stress that alter the regulation of autoreactive lymphocytes. Attacks of allergic rhinitis are associated with increased risk for relapse in those with Graves' disease, most likely because of the Th2-dominant effects of cytokines produced during the attack.[82] Exogenous cytokines given therapeutically, particularly interferon-alpha (IFN-α), exacerbate preexisting thyroid and other types of autoimmunity and lead to the development of autoimmune hypothyroidism in predisposed individuals.[83] Other immunologically active agents can cause Graves' disease, particularly during the recovery phase after administration of lymphocyte-depleting monoclonal antibodies given to patients with multiple sclerosis,[84] possibly by deviating the immune response to a Th2-predominant phase. The roles of toxins and pollutants remain underexplored, although the adverse effects of smoking on Graves' disease and ophthalmopathy provide a clear example that these factors could be important.[85]

T Cell–Mediated Responses

Many studies have been performed to characterize the circulating T cell population in autoimmune thyroid disease, but because the functional consequences of alterations in T cell phenotype are still not clear, particularly within this lymphocyte compartment, the meaning of any changes is open to debate. Although complete consensus has not been achieved, it seems that CD8+ T cell numbers are decreased in active Hashimoto's thyroiditis and in Graves' disease, with an increase in activated T cells expressing markers such as HLA-DR.[86] Both CD4+ and CD8+ T cells occur in the thyroid lymphocytic infiltrate, with a preponderance of activated CD4+ cells.[87,88]

Attention has focused on possible clonal restriction of intrathyroidal T cells, as shown by limited usage of the V gene families encoding the α chain of the TCR.[89] Although this concept seems plausible in the earliest stages of an autoimmune response, by the time that disease is recognizable clinically, multiple antigens and epitopes are responsible for T cell autoreactivity (so-called spreading of the immune response), and such restriction therefore would not be expected; little evidence of TCR restriction is apparent when IL-2 receptor–positive (and hence recently activated) intrathyroidal T cells in Graves' disease are analyzed.[90] However, restricted V gene usage by CD8+ T cells seen in Hashimoto's thyroiditis could reflect clonal expansion of cytotoxic populations.[91] Certainly, cytotoxic T cells have been cloned from this population.[92] These cells have the $\alpha\beta$ TCR, but a second cytotoxic population with $\gamma\delta$ TCRs has also been identified in Graves' disease; the nature of the thyroid surface autoantigen and the mode of its presentation to these T cells are unknown.[93]

A wide array of cytokines, including IL-2, IFN-γ, tumor necrosis factor-alpha (TNF-α), IL-4, IL-6, IL-10, IL-12, IL-13, and IL-15, are produced by the lymphocytic infiltrate in autoimmune thyroid disease, with some variations noted between patients and yet no predominance of a Th1 or Th2 response.[94] Once again, this situation could reflect the late stage of disease and the mixed cell populations that have been analyzed in such studies. Ideally, one would wish to examine only thyroid autoantigen–specific CD4+ T cells to determine the pattern of helper T cell cytokine production, but establishing such clones has been difficult, and the very process of expanding these cells in vitro might well distort their behavior. Weak in vitro responses to TG, TPO, and TSHR, used as whole antigen or as putative peptide epitopes, have been detected in circulating and intrathyroidal T cell populations in assays of proliferation, secretion of migration inhibition factor, or B cell helper activity as readouts.[30,50,51,58,59] Attempts to define thyroid antigen–specific suppressor T cells with such systems have also been made, but the suppressor cell defects that such assays have suggested in autoimmune thyroid disease[95] have been disputed on grounds of specificity and the nonphysiologic nature of the assay systems.[96]

B Cell Responses

TG and TPO antibodies occur, often in very high concentrations, in patients with Hashimoto's thyroiditis and primary myxedema (Fig. 8-8); in patients without circulating antibodies, they can be detected by culture of intrathyroidal lymphocytes.[97] These antibodies are less common but still frequent in Graves' disease, whereas TPO rather than TG antibodies are frequent in postpartum thyroiditis.[6] Both antibodies show partial restriction to the IgG1 and IgG4 subclass and κ light chain restriction of TPO antibodies.[53,98] The pathogenic role of TG antibodies is unclear because the epitopes on the antigen are too widely spaced to allow bound autoantigen to cross-link and thus fix complement, but these antibodies can mediate ADCC, at least in vitro.[98] In contrast, TPO antibodies do fix complement, and immunohistochemical evidence has established the formation of terminal complement complexes within the thyroid in autoimmune thyroid disease.[99] Because TPO is located at the apical surface and within the thyroid cell cytoplasm, it seems that under normal circumstances, TPO antibodies do not gain access to their autoantigen, which accounts for the euthyroidism seen in healthy individuals with TPO antibodies and in neonates born to mothers with high levels of TPO antibodies. Cell-mediated injury may be necessary for TPO antibodies to gain access to their antigen and become pathogenic. For instance, cytokines such as IL-1α could induce dissociation of the junctional complexes between thyroid cells within a follicle (see Fig. 8-8).[100]

Thyroid-stimulating antibodies (TSAbs) directed against the TSHR are the hallmark of Graves' disease, and the best antibody assays currently have a sensitivity of up to 99%. These antibodies are often κ chain restricted and of the IgG1 subclass,[101,102] which suggests origin from a small number of B cell clones. It is now established that TSAbs also occur in a small proportion of patients with autoimmune hypothyroidism, but their effects are obscured by TSHR-blocking antibodies and destructive processes.[103] In some patients, fluctuation in the relative proportion of the two types of TSHR antibody may produce a confusing clinical picture of alternating hyperthyroidism and hypothyroidism, and such fluctuation also may occur after pregnancy.[104] Blocking antibodies have been found in 10% to 20% of patients with autoimmune hypothyroidism, and in Asian populations, they seem to be most closely associated with atrophic rather than goitrous thyroiditis.[105] In whites, however, they appear in Hashimoto's thyroiditis as well, and in such patients, the goiter is most likely to be the result of lymphocytic infiltration.[106] The existence of separate populations of growth-stimulating and growth-inhibiting immunoglobulins, operating independently of the TSHR, remains disputed.[107,108] In Graves' disease at least, it is TSAbs that mediate goitrogenesis.

Pathogenic Mechanisms

Graves' disease clearly results from the action of TSAbs, primarily via the cAMP pathway, although other signaling pathways may be used by TSHR antibodies in some patients, which suggests a subdivision based on the effector function of these antibodies.[109] TSAbs also increase the vascularity of the Graves' thyroid by enhancing local expression of vascular endothelial growth factor and its receptor.[110] In around 15% of patients with Graves' disease who are treated with antithyroid drugs, hypothyroidism supervenes years later, thus indicating that similar destructive mechanisms operate in Graves' disease and autoimmune hypo-

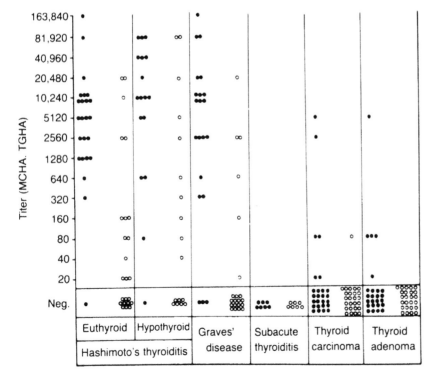

FIGURE 8-8. Titers of microsomal/thyroid peroxidase (TPO) hemagglutination antibodies (MCHAs), shown as *solid circles*, and thyroglobulin hemagglutination antibodies (TGHAs) in various thyroid diseases. (From Amino N, Hagan SR, Yamada N, Refetoff S: Measurement of circulating thyroid microsomal antibodies by the tanned red cell haemagglutination technique: its usefulness in the diagnosis of autoimmune thyroid disease. Clin Endocrinol 5:115–126, 1976.)

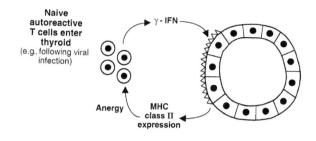

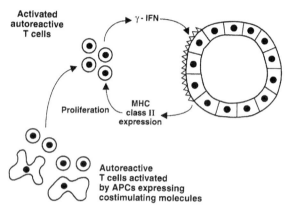

FIGURE 8-9. Alternative outcomes after major histocompatibility complex (MHC) class II expression by thyroid cells. Naïve T cells require costimulation for activation, and anergy can be induced by interaction with the MHC class II molecule/antigenic epitope alone (*upper panel*, peripheral tolerance). If T cells receive costimulation from classic antigen-presenting cells (APCs), class II expression by thyroid cells can enhance the T cell response (*lower panel*).

thyroidism. These shared pathogenic mechanisms are detailed after consideration of the role of thyroid follicular cells as APCs.

The discovery that thyroid cells express MHC class II molecules in autoimmune thyroid disease, but not under normal circumstances, led to the suggestion that such expression could permit thyroid autoantigen presentation, which in turn could initiate or exacerbate disease.[111] It is now clear that thyroid cells generally express class II molecules only after stimulation with IFN-γ, which implies that a T cell infiltrate must precede such expression, so class II expression is a secondary event and transgenic expression of class II molecules on thyroid cells in mice alone does not induce EAT.[112] Furthermore, thyroid cells do not express B7-1 or B7-2 costimulatory molecules and therefore can act as APCs only for T cells that no longer require such costimulation, in general those that have been activated previously. In vitro experiments confirm that thyroid cells can act as APCs under such circumstances, but they also are able to induce anergy in naïve T cells that require costimulation[113] (see Fig. 8-3). Teleologically, MHC class II expression is likely to be an important means of ensuring peripheral T cell tolerance under normal circumstances, but such expression is damaging under conditions of thyroid autoimmunity (Fig. 8-9). Class II expression is more readily induced by IFN-γ in Graves' thyroid cells than in those from multinodular goiter, thus suggesting a genetically regulated component to this response.[114]

Cytokines have a large number of other effects on thyroid cells that might be of pathogenic relevance. As well as adversely affecting thyroid growth and function, a number of immunologically important molecules are expressed by thyroid cells in response to cytokines that are known to be produced locally by the infiltrating leukocytes in Graves' disease and autoimmune hypothyroidism[94] (Fig. 8-10). Expression of ICAM-1, LFA-3, CD40, and MHC class I molecules is enhanced by IL-1, TNF, and IFN-γ, and this response increases the ability of cytotoxic T cells to mediate lysis.[94] A complex series of interactions, including secretion of chemokines, is important in allowing lymphocytes to enter the thyroid and in some cases to develop tertiary lymphoid structures within the gland.[115] Thyroid cell destruction is mediated both by perforin-containing T cells, which accumulate in the thyroid,[116] and by Fas-dependent mechanisms.[117] A unique type of suicide has been suggested by reports that IL-1β–stimulated thyroid cells in Hashimoto's thyroiditis express FasL, which could lead to self-ligation with Fas and thus cell death,[117] but these findings have not been reproduced consistently, and the final outcome of Fas ligation depends on a complex regulatory pathway that might also involve the death ligand TRAIL.[118] Cytokines and other toxic molecules such as nitric oxide and reactive oxygen metabolites probably also contribute directly to cell-mediated tissue injury.

Humoral immunity most likely exacerbates cell-mediated damage in a secondary fashion, both by direct complement fixation (for TPO antibodies) and by ADCC.[98,119] These effects occur in addition to the inhibitory effects of TSHR-blocking antibodies on thyroid cell function. Thyroid cells increase their expression of a number of regulatory proteins (CD46, CD55, CD59) in response to cytokines, and these proteins prevent cell death in the face of widespread complement damage in autoimmune thyroid disease.[87,120] Nonetheless, a sublethal complement attack, initiated via the classic or alternative pathway, impairs the metabolic function of thyroid cells and induces them to secrete IL-1, IL-6, reactive oxygen metabolites, and prostaglandins, all of which could enhance the autoimmune response.[121] As well as T and B cells, dendritic cells and monocytes/macrophages accumulate in the thyroid, where they presumably play a major role as APCs that are capable of providing costimulatory signals. Besides acting as APCs, these cells are important sources of cytokines, as shown by the inhibition of thyroid cell growth by IL-1 and IL-6 derived from dendritic cells.[122] An additional group of inflammatory cells, namely, NK-like T cells, has been identified in the thyroid infiltrate, in turn suggesting a role for lipid-containing molecules in thyroid autoimmunity.[123]

Natural History and Response to Treatment

The natural history of subclinical hypothyroidism, present in many cases of focal thyroiditis, is now well established from epidemiologic surveys: The presence of thyroid autoantibodies in addition to this biochemical picture confers a considerable future risk for permanent hypothyroidism—much greater than the presence of autoantibodies alone.[124] Around a quarter of patients with postpartum thyroiditis progress to permanent hypothyroidism,[6] but as in the case of subclinical hypothyroidism, it is unclear which factors predispose to this outcome. One speculation is that maternal microchimerism, caused by the transfer of fetal cells bearing paternal antigens at delivery, leads to the enhancement of any ongoing autoimmune response, and the most severe disease therefore would accompany the greatest cell transfer. Certainly, evidence for intrathyroidal fetal microchimerism in autoimmune thyroid disease is growing.[125] Hormonal disturbances during and after pregnancy also may be involved in these changes, as postpartum thyroiditis has been associated with low cortisol levels in the last trimester.[126]

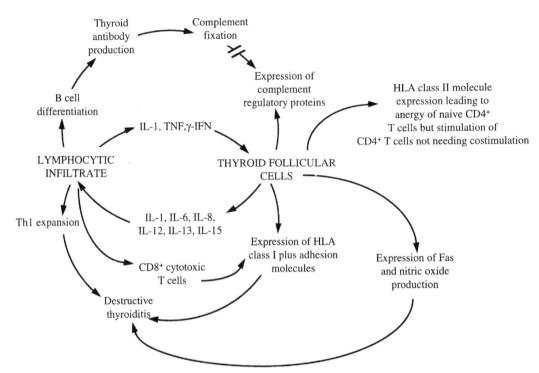

FIGURE 8-10. Interaction between thyroid cells and the immune system via cytokines. Expression of complement regulatory proteins in response to interleukin-1 (IL-1), tumor necrosis factor (TNF), and interferon-γ (IFN-γ) will protect against complement-mediated injury, and class II expression may induce T cell anergy under appropriate conditions; the other cytokine-induced events will amplify the autoimmune process. (From Weetman AP, Ajjan RA, Watson PF: Cytokines and Graves' disease. Baillieres Clin Endocrinol Metab 11:481–497, 1997.)

Spontaneous resolution of Graves' disease and autoimmune hypothyroidism does occur but seems unusual, and thus far, no prospective study has fully established whether any remission is permanent rather than temporary. However, patients with autoimmune hypothyroidism and TSHR-blocking antibodies seem particularly likely to enter remission after T_4 treatment, although no consensus has been reached on whether this remission is associated with decreases in antibody levels.[105,127] Intermittent exposure to a crucial environmental agent could explain some remissions, and it is noteworthy that many animal models of EAT spontaneously remit. One potential factor that has recently been tried therapeutically is selenium: supplementation with this trace element appears to lower TPO antibody levels.[128]

Treatment with antithyroid drugs (carbimazole, methimazole, and propylthiouracil) for Graves' disease leads to a decline in TSAbs and other thyroid antibodies and a decline in the severity of thyroiditis, as well as other immunologic changes (Table 8-6). This may occur because antithyroid drugs inhibit the release of proinflammatory molecules by thyroid cells, which would explain both the altered immune response during treatment and its thyroid specificity.[121]

Radioiodine therapy is followed after 3 to 6 months by a striking rise in thyroid autoantibodies, and the possibility of differential effects on TSAbs and TSHR-blocking antibodies could explain transient thyroid dysfunction at this time. Thyroid-associated ophthalmopathy may worsen transiently after radioiodine treatment in some patients.[129] Both events may be related to the release of thyroid autoantigens or radiation effects on T cell subpopulations, inasmuch as activated T cells increase in the circulation weeks after ^{131}I administration.[130]

Undoubtedly, improved understanding of the immunologic basis of Graves' disease ultimately will lead to immunologically based treatment aimed at reinducing tolerance to TSHR. Pilot

Table 8-6. Immunologic Effects of Antithyroid Drugs

In Vivo

Reduction in levels of TSHR, TG, and TPO antibodies but not nonthyroid autoantibodies

Reduction in thyroid lymphocytic infiltration in Graves' disease and experimental/spontaneous autoimmune thyroiditis in animals

Reversal of thymic hyperplasia

Restoration of elevated circulating levels of activated and CD69+ T cells and increased CD4/CD8 ratio

Reduction in circulating levels of soluble markers of immune response (terminal complement complexes, CD8, ICAM-1)

In Vitro

Suppression of immunoglobulin synthesis

Oxygen metabolite scavenger

Enhanced IL-2 production and T-cell proliferation

Suppression of IL-1, IL-6, and prostaglandin synthesis by thyroid cells

Variable effects on thyroid cell surface expression of MHC molecules

ICAM-1, Intercellular adhesion molecule-1; *IL*, interleukin; *MHC*, major histocompatibility complex; *TG*, thyroglobulin; *TPO*, thyroid peroxidase; *TSHR*, thyroid-stimulating hormone receptor.

studies have been performed to assess the potential for oral tolerance with the use of TG,[131] and it is possible that any such treatment might have benefit for ophthalmopathy as well. On the other hand, T_4 is such a simple treatment for autoimmune hypothyroidism that, at present, novel treatments are most unlikely.

Relation to Other Diseases

Thyroiditis and thyroid antibodies are found in a quarter to a third of patients with thyroid cancer, and such patients have an improved prognosis.[132] Preexisting Hashimoto's thyroiditis is the major risk factor for the development of primary thyroid lymphoma.[133] Other novel associations have been suggested by studies that show an increased frequency of autoimmune thyroiditis in women with breast cancer,[134] infertility and persistent miscarriage,[135] and depression.[136] In all these examples, the reasons for the links with thyroid autoimmunity remain unclear. Finally, autoimmune thyroid disease is associated with many other autoimmune diseases and is a well-recognized component of autoimmune polyglandular syndrome type 2, as well as a minor component of the type 1 syndrome.[137-139]

Summary

Autoimmune thyroid disease is the result of a complex interaction between genetic and environmental factors, many of which remain to be defined; it leads to failure of one or more mechanisms responsible for controlling thyroid-reactive T and B cells. Such cells are probably present, to a greater or lesser extent, in all individuals, with disease resulting only when the autoreactive lymphocytes are able to escape tolerance or ignorance. Both cell-mediated and humoral immune responses contribute to tissue injury in autoimmune hypothyroidism; in Graves' disease, production of TSAbs leads to hyperthyroidism. The thyroid cell interacts with the immune system at a number of points in the development of autoimmunity, and many of these interactions appear to exacerbate the disease process. The multistep development of disease suggests that it will be possible to restore normal tolerance and treat Graves' disease immunologically with novel agents directed at the interaction between T cells and APCs or at immunoregulatory T cell subsets.

REFERENCES

1. Rose NR, Witebsky E: Changes in the thyroid glands of rabbits following active immunization with rabbit thyroid extracts, J Immunol 76:417–427, 1956.
2. Roitt IM, Doniach D, Campbell PN, et al: Autoantibodies in Hashimoto's disease (lymphadenoid goitre), Lancet 2:820–821, 1956.
3. Adams DD: The presence of an abnormal thyroid-stimulating hormone in the serum of some thyrotoxic patients, J Clin Endocrinol Metab 18:699–712, 1958.
4. Okayasu I, Hara Y, Nakamura K, et al: Racial and age-related differences in incidence and severity of focal autoimmune thyroiditis, Anat Pathol 101:698–702, 1993.
5. Jacobson DL, Gange SJ, Rose NR, et al: Epidemiology and estimated population burden of selected autoimmune diseases in the United States, Clin Immunol Immunopathol 84:223–243, 1997.
6. Stagnaro-Green A: Postpartum thyroiditis, J Clin Endocrinol Metab 87:4042–4047, 2002.
7. LiVolsi VA: Pathology of thyroid disease. In Falk SA, editor: Thyroid Disease: Endocrinology, Surgery, Nuclear Medicine and Radiotherapy, New York, 1990, Raven Press, pp 127–175.
8. Mizukami Y, Michigishi T, Kawato M, et al: Thyroid function and histologic correlations in 601 cases, Hum Pathol 23:980–988, 1991.
9. Hayashi Y, Tamai H, Fukata S, et al: A long term clinical, immunological, and histological follow-up study of patients with goitrous chronic lymphocytic thyroiditis, J Clin Endocrinol Metab 61:1172–1177, 1985.
10. Weetman AP, McGregor AM, Wheeler MH, et al: Extrathyroidal sites of autoantibody synthesis in Graves' disease, Clin Exp Immunol 56:330–336, 1984.
11. Goodnow CC, Sprent J, Fazekas de St Groth B, et al: Cellular and genetic mechanisms of self tolerance and autoimmunity, Nature 435:590–597, 2005.
12. Garcia KC, Teyton L, Wilson IA: Structural basis of T cell recognition, Annu Rev Immunol 17:369–397, 1999.
13. Delves PJ, Roitt IM: The immune system, N Engl J Med 343:37–49, 2000.
14. Sansom DM, Manzotti CN, Zheng Y: What's the difference between CD80 and CD86? Trends Immunol 24:314–319, 2003.
15. Frauwirth KA, Thompson CB: Activation and inhibition of lymphocytes by costimulation, J Clin Invest 109:295–299, 2002.
16. Jiang H, Chess L: Regulation of immune responses by T cells, N Engl J Med 354:1166–1176, 2006.
17. Bettelli E, Oukka M, Kuchroo V: T$_H$-17 cells in the circle of immunity and autoimmunity, Nature Immunol 8:345–350, 2007.
18. Perussia B, Loza MJ: Linear "2-0-1" lymphocyte development: hypotheses on cellular bases for immunity, Trends Immunol 24:235–241, 2003.
19. Beverley PCL: Primer: making sense of T-cell memory, Nature 4:43–49, 2008.
20. D'Ambrosio D, Sinigaglia F, Adorini L: Special attractions for suppressor T cells, Trends Immunol 24:122–126, 2003.

21. Sakaguchi S, Yamaguchi T, Nomura T, et al: Regulatory T cells and immune tolerance, Cell 133:775–787, 2008.
22. Hirsh MI, Junger WG: Roles of heat shock proteins and gamma-delta T cells in inflammation, Am J Respir Cell Mol Biol 39:509–513, 2008.
23. Matsuda F, Honjo T: Organization of the human immunoglobulin heavy-chain locus, Adv Immunol 62:1–29, 1996.
24. Laver WG, Air GM, Webster RG, et al: Epitopes on protein antigens: misconceptions and realities, Cell 61:553–556, 1990.
25. MacKay IR, Rosen FS: Tolerance and autoimmunity, N Engl J Med 344:655–664, 2001.
26. Cheng MH, Shum AK, Anderson MS: What's new in the Aire? Trends Immunol 28:321–327, 2007.
27. Goodnow CC: Balancing immunity and tolerance: deleting and tuning lymphocyte repertoires, Proc Natl Acad Sci U S A 93:2264–2271, 1996.
28. Cone RE, Malley A: Soluble, antigen-specific T-cell proteins: T-cell-based humoral immunity? Immunol Today 17:318–322, 1996.
29. Goldschneider I, Cone RE: A central role for peripheral dendritic cells in the induction of acquired thymic tolerance, Trends Immunol 24:77–81, 2003.
30. Weetman AP, McGregor AM: Autoimmune thyroid disease: further developments in our understanding, Endocr Rev 15:788–830, 1994.
31. Ando T, Imaizumi M, Graves P, et al: Induction of thyroid-stimulating hormone receptor autoimmunity in hamsters, Endocrinology 144:671–680, 2003.
32. Schwarz-Lauer L, Pichurin PN, Chen C-R: The cysteine-rich amino terminus of the thyrotropin receptor is the immunodominant linear antibody epitope in mice immunized using naked deoxyribonucleic acid or adenovirus vectors, Endocrinology 144:1718–1725, 2003.
33. Wick G, Cole R, Dietrich H, et al: The obese strain of chickens with spontaneous thyroiditis as a model for Hashimoto disease. In Cohen IR, Miller A, editors: Autoimmune Disease Models, San Diego, CA, 1994, Academic Press, pp 107–122.
34. Kong Y-C, Lomo LC, Mott RW, et al: HLA-DRB1 polymorphism determines susceptibility to autoimmune thyroiditis in transgenic mice: definitive association with HLA-DRB1*0301 (DR3) gene, J Exp Med 184:1167–1172, 1996.
35. Barin JG, Talor MV, Sharma RB, et al: Iodination of murine thyroglobulin enhances autoimmune reactivity in the NOD.H2^{h4} mouse, Clin Exp Immunol 142:251–259, 2005.
36. Rennie DP, McGregor AM, Keast D, et al: The influence of methimazole on thyroglobulin-induced autoimmune thyroiditis in the rat, Endocrinology 112:326–330, 1983.
37. Penhale WJ, Young PR: The influence of the normal microbial flora on the susceptibility of rats to experimental autoimmune thyroiditis, Clin Exp Immunol 72:288–292, 1988.
38. Okayasu I, Kong YM, Rose NR: Effect of castration and sex hormones on experimental autoimmune

thyroiditis, Clin Immunol Immunopathol 20:240–245, 1981.
39. Quaratino S, Badami E, Pang YY, et al: Degenerate self-reactive human T-cell receptor causes spontaneous autoimmune disease in mice, Nature Med 10:920–926, 2004.
40. Yu S, Maiti PK, Dyson M, et al: B cell-deficient NOD.H-2h4 mice have CD4$^+$ CD25$^+$ T regulatory cells that inhibit the development of spontaneous autoimmune thyroiditis, J Exp Med 203:349–358, 2006.
41. McLachlan S, Nagayama Y, Rapoport B: Insight into Graves' hyperthyroidism from animal models, Endocrine Reviews 26:800–832, 2005.
42. Akkaraju S, Canaan K, Goodnow CC: Self-reactive B cells are not eliminated or inactivated by autoantigen expressed on thyroid epithelial cells, J Exp Med 186:2005–2012, 1997.
43. Malthiery Y, Lissitzky S: Primary structure of human thyroglobulin deduced from the sequence of its 8848-base complementary DNA, Eur J Biochem 105:491–498, 1987.
44. Carayanniotis G, Rao VP: Searching for pathogenic epitopes in thyroglobulin: parameters and caveats, Immunol Today 18:83–88, 1997.
45. Nye L, Pontes de Carvalho L, Roitt I: Restriction in the response to autologous thyroglobulin in the human, Clin Exp Immunol 41:252–263, 1980.
46. Bresler HS, Burek CL, Hoffman WH, et al: Autoantigenic determinants on human thyroglobulin: II. Determinants recognized by autoantibodies from patients with chronic autoimmune thyroiditis compared to autoantibodies from healthy subjects, Clin Immunol Immunopathol 54:76–86, 1990.
47. Prentice L, Kiso Y, Fukuma N, et al: Monoclonal thyroglobulin autoantibodies: variable region analysis and epitope recognition, J Clin Endocrinol Metab 80:977–986, 1995.
48. Tomer Y: Anti-thyroglobulin autoantibodies in autoimmune thyroid diseases: cross-reactive or pathogenic? Clin Immunol Immunopathol 82:3–11, 1997.
49. McLachlan SM, Rapoport B: The molecular biology of thyroid peroxidase: cloning, expression, and role as autoantigen in autoimmune thyroid disease, Endocr Rev 13:192–206, 1992.
50. Tandon N, Freeman M, Weetman AP: T cell responses to synthetic thyroid peroxidase peptides in autoimmune thyroid disease, Clin Exp Immunol 86:56–60, 1991.
51. Fisfalen M-E, Soliman M, Okamoto Y, et al: Proliferative responses of T cells to thyroid antigens and synthetic thyroid peroxidase peptides in autoimmune thyroid disease, J Clin Endocrinol Metab 80:1597–1604, 1995.
52. Hamada N, Jaeduck N, Portman L, et al: Antibodies against denatured and reduced thyroid microsomal antigen in autoimmune thyroid disease, J Clin Endocrinol Metab 64:230–238, 1987.
53. McIntosh R, Watson P, Weetman A: Somatic hypermutation in autoimmune thyroid disease, Immunol Rev 162:219–231, 1998.

54. Chazenbalk GD, Portolano S, Russo D, et al: Human organ-specific autoimmune disease. Molecular cloning and expression of an autoantibody gene repertoire for a major autoantigen reveals an antigenic immunodominant region and restricted immunoglobulin gene usage in the target organ, J Clin Invest 92:62–74, 1993.
55. Vassart G, Dumont JE: The thyrotropin receptor and the regulation of thyrocyte function and growth, Endocr Rev 13:596–611, 1992.
56. Chen C-R, Pichurin P, Nagayama Y, et al: The thyrotropin receptor autoantigen in Graves disease is the culprit as well as the victim, J Clin Invest 111:1897–1904, 2003.
57. Bahn RS, Dutton CM, Natt N, et al: Thyrotropin receptor expression in Graves' orbital adipose/connective tissues: potential autoantigen in Graves' ophthalmopathy, J Clin Endocrinol Metab 83:998–1002, 1998.
58. Tandon N, Freeman MA, Weetman AP: T cell responses to synthetic TSH receptor peptides in Graves' disease, Clin Exp Immunol 89:468–473, 1992.
59. Martin A, Nakashima M, Zhou A, et al: Detection of major T cell epitopes on human thyroid stimulating hormone receptor by overriding immune heterogeneity in patients with Graves' disease, J Clin Endocrinol Metab 82:3361–3366, 1997.
60. Schott M, Scherbaum WA, Morgenthaler NG: Thyrotropin receptor autoantibodies in Graves' disease, Trends Endocrinol Metab 16:243–248, 2005.
61. Sanders J, Evans M, Premawardhana LDKE, et al: Human monoclonal thyroid stimulating autoantibody, Lancet 362:126–128, 2003.
62. Raspe E, Costagliola S, Ruf J, et al: Identification of the thyroid Na^+/I^- symporter in the sera of patients with autoimmune thyroid disease, Biochem Biophys Res Commun 224:399–405, 1996.
63. Ajjan RA, Findlay C, Metcalfe RA, et al: The modulation of the human sodium iodide symporter activity by Graves' disease sera, J Clin Endocrinol Metab 83:1217–1221, 1998.
64. Benvenga S, Trimarchi F, Robbins J: Circulating thyroid hormone autoantibodies, J Endocrinol Invest 10:605–610, 1987.
65. Brix TH, Kyvik KO, Hegedüs L: What is the evidence of genetic factors in the etiology of Graves' disease? A brief review, Thyroid 8:627–635, 1998.
66. Zeitlin AA, Simmonds MJ, Gough SCL: Genetic developments in autoimmune thyroid disease: an evolutionary process, Clin Endocrinol 68:671–682, 2008.
67. Yanagawa T, Hidaka Y, Guimaraes V, et al: CTLA-4 gene polymorphism associated with Graves' disease in Caucasian population, J Clin Endocrinol Metab 80:41–45, 1995.
68. Kavvoura FK, Akamizu T, Awata T, et al: Cytotoxic T-lymphocyte associated antigen 4 gene polymorphisms and autoimmune thyroid disease: a meta-analysis, J Clin Endocrinol Metab 92:3162–3170, 2007.
68a. Taylor JC, Gough SC, Hunt PJ, et al: A genome-wide screen in 1119 relative pairs with autoimmune thyroid disease, J Clin Endocrinol Metab 91:646–653, 2006.
69. Velaga MR, Wilson V, Jennings CE, et al: The codon 620 tryptophan allele of the lymphoid tyrosine phosphatase (LYP) gene is a major determinant of Graves' disease, J Clin Endocrinol Metab 89:5862–5865, 2004.
70. Brand OJ, Lowe CE, Franklyn JA, et al: Association of the interleukin-2 receptor alpha (IL-2Ralpha)/CD25 gene region with Graves' disease using a multilocus test and tag SNPs, Clin Endocrinol 66:508–512, 2007.
71. Kochi Y, Yamada R, Suzuki A, et al: A functional variant in FCRL3, encoding Fc receptor-like 3, is associated with rheumatoid arthritis and several autoimmunities, Nature Genetics 37:478–485, 2005.
72. Simmonds MJ, Heward JM, Carr-Smith J, et al: Contribution of single nucleotide polymorphisms within FRCL3 and MAP3K7IP2 to the pathogenesis of Graves' disease, J Clin Endocrinol Metab 91:1056–1061, 2005.
73. Dechairo BM, Zabaneh D, Collins J, et al: Association of the TSHR gene with Graves' disease: the first disease specific locus, Eur J Human Genetics 13:1223–1230, 2005.
74. Benvenga S, Trimarchi F: Changed presentation of Hashimoto's thyroiditis in north-eastern Sicily and Calabria (Southern Italy) based on a 31 year experience, Thyroid 18:429–441, 2008.
75. Papanastiou L, Alebizaki M, Piperingos G, et al: The effect of iodine administration on the development of thyroid autoimmunity in patients with non-toxic goiter, Thyroid 10:493–496, 2000.
76. Huysmans DAKC, Hermus ADRMM, Edelbroek MAL, et al: Autoimmune hyperthyroidism occurring late after radioiodine treatment for volume reduction of large multinodular goiters, Thyroid 7:535–538, 1997.
77. Völzke H, Werner A, Wallaschofski H, et al: Occupational exposure to ionizing radiation is associated with autoimmune thyroid disease, J Clin Endocrinol Metab 90:4587–4592, 2005.
78. Tomer Y, Davies TF: Infection, thyroid disease, and autoimmunity, Endocr Rev 14:107–120, 1993.
79. Bartalena L, Bogazzi F, Percori F, et al: Graves' disease occurring after subacute thyroiditis: report of a case and review of the literature, Thyroid 6:345–348, 1996.
80. Kondrashova A, Viskari H, Haapla A-M, et al: Serological evidence of thyroid autoimmunity among schoolchildren in two different socioeconomic environments, J Clin Endocrinol Metab 93:729–734, 2008.
81. Chiovato L, Pinchera A: Stressful life events and Graves' disease, Eur J Endocrinol 134:680–682, 1996.
82. Sato A, Takemura Y, Yamada T, et al: A possible role of immunoglobulin E in patients with hyperthyroid Graves' disease, J Clin Endocrinol Metab 84:3602–3605, 1999.
83. Carella C, Mazziotti G, Amato G, et al: Interferon-α related thyroid disease: pathophysiological, epidemiological and clinical aspects, J Clin Endocrinol Metab 88:3656–3661, 2004.
84. Coles A, Wing M, Smith S, et al: Pulsed monoclonal antibody treatment and autoimmune thyroid disease in multiple sclerosis, Lancet 354:1691–1695, 1999.
85. Krassas GE, Wiersinga W: Smoking and autoimmune thyroid disease: the plot thickens, Eur J Endocrinol 154:777–780, 2006.
86. Iwatani Y, Amino N, Hidaka Y, et al: Decreases in $\alpha\beta$ T cell receptor negative T cells and $CD8^+$ cells, and an increase in $CD4^+$, $CD8^+$ cells in active Hashimoto's disease and subacute thyroiditis, Clin Exp Immunol 87:444–449, 1992.
87. Aichinger G, Fill H, Wick G: In situ immune complexes, lymphocyte subpopulations, and HLA-DR positive epithelial cells in Hashimoto's thyroiditis, Lab Invest 52:132–140, 1985.
88. Ueki YM, Eguchi K, Otsubo T, et al: Phenotypic analysis of concanavalin-A-induced suppressor cell dysfunction of thyroidal lymphocytes from patients with Graves' disease, J Clin Endocrinol Metab 67:1018–1024, 1988.
89. Davies TF, Martin A, Concepcion ES, et al: Evidence for selective accumulation of intrathyroidal T lymphocytes in human autoimmune thyroid disease based on T cell receptor V gene usage, J Clin Invest 89:157–162, 1992.
90. McIntosh RS, Tandon N, Pickerill AP, et al: IL-2 receptor positive intrathyroidal lymphocytes in Graves' disease: analysis of Vα transcript microheterogeneity, J Immunol 91:3884–3893, 1993.
91. McIntosh RS, Watson PF, Weetman AP: Analysis of T cell receptor Vα repertoire in Hashimoto's thyroiditis: evidence for the restricted accumulation of $CD8^+$ T cells in the absence of $CD4^+$ T cell restriction, J Clin Endocrinol Metab 82:1140–1146, 1997.
92. MacKenzie WA, Davies TF: An intrathyroidal T-cell clone specifically cytotoxic for human thyroid cells, Immunology 61:101–103, 1987.
93. Catalfamo M, Roura-Mir C, Sospedra M, et al: Self-reactive cytotoxic $\gamma\delta$ T lymphocytes in Graves' disease specifically recognize thyroid epithelial cells, J Immunol 156:804–811, 1996.
94. Ajjan RA, Watson PF, Weetman AP: Cytokines in Graves' disease. In Rapoport B, McLachlan SM, editors: Graves' Disease: Pathogenesis and Treatment, Norwell, MA, 2000, Kluwer Academic Publishers, p 79.
95. Volpe R: Immunoregulation in autoimmune thyroid disease, Thyroid 4:373–377, 1994.
96. Martin A, Davies TF: T cells in human autoimmune thyroid disease: emerging data shows lack of need to invoke suppressor T cell problems, Thyroid 2:247–261, 1992.
97. Baker JR, Saunders NB, Tseng YC, et al: Seronegative Hashimoto thyroiditis with thyroid autoantibody production localized to the thyroid, Ann Intern Med 108:26–30, 1988.
98. Weetman AP, Black CM, Cohen SB, et al: Affinity purification of IgG subclasses and the distribution of thyroid autoantibody reactivity in Hashimoto's thyroiditis, Scand J Immunol 30:73–82, 1989.
99. Weetman AP, Cohen SB, Oleesky DA, et al: Terminal complement complexes and C1/C1 inhibitor complexes in autoimmune thyroid disease, Clin Exp Immunol 77:25–30, 1989.
100. Rebufaat SA, Nguyen B, Robert B, et al: Antithyroperoxidase antibody-dependent cytotoxicity in autoimmune thyroid disease, J Clin Endocrinol Metab 93:929–932, 2008.
101. Williams RC, Marshall NJ, Kilpatrick K, et al: Kappa/lambda immunoglobulin distribution of Graves' thyroid stimulating antibodies: simultaneous analysis of Cλ gene polymorphisms, J Clin Invest 82:1306–1312, 1988.
102. Weetman AP, Yateman ME, Ealey PA, et al: Thyroid-stimulating antibody activity between different immunoglobulin G subclasses, J Clin Invest 86:723–727, 1990.
103. Kohn LD, Suzuki K, Hoffman WH, et al: Characterization of monoclonal thyroid-stimulating and thyrotropin binding-inhibiting autoantibodies from a Hashimoto's patient whose children had intrauterine and neonatal thyroid disease, J Clin Endocrinol Metab 82:3998–4009, 1997.
104. Kung AWC, Jones BM: A change from stimulatory to blocking antibody activity in Graves' disease during pregnancy, J Clin Endocrinol Metab 83:514–518, 1998.
105. Cho BY, Kim WB, Chung JH, et al: High prevalence and little change in TSH receptor blocking antibody titres with thyroxine and antithyroid drug therapy in patients with non-goitrous autoimmune thyroiditis, Clin Endocrinol 43:465–471, 1995.
106. Kraiem Z, Lahat N, Glaser B, et al: Thyrotrophin receptor blocking antibodies: incidence, characterization and in vivo synthesis, Clin Endocrinol 27:409–421, 1987.
107. Drexhage HA: Autoimmunity and thyroid growth: where do we stand? Eur J Immunol 135:39–45, 1996.
108. Vitti P, Chiovato L, Tonacchera M, et al: Failure to detect thyroid growth-promoting activity in immunoglobulin G of patients with endemic goiter, J Clin Endocrinol Metab 78:1020–1025, 1994.
109. Di Cerbo A, Di Paola R, Bonati M, et al: Subgroups of Graves' patients identified on the basis of the biochemical activities of their immunoglobulins, J Clin Endocrinol Metab 80:2785–2790, 1995.
110. Sato K, Yamazaki K, Shizume K, et al: Stimulation by thyroid-stimulating hormone and Graves' immunoglobulin G of vascular endothelial growth factor mRNA expression in human thyroid follicles in vitro and flt mRNA expression in the rat thyroid in vivo, J Clin Invest 96:1295–1302, 1995.
111. Bottazzo GF, Pujol-Borrell R, Hanafusa T, et al: Role of aberrant HLA-DR expression and antigen presentation in induction of endocrine autoimmunity, Lancet 2:1115–1119, 1983.
112. Kimura H, Kimura M, Tzou S-C, et al: Expression of class II major histocompatiblity complex molecules on thyrocytes does not cause spontaneous thyroiditis but mildly increases its severity after immunization, Endocrinol 146:1154–1162, 2005.
113. Marelli-Berg F, Weetman AP, Frasca L, et al: Antigen presentation by epithelial cells induces anergic immunoregulatory $CD45R0^+$ T cells and deletion of $CD45RA^+$T cells, J Immunol 159:5853–5861, 1997.
114. Sospedra M, Obiols G, Babi LFS, et al: Hyperinducibility of HLA class II expression of thyroid follicular cells from Graves' disease, J Immunol 154:4213–4222, 1995.
115. Marinkovic T, Garin A, Yokota Y, et al: Interaction of mature $CD3^+CD4^+$ T cells with dendritic cells triggers the development of tertiary lymphoid structures in the thyroid, J Clin Invest 116:2622–2632, 2006.
116. Wu Z, Podack ER, McKenzie JM, et al: Perforin expression by thyroid-infiltrating T cells in autoimmune thyroid disease, Clin Exp Immunol 98:470–477, 1994.
117. Giordano C, Stassi G, De Maria R, et al: Potential involvement of Fas and its ligand on the pathogenesis of Hashimoto's thyroiditis, Science 275:960–963, 1997.

118. Bretz JD, Baker JR Jr: Apoptosis and autoimmune thyroid disease: following a TRAIL to destruction? Clin Endocrinol 55:1–11, 2001.

119. Chiovato L, Bassi P, Santini F, et al: Antibodies producing complement-mediated thyroid cytotoxicity in patients with atrophic or goitrous autoimmune thyroiditis, J Clin Endocrinol Metab 77:1700–1705, 1993.

120. Tandon N, Yan SL, Morgan BP, et al: Expression and function of multiple regulators of complement activation in autoimmune thyroid disease, Immunology 84:643–647, 1994.

121. Weetman AP, Tandon N, Morgan BP: Antithyroid drugs and release of inflammatory mediators by complement-attacked thyroid cells, Lancet 340:633–636, 1992.

122. Simons PJ, Delemarre FGA, Drexhage HA: Antigen-presenting dendritic cells as regulators of the growth of thyrocytes: a role of interleukin-1β and interleukin-6, Endocrinology 139:3148–3156, 1998.

123. Roura-Mir C, Catálfamo M, Cheng T-Y, et al: CD1a and CD1c activate intrathyroidal T cells during Graves' disease and Hashimoto's thyroiditis, J Immunol 174:3773–3780, 2005.

124. Vanderpump MPJ, Tunbridge WMG, French JM, et al: The incidence of thyroid disorders in the community: a twenty-year follow-up of the Whickham survey, Clin Endocrinol 43:55–68, 1995.

125. Ando T, Davies TF: Postpartum autoimmune thyroid disease: the potential role of fetal michochimerism, J Clin Endocrinol Metab 88:2965–2971, 2003.

126. Kokandi AA, Parkes AB, Premawardhana LDKE, et al: Association of postpartum thyroid dysfunction with antepartum hormonal and immunological changes, J Clin Endocrinol Metab 88:1126–1132, 2003.

127. Takasu N, Yamada Y, Takasu M, et al: Disappearance of thyrotropin-blocking antibodies and spontaneous recovery from hypothyroidism in autoimmune thyroiditis, N Engl J Med 326:513–518, 1992.

128. Turker O, Kumanlioglu K, Karapolat I, et al: Selenium treatment in autoimmune thyroiditis: 9-month follow-up with variable doses, J Endocrinol 190:151–156, 2006.

129. Bartalena L, Marcocci C, Bogazzi F, et al: Relation between therapy for hyperthyroidism and the course of Graves' ophthalmopathy, N Engl J Med 338:73–78, 1998.

130. Teng WP, Stark R, Munro AJ, et al: Peripheral blood T cell activation after radioiodine treatment for Graves' disease, Acta Endocrinol 122:233–240, 1990.

131. Lee S, Scherberg N, DeGroot LJ: Induction of oral tolerance in human autoimmune thyroid disease, Thyroid 8:229–234, 1998.

132. Baker JR Jr, Fosso CK: Immunological aspects of cancers arising from thyroid follicular cells, Endocr Rev 13:729–746, 1993.

133. Thieblemont C, Mayer A, Dumontet C, et al: Primary thyroid lymphoma is a heterogeneous disease, J Clin Endocrinol Metab 87:105–111, 2002.

134. Giani C, Fierabracci P, Bonacci R, et al: Relationship between breast cancer and thyroid disease: relevance of autoimmune thyroid disorders in breast malignancy, J Clin Endocrinol Metab 81:990–994, 1996.

135. Prummel MF, Wiersinga W: Thyroid autoimmunity and miscarriage, Eur J Endocrinol 150:751–755, 2004.

136. Pop VJ, Maartens LH, Leusink G, et al: Are autoimmune thyroid dysfunction and depression related? J Clin Endocrinol Metab 83:3194–3197, 1998.

137. Jenkins RC, Weetman AP: Disease associations with autoimmune thyroid disease, Thyroid 12:975–986, 2002.

138. Cetani F, Barbesino G, Borsari S, et al: A novel mutation of the autoimmune regulator gene in an Italian kindred with autoimmune polyendocrinopathy-candidiasis-ectodermal dystrophy, acting in a dominant fashion and strongly cosegregating with hypothyroid autoimmune thyroiditis, J Clin Endocrinol Metab 86:4747–4752, 2001.

139. Dittmar M, Kahaly GJ: Polyglandular autoimmune syndromes: immunogenetics and long-term follow-up, J Clin Endocrinol Metab 88:2983–2992, 2003.

Chapter 9

GRAVES' DISEASE

MICHELE MARINÒ, LUCA CHIOVATO, and ALDO PINCHERA

Toxic diffuse goiter, commonly referred to as *Graves' disease*, is a uniquely human disease and since its first descriptions has stimulated and puzzled clinicians and scientists. In its classic form, it is characterized by excessive production of hormones by the thyroid gland (hyperthyroidism) and by its diffuse enlargement. Graves' disease is often (but not always) associated with a unique eye inflammatory disorder, named *Graves' orbitopathy* or *ophthalmopathy*. When present, Graves' orbitopathy makes the diagnosis of Graves' disease almost unmistakable. Other more rarely associated features are a localized infiltrative dermopathy (pretibial myxedema) and the so-called Graves' acropachy.

Graves' disease is now universally classified among the autoimmune organ-specific diseases because it fulfills all the criteria required for this definition (Table 9-1). The main pathogenic mechanism is stimulation of growth and function of the thyroid gland by circulating antibodies directed against the thyroid-stimulating hormone (TSH) receptor (TSHR), thereby mimicking the effects of TSH. Thus TSHR is the major autoantigen of Graves' disease.

In spite of major basic and clinical advancements, the ultimate cause of Graves' disease is poorly known. However, we are beginning to understand how the influence of the genetic background and environmental factors contribute to disrupt immune tolerance leading to expansion of the immune response to TSHR.

Several clinical and laboratory features as well as imaging techniques are helpful for diagnosing Graves' disease. On the therapeutic side, the clinician can take advantage of several available options when treatment is being planned. The decision-making process is now supported by the experience derived from a large body of clinical data.

Historical Notes

Graves' disease is the eponym by which a syndrome characterized by diffuse goiter and hyperthyroidism is recognized in English-speaking countries. Robert James Graves (Fig. 9-1) was a brilliant and productive Irish physician who contributed in many ways to the development of medical science of his time.[1] Credit for his prominent position is probably due to his description in 1835 of "... three cases of violent and long palpitations in females, in each of which the same peculiarity presented ... enlargement of the thyroid gland", which was the first report of toxic diffuse goiter.[2] However, Caleb Hillier Parry, a less renowned physician of Bath, England, had described a similar syndrome earlier, in 1825: "There is one malady which I have in five cases seen coincident with what appears to be enlargement of the heart, and which, so far as I know has not been noticed in that connection by medical writers. This malady to which I allude is enlargement of the thyroid gland".[3] He also described protrusion of the eyes as a feature of the syndrome. Even earlier than that, in 1805, the Italian Giuseppe Flajani in Rome had reported two cases of diffuse swelling of the neck accompanied by palpitations.[4] He failed to recognize the thyroidal origin of

Table 9-1. Criteria for Organ-Specific Autoimmune Diseases and Their Presence in Graves' Disease

Criteria	Present in Graves' Disease
Lymphocytic infiltration of the target organ	Yes
Identification of the specific antigen(s)	Yes
Production of humoral and/or cellular autoimmune responses (or both) in animals sensitized by autologous antigen	Yes
Presence of organ-specific lesions in autosensitized animals	Yes
Association with other autoimmune diseases	Yes

the swelling and named it "bronchocele." In 1840, in Germany, Carl A. von Basedow described "*Exophthalmos durch Hypertrophie del Zellgewebes in der Augenhohle*," or exophthalmos caused by hypertrophy of the cellular tissue of the orbit.[5] This was in fact the first description of the complete syndrome that included the triad exophthalmos, goiter, and palpitations. Von Basedow was struck by the prominence of the eye changes and made exophthalmos the hallmark of the disease. His descriptions were widely disseminated at the time, so that in most non-English-speaking European countries, the disease is still called *Basedow's disease*. In 1880, Ludwig Rehn performed the first thyroidectomy for toxic diffuse goiter, and in 1909, Kocher was awarded the Nobel Prize for his innovations in thyroid surgery.[6] In 1886, Moebius proposed that exophthalmic goiter was due to an excessive function of the thyroid gland.[6] In 1911, Marine proposed treatment of Graves' disease with iodine in the form of Lugol's solution.[7] In the early 1940s, the antithyroid drugs thioureas were described,[8] and Astwood introduced them into clinical use for the control of thyrotoxicosis.[9] At the same time, physicists and physicians in Boston and in Berkeley started to treat thyrotoxic patients with radioiodine (^{131}I).[10] In the span of just a few years, the two mainstays of modern treatment of Graves' disease were initiated. The following decade was marked by the discovery in 1956 of the long-acting thyroid stimulator (LATS) by Adams and Purves[11] and by the subsequent identification of this stimulator as an antibody, thereby forming the basis for our current understanding of the pathogenic mechanisms of Graves' disease. Cloning of TSHR[12,13] is only the most recent and will certainly not be the last memorable event in the uncovering of a disease that has paralleled the development of modern medicine across 2 centuries.

Epidemiology

Graves' disease is a relatively prevalent disorder, and it is the most frequent cause of thyrotoxicosis in iodine-sufficient countries.[14]

Several studies have attempted estimating the exact frequency of Graves' disease in the general population. However, comparison of surveys is difficult because of the use of different criteria in population sampling, because of ethnic differences, and because diagnostic tools have changed over the years. In the United States, a large survey performed in the 1970s estimated the prevalence of Graves' disease to be 0.4%.[15] A similar prevalence (0.6%) was found in the Pescopagano study in Italy.[16] The Whickham survey in the United Kingdom suggested a prevalence of 1.1% to 1.6% (i.e., about threefold to fourfold higher) for thyrotoxicosis of all causes, of which Graves' disease was presumably the most frequent.[17,18] A recent study performed in

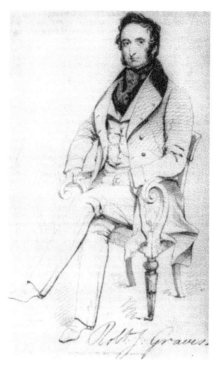

FIGURE 9-1. Portrait of Dr. Robert J. Graves. (From Taylor S: Robert Graves. The Golden Years of Irish Medicine. New York: Royal Society of Medicine Services, 1989.)

Sweden has shown an incidence of Graves' disease of approximately 25 cases/100,000 per year, which is relatively high compared with other studies, a possible interpretation of which is a high iodine intake of the selected population (see later discussion).[19] Overall, a meta-analysis of various studies has estimated the general prevalence of the disorder to be about 1%,[20] which makes it one of the most frequent clinically relevant autoimmune disorders.

The dietary iodine supply appears to be a major factor in determining the frequency of Graves' disease.[21-28] For example, iodine supplementation of previously iodine-deficient Tasmania induced a threefold increase in the incidence of hyperthyroidism in 3 years.[21] Although the increase was mainly due to iodine-induced thyrotoxicosis in patients with autonomously functioning nodules or goiters, it was also shown that LATSs or LATS protectors were present in a number of cases of thyrotoxicosis in the early supplementation period, thus suggesting that some of the iodine-induced cases of hyperthyroidism might have been due to Graves' disease. Since the Tasmanian report, outbursts of iodine-induced thyrotoxicosis have been reported in many countries after the implementation of iodine supplementation programs.[22-28] Thyrotoxicosis occurred primarily in older people with preexisting nodular goiter. However, in a study performed in Switzerland, a slight and transient increase in the incidence of Graves' disease was noted after stepwise, full iodine supplementation (Fig. 9-2).[23] Similar increases in the incidence of thyrotoxicosis have been reported in Sweden (16.6/100,000),[24] New Zealand (15/100,000),[25] Britain (23/100,000),[26] and Denmark[27], in the latter population especially in younger age groups.[28] Population-based studies also show differences in the incidence of Graves' disease in populations with different but relatively constant iodine intake. Nevertheless, this corresponds to a higher frequency of nonautoimmune thyrotoxicosis in iodine-deficient areas. Thus, by comparing two genetically similar populations

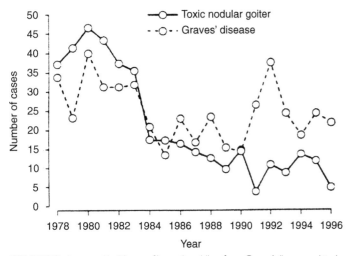

FIGURE 9-2. Increased incidence of hyperthyroidism from Graves' disease and toxic nodular goiter in Switzerland after the introduction of iodine supplementation. (Modified from Burgi H, Kohler M, Morselli B: Thyrotoxicosis incidence in Switzerland and benefit of improved iodine supply. Lancet 352:1034, 1998.)

that differed in terms of iodine intake (iodine-sufficient Iceland versus iodine-deficient East Jutland in Denmark), it was found that the incidence of Graves' hyperthyroidism was slightly higher in the iodine-sufficient (20/100,000 inhabitants/year) than in the iodine-deficient population (15/100,000/year), but that the incidence of thyrotoxicosis of all causes was greater in the iodine-deficient (39/100,000/year) than in the iodine-sufficient (23/100,000/year) population.[14] Clearly, these findings show that fear of an increased incidence of Graves' disease should not prevent the implementation of iodine supplementation programs.

Although ethnic differences in susceptibility to Graves' disease are likely to exist, they have not been consistently investigated in comparative studies. As with many other autoimmune disorders, Graves' disease is about fivefold more prevalent in women than men. The reasons for this observation are understood only in part, but some hypotheses will be discussed later. The annual incidence is clearly and consistently related to age, with peaks in the fourth to sixth decades of life,[28] although Graves' disease can be observed in people of any age, including children.

Etiology

Most of the pathogenic mechanisms of Graves' disease have been clarified since the first description of LATS.[11] It is now well established that Graves' disease is an organ-specific autoimmune disorder, with involvement of both T-cell and B-cell–mediated immunity against thyroid antigens. TSHR is the main antigen involved, and circulating autoantibodies against TSHR (TSH receptor antibodies [TRAbs]) that are capable of stimulating the receptor are responsible for the most distinctive features of the disease, namely hyperthyroidism and goiter. Nevertheless, in spite of advancements in understanding the pathogenic mechanisms of Graves' disease, the ultimate cause of the disease remains elusive. The majority of investigators share the opinion that Graves' disease is a multifactorial disease caused by a complex interplay of genetic, hormonal, and environmental influences that lead to the loss of immune tolerance to thyroid antigens and to the initiation of a sustained autoimmune reaction.

GENETICS OF GRAVES' DISEASE

It is common for endocrinologists to observe familial clustering of Graves' disease by simply eliciting the family history of patients. Besides this common knowledge, a body of evidence indicates the existence of a genetic predisposition to Graves' disease.

The strongest data in support of a genetic predisposition to Graves' disease comes from twin studies.[29,30] Dizygotic twins share on average 50% of their genome, whereas monozygotic twins share 100%. Moreover, twins are likely to share environmental factors more than any other kind of siblings. Several large twin studies have reported greater concordance rate of Graves' disease in monozygotic than in dizygotic twins.[29] Data obtained with modern diagnostic tools have shown a relatively low (~17% to 35%), but still significant, concordance in monozygotic twins.[29,30] These findings clearly show a genetic influence, possibly characterized by low penetrance of the genes involved.

Another tool widely used to establish the existence of a genetic predisposition to any condition is family studies, in which the prevalence of the disease in relatives of index cases is compared with the prevalence in the general population. Early family studies showed a high prevalence of Graves' disease and other thyroid abnormalities in first-degree relatives of patients with Graves' disease and Hashimoto's thyroiditis.[31,32] The prevalence of circulating thyroid autoantibodies in siblings of patients was as high as 56% in some studies,[31] which suggested a dominant mode of inheritance. These observations have been consistently confirmed in highly selected populations,[33] but the results may not be applicable to the general population because of ascertainment bias. In an extensive segregation analysis with randomly ascertained probands, circulating antibodies were found in only 25% of the offspring of positive parents and in 14% of the offspring of negative parents, thus suggesting a multigenic model with less than 100% penetrance for the antibody trait.[34] With the exception of very early studies, the prevalence of overt Graves' disease has been found to be relatively low in siblings of patients.[33,36] However, initial abnormalities in thyroid function compatible with subclinical hyperthyroidism or hypothyroidism have been reported.[33,35] Villanueva et al. found that 36% of Graves' patients with ophthalmopathy have a family history of either Graves' disease or autoimmune thyroiditis, which in 23% of the cases affected first-degree relatives.[37] Autoimmune thyroiditis is frequently observed in siblings of probands with Graves' disease, as well as the contrary,[33,37] suggesting that the two diseases may share some susceptibility genes that predispose to thyroid autoimmunity, but that the full expression of the phenotype depends on other genes and/or on environmental factors. Other organ-specific, non-thyroid-related autoimmune diseases may also be more prevalent in relatives of patients with Graves' disease.[33]

These data and those obtained in twin studies are indicative of a complex multigenic pattern of inheritance of Graves' disease. Some of the components of the phenotype, such as the presence of circulating antithyroglobulin and antithyroperoxidase antibodies, may be inherited in a dominant fashion with high penetrance.[33] However, these genetic determinants do not appear to be sufficient for full expression of the disease. Clearly, other genes must be involved, which is in line with the complexity of the inheritance observed. Also, it appears from epidemiologic and experimental data that environmental factors (reviewed later in this chapter) play an important role by modulating the effect of an inherited predisposition. Based on the above evidence, a

Table 9-2. Genetic Determinants Associated With Graves' Disease

Gene	Possible Mechanism	Evidence in Favor of an Association
HLA-DR	Altered antigen presentation	Fair
CD40	Altered antigen presentation	Fair
CTLA-4	Altered antigen presentation	Good
PTPN22	Altered T-cell activation	Fair
Thyroglobulin	Loss of tolerance	Good
TSH-R	Loss of tolerance	Poor

number of genes or loci have been investigated as candidates for predisposing factors (Table 9-2).[33,38]

Genes Predisposing to Graves' Disease

In the last 20 years, the impressive advancement of biomedical research has allowed a remarkable expansion in genetics, which has led to the identification of several genes involved in the predisposition to Graves' disease.[33,38] Linkage, association, and candidate genes analyses, as well as whole-genome screening, have all been used to accomplish this goal. Based on the data available, genetic susceptibility to thyroid autoimmunity in general and to Graves' disease in particular seems to be determined by a combination of a number of genes, some which most likely still remain to be identified.[33,38,39]

1: The HLA Complex

The HLA complex, which is located on the short arm of human chromosome 6, contains the sequence encoding about a hundred genes, most of which are involved in regulation of the immune response.[40-42] The HLA genes are classically grouped into three major classes. Class I includes histocompatibility genes expressed on the surface of most cells (HLA-A, HLA-B, and HLA-C). Class II includes histocompatibility genes expressed exclusively on the surface of leukocytes and immune cells (HLA-DR). Class III includes a heterogeneous group of genes encoding molecules involved in the immune response, such as some complement factors, cytokines, and lymphocyte surface molecules. Other genes in this class are not clearly related with immunity. Most genes of the HLA complex are highly polymorphic, which makes them excellent candidates for disease susceptibility.

Experimental thyroiditis in the mouse was the first autoimmune disease to be associated with HLA.[43,44] Early population studies in humans indicated an association of Graves' disease with HLA-B8 and a relative risk of 3.9 in white patients.[45] Subsequent studies also suggested an influence of that haplotype on the clinical course of the disease.[33,44] However, HLA-DR3 (HLA-DRB1*03) was later shown to increase the risk to a greater extent and was considered to be the true determinant of the disease because it was in linkage disequilibrium with the B8 allele.[33] Among Caucasians, HLA-DQA1*0501 was found to confer a relatively high risk within DR3 itself.[33,44] This allele is in linkage disequilibrium with both B8 and DR3 and gives a relative risk of 3 to 4 for Graves' disease in the white population. Sequencing of the DRβ-1 chain of HLA-DR3 allowed the identification of Arg74 as the critical amino acid conferring susceptibility to Graves' disease.[33,44]

Different haplotypes seem to be involved in ethnic groups other than Caucasians: DQ3 in patients of African descent and Bw46 in those of Asian descent, although the data available are limited and have not always been reproducible.[33,44]

In general, HLA associations have been shown to confer a relatively low risk, even with alleles that have a high prevalence in the general population. Thus linkage analysis, a powerful tool for mapping essential predisposition genes, has been negative when the HLA region was examined using different polymorphisms at the same locus.[33,44] Overall, it seems that the HLA locus explains a small fraction of the total genetic predisposition, but it is neither the major nor the only determinant, although it represents an established risk-increasing factor.

2: CD40

CD40, a member of the tumor necrosis factor receptor family, is expressed in B cells and other antigen-presenting cells and is involved in B-cell activation and proliferation, antibody secretion, immunoglobulin class switching, affinity maturation and generation of memory cells.[46] Linkage studies have shown an association of the CD40 gene with Graves' disease and the subsequent sequencing of the gene led to the identification of a C/T polymorphism at the 5′ untranslated region of CD40 strongly associated with Graves' disease.[33] This polymorphism influences the translational efficiency of the gene, which may have functional consequences in the CD40 protein.

3: CTLA-4

CTLA-4 is a T-lymphocyte surface protein with a major role in down-regulation of the immune response.[47] Several studies have provided evidence that CTLA-4 is linked to Graves' disease, autoimmune thyroiditis, and to the production of autoantibodies against thyroid antigens.[33,44-48] Several variants of the CTLA-4 gene have been implicated in its possible causative role in Graves' disease, among which a CTLA-4 polymorphism at position 60 was found to be the most suitable candidate in a large comprehensive analysis, the functional relevance of the polymorphism being possibly due to a reduced mRNA expression encoding the soluble form of the molecule.[47] Nevertheless, a subsequent study did not confirm these data.[48] Although CTLA-4 seems to be a genetic determinant of Graves' disease, the causative variant remains to be identified with certainty, and it is possible that a haplotype consisting of more than one variant is responsible for the association.[33]

4: The Protein Tyrosine Phosphatase 22 (PTPN22) Gene

PTPN22 is a powerful inhibitor of T-cell activation.[49] A single nucleotide polymorphism at codon 620 associated with other autoimmune diseases was found to be associated with both Graves' disease and autoimmune thyroiditis, with significant ethnic differences in the association.[49,50]

5: Thyroglobulin

Thyroglobulin is the precursor of thyroid hormones and a major autoantigen in thyroid autoimmunity. Recent wide genome screens have provided evidence for a strong linkage between a locus on chromosome 8q24, where the thyroglobulin gene is located, and autoimmune thyroid diseases.[33,51] Sequence analysis of the thyroglobulin gene has shown numerous single nucleotide missense polymorphism, suggesting that amino acid variants in the Tg proteins may contribute the pathogenesis of autoimmune thyroid diseases, including Graves' disease.[33,52]

6: TSH-R

Despite the central role of TSH-R in the pathogenesis of Graves' disease, the association of the disease with the gene encoding the receptor remains controversial.[33] Although three common missense single nucleotide polymorphisms have been found to be associated with Graves' disease, these associations were not always confirmed by other studies. The extent of the contribution of the TSH-R gene remains to be established.[33]

7: Other Genes

In the search for genetic determinants of Graves' disease, several other genes have been studied over the years, namely genes involved in the immune response. The immunoglobulin genes were studied extensively, but conflicting results were observed in association studies.[33] Other candidate immunoregulatory genes that have been studied include interleukin 1 (IL-1), IL-1 receptor antagonist, tumor necrosis factor receptor 2 (TNF-2), and interferon γ (INF-γ). None of these genes showed significant associations with Graves' disease.[33] Additional loci have been linked in families with Graves' disease, including one on chromosome 14q31 (GD-1), one on chromosome 20 (GD-2), and one on chromosome Xq21-22 (GD-3).[33]

ENVIRONMENTAL FACTORS AND GRAVES' DISEASE

The relative low penetrance in twins and first-degree relatives of patients with Graves' disease suggests that environmental factors must play a major role in inducing the disease in genetically susceptible individuals.[33,53,54] Several studies have shown that various nongenetic factors may in fact contribute to the development of Graves' disease.

Infections

Over the years, both experimental and epidemiologic evidence has suggested that infections could play a role in the pathogenesis of Graves' disease.[54,55] Seasonal and geographic variations in the incidence of the disease have been reported,[56,57] although seasonal variations have not been confirmed in other studies.[58] Blood group nonsecretors, who are more prone than secretors to infections, are more frequently found among patients with Graves' disease than in controls.[59] This observation has been interpreted as indirect evidence that infectious pathogens may be involved in the etiology of Graves' disease, although a direct genetic effect of the secretor status could also explain these results. Evidence of a recent viral infection has been reported in a high percentage of patients with Graves' disease.[54,55]

Molecular mimicry has been invoked to explain the association between infections and Graves' disease.[60] Molecular mimicry is based on the hypothesis that cross-reactions of some microbial antigens with a self-antigen may cause an immune response to autoantigens. In Graves' disease, the pathogen *Yersinia enterocolitica* has been thoroughly studied after reports of association of this microbe with the disease. A high prevalence of circulating antibodies against *Y. enterocolitica* has been observed in patients with Graves' disease, and *Yersinia* antibodies were found to interact with thyroid structures.[61-63] In a recent study from Denmark, it was shown that the occurrence of IgA and IgG antibodies against *Yersinia* not only is more frequent in Graves' patients than in case controls but also in twins with Graves' disease compared with their discordant twins.[64] Saturable binding sites for TSH have been found in *Yersinia* and were also recognized by TRAbs from patients with Graves' disease.[65,66] In animals immunized with *Yersinia* proteins, antibodies developed against human thyroid epithelial cells and TSHR.[67,68] Overall, the affinity of these cross-reactive antibodies to the thyroid was low, and immune responses were transient. Low-affinity binding sites for TSH have also been found in other bacteria, including some

species of *Leishmania* and *Mycoplasma*.[53,54] However, it must be noted that thyroid autoimmunity does not develop in most patients with *Yersinia* infections,[69] so the evidence in favor of *Yersinia* infections as a precipitating cause of Graves' disease awaits confirmation.

Viruses could theoretically trigger autoimmunity through several mechanisms, including interactions with autoantigens, permanent expression of viral proteins on the surface of epithelial cells, aberrant induction of HLA antigens on epithelial cells (see later), and molecular mimicry.[60,70] In 1989, the presence of retroviral (HIV-1 glycosaminoglycan protein) sequences in the thyroid and peripheral mononuclear cells of patients with Graves' disease was reported,[71] but viral sequences were not found in control thyroids. This finding, however, remained isolated and was not confirmed in subsequent studies.[72,73] Human foamy virus antigens were shown by immunofluorescence to be present in the thyroid of patients with Graves' disease.[74] Again, further studies using more specific and sensitive techniques failed to identify foamy virus DNA and antiviral antibodies in the blood of affected subjects.[75,76] Homology between another HIV-1 protein (Nef) and human TSHR has also been reported, although sera from patients with Graves' disease did not react with the peptide bearing the highest degree of homology.[77] Another retroviral protein, p15E, has been isolated from the thyroids of patients with Graves' disease but not from control glands.[78] In this regard, it is worthwhile emphasizing that retroviral-like proteins, including p15E, are encoded by the normal human genome. Although their function is unclear, they may be expressed in many epithelial tissues under certain conditions such as inflammation and may modulate but not initiate the immune response.[79] The finding of retroviral sequences or proteins in the glands of patients with Graves' disease may therefore represent a secondary rather than a causative phenomenon. Circulating antibodies against another retroviral particle, namely HIAP-1, have been found in as many as 87.5% of patients with Graves' disease as compared with 10% to 15% of controls,[80] but HIAP-1 particles were not detected when human T cells were co-cultured with Graves' thyrocytes.[81]

A highly speculative hypothesis has been raised that involves superantigens.[55,60] Superantigens are endogenous or exogenous proteins, such as microbial proteins, capable of stimulating a strong immune response through molecular interactions with nonvariant parts of the T-cell receptor and the HLA class II proteins. Through this mechanism, superantigens are in theory capable of stimulating the expansion of autoreactive T cells and therefore of driving an autoimmune response.[55,60] Such a mechanism has been suggested in rheumatoid arthritis, and a similar mechanism was proposed for Graves' disease. In vitro superantigen stimulation of glands with autoimmune thyroid disease induced expression of HLA class II molecules on thyrocytes, and this phenomenon was IFN-γ dependent.[82] The interpretation of this observation was that superantigen-reactive T cells exist among the lymphocytes infiltrating the thyroid in autoimmune thyroid disease, and that these lymphocytes may have been activated after exposure to extrinsic superantigens.

The most recent hypothesis, the so-called "hygiene hypothesis of autoimmunity," implies that infections may protect from, rather than precipitate, autoimmune diseases. Exposure of the immune system to infective agents may somehow allow better control of autoimmune responses. In this regard, improved living standards have been associated with decreased exposure to infections and an increased risk of autoimmune diseases. Kondrashova et al. reported a much reduced prevalence of thyroid autoantibodies in the lower-economic population, which may suggest the hygiene hypothesis may apply to thyroid autoimmune diseases.[83] Further studies are needed to investigate whether this is in fact the case.

In summary, although epidemiologic evidence indicates that infection may play an important role as a causative or protective factor in Graves' disease, we are still lacking definitive identification of the etiologic organism(s) and a reasonable explanation for microbes to precipitate or protect from the disorder.

Stress

The suggestion that psychological stress may be a precipitating factor in Graves' disease has been made as early as the first description of the disease.[3] The occurrence of stressful events before the onset of Graves' disease is a recurrent impression among clinicians, and by the end of the 19th century, Graves' disease was considered to be a result of prolonged emotional disturbances. In cross-sectional questionnaire-based studies, some investigators have shown an increased prevalence of stressful life events in the months preceding the onset of Graves' disease.[84-87] However, some of the recorded events (such as arguments with spouses and in the workplace) could have been influenced by the behavior of patients with a yet undetected hyperthyroidism and therefore be a consequence rather than a cause of the disease. Other events, however, were largely independent of the patient's behavior, such as unemployment and financial difficulties. In some studies, patients were asked to rate the stressfulness of life events, and patients with Graves' disease ranked such events more stressful than did controls.[84] Thus it is possible that the perception of life events is different in hyperthyroid patients. In cross-sectional studies, an increase in the prevalence of Graves' disease was reported during World War II in Germany but not during the civil unrest in Ireland or during the German occupation of Belgium, which suggests that the stressful events of personal life may be more important than "social stress."[84] On the other hand, chronic stress due to panic disorder was not associated with the occurrence of Graves' disease.[88] Stress is associated with increased adrenocorticotropic hormone (ACTH) and cortisol secretion, which can in turn determine immune suppression, but additional non-ACTH-related immunosuppressive phenomena also occur.[89,90] Recovery from such immune suppression can be associated with rebound immune hyperactivity, which could precipitate autoimmunity. The best example of such a phenomenon is perhaps the well-documented immune suppression of pregnancy, which can be followed by new or recurrent onset of autoimmune disorders, including Graves' disease (see later discussion).[91]

In summary, limited but significant evidence indicates that stress may be a contributing factor in the etiology of Graves' disease, probably in connection with other predisposing factors. The available studies are all retrospective and therefore carry a number of possible biases. Worried patients sick with hyperthyroidism may be more prone to recall upsetting events, and subclinical undetected thyrotoxicosis present before clinical diagnosis may alter the perception of life events and even the behavior of patients. Unfortunately, prospective studies addressing the problem of stress and Graves' disease and its interplay with genetic factors are not available to date.

Gender

Graves' disease is typically but not exclusively a disease of women. In most series, the female-to-male ratio ranges from 5 to 10 at any age,[16,17] although the difference may be smaller

during childhood.[92] The reason for the disproportionate prevalence of Graves' disease in women is not known, but genetic and nongenetic factors must play a role. A number of studies indicate a stronger immune system in women.[93,94] Autoimmune phenomena and diseases are in general more prevalent in women.[93,94] A large body of evidence clearly indicates the existence of sexual dimorphism in normal and abnormal immune responses in spontaneous and experimental animal models, including models of autoimmune thyroiditis.[93,94] In these models, male hormones appear to down-regulate immunity and therefore protect animals from autoimmunity, whereas the effect of estrogen is not always unequivocal. Despite the evidence obtained from animal studies, little evidence in the literature supports a role for sex hormones in the high prevalence of Graves' disease in women.[93,94] Women with normal baseline levels of estrogen, but with an increased sensitivity to the hormone as shown by the presence of melasma, had a higher prevalence of thyroid autoimmune disorders.[95] However, a clear association between exogenous estrogen administration and Graves' disease has never been reported. Moreover, thyroid autoimmunity is often found in patients with Turner's syndrome, who typically have low estrogen levels.[96] Conversely, male patients with primary hypogonadism such as in Klinefelter's syndrome do not show a higher incidence of Graves' disease or Hashimoto's thyroiditis.[97] In these human conditions, however, the chromosomal abnormality probably plays an important role that is largely independent of sex hormone levels.

Pregnancy is an important risk factor, and it is well recognized that in any woman the risk of development of Graves' disease increases fourfold to eightfold in the postpartum year.[91] The abrupt fall in the level of pregnancy-associated immunosuppressive factors immediately after delivery (rebound immunity) is likely to be the mechanism responsible for the precipitation of Graves' disease.[91] Nevertheless, in a recent retrospective study it was found that the relative frequencies of postpartum onset of Graves' disease were similar in relation of increasing parity, which would not support a role of the postpartum period as a major risk factor for the first appearance of Graves' disease.[98] On the other hand, it was also shown by the same group that the postpartum period is indeed a risk factor for relapse of Graves' thyrotoxicosis after withdrawal of antithyroid drugs.[99] The factors involved in the immune alterations of the postpartum period may include but are not limited to estrogen and progestin.[91,100]

Besides sex hormones, factors on the X chromosome could explain the epidemiologic evidence of a female preponderance in Graves' disease. A linkage analysis in families with Graves' disease has located a putative Graves' disease susceptibility locus on the long arm of the X chromosome.[33] Although most X-linked disorders are expressed phenotypically only in men, it is possible that a gene with a dose-dependent effect may determine more relevant clinical effects in women. This finding could help explain the higher incidence of Graves' disease observed in women and, possibly, in patients with Turner's syndrome. Inactivation of the X chromosome, an epigenetic phenomenon, has also been suggested to be involved in the female predisposition to thyroid autoimmunity, and recently it was shown that this phenomenon is more frequently observed in patients with Graves' disease or autoimmune thyroiditis than in healthy controls.[101]

Smoking

A number of studies have provided evidence for an association between smoking and thyroid diseases, including Graves' disease.[102,103] Retrospective analysis shows that in smokers there is an increased risk of Graves' disease and ophthalmopathy, as well as of relapse of hyperthyroidism following anti-thyroid drug withdrawal, which is more pronounced in the female gender. The findings may be explained both by a direct action of smoking metabolites on the immune system or by damage induced by smoking metabolites on thyrocytes, which may determine exposure of thyroid antigens to the immune system.

Thyroid Damage

There are reports of Graves' disease appearing after ethanol injections performed for treatment of autonomous thyroid nodules, which has been interpreted as due to the massive release of thyroid antigens, thereby triggering an autoimmune response to TSH-R in predisposed individuals.[104] Furthermore, and possibly because of similar pathogenetic mechanisms (i.e., massive release of thyroid antigens), Graves' disease or simply serum TRAb have been reported to appear following radioiodine treatment for toxic adenoma or toxic nodular goiter.[105] We observed a patient with Graves' disease that appeared after a neck injury (unpublished observation), which in theory may also reflect release of thyroid antigens.

Pathology

It is now rare to observe the full pathologic changes that occur in the thyroid glands of untreated patients.[106] On gross pathology the gland is significantly enlarged, with a smooth and hyperemic surface. A prominent pyramidal lobe is often visible, and the contour of the gland is irregular with multiple lobulations. Microscopically, both hypertrophy and hyperplasia are found. Follicles are small, with scanty colloid as a result of ongoing thyroid hormone secretion. The follicular epithelium presents a columnar aspect, with even a pseudopapillary appearance. Blood vessels are large and congested. Various degrees of lymphocytic infiltration can be found between the follicles. T cells predominate in the interstitium, whereas B cells and plasma cells predominate in the occasional lymphoid follicles. On electron microscopy, the cellular hyperactivity is demonstrated by an increase in the Golgi reticulum and the number of mitochondria and by the presence of prominent microvilli. With longstanding Graves' disease, distinct nodularities with an adenomatous appearance may develop, and the lymphocytic infiltrate may become more prominent and resemble chronic thyroiditis.

This pathologic picture of active Graves' disease is dramatically changed by antithyroid drugs and iodine treatment, which is now universally performed before surgery. Vascularity and vascular congestion are much less pronounced, and the follicles can be larger.[106]

Pathogenesis of Graves' Disease

Although the ultimate cause of Graves' disease is still unknown, over the years a large body of evidence has accumulated and provided important insight into the immune mechanisms that eventually lead to the clinical manifestations of the disease. Since their first description in 1956,[11] much attention has been devoted to the study of TRAbs. It has also been recognized that although TRAbs are the ultimate cause of both goiter and hyperthyroidism, the nature of the immune dysfunction involves many aspects of the immune system, including changes in both B-cell and

T-cell function. The follicular cell per se may also play an independent role.

ROLE OF TSH RECEPTOR ANTIBODIES
Nomenclature

The nomenclature of TRAbs is complex and largely dependent on the assay used to detect these antibodies in serum.[107-111] Assays measuring displacement of radiolabeled TSH from its receptor by serum immunoglobulins detect TRAbs regardless of their functional activity. These antibodies have been termed *TSH-binding inhibitory immunoglobulins* (TBIIs). Assays for TSAbs use cellular systems carrying a functional TSHR and detect the release of cyclic adenosine monophosphate (cAMP) in the culture medium upon challenge with serum or purified immunoglobulins.[107-111] These antibodies are essentially the cause of hyperthyroidism in Graves' disease. In the same bioassay system, antibodies with blocking activity on the TSHR (TBAbs) can be detected.[107-112] These antibodies characterize a subset of patients with atrophic autoimmune thyroiditis and hypothyroidism, but they can also occasionally be found in patients with Graves' disease, in combination with TSAbs.[112]

Major Autoantigen in Graves' Disease: Structure-Function Relationship of the TSHR

Definitive proof that TSHR is the target of TSAbs came from the cloning of this protein in the late 1980s.[12,13,107-109] The receptor is a member of the G protein–coupled receptor superfamily. Its structure includes seven hydrophobic transmembrane domains, an extracellular N-terminal domain (ectodomain), and an intracellular C-terminal domain. Heavy glycosylation of the extracellular domain accounts for about 20% of its molecular weight of 84 kD. The primary structure of the protein consists of 744 residues. The gene is located on chromosome 14q31 and is formed by 10 exons that yield a single polypeptide. Shedding of the N-terminal extracellular 310 amino-acid residues (the so-called A subunit) may either initiate or amplify the immune response against TSHR, being immunoreactive epitopes partially sterically hindered on the holoreceptor on the plasma membrane.[108,113,114] Binding sites for TSH and TRAbs are located in the extracellular domain and are mainly conformational.[107,108] The major epitopes for TSAbs are located in the extreme N-terminal portion, whereas those for TBABs are mainly, but not exclusively, in the C-terminal portion of the extracellular domain, closer to the cell membrane.[107,108,115-118] However, this should not be taken as a paradigm, especially since TBABs are more diverse and spread over the receptor extracellular domain.[108] In fact, TRAbs are to some extent heterogeneous for epitope recognition, possibly due to epitope spreading during the immune response.[108] Whether and to what extent glycosylation and dimerization of TSH receptor affects its recognition by antibodies is uncertain.[108]

Assays for TSH Receptor Antibody

The pioneering era of bioassays in vivo for TRAbs[11,119] has been superseded by the present period, in which a number of in vitro assays are more readily performed by many laboratories and provide more reproducible and reliable measures of TRAb levels in the serum of patients. The radioreceptor assay uses TSHR from various sources: porcine or human recombinant TSHR from transfected cell lines.[120-126] Although assay design varies in all these methods, they all rely on displacement of labeled TSH from solubilized TSHR from the serum of patients. Studies in

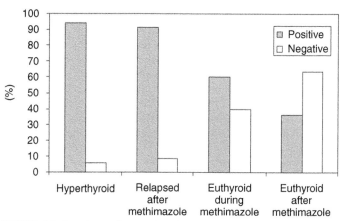

FIGURE 9-3. Prevalence of serum thyroid-stimulating antibody tests in Chinese hamster ovary cells transfected with recombinant human thyroid-stimulating hormone (TSH) receptor (CHO-R). Serum IgG was purified from untreated and treated patients with Graves' disease. (Modified from Vitti P, Elisei R, Tonacchera M et al: Detection of thyroid-stimulating antibody using Chinese hamster ovary cells transfected with cloned human thyrotropin receptor. J Clin Endocrinol Metab 76:499–503, 1993.)

hyperthyroid patients with Graves' disease show positive TBII tests with these methods in 75% to 95% of patients. The recently designed second-generation radioreceptor assay attains even higher sensitivity while maintaining high specificity (99%)[126] and is commonly used by the majority of laboratories for the routine detection of TRAb. An enzyme-linked assay is also available.[127] Radioreceptor assays do not require permanent cell cultures; they are the most readily available (also commercially) and are therefore the most frequently used in clinical practice. The TBII test, however, does not give information on the functional properties of the antibody detected and can be positive in the presence of TBAb.

The functional stimulating properties of TRAbs can be studied by in vitro bioassays based on the measurement of cAMP production from cells with a functional TSHR.[120] Human thyroid follicular cells,[128] a rat thyroid cell strain (FRTL-5),[129,130] and Chinese hamster ovary cells stably transfected with human TSHR (CHO-R)[131-133] have all been used for this purpose. With these assays, TSAb can be detected in more than 90% of patients with untreated Graves' disease (Fig. 9-3). The system using CHO-R cells has some advantages over the others: it is slightly more sensitive and relies on easier culture conditions, which also makes it more reproducible in different laboratories. As stated previously, the bioassays have the advantage of giving information on the functional properties of TRAbs and, in a modification of the assay, can also identify TBAbs.[112,133] However, they require permanent cell culture equipment and pre-purification of the immunoglobulin fraction of serum, which makes these assays not readily available to routine endocrine laboratories. The latter problem has been overcome by very sensitive assays in which activation of a transfected firefly luciferase gene produces chemiluminescence in response to TSHR stimulation by whole serum.[134,135] Even more recently, a coated-tube assay which discriminates TSAb from TBAb was developed.[136] The assay is based on the use of a chimeric receptor, where a TSAb epitope 8-165 is replaced by comparable LH receptor residues. Binding of radiolabeled TSH to this chimera can be inhibited by sera containing TBAb up to 95%.

Thyroid-Stimulating Antibody in the Pathogenesis and Natural History of Graves' Disease

Historically, the identification of TSAbs as the cause of hyperthyroidism and goiter in Graves' disease came from the demonstration of a stimulating factor in the sera of hyperthyroid patients with a half-life much longer than that of TSH (LATS).[11] Subsequently this factor was shown to be an autoantibody.[137-139] TSAbs were shown to interact with TSHR in that they act as a potent agonist and thus cause hyperfunction of the thyroid gland.[107-110] Definitive proof that TRAbs interact with TSHR eventually came from studies with the cloned protein.[107-110] A clear-cut demonstration of the role of TSAb in the pathogenesis of hyperthyroidism is provided by the observation that the transplacental transfer of antibodies from TSAb-positive pregnant mothers to the fetus may cause a form of transient neonatal thyrotoxicosis that vanishes with the disappearance of TSAb from the serum of the newborn.[140]

TSAbs are oligo- or pauciclonal, and this observation has suggested a primary defect at the B-cell level.[107-110] TSAbs appear to be produced mainly by thyroid-infiltrating lymphocytes and lymphocytes in the draining lymph nodes.[141] Synthesis by peripheral blood lymphocytes has been documented as well.[142-144] As mentioned earlier, TSAbs can be detected in more than 90% of patients with untreated Graves' disease hyperthyroidism.[120-126] The observation of a small proportion of patients with undetectable TBIIs or TSAbs has been attributed to the occurrence of these autoantibodies at a serum level too low to be detected by current methods. Alternatively, restricted intrathyroidal production of TRAbs has been hypothesized.[145] A positive correlation between TSAb levels and serum triiodothyronine (T_3) levels, serum thyroglobulin levels, and goiter size has been observed.[107-110]

TRAb levels usually fall during long-term treatment with antithyroid drugs.[146,147] This phenomenon has been attributed to an immunosuppressive effect of antithyroid drugs,[148] but it could also result from the correction of thyrotoxicosis or even reflect the natural history of the disease.

OTHER ANTIGENS

In addition to TRAbs, autoantibodies against thyroglobulin and thyroperoxidase are commonly found in patients with Graves' disease, although autoimmunity against these two antigens is generally believe to be a secondary phenomenon with no pathogenetic implications. A possible role in the pathogenesis of Graves' disease, especially of its extrathyroidal manifestations (e.g., Graves' ophthalmopathy), was recently attributed to the insulin-like growth factor 1 receptor (IGF1-R). The receptor is expressed in thyroid epithelial cells as well as in orbital fibroblasts, and autoantibodies against the receptor have been detected in patients with Graves' disease.[149] Whether autoimmunity against IGF1-R has any role in the pathogenesis of the disease is under investigation.

ROLE OF CELLULAR IMMUNITY

The primary requirement for a specific autoimmune (either humoral or cell-mediated) response is an antigen-specific T cell.[150] Activation of T cells requires presentation of antigenic peptides in the context of HLA molecules. This task is accomplished by a specialized subset of immune cells called *professional antigen-presenting cells*. Once activated, helper (CD4+) T cells can be subdivided into two functional subtypes according to their cytokine production pattern[150,151]: the T_H1 subset, mainly involved in delayed-type hypersensitivity reactions, and the T_H2 subset, prominently involved in humoral immune responses. T_H1 cells produce tumor necrosis factor-β, IFN-γ, and IL-2; T_H2 cells secrete mainly IL-4, IL-5, IL-6, and IL-13. T_H1 cells have been implicated in organ-specific autoimmune diseases, an action that seem to be exerted especially by the so-called T_H17 subtype, which among T_H1 cells produces uniquely IL-17.[152] The subset of T lymphocytes primarily activated by specific antigens and the cytokine milieu produced by antigen-presenting cells determine the direction of the immune response toward a T_H1 cell-mediated tissue-damaging reaction, a more prominent humoral reaction (T_H2 mediated), or a balance of the two.[152]

Studies of patients with Graves' disease showed activated T cells both in the peripheral circulation and in the thyroid gland.[153-155] T cells infiltrating the thyroid gland in Graves' disease have been studied by surface monoclonal antibody phenotyping. The percentage of $CD8^+$ (suppressor/cytotoxic) T cells was found to be much lower in Graves' disease than in Hashimoto's thyroiditis.[156-159] The phenotype of the $CD4^+$ (helper/inducer) T-cell population was predominantly composed of memory cells.[160,161] Further studies involved cloning of infiltrating T cells. Most of the resulting T-cell lines belonged to the memory ($CD4^+$, $CD29^+$) subtype and responded with significant growth and/or cytokine production to challenge with autologous thyroid follicular cells or thyroid antigens.[162-166]

As assessed by their cytokine profile, intrathyroidal T cells were found to be predominantly of the T_H1 subtype,[158,167] and this pattern was also true for TSHR-responsive clones.[168] This finding is somewhat unexpected in a disease such as Graves' disease, which is mainly characterized by the action of TSAbs producing thyroid hyperfunction and follicular cell growth. However, it is worthwhile noting that T_H1 cells may also induce antibody production through secretion of IL-10, which in turn activates B cells.[141] In keeping with this sequence of events, TRAbs of Graves' disease are more often of the IgG1 subclass,[151] which is selectively induced by T_H1 cells. A significant proportion of T_H0 (uncommitted) cells were also detected among TSHR autoreactive T cells.[168]

The basis for an organ-specific autoimmune process is the interaction of antigen-specific T cells with the target tissue itself in a way that leads to selection and clonal expansion of autoreactive cells. The specificity of this interaction is provided by the immense variability in mature T-cell antigen receptors caused by the somatic rearrangement of their variable (V) chain with the constant (C) and the junction (J) regions.[169,170] When an immune response is initiated, T cells carrying the individual receptor specific for the antigen involved are stimulated and clonally expanded. In keeping with this concept, restricted use of T-cell receptor Vα and Vβ genes was observed in T lymphocytes obtained by fine-needle aspiration of Graves' disease thyroids.[171] When surgically obtained specimens of thyroids with Graves' disease have been examined, selective use of T-cell receptor Vα and Vβ genes has been confirmed in some[172-175] but not all studies.[176,177] These observations indicate that a highly selective response to thyroid autoantigens is elicited in the thyroid glands of patients with Graves' disease during the initial phase of the disease. Afterward, spreading of the autoimmune response occurs and leads to less restricted T-cell receptor gene usage.

The antigen specificity of autoreactive T cells has also been tested. Initial studies with thyroid follicular cells in culture or with their subcellular fractions suffered from contamination with thyroid autoantigens other than TSHR, so that the antigen specificity of T cells was questionable. Indeed, thyroid peroxidase–specific and thyroglobulin-specific T cells also exist within the thyroid gland of patients with Graves' disease.[168] Since the cloning of TSHR cDNA, however, a number of laboratories have searched for TSHR-specific T-cell clones and investigated their role in thyroid autoimmunity and Graves' disease. Studies using TSHR peptides identified specific responses and showed positive stimulation indexes of peripheral blood mononuclear cells from patients with Graves' disease, as well as from healthy controls.[173] Considerable effort has also been expended in identifying immunodominant T-cell epitopes on the TSHR. Four distinct peptides were recognized by lymphocytes from most patients with Graves' disease in one study.[178] More recently, another set of immunodominant peptides has been described.[179] It is possible that HLA haplotypes and other poorly understood factors play a role in determining which epitope is immunodominant in individual patients. Overall, these observations show that immunodominant T cell–dependent epitopes exist within the TSHR, and that these epitopes may be at least in part shared by different patients. Identification of T cell–dependent epitopes would be important in efforts to design immunologic approaches to the treatment of Graves' disease, such as tolerizing vaccines or antigen-specific lymphocyte deletion.

Unlike in destructive autoimmune processes such as autoimmune thyroiditis, the network of factors and substances released by lymphocytes or macrophages should not play a major role in the pathogenesis of a disease such as Graves' disease, in which autoantibodies have a more important role. Nevertheless, recent studies have underscored the possibility that chemokines may also be of some importance in Graves' disease.[180] Chemokines are a group of peptides that induce chemotaxis of different leukocyte subtypes. Their major function is the recruitment of leukocytes to inflammation sites. In the last few years, experimental evidence has accumulated supporting the concept that IFN-γ inducible chemokines (CXCL9, CXCL10, and CXCL11) and their receptor, CXCR3, play an important role in the initial stage of autoimmune disorders involving endocrine glands. After IFN-γ stimulation, endocrine cells secrete CXCL10, which recruits T_H1 helper lymphocytes expressing CXCR3 and secreting IFN-γ, thus perpetuating the autoimmune inflammation. In Graves' disease, serum levels of CXCL10 are higher in newly diagnosed hyperthyroid patients and decrease when euthyroidism is restored, which may be related to the active inflammatory phase of the disease.[180]

ROLE OF THYROID FOLLICULAR CELLS

Whether primary defects in the thyroid gland contribute to the pathogenesis of thyroid autoimmunity has been pondered since the mid-1980s.[181-183] The observation that thyroid cells from patients with Hashimoto's thyroiditis and Graves' disease express HLA class II antigen (DR), which is usually expressed by professional antigen-presenting cells, led to the hypothesis that aberrant expression of these molecules on thyroid cells could initiate thyroid autoimmunity via direct thyroid autoantigen presentation.[184,185] It was later suggested that expression of HLA class II molecules on thyroid cells is a secondary rather than a primary phenomenon, determined by the cytokines released by the lymphocytic infiltrate.[186,188] Thyroidal HLA-DR expression can be induced by cytokines such as IFN-γ, which is able to induce thyroiditis when administered to susceptible mice and to predisposed human subjects.[186,187] In addition, overexpression of IFN-γ in transgenic mice results in hypothyroidism due to disruption of the thyroid structure.[189,190] However, IFN-γ may not be the sole determinant; its genetic disruption reduced the severity of experimental thyroiditis but did not abrogate it.[191] Moreover, in experimental models of thyroiditis, HLA class II expression appeared to be a late phenomenon that is present only after the infiltrate has appeared, although such observations may depend on the sensitivity of the detecting system used.[192,193] Thus it would appear that HLA class II antigen expression is probably not a primary mechanism leading to Graves' disease, but rather it is important for perpetuation and enhancement of the autoimmune reaction. In this regard, thyroid cells have been shown to be capable of stimulating T lymphocytes both in the presence and in the absence of professional antigen-presenting cells.[194,195] Co-culture of peripheral blood mononuclear cells from Graves' disease patients with homologous thyrocytes induced T-cell activation[182] as well as IFN-γ production and HLA class II antigen expression on thyroid cells.[196] There is evidence that genetic manipulation of HLA class II molecules may affect the susceptibility to the development of experimental autoimmune thyroiditis in mice,[197] but such a phenomenon has not been tested in Graves' disease. In a recent study, some of the HLA-DR natural ligands in Graves'-affected thyroid tissue were identified as thyroglobulin peptide, and it was suggested that binding between HLA-DR and thyroglobulin or thyroglobulin fragments may be involved in the maintenance of the autoimmune inflammatory process.[198]

Local production of chemokines by thyrocytes has been shown, which may be responsible for recruitment of immune cells.[199] As mentioned previously, high levels of CXCL10 are present in the serum of Grave's patients.[180] Professional antigen-presenting cells, such as dendritic cells, macrophages, and even B cells, also exist within the thyroid lymphocytic infiltrate in close relationship with thyrocytes and are involved in thyroid autoantigen presentation.[200,201]

Professional antigen-presenting cells express on their surface a family of co-stimulatory proteins named *B7* that interact with molecules (CD28 and CTLA-4) on the surface of helper (CD4⁺) T cells during antigen presentation.[202] This co-stimulatory process is critical for determining the direction of the immune response, because its absence may result in anergy and/or deletion of antigen-specific T cells. The B7-1 and B7-2 molecules are not expressed on thyroid cells derived from patients with Graves' disease,[203] which suggests that these cells must rely on other co-stimulatory factors, possibly from professional antigen-presenting cells.[202] Co-stimulatory molecules may also influence the resulting T_H1 or T_H2 T-cell phenotype.[150] In this regard, studies on antigen presentation indicate that in the absence of co-stimulatory signals, such as those provided by B7 molecules, HLA class II expression by thyroid cells will lead to continued activation of T cells if the immune response has already been established by professional antigen-presenting cells, whereas it will induce peripheral tolerance of naive, not previously stimulated T cells.[203]

ANIMAL MODELS OF GRAVES' DISEASE

No spontaneous animal diseases mimicking human Graves' disease have been reported, and the absence of such an animal model has slowed the acquisition of knowledge on processes leading to this condition. Experimental immunization with soluble forms of TSHR has led only to antibodies deprived of stimulating activity that did not cause hyperthyroidism in the immunized animals. More recently, a different approach has been successful in inducing hyperthyroidism and goiter, thereby allowing researchers to gain some insights into the pathogenesis of Graves' disease, especially concerning antigen presentation,

the role of T cells and of humoral immunity, and the production of TSH-R monoclonal antibodies.[204-207] In this model, mice are immunized by injecting living cells (professional or nonprofessional antigen-presenting cells) expressing TSHR or by DNA vaccination with TSHR cDNA in plasmid or adenovirus vectors.

Clinical Aspects of Graves' Disease

The hallmarks of Graves' disease are a diffuse goiter associated with the symptoms and signs of thyrotoxicosis and the typical orbitopathy.[208] More rarely, pretibial myxedema and acropachy are present. The onset of symptoms is usually gradual over a period of weeks to months, but it can be abrupt in some cases. In other cases, mild symptoms can exist for years before a diagnosis is made.

Although some symptoms of the syndrome are almost unique to Graves' disease, many are entirely due to thyrotoxicosis and are therefore common to other thyroid disorders but are usually more prominent and severe. Among the distinctive symptoms, ophthalmopathy and pretibial myxedema are most helpful in establishing the correct diagnosis.

CLINICAL MANIFESTATIONS OF GRAVES' HYPERTHYROIDISM

Thyrotoxic symptoms of Graves' disease do not differ from those seen in thyrotoxicosis of other causes (Table 9-3).[209] Most organs are sensitive to thyroid hormone action and are therefore altered by thyroid hormone excess. Symptoms of thyrotoxicosis consequently encompass a wide range of manifestations, each contributing to a clinical picture that can rarely be mistaken when all its components are present. However, the spectrum of manifestations of thyrotoxicosis may range widely from the classic picture to more subtle signs and symptoms, which depends on many variables, including age at onset, duration of thyrotoxicosis, severity of thyrotoxicosis, and possibly, poorly understood individual factors.

Thyroid

The thyroid gland is usually symmetrically enlarged (Fig. 9-4), although nodular glands can be seen, especially in geographic areas of iodine deficiency, where nodular goiter often preexisted. Sometimes true nodules are difficult to distinguish from the lobulations typical of a hyperplasic gland. Goiter size is widely variable, and some patients can even have a gland of normal size. Large goiters can be associated with engorgement of the jugular veins and a positive Pemberton sign (swelling of the jugular veins

Table 9-3. Symptoms of Hyperthyroidism and Their Frequency

Symptom	Frequency (%)
Nervousness	80-95
Fatigue	50-80
Palpitations	65-95
Dyspnea	65-80
Weight loss	50-85
Heat intolerance	40-90
Fatigability	45-85
Oligomenorrhea	45-80
Increased appetite	10-65
Sweating	50-90
Diarrhea	8-33
Eye signs	50-60

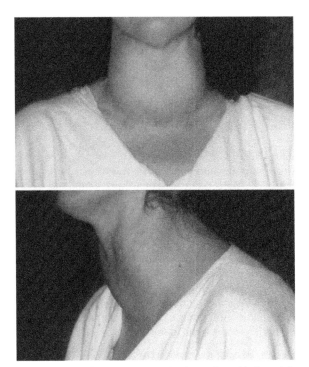

FIGURE 9-4. Large, diffuse symmetrical goiter in a patient with Graves' disease.

upon elevation of the arms). By palpation, the consistency of the gland is generally firm, although softer than in Hashimoto's thyroiditis. Thrills and bruits resulting from increased blood flow may be present on the gland, especially in the early phases of the disease and with a large goiter.

Skin and Appendages

The skin of a thyrotoxic patient is warm, thin, and moist; palmar erythema is common. Dermatographism and pruritus are often reported, but their significance is unclear.[210] Urticaria may also be associated. Vitiligo is frequent, being not a consequence of thyrotoxicosis but rather an associated independent skin autoimmune disease.[211] The hair is friable, diffuse alopecia of mild degree is often observed, but alopecia areata is rare. Nails are soft and friable with longitudinal striations, and onycholysis (detachment of the nail from the ungual bed) is observed in long-lasting cases. Pretibial myxedema and thyroid acropachy, described elsewhere in this chapter, can also be seen.

Cardiovascular System

Heart-related symptoms are a frequent initial complaint in patients with Graves' disease.[212,213] The most common are tachycardia and palpitations. Signs and symptoms of heart failure may also develop, and edema of the lower extremities is often found in elderly patients. The heart and vascular system are major targets of thyroid hormones, which explains the high prevalence of cardiovascular symptoms in thyrotoxic patients with Graves' disease. Cardiac complications may be a major concern in the care of these patients. Thyrotoxicosis causes an increase in both inotropism and chronotropism of the heart. Overall, vascular resistance is decreased because of peripheral vasodilatation. The net effect of these changes is increased cardiac output, which is the major pathophysiologic event. Increased cardiac workload causes increased oxygen consumption, which in turn can precipitate angina pectoris in the presence of preexisting coronary artery disease. Peripheral edema can be observed in the absence

of overt heart failure. Dyspnea on exertion or at rest and chest pain may also be present and are prominent features of thyrotoxic heart disease.

On physical examination, the heart of a thyrotoxic patient is characterized by resting tachycardia. Heart sounds are accentuated. A systolic murmur may be heard on the precordium, sometimes related to associated mitral valve prolapse. Arrhythmias can range from sporadic premature beats to atrial fibrillation.

Electrocardiographic findings are nonspecific and include sinus tachycardia with ST elevation, QT shortening, and PR prolongation. Atrial fibrillation or flutter can occur in up to 10% to 15% of patients, especially if elderly. Ischemic changes can be found when underlying coronary artery disease is present. The observation of reversible heart failure in younger patients with thyrotoxicosis has raised the question whether a distinct thyrotoxic cardiomyopathy exists in the absence of preexisting detectable heart disease.[212,213] Technically, the high-output heart failure typically observed in these cases may not be due to "failure" of the heart pump, but instead only to the changes in the peripheral circulation induced by vasodilatation and sodium-water retention. However, long-lasting tachyarrhythmias have been shown to impair the contractility of cardiac myocytes, and this mechanism has been proposed for the thyrotoxicosis-induced heart failure observed in young patients.[214] In most cases, however, cardiac complications occur in elderly patients in whom underlying heart disease is likely to exist. In this setting, heart failure occurs mainly in the presence of atrial fibrillation or ischemic heart disease.[212,213]

Gastrointestinal Tract

Increased appetite associated with weight loss is a very common complaint and is due to increased catabolism. Increased gastrointestinal motility of the bowel leads to frequent bowel movements and, less often, to diarrhea.[215] These symptoms can be associated with some degree of malabsorption and steatorrhea, which can contribute to weight loss.[216] Atrophic gastritis and/or celiac disease of autoimmune origin may be associated with Graves' disease.[211] Major toxic effects of thyroid hormone on the liver have not been reported. Nonetheless, mild elevations of liver enzymes are often detected in thyrotoxic patients.[217] Thyrotoxicosis-induced liver function abnormalities can last for months and need to be taken into account when examining patients during treatment with antithyroid drugs, because they can be mistaken for adverse reactions to thionamides.

Nervous System

Psychic and nervous symptoms are a prominent and relevant part of the clinical picture.[218] Insomnia and irritability are the most frequent complaints. Patients appear restless and agitated, and logorrhea is often present and becomes clearly evident during history taking. Concentration ability is also decreased. This picture may sometimes confound the physician, and manic disorders have initially been diagnosed in many patients with Graves' disease. Fatigability and asthenia are often present and are important in differentiation from true manic or bipolar disorders. In some cases, nervous signs take the form of "apathetic thyrotoxicosis" with severe apathy, lethargy, and pseudodementia, a profile more commonly observed in elderly patients.[219] In rare cases, true psychoses can be precipitated by thyrotoxicosis and improve with restoration of euthyroidism.[218]

The peripheral nervous system is also deeply affected.[220,221] Fine distal tremor is an almost universal finding and can also be observed on protrusion of the tongue or at the eyelids. Deep tendon reflexes are brisk, with a shortened relaxation time. Clonus can be sometimes elicited. The characteristic stare of a thyrotoxic patient is due to autonomic hyperstimulation of the elevator muscle of the lid and can also be found in the absence of Graves' ophthalmopathy. True thyrotoxic neuropathy has occasionally been reported and is characterized by areflexic flaccid quadriparesis.[220,221]

Muscles

Thyrotoxic patients frequently report muscle weakness and easy exhaustion. In more severe cases, atrophy of variable degree can occur in the setting of a more general wasting syndrome. Specific diseases of the muscle can be associated with Graves' disease. Less than 1% of patients with Graves' disease have classic myasthenia gravis, although ocular myasthenia gravis may be more frequent in these patients.[222-225] Conversely, about 3% of patients with myasthenia gravis have Graves' disease.[223] The pathogenic significance of this association is not known, but it is interesting that the two prototypic diseases characterized by cell surface-receptor autoimmunity can occur together. Recognition of this association is clinically important because thyrotoxic myopathy can worsen the muscular symptoms of myasthenia. Moreover, it is important to correctly distinguish the ocular manifestations of the two disorders (they both cause diplopia), because the treatment is different. Therefore, when the degree of ocular muscle dysfunction in a patient with Graves' disease is disproportionate to the degree of proptosis and inflammatory changes, clinical and serologic (anti–acetylcholine receptor antibodies) tests for myasthenia gravis are warranted.

In some patients, Graves' disease thyrotoxicosis can precipitate crises of periodic hypokalemic paralysis.[226] The syndrome is in all regards identical to familial periodic paralysis, but thyrotoxicosis of various causes is invariably present. The reason for the more frequent association with Graves' disease may merely be that Graves' disease is the most frequent cause of severe and long-lasting thyrotoxicosis in susceptible populations. Periodic hypokalemic paralysis is much more frequent in Asian subjects, in whom an association with certain HLA haplotypes has been observed,[227] but it has also been reported in white and Native American patients.[226] Mutations of ionic (potassium) channel genes have been shown to be responsible for some cases of hypokalemic paralysis in thyrotoxic patients.[228] Effective treatments include potassium replacement, β-blocking agents, and rapid correction of thyrotoxicosis. Relapse of the hypokalemic crisis has occasionally been reported in patients after definitive treatment of the thyrotoxicosis, but it is rare.[226]

Skeletal System

Thyrotoxicosis is known to be associated with an increased rate of bone remodeling.[229-231] The disproportionate increase in bone resorption over new bone formation leads to net bone loss, and consequently hyperthyroid patients have a reduced bone mass. Bone density improves after attainment of euthyroidism, but it often remains below the normal range. The degree of osteoporosis depends on the duration of hyperthyroidism and the coexistence of other risk factors for osteoporosis. Hence postmenopausal women with a history of hyperthyroidism have an increased risk of fractures, and hyperthyroid women are found more frequently among women with fractures.[229-231] The consequences of this effect of thyrotoxicosis on public health have been demonstrated in a large epidemiologic survey showing that fracture-related mortality is significantly increased among women with a history of hyperthyroidism.[232] Mild hypercalcemia and increased levels

of bone turnover markers can be observed in thyrotoxic patients. Their levels are closely correlated with those of serum thyroid hormones and return to normal after correction of thyrotoxicosis.[229-231] It has been recently found that the effects of thyrotoxicosis on bone may reflect the loss of a protective action that TSH exerts via the TNF-α pathway, rather than (or in addition to) a direct action of thyroid hormones on bone.[233-236]

Hematopoietic System

Mild leukopenia with relative lymphocytosis is a relatively common finding in patients with thyrotoxic Graves' disease, which needs to be distinguished from antithyroid drug–induced leucopenia or agranulocytosis.[237] Normocytic anemia is rare, but it can occur.[238] Pernicious anemia occurs in a small minority of patients with Graves' disease, but circulating autoantibodies to gastric parietal cells are found in a much higher percentage of cases and are a sign of associated gastric autoimmunity.[211,239] Aplastic anemia has also been reported.[240] Graves' disease is occasionally associated with autoimmune thrombocytopenic purpura, but nonimmunologic alterations in hemostasis have also been reported.[211] Increases in factor VIII levels and fibrinogen have been reported most consistently, but the clinical relevance of these findings is unknown.[241]

Reproductive System

Females

In severe thyrotoxicosis, the menstrual cycle is often deranged and characterized by oligomenorrhea or amenorrhea.[242-244] As a consequence of impaired ovulation, fertility is decreased, but pregnancy can still occur. The mechanisms for these alterations are poorly understood, but they almost exclusively occur in women with severe weight loss. In women (and in men) with thyrotoxicosis, sex hormone–binding globulin (SHBG) is increased, but the physiologic consequences of this increase are unclear.[245] Thyrotoxicosis in pregnancy is associated with an increased incidence of miscarriage, low-birth-weight infants, and preeclampsia (see later discussion).

Males

Gynecomastia may develop in men, and erectile dysfunction and reduced sperm count are not infrequent.[246] Other features suggesting estrogenic excess include spider angiomas and reduced libido. Total testosterone is increased as a result of increased SHBG concentrations, but unbound and bioavailable testosterone levels remain in the normal range. The circulating estradiol level is increased, probably because of increased peripheral aromatization of testosterone. All these changes are fully reversible with treatment of thyrotoxicosis and require no other specific treatment. Treatment of reduced libido with testosterone may result in worsening of gynecomastia.

Metabolic Changes

Significant weight loss with normal or increased caloric intake is a hallmark of thyrotoxicosis.[247] It is explained by an increased metabolic rate, with increased heat production as a net result. Mitochondrial oxygen consumption is increased by thyroid hormones in almost every tissue. Increased mitochondrial activity and numbers were also shown in several tissues in experimental thyrotoxicosis. The use of oxygen by mitochondria is inefficient in experimental thyrotoxicosis in that fewer molecules of high-energy substrates are produced per molecule of oxygen used. A widespread increase in the use of ATP by cation transporters in tissues has been proposed to explain the increased energy use, although this point is controversial.[247,248] Whatever the mechanism, increased heat production and dispersion are manifested as a moderate rise in body temperature that is partially compensated for by increased sweating, heat intolerance, and weight loss.[247]

Peripheral utilization of carbohydrates is increased in thyrotoxicosis, in keeping with the enhanced energy consumption, and the primary mechanism seems to be an increased cellular transport of glucose.[249] Thyrotoxicosis, however, also causes some degree of insulin resistance.[249] Consequently, diabetes mellitus may be exacerbated by thyrotoxicosis. Type I diabetes mellitus can be associated with Graves' disease within polyglandular autoimmune syndromes.[211]

Serum cholesterol and triglyceride levels are decreased in thyrotoxicosis, mainly because of a decrease in low-density lipoproteins (LDLs), in spite of an increase of hepatic lipogenesis.[250,251] This reduction in lipids can result from the decrease in total body fat as a consequence of weight loss, but specific actions of thyroid hormones on lipid metabolism have also been described. Cholesterol conversion to bile acid in the liver is enhanced, and LDL receptor number on adipocytes is increased as well.[250] These phenomena may account for the increased turnover of cholesterol and triglycerides. Thyroid function may alter adipokines, a number of biologically active substances produced by adipocyte with different physiologic functions, which include leptin, adiponectin, and resistin.[251,252] Thyrotoxicosis was reported to be associated with elevated serum levels of adiponectin, but the finding was not confirmed.[251-254] Serum leptin and resistin seem to be unaffected by thyrotoxicosis.[251-254]

Protein metabolism is altered during thyrotoxicosis, with both increased protein synthesis and degradation. In most cases, however, degradation predominates and causes negative nitrogen balance. This imbalance can be partly controlled by adequate calories and protein intake.[247]

DISTINCTIVE MANIFESTATIONS OF GRAVES' DISEASE

Graves' Ophthalmopathy

Graves' ophthalmopathy is the clinical manifestation of an inflammatory disorder of the orbit and is almost exclusively associated with Graves' disease.[255,256] The many aspects of this puzzling disorder are examined in detail elsewhere in this book. The prominence of the signs of Graves' ophthalmopathy makes this feature the most striking physical finding in some patients (Fig. 9-5). Most of the manifestations of Graves' ophthalmopathy are related to its central pathophysiologic event, an increase in the volume of retro-orbital tissue because of inflammation. As a consequence, the eye bulb is pushed forward and proptosis or exophthalmos results. Venous congestion causes swelling and edema of the periorbital tissue. Inflammatory changes also involve the extraocular muscles and may cause diplopia. The eyes are protruding, often asymmetrically. Lid retraction is seen and can be worsened by the concurrent thyrotoxicosis. Edema and swelling of the lids are also typical. The conjunctival mucosa is injected and edematous (chemosis). Lagophthalmos (incomplete palpebral closure) and lacrimal gland dysfunction may combine to cause drying of the mucosal and corneal surfaces and consequently irritation and (less often) corneal ulceration.

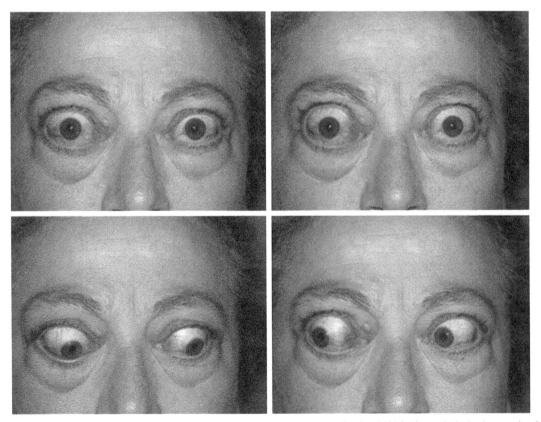

FIGURE 9-5. Typical ophthalmopathy in a patient with Graves' disease. Proptosis, inflammatory signs (conjunctival injection, palpebral edema and redness, lacrimal gland edema), and eyelid retraction are quite evident.

Photophobia, burning sensation, retrobulbar pain, tearing, and a sandy sensation are common symptoms and may initially mislead clinicians into making a diagnosis of conjunctivitis. Optic neuropathy resulting from optic nerve compression by inflamed and swollen extraocular muscles at the orbital apex may occur in the most severe cases and cause reduction or loss of vision. When the proptosis is extremely severe, subluxation of the bulb outside the orbit may occur and pose an immediate threat to visual function.

Clinical signs or symptoms of ophthalmopathy are present in about 50% of Graves' patients, with a wide variability of its degree of severity.[255,256] When present, the onset of Graves' ophthalmopathy coincides with the onset of thyrotoxicosis in about 40% of cases, follows it in another 40%, and precedes it in 20%.[255,256] Even when the onset of the two disorders does not coincide, each occurs within 18 months from the onset of the first manifestation. As reported later in the chapter, the presence of ophthalmopathy may affect the choice of treatment of hyperthyroidism in patients with Graves' disease.[257]

Pretibial (or Localized) Myxedema and Thyroid Acropachy

When von Basedow first described his cases of Graves' disease,[5] he also reported a puzzling manifestation of the skin characterized by a nonpitting swelling of the pretibial areas, brownish and reddish in color, well delimited, and containing little free fluid. This manifestation of unknown pathogenesis is relatively rare in patients with Graves' disease and is almost invariably observed only when Graves' ophthalmopathy is also present.[258] Although most frequently localized to the pretibial regions, it has also been observed on the forearms and other areas.[258] Different degrees

of severity have been described (Fig. 9-6). *Diffuse pretibial myxedema* refers to the mildest form, with only superficial diffuse edema. Localized areas of more prominent infiltration that assume a papular aspect characterize the *nodular form*. In the most severe forms, *elephantiasis* occurs with extensive swelling and sometimes ulceration.

Histopathologic studies have shown that the swelling is caused by the inordinate accumulation of hyaluronic acid in the subcutaneous layers of the involved areas, strikingly similar to the diffuse myxedematous changes of hypothyroidism but also to some extent to the changes in orbital tissues in Graves' ophthalmopathy. A lymphocytic infiltrate may be observed, but it is by no means a constant finding. The origin of the mucinous material (hyaluronic acid) appears to be the skin fibroblast.[258]

The cause of pretibial myxedema is unknown, as is its relationship to the pathogenetic events of Graves' disease.[258,259] Most experts in the field agree that pretibial myxedema is another autoimmune manifestation of Graves' disease, because of their association and of the almost invariable presence of serum TRAbs in patients with myxedema.[258,259] T-cell receptor V chain restriction has been observed in the lymphocytic infiltration of patients with early pretibial myxedema and suggests the presence of an ongoing antigen-specific immune response.[260] As for Graves' ophthalmopathy, TSHR is the obvious candidate antigen.[258] Using patients' serum as a tool, putative TSH-binding sites on pretibial fibroblasts were detected.[261] In addition, expression of TSHR mRNA and TSHR immunoreactivity in human fibroblasts from the pretibial region were found, as well as immunoreactivity for TSHR in pretibial connective tissue from patients with myxedema, but not from normal subjects.[262-264] In contrast, thy-

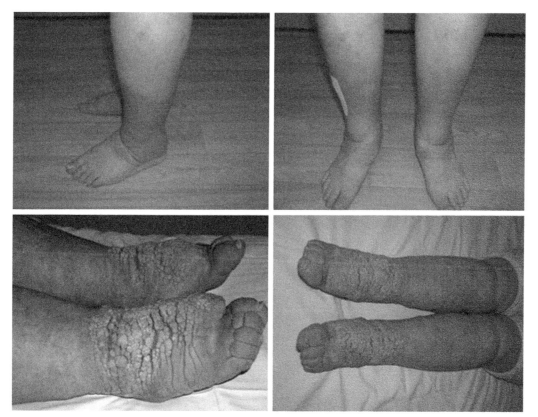

FIGURE 9-6. Two variants of pretibial myxedema patients with Graves' disease. *Upper panel:* A classical form of pretibial myxedema: The skin of the pretibial area appears swollen, reddened, and typically wrinkled and takes the appearance of orange skin. *Lower panel:* Elephantiasic pretibial myxedema: The skin appears severely thickened with fibromatous-like lesions; inflammation is extended up to the knees.

roglobulin, another candidate antigen which may contribute to the pathogenesis of Graves' ophthalmopathy by reaching orbital tissues from the thyroid,[265] was not found in pretibial myxedema (Marinò et al., unpublished). In summary, the pathogenesis of pretibial myxedema, similar to that of Graves' ophthalmopathy, remains obscure, although most studies support the hypothesis of an autoimmune disorder because of the ectopic expression of thyroidal antigens or the presence of cross-reacting antigens localized to restricted regions of the human skin.

Thyroid acropachy is another rare manifestation of Graves' disease that is observed most often in long-lasting and usually severe forms of Graves' ophthalmopathy and pretibial myxedema; it is almost invariably associated with the presence of serum TRAbs.[258,266] Thyroid acropachy is characterized by clubbing and soft tissue swelling of the last phalanx of the fingers and toes, all changes that are similar to those observed in chronic respiratory insufficiency. The overlying skin is often discolored and thickened. Microscopically, increased glycosaminoglycan deposition in the skin is observed. Subperiosteal new bone formation is also present. Again, the pathogenesis and the link with the immunologic changes of Graves' disease are unknown, being the most "popular" hypothesis similar to those formulated for Graves' ophthalmopathy and pretibial myxedema.[258,266] The disease develops without symptoms over a period of years, and it often goes unnoticed by the patient. This manifestation of Graves' disease is harmless and asymptomatic and generally requires no treatment.

CLINICAL DIAGNOSIS

The typical patient with Graves' disease complains of palpitations, nervousness, weight loss, and increased appetite. The patient appears restless, anxious, and logorrheic. On physical examination, the eye signs of Graves' ophthalmopathy, proptosis and lid lag, are often immediately detected and contribute to the "frightened" appearance of the patient. A symmetrical goiter is often present on inspection and almost always palpable. The skin is moist and warm, thin and smooth. The typical fine distal tremor is easily observed and readily distinguished from other forms of tremor. Examination of the cardiovascular system shows tachycardia with loud heart sounds. Premature beats are frequent, and complete arrhythmia from atrial fibrillation is sometimes present. In its classic form, the diagnosis of Graves' disease is readily made on clinical grounds before any laboratory test is performed. Infrequent but significant exceptions to this rule include the coexistence of nodules, which may suggest toxic nodular goiter, or nonthyroidal diseases, which may blunt or confuse the clinical picture. Graves' disease at its very beginning may produce a mild clinical picture and can be difficult to recognize in otherwise healthy people. In some cases, the thyroid may not be enlarged and ophthalmopathy may be absent or clinically undetectable. Symptoms of hyperthyroidism may be less evident in elderly people, who often have the apathetic variant of thyrotoxicosis. For these reasons and to establish a thorough baseline assessment of the patient, the clinical diagnosis must be supported by an accurate laboratory workup.

LABORATORY DIAGNOSIS

Hormone Measurements

Although laboratory assessment of thyroid function is treated in detail elsewhere in this book, it seems appropriate to review in this section the mainstays of the diagnosis of Graves' hyperthyroidism. Suspicion of hyperthyroidism can be confirmed by thyroid hormone measurements. TSH is the single most useful test in confirming the presence of thyrotoxicosis.[267] By sensitive assays, TSH should be undetectable or low in all patients with thyrotoxicosis of thyroidal origin. Low TSH levels can also be observed in a number of conditions such as nonthyroidal illnesses or endogenous or exogenous corticosteroid excess. Therefore, parallel measurement of thyroid hormone levels is recommended in all patients for a correct interpretation of a low TSH level. Total thyroxine (TT_4) and triiodothyronine (TT_3) measurements are relatively inexpensive and reliable, but they can yield high values in otherwise euthyroid subjects with conditions characterized by increased levels of serum thyroxine-binding globulin (TBG), most commonly pregnancy, oral contraceptive use, and chronic liver disease.[267] Familial excess of TBG and familial dysalbuminemic hyperthyroxinemia are rare disorders that also cause elevated TT_4 levels.[268] Free thyroid hormone measurements, although not completely devoid of flaws, are therefore more satisfactory but more expensive.[267] In most iodine-sufficient countries, a single free thyroxine (FT_4) measurement is sufficient to confirm or reject the suspicion of thyrotoxicosis. After the TSH level, FT_4 is the test most often used in North America for thyroid function screening and therefore the one that most clinicians are familiar with. However, in iodine-deficient countries, a significant proportion of hyperthyroid patients (up to 12%) may have normal FT_4 levels with elevated free T_3 (FT_3) levels, a condition termed T_3 toxicosis.[267] Conversely, FT_4 can be falsely elevated in conditions causing reduced peripheral conversion of T_4 to T_3, such as amiodarone administration or high-dose propranolol treatment. In our practice, we initially measure both FT_4 and FT_3 levels together with TSH, with little additional expense, to obtain a complete baseline assessment of thyroid function status. Circulating thyroglobulin concentrations are high in hyperthyroidism and low in factitious thyrotoxicosis. Measurement of thyroglobulin in serum is therefore useful in the differential diagnosis of thyrotoxicosis in patients with no goiter or ophthalmopathy.[269]

Circulating Autoantibodies

Although by no means necessary, tests for circulating thyroglobulin (TgAb) and thyroid peroxidase (TPOAb) antibodies may be useful in confirming the presence of thyroid autoimmunity. TPOAbs can be detected by commercial radioimmunoassays in up to 90% of patients with untreated Graves' disease,[270,271] whereas TgAbs are less frequently positive, in about 50% to 60% of cases, depending on the sensitivity of the method used.[272,273] Both antibodies can be detected in a relatively high percentage (up to 25%) of normal subjects, especially elderly women or in patients with other nonautoimmune thyroid disorders such as nodular goiter or thyroid carcinoma.[273,274] Therefore, tests for TPOAb and TgAb have limited diagnostic value and must be considered complementary to the diagnosis.

TRAb assay is very specific and sensitive for hyperthyroid Graves' disease. Up to 98% of untreated patients are positive with second-generation radioreceptor assays, with very few false-positive results.[126] The radioreceptor test for TRAb is widely available in commercial laboratories but quite expensive. It is needed in selected situations in which confirmation of the nature of thyrotoxicosis is required or when the clinical picture or thyroid function tests are not clear. These situations include the differential diagnosis of thyrotoxicosis in pregnancy, the nodular variants of Graves' disease, which must be differentiated from toxic nodular goiter,[275] and patients with exophthalmos without thyrotoxicosis (euthyroid Graves' disease).[224]

Table 9-4. Causes of Thyrotoxicosis and Features Different*
From Those of Graves' Disease

Cause	Distinctive Feature
Toxic nodular goiter	"Hot" nodule/s at thyroid scan
	Nodules at thyroid ultrasound
	Undetectable TRAb
Subacute thyroiditis	Low RAIU
	Neck pain
	Elevated indexes of inflammation
	Undetectable TRAb
Painless thyroiditis	Low RAIU
	Undetectable TRAb
Factitious thyrotoxicosis	Low RAIU
	Low serum thyroglobulin
	Undetectable TRAb
Struma ovarii	Low thyroid RAIU
	Positive abdominal RAIU
	Undetectable TRAb
Amiodarone-induced thyrotoxicosis	Low RAIU
	High urinary iodine
	Undetectable TRAb
Central hyperthyroidism	Inappropriately normal or high TSH
	Undetectable TRAb
TSH receptor activating mutations	Undetectable TRAb
Vesicular mole	Undetectable TRAb
Choriocarcinoma	Undetectable TRAb
Metastatic follicular thyroid cancer	Undetectable TRAb

*Generally but not always different.

Thyroid Radioiodine Uptake and Scanning

Before the introduction of accurate thyroid hormone and TSH measurements, a radioactive iodine uptake (RAIU) test was always required for the evaluation of thyrotoxicosis. Normal ranges for RAIU vary according to the status of iodine supply in the population.[276,277] In iodine-replete countries, the upper limit of normal RAIU 24 hours after the administration of a tracer dose of radioiodine is around 25%, whereas it may reach 40% in areas with mild to moderate iodine deficiency. In patients with Graves' disease, a high value is always found after 24 hours, and in some cases the value after 3 or 6 hours can be even higher as a consequence of the rapid iodine turnover typical of Graves' disease glands. The RAIU test is not readily available as an office-based approach and is not always required. It can be very useful, however, to rule out silent or subacute thyroiditis, factitious thyrotoxicosis, and type II amiodarone-induced thyrotoxicosis[278] (Table 9-4). RAIU results can also be used before radioiodine treatment of hyperthyroidism to calculate the dose needed (see relevant heading). RAIU, like any other radioisotopic in vivo procedure, is absolutely contraindicated during pregnancy.

Thyroid imaging with radioisotopes can be performed with radioiodine at the time that RAIU is performed or by using pertechnetate 99m (Fig. 9-7A). Thyroid scanning in Graves' disease is useful when coexisting nodules are detected by palpation and their functional status needs to be evaluated.

Thyroid Ultrasound

The thyroid gland is an excellent candidate for ultrasound studies, given its superficial anatomic location and the presence of a high number of liquid-solid interfaces (virtually one at every follicle/colloid-lining surface), which in normal conditions produce high reflectivity. Although the equipment is still relatively quite costly, it is now affordable at the office level and requires little maintenance. Thyroid ultrasound is an invaluable

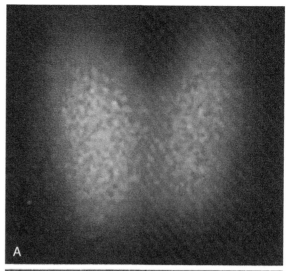

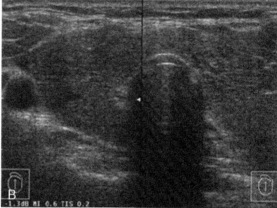

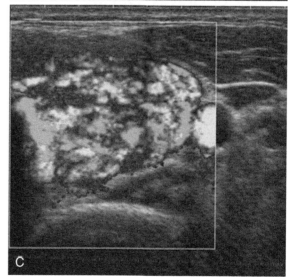

FIGURE 9-7. Thyroid scanning **(A)**, ultrasound **(B)**, and color flow Doppler **(C)** findings in Graves' disease. **A,** An enlarged thyroid with diffuse homogeneous and active uptake is observed at Pertechnetate 99m scanning. **B,** The thyroid is enlarged, and the tissue appears diffusely hypoechoic. **C,** Markedly increased signals show the diffuse increase in thyroid vascularity.

tool in the diagnosis of thyroid nodular disorders and has become more and more an extension of the physical examination for many endocrinologists. Its application to non-nodular disorders of the thyroid has come from early observations of typical changes of the gland's echoic structure in thyroid autoimmune diseases.[279] In hyperthyroid Graves' disease, the echoic pattern undergoes diffuse changes. The tissue, possibly because of the reduction in colloid content, the increase in thyroid vascularity, and the lymphocytic infiltrate, becomes typically hypoechoic (Fig. 9-7B). This pattern is similar to the one observed in chronic thyroiditis and, when diffuse, is almost pathognomonic of thyroid autoimmunity.[280] Therefore, thyroid ultrasound can be useful during the evaluation of thyrotoxicosis to confirm the suspicion of thyroid autoimmunity. Thyroid ultrasound also allows accurate measurement of thyroid size,[281] information that can help in the decision-making process when definitive treatment is being planned (see later). Moreover, careful definition of coexisting nodules can be obtained when needed. Therefore, thyroid ultrasonography provides very useful information in the initial evaluation of patients with Graves' disease, although it is seldom strictly required for purely diagnostic purposes.

Color flow Doppler (CFD) techniques have been applied to the study of glands with Graves' disease. CFD allows semiquantitative measurement of blood flow to the thyroid gland.[282] In untreated Graves' disease, a distinct CFD pattern characterized by markedly increased signals with a patchy distribution is usually observed (Fig. 9-7C). This pattern, in conjunction with a hypoechoic pattern, allows distinction from Hashimoto's thyroiditis. In this setting, CFD studies of the thyroid gland can be useful in distinguishing hyperthyroidism of Graves' disease from thyrotoxicosis of other causes, such as amiodarone-induced thyrotoxicosis, subacute thyroiditis, painless thyroiditis and factitious thyrotoxicosis. For this reason, CFD evaluation may become a valid substitute for RAIU when these conditions are included in the differential diagnosis.

Treatment of Graves' Disease

Etiologic treatment of Graves' disease is not available at present. Therefore, the major aim of current methods is correction of thyrotoxicosis in all cases and treatment of Graves' ophthalmopathy when present and severe (detailed elsewhere in this textbook). Additional goals include relief of compressive symptoms from large goiters.

Correction of thyroid hormone overproduction can be obtained by inhibition of its synthesis or release or by ablation of thyroid tissue via surgery or radioiodine. In addition, the peripheral metabolism of thyroid hormone can be altered in a favorable way by available drugs.

Selection of the treatment option from among those available should be made after careful consideration of the many variables inherent in any given patient, but there is room for the patient's choice in most cases. The patient should therefore participate in the choice of treatment, after thorough information on the therapeutic alternatives.

OVERVIEW OF THERAPEUTIC TOOLS IN GRAVES' DISEASE THYROTOXICOSIS

Thionamides

Clinical Pharmacology

Thionamides (methimazole, carbimazole, and propylthiouracil) were first described and introduced into clinical practice in the early 1940s.[9] The major action of thionamides is to inhibit the organification of iodine and coupling of iodotyrosines, thus blocking the synthesis of thyroid hormones.[237,283] Carbimazole is not active as it is, but it is almost completely converted to

Table 9-5. Pharmacologic Properties of Thionamides: Comparison Between Methimazole and Propylthiouracil

Property	Methimazole	Propylthiouracil
Relative potency	>10 (up to 50)	I
Administration route	PO	PO
Absorption	Almost complete	Almost complete
Binding to serum proteins	Negligible	75%
Serum half-life (hours)	4-6	I-2
Duration of action (hours)	>24	12-24
Transplacental passage	Low	Lower
Levels in breast milk	Low	Lower
Inhibition of deiodinase	No	Yes

methimazole in the body, and their effects are comparable. Propylthiouracil has the additional effect of partially inhibiting the conversion of T_4 to T_3 in peripheral tissues, but this effect is of limited clinical value. Methimazole is at least 10 times more potent than propylthiouracil. The pharmacologic properties of the two major thionamides are compared in Table 9-5.

Both methimazole and propylthiouracil are very effective in controlling hyperthyroidism, and their side-effect record is quite similar, thus making the choice between the two drugs largely a matter of personal preference and local availability. Antithyroid drugs do not block the release of preformed thyroid hormones, so euthyroidism is not obtained until intrathyroidal hormone and iodine stores are depleted. This process requires 1 to 6 weeks, depending on factors such as disease activity, initial levels of circulating thyroid hormones, and intrathyroidal hormone and iodine stores. Large goiters with abundant deposits of thyroid hormone, especially when iodine excess is present, often show a delayed response to thionamides.

The main problem with thionamide treatment is the high relapse rate of thyrotoxicosis after discontinuation of even long-term treatment. Although remission rates on the order of 50% to 60% within 1 year after withdrawal of thionamides have been reported in a few series,[284] in most studies hyperthyroidism recurred in 50% to 80% of patients, depending on the duration of the follow-up period.[285-288] Remission rates have been decreasing in the last decades, possibly as a result of increased iodine supply in the diet.[289,290] A practical problem is that no single test or combination of tests will accurately separate patients who will relapse from those who will not. Size of the goiter before or during antithyroid drug treatment, HLA-DR3 typing, TRAb or TPOAb levels, serum thyroglobulin concentrations, thyroid echogenicity by ultrasound, circulating activated T cells, T-cell subset ratios, and presence of Graves' ophthalmopathy, have all been indicated as significant pretreatment risk factors for relapse, but none has the required sensitivity or specificity to predict the outcome in individual patients. The presence of a large goiter seems to be the most significant predictor of future hyperthyroidism relapse[287] (Fig. 9-8). Similar considerations apply during treatment to parameters such as T_3 suppression of ^{99m}Tc uptake, the thyrotropin-releasing hormone test, and the T_3/T_4 ratio at the time of discontinuation of thionamide therapy.[286,287,291-297] In children, a longer initial duration of euthyroid state with antithyroid drugs seems to be the only variable related to the risk of relapse.[288] Regardless of age, a good predictor of relapse of hyperthyroidism is a positive TSAb test before discontinuation of medical treatment. However, even when TSAbs disappear, the chances of relapse are still high, ranging from 20% to 50%.

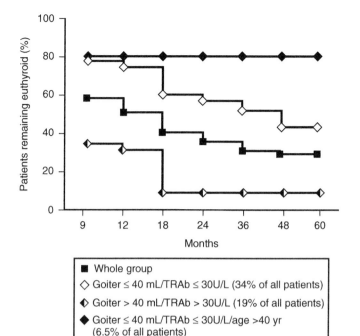

FIGURE 9-8. Effect of goiter size and thyroid-stimulating hormone receptor antibody (TRAb) level at the time of antithyroid drug discontinuation on the incidence of relapses of hyperthyroidism in a cohort of patients with Graves' disease. (Modified from Vitti P, Rago T, Chiovato L et al: Clinical features of patients with Graves' disease undergoing remission after antithyroid drug treatment. Thyroid 7:369–375, 1997.)

Most relapses of hyperthyroidism occur within 3 to 6 months after medical therapy is discontinued, and more than two thirds of patients who relapse will do so within 2 years. However, hyperthyroidism can also recur much later. Late evolution to primary hypothyroidism can be observed as well, mainly in patients who remain euthyroid after discontinuation of therapy.[298,299] Relapse of hyperthyroidism after a full cycle of thionamides is a strong indication for alternative treatments such as radioiodine or thyroidectomy, but a second course of the drug can be given, for example, to adolescents, while bearing in mind that people who have relapsed once are more likely to do so after a second cycle.

Minor side effects of thionamides have been reported in 1% to 15% of patients, but the average appears to be 6%. Pruritus, skin rash, and much less commonly, urticaria are the most prominent manifestations.[283] Arthralgias have also been reported. These side effects frequently resolve spontaneously despite continued therapy. However, when any of them occur, it is generally advisable to replace one thionamide with the other, although cross-sensitivity to these drugs may occur. Antihistamine drugs can be used to control mild side effects. Slight elevations in liver enzyme levels have often been reported, and sometimes it is difficult to distinguish this effect of thionamides from the effect of thyrotoxicosis itself. When detected, serious alterations in liver function test results must be monitored closely because toxic hepatitis may develop suddenly.

Serious side effects are uncommon with thionamides and are observed in approximately 3 of every 1000 patients.[283,300] Agranulocytosis (granulocyte count <500/mm³) may be observed with both methimazole and propylthiouracil. Agranulocytosis has been reported more frequently in elderly patients, but it can occur at any age. It is most often detected within the first 3 to 4 months after starting therapy. Agranulocytosis may develop so suddenly that even weekly white blood cell counts may not

detect it. Agranulocytosis is typically initially manifested by fever and evidence of infections, most often in the upper respiratory tract. Instructing all patients taking antithyroid drugs to report these symptoms immediately is probably the safest measure for immediate detection of this complication. Routine white blood cell counts should be performed in all patients before initiation of treatment, because mild leukopenia is common in Graves' disease and needs to be distinguished from a drug reaction. In addition to prompt discontinuation of the antithyroid drug, treatment of agranulocytosis includes the administration of broad-spectrum antibiotics and growth factors to stimulate bone marrow. Patients usually recover within 2 to 3 weeks, but some deaths have been reported from this complication.

Cholestatic (mostly observed with methimazole) or necrotic (mostly observed with propylthiouracil) hepatitis is another rare but severe complication of thionamide treatment, being associated with significant mortality and sometimes requiring liver transplantation.[283,300] Vasculitis and lupus-like syndromes are even rarer. In the presence of a major adverse reaction to thionamides, such as agranulocytosis, hepatitis, or vasculitis, prompt withdrawal of the drug is mandatory. The risk of cross-reactivity is such that switching from methimazole to propylthiouracil or vice versa is not recommended when side effects are severe, so alternative treatments of thyrotoxicosis must be sought.

Treatment Strategies

The purpose of treatment of Graves' disease hyperthyroidism with antithyroid drugs is to achieve stable euthyroidism. Antithyroid drugs can be used either as preparatory treatment before surgery or radioiodine or as a primary management tool of the disease in an attempt to induce long-term remission of thyrotoxicosis. A direct effect of methimazole and propylthiouracil on the immune system has been proposed to explain the observation that a minority of patients experience long-lasting remissions of Graves' disease thyrotoxicosis after withdrawal of these drugs.[148] This view is suggested by the following lines of evidence. In some follow-up studies, patients treated with antithyroid drugs had a higher remission rate than did those to whom β-blockers alone were administered,[148] but randomized studies have never been performed. Treatment of Graves' disease with antithyroid drugs is followed by a fall in the levels of circulating TRAb, AbTg, and AbTPO,[146,301-303] although this effect is not dose dependent.[284] In vitro experiments have suggested a down-regulating effect of methimazole on antigen presentation,[304] and in vivo studies have shown that the drug is able to reduce the severity of experimental thyroiditis.[305,306] Despite these observations, the immunosuppressive effect of thionamides remains controversial. A decrease in circulating thyroid antibody titer has also been observed in hyperthyroid patients treated with perchlorate, a drug with different pharmacologic properties.[307] Restoration of euthyroidism per se might be responsible for the decrease in thyroid autoantibodies, through a direct effect of thyroid hormone on the immune system.[308] The natural history of the disease, which like that of many other autoimmune disorders is characterized by cycles of spontaneous relapse and remission, could also explain the reduction in thyroid autoantibody titers. In other words, a course of 12 to 24 months of thionamides would merely be a way of keeping the patient euthyroid while waiting for the autoimmune process to subside or even vanish.

Thionamide treatment is usually started with high doses (20 to 40 mg/day of methimazole or 200 to 400 mg/day of propylthiouracil). Doses of methimazole above 40 mg/day are rarely necessary. When long-term thionamide treatment is planned, one of two treatment strategies is currently used:

1. Maintenance of euthyroidism with the minimum effective dose throughout the trial period, with thyroid function tests performed every 1 to 3 months. The minimum dose capable of maintaining euthyroidism is derived by "back-titration" every 4 to 6 weeks.
2. Administration of fixed, relatively high doses of thionamide in combination with levothyroxine to prevent iatrogenic hypothyroidism, the so-called block-and-replace regimen.

With both schemes, patients should be kept completely euthyroid, with serum TSH levels within the normal range.

The second protocol was proposed because of the supposed immunosuppressive effect of higher doses of thionamides and because of studies suggesting a greater remission rate of hyperthyroidism in Graves' patients treated with high doses of thionamides (60 versus 15 mg of methimazole per day).[309] The addition of levothyroxine supposedly provides an extra advantage, and very high remission rates were reported in Japanese patients treated with methimazole for 6 months and then given a combination of methimazole and levothyroxine for an additional year, followed by levothyroxine alone for 3 years.[309,310] However, the latter results have not been reproduced by a number of subsequent studies.[301-315] In a prospective randomized trial of low (10 mg/day) versus moderately high (40 mg/day) doses of methimazole, no advantages were observed in terms of a decrease in TRAb titer or the rate of relapse of hyperthyroidism.[284] The rate of adverse reactions was greater in the group of patients receiving methimazole at 40 mg/day. Thus at present, the block-and-replace regimen has no proven advantage, although one point in favor of it is that it probably requires less testing. The block-and-replacement strategy can also be useful in rare patients who experience changes from hyperthyroidism to hypothyroidism and vice versa after minimal changes in the dosage of antithyroid drugs ("brittle hyperthyroidism"). In these unusual patients, maintenance of euthyroidism is difficult with antithyroid drugs alone.

Regardless of the chosen regimen, treatment is maintained for 12 to 24 months, after which thionamide therapy is usually discontinued. Indefinite treatment even with low doses of thionamides is not a common practice.

In summary, thionamide treatment of Graves' disease thyrotoxicosis has the major advantages of not causing permanent hypothyroidism and of limiting exposure to radiation. It is, however, associated with a very high failure rate, and in many cases it is only a way to delay thyroid ablation by radioiodine or surgery.

Iodine and Iodine-Containing Compounds

Inorganic iodine given in pharmacologic doses (as Lugol's solution or as saturated solution of potassium iodide [SSKI]) decreases its own transport into the thyroid, inhibits iodine organification (the Wolff-Chaikoff effect), and blocks the release of T_4 and T_3 from the gland.[316] As an additional advantage, iodine sharply decreases the vascularity of the thyroid in Graves' disease.[317,318] These effects are, however, transient and last a few days or weeks, after which the antithyroid action of pharmacologic iodine is lost and thyrotoxicosis recurs or may worsen. Therefore, iodine therapy is now used only for short periods in the preparation of patients for surgery, after euthyroidism has already been achieved and maintained with thionamides. Iodine is also used in the management of severe thyrotoxicosis (thyroid storm) because of

its ability to inhibit thyroid hormone release acutely. The usual dose of Lugol's solution is 3 to 5 drops three times a day, and that of SSKI is 1 to 3 drops three times daily.

Oral cholecystographic agents (iopanoic acid and sodium ipodate) produce a very rapid fall in the serum concentration of thyroid hormones.[319-321] These agents act through a dual mechanism: virtually complete inhibition of the peripheral conversion of T_4 to T_3 and prevention of thyroid hormone secretion because of the inorganic iodine released from the drug.[322,323] The first action is the predominant one and makes these drugs highly effective when rapid management of thyrotoxicosis is needed. The rate of fall in T_3 levels after treatment is started approaches the physiologic half-life of the hormone, approximately 1 day. Although early reports suggested that these iodinated compounds could be successfully used as a primary therapy for hyperthyroidism in doses of 0.5 to 1 g/day, they proved to be of limited value in long-term treatment because of the escape of thyroid hormone synthesis from the blocking effect of iodine.[324-326] Moreover, they provide the thyroid with a load of iodine, which may make the use of radioiodine unfeasible for some weeks. Therefore, these agents are ideally used in emergency situations when rapid control of thyrotoxicosis is needed, in preparation for thyroid surgery, or while waiting for the effect of radioiodine therapy. In the latter case, they may also be used to prevent or correct the transient thyrotoxicosis caused by the release of preformed thyroid hormone, as it can occur after radioiodine treatment.

Perchlorate

Perchlorate inhibits active transport of iodine into the thyroid.[327] Side effects (gastric irritation) and adverse effects (aplastic anemia) are not infrequent and preclude the use of perchlorate in the long-term management of Graves' disease thyrotoxicosis.[328] In conjunction with thionamides, perchlorate has been successfully used as a tool for depleting the thyroidal iodine overload in amiodarone-induced hyperthyroidism.[329]

Lithium

It has been reported that the use of lithium may be beneficial in Graves' patients undergoing radioiodine therapy.[330] If given on the day of thionamide withdrawal (5 days before radioiodine) for 19 days, lithium has been found to reduce markedly the extent of thyrotoxicosis either due to thionamide withdrawal before radioiodine or to radioiodine itself after its administration. The dosage used was 900 mg/day, but even doses of 450 mg/day seem to be effective. The effects of lithium possibly reflect a direct inhibitory action on hormone release or on intrathyroidal iodine turnover. In the patients treated with this type of therapy, no adverse effects have been reported, even though psychic effects are in theory possible.[331]

β-Adrenergic Antagonist Drugs

Many of the manifestations of thyrotoxicosis, especially those in the cardiovascular system, are due to hyperactivity or hypersensitivity of the sympathetic nervous system. Blockade of β-adrenergic receptors thus ameliorates the manifestations of thyrotoxicosis that are related to sympathetic action, such as tachycardia, palpitation, tremor, and anxiety.[332] This effect is much faster than that obtained with thionamides, and for this reason β-blockers are important in the early management of thyrotoxicosis. β-Adrenergic antagonists do not affect thyroid hormone synthesis and release or their action at the level of many tissues, such as bone. These drugs should not be used alone in Graves' disease thyrotoxicosis, except for short periods before and/or after radioiodine therapy. Since the introduction of propranolol, a number of new agents became available with a longer duration (atenolol, metoprolol, and nadolol) or with greater cardioselectivity (atenolol, metoprolol, bisoprolol). None of these drugs seems to have an advantage over the others, and the choice largely depends on the personal experience of the physician. Propranolol has the additional advantage of mild inhibition of the peripheral conversion of T_4 to T_3,[333] but the real clinical advantage provided by this pharmacologic property is unclear. The usual contraindications to β-adrenergic antagonists, such as asthma, should be taken into account. β-Blocker use can be rapidly tapered and discontinued once stable euthyroidism is obtained with thionamides, radioiodine, or surgery.

Glucocorticoids

Glucocorticoids in high doses inhibit the peripheral conversion of T_4 to T_3. In Graves' disease thyrotoxicosis, glucocorticoids appear to decrease T_4 secretion by the thyroid, possibly by immune suppression, but the efficiency and duration of this effect are unknown. Because of the significant side effects associated with the long-term use of glucocorticoids and the effectiveness of alternative treatments, use of these drugs in the management of Graves' hyperthyroidism is not justified. On the contrary, the immunosuppressive effect of glucocorticoids in high doses is commonly exploited in the treatment of ophthalmopathy and dermopathy of Graves' disease. In severe thyrotoxicosis or thyroid storm, short-term glucocorticoid administration may be used as a general supportive treatment.

Radioiodine

Radioactive isotopes of iodine were initially used in the treatment of Graves' disease in the 1940s.[10] Among different radioactive isotopes, ^{131}I is the agent of choice in the treatment of thyroid hyperfunction because of its half-life and its favorable emission profile. After oral administration, radioiodine is completely absorbed, rapidly concentrated, oxidized, and organified by thyroid follicular cells—exactly the same fate of [127]I (the stable isotope). Thyroid cells are destroyed by the ionizing effects of β particles with an average path length of 1 to 2 mm. One microcurie of ^{131}I retained per gram of thyroid tissue delivers approximately 70 to 90 rad. The early biologic effects of radioiodine include necrosis of follicular cells and vascular occlusion, which fully develop over a period of weeks to months after a single dose of radioiodine. As a consequence, control of hyperthyroidism requires at least weeks or months to be achieved. Long-term effects include shorter survival, impaired replication of surviving cells with atrophy and fibrosis, and a chronic inflammatory response resembling Hashimoto's thyroiditis. These later effects account for the development of hypothyroidism even years after treatment.[334]

Treatment Strategies

In Graves' disease, the goal of radioiodine therapy is to destroy enough thyroid tissue to cure thyrotoxicosis with one dose of ^{131}I, possibly given in a single session. Three outcomes of radioiodine treatment are possible:

1. The patient is rendered stably euthyroid. Achievement of euthyroidism was once considered the "success" situation, but it might not be the ideal outcome in patients with coexistent Graves' ophthalmopathy, in whom greater thyroid antigen ablation may be desirable.

2. The patient remains thyrotoxic. This result is, of course, a failure and requires a second treatment.

3. The patient becomes permanently hypothyroid. This outcome is now considered an acceptable consequence of radioiodine treatment, because correction of hypothyroidism with levothyroxine is easy, safe, and inexpensive.

In any patient with Graves' disease who receives radioiodine, the likelihood of these possible outcomes depends on the amount of radioiodine that is delivered and retained by the thyroid tissue and on other incompletely understood individual factors. The latter make it impossible to predict a successful dose in every single patient. The dose of radioiodine to be administered is most often calculated on the basis of thyroid size and uptake of ^{131}I and is determined by using the following equation[335]:

$$\text{Dose (mCi)} = \text{estimated thyroid weight (g)} \times \text{planned dose} \\ (\mu Ci/g)/\text{fractional 24-hour radioiodine} \\ \text{uptake} \times 1000$$

The planned dose varies according to the aim of treatment and ranges from 80 to 200 μCi/g in different centers. In some centers, standard fixed doses are given. Lower doses result in a lower rate of early (within 1 year) hypothyroidism, but at the expense of a higher rate of recurrent or persistent thyrotoxicosis and thus the necessity of a second or, less frequently, a third dose. Even patients given a lower dose and remaining euthyroid in the first year have a high incidence of late-onset hypothyroidism. The cumulative incidence of post-radioiodine hypothyroidism steadily increases at a rate of 2% to 3% new cases per year. The overall incidence of post-radioiodine hypothyroidism approaches a total of 40% at 5 years and 60% or more at 10 years.[336] Therefore, in many centers, including our own, the strategy of radioiodine treatment is to give a dose of radioiodine that ensures cure in the highest number of patients while being aware that most of the "cured" patients will eventually become hypothyroid. Hypothyroidism should be regarded as a common outcome of radioiodine treatment rather than a true complication, and it can be easily and economically controlled with levothyroxine substitution treatment. Further arguments can be made in favor of this approach. Recurrence of thyrotoxicosis can rarely occur, even in patients who were euthyroid after the first dose of radioiodine. These recurrences are psychologically disturbing for the patient and may carry additional cardiovascular risk, especially in the elderly. Moreover, in some centers, treatment of moderate to severe Graves' ophthalmopathy, when needed, is delayed until permanent correction of thyrotoxicosis is achieved, so rapid attainment of this goal is desirable.

With the use of relatively high delivered doses of ^{131}I, 150 to 200 μCi/g of estimated thyroid weight, nearly 70% of patients are cured after one dose of ^{131}I, 25% require a second dose, and rare patients need a third or fourth dose. Large goiter size, rapid iodine turnover, and adjunctive therapy with antithyroid drugs too soon after radioiodine are associated with a higher rate of persistence of hyperthyroidism, but other individual factors are also likely to exist. The decision to give a second dose of ^{131}I is not usually made before 6 to 12 months after the first one, when firm demonstration of persistence of thyrotoxicosis can be obtained. Transient hypothyroidism may be observed in the first 6 months after ^{131}I therapy. To correctly detect these cases, levothyroxine substitution should be initiated at submaximal doses so that TSH can be rechecked 2 to 4 months later; if high, the hypothyroidism is very likely to be permanent.

Short-Term Adverse Effects of Radioiodine

Transient exacerbation of mild to moderate preexisting Graves' ophthalmopathy may occur in the first few months after radioiodine therapy,[337] although this experience is not shared by all investigators, and the effect may be due to untreated hypothyroidism, according to others.[338] Because worsening of ophthalmopathy is transient and effectively controlled with a short course of oral corticosteroids, the presence of mild to moderate ophthalmopathy is not a contraindication to the use of radioiodine.[337] When severe Graves' ophthalmopathy is present, specific treatment with high-dose oral or intravenous corticosteroids and/or external radiation therapy should be started soon after radioiodine treatment.

Radioiodine treatment causes a radiation-induced acute thyroiditis that can rarely be clinically manifested 3 or 4 days after administration of the isotope by pain and swelling in the neck. This side effect is benign and self-limited and can be treated with a short course of antiinflammatory drugs. The destruction of thyroid tissue after radioiodine treatment also induces the release of preformed thyroid hormone from the gland, which can result in reexacerbation of thyrotoxicosis in the weeks after the procedure. To prevent this phenomenon by depleting intrathyroidal stores of hormones, a few months' course of thionamide is often given and discontinued 3 to 8 days before radioiodine administration. True relapses of hyperthyroidism after thionamide withdrawal in preparation for ^{131}I administration may also occur and account for the increase in thyroid hormone levels observed after radioiodine administration.[339] Because the effect of radioiodine is relatively delayed, several months may be required for complete control of the thyrotoxicosis. While waiting for the effect of radioiodine, a short course of antithyroid drugs can be initiated 2 weeks after treatment and the dose smoothly tapered in the following months. Earlier thionamide treatment has been associated with a higher rate of radioiodine failure. Alternatively, iopanoic acid or sodium ipodate can be administered a few days after the administration of radioiodine. This form of treatment has the advantage of rapidly controlling both thyrotoxicosis from radiation thyroiditis and transient relapse of hyperthyroidism. As mentioned earlier, lithium is another valid alternative.

Potential Long-Term Risks of Radioiodine

Radioisotope treatment of a benign disorder such as Graves' disease may raise concern regarding possible carcinogenic effects and the risk of genetic damage (i.e., the risk of causing germline mutations in the offspring of patients treated during the childbearing years). Although external head and neck irradiation is undoubtedly associated with an increased rate of thyroid carcinoma,[340,341] no association between radioiodine treatment for hyperthyroidism and thyroid cancer was found in large epidemiologic studies.[336] Similarly, no evidence has indicated that radioiodine therapy for hyperthyroidism increases the patient's risk for leukemia or solid tumors.[336] A minimal increase in the risk of gastric cancer 10 years or more after treatment was found in a survey in Sweden[342] but not in large epidemiologic studies in the United Kingdom[336] and the United States.[343] No association between radioiodine treatment of hyperthyroidism and congenital abnormalities in subsequent offspring has been observed.[344] In addition, no evidence of chromosome damage was found in one recent study in children and adolescents given radioactive iodine for thyroid carcinoma.[345] A rough estimate of the dose to the ovaries is about 0.2 rad/mCi of administered [131]I. Thus the dose to the ovaries in a patient receiving 10 mCi of

radioiodine is similar to that received from a barium enema or intravenous pyelography. It has been calculated that if a genetic risk induced by ^{131}I really does exist, the risk would be only 0.003% per rad of parental gonadal exposure and therefore a very small fraction of the spontaneous incidence of genetic disorders.[346] Increased risks of all-cause and circulatory deaths versus age- and period-specific mortality were reported but found to be associated with mild hypothyroidism prior to thyroxine therapy rather than to radioiodine treatment per se.[347] The experience accumulated in more than 50 years of radioiodine treatment of hyperthyroidism has shown that potential long-term risks are absent or negligible in the adult population. Unfortunately, no large studies are available on such risks in the pediatric population. Data from populations exposed to radioactive isotopes after the Chernobyl accident indicate that in infancy the thyroid is much more susceptible to radioiodine-induced carcinogenesis.[348,349] These observations are based on data that are very skewed with regard to the amount and duration of exposure to the radioactive fallout and therefore cannot be extrapolated to the therapeutic use of radioiodine. The Cooperative Thyrotoxicosis Therapy Follow-up Study showed that thyroid cancer develops in children treated with low but not with high doses of [131]I.[350] Therefore, it has been recently suggested to treat children with doses higher than those given to adults for Grave's hyperthyroidism.[351] Nevertheless, because of concerns and uncertainties especially for the risk of cancer of other organs, there is still no consensus for recommending radioiodine treatment for persons younger than 16 to 18 years.

Surgery

The aim of surgical treatment in Graves' hyperthyroidism is to reduce the excessive secretion of thyroid hormones and prevent relapse of thyrotoxicosis by removal of enough thyroid tissue. Subtotal thyroidectomy has for a long time been the choice of surgery for Graves' disease. The classic procedure consists of removing the bulk of the gland, with a few grams of tissue left in both lobes. With subtotal thyroidectomy, many patients remain euthyroid but are exposed to the risk of future relapse of thyrotoxicosis. A significant number of patients treated with subtotal thyroidectomy also become hypothyroid[352] (Fig. 9-9).

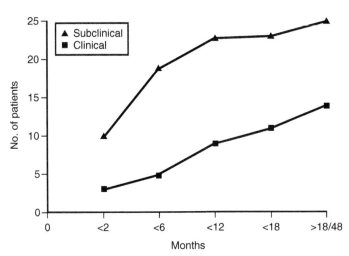

FIGURE 9-9. Prevalence of subclinical and clinical hypothyroidism in a cohort of patients with Graves' disease treated by subtotal thyroidectomy. (Modified from Miccoli P, Vitti P, Rago T et al: Surgical treatment of Graves' disease: subtotal or total thyroidectomy? Surgery 120:1020–1025, 1996.)

Therefore, lifelong surveillance is needed after subtotal thyroidectomy. Near-total thyroidectomy consists of the removal of most thyroid tissue, with only subcentimeter fragments left in sensitive regions, such as around the laryngeal recurrent nerve or the parathyroid glands. Near-total thyroidectomy has more recently been performed in patients with Graves' disease and results in a higher rate of hypothyroidism but a much smaller incidence of recurrent hyperthyroidism.[352,353] Because of the very low risk of relapse of thyrotoxicosis, near-total thyroidectomy has become the preferred operation in specialized centers.[352] Total thyroidectomy (e.g., removal of all visible thyroid tissue) may have the additional advantage of removing virtually all thyroidal autoantigens, and thus it might have a positive influence on the course of Graves' ophthalmopathy when present.[354]

Preparation of the patient for thyroid surgery is of paramount importance. A course of thionamide treatment is recommended to restore and maintain euthyroidism and to deplete intrathyroidal stores of hormones that could be released during surgery. The preoperative administration (10 days) of inorganic iodine induces involution of the gland and a reduction in vascularity.[317] Another approach has been proposed, namely, preparation with propranolol and iodine alone, which allows earlier surgery. In the absence of a real need for rapid surgery, however, this approach should be discouraged because it exposes patients to unnecessary risks. When emergency surgery is needed, oral cholecystographic agents represent the fastest way to obtain euthyroidism.

Besides the common nonspecific complications of surgery and anesthesia, thyroid surgery exposes patients to certain specific complications, including thyroid storm (which is now extremely rare), bleeding, injury to the recurrent laryngeal nerve, and hypoparathyroidism. In particular, the risk of laryngeal nerve injury and hypoparathyroidism cannot be disregarded. The incidence of these complications depends on the skill and experience of the surgeon and may range from 2% in specialized centers with wide experience in thyroid surgery up to 10% to 15% in some series.[354-359]

As stated earlier, these two potential complications need to be carefully explained to the patient when the discussion of treatment options is started. Postoperative thyroid function largely depends on the extent of thyroidectomy and duration of follow-up. Insufficient tissue removal results in persistent hyperthyroidism or in later relapse of hyperthyroidism, which may occur in 5% to 10% of patients within 5 years and in up to 40%

within 30 years after limited thyroidectomy. Recurrence of hyperthyroidism is particularly undesirable, because a second operation is technically more difficult than the first one and involves a higher risk of complications. With few exceptions, therefore, such patients should be treated with radioiodine. Extensive thyroidectomy results in postoperative thyroid failure, which always occurs after total and near-total thyroidectomy and often after subtotal thyroidectomy. In the first year after surgery, hypothyroidism has been reported in percentages of patients ranging from 5% to 60%.[352] Late-onset cases develop in an additional 1% to 3% per year. Hypothyroidism is easily and economically treated with levothyroxine replacement therapy, so thyroid failure after thyroidectomy for Graves' hyperthyroidism should not be considered a real complication.

MAKING THE CHOICE OF TREATMENT

In the preceding paragraphs, the possible therapeutic tools for Graves' disease thyrotoxicosis (antithyroid drugs, radioiodine, and surgery) have been examined. Some of them represent alternatives to the others. It is therefore important to discuss the relevant variables that will guide both the patient and the clinician in the choice of the best option for each particular case. General advantages and disadvantages of three major tools for the treatment of Graves' disease hyperthyroidism are listed in Table 9-6. Scientific evidence collected over the past 50 years or so is of invaluable help in making the correct decision. In many cases, the choice is in fact guided by preference, by personal experience of both the patient and the physician, or by environmental conditions (for example, the lack of an experienced surgeon or a well-equipped nuclear medicine facility). A survey of practice in Europe showed that a large majority of European endocrinologists still preferred medical treatment with thionamides in many cases of Graves' hyperthyroidism, including the most typical one, a woman in her forties with a medium-sized goiter. Ninety-five percent of European endocrinologists would have chosen this approach in a younger patient (e.g., a 19-year-old woman).[360] In contrast, when the same questionnaire was given to North American endocrinologists, 69% selected radioiodine for the older patient, and 27% chose it for the 19-year-old hyperthyroid female.[361] In both groups, thyroidectomy was not considered adequate in small to medium-sized goiters. Such wide differences in the perception of the best option for the treatment of Graves' disease not only reflect different traditions and experiences worldwide but also the fact

Table 9-6. Advantages and Disadvantages of Available Treatment Modalities for Graves' Disease Thyrotoxicosis

Treatment Modality	Advantages	Disadvantages
Radioiodine	Definitive treatment of thyrotoxicosis Rare, mild and transient side effects No surgical risks Easy to perform Fast	Delayed control of thyrotoxicosis Lower efficacy in large goiters Radiation hazard (?) Possible appearance of ophthalmopathy Worsening of a preexisting ophthalmopathy Possible requirement of glucocorticoids to prevent appearance of worsening of ophthalmopathy High cost
Thyroidectomy	Definitive treatment of thyrotoxicosis No radiation hazards Removal of large goiters Fast	Hypoparathyroidism (0.9%-2%) Recurrent laryngeal nerve damage (0.1%-2%) Bleeding/infections/anesthesia Scarring High cost
Thionamides	No radiation hazards No surgical risks No permanent hypothyroidism Low cost	Frequent relapses Requires frequent testing Side effects and adverse reactions

that none of the available options has a clear-cut advantage over the others.

In a typical uncomplicated Graves' disease case, for example, a middle-aged woman with a medium-sized goiter and mild Graves' ophthalmopathy, it is reasonable to offer the patient a trial of antithyroid drugs in an attempt to obtain persistent remission of hyperthyroidism, with the knowledge that this result will be obtained in a small, albeit significant minority of cases. At the same time, the patient can also be presented with the possibility of definitive treatment of hyperthyroidism with radioiodine and should receive an explanation regarding the fact that the most likely result will be permanent hypothyroidism. In many cases, however, this basic approach to the treatment of hyperthyroidism must be modified in light of other factors, which makes the choice of treatment somewhat less optional.

Age

Although radioiodine has been effectively used in adolescents and young adults with no adverse effects,[362,363] because of the lack of studies on the long-term effects of radioiodine, we usually exert caution in this situation, and our primary choice for treatment is antithyroid drugs, at least until the patient is 20 years old or so. Thyroidectomy may also be advised in children and adolescents who are allergic or noncompliant with antithyroid drugs. However, subtotal thyroidectomy may be more hazardous in children, in whom acute complications are reported in 16% to 35% and permanent complications in up to 8%.[364,365]

In women in the reproductive age, pregnancy must be delayed for at least 4 months after radioiodine administration and possibly for 1 year.[366] Therefore, the treatment plan should be designed with the patient according to her family plans, with antithyroid drug treatment being relatively safe and effective during pregnancy (see later heading).

Opposite considerations can be made in elderly subjects, in whom faster definitive correction of hyperthyroidism may be warranted. Relapse of hyperthyroidism after antithyroid drug treatment increases the cardiovascular risk in elderly patients, and surgery may present excessive risks in these patients. Therefore, radioiodine can be considered the best choice in the elderly.

Goiter Size and Associated Nodular Thyroid Disease

Large goiters are relatively resistant to ^{131}I and often require multiple treatments before correction of hyperthyroidism. Moreover, radioiodine only induces partial and slow shrinkage of the goiter. Therefore, when the patient has a large goiter, especially if compressive symptoms are present, surgery is the best choice of treatment, provided that an experienced surgeon is available.

Surgery is also recommended when Graves' disease is superimposed on endemic goiters with multiple cold nodules, which are not expected to respond with shrinkage to radioiodine. Finally, surgery is mandatory when a suspicion of malignancy cannot be ruled out in an associated single cold nodule, regardless of the size of the goiter.

Graves' Ophthalmopathy

The possible untoward effects of radioiodine on preexisting mild or moderate Graves' ophthalmopathy have been considered previously. The presence of severe Graves' ophthalmopathy requiring active treatment may modify the clinical approach. In a recent survey, most European thyroidologists chose antithyroid drug treatment in an index case with severe ophthalmopathy,[367] which implies that most of them were concerned with a possible worsening of Graves' ophthalmopathy after radioiodine treatment. The fact that thionamide treatment does not appear to be associated with worsening of ophthalmopathy was also responsible for this choice. As an alternative option, prompt definitive treatment of thyrotoxicosis by radioiodine or surgery may be warranted in the hope that the ongoing autoimmune process in the thyroid gland may drive the one in the orbit and that removal of possible cross-reacting thyroidal antigen(s) may improve orbital autoimmunity. In this regard, evidence in patients with differentiated thyroid carcinoma and coexistent thyroid autoimmunity indicates that successful removal of the thyroid by total thyroidectomy and radioiodine ablation is followed by the disappearance of autoantibodies.[368] Indeed, it has been recently reported a more beneficial outcome to glucocorticoid treatment in patients with Graves' ophthalmopathy treated by total thyroid ablation (near-total thyroidectomy followed by radioiodine ablation) compared with patients treated with thyroidectomy not followed by radioiodine.[354]

Relapses of thyrotoxicosis after discontinuation of treatment with antithyroid drugs are also frequent and may result in exacerbation of the orbital inflammatory process. Therefore, in these cases we usually advise rapid ablation of the thyroid with radioiodine or surgery, closely followed by the appropriate treatment of Graves' ophthalmopathy.

Concurrent Nonthyroidal Illnesses

The presence of nonthyroidal illnesses, especially heart disease, requires special attention in the choice of treatment of Graves' thyrotoxicosis. In these patients, surgery may be contraindicated or involve excessive risk, and relapses of thyrotoxicosis can worsen the concurrent heart disease. For these reasons, radioiodine is the therapeutic tool of choice, preceded by accurate short-term antithyroid drug preparation and followed by protection from post-radioiodine thyrotoxicosis by thionamides, iopanoic acid (see following discussion), or lithium. A similar approach can be taken with other nonthyroidal disorders that can be affected by thyroid function status, such as diabetes and severe psychiatric diseases, although in the latter conditions thyroidectomy can be advised as well.

Patient's Choice and Environmental Factors

From the preceding, it is apparent that only rarely is the choice of one treatment modality mandatory. As a consequence, the patient can often be directly involved in the decision-making process after complete information on advantages and disadvantages. For example, some patients may have a disproportionate perception and fear of the meaning of "treatment with radioactive compounds." In other cases, the presence of a goiter is perceived as disfiguring, and the patient may require surgery for cosmetic purposes. Yet other patients may be reluctant to undergo long-term drug therapy or may wish to solve the problem quickly. Other considerations that must be taken into account when selecting the treatment modality are the availability of an experienced surgeon and/or an experienced nuclear medicine facility. In some countries, restrictive legislation makes administration of sufficient doses of radioiodine more difficult.

SPECIAL SITUATIONS
Graves' Disease and Pregnancy

A higher incidence of abortion, preterm delivery, low-birth-weight infants, and neonatal mortality is seen in pregnancies complicated by maternal hyperthyroidism.[369] Besides fetal complications, hyperthyroidism may also cause maternal complications such as heart failure, eclampsia, and thyroid storm during delivery. Recognition of thyrotoxicosis during gestation or before a planned pregnancy warrants immediate and appropriate treatment inasmuch as pregnancies in which hyperthyroidism is fully controlled have excellent outcomes in mothers with Graves' disease.[369] It should also be added that for this reason pregnancy is not contraindicated in patients with Graves' disease, and conversely, thyrotoxicosis is not a reason for recommending abortion.

When Graves' disease is diagnosed in a woman planning pregnancy, pregnancy can be allowed after restoration of euthyroidism with thionamide drugs and treatment continued during pregnancy (see later). Alternatively, the radioiodine option can be offered because of a lack of evidence of an association between ^{131}I treatment of hyperthyroidism and congenital abnormalities in subsequent offspring. Current guidelines recommend that pregnancy be delayed for at least 4 months after radioiodine therapy,[369] but in a conservative approach, we usually advise the patient to wait for 1 year, when thyroid function is fully normalized and the outcome of treatment is clear.

Thyroidectomy may also be considered as an alternative because of more rapid restoration of euthyroidism.

Radioiodine therapy is absolutely contraindicated during pregnancy because it may result in congenital hypothyroidism and may cause malformations. Surgery is restricted to exceptional cases.

Thionamides are the first choice for treatment in a pregnant woman with Graves' disease. Clinical improvement with thionamides occurs after the first week, and euthyroidism may be reached after 2 to 4 weeks of therapy. Both propylthiouracil and methimazole have been used in pregnancy and are equally effective in the management of hyperthyroidism in this setting.[237,369,370] In the United States, propylthiouracil has traditionally been preferred to methimazole because of methimazole's purported increased passage across the placenta and breast epithelium, and because of a reported association between methimazole use and aplasia cutis (see following). However, methimazole or its precursor, carbimazole, are used widely throughout the world to treat pregnant women. In the only in vivo human study to formally examine the possible placental transfer of propylthiouracil and methimazole, pregnant women ingested ^{35}S-labeled compounds 2 hours before the elective termination of pregnancies in gestational age of 8 to 20 weeks.[371] The ratio of fetal serum or cord blood drug levels to maternal blood levels was substantially higher for methimazole or carbimazole (0.72 to 1) than for propylthiouracil (0.27 to 0.35). The differences were attributed to the known disparity in drug binding to albumin (propylthiouracil > methimazole) and in lipid solubility, as well as to possible differences in maternal/fetal volumes of distribution, excretion, and metabolism. More recently, a study using isolated perfused human placentas found no difference in the rate or extent of transplacental passage between propylthiouracil and methimazole.[372] Although it is uncertain whether this in vitro model is completely representative of in vivo events, a lack of a difference in placental transfer of propylthiouracil and methimazole is consistent with clinical observations showing similar fetal outcomes with either drug, in terms of thyroid function and congenital anomalies, and with data showing that cord blood propylthiouracil levels were similar to or higher than simultaneously obtained maternal serum propylthiouracil levels.[372]

Aplasia cutis is a congenital localized absence of skin that occurs spontaneously in approximately 1 in 2000 births.[373] Some cases of aplasia cutis (and also of other malformations) have been reported in the offspring of mothers who had taken methimazole during pregnancy, suggesting a possible association between methimazole and aplasia cutis.[237,369,370] Nevertheless, there is no definitive proof that methimazole is actually responsible for the condition, and considering the extreme rarity of this association, the fear of aplasia cutis should not prevent the use of methimazole during pregnancy, especially in those countries where propylthiouracil is not promptly available. Additional congenital malformations in newborns exposed to methimazole during the first trimester of pregnancy are choanal and esophageal atresia, minor facial abnormalities, and psychomotor delay, which either isolated or associated in rare cases with aplasia cutis define a condition named *methimazole embryopathy*.[237,369,370] As for isolated aplasia cutis, there is no proof that methimazole is responsible for these malformations, which therefore should not prevent the use of the drug during pregnancy. In a hyperthyroid pregnant women, the first priority should always be the control of hyperthyroidism, regardless of the drug. Nevertheless, because there are no case reports of aplasia cutis in association with propylthiouracil, when promptly available, propylthiouracil might still be preferred by some physicians.

Treatment with thionamides should be monitored so that maternal FT4 is kept in the high normal range. This level will ensure fetal euthyroidism inasmuch as FT4 levels in the mother's serum are correlated with fetal FT4 levels, as assessed in cord blood.[374] A low TSH level is not a reliable index to judge the adequacy of treatment, because it may not reflect changes in thyroid function as promptly as FT4 does, but it is important to test it because a high level always indicates insufficient treatment and should prompt adjustment of the thionamide dose. Because of the immunosuppressive effect of pregnancy, partial and transient remission of Graves' disease may occur in the second and third trimesters and allow a reduction and even discontinuation of thionamide treatment (Fig. 9-10). On the other hand, relapse of hyperthyroidism is frequent in the postpartum period.[99]

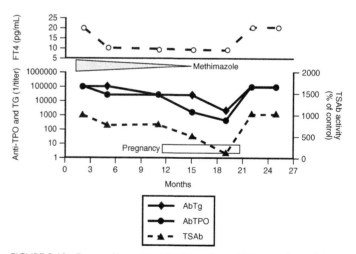

FIGURE 9-10. Course of hyperthyroidism in a patient with Graves' disease before, during, and after pregnancy. The immunosuppressive effect of pregnancy is shown by the reduction in serum antithyroid peroxidase (TPOAb) and antithyroglobulin (TgAb) titers and by the disappearance of serum antithyroid-stimulating hormone receptor antibodies (TSAb) during the third trimester of pregnancy, which allowed discontinuation of methimazole (MMI) treatment *(lower panel)*. Serum free thyroxine (FT4) remained within the normal range without treatment *(upper panel)*, until a relapse of the autoimmune process (shown by an increase in the titer of the three antibodies) caused a relapse of thyrotoxicosis shortly after the end of pregnancy.

The block-and-replace regimen is not recommended in pregnancy, because much more thionamide than levothyroxine will cross the placenta and cause fetal hypothyroidism. Iodine is avoided because of the risk of fetal hypothyroidism and goiter caused by the greater sensitivity of the fetal thyroid to the Wolff-Chaikoff effect. The use of β-blockers is controversial in pregnancy, but most authorities will not recommend them, at least for prolonged periods.

Both methimazole and propylthiouracil are secreted in breast milk (methimazole more than propylthiouracil) in small amounts.[237,369,370] However, maternal treatment with thionamides during lactation appears to be safe, whether it is continued after gestation or initiated in the postpartum period. For methimazole, doses of up to 20 mg daily have been documented not to affect infants' thyroid function.[375] For propylthiouracil, data available are scanty, and relatively low doses are therefore recommended. Whatever the drug, a mother should take her drug dose just after breastfeeding, which should provide a 3- to 4-hour interval before she lactates again. Although maternal hormone levels must be monitored with appropriate antithyroid drug adjustment, it appears that the child's thyroid function does not need to be checked regularly as long as somatic and mental development are progressing normally.

Surgical treatment is only occasionally indicated and may be considered in cases of poor compliance, severe drug allergy, very large goiter, associated thyroid malignancy, or the necessity of using high doses of thionamides to maintain euthyroidism. When needed, thyroidectomy is most safely performed in the second trimester. Complications of surgery, such as vocal cord paralysis or hypoparathyroidism, are disabling, and the latter may be difficult to treat during pregnancy. Levothyroxine therapy for the mother should be promptly initiated postoperatively.

Neonatal and Fetal Transfer Thyrotoxicosis

Immunoglobulins cross the placenta, and maternal TSAbs can also do so (Fig. 9-11). Because of this phenomenon, neonatal thyrotoxicosis may occur in association with maternal Graves' disease.[376] Mothers who have had Graves' disease and are euthyroid after thyroidectomy or radioiodine treatment may still have circulating TSAbs capable of causing neonatal thyrotoxicosis. Therefore, this possibility should be considered in all pregnant women with a current or past history of Graves' disease. Because of its pathogenesis, neonatal transfer thyrotoxicosis is always transient and spontaneously remits once maternal TSAbs disappear from the circulation, but it can cause acceleration of growth and craniosynostosis. Tachycardia, jaundice, heart failure, and failure to thrive characterize neonatal thyrotoxicosis. Onset may be delayed for a few days after delivery, until maternal thionamides clear, or rarely for a few weeks when an admixture of TBAbs and TSAbs is present in the serum. In mothers with high-titer TRAb in serum, testing for these antibodies in fetal cord blood can be performed at the time of delivery to predict the onset of neonatal thyrotoxicosis.[377]

Neonatal transfer thyrotoxicosis requires prompt treatment in close collaboration with a neonatologist. Thionamides, methimazole (0.5 to 1 mg/kg/day) or propylthiouracil (5 to 10 mg/kg/day), must be administered every 8 hours. Propranolol may be added to slow the heart rate and reduce hyperactivity. Iodine (1 drop of Lugol's solution, equivalent to 8 mg of iodine every 8 hours) is also used in addition to thionamides to inhibit the release of preformed thyroid hormones. As an alternative form of treatment, sodium ipodate alone, 0.5-g doses every 3 days, has been reported to rapidly normalize serum T_4 and T_3 in thyrotoxic neonates.[378] In severely ill infants, glucocorticoids may be added as a general supportive measure and to block conversion of T_4 to T_3.

When hyperthyroidism occurs during fetal life, the diagnosis is suggested by a heart rate over 160 beats per minute after 22 weeks of gestation. The diagnosis can be confirmed by fetal cord blood sampling, but this procedure is risky, with a 1% chance of fetal loss.[377] In utero treatment of hyperthyroidism may be accomplished by giving antithyroid drugs to the mother. The dose of thionamide should be adjusted to maintain a fetal heart rate of about 140 beats/min.

Graves' Disease in Childhood and Adolescence

Graves' disease may occur in childhood, but it is rarely seen before 10 years of age. Most cases occur around puberty, between the ages of 11 and 15. The clinical findings are often impressive, with prominent neuropsychological manifestations and an acceleration of growth that can result in premature ossification of bone end plates and reduced final height. Antithyroid drugs, radioiodine, and surgery have all been successfully used in children.[363] Radioiodine has been shown to be effective in children with hyperthyroidism,[362] but its long-range potential for radiation oncogenesis and gonadal damage remains to be established. Long-term follow-up studies of radioiodine therapy in children, that is, in patients who have a 60- to 70-year life expectancy, are still limited, although some authors consider this form of treatment safe.[351,363] Given the above considerations, most children are treated with thionamides for long periods (3 to 4 years) in an attempt to induce stable remission or until they reach an age when radioiodine treatment or surgery is more suitable (usually 18 to 20 years of age). Long-term courses of therapy imply close medical supervision and parental involvement because compliance may be low in this age group.

Thyroidectomy is rarely performed in children and adolescents, because permanent complications occur at a relatively higher rate in this age group and have a greater impact on devel-

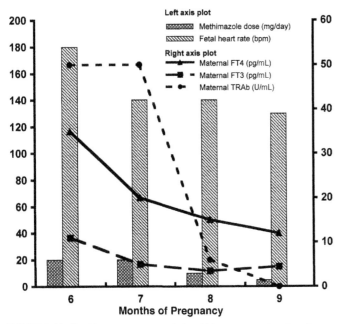

FIGURE 9-11. Fetal heart rate, maternal thyroid hormone, and maternal serum thyroid-stimulating hormone receptor antibodies (TRAb) during methimazole (MMI) treatment in a woman in whom Graves' disease was diagnosed at the sixth month of pregnancy. *FT3,* Free triiodothyronine; *FT4,* free thyroxine.

Table 9-7. Distinctive Initial Symptoms of Thyrotoxicosis in the Elderly (Apathetic Thyrotoxicosis)

Tachycardia	Depression
Congestive heart failure	Lethargy
Atrial fibrillation	Agitation and anxiety
Weight loss associated with anorexia	Confusion up to dementia
Muscle wasting and weakness	Osteoporosis up to bone fractures

opmental age. Nevertheless, very large goiters or poor compliance with antithyroid drug therapy may be an indication for surgical treatment.

Hyperthyroidism in the Elderly With Heart Disease

In the elderly, hyperthyroidism and cardiac disease are often associated. Hyperthyroid symptoms may be quite different in aged patients, and symptoms related to adrenergic hyperactivity such as hyperactive reflexes, increased sweating, heat intolerance, tremor, nervousness, and increased appetite are found less frequently than in younger patients[379] (Table 9-7). Weight loss is more often associated with anorexia, depression, and lethargy than with decreased appetite.[380] Overall, these findings justify the expression "apathetic thyrotoxicosis." Graves' ophthalmopathy has been reported to be more severe in the elderly, when present.[381]

Hyperthyroidism may precipitate heart failure or may worsen preexisting heart conditions. Atrial fibrillation is found in 30% to 60% of patients at diagnosis.[379,380] Therefore, special attention should be put into rapidly controlling hyperthyroidism, avoiding relapses, and preventing additional heart complications. When heart disease is already present at the time of diagnosis, the treatment plan should be particularly cautious and include (1) prompt restoration of euthyroidism with antithyroid drugs while independently addressing the heart disease; (2) administration of β-adrenergic antagonists; (3) definitive, ablative treatment of hyperthyroidism with radioiodine; (4) protection of the heart from the possible radioiodine-induced transient thyrotoxicosis with β-adrenergic antagonists (immediately) and/or oral cholecystographic agents (2 weeks after radioiodine) or lithium; (5) resumption of thionamide therapy 2 weeks after radioiodine administration to control hyperthyroidism while waiting for the complete effect of radioiodine; (6) strict control of thyroid function in the next 12 months; (7) cautious tapering of antithyroid drug doses until discontinuation; and (8) correction of hypothyroidism with the minimal amount of levothyroxine needed to maintain serum TSH in the normal range.

TREATMENT OF PRETIBIAL MYXEDEMA

In most cases, pretibial myxedema causes little discomfort, but it can be disfiguring in others. Itching may also be a dominant symptom. Application of occlusive dressings with topical high-potency corticosteroids appears to be an effective treatment.[382] Alternative treatment modalities include local injections of corticosteroids or hyaluronidase.[383] The treatment needs to be repeated from time to time because the disease is characterized by a course of remissions and relapses. Eventually, stable remis-

sions are obtained in most cases. In more severe cases, surgical excision of pseudotumorous or polypous forms has been performed with success.[384,385] Systemic treatment has included plasmapheresis and high-dose corticosteroids.[382] Plasmapheresis is effective, but its favorable effects are transient when used alone without long-term immunosuppression. High-dose intravenous immunoglobulins have been used as well in uncontrolled studies, but this treatment is very expensive and offers no advantages over corticosteroids.

THYROID STORM

Thyroid storm is an acute and severe life-threatening complication of thyrotoxicosis characterized by manifestations of severe hypermetabolism with high fever, tachyarrhythmias, profuse sweating, diarrhea and vomiting, confusion, delirium, and coma.[385] Congestive heart failure is often a relevant part of the picture. Thyroid storm occurs in patients with poor nutritional status and longstanding thyrotoxicosis, most often Graves' disease, either not recognized or not adequately treated. Although the cause is thought to be an abrupt release of large quantities of stored thyroid hormones into the circulation, in many cases the mechanism cannot be found. Before the use of antithyroid drugs, thyroid surgery and radioiodine therapy were relatively common causes of thyroid storm. Infections, trauma, surgical distress, metabolic disorders, and pulmonary and cardiovascular diseases are among the other factors that may precipitate a thyroid storm. Thyroid storm used to be much more frequent in the past and was associated with very high mortality, up to 75%.[386]

True thyroid storm is an extremely rare event nowadays. However, less severe forms of thyrotoxic crisis are not exceptional and may be a medical emergency requiring prompt recognition and adequate treatment. Underlying nonthyroidal illnesses should be promptly recognized and specifically treated. Normalization of body temperature may require the use of cooling blankets and/or pharmacologic agents such as acetaminophen, chlorpromazine, or meperidine. Intravenous corticosteroids are beneficial in sustaining the peripheral circulation and preventing shock. Supportive measures such as oxygen and intravenous fluids should be given in case of hypoxia or dehydration. All means should be used to reduce the levels of circulating thyroid hormone. Inhibition of the synthesis and release of thyroid hormones can be achieved with the use of thionamides and iodine, but this effect is delayed and therefore not sufficient, although they are necessary. Inhibition of the peripheral conversion of T_4 to T_3 by iodinated contrast agents is probably the fastest way to obtain a significant reduction in circulating T_3. Block of the peripheral effects of thyroid hormones by β-adrenergic antagonists (propranolol, metoprolol, atenolol) is also indicated. Removal of excess thyroid hormones from the circulation by plasmapheresis, peritoneal dialysis, extracorporeal resin perfusion, or charcoal plasma perfusion have all been reported in extreme situations. All drugs should be used in maximal doses. Patients require continuous monitoring of the electrocardiogram and an intravenous line to administer fluids and drugs. Alternatively, drugs can be delivered by nasogastric tube.

REFERENCES

1. Taylor S: Robert Graves. The Golden Years of Irish Medicine, New York, 1989, Royal Society of Medicine Services.
2. Graves RJ: Newly observed affection of the thyroid, London Med Surg J 7:515–523, 1835.
3. Parry CH: Collections from the Unpublished Medical Writings of the Late Caleb Hillier Parry, London, 1825, Underwood.
4. Flajani G: Sopra un tumor freddo nell'anterior parte del collo detto broncocele, [Collezione d'osservazioni e riflessioni di chirurgia.] 3:270–273, 1802.
5. von Basedow KA: Exophthalmos durch hypertrophie des zellgewebes in der Augenhole, Wochenschr Ges Heilk Berl 6:197, 1840.

6. Hennemannn G: Historical aspects about the development of our knowledge of morbus Basedow, J Endocrinol Invest 14:617–624, 1991.
7. Medvei VC: History of Clinical Endocrinology, New York, 1992, Parthenon.
8. MacKenzie JB, MacKenzie CG, McCollum EV: The effect of sulfanylguanidine on the thyroid in the rat, Science 94:518–519, 1941.
9. Astwood EB: Treatment of hyperthyroidism with thiourea and thiouracil, JAMA 122:78, 1943.
10. Sawin CT, Becker DV: Radioiodine and the treatment of hyperthyroidism: the early history, Thyroid 7:163–176, 1997.
11. Adams DD, Purves HD: Abnormal responses in the assay of thyrotropin, Proc Univ Otago Med Sch 34:11–12, 1956.
12. Nagayama Y Kaufman KD, Seto P, Rapoport B: Molecular cloning, sequence and functional expression of the cDNA for the human thyrotropin receptor, Biochem Biophys Res Commun 165:1184–1190, 1989.
13. Parmentier M, Libert F, Maenhaut C, et al: Molecular cloning of the thyrotropin receptor, Science 246:1620–1622, 1989.
14. Laurberg P, Pedersen KM, Vestergaard H, et al: High incidence of multinodular toxic goitre in the elderly population in a low iodine intake area vs. high incidence of Graves' disease in the young in a high iodine intake area: comparative surveys of thyrotoxicosis epidemiology in East-Jutland Denmark and Iceland, J Intern Med 229:415–420, 1991.
15. Furszyfer J, Kurland LT, McConahey WM, et al: Epidemiologic aspects of Hashimoto's thyroiditis and Graves' disease in Rochester Minnesota (1935–1967), with special reference to temporal trends, Metabolism 21:197–204, 1972.
16. Aghini-Lombardi F, Antonangeli L, Martino E, et al: The spectrum of thyroid disorders in an iodine-deficient community: the Pescopagano survey, J Clin Endocrinol Metab 84:561–566, 1999.
17. Tunbridge W, Evered DC, Hall R, et al: The spectrum of thyroid disease in a community: the Whickham survey, Clin Endocrinol (Oxf) 7:481–493, 1977.
18. Vanderpump MP, Tunbridge WM, French JM, et al: The incidence of thyroid disorders in the community: a twenty-year follow-up of the Whickham Survey, Clin Endocrinol (Oxf) 43:55–68, 1995.
19. Abraham-Nordling M, Törring O, Lantz M, et al: Incidence of hyperthyroidism in Stockholm, Sweden, 2003–2005, Eur J Endocrinol 158:823–827, 2008.
20. Jacobson DL, Gange SJ, Rose NR, et al: Epidemiology and estimated population burden of selected autoimmune diseases in the United States, Clin Immunol Immunopathol 84:223–243, 1997.
21. Connolly RJ, Vidor GI, Stewart JC: Increase in thyrotoxicosis in endemic goitre area after iodination of bread, Lancet 1:500–502, 1970.
22. Stanbury JB, Ermans AE, Bourdoux P, et al: Iodine-induced hyperthyroidism: occurrence and epidemiology, Thyroid 9:83–100, 1998.
23. Burgi H, Kohler M, Morselli B: Thyrotoxicosis incidence in Switzerland and benefit of improved iodine supply, Lancet 352:1034, 1998.
24. Lundgren E, Christensen Borup S: Decreasing incidence of thyrotoxicosis in an endemic goitre inland area of Sweden, Clin Endocrinol 33:133–138, 1990.
25. Brownlie BE, Wells JE: The epidemiology of thyrotoxicosis in New Zealand: incidence and geographical distribution in north Canterbury, 1983–1985, Clin Endocrinol (Oxf) 33:249–259, 1990.
26. Barker DJP, Phillips DIW: Current incidence of thyrotoxicosis and past prevalence of goitre in 12 British towns, Lancet 2:567–570, 1984.
27. Laurberg P, Jørgensen T, Perrild H, et al: The Danish investigation on iodine intake and thyroid disease, DanThyr: status and perspectives, Eur J Endocrinol 155:219–228, 2006.
28. Bülow Pedersen I, Laurberg P, Knudsen N, et al: Increase in incidence of hyperthyroidism predominantly occurs in young people after iodine fortification of salt in Denmark, J Clin Endocrinol Metab 2006, 91:3830–3834, 2006.
29. Brix TH, Kyvik KO, Christensen K, et al: Evidence for a major role of heredity in Graves' disease: a population-based study of two Danish twin cohorts, J Clin Endocrinol Metab 86:930–934, 2001.
30. Ringold DA, Nicoloff JT, Kesler M, et al: Further evidence for a strong genetic influence on the development of autoimmune thyroid disease: the California twin study, Thyroid 12:647–653, 2002.
31. Hall R, Stanbury JB: Familial studies of autoimmune thyroiditis, Clin Exp Immunol 2:719–725, 1967.
32. Hall RO, Owen SG, Smart GA: Evidence for a genetic predisposition to formation of thyroid autoantibodies, Lancet ii:187–190, 1960.
33. Jacobson EM, Tomer Y: The genetic basis of thyroid autoimmunity, Thyroid 17:949–961, 2007.
34. Hall R, Dingle PR, Roberts DF: Thyroid antibodies: a study of first-degree relatives, Clin Genet 3:319–324, 1972.
35. Tamai H, Ohsako N, Takeno K, et al: Changes in thyroid function in euthyroid subjects with family history of Graves' disease; a follow up study of 69 patients, J Clin Endocrinol Metab 51:1123–1128, 1980.
36. Villanueva R, Greenberg DA, Davies TF, et al: Sibling recurrence risk in autoimmune thyroid disease, Thyroid 13:761–764, 2003.
37. Villanueva R, Inzerillo AM, Tomer Y, et al: Limited genetic susceptibility to severe Graves' ophthalmopathy: no role for CTLA-4 but evidence for an environmental etiology, Thyroid 10:791–798, 2000.
38. Ban Y, Tomer Y: Susceptibility genes in thyroid autoimmunity, Clin Dev Immunol 12:47–58, 2005.
39. Tomer Y, Menconi F, Davies TF, et al: Dissecting genetic heterogeneity in autoimmune thyroid diseases by subset analysis, J Autoimmun 29:69–77, 2007.
40. Vladutiu AO, Rose NR: Autoimmune murine thyroiditis: relation to histocompatibility (H-2) type, Science 174:1137–1139, 1971.
41. Farid NR, Barnard JM, Marshall WH: The association of HLA with autoimmune thyroid disease in Newfoundland. The influence of HLA homozygosity in Graves' disease, Tissue Antigens 8:181–189, 1976.
42. Irvine WJ, Gray RS, Morris PJ, et al: Correlation of HLA and thyroid antibodies with clinical course of thyrotoxicosis treated with antithyroid drugs, Lancet 2:898–900, 1977.
43. Tomer Y, Davies TF: Searching for the autoimmune thyroid disease susceptibility genes: from gene mapping to gene function, Endoc Rev, 24:694–717, 2003.
44. Jacobson EM, Huber A, Tomer Y: The HLA gene complex in thyroid autoimmunity: from epidemiology to etiology. J Autoimmun 30:58–62, 2008.
45. Farid NR, Barnard JM, Marshall WH: The association of HLA with autoimmune thyroid disease in Newfoundland. The influence of HLA homozygosity in Graves' disease, Tissue Antigens 8:181–189, 1976.
46. Banchereau J, Bazan F, Blanchard D, et al: The CD40 antigen and its ligand, Annu Rev Immunol 12:881–922, 1994.
47. Teft WA, Kirchhof MG, Madrenas J: A molecular perspective of CTLA-4 function, Annu Rev Immunol 24:65–97, 2006.
47a.Tomer Y, Greenberg DA, Barbesino G, et al: CTLA-4 and not CD28 is a susceptibility gene for thyroid autoantibody production, J Clin Endocrinol Metab 86:1687–1693, 2001.
47b.Ueda H, Howson JM, Esposito L, et al: Association of the T-cell regulatory gene CTLA4 with suceptibility to autoimmune disease, Nature 423:506–511, 2003.
48. Mayans S, Lackovic K, Nyholm C, et al: CT60 genotype does not affect CTLA-4 isoform expression despite association to T1D and AITD in northern Sweden, BMC Med Genet 8:3, 2007.
49. Velaga MR, Wilson V, Jennings CE, et al: The codon 620 tryptophan allele of the lymphoid tyrosine phosphatase (LYP) gene is a major determinant of Graves' disease, J Clin Endocrinol Metab 89:5862–5865, 2004.
50. Criswell LA, Pfeiffer KA, Lum RF, et al: Analysis of families in the multiple autoimmune disease genetics consortium (MADGC) collection: the PTPN22 620W allele associates with multiple autoimmune phenotypes, Am J Hum Genet 76:561–571, 2005.
51. Tomer Y, Greenberg DA, Conception E, et al: Thyroglobulin is a thyroid specific gene for the familial autoimmune diseases, J Clin Endocrinol Metab 87:404–407, 2002.
52. Ban Y, Greenberg DA, Concepcion E, et al: Amino acid substitutions in the thyroglobulin gene are associated with susceptibility to human and murine autoimmune thyroid disease, Proc Natl Acad Sci U S A 100:15119–15124, 2003.
53. Prummel MF, Strieder T, Wiersinga WM: The environment and autoimmune thyroid diseases, Eur J Endocrinol 150:605–618, 2004.
54. Brix TH, Christensen K, Niels VH, et al: Genetic versus environment in Graves' disease—a population based twin study, Thyroid 7(suppl):13, 1997.
55. Tomer Y, Davies TF: Infection, thyroid disease and autoimmunity, Endocr Rev 14:107–120, 1993.
56. Phillips DI, Barker DJ, Rees SB, et al: The geographical distribution of thyrotoxicosis in England according to the presence or absence of TSH-receptor antibodies, Clin Endocrinol (Oxf) 23:283–287, 1985.
57. Cox SP, Phillips DIW, Osmond C: Does infection initiate Graves disease? A population based 10 year study, Autoimmunity 4:43–49, 1989.
58. Facciani JM, Kazim M: Absence of seasonal variation in Graves disease, Ophthalm Plast Reconstr Surg 16:67–71, 2000.
59. Toft AD, Blackwell CC, Saadi AT, et al: Secretor status and infection in patients with Grave's disease, Autoimmunity 7:279–289, 1990.
60. Prabhkar BS, Bhan RS, Smith TJ: Current perspective on the pathogenesis of Graves disease and ophthalmopathy, Endocr Rev 24:802–835, 2003.
61. Shenkman L, Bottone EJ: Antibodies to Yersinia enterocolitica in thyroid disease, Ann Intern Med 85:735–739, 1976.
62. Lidman K, Eriksson U, Norberg R, et al: Indirect immunofluorescence staining of human thyroid by antibodies occurring in Yersinia enterocolitica infections, Clin Exp Immunol 23:429–435, 1976.
63. Bech K: Yersinia enterocolitica and thyroid autoimmunity, Autoimmunity 7:291–294, 1990.
64. Brix TH, Hansen PS, Hegedüs L, et al: Too early to dismiss Yersinia enterocolitica infection in the aetiology of Graves' disease. Evidence from a twin case-control study, Clin Endocrinol 2008 (in press).
65. Weiss M, Ingbar SH, Winblad S, et al: Demonstration of a saturable binding site for thyrotropin in Yersinia enterocolitica, Science 219:1331–1333, 1983.
66. Heyma P, Harrison LC, Robinsk-Browne R: Thyrotrophin (TSH) binding sites on Yersinia enterocolitica recognized by immunoglobulins from humans with Graves' disease, Clin Exp Immunol 64:249–254, 1986.
67. Wenzel BE, Heesemann J, Heufelder A, et al: Enteropathogenic Yersinia enterocolitica and organ-specific autoimmune diseases in man, Contrib Microbiol Immunol 12:80–88, 1991.
68. Luo G, Fan JL, Seetharamaiah GS, et al: Immunization of mice with Yersinia enterocolitica leads to the induction of antithyrotropin receptor antibodies, J Immunol 151:922–928, 1993.
69. Lindholm H, Visakorpi R: Late complications after a Yersinia enterocolitica epidemic: a follow up study, Ann Rheum Dis 50:694–696, 1991.
70. Kohn LD, Napolitano G, Singer DS, et al: Graves' disease: a host defense mechanism gone awry, Int Rev Immunol 19:633–664, 2000.
71. Ciampolillo A, Mirakian R, Schulz T, et al: Retrovirus-like sequences in Graves' disease: implications for human autoimmunity, Lancet 1:1096–1099, 1989.
72. Humphrey M, Baker JJ, Carr FE, et al: Absence of retroviral sequences in Graves' disease, Lancet 337:17–18, 1991.
73. Fierabracci A, Upton CP, Hajibagheri N, et al: Lack of detection of retroviral particles (HIAP-1) in the H9 T cell line co-cultured with thyrocytes of Graves' disease, J Autoimmun 16:457–462, 2001.
74. Wick G, Grubeck-Loebenstein B, Trieb K, et al: Human foamy virus antigens in thyroid tissue of Graves' disease patients, Int Arch Allergy Immunol 99:153–156, 1992.
75. Schweizer M, Turek R, Reinhardt M, et al: Absence of foamy virus DNA in Graves' disease, AIDS Res Hum Retroviruses 10:601–605, 1994.
76. Schweizer M, Turek R, Hahn H, et al: Markers of foamy virus infections in monkeys, apes, and accidentally infected humans: Appropriate testing fails to confirm suspected foamy virus prevalence in humans, AIDS Res Hum Retroviruses 11:161–170, 1995.
77. Burch HB, Nagy EV, Lukes YG, et al: Nucleotide and amino acid homology between the human thyrotropin receptor and HIV-1 nef protein: identification and functional analysis, Biochem Biophys Res Commun 181:498–505, 1991.

78. Tas M, de Haan-Meulman M, Kabel PJ, et al: Defects in monocyte polarization and dendritic cell clustering in patients with Graves' disease. A putative role for a non-specific immunoregulatory factor related to retroviral p15E, Clin Endocrinol 34:441–448, 1991.
79. Leib-Mosch C, Bachmann M, Brack-Werner R, et al: Expression and biological significance of human endogenous retroviral sequences, Leukemia 6(suppl):72–75, 1992.
80. Jaspan JB, Luo H, Ahmed B, et al: Evidence for a retroviral trigger in Graves' disease, Autoimmunity 20:135–142, 1995.
81. Fierabracci A, Upton CP, Hajibagheri N, et al: Lack of detection of retroviral particles (HIAP-1) in the H9 T cell line co-cultured with thyrocytes of Graves' disease, J Autoimmunity 16:457–462, 2001.
82. Fierabracci A, Hammond L, Lowdell M, et al: The effect of staphylococcal enterotoxin B on thyrocyte HLA molecule expression, J Autoimmun 12:305–314, 1999.
83. Kondrashova A, Viskari H, Haapala A-M, et al: Serological evidence of thyroid autoimmunity among schoolchildren in two different socioeconomic environments, J Clin Endocrinol Metab 93:729–734, 2008.
84. Chiovato L, Pinchera A: Stressful life events and Graves' disease, Eur J Endocrinol 134:680–682, 1996.
85. Bagnasco M, Bossert I, Pesce G: Stress and autoimmune thyroid diseases, Neuroimmunomodulation 2006 13:309–317, 2007.
86. Mizokami T, Wu Li A, El-Kaissi S, et al: Stress and thyroid autoimmunity, Thyroid 14:1047–1055, 2004.
87. Dayan CM: Stressful life events and Graves' disease revisited, Clin Endocrinol 55:15–19, 2001.
88. Chiovato L, Marino M, Perugi G, et al: Chronic recurrent stress due to panic disorder does not precipitate Graves' disease, J Endocrinol Invest 21:758–764, 1998.
89. Stein SP, Keller SE, Schleifer SJ: Stress and immunomodulation: the role of depression and neuroendocrine function, J Immunol 135(suppl):827–833, 1985.
90. Ziemssen T, Kern S: Psychoneuroimmunology—cross-talk between the immune and nervous systems, J Neurol Suppl 2:II8–11, 2007.
91. Amino N, Tada H, Hidaka Y: Postpartum autoimmune thyroid syndrome: a model of aggravation of autoimmune disease, Thyroid 9:705–713, 1999.
92. Wong GW, Kwok MY, Ou Y: High incidence of juvenile Graves' disease in Hong Kong, Clin Endocrinol (Oxf) 43:697–700, 1995.
93. Zandman-Goddard G, Peeva E, Shoenfeld Y: Gender and autoimmunity, Autoimmun Rev 2007, 6:366–372, 2007.
94. Chiovato L, Lapi P, Fiore E, et al: Thyroid autoimmunity and female gender, J Endocrinol Invest 16:384–391, 1993.
95. Lutfi RJ, Fridmanis M, Misiunas AL, et al: Association of melasma with thyroid autoimmunity and other thyroidal abnormalities and their relationship to the origin of the melasma, J Clin Endocrinol Metab 61:28–31, 1985.
96. Chiovato L, Larizza D, Bendinelli G, et al: Autoimmune hypothyroidism and hyperthyroidism in patients with Turner's syndrome, Eur J Endocrinol 134:568–575, 1996.
97. Vallotton MB, Forbes AP: Autoimmunity in gonadal dysgenesis and Klinefelter's syndrome, Lancet 1:648–651, 1967.
98. Rotondi M, Pirali B, Lodigiani S, et al: The postpartum period and the onset of Graves' disease: an overestimated risk factor, Eur J Endocrinol 159:161–165, 2008.
99. Rotondi M, Cappelli C, Pirali B, et al: The effect of pregnancy on subsequent relapse from Graves' disease following a successful course of anti-thyroid drug therapy, J Clin Endocrinol Metab 2008 (in press).
100. Davies TF: The thyroid immunology of the postpartum period, Thyroid 9:675–684, 1999.
101. Yin X, Latif R, Tomer Y, et al: Thyroid epigenetics: X chromosome inactivation in patients with autoimmune thyroid disease, Ann N Y Acad Sci 1110:193–200, 2007.
102. Bartalena L: Smoking and Graves' disease, J Endocrinol Invest 25:402, 2002.
103. Holm IA, Manson JE, Michels KB, et al: Smoking and other lifestyle factors and the risk of Graves' hyperthyroidism, Arch Intern Med 165:1606–1611, 2005.
104. Monzani F, Del Guerra P, Caraccio N, et al: Appearance of Graves' disease after percutaneous ethanol injection for the treatment of hyperfunctioning thyroid adenoma, J Endocrinol Invest 20:294–298, 1977.
105. Chiovato L, Santini F, Vitti P, et al: Appearance of thyroid stimulating antibody and Graves' disease after radioiodine therapy for toxic nodular goitre, Clin Endocrinol (Oxf) 40:803–806, 1994.
106. LiVolsi VA: The pathology of autoimmune thyroid disease: a review, Thyroid 4:333–339, 1994.
107. Davies TF, Ando T, Lin RY, et al: Thyrotropin receptor-associated diseases: from adenomata to Graves disease, J Clin Invest 115:1972–1983, 2005.
108. Rapoport B, McLachlan SM: The thyrotropin receptor in Graves' disease, Thyroid 17:911–922, 2007.
109. Rapoport B, Chazenbalk GD, Jaume JC, et al: The thyrotropin (TSH) receptor: interaction with TSH and autoantibodies, Endocr Rev 19:673–716, 1998.
110. Rees Smith B, McLachlan SM, Furmaniak J: Autoantibodies to the thyrotropin receptor, Endocr Rev 9:106–121, 1988.
111. McKenzie JM, Zakarija M: Clinical review 3: the clinical use of thyrotropin receptor antibody measurements, J Clin Endocrinol Metab 69:1093–1096, 1989.
112. Chiovato L, Vitti P, Bendinelli G, et al: Detection of antibodies blocking thyrotropin effect using Chinese hamster ovary cells transfected with the cloned human TSH receptor, J Endocrinol Invest 17:809–816, 1994.
113. Chazenbalk GD, Pichurin P, Chen CR, et al: Thyroid-stimulating autoantibodies in Graves disease preferentially recognize the free A subunit, not the thyrotropin holoreceptor, J Clin Invest 110:209–217, 2002.
114. Chen CR, Pichurin P, Nagayama Y, et al: The thyrotropin receptor autoantigen in Graves disease is the culprit as well as the victim, J Clin Invest 111:1897–1904, 2003.
115. Chen CR, Tanaka K, Chazenbalk GD, et al: A full biological response to autoantibodies in Graves' disease requires a disulfide-bonded loop in the thyrotropin receptor N terminus homologous to a laminin epidermal growth factor-like domain, J Biol Chem 276:14767–14772, 2001.
116. Cundiff JG, Kaithamana S, Seetharamaiah GS, et al: Studies using recombinant fragments of human TSH receptor reveal apparent diversity in the binding specificities of antibodies that block TSH binding to its receptor or stimulate thyroid hormone production, J Clin Endocrinol Metab 86:4254–4260, 2001.
117. Tahara K, Ishikawa N, Yamamoto K, et al: Epitopes for thyroid stimulating and blocking autoantibodies on the extracellular domain of the human thyrotropin receptor, Thyroid 7:867–877, 1997.
118. Schwarz-Lauer L, Chazenbalk GD, Mclachlan SM, et al: Evidence for a simplified view of autoantibody interactions with the thyrotropin receptor, Thyroid 12:115–120, 2002.
119. McKenzie JM: Delayed thyroid response to serum from thyrotoxic patients, Endocrinology 62:865–868, 1958.
120. Schott M, Scherbaum WA, Morgenthaler NG: Thyrotropin receptor autoantibodies in Graves' disease, Trends Endocrinol Metab 16:243–248, 2005.
121. Shewring G, Smith BR: An improved radioreceptor assay for TSH receptor antibodies, Clin Endocrinol (Oxf) 17:409–417, 1982.
122. Southgate K, Creagh F, Teece M, et al: A receptor assay for the measurement of TSH receptor antibodies in unextracted serum, Clin Endocrinol (Oxf) 20:539–548, 1984.
123. Filetti S, Foti D, Costante G, et al: Recombinant human TSH receptor in a radioreceptor assay for the measurement of TSH receptor autoantibodies, J Clin Endocrinol Metab 72:1096–1101, 1991.
124. Costagliola S, Swillens S, Niccoli P, et al: Binding assay for thyrotropin receptor autoantibodies using the recombinant receptor protein, J Clin Endocrinol Metab 75:1540–1544, 1992.
125. Ludgate M, Costagliola S, Danguy D, et al: Recombinant TSH-receptor for determination of TSH-receptor-antibodies, Exp Clin Endocrinol 100:73–74, 1992.
126. Costagliola S, Morgenthaler NG, Hoermann R, et al: Second generation assay for thyrotropin receptor antibodies has superior diagnostic sensitivity for Graves' disease, J Clin Endocrinol Metab 84:90–97, 1999.
127. Bolton J, Sanders J, Oda Y, et al: Measurement of thyroid-stimulating hormone receptor autoantibodies by ELISA, Clin Chem 45:2285–2287, 1999.
128. Rapoport B, Greenspan FS, Filetti S, et al: Clinical experience with a human thyroid cell bioassay for thyroid-stimulating immunoglobulin, J Clin Endocrinol Metab 58:332–338, 1984.
129. Vitti P, Valente WA, Ambesi-Impiombato FS, et al: Graves' IgG stimulation of continuously cultured rat thyroid cells: a sensitive and potentially useful clinical assay, J Endocrinol Invest 5:179–182, 1982.
130. Vitti P, Rotella CM, Valente WA, et al: Characterization of the optimal stimulatory effects of Graves' monoclonal and serum immunoglobulin G on adenosine 3′,5′-monophosphate production in fRTL-5 thyroid cells: a potential clinical assay, J Clin Endocrinol Metab 57:782–791, 1983.
131. Ludgate M, Perret J, Parmentier M, et al: Use of the recombinant human thyrotropin receptor (TSH-R) expressed in mammalian cell lines to assay TSH-R autoantibodies, Mol Cell Endocrinol 73:R13–R18, 1990.
132. Vitti P, Elisei R, Tonacchera M, et al: Detection of thyroid-stimulating antibody using Chinese hamster ovary cells transfected with cloned human thyrotropin receptor, J Clin Endocrinol Metab 76:499–503, 1993.
133. Morgenthaler NG, Pampel I, Aust G, et al: Application of a bioassay with CHO cells for the routine detection of stimulating and blocking autoantibodies to the TSH-receptor, Horm Metab Res 30:162–168, 1998.
134. Watson PF, Ajjan RA, Phipps J, et al: A new chemiluminescent assay for the rapid detection of thyroid stimulating antibodies in Graves' disease, Clin Endocrinol (Oxf) 49:577–581, 1998.
135. Evans C, Morgenthaler NG, Lee S, et al: Development of a luminescent bioassay for thyroid stimulating antibodies, J Clin Endocrinol Metab 84:374–377, 1999.
136. Minich WB, Lenzner C, Bergmann A, et al: A coated tube assay for the detection of blocking thyrotropin receptor autoantibodies, J Clin Endocrinol Metab 89:352–356, 2004.
137. McKenzie JM: The gamma globulin of Graves' disease: thyroid stimulation by fraction and fragment, Trans Assoc Am Physicians 78:174–186, 1965.
138. Kriss JP, Pleshakov V, Rosenblum AL, et al: Studies on the pathogenesis of the ophthalmopathy of Graves' disease, J Clin Endocrinol Metab 27:582–593, 1967.
139. Pinchera A, Liberti P, De Santis R, et al: Relationship between the long-acting thyroid stimulator and circulating thyroid antibodies in Graves' disease, J Clin Endocrinol Metab 27:1758–1760, 1967.
140. McKenzie JM, Zakarija M: Fetal and neonatal hyperthyroidism and hypothyroidism due to maternal TSH receptor antibodies, Thyroid 2:155–159, 1992.
141. Leovey A, Nagy E, Balazs G, et al: Lymphocytes resided in the thyroid are the main source of TSH-receptor antibodies in Basedow's-Graves' disease? Exp Clin Endocrinol 99:147–150, 1992.
142. McLachlan SM, Dickinson AM, Malcolm A, et al: Thyroid autoantibody synthesis by cultures of thyroid and peripheral blood lymphocytes. I: Lymphocyte markers and response to pokeweed mitogen, Isr J Med Sci 52:45–53, 1983.
143. Okuda J, Akamizu T, Sugawa H, et al: Preparation and characterization of monoclonal antithyrotropin receptor antibodies obtained from peripheral lymphocytes of hypothyroid patients with primary myxedema, J Clin Endocrinol Metab 79:1600–1604, 1994.
144. Morgenthaler NG, Kim MR, Tremble J, et al: Human immunoglobulin G autoantibodies to the thyrotropin receptor from Epstein-Barr virus–transformed B lymphocytes: characterization by immunoprecipitation with recombinant antigen and biological activity, J Clin Endocrinol Metab 81:3155–3161, 1996.
145. Sugenoya A, Kobayashi S, Kasuga Y, et al: Evidence of intrathyroidal accumulation of TSH receptor antibody in Graves' disease, Acta Endocrinol (Copenh) 126:416–418, 1992.
146. Pinchera A, Liberti P, Martino E, et al: Effects of antithyroid therapy on the long-acting thyroid stimulator and the antithyroglobulin antibodies, J Clin Endocrinol 29:231–289, 1969.
147. Fenzi GF, Hashizume K, Roudeboush CP, et al: Changes in thyroid-stimulating immunoglobulins during antithyroid therapy, J Clin Endocrinol Metab 48:572–576, 1979.
148. Weetman AP, McGregor AM, Hall R: Evidence for an effect of antithyroid drugs on the natural history of Graves' disease, Clin Endocrinol 21:163–172, 1984.
149. Tsui S, Naik V, Hoa N, et al: Evidence for an association between thyroid-stimulating hormone and insulin-like

growth factor 1 receptors: a tale of two antigens implicated in Graves' disease, J Immunol 181:4397–4405, 2008.

150. Romagnani S: Regulation of the T cell response, Clin Exp Allergy 2006 11:1357–1366, 2006.

151. Abbas AK, Murphy KM, Sher A: Functional diversity of T lymphocytes, Nature 383:787–793, 1996.

152. Dardalhon V, Korn T, Kuchroo VK, et al: Role of Th1 and Th17 cells in organ-specific autoimmunity, J Autoimmun 2008 (in press).

153. Jackson RA, Haynes BF, Burch WM, et al: Ia+ T cells in new onset Graves' disease, J Clin Endocrinol Metab 59:187–190, 1984.

154. Matsunaga M, Eguchi K, Fukuda T, et al: Class II major histocompatibility complex antigen expression and cellular interactions in thyroid glands of Graves' disease, J Clin Endocrinol Metab 62:723–728, 1986.

155. Zeki K, Fujihira T, Shirakawa F, et al: Existence and immunological significance of circulating Ia+ T cells in autoimmune thyroid diseases, Acta Endocrinol (Copenh) 115:282–288, 1987.

156. McLachlan SM, Pegg CA, Atherton MC, et al: Subpopulations of thyroid autoantibody secreting lymphocytes in Graves' and Hashimoto thyroid glands, Clin Exp Immunol 65:319–328, 1986.

157. Aozasa M, Amino N, Iwatani Y, et al: Separation and analysis of mononuclear cells infiltrating the thyroid of patients with Graves' disease, Clin Immunol Immunopathol 43:343–353, 1987.

158. Mariotti S, del Prete GF, Mastromauro C, et al: The autoimmune infiltrate of Basedow's disease: analysis of clonal level and comparison with Hashimoto's thyroiditis, Exp Clin Endocrinol 97:139–146, 1991.

159. Martin A, Davies TF: T cells and human autoimmune thyroid disease: emerging data show lack of need to invoke suppressor T-cell problems, Thyroid 2:247–261, 1992.

160. Ueki Y, Eguchi K, Otsubo T, et al: Phenotypic analyses and concanavalin-A-induced suppressor cell dysfunction of intrathyroidal lymphocytes from patients with Graves' disease, J Clin Endocrinol Metab 67:1018–1024, 1988.

161. Martin A, Goldsmith NK, Friedman EW, et al: Intrathyroidal accumulation of T cell phenotypes in autoimmune thyroid disease, Autoimmunity 6:269–281, 1990.

162. Londei M, Bottazzo GF, Feldmann M: Human T-cell clones from autoimmune thyroid glands: specific recognition of autologous thyroid cells, Science 228:85–89, 1985.

163. Mackenzie WA, Davies TF: An intrathyroidal T-cell clone specifically cytotoxic for human thyroid cells, Immunology 61:101–103, 1987.

164. Mackenzie WA, Schwartz AE, Friedman EW, et al: Intrathyroidal T cell clones from patients with autoimmune thyroid disease, J Clin Endocrinol Metab 64:818–824, 1987.

165. Fisfalen ME, DeGroot LJ, Quintans J, et al: Microsomal antigen–reactive lymphocyte lines and clones derived from thyroid tissue of patients with Graves' disease, J Clin Endocrinol Metab 66:776–784, 1988.

166. Dayan CM, Londei M, Corcoran AE, et al: Autoantigen recognition by thyroid-infiltrating T cells in Graves' disease, Proc Natl Acad Sci U S A 88:7415–7419, 1991.

167. Watson PF, Pickerill AP, Davies R, et al: Analysis of cytokine gene expression in Graves' disease and multinodular goiter, J Clin Endocrinol Metab 79:355–360, 1994.

168. Fisfalen ME, Palmer EM, Van Seventer GA, et al: Thyrotropin-receptor and thyroid peroxidase–specific T cell clones and their cytokine profile in autoimmune thyroid disease, J Clin Endocrinol Metab 82:3655–3663, 1997.

169. Davis MM, Bjorkman PJ: T-cell antigen receptor genes and T-cell recognition, Nature 334:395–402, 1988.

170. Weiss A: Structure and function of the T cell antigen receptor, J Clin Invest 86:1015–1022, 1990.

171. Davies TF, Concepcion ES, Ben-Nun A, et al: T-cell receptor V gene use in autoimmune thyroid disease: direct assessment by thyroid aspiration, J Clin Endocrinol Metab 76:660–666, 1993.

172. Davies TF, Martin A, Concepcion ES, et al: Evidence of limited variability of antigen receptors on intrathyroidal T cells in autoimmune thyroid disease, N Engl J Med 325:238–244, 1991.

173. Tandon N, Freeman MA, Weetman AP: T cell response to synthetic TSH receptor peptides in Graves' disease, Clin Exp Immunol 89:468–473, 1992.

174. Heufelder AE, Wenzel BE, Scriba PC: Antigen receptor variable region repertoires expressed by T cells infiltrating thyroid, retroorbital, and pretibial tissue in Graves' disease, J Clin Endocrinol Metab 81:3733–3739, 1996.

175. Nakashima M, Kong YM, Davies TF: The role of T cells expressing TcR V beta 13 in autoimmune thyroiditis induced by transfer of mouse thyroglobulin-activated lymphocytes: Identification of two common CDR3 motifs, Clin Immunol Immunopathol 80:204–210, 1996.

176. McIntosh RS, Watson PF, Pickerill AP, et al: No restriction of intrathyroidal T cell receptor V alpha families in the thyroid of Graves' disease, Clin Exp Immunol 91:147–152, 1993.

177. Caso-Pelaez E, McGregor AM, Banga JP: A polyclonal T cell repertoire of V-alpha and V-beta T cell receptor gene families in intrathyroidal T lymphocytes of Graves' disease patients, Scand J Immunol 41:141–147, 1995.

178. Martin A, Nakashima M, Zhou A, et al: Detection of major T cell epitopes on human thyroid stimulating hormone receptor by overriding immune heterogeneity in patients with Graves' disease, J Clin Endocrinol Metab 82:3361–3366, 1997.

179. Inaba H, Martin W, De Groot AS, et al: Thyrotropin receptor epitopes and their relation to histocompatibility leukocyte antigen-DR molecules in Graves' disease, J Clin Endocrinol Metab 91:2286–2294, 2006.

180. Rotondi M, Chiovato L, Romagnani S, et al: Role of chemokines in endocrine autoimmune diseases, Endocr Rev 28:492–520, 2007.

181. Bottazzo GF, Todd I, Pujol BR: Hypotheses on genetic contributions to the etiology of diabetes mellitus, Immunol Today 5:230, 1984.

182. Davies TF: Co-culture of human thyroid monolayer cells and autologous T cells: impact of HLA class II antigen expression, J Clin Endocrinol Metab 61:418–422, 1985.

183. Weetman AP: The potential immunological role of the thyroid cell in autoimmune thyroid disease, Thyroid 4:493–499, 1994.

184. Hanafusa T, Pujol BR, Chiovato L, et al: Aberrant expression of HLA-DR antigen on thyrocytes in Graves' disease: relevance for autoimmunity, Lancet 2:1111–1115, 1983.

185. Bottazzo GF, Pujol BR, Hanafusa T, et al: Role of aberrant HLA-DR expression and antigen presentation in induction of endocrine autoimmunity, Lancet 2:1115–1119, 1983.

186. Jansson R, Karlsson A, Forsum U: Intrathyroidal HLA-DR expression and T lymphocyte phenotypes in Graves' thyrotoxicosis, Hashimoto's thyroiditis and nodular colloid goiter, Clin Exp Immunol 58:264–272, 1984.

187. Aichinger G, Fill H, Wick G: In situ immune complexes, lymphocyte subpopulations, and HLA-DR-positive epithelial cells in Hashimoto thyroiditis, Lab Invest 52:132–140, 1985.

188. Kawakami Y, Kuzuya N, Watanabe T, et al: Induction of experimental thyroiditis in mice by recombinant interferon gamma administration, Acta Endocrinol (Copenh) 122:41–48, 1990.

189. Tomer Y, Blackard JT, Akeno N: Interferon alpha treatment and thyroid dysfunction, Endocrinol Metab Clin North Am 36:105110–105166, 2007.

190. Caturegli P, Hejazi M, Suzuki K, et al: Hypothyroidism in transgenic mice expressing IFN-gamma in the thyroid, Proc Natl Acad Sci U S A 97:1719–1724, 2000.

191. Alimi E, Huang S, Brazillet MP, et al: Experimental autoimmune thyroiditis (EAT) in mice lacking the IFN-gamma receptor gene, Eur J Immunol 28:201–208, 1998.

192. Voorby HAM, Kabel PJ, De Haan M, et al: Dendritic cells and class II MHC expression on thyrocytes during the autoimmune thyroid disease of the BB rat, Clin Immunol Immunopathol 55:9–22, 1990.

193. Davies TF: The complex role of epithelial cell MHC class II antigen expression in autoimmune thyroid disease, Autoimmunity 8:87–89, 1990.

194. Londei M, Lamb JR, Bottazzo GF, et al: Epithelial cells expressing aberrant MHC class II determinants can present antigen to cloned human T cells, Nature 312:639–641, 1984.

195. Kimura H, Davies TF: Thyroid-specific T cells in the normal Wistar rat. II: T cell clones interact with cloned Wistar rat thyroid cells and provide direct evidence for autoantigen presentation by thyroid epithelial cells, Clin Immunol Immunopathol 58:195–206, 1991.

196. Eguchi K, Otsubo T, Kawabe K, et al: The remarkable proliferation of helper T cell subset in response to autologous thyrocytes and intrathyroidal T cells from patients with Graves' disease, Isr J Med Sci 70:403–410, 1987.

197. Kong YC, Flynn JC, Wan Q, et al: HLA and H2 class II transgenic mouse models to study susceptibility and protection in autoimmune thyroid disease, Autoimmunity:36:397–404, 2003.

198. Muixi L, Carrascal M, Alvarez I, et al: Thyroglobulin peptides associate in vivo in autoimmune thyroid glands, J Immunol 181:795–807, 2008.

199. Romagnani P: Rotondi M, Lazzeri E, et al: Expression of IP-10/CXCL10 and MIG/CXCL9 in the thyroid and increased levels of IP-10/CXCL10 in the serum of patients with recent onset Graves' disease, Am J Pathol 161:195–206, 2002.

200. Hutchings P, Rayner DC, Champion BR, et al: High efficiency antigen presentation by thyroglobulin-primed murine spleen B cells, Eur J Immunol 17:393–398, 1987.

201. Kabel PJ, Voorbij HA, De Haan M, et al: Intrathyroidal dendritic cells, J Clin Endocrinol Metab 66:199–207, 1988.

202. Salmaso C, Olive D, Pesce G, et al: Costimulatory molecules and autoimmune thyroid diseases, Autoimmunity 35:159–167, 2002.

203. Battifora M, Pesce G, Paolieri F, et al: B7.1 costimulatory molecule is expressed on thyroid follicular cells in Hashimoto's thyroiditis, but not in Graves' disease, J Clin Endocrinol Metab 83:4130–4139, 1998.

204. Weetman AP, McGregor AM: Autoimmune thyroid disease: further developments in our understanding, Endocr Rev 15:788–830, 1994.

205. Shimojo N, Kohno Y, Yagamuchi K, et al: Induction of Graves-like disease in mice by immunization with fibroblasts transfected with the thyrotropin receptor and a class II molecule, Proc Natl Acad Sci U S A 93:11074–11079, 1996.

206. McLachlan SM, Nagayama Y, Rapoport B: Insight into Graves' hyperthyroidism from animal models, Endocr Rev 26:800–832, 2005.

207. Nagayama Y: Graves' animal models of Graves' hyperthyroidism, Thyroid 17:981–988, 2007.

208. Brent GA: Graves' disease, N Engl J Med 358:2594–2605, 2008.

209. Cooper DS: Hyperthyroidism, Lancet 362:459–468, 2003.

210. Leznoff A, Sussman GL: Syndrome of idiopathic chronic urticaria and angioedema with thyroid autoimmunity: a study of 90 patients, J Allergy Clin Immunol 84:66–71, 1989.

211. Betterle C, Dal Pra C, Mantero F, et al: Autoimmune adrenal insufficiency and autoimmune polyendocrine syndromes: autoantibodies, autoantigens, and their applicability in diagnosis and disease prediction, Endocr Rev 23:327–364, 2002.

212. Kahaly GJ, Dillmann WH: Thyroid hormone action in the heart, Endocr Rev 26:704–728, 2005.

213. Klein I, Danzi S: Thyroid disease and the heart, Circulation 116:1725–1735, 2007.

214. Klein I, Ojamaa K: Thyrotoxicosis and the heart, Endocrinol Metab Clin North Am 27:51–62, 1998.

215. Shafer RB, Prentiss RA, Bond JH: Gastrointestinal transit in thyroid disease, Gastroenterology 86:852–855, 1984.

216. Thomas FB, Caldwell JH, Greenberger NJ: Steatorrhea in thyrotoxicosis. Relation to hypermotility and excessive dietary fat, Ann Intern Med 78:669–675, 1973.

217. Kubota S, Amino N, Matsumoto Y, et al: Serial changes in liver function tests in patients with thyrotoxicosis induced by Graves' disease and painless thyroiditis, Thyroid 18:283–287, 2008.

218. Bunevicius R, Prange AJ Jr: Psychiatric manifestations of Graves' hyperthyroidism: pathophysiology and treatment options, CNS Drugs 20:897–909, 2006.

219. Mariotti S, Franceschi C, Cossarizza A, et al: The aging thyroid, Endocr Rev 16:686–715, 1995.

220. Feibel JH, Campa JF: Thyrotoxic neuropathy (Basedow's paraplegia), J Neurol Neurosurg Psychiatry 39:491–497, 1976.

221. Pandit L, Shankar SK, Gayathri N, et al: Acute thyrotoxic neuropathy—Basedow's paraplegia revisited, J Neurol Sci 155:211–214, 1998.

222. Marino M, Ricciardi R, Pinchera A, et al: Mild clinical expression of myasthenia gravis associated with autoimmune thyroid diseases, J Clin Endocrinol Metab 82:438–443, 1997.

223. Marino M, Barbesino G, Manetti L, et al: Mild clinical expression of myasthenia gravis associated with autoimmune thyroid disease (letter), J Clin Endocrinol Metab 82:3905–3906, 1997.

224. Marinò M, Barbesino G, Pinchera A, et al: Increased frequency of euthyroid ophthalmopathy in patients with Graves' disease associated with myasthenia gravis, Thyroid 10:799–802, 2000.

225. Kanazawa M, Shimohata T, Tanaka K, et al: Clinical features of patients with myasthenia gravis associated with autoimmune diseases, Eur J Neurol 14:1403–1404, 2007.

226. Kung AW: Clinical review: thyrotoxic periodic paralysis: a diagnostic challenge, J Clin Endocrinol Metab 91:2490–2495, 2006.

227. Tamai H, Tanaka K, Komaki G, et al: HLA and thyrotoxic periodic paralysis in Japanese patients, J Clin Endocrinol Metab 64:1075–1078, 1987.

228. Dias Da Silva MR, Cerutti JM, Arnaldi LA, et al: A mutation in the KCNE3 potassium channel gene is associated with susceptibility to thyrotoxic hypokalemic periodic paralysis, J Clin Ebndocrinol Metab 87:4879–4880, 2002.

229. Painter SE, Kleerekoper M, Camacho PM: Secondary osteoporosis: a review of the recent evidence, Endocr Pract 12:436–445, 2006.

230. Vestergaard P, Mosekilde L: Hyperthyroidism, bone mineral, and fracture risk—a meta-analysis, Thyroid 585–593, 2003.

231. Wexler JA, Sharretts J: Thyroid and bone, Endocrinol Metab Clin North Am 36:673–705, 2007.

232. Franklyn JA, Maisonneuve P, Sheppard MC, et al: Mortality after the treatment of hyperthyroidism with radioactive iodine, N Engl J Med 338:712–718, 1998.

233. Abe E, Marians RC, Yu W, et al: TSH is a negative regulator of skeletal remodeling, Cell 115:151–162, 2003.

234. Sun L, Vukicevic S, Baliram R, et al: Intermittent recombinant TSH injections prevent ovariectomy-induced bone loss, Proc Natl Acad Sci U S A 105:4289–4294, 2008.

235. Zaidi M, Sun L, Davies TF, et al: Low TSH triggers bone loss: fact or fiction? Thyroid 16:1075–1076, 2006.

236. Hase H, Ando T, Eldeiry L, et al: TNF alpha mediates the skeletal effects of thyroid-stimulating hormone, Proc Natl Acad Sci U S A 103:12849–12854, 2006.

237. Cooper DS: Antithyroid drugs, N Engl J Med 352:905–917, 2005.

238. Fein HG, Rivlin RS: Anemia in thyroid diseases, Med Clin North Am 59:1133–1145, 1975.

239. Sibilla R, Santaguida MG, Virili C, et al: Chronic unexplained anaemia in isolated autoimmune thyroid disease or associated with autoimmune related disorders, Clin Endocrinol (Oxf) 68:640–645, 2008.

240. Aydin Y, Berker D, Ustün I, et al: A very rare cause of aplastic anemia: Graves disease, South Med J 101:666–667, 2008.

241. Erem C, Ersoz HO, Karti SS, et al: Blood coagulation and fibrinolysis in patients with hyperthyroidism, J Endocrinol Invest 25:345–350, 2002.

242. Krassas GE: Thyroid disease and female reproduction, Fertil Steril 74:1063–1070, 2000.

243. Koutras DA: Disturbances of menstruation in thyroid disease, Ann N Y Acad Sci 816:280–284, 1997.

244. Chiovato L, Lapi P, Fiore E, et al: Thyroid autoimmunity and female gender, J Endocrinol Invest 16:384–391, 1993.

245. Pugeat M, Crave JC, Tourniaire J, et al: Clinical utility of sex hormone-binding globulin measurement, Horm Res 45:148–155, 1996.

246. Meikle AW: The interrelationships between thyroid dysfunction and hypogonadism in men and boys, Thyroid 14(Suppl 1):S17–25, 2004.

247. Kim B: Thyroid hormone as a determinant of energy expenditure and the basal metabolic rate, Thyroid 18:141–144, 2008.

248. Simonides WS, van Hardeveld C: Thyroid hormone as a determinant of metabolic and contractile phenotype of skeletal muscle, Thyroid 18:205–216, 2008.

249. Chidakel A, Mentuccia D, Celi FS: Peripheral metabolism of thyroid hormone and glucose homeostasis, Thyroid 15:899–903, 2005.

250. Duntas LH: Thyroid disease and lipids, Thyroid 12:287–293, 2002.

251. Cachefo A, Boucher P, Vidon C, et al: Hepatic lipogenesis and cholesterol synthesis in hyperthyroid patients, J Clin Endocrinol Metab 86:5353–5357, 2001.

252. Iglesias P, Díez JJ: Influence of thyroid dysfunction on serum concentrations of adipocytokines, Cytokine 40:61–70, 2007.

253. Feldt-Rasmussen U: Thyroid and leptin, Thyroid 17:413–419, 2007.

254. Santini F, Marsili A, Mammoli C, et al: Serum concentrations of adiponectin and leptin in patients with thyroid dysfunctions, J Endocrinol Invest 27:RC5–7, 2004.

255. Bartalena L, Pinchera A, Marcocci C: Management of Graves' ophthalmopathy: reality and perspectives, Endocr Rev 21:168–199, 2000.

256. Bartalena L, Wiersinga WM, Pinchera A: Graves' ophthalmopathy: state of the art and perspectives, J Endocrinol Invest 27:295–301, 2004.

257. Marcocci C, Pinchera A, Marinò M: A treatment strategy for Graves' orbitopathy, Nat Clin Pract Endocrinol Metab 3:430–436, 2007.

258. Fatourechi V: Pretibial myxedema: pathophysiology and treatment options, Am J Clin Dermatol 6:295–309, 2005.

259. Rapoport B, Alsabeh R, Afterggod D, et al: Elephantiasic pretibial myxedema: insight into and a hypothesis regarding the pathogenesis of the extrathyroidal manifestations of Graves' disease, Thryoid 10:629–630, 2000.

260. Heufelder AE, Bahn RS, Scriba PC: Analysis of T-cell antigen receptor variable region gene usage in patients with thyroid-related pretibial dermopathy, J Invest Dermatol 105:372–378, 1995.

261. Chang TC, Wu SL, Hsiao YL, et al: TSH and TSH receptor antibody–binding sites in fibroblasts of pretibial myxedema are related to the extracellular domain of entire TSH receptor, Clin Immunol Immunopathol 71:113–120, 1994.

262. Heufelder AE, Dutton CM, Sarkar G, et al: Detection of TSH receptor RNA in cultured fibroblasts from patients with Graves' ophthalmopathy and pretibial dermopathy, Thyroid 3:297–300, 1993.

263. Stadlmayr W, Spitzweg C, Bichlmair AM, et al: TSH receptor transcripts and TSH receptor–like immunoreactivity in orbital and pretibial fibroblasts of patients with Graves' ophthalmopathy and pretibial myxedema, Thyroid 7:3–12, 1997.

264. Daumerie C, Ludgate M, Costagliola S, et al: Evidence for thyrotropin receptor immunoreactivity in pretibial connective tissue from patients with thyroid-associated dermopathy, Eur J Endocrinol 146:35–38, 2002.

265. Marinò M, Chiovato L, Lisi S, et al: Role of thyroglobulin in the pathogenesis of Graves' ophthalmopathy: the hypothesis of Kriss revisited, J Endocrinol Invest 27:230–236, 2004.

266. Fatourechi V, Bartley GB, Eghbali-Fatourechi GZ, et al: Graves' dermopathy and acropachy are markers of severe Graves' ophthalmopathy, Thyroid 13:1141–1144, 2003.

267. Dufour DR: Laboratory tests of thyroid function: uses and limitations, Endocrinol Metab Clin North Am 36:579–594, 2007.

268. Grüters A: Thyroid hormone transporter defects, Endocr Dev 10:118–126, 2007.

269. Mariotti S, Martino E, Cupini C, et al: Low serum thyroglobulin as a clue to the diagnosis of thyrotoxicosis factitia, N Engl J Med 307:410–412, 1982.

270. Mariotti S, Caturegli P, Piccolo P, et al: Antithyroid peroxidase autoantibodies in thyroid diseases, J Clin Endocrinol Metab 71:661–669, 1990.

271. McLachlan SM, Rapoport B: Thyroid peroxidase as an autoantigen, Thyroid 17:939–994, 2007.

272. McLachlan SM, Rapoport B: Why measure thyroglobulin autoantibodies rather than thyroid peroxidase autoantibodies? Thyroid 14:510–520, 2004.

273. Mariotti S, Barbesino G, Caturegli P, et al: Assay of thyroglobulin in serum with thyroglobulin autoanti-

bodies: an unobtainable goal? J Clin Endocrinol Metab 80:468–472, 1995.

274. Mariotti S, Sansoni P, Barbesino G, et al: Thyroid and other organ-specific autoantibodies in healthy centenarians, Lancet 339:1506–1508, 1992.

275. Macchia E, Concetti R, Borgoni F, et al: Assays of TSH-receptor antibodies in 576 patients with various thyroid disorders: Their incidence, significance and clinical usefulness, Autoimmunity 3:103–112, 1989.

276. Pittman JA Jr, Dailey GE 3d, Beschi RJ: Changing normal values for thyroidal radioiodine uptake, N Engl J Med 280:1431–1434, 1969.

277. O'Hare NJ, Murphy D, Malone JF: Thyroid dosimetry of adult European populations, Br J Radiol 71:535–543, 1998.

278. Martino E, Bartalena L, Mariotti S, et al: Radioactive iodine thyroid uptake in patients with amiodarone-iodine–induced thyroid dysfunction, Acta Endocrinol (Copenh) 119:167–173, 1988.

279. Gutekunst R, Hafermann W, Mansky T, et al: Ultrasonography related to clinical and laboratory findings in lymphocytic thyroiditis, Acta Endocrinol (Copenh) 121:129–135, 1989.

280. Vitti P: Grey scale thyroid ultrasonography in the evaluation of patients with Graves' disease, Eur J Endocrinol 142:22–24, 2000.

281. Vitti P, Martino E, Aghini-Lombardi F, et al: Thyroid volume measurement by ultrasound in children as a tool for the assessment of mild iodine deficiency, J Clin Endocrinol Metab 79:600–603, 1994.

282. Bogazzi F, Vitti P: Could improved ultrasound and power Doppler replace thyroidal radioiodine uptake to assess thyroid disease? Nat Clin Pract Endocrinol Metab 4:70–71, 2008.

283. Cooper DS: Antithyroid drugs, N Engl J Med 311:1353–1362, 1984. Review.

284. Reinwein D, Benker G, Lazarus JH, et al: A prospective randomized trial of antithyroid drug dose in Graves' disease therapy. European Multicenter Study Group on Antithyroid Drug Treatment, J Clin Endocrinol Metab 76:1516–1521, 1993.

285. Hedley AJ, Young RE, Jones SJ, et al: Antithyroid drugs in the treatment of hyperthyroidism of Graves' disease: long-term follow-up of 434 patients. Scottish Automated Follow-Up Register Group, Clin Endocrinol (Oxf) 31:209–218, 1989.

286. Schleusener H, Schwander J, Fischer C, et al: Prospective multicentre study on the prediction of relapse after antithyroid drug treatment in patients with Graves' disease [published erratum appears in Acta Endocrinol (Copenh) 1989 Aug;121(2):304]. Acta Endocrinol (Copenh) 120:689–701, 1989.

287. Vitti P, Rago T, Chiovato L, et al: Clinical features of patients with Graves' disease undergoing remission after antithyroid drug treatment, Thyroid 7:369–375, 1997.

288. Kaguelidou F, Alberti C, Castanet M, et al: Predictors of Autoimmune Hyperthyroidism Relapse in Children after Discontinuation of Antithyroid Drug Treatment, J Clin Endocrinol Metab 2008 Jul 15. [Epub ahead of print].

289. Wartofsky L: Low remission after therapy for Graves disease. Possible relation of dietary iodine with antithyroid therapy results, JAMA 226:1083–1088, 1973.

290. Solomon BL, Evaul JE, Burman KD, et al: Remission rates with antithyroid drug therapy: continuing influence of iodine intake? Ann Intern Med 107:510–512, 1987.

291. Davies TF, You FP, Evered DC, et al: Value of thyroid-stimulating-antibody determinations in predicting short-term thyrotoxic relapse in Graves' disease, Lancet 1:1181–1182, 1977.

292. Eshoj O, Kvetny J, Mogensen EF, et al: Prediction of the course of Graves' disease after medical antithyroid treatment, Acta Med Scand 217:225–228, 1985.

293. Nagataki S: Prediction of relapse in Graves' disease, Ann Acad Med Singapore 15:486–491, 1986.

294. Weetman AP, Ratanachaiyavong S, Middleton GW, et al: Prediction of outcome in Graves' disease after carbimazole treatment, Q J Med 59:409–419, 1986.

295. Wilson R, McKillop JH, Henderson N, et al: The ability of the serum thyrotrophin receptor antibody (TRAb) index and HLA status to predict long-term remission of thyrotoxicosis following medical therapy for Graves' disease, Clin Endocrinol (Oxf) 25:151–156, 1986.

296. Talbot JN, Duron F, Feron R, et al: Thyroglobulin, thyrotropin and thyrotropin binding inhibiting immunoglobulins assayed at the withdrawal of antithyroid drug therapy as predictors of relapse of Graves' disease within one year, J Endocrinol Invest 12:589–595, 1989.

297. Ikenoue H, Okamura K, Sato K, et al: Prediction of relapse in drug-treated Graves' disease using thyroid stimulation indices, Acta Endocrinol (Copenh) 125:643–650, 1991.

298. Lamberg BA, Salmi J, Wagar G, et al: Spontaneous hypothyroidism after antithyroid treatment of hyperthyroid Graves' disease, J Endocrinol Invest 4:399–402, 1981.

299. Feldt-Rasmussen U, Schleusener H, Carayon P: Meta-analysis evaluation of the impact of thyrotropin receptor antibodies on long term remission after medical therapy of Graves' disease, J Clin Endocrinol Metab 78:98–102, 1994.

300. Romaldini JH, Werner MC, Bromberg N, et al: Adverse effects related to antithyroid drugs and their dose regimen, Exp Clin Endocrinol 97:261–264, 1991.

301. Davies TF, Yeo PP, Evered DC, et al: Value of thyroid-stimulating-antibody determinations in predicting short-term thyrotoxic relapse in Graves' disease, Lancet 1:1181–1182, 1977.

302. McGregor AM, Petersen MM, McLachlan SM, et al: Carbimazole and the autoimmune response in Graves' disease, N Engl J Med 303:302–304, 1980.

303. Marcocci C, Chiovato L, Mariotti S, et al: Changes of circulating thyroid autoantibody levels during and after the therapy with methimazole in patients with Graves' disease, J Endocrinol Invest 5:13–19, 1982.

304. Weetman AP, McGregor AP, Hall R: Methimazole inhibits thyroid autoantibody production by an action on accessory cells, Clin Immunol Immunopathol 28:39–45, 1983.

305. Weiss I, Davies TF: Inhibition of immunoglobulin-secreting cells by antithyroid drugs, J Clin Endocrinol Metab 53:1223–1228, 1981.

306. Rennie DP, McGregor AM, Keats D, et al: The influence of methimazole on thyroglobulin-induced autoimmune thyroiditis in the rat, Endocrinology 112:326–330, 1983.

307. Wenzel KW, Lente JR: Similar effects of thionamide drugs and perchlorate on thyroid-stimulating immunoglobulins in Graves' disease: evidence against an immunosuppressive action of thionamide drugs, J Clin Endocrinol Metab 58:62–69, 1984.

308. Mariotti S, Pinchera A: Role of the immune system in the control of thyroid function. In Greer MA, editor: The Thyroid Gland, New York, 1990, Raven, pp 147–218.

309. Hashizume K, Ichikawa K, Sakurai A, et al: Administration of thyroxine in treated Graves' disease—effects on the level of antibodies to thyroid stimulating hormone receptors and on the risk of recurrence of hyperthyroidism, N Engl J Med 324:947–953, 1991.

310. Romaldini JH, Bromberg N, Werner RS, et al: Comparison of effects of high and low dosage regimens of antithyroid drugs in the management of Graves' hyperthyroidism, J Clin Endocrinol Metab 57:563–570, 1983.

311. Weetman AP, Pickerill AP, Watson P, et al: Treatment of Graves' disease with the block-replace regimen of antithyroid drugs: The effect of treatment duration and immunogenetic susceptibility on relapse, Q J Med 87:337–341, 1994.

312. Tamai H, Hayaki I, Kawai K, et al: Lack of effect of thyroxine administration on elevated thyroid stimulating hormone receptor antibody levels in treated Graves' disease patients, J Clin Endocrinol Metab 80:1481–1484, 1995.

313. Rittmaster RS, Zwicker H, Abbott EC, et al: Effect of methimazole with or without exogenous L-thyroxine on serum concentrations of thyrotropin (TSH) receptor antibodies in patients with Graves' disease, J Clin Endocrinol Metab 81:3283–3288, 1996.

314. Rizvi A, Crapo LM: Failure of thyroxine therapy for Graves disease (letter), Ann Intern Med 124:694, 1996.

315. Rittmaster RS, Abbott EC, Douglas R, et al: Effect of methimazole, with or without L-thyroxine, on remission rates in Graves' disease, J Clin Endocrinol Metab 83:814–818, 1998.

316. Emerson CH, Anderson AJ, Howard WJ, et al: Serum thyroxine and triiodothyronine concentrations during iodide treatment of hyperthyroidism, J Clin Endocrinol Metab 40:33–36, 1975.

317. Marigold JH, Morgan AK, Earle DJ, et al: Lugol's iodine: its effect on thyroid blood flow in patients with thyrotoxicosis, Br J Surg 72:45–47, 1985.

318. Chang DC, Wheeler MH, Woodcock JP, et al: The effect of preoperative Lugol's iodine on thyroid blood flow in patients with Graves' hyperthyroidism, Surgery 102:1055–1061, 1987.

319. Burgi H, Wimpfheimer C, Burger A, et al: Changes of circulating thyroxine, triiodothyronine and reverse tri-iodothyronine after radiographic contrast agents, J Clin Endocrinol Metab 43:1203–1210, 1976.

320. Wu SY, Chopra IJ, Solomon DH, et al: Changes in circulating iodothyronines in euthyroid and hyperthyroid subjects given ipodate (Oragrafin), an agent for oral cholecystography, J Clin Endocrinol Metab 46:691–697, 1978.

321. Bogazzi F, Bartalena L, Cosci C, et al: Treatment of type II amiodarone-induced thyrotoxicosis by either iopanoic acid or glucocorticoids: a prospective, randomized study, J Clin Endocrinol Metab 88:1999–2002, 2003.

322. Robuschi G, Manfredi A, Salvi M, et al: Effect of sodium ipodate and iodide on free T$_4$ and free T$_3$ concentrations in patients with Graves' disease, J Endocrinol Invest 9:287–291, 1986.

323. Laurberg P, Boye N: Inhibitory effect of various radiographic contrast agents on secretion of thyroxine by the dog thyroid and on peripheral and thyroidal deiodination of thyroxine to tri-iodothyronine, J Endocrinol 112:387–390, 1987.

324. Wu SY, Shyh TP, Chopra IJ, et al: Comparison of sodium ipodate (Oragrafin) and propylthiouracil in early treatment of hyperthyroidism, J Clin Endocrinol Metab 54:630–634, 1982.

325. Shen DC, Wu SY, Chopra IJ, et al: Long-term treatment of Graves' hyperthyroidism with sodium ipodate, J Clin Endocrinol Metab 61:723–727, 1985.

326. Martino E, Balzano S, Bartalena L, et al: Therapy of Graves' disease with sodium ipodate is associated with a high recurrence rate of hyperthyroidism, J Endocrinol Invest 14:847–851, 1991.

327. DeGroot LJ, Buhler U: Effect of perchlorate and methimazole on iodine metabolism, Acta Endocrinol (Copenh) 68:696–706, 1971.

328. Barzilai D, Sheinfeld M: Fatal complications following use of potassium perchlorate in thyrotoxicosis. Report of two cases and a review of the literature, Isr J Med Sci 2:453–456, 1966.

329. Bartalena L, Brogioni S, Grasso L, et al: Treatment of amiodarone-induced thyrotoxicosis, a difficult challenge: results of a prospective study, J Clin Endocrinol Metab 81:2930–2933, 1996.

330. Bogazzi F, Bartalena L, Campomori A, et al: Treatment with lithium prevents serum thyroid hormone increase after thionamide withdrawal and radioiodine therapy in patients with Graves' disease, J Clin Endocrinol Metab 87:4490–4495, 2002.

331. Bogazzi F, Martino E, Bartalena L: Antithyroid drug treatment prior to radioiodine therapy for Graves' disease: yes or no? J Endocrinol Invest 26:174–176, 2003.

332. Henderson JM, Portmann L, Van Melle G, et al: Propranolol as an adjunct therapy for hyperthyroid tremor, Eur Neurol 37:182–185, 1997.

333. Wiersinga WM: Propranolol and thyroid hormone metabolism, Thyroid 1:273–277, 1991.

334. Dobyns BM, Vickery AL, Maloof F, et al: Functional and histologic effects of therapeutic doses of radioiodine therapy for hyperthyroidism, J Clin Endcrinol Metab 13:548, 1953.

335. Beierwaltes WH: The treatment of hyperthyroidism with iodine-131, Semin Nucl Med 8:95–103, 1978.

336. Franklyn JA, Daykin J, Drolc Z, et al: Long-term follow-up of treatment of thyrotoxicosis by three different methods, Clin Endocrinol (Oxf) 34:71–76, 1991.

337. Bartalena L, Marcocci C, Bogazzi F, et al: Relation between therapy for hyperthyroidism and the course of Graves' ophthalmopathy, N Engl J Med 338:73–78, 1998.

338. Perros P, Kendall-Taylor P, Neoh C, et al: A prospective study of the effects of radioiodine therapy for hyperthyroidism in patients with minimally active Graves' ophthalmopathy, J Clin Endocrinol Metab 90:5321–5323, 2005.

339. Burch HB, Solomon BL, Wartofsky L, et al: Discontinuing antithyroid drug therapy before ablation with radioiodine in Graves' disease, Ann Intern Med 121:553–559, 1994.

340. Block MA, Miller MJ, Horn RC Jr: Carcinoma of the thyroid after external radiation to the neck in adults, Am J Surg 118:764–769, 1969.

341. Ron E, Saftlas AF: Head and neck radiation carcinogenesis: epidemiologic evidence, Otolaryngol Head Neck Surg 115:403–408, 1996.

342. Hall P, Holm LE: Late consequences of radioiodine for diagnosis and therapy in Sweden, Thyroid 7:205–208, 1997.

343. Ron E, Doody MM, Becker DV, et al: Cancer mortality following treatment for adult hyperthyroidism. Cooperative Thyrotoxicosis Therapy Follow-up Study Group, JAMA 280:347–355, 1998.

344. Graham GD, Burman KD: Radioiodine treatment of Graves' disease. An assessment of its potential risks, Ann Intern Med 105:900–905, 1986.

345. Federico G, Boni G, Fabiani B, et al: No evidence of chromosome damage in children and adolescents with differentiated thyroid carcinoma after receiving ^{131}I radiometabolic therapy, as evaluated by micronucleus assay and microarray analysis, Eur J Nucl Med Mol Imaging. 2008 (in press).

346. Hennemann G, Krenning EP, Sankaranarayanan K: Place of radioactive iodine in treatment of thyrotoxicosis, Lancet 1:1369–1372, 1986.

347. Franklyn JA, Sheppard MC, Maisonneuve P: Thyroid function and mortality in patients treated for hyperthyroidism, JAMA 294:71–80, 2005.

348. Baverstock K, Egloff B, Pinchera A, et al: Thyroid cancer after Chernobyl, Nature 359:21–22, 1992.

349. Pacini F, Vorontsova T, Demidchik EP, et al: Post-Chernobyl thyroid carcinoma in Belarus children and adolescents: comparison with naturally occurring thyroid carcinoma in Italy and France, J Clin Endocrinol Metab 82:3563–3569, 1997.

350. Dobyns BM, Sheline GE, Workman JB, et al: Malignant and benign neoplasms of the thyroid in patients treated for hyperthyroidism: a report of the Cooperative Thyrotoxicosis Therapy Follow-Up Study, J Clin Endocrinol Metab 38:976–998, 1974.

351. Rivkees SA, Dinauer C: An optimal treatment for pediatric Graves' disease is radioiodine, J Clin Endocrinol Metab 92:797–800, 2007.

352. Miccoli P, Vitti P, Rago T, et al: Surgical treatment of Graves' disease: subtotal or total thyroidectomy? Surgery 120:1020–1025, 1996.

353. Kasuga Y, Sugenoya A, Kobayashi S, et al: Clinical evaluation of the response to surgical treatment of Graves' disease, Surg Gynecol Obstet 170:327–330, 1990.

354. Menconi F, Marinò M, Pinchera A, et al: Effects of total thyroid ablation versus near-total thyroidectomy alone on mild to moderate Graves' orbitopathy treated with intravenous glucocorticoids, J Clin Endocrinol Metab 92:1653–1658, 2007.

355. Baeza A, Aguayo J, Barria M, et al: Rapid preoperative preparation in hyperthyroidism, Clin Endocrinol (Oxf) 35:439–442, 1991.

356. Tomaski SM, Mahoney EM, Burgess LP, et al: Sodium ipodate (Oragrafin) in the preoperative preparation of Graves' hyperthyroidism, Laryngoscope 107:1066–1070, 1997.

357. Max MH, Scherm M, Bland KI: Early and late complications after thyroid operations, South Med J 76:977–980, 1983.

358. Kasemsuwan L, Nubthuenetr S: Recurrent laryngeal nerve paralysis: a complication of thyroidectomy, J Otolaryngol 26:365–367, 1997.

359. Pattou F, Combemale F, Fabre S, et al: Hypocalcemia following thyroid surgery: incidence and prediction of outcome, World J Surg 22:718–724, 1998.

360. Glinoer D, Hesch D, Lagasse R, et al: The management of hyperthyroidism due to Graves' disease in Europe in 1986. Results of an international survey, Acta Endocrinol Suppl 285:3–23, 1987.

361. Wartofsky L, Glinoer D, Solomon B, et al: Differences and similarities in the treatment of diffuse goiter in Europe and the United States, Exp Clin Endocrinol 97:243–251, 1991.

362. Freitas JE, Swanson DP, Gross MD, et al: Iodine-131: optimal therapy for hyperthyroidism in children and adolescents? J Nucl Med 20:847–850, 1979.

363. Rivkees SA, Sklar C, Freemark M: Clinical review 99: the management of Graves' disease in children, with special emphasis on radioiodine treatment, J Clin Endocrinol Metab 83:3767–3776, 1998.

364. Waldhausen JH: Controversies related to the medical and surgical management of hyperthyroidism in children, Semin Pediatr Surg 6:121–127, 1997.

365. Witte J, Goretzki PE, Roher HD: Surgery for Graves' disease in childhood and adolescence, Exp Clin Endocrinol Diabetes 105:58–60, 1997.

366. Lazarus JH: Guidelines for the use of radioiodine in the management of hyperthyroidism: a summary. Prepared by the Radioiodine Audit Subcommittee of the Royal College of Physicians Committee on Diabetes and Endocrinology, and the Research Unit of the Royal College of Physicians, J R Coll Physicians Lond 29:464–469, 1995.

367. Weetman AP, Wiersinga WM: Current management of thyroid-associated ophthalmopathy in Europe. Results of an international survey, Clin Endocrinol (Oxf) 49:21–28, 1998.

368. Chiovato L, Latrofa F; Braverman LE, et al: Disappearance of humoral thyroid autoimmunity after complete removal of thyroid antigens, Ann Int Med 139:346–351, 2003.

369. Abalovich M, Amino N, Barbour LA, et al: Management of thyroid dysfunction during pregnancy and postpartum: an Endocrine Society Clinical Practice Guideline, J Clin Endocrinol Metab 92(8 Suppl):S1–47, 2007.

370. Chattaway JM, Klepser TB: Propylthiouracil versus methimazole in treatment of Graves' disease during pregnancy, Ann Pharmacother 41:1018–1022, 2007.

371. Marchant B, Brownlie BE, Hart DM, et al: The placental transfer of propylthiouracil, methimazole and carbimazole, J Clin Endocrinol Metab 45:1187–1193, 1977.

372. Cheron RG, Kaplan MM, Larsen PR, et al: Neonatal thyroid function after propylthiouracil therapy for maternal Graves' disease, N Engl J Med 304:525–528, 1981.

373. Ribuffo D, Costantini M, Gullo P, et al: Aplasia cutis congenita of the scalp, the skull, and the dura, Scand J Plast Reconstr Surg Hand Surg 37:176–180, 2003.

374. Santini F, Chiovato L, Ghirri P, et al: Serum iodothyronines in the human fetus and the newborn: evidence for an important role of placenta in fetal thyroid hormone homeostasis, J Clin Endocrinol Metab 84:493–498, 1999.

375. Lamberg BA, Ikonen E, Osterlund K, et al: Antithyroid treatment of maternal hyperthyroidism during lactation, Clin Endocrinol (Oxf) 21:81–87, 1984.

376. Zakarija M, McKenzie JM: Pregnancy-associated changes in the thyroid-stimulating antibody of Graves' disease and the relationship to neonatal hyperthyroidism, J Clin Endocrinol Metab 57:1036–1040, 1983.

377. Tamaki H, Amino N, Takeoka K, et al: Prediction of later development of thyrotoxicosis or central hypothyroidism from the cord serum thyroid-stimulating hormone level in neonates born to mothers with Graves' disease, J Pediatr 115:318–321, 1989.

378. Karpman BA, Rapoport B, Filetti S, et al: Treatment of neonatal hyperthyroidism due to Graves' disease with sodium ipodate, J Clin Endocrinol Metab 64:119–123, 1987.

379. Trivalle C, Doucet J, Chassagne P, et al: Differences in the signs and symptoms of hyperthyroidism in older and younger patients, J Am Geriatr Soc 44:50–53, 1996.

380. Martin FI, Deam DR: Hyperthyroidism in elderly hospitalised patients. Clinical features and treatment outcomes, Med J Aust 164:200–203, 1996.

381. Perros P, Crombie AL, Matthews JN, et al: Age and gender influence the severity of thyroid-associated ophthalmopathy: a study of 101 patients attending a combined thyroid-eye clinic, Clin Endocrinol (Oxf) 38:367–372, 1993.

382. Kriss JP, Pleshakov V, Rosenblum A, et al: Therapy with occlusive dressings of pretibial myxedema with fluocinolone acetonide, J Clin Endocrinol Metab 27:595–604, 1967.

383. Lang PG, Sisson JC, Lynch PJ: Intralesional triamcinolone therapy for pretibial myxedema, Arch Dermatol 111:197–202, 1975.

384. Derrick EK, Tanner B, Price ML: Successful surgical treatment of severe pretibial myxoedema, Br J Dermatol 133:317–318, 1995.

385. Pingsmann A, Ockenfels HM, Patsalis T: Surgical excision of pseudotumorous pretibial myxedema, Foot Ankle Int 17:107–110, 1996.

386. Wartofsky L: Treatment options for hyperthyroidism, Hosp Pract 31:69–73, 76–78, 81–84, 1996.

Chapter 10

GRAVES' OPHTHALMOPATHY

HENRY B. BURCH and REBECCA S. BAHN

Graves' ophthalmopathy occurs as a spectrum of disease ranging from subclinical enlargement of the extraocular muscles in most patients with this condition to disfiguring and vision-threatening involvement of the entire orbit in an unfortunate few. Although the diagnosis of ophthalmopathy in patients with Graves' disease may precede, accompany, or follow that of hyperthyroidism, eye involvement generally is diagnosed concurrently with or after the diagnosis of thyrotoxicosis[1-5] (Fig. 10-1).

The concept of a pathophysiologic link between Graves' thyrotoxicosis and ophthalmopathy has been challenged on the basis of the existence of patients with euthyroid ophthalmopathy or unilateral eye disease and a poor numeric correlation between thyroid-stimulating antibody levels and the presence of eye disease. However, these arguments have been superseded by the demonstration of subtle thyroid abnormalities in most "euthyroid" ophthalmopathy patients,[6,7] the finding of contralateral eye muscle abnormalities in most patients with apparent unilateral

disease,[1] and the demonstration of a definite qualitative association between the severity of ophthalmopathy and other peripheral manifestations of Graves' disease and thyroid-stimulating antibody titers.[8,9]

Studies investigating the pathogenesis of Graves' ophthalmopathy have served to expand the understanding of ophthalmopathy beyond early purely mechanical descriptions. These efforts have focused on the identification of orbital fibroblasts as active participants in the retrobulbar immune response and on the elucidation of immune mechanisms responsible for the activation of these cells. In addition, recent studies have identified thyrotropin (the thyroid-stimulating hormone receptor [TSHR]) as an important orbital autoantigen.

Management of Graves' ophthalmopathy requires a carefully integrated approach involving the endocrinologist and the ophthalmologist, with the goal of preserving the patient's vision and restoring favorable self-perception and quality of life.[10] In this chapter, we provide an examination of the present state of knowledge regarding the pathogenesis of Graves' ophthalmopathy and an up-to-date review of current methods in the diagnosis and management of this disorder.

Epidemiology

Clinically evident ophthalmopathy occurs in 10% to 25% of unselected patients with Graves' disease if lid signs are excluded as a diagnostic feature, in 30% to 45% if lid signs are included,[3,11] and in approximately 70% of patients without overt eye disease if computed tomography (CT) or increased intraocular pressure on upgaze is used to establish the diagnosis.[12-15] Magnetic resonance imaging (MRI) reveals extraocular muscle enlargement in 71% of patients without overt findings on physical examination.[16] Fortunately, fewer than 5% of patients with Graves' disease have severe ophthalmopathy.[17] The age-adjusted incidence of Graves' ophthalmopathy in the population of Olmsted County, Minnesota, was found to be 16 cases per 100,000 population per year for women and 2.9 for men.[18] A bimodal distribution was noted, with peak incidence in the age groups 40 to 44 years and 60 to 64 years in women and 45 to 49 years and 65 to 69 years in men. Additional peripheral manifestations of Graves' disease such as dermopathy and acropachy occur with lower frequency. Thyroid dermopathy is found in 4% to 15% of patients with clinically evident Graves' ophthalmopathy, and 7% of dermopathy patients will also have thyroid acropachy.[4]

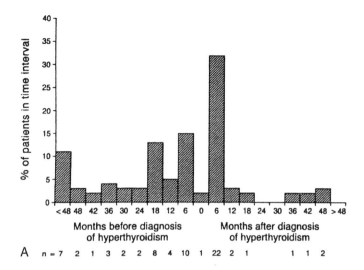

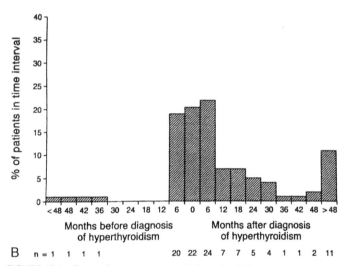

FIGURE 10-1. Onset of eye symptoms and diagnosis of Graves' ophthalmopathy relative to the time of diagnosis of hyperthyroidism (0 on the horizontal axis). **A,** The number of patients who first experienced eye symptoms within a given 6-month period is expressed as a percentage of the entire group. **B,** The number of patients in whom Graves' ophthalmopathy was first diagnosed within a given 6-month period. (From Bartley GB, Fatourechi V, Kadrmas EF, et al: The chronology of Graves' ophthalmopathy in an incidence cohort. Am J Ophthalmol 121:426–434, 1996. Published with permission from the American Journal of Ophthalmology. Copyright by the Ophthalmic Publishing Company.)

Pathogenesis

MECHANICAL FACTORS

Orbital imagining in Graves' ophthalmopathy reveals an increase in the volume of soft tissue within the orbit, including the extraocular muscles and adipose and connective tissues. The bones of the orbit are unyielding in response to the pressure generated by this increase in tissue volume. Therefore, forward displacement of the globe, or proptosis, may result and can serve as a natural means of orbital decompression. The degree of proptosis is limited, to varying degrees, by the orbital septum and tethering action of the extraocular muscles on the globe. Although CT scans show that the increased volume of orbital tissues is due to enlargement of both the orbital fat and the extraocular muscles in most patients, some patients appear to have predominantly adipose tissue or extraocular muscle involvement.[19] In addition, the orbital fatty tissue volume appears to be more closely cor-

related with the degree of proptosis than is the extraocular muscle volume. Besides resulting in forward displacement of the globe, the increase in orbital tissue volume causes impairment of venous and lymphatic outflow from the orbit, leading to periorbital and conjunctival edema.

PREDISPOSING INFLUENCES

Genetic Influence

The autoimmune thyroid diseases, including Graves' disease and Hashimoto's thyroiditis, are genetically complex and develop as a result of interactions between susceptibility genes and nongenetic factors. Studies performed in the past decade have identified several genes that either contribute directly to the development of these diseases or appear to be linked to important susceptibility genes.[20-23] However, no unique gene associations distinct from those predisposing to Graves' disease itself have been convincingly identified in patients with severe ophthalmopathy. A study of the families of 114 consecutive patients with Graves' ophthalmopathy did not support a major role for familial factors in the development of severe ophthalmopathy.[24] These findings suggest that environmental factors, rather than major susceptibility genes, are likely to predispose certain individuals with Graves' disease to the development of ophthalmopathy.

Tobacco Smoking

A striking association between cigarette smoking and Graves' ophthalmopathy has been noted in several studies. One group of researchers found that current smokers or ex-smokers represented 64% of patients with Graves' disease and ophthalmopathy, compared with 47.9% of those without overt ophthalmopathy, 23.6% of patients with toxic nodular goiter, 30.4% of individuals with nontoxic goiter, 33.5% of patients with Hashimoto's thyroiditis, and 27.8% of normal controls[25] (Fig. 10-2). These effects do not appear to be related to behavioral changes associated with thyrotoxicosis, nor do they seem to be due to differences in the age, gender, or educational background of the study patients and their controls.[26] Although the mechanisms underlying this association remain unknown, smokers have larger thyroids and higher thyroglobulin levels than do nonsmokers. Other contributors might include the effect of orbital hypoxia[27] or the action of free radicals contained in tobacco smoke on orbital fibroblast proliferation.[28] Smokers have lower levels of interleukin-1 receptor antagonists than do nonsmokers,[29] which could lead to enhanced negative effects of interleukin-1 on the orbital inflammatory process.[30] Smokers in one study were more likely to experience aggravation of ophthalmopathy after radioiodine therapy than were nonsmokers.[17,31] Finally, smoking was shown to adversely influence the course of the eye disease during treatment with corticosteroids and orbital radiotherapy.[32] The strong association between smoking and ophthalmopathy might provide important clues to the pathogenesis of this disorder in at least a subset of patients.

Age and Gender

Patient age and gender may also affect the prevalence and severity of Graves' ophthalmopathy. The female-to-male ratio in series of ophthalmopathy patients has ranged from 1.8 to 1 to 2.8 to 1, which is considerably lower than the ratio of 8 to 1 generally cited for Graves' disease in general.[33] Men also appear to be disproportionately represented among patients with severe ophthalmopathy. One study found a female-to-male ratio of 9.3

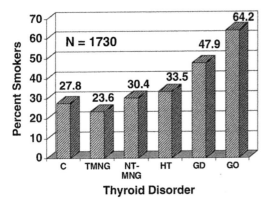

FIGURE 10-2. The prevalence of past and present cigarette smokers among patients with various thyroid disorders. Percentages shown (on the vertical axis) represent the prevalence of cigarette smokers in the group. Normal controls (C), toxic nodular goiter (TMNG), nontoxic goiter (NT-MNG), Hashimoto's thyroiditis (HT), Graves' disease without eye involvement (GD), and Graves' disease with ophthalmopathy (GO) are shown. Smokers represented significantly increased proportions among patients with diagnoses of Graves' disease and Graves' ophthalmopathy. (From Burch HB, Wartofsky L: Graves' ophthalmopathy: current concepts regarding pathogenesis and management. Endocr Rev 14:747–793, © 1993, The Endocrine Society.)

to 1 in patients with mild disease, 3.2 to 1 in patients with moderate disease, and 1.4 to 1 in patients with severe ophthalmopathy.[34]

Therapy for Thyrotoxicosis

An area of considerable controversy concerns the impact of the choice of therapy for hyperthyroidism on the subsequent course of ophthalmopathy in Graves' disease.[35-37] Several retrospective studies have examined this issue, often with conflicting results.[3] More recently, prospective trials have focused on this area.[38-42] Two studies allow a direct comparison between the effects of radioiodine, thyroidectomy, or antithyroid drug therapy.[39,42] In the first of these studies, 114 patients aged 35 to 55 years were randomized to receive radioiodine, thyroidectomy, or methimazole.[39] As assessed with an ophthalmopathy index, new or worsened eye involvement occurred in 10% of patients treated medically, 16% of those treated surgically, and 33% of those treated with [131]I. Interpretation of this small study was hampered by a higher prevalence of cigarette smokers among the radioiodine-treated patients, a period of hypothyroidism before thyroid hormone therapy was started in patients treated with radioiodine, and a requirement for multiple doses of radioiodine in nearly half the patients receiving this therapy, which suggests both refractory disease and a mechanism by which repeated release of thyroid antigen may have contributed to the autoimmune response.[1,43] However, these authors later showed that elevated TSH levels after ^{131}I treatment did not correlate with worsening eye status,[44,45] and that eye changes in smokers were no more frequent than eye changes in nonsmokers. Finally, the authors noted that most patients receiving multiple doses of ^{131}I had worsening of eye status before the second dose of radioiodine was given.[46]

Another randomized trial compared eye changes in 150 patients treated with radioiodine, 148 patients receiving methimazole alone, and a third group of 145 patients receiving both radioiodine and prophylactic prednisone.[42] Patients were monitored for 1 year and were assessed for change by largely objective criteria, as well as an activity score and patient self-assessment. The groups were similar with regard to percentages of smokers

or patients with preexisting ophthalmopathy. Hypothyroidism or persistent hyperthyroidism was corrected within 2 to 3 weeks of testing performed every 1 to 2 months. Worsening of eye disease occurred within 6 months after radioiodine therapy in 15% of patients versus 2.7% of patients who received antithyroid drugs alone. Seventy-four percent of the patients who experienced worsening eye status after radioiodine therapy had preexisting ophthalmopathy. The eye changes that occurred were largely mild and returned to baseline within 2 to 3 months in 65% of cases. However, eight patients (5%) in the radioiodine group required orbital radiation or high-dose corticosteroids as compared with one patient in the methimazole group and no patients in the combined prednisone and radioiodine group. Patients who had preexisting ophthalmopathy and those who were smokers were more likely to have progression after radioiodine administration.

A logical interpretation of the two prospective controlled studies in this area is that patients with Graves' disease who are treated with radioiodine therapy have an increased risk for worsening eye status compared with those who are treated with antithyroid drugs alone. An alternative explanation for these findings is that patients who are treated with antithyroid drugs experience beneficial effects from this therapy[47] rather than harmful effects from the radioiodine.[48] In any event, the ocular worsening that was noted was generally mild, reversible, and short-lived. Patients with preexisting eye disease and those who smoke or have severe thyrotoxicosis appear to be more likely to experience this complication, but concurrent use of corticosteroids negates this risk.[1,49,50]

Despite continuing uncertainty concerning the use of radioiodine thyroid ablation, results of these studies appear to have influenced management practices in patients with Graves' hyperthyroidism. A recent survey of members of the European Thyroid Association revealed that 60% of respondents believe that their choice of therapy would be influenced by the presence of ophthalmopathy, two thirds of whom would avoid radioiodine in the presence of severe eye disease.[51] However, many members of this organization would not chose radioiodine as the first therapy even in the absence of eye disease.[52]

The authors use an approach that is tailored to the individual patient. Thyrotoxicosis in patients without ophthalmopathy or with mild inactive ophthalmopathy generally is managed with radioiodine without concurrent corticosteroids. Patients with active eye disease are managed with antithyroid drugs alone or the combined use of radioiodine and corticosteroids (commencing with 0.3 to 0.5 mg of prednisone/kg bw per day orally 1 to 3 days after radioiodine and tapering the dose until withdrawal about 3 months later).[1] Near-total thyroidectomy is occasionally the treatment of choice, such as in a patient who is allergic to thionamides and has progressive ophthalmopathy. Thyroidectomy and total thyroid ablation share the theoretical advantage of removing thyroid antigen, which could potentially serve to bolster the autoimmune response directed against this antigen. However, evidence at present is insufficient to support this as a routine approach. The most important factors in prevention or successful treatment for Graves' eye disease appear to be early and accurate control of hyperthyroidism (with avoidance of subsequent hypothyroidism) with the use of radioiodine, antithyroid drugs, or surgery, and counseling the patient to refrain from smoking.[1,17] Frequent monitoring of thyroid status (every 4 to 6 weeks) is important in the initial stages of treatment to ensure that euthyroidism is restored promptly and maintained stably.[1]

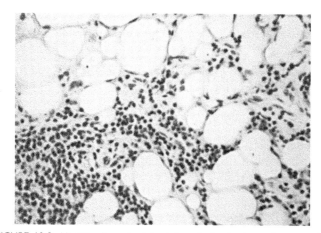

FIGURE 10-3. Hematoxylin-eosin–stained, formalin-fixed retro-ocular connective tissue (obtained from a patient with severe Graves' ophthalmopathy during orbital decompression surgery). Mononuclear cell infiltration is present throughout the retro-ocular connective tissue (∞160).

THE ORBITAL AUTOIMMUNE RESPONSE

The autoimmune response within the orbit can be dissected into contributions from constituent cells of the inflamed orbit, including extraocular myocytes, connective tissue (fibroblasts, adipocytes, and intercellular matrix), and "professional" immune effector cells and their products.[2,3,53] Histologic analysis has revealed largely intact muscle fibers, an expanded extracellular compartment, and infiltration by macrophages, activated T lymphocytes, and to a lesser extent B lymphocytes, as well as natural killer cells[54] (Fig. 10-3). Further characterization of the activated retro-ocular T lymphocytes reveals increases in both CD4+ and CD8+ lymphocytes and restriction in the T cell receptor repertoire.[55] T cell phenotyping has shown the presence of Th1[56] or Th2[57] profiles for cytokine gene expression or no clear preponderance of either phenotype.[58,59] Additional evidence suggests that the profile that is found might depend on the stage of disease, Th1 being predominant in early disease and the Th2 profile appearing in later stages.[60] Enlargement of the connective tissue compartment can be ascribed in part to a proliferation of retro-ocular fibroblasts and an attendant increase in the secretion of hydrophilic glycosaminoglycans by these cells.[53] In addition, recent studies suggest that adipogenesis is active in the orbits of patients with Graves' ophthalmopathy and results in expansion of the orbital adipose tissues.[2,61,62] The increase in orbital tissue volume caused by edema and increased orbital fat causes forward displacement of the globe and venous compression, followed by orbital congestion and further edema.

ORBITAL IMMUNE TARGETS

Although extraocular muscle enlargement and subsequent fibrosis play a central role in the mechanics of Graves' ophthalmopathy, the retro-ocular fibroblast and the embryologically related preadipocyte may have a greater role in the molecular events contributing to orbital autoimmunity. Retro-ocular CD8+ T cells proliferate in response to autologous retro-ocular fibroblasts but not eye muscle extracts, which suggests that fibroblasts might contain antigenic targets for activated T lymphocytes.[63] Similar results were found recently with the use of retro-ocular CD4+ T cells against autologous orbital fibroblast protein.[64] Retro-ocular fibroblasts respond to various cytokines with proliferation, release of glycosaminoglycan, and expression of several immunomodulatory proteins, including HLA class II molecules,

lymphocyte adhesion molecules such as intercellular adhesion molecule-1, and heat shock proteins.[2,53] Orbital fibroblasts also appear to have unique characteristics and responses to cytokines that facilitate their participation in the autoimmune response, as opposed to fibroblasts derived from other sources.[65-67]

Coexpression of thyroid autoantigen in the retro-ocular tissue has received considerable attention in studies investigating the pathogenesis of Graves' ophthalmopathy. Investigators in studies of this sort have difficulty distinguishing a secondary immune response against previously sequestered antigens released during tissue damage from a primary autoimmune response. It now is generally believed that antibodies against such retro-ocular proteins as the 64 kDa extraocular muscle protein,[68] protein 1D,[69] and the 23 kDa fibroblast protein[70] are secondary phenomena.

Because the autoimmune response against the TSHR is responsible for the hyperthyroidism of Graves' disease, numerous studies have examined retro-ocular tissue for expression of the TSHR or antigenically related proteins. Most studies show at least a low level of TSHR gene expression in retro-ocular fibroblasts,[71,72] preadipocytes, or retro-orbital fat[73,74] and either a TSHR or an antigenically related protein in these cells.[75-77] In addition, some studies have found higher levels of TSHR gene expression in Graves' orbital adipose tissues than in normal orbital tissues or tissues from Graves' patients with inactive eye disease.[73,78,79] Insight into the role of TSHR as a thyroid and orbital antigen has come from animal models of Graves' disease, including one in which increased TSHR expression was noted in the orbits of mice vaccinated with TSHR cDNA or receiving T cells that were primed in animals immunized with a TSHR fusion protein.[80] Recent studies of cultured orbital preadipocytes have shown enhanced TSHR expression following stimulation of adipogenesis in these cells,[81] suggesting a link between increased TSHR antigen expression and the expanded orbital adipose tissues characteristic of the disease.[62] A current model for the pathogenesis of Graves' ophthalmopathy is shown in Fig. 10-4.

History and Examination

In diagnosing the clinical features of Graves' ophthalmopathy, it is helpful for the physician to be familiar with a problem-focused ophthalmic history and examination.[82,83]

HISTORY OF THE PRESENT ILLNESS

A complete eye history should be taken for each new patient with Graves' disease at the initial evaluation and periodically thereafter. Does the patient have frequent injection, tearing, foreign body sensation, or photophobia from exposure keratitis? Is diplopia present, and if so, is it intermittent or constant? Has the patient experienced visual blurring or blind spots (scotomas)? If visual blurring is present, is it relieved by blinking, such as occurs with dryness, or by covering one eye, as occurs with unilateral neuropathy or extraocular muscle dysfunction? Is pain or a sense of pressure felt behind the eyes? Does the patient smoke?

THE PAST OPHTHALMIC HISTORY

Patients should be questioned about previous ophthalmic surgical procedures or treatments to help determine whether recent eye complaints are related to previous disorders. Specifically, has the patient undergone cataract extraction, strabismus operations, retinal detachment repair, or laser surgery? Some patients with

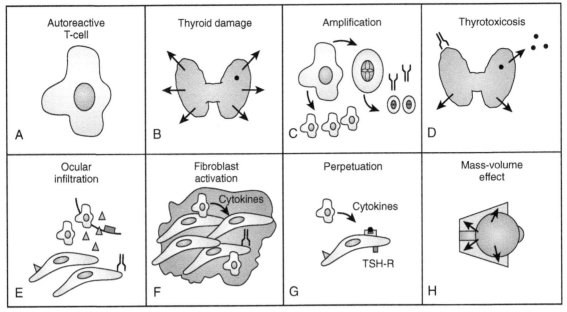

FIGURE 10-4. The authors' current concept of the pathogenesis of Graves' ophthalmopathy. **A,** In the presence of a permissive immunogenetic milieu and given appropriate environmental stimuli, autoreactive T cells directed against thyroid antigens emerge. **B,** Thyroid damage releases thyroid antigens, including the thyroid-stimulating hormone receptor (TSHR), thyroglobulin, and thyroid peroxidase. **C,** Release of thyroid antigens leads to further activation of autoreactive T lymphocytes, which results in amplification of both the cellular and humoral immune response against thyroid antigens. **D,** Thyrotoxicosis results from activation of the TSHR by circulating antibodies against this receptor. **E,** Circulating activated T lymphocytes infiltrate the orbit in response to the elaboration of specific lymphocyte adhesion molecules by orbital connective tissue cells. **F,** Activated T lymphocytes synthesize and release cytokines that stimulate fibroblasts to proliferate and to produce glycosaminoglycans. In addition, orbital preadipocytes are stimulated to differentiate into adipocytes that express increased levels of TSHR. **G,** Presentation of thyroid-eye cross-reactive antigens, such as hTSHR, leads to further activation of the local autoimmune response within the orbit. Enhanced orbital fat cell production and local edema caused by glycosaminoglycan-associated hydrophilic forces result in increased orbital tissue volume. **H,** The resulting mass-volume mismatch within the orbit produces venous congestion and forward displacement of the globe and leads to periorbital and conjunctival edema, extraocular muscle dysfunction, and proptosis.

a history of strabismus might not recall that they had crossed eyes during childhood or had extraocular muscle surgery; this historical detail may imply the presence of amblyopia (lazy eye), of which many patients are surprisingly unaware until unrelated ophthalmic problems develop in adulthood. A history of ocular trauma or treatment for glaucoma is of obvious importance, and the past or present use of topical ophthalmic medications, several of which have systemic side effects, should be recorded.

EXAMINATION OF THE EYE: AN OPHTHALMIC EVALUATION FOR THE NONOPHTHALMOLOGIST

Objective measurement and recording of eye findings are essential for assessing both the severity of ophthalmopathy and the response to therapy.[84] In addition, an assessment of disease activity and the patient's self-assessment of the disease state are important.[85] The following nine areas should be included in the eye evaluation.

Visual Acuity

Visual acuity usually is measured as a Snellen fraction (e.g., 20/30) for distance vision. During bedside or office examinations, however, one may use a near-vision acuity card, several of which are commercially available. In the absence of a standardized card, the patient may be asked to read any available printed material, for example, the smallest type possible in a newspaper; the size of the print can be recorded, or the material itself can be taped in the patient's record. Of course, patients should wear their glasses when visual acuity is being checked. Because loss of color perception can be an early sign of optic neuropathy, color vision evaluation is an important diagnostic test.[86,87] One

simple method for detecting possible early optic neuropathy is to check whether the patient perceives a difference between the two eyes in the color intensity of a red object; the top of a bottle of mydriatic eye drops is commonly used for this purpose. More advanced color vision testing should be performed by an ophthalmologist.

Pupils

Direct and consensual pupillary responses should be checked. An afferent pupillary defect (Marcus Gunn pupil) may indicate optic neuropathy.

Eyelids

Upper eyelid retraction is a common finding in patients with Graves' ophthalmopathy.[5,88-90] Early in the course of Graves' disease, eyelid malposition may result from increased sympathetic activity. With chronicity, the eyelid retractors (levator palpebrae superioris and Müller's muscle) become hypertrophic, eventually fibrotic, and adherent to orbital tissues.[91] Lid retraction may be unilateral or bilateral and may be subtle in some instances. The upper lid usually rests 1 to 2 mm below the junction of the cornea and sclera; therefore, if the white of the eye is seen above the corneoscleral limbus, eyelid retraction of at least 1.5 mm is present. The level of the lower eyelid is typically at the inferior corneoscleral limbus. Lower eyelid retraction is a less constant and specific finding and usually is not seen in patients with Graves' ophthalmopathy without concomitant retraction of the upper lids. Lid lag (Figs. 10-5 and 10-6), which is diagnosed by asking the patient to look down and then observing delayed or restricted excursion of the upper eyelids as they follow the globes, and lagophthalmos (Fig. 10-7), which is an inability to

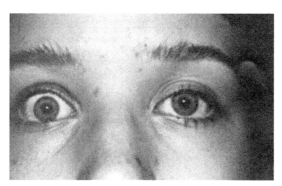

FIGURE 10-5. Right upper eyelid retraction in a patient with Graves' ophthalmopathy.

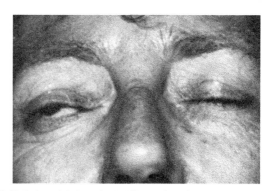

FIGURE 10-7. Lagophthalmos (an inability to close the eyelids completely) often causes exposure keratopathy (dryness of the cornea and conjunctiva).

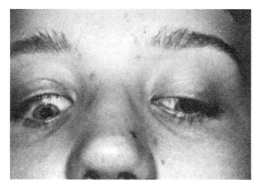

FIGURE 10-6. Lid lag of the right upper eyelid, a common sign of Graves' ophthalmopathy.

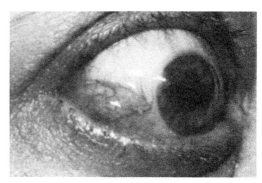

FIGURE 10-8. Chemosis (conjunctival edema) and focal injection (conjunctival blood vessel dilation) over the lateral rectus muscle insertion in a patient with Graves' ophthalmopathy.

close the eyelids completely, are additional stigmata of Graves' ophthalmopathy. Eyelid retraction, lid lag, and lagophthalmos frequently interfere with the maintenance of an adequate tear film on the eye. Results include ocular irritation and dryness, reflex tearing, photophobia, and corneal scarring or even ulceration in severe cases.

Conjunctiva and Cornea

The conjunctiva is the clear, thin tissue that covers the sclera. It is normally transparent, except for the small blood vessels that course within it. In Graves' ophthalmopathy, the conjunctiva may become hyperemic (usually termed **injection**) or edematous (chemosis) from exposure or from decreased venous drainage secondary to orbital suffusion. A characteristic conjunctival finding in patients with Graves' eyes is focal injection over the insertions of the lateral or medial rectus muscles (Fig. 10-8). Engorged blood vessels do not extend to the corneoscleral limbus.

The cornea normally appears transparent and lustrous. Dryness resulting from exposure is difficult to detect without slit-lamp biomicroscopy. Corneal ulceration, which is an ophthalmic emergency, usually can be seen grossly with a penlight and typically is accompanied by severe pain.[92]

Exophthalmometry

Proptosis may be quantitated with an exophthalmometer, an instrument that measures the position of the globes in relation to the lateral orbital rim. The device is easy to use and is helpful in documenting the results of treatment. Exophthalmometry measurements in most adult eyes are 22 mm or less, and the difference between the patient's two eyes usually does not exceed 2 mm.[93] Caucasians tend to have Hertel exophthalmometry measurements of less than 18 to 20 mm, which is higher than that of Asians (16 to 18 mm) and lower than those seen in many blacks (20 to 22 mm).[94-96]

Ocular Motility

The range of movement should be evaluated for each eye separately and then for the eyes together, during which time the patient should be asked to state whether double vision is noted. Diplopia is most likely to occur in upgaze or in the extremes of lateral gaze because of restriction of the inferior or medial recti. Any or all of the extraocular muscles may be involved in Graves' ophthalmopathy, however, and unusual patterns of strabismus may occur (Fig. 10-9).

Visual Fields

As was noted earlier, scotomas may appear in the visual field from optic neuropathy. Gross visual field defects may be detected with careful confrontation testing. An Amsler grid, a handheld card with a pattern of perpendicular crossed lines, may be used in the office or at the bedside as a simple screening tool. Formal perimetry testing should be performed by an ophthalmologist.

Ophthalmoscopy

Examination of the posterior pole of the retina may show a swollen optic disk from the compressive optic neuropathy or choroidal folds (a slat-like, corrugated pattern) that occasionally accompany mechanical orbital processes. Visually significant disorders such as opacities of the ocular media (corneal irregularities or cataracts) or macular degeneration also may be noted easily with the direct ophthalmoscope.

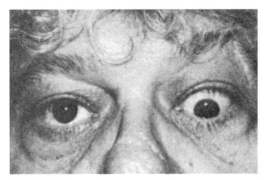

FIGURE 10-9. Hypotropia of the left eye secondary to contraction of the left inferior rectus muscle in Graves' ophthalmopathy. Unusual patterns of strabismus are characteristic of both Graves' ophthalmopathy and myasthenia gravis, diseases that may occur concomitantly.

Disease Activity

It is useful to classify patients with Graves' ophthalmopathy as to whether they have active or inactive disease, as patients with active disease are more likely to respond to immunosuppressive therapy.[1] This can be accomplished by using the Clinical Activity Score (CAS), which most commonly is a scale consisting of seven items, including spontaneous retrobulbar pain, pain on attempted upgaze or downgaze, redness of the eyelids, redness of the conjunctivae, swelling of the eyelids, inflammation of the caruncle and/or plica, and conjunctival edema. Patients who have a CAS ≥3/7 of these items should be considered to have active disease.[1]

FORMAL OPHTHALMOLOGY TESTING

Patients with positive findings in any of the above areas (i.e., most patients with Graves' ophthalmopathy, except the mildest cases) should be referred to an ophthalmologist for additional testing, which may include color vision testing, perimetry (visual fields), measurement of intraocular pressure, and slit-lamp biomicroscopy. It is important to refer urgently any patient with Graves' ophthalmopathy who experiences unexplained deterioration in vision, change in intensity or quality of color vision, globe subluxation, corneal opacity, disk swelling, or corneal exposure when eyelids are closed.[1]

Subtle evidence of optic neuropathy may be assessed with visual-evoked potentials,[97] color vision testing, or automated perimetry. A Farnsworth-Munsell panel detects subtle acquired color vision defects better than do most pseudoisochromatic color plate systems designed to evince congenital color vision abnormalities.[98] It is important to remember that approximately 7% to 8% of the male population has some degree of congenital red-green color "blindness." Measurement of extraocular muscle dysfunction relies on the Maddox rod test, the alternate cover test, the Hess chart, or the Lancaster red-green test. Exposure keratitis may be detected by slit-lamp examination with rose bengal or fluorescein staining.

Differential Diagnosis

Each major manifestation of Graves' ophthalmopathy has an associated differential diagnosis. The combination of more than one finding, such as lid retraction and proptosis, or the finding of biochemical thyroid dysfunction increases the likelihood that one is dealing with a manifestation of Graves' disease.[99]

Table 10-1. Differential Diagnosis of Proptosis

Endocrine	Granulomatous
Graves' ophthalmopathy	Sarcoidosis
Cushing's syndrome	Wegener's granulomatosis
Orbital neoplasms	Infectious
Primary neoplasms	Orbital cellulitis
Hemangioma	Syphilis
Lymphoma	Mucormycosis
Optic nerve glioma	Parasitic
Choroidal melanoma	Vascular
Lacrimal gland tumors	Carotid-cavernous fistula
Meningioma	Miscellaneous
Rhabdomyosarcoma	Lithium therapy
Extension of paranasal sinus tumors	Cirrhosis
Metastatic disease	Obesity
Melanoma	Amyloidosis
Breast carcinoma	Dermoid and epidermoid cysts
Lung carcinoma	Foreign body
Kidney	
Prostate	
Inflammatory	
Orbital pseudotumor	
Orbital myositis	

Visual loss caused by optic neuropathy in Graves' ophthalmopathy needs to be distinguished from that resulting from exposure keratitis, cataracts, macular degeneration, intracranial or orbital tumors, diabetic retinopathy, or psychogenic causes. The differential diagnosis for eyelid retraction includes neurogenic, myogenic, and mechanical causes.[100] Pseudoretraction of an eyelid may occur in response to aponeurogenic ptosis in the normal appearing contralateral eye.[100,101] Proptosis measurements may be affected by systemic nonthyroidal illness, with recession of the orbit in wasting disorders and forward protrusion in obesity. Proptosis of up to 25 mm has been described as a familial trait.[102] The differential diagnosis for proptosis is reviewed in Table 10-1.

Extraocular muscle enlargement may be seen with orbital malignancies, orbital "pseudotumor," and other inflammatory conditions, including sarcoidosis and Wegener's granulomatosis.[3] Vascular anomalies of the orbit that can simulate the clinical features of Graves' ophthalmopathy include dural-cavernous sinus fistulas (low-flow shunts), carotidcavernous sinus fistulas (high-flow shunts),[103] and orbital varices. Historical features and appropriate radiographic studies usually facilitate proper diagnosis. Myasthenia gravis may cause both eyelid malposition and extraocular muscle dysfunction and can be confused with or may add to the severity of Graves' ophthalmopathy. Patients with ocular myasthenia are more likely to have an associated autoimmune thyroid disease and are less likely to be anticholinesterase antibody positive than are patients with generalized myasthenia.[104]

Natural History

The natural history of Graves' ophthalmopathy is characterized by a period of progression over a span of 3 to 6 months, a plateau phase, and then gradual improvement. Individual components of ophthalmopathy have differing natural histories. Lid retraction is unlikely to be present at long-term follow-up, and soft tissue changes such as chemosis and lid edema improve or resolve in the vast majority of patients over short-term follow-up. Strabismus regresses spontaneously in only 30% to 40% of patients without specific therapy, and proptosis persists to some degree in up to 90% of carefully monitored individuals.[3] A recent follow-up survey of an incidence cohort of patients with Graves' ophthalmopathy at a mean of 9.4 years after initial eye examination revealed that 10% had experienced diplopia within the preceding 4 weeks, and 32.6% experienced ocular discomfort within the previous 4 weeks. Sixty-one percent of patients believed that their eyes had not returned to baseline, and 37.9% were dissatisfied with the appearance of their eyes.[105] Another study found that among 59 patients with mild Graves' ophthalmopathy who did not receive disease-modifying eye therapy and who were monitored for a median of 12 months, 64% showed spontaneous improvement, 22% showed no change, and 13.5% showed deterioration.[106]

Therapy

The vast majority of patients with Graves' ophthalmopathy experience a mild self-limited disease course that has only minor impact on daily life and requires only local measures for symptomatic improvement. These patients generally have minor lid retraction (<2 mm), mild soft tissue involvement, exophthalmos <3 mm above normal for race and gender, transient or no diplopia, and corneal exposure responsive to lubricants.[1] Other patients with more severe signs and symptoms that affect their daily lives to a significant extent may benefit from immunosuppressive therapy (if active) or surgical intervention (generally done in inactive disease). Patients with dysthyroid optic neuropathy or corneal breakdown warrant immendiate treatment. For all patients, it is important to restore thyroid hormone levels to normal before any type of orbital surgery is performed. The single exception to this rule is when sight-threatening ophthalmopathy threatens vision and requires urgent orbital decompression. The effect of ophthalmopathy on the selection of therapy for thyrotoxicosis was discussed earlier in the chapter under the heading "Therapy for Thyrotoxicosis."

LOCAL MEASURES

Mild symptoms resulting from corneal drying are treated effectively by instilling methylcellulose-containing eye drops and taping the eyelids shut at night to prevent nocturnal corneal drying.[107] Worsening of diplopia and soft tissue changes at night results from dependent edema, which often responds to elevation of the head. The use of sunglasses or tinted lenses can assist in decreasing photophobia. Prisms are occasionally useful for the correction of mild diplopia. In a recent survey of members of the European Thyroid Association on management of an index case of ophthalmopathy, 76% of respondents recommended methylcellulose eye drops, 21% would use diuretics to decrease ocular edema, and 18% would recommend prisms to correct diplopia.[108] The topical use of guanethidine eye drops to correct lid retraction has been associated with local irritation and variable effectiveness[109] and is rarely encouraged today.

IMMUNOMODULATORY THERAPY

Corticosteroids

Corticosteroids have been used for nearly 50 years in the treatment of Graves' ophthalmopathy. These agents have both antiinflammatory and immunomodulatory effects and may inhibit the synthesis and release of glycosaminoglycan by fibroblasts.[110-112] In general, corticosteroid therapy provides rapid relief from the pain, injection, and conjunctival edema associated

with inflammatory soft tissue changes in patients with active Graves' ophthalmopathy. Corticosteroid therapy, especially when given intravenously,[1] is also highly effective in the treatment of compressive optic neuropathy, with most patients showing at least some improvement.[1] Regression in proptosis and ophthalmoplegia has been reported, but such regression occurs to a lesser extent and with a greater likelihood of exacerbation after drug withdrawal.[1]

Oral corticosteroid therapy generally is initiated at a relatively high dose, such as 40 to 80 mg of prednisone per day.[1] After 2 to 4 weeks, the daily dose is tapered by 2.5 to 10.0 mg every 2 to 4 weeks. In many instances, drug withdrawal results in exacerbation, which requires increased dosage and slowing of the rate of subsequent taper.[113,114] Improvement in soft tissue inflammation begins within 1 to 2 days, and typical courses range from 3 to 12 months. Side effects associated with high-dose corticosteroid therapy may include gastrointestinal irritation, weight gain, psychosis, osteoporosis, and glucose intolerance.[1]

The use of depot subconjunctival or retrobulbar corticosteroid injections has been advocated as a means of attaining a high local concentration of drug and minimizing systemic side effects.[115,116] However, the risk,[117] patient discomfort, and lack of benefit beyond conventional regimens[115] limit the utility of this approach.

Pulse therapy with intravenous methylprednisolone has been studied in patients with Graves' ophthalmopathy. Using three doses of 500 mg on alternate days intravenously, followed by an oral regimen, one study found clinical improvement in 83% of the patients studied.[118] Similar results have been found by others, including one study consisting of five patients with optic neuropathy.[119] A recent randomized trial compared pulse therapy with methylprednisolone versus oral prednisolone and found that intravenous pulse therapy was more effective and better tolerated than the oral regimen.[120] While using weekly infusions of 500 mg methylprednisolone for 6 weeks, followed by 250 mg weekly for an additional 6 weeks, the authors noted improved disease activity and severity relative to the oral regimen. One important caveat regarding this approach is that the cumulative dose of intravenous methylprednisolone must not exceed 6 to 8 g, because higher doses have been associated with fatal hepatic dysfunction due to either direct toxicity or activation of autoimmune liver disease when these medications are discontinued.[121]

Predictors of clinical response to corticosteroids include high scores on a disease activity scale,[122] signal intensity on T1-weighted MRI (signal intensity [SI] of extraocular muscle: SI of cerebral substantia nigra $\geq 2.15:1$),[123,124] orbital uptake of radiolabeled somatostatin analogues,[125,126] and duration of disease (<18 months).

Combined use of corticosteroids with other forms of immunomodulatory therapy such as orbital radiation or cyclosporine is detailed in the relevant sections below.

Cyclosporine

Cyclosporine inhibits helper T cell proliferation and cytokine production, prevents cytotoxic T cell activation, and suppresses immunoglobulin production by B lymphocytes.[127] Two prospective randomized trials have examined the efficacy of cyclosporine in Graves' ophthalmopathy.[128,129] In one study,[128] patients who were receiving prednisone alone were compared with those who were given both prednisone and cyclosporine, and changes in an activity score were used to monitor therapy. Combined therapy resulted in a more rapid fall in activity score and a greater decrease in extraocular muscle thickness as seen on CT. Recurrences were seen after corticosteroid therapy was stopped in nearly half the patients in the prednisone-alone group as compared with only 5% in the combined treatment group. In a second study,[129] cyclosporine and prednisone were compared directly as single-agent therapies, and patients who failed either drug alone were given combination therapy. Prednisone was superior to cyclosporine as single-agent therapy, but nearly 60% of patients who did not respond to either drug alone subsequently improved with combined therapy. Despite this apparent efficacy, the high cost of cyclosporine and the requirement for frequent drug monitoring, together with an extensive side effect profile, limit the utility of this drug in clinical practice.

Somatostatin Analogue Therapy

The presence of somatostatin receptors on the surface of activated lymphocytes has been suggested as the explanation for orbital uptake of radiolabeled somatostatin analogues[126] and has provided a rationale for the therapeutic use of octreotide and lanreotide in Graves' ophthalmopathy. Despite findings of clinical improvement in nonrandomized trials, two recent randomized controlled trials utilizing a long-acting release formulation of octreotide showed minimal beneficial effect,[130,131] and a third randomized trial noted slight improvement in fissure width measurement in patients with lid retraction, with no other clinical benefit.[132]

Plasmapheresis

The utility of removal of circulating immunoglobulins by plasmapheresis in ophthalmopathy patients has been examined in several small studies. However, interpretation of the results of these studies is hampered by the lack of controls and the concurrent use of immunosuppressive therapy.

Orbital Radiotherapy

The rationale for the use of orbital radiation therapy in Graves' ophthalmopathy involves the marked radiosensitivity of the lymphocyte, thought to be a primary effector in this disorder. Radiation to the orbits generally is administered at 20 Gy (2000 rad) calculated at the midline and delivered by lateral ports angled 5 degrees posteriorly to prevent inclusion of the anterior chamber and retina. Therapy is delivered in 10 fractions over a 2-week period. Several European centers have used a lower total dosage effectively.[133,134] A beneficial effect has been reported within 1 to 4 weeks after the start of therapy[135] and can continue for as long as 12 months after completion.

In a review of 14 uncontrolled studies of orbital radiotherapy in Graves' ophthalmopathy, orbital radiation appeared to be well tolerated and seemed to provide benefit in approximately two thirds of treated patients.[1] The largest single-center experience involved more than 300 patients treated with megavoltage irradiation, one third of whom received concurrent corticosteroid therapy.[136,137] After orbital irradiation, 80% of patients exhibited improvement in soft tissue changes, 51% had recession of proptosis, 56% had improvement in eye muscle function, and 67% had improvement in vision. Despite this improvement, 29% of patients required one or more eye surgeries after orbital irradiation, most of which were performed to correct strabismus. It has been suggested that rather than obviating the need for corrective surgery, radiation might shorten the interval until stabilization of disease, thereby allowing earlier surgical intervention.

A randomized double-blind trial comparing orbital irradiation with prednisone in patients with Graves' ophthalmopathy showed that although these two therapies yielded similar results,

orbital irradiation had fewer side effects.[138] In another study, the combination of orbital irradiation and corticosteroid therapy was deemed to be superior to medical therapy alone.[139] These authors found that 26 of 36 (72%) patients who were treated with concurrent corticosteroids and orbital irradiation experienced a good or excellent response, as compared with only 3 of 12 (25%) patients who were treated with steroids alone.

A study in which patients were used as their own controls found little effectiveness of orbital radiotherapy alone in the treatment of Graves' ophthalmopathy.[140] In this prospective, randomized, double-blind, placebo-controlled study, the authors were unable to demonstrate any clinically significant beneficial effect of this treatment in patients with moderately severe disease. Prummel and colleagues examined the use of orbital irradiation in 88 patients with mild ophthalmopathy who were randomized to receive actual or sham irradiation.[141] Among treated patients, 57% showed improvement in one or two major criteria such as duction and diplopia, compared with only 27% of patients receiving sham irradiation. No apparent effect on overall quality of life, cost of management, progression to severe disease, or need for corrective surgery was noted in treated patients. Although none of the trials examining orbital irradiation show sustained benefit, it is possible that orbital radiotherapy may be of benefit for selected patients, especially those with particularly active or severe disease, but this remains to be demonstrated.[142]

Side effects of orbital irradiation include temporary hair loss at the temples and transient worsening of soft tissue changes. Rare cases of retinopathy and cataracts have been described after orbital irradiation, and this underscores the importance of reliance on a center in which staff members have expertise with this application.[143,144] Diabetic retinopathy is considered a contraindication to orbital irradiation because this condition increases vascular susceptibility to radiation damage.[140]

Other Immunomodulatory Therapy

B cell depletion therapy with such drugs as rituximab has been found to provide benefit for patients with rheumatologic disease, and several small uncontrolled studies have applied this therapy to patients with Graves' disease with and without active ophthalmopathy. Salvi and colleagues treated nine Graves' disease patients with rituximab at 2-week intervals for 16 weeks.[145] Seven patients had active ophthalmopathy, and the remaining two had mild lid changes alone. Improvement in the clinical activity score occurred in all seven patients with active eye disease, with the change from a mean CAS of 4.7 to 1.8 after 30 weeks of follow-up.[145] It is interesting to note that thyroid-stimulating hormone (TSH) receptor antibody titers did not change significantly during rituximab therapy. El Fassi and colleagues noted subjective and objective improvement in active ophthalmopathy in two patients treated with retuximab therapy at weekly intervals for 4 weeks.[146] These same authors noted higher thyrotoxicosis remission rates in Graves' disease patients treated with rituximab compared with untreated patients in a nonrandomized study—an effect that was unrelated to changes in TSH receptor antibody titers.[147] Adverse effects, including fever, nausea, and a serum sickness–like response requiring corticosteroids, were common with rituximab therapy.

Additional immune therapy for active Graves' ophthalmopathy has included azathioprine, cyclophosphamide, ciamexon, pentoxifylline, and intravenous immunoglobulin, all used with no benefit or no clear advantage noted over conventional therapy.[3]

NONIMMUNOMODULATORY THERAPY

Nonimmunomodulatory therapy for Graves' ophthalmopathy, including local injection of botulinum toxin,[148] bromocriptine,[149] metronidazole,[150] and acupuncture, has been tested with varying results.[151]

SURGICAL TREATMENT FOR GRAVES' OPHTHALMOPATHY

A tripartite approach is used most commonly in surgical treatment for Graves' ophthalmopathy: orbital decompression to relieve optic neuropathy or proptosis, extraocular muscle surgery to reduce diplopia, and eyelid procedures to treat retraction and cosmetic disfigurement.[152,153] In general, surgical intervention is performed in inactive disease to relieve significant proptosis or diplopia.[1] However, orbital decompression sometimes is performed when the disease is active in patients who are intolerant or nonresponsive to immunosuppressive therapy.[154] Although only a small fraction of patients with Graves' disease require operative intervention, some patients with severe ophthalmopathy need multiple procedures to achieve satisfactory functional and aesthetic results.[155]

Orbital Decompression

The orbit is decompressed by removal of one or more of its bony walls, which expands the eye socket and increases the potential space for orbital contents.[156] Indications for this procedure include optic neuropathy, severe proptosis (which in some patients may cause subluxation of the globe anterior to the lids), vision-threatening ocular exposure, debilitating retrobulbar and periorbital pain, and intolerable corticosteroid side effects.[1] Additionally, because some extraocular muscle procedures used in patients with Graves' ophthalmopathy may worsen exophthalmos, preliminary orbital decompression may be useful in those with severe proptosis. Finally, orbital expansion may be considered in some patients who do not have functional ocular disease but desire enhanced cosmesis.[157]

Optic neuropathy is the most common indication for orbital decompression. In most instances, the optic nerve is compressed by the enlarged or noncompliant extraocular muscles at the crowded orbital apex[158,159] (Fig. 10-10); in some patients, however, the muscles are of essentially normal size. Through removal of one or more walls of the bony orbit, pressure on the nerve is reduced. Numerous approaches to orbital decompression have been described; variations include the number of walls removed (one, two, three, or four) and the avenue used for surgical access: lateral, medial, transpalpebral, transantral, transcranial, through a bicoronal incision, endoscopically, or through a combination of procedures.[157] Transantral orbital decompression with removal of a portion of the medial wall and the orbital floor has been the preferred method at the Mayo Clinic over the past 25 years.[160] Potential complications of orbital decompression include worsened diplopia, hypoglobus, numbness in the distribution of the infraorbital nerve, eyelid malposition, nasolacrimal duct obstruction, cerebrospinal fluid leakage, meningitis, and even death in rare instances.

It is important to recognize that patients with optic neuropathy often have less exophthalmos than do patients without optic nerve compromise because proptosis may function as the body's way of "autodecompressing" the orbit. Needle aspiration of the orbital contents, previously recommended as a preliminary adjunct to orbital decompression, should be avoided.

Extraocular Muscle Surgery

Diplopia resulting from extraocular muscle involvement in Graves' ophthalmopathy is often difficult to treat. When the disease is active, ocular alignment may vary from hour to hour and can preclude prism spectacle correction or surgical repair. If the disease is inactive and double vision cannot be corrected with glasses, strabismus surgery is indicated.[161] Because the underlying problem is usually a restrictive myopathy (not paralysis, as older reports suggested) from tight, hypertrophied, and eventually fibrotic muscles, strabismus procedures for Graves' ophthalmopathy most frequently involve weakening the muscles by recessing their insertions onto the globe. The goal of surgery is to allow single vision in primary (straight ahead) gaze, as well as in the reading position; postoperative diplopia in the extremes of lateral gaze or in upgaze is common and does not signify an unsuccessful procedure.

Eyelid Surgery

Eyelid surgery for Graves' ophthalmopathy typically is performed after orbital decompression and strabismus procedures, if either or both are needed[162] (Figs. 10-11 and 10-12). The retractors of the upper eyelid, the levator palpebrae superioris and Müller's

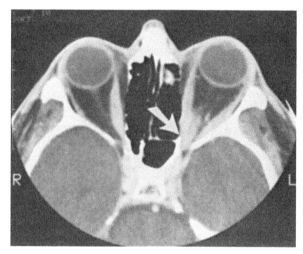

FIGURE 10-10. Computed tomography is useful to demonstrate fusiform enlargement of the extraocular muscles in Graves' ophthalmopathy. In the left orbital apex, the optic nerve is compressed by the hypertrophied muscles (arrow).

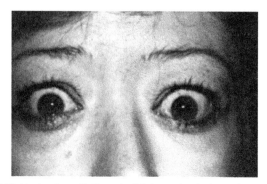

FIGURE 10-11. A patient with Graves' ophthalmopathy who has undergone bilateral transantral orbital decompression and strabismus surgery. Treatment for upper eyelid retraction is indicated both to reduce ocular exposure and to enhance cosmesis.

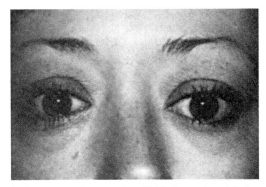

FIGURE 10-12. A patient after recession of Müller's muscle and the levator palpebrae superioris muscle in each upper eyelid.

muscle, undergo pathologic changes similar to those seen in the extraocular muscles. Upper lid retraction is relieved by weakening (recessing) the muscles; lower lid retraction is treated with analogous procedures, although spacers of hard palate mucosa, tarsus, donor sclera, or cartilage often are grafted into the lids

to counteract the tendency of gravity to pull the lids inferiorly during the postoperative period. Blepharoplasty (removal of excess eyelid and orbital tissue that prolapses anteriorly from the increase in orbital volume) may be of additional cosmetic value in selected patients.

Summary

Through judicious application of the diagnostic and multidisciplinary therapeutic measures outlined in this chapter, most patients with severe Graves' ophthalmopathy will be given comfortable functional eyes and will achieve satisfactory cosmesis. Early assessment of the patient's priorities and expectations serves as a key element in the alignment of patient and physician goals for successful therapy.

Acknowledgment

The authors wish to thank Drs. Colum Gorman and George Bartley for their valuable contributions to earlier editions of this chapter.

REFERENCES

1. Bartalena L, Baldeschi L, Dickinson A, et al: Consensus statement of the European group on Graves' orbitopathy (EUGOGO) on management of Graves' orbitopathy, Thyroid 18:333–346, 2008.
2. Bahn RS: Clinical Review 157: pathophysiology of Graves' ophthalmopathy: the cycle of disease, J Clin Endocrinol Metab 88(5):1939–1946, 2003 May.
3. Burch HB, Wartofsky L: Graves' ophthalmopathy: current concepts regarding pathogenesis and management, Endocr Rev 14:747–793, 1993.
4. Gorman CA: Temporal relationship between onset of Graves' ophthalmopathy and diagnosis of thyrotoxicosis, Mayo Clin Proc 58:515–519, 1983.
5. Bartley GB, Fatourechi V, Kadrmas EF, et al: The chronology of Graves' ophthalmopathy in an incidence cohort, Am J Ophthalmol 121:426–434, 1996.
6. Salvi M, Zhang Z-G, Haegert D, et al: Patients with endocrine ophthalmopathy not associated with overt thyroid disease have multiple thyroid immunological abnormalities, J Clin Endocrinol Metab 70:89–94, 1990.
7. Kasagi K, Konishi J, Iida Y, et al: Scintigraphic findings of the thyroid in euthyroid ophthalmic Graves' disease, J Nucl Med 35:811–817, 1994.
8. Morris JC, Hay ID, Nelson RE, et al: Clinical utility of thyrotropin receptor antibody assays: comparison of radioreceptor and bioassay methods, Mayo Clin Proc 63:707, 1988.
9. Chang TC, Chang TJ, Change CC, et al: TSH and TSH receptor antibody-binding sites in pretibial myxedema are related to the extracellular domain of entire TSH receptor, Clin Immunol Immunopathol 71:113–120, 1994.
10. Terwee C, Wakelkamp I, Tan S, et al: Long-term effects of Graves' ophthalmopathy on health-related quality of life, Eur J Endocrinol 146:751–757, 2002.
11. Werner SC, Coelho B, Quimby EH: Ten year results of I-131 therapy in hyperthyroidism, Bull N Y Acad Med 33:783–806, 1957.
12. Forbes G, Gorman CA, Brennan MD, et al: Ophthalmopathy of Graves' disease: computerized volume measurements of the orbital fat and muscle, Am J Neuroradiol 7:651–656, 1986.
13. Chang TC, Huang KM, Chang TJ, et al: Correlation of orbital computed tomography and antibodies in patients with hyperthyroid Graves' disease, Clin Endocrinol 32:551–558, 1990.
14. Gamblin GT, Harper DG, Galentine P, et al: Prevalence of increased intraocular pressure in Graves' disease—evidence of frequent subclinical ophthalmopathy, N Engl J Med 308:420–424, 1983.

15. Gamblin GT, Galentine PG, Eil C: Intraocular pressure and thyroid disease. In Gorman CA, Campbell RJ, Dyer JA, editors: The Eye and Orbit in Thyroid Disease, New York, 1984, Raven Press, pp 155–166.
16. Villadolid MC, Nagataki S, Uetani M, et al: Untreated Graves' disease patients without clinical ophthalmopathy demonstrate a high frequency of extraocular muscle (EOM) enlargement by magnetic resonance, J Clin Endocrinol Metab 80:2830–2833, 1995.
17. Wiersinga WM, Bartalena L: Epidemiology and prevention of Graves' ophthalmopathy, Thyroid 12:855–860, 2002.
18. Bartley GB, Fatourechi V, Kadrmas EF, et al: The incidence of Graves' ophthalmopathy in Olmsted County, Minnesota, Am J Ophthalmol 120:511–517, 1995.
19. Anderson RL, Tweeten JP, Patrinely JR, et al: Dysthyroid optic neuropathy without extraocular muscle involvement, Ophthalmic Surg 20:568–574, 1989.
20. Ban Y, Davies TF, Greenberg DA, et al: The influence of human leukocyte antigen (HLA) genes on autoimmune thyroid disease (AITD): results of studies in HLA-DR3 positive AITD families, Clin Endocrinol 57:81–88, 2002.
21. Kouki T, Gardine CA, Yanagawa T, et al: Relation of three polymorphisms of the CTLA-4 gene in patients with Graves' disease, J Endocrinol Invest 25:208–213, 2002.
22. Tomer Y: Genetic dissection of familial autoimmune thyroid disease using whole genome screening, Autoimmun Rev 1:198–204, 2002.
23. Brix TH, Kyvik KO, Hegedus L: What is the evidence of genetic factors in the etiology of Graves' disease? A brief review, Thyroid 8:727–734, 1998.
24. Villanueva R, Inzerillo AM, Tomer Y, et al: Limited genetic susceptibility to severe Graves' ophthalmopathy: no role for CTLA-4 but evidence for an environmental etiology, Thyroid 10:791–798, 2000.
25. Bartalena L, Martino E, Marcocci C, et al: More on smoking habits and Graves' ophthalmopathy, J Endocrinol Invest 12:733–737, 1989.
26. Prummel MF, Wiersinga WM: Smoking and risk of Graves' disease, JAMA 269:479–482, 1993.
27. Metcalfe RA, Weetman AP: Stimulation of extraocular muscle fibroblasts by cytokines and hypoxia: possible role in thyroid-associated ophthalmopathy, Clin Endocrinol (Oxf) 40:67–72, 1994.
28. Burch HB, Lahiri S, Bahn R, et al: Superoxide radical production stimulates human retroocular fibroblast proliferation in Graves' ophthalmopathy, Exp Eye Res 65:311–316, 1997.

29. Hofbauer LC, Muhlberg T, Konig A, et al: Soluble interleukin-1 receptor antagonist serum levels in smokers and nonsmokers with Graves' ophthalmopathy undergoing orbital radiotherapy, J Clin Endocrinol Metab 82:2244–2247, 1997.
30. Tan GH, Dutton CM, Bahn RS: Interleukin-1 (IL-1) receptor antagonist and soluble IL-1 receptor inhibit IL-1-induced glycosaminoglycan production in cultured human orbital fibroblasts from patients with Graves' ophthalmopathy, J Clin Endocrinol Metab 81:449–452, 1996.
31. Bartalena L, Marcocci C, Tanda ML, et al: Cigarette smoking and treatment outcomes in Graves ophthalmopathy, Ann Intern Med 129:632–635, 1998.
32. Eckstein A, Quadbeck B, Mueller G, et al: Impact of smoking on the response to treatment of thyroid associated ophthalmopathy, Br Med J 87:773–776, 2003.
33. Vanderpump MP, Tunbridge WM, French JM, et al: The incidence of thyroid disorders in the community: A twenty-year follow-up of the Whickham survey, Clin Endocrinol (Oxf) 43:55–68, 1995.
34. Perros P, Kendall-Taylor P: Pathogenetic mechanisms in thyroid-associated ophthalmopathy, J Intern Med 231:205–211, 1992.
35. Gorman CA: Therapeutic controversies: radioiodine therapy does not aggravate Graves' ophthalmopathy, J Clin Endocrinol Metab 80:340–342, 1995.
36. Pinchera A, Bartalena L, Marcocci C: Therapeutic controversies: radioiodine may be bad for Graves' ophthalmopathy, J Clin Endocrinol Metab 80:342–345, 1995.
37. Wartofsky L: Therapeutic controversies: summation, commentary, and overview: concerns over aggravation of Graves' ophthalmopathy by radioactive iodine treatment and the use of retrobulbar radiation therapy, J Clin Endocrinol Metab 80:347–349, 1995.
38. Bartalena L, Marcocci C, Bogazzi F, et al: Use of corticosteroids to prevent progression of Graves' ophthalmopathy after radioiodine therapy for hyperthyroidism, N Engl J Med 321:1349–1352, 1989.
39. Tallstedt L, Lundell G, Tarring O, et al: Occurrence of ophthalmopathy after treatment for Graves' hyperthyroidism, N Engl J Med 326:1733–1738, 1992.
40. Kung AW, Cheng A, Yau CC: The incidence of ophthalmopathy after radioiodine therapy for Graves' disease: prognostic factors and the role of methimazole, J Clin Endocrinol Metab 79:542–546, 1994.
41. Fernandez-Sanchez JR, Vara-Thorbeck R, Garbin-Fuentes I, et al: Graves' ophthalmopathy after subtotal thyroidectomy and radioiodine therapy, Br J Surg 80:1134–1136, 1993.

42. Bartalena L, Pinchera A, Martino E, et al: Relation between therapy for hyperthyroidism and the course of Graves' ophthalmopathy, N Engl J Med 338:73–78, 1998.

43. Mendlovic DB, Saeed Zafar M: Ophthalmopathy after treatment for Graves' hyperthyroidism, N Engl J Med 327:1320, 1992.

44. Torring O, Hamberger B, Saaf M, et al: Graves' hyperthyroidism: treatment with antithyroid drugs, surgery, or radioiodine: a prospective, randomized study: Thyroid Study Group, J Clin Endocrinol Metab 81:2986–2993, 1996.

45. Tallstedt L, Lundell G: Radioiodine treatment, ablation, and ophthalmopathy: a balanced perspective, Thyroid 7:241–245, 1997.

46. Tallstedt L: Ophthalmopathy after treatment for Graves' hyperthyroidism, N Engl J Med 327:1321, 1992.

47. Wartofsky L: Has the use of antithyroid drugs for Graves' disease become obsolete? Thyroid 3:335–344, 1993.

48. Wiersinga WM: Preventing Graves' ophthalmopathy, N Engl J Med 338:121–122, 1998.

49. Bartalena L, Marcocci C, Bogazzi F, et al: Use of corticosteroids to prevent progression of Graves' ophthalmopathy after radioiodine therapy for hyperthyroidism, N Engl J Med 321:1349–1352, 1989.

50. Bartalena L, Pinchera A, Martino E, et al: Relation between therapy for hyperthyroidism and the course of Graves' ophthalmopathy, N Engl J Med 338:73–78, 1998.

51. Weetman AP, Wiersinga WM: Current management of thyroid-associated ophthalmopathy in Europe: results of an international survey, Clin Endocrinol (Oxf) 49:21–28, 1998.

52. Wartofsky L, Glinoer D, Solomon B, et al: Differences and similarities in the diagnosis and treatment of Graves' disease in Europe, Japan, and the United States, Thyroid 1:129–135, 1991.

53. Bahn RS, Heufelder AE: Pathogenesis of Graves' ophthalmopathy, N Engl J Med 329:1468–1475, 1993.

54. Delemarre FG, Drexhage HA, Simons PJ: Histomorphological aspects of the development of thyroid autoimmune diseases: consequences for our understanding of endocrine ophthalmopathy, Thyroid 6:369–377, 1996.

55. Heufelder AE, Scriba PC, Wenzel BE: Antigen receptor variable region repertoires expressed by T cells infiltrating thyroid, retroorbital, and pretibial tissue in Graves' disease, J Clin Endocrinol Metab 81:3733–3739, 1996.

56. de Carli M, del Prete G, Romagnani S, et al: Cytolytic T cells with Th1-like cytokine profile predominate in retroorbital lymphocytic infiltrates of Graves' ophthalmopathy, J Clin Endocrinol Metab 77:1120–1121, 1993.

57. McLachlan SM, Rapoport B, Prummel MF: Cell-mediated or humoral immunity in Graves' ophthalmopathy?: Profiles of T-cell cytokines amplified by polymerase chain reaction from orbital tissue, J Clin Endocrinol Metab 78:1070–1074, 1994.

58. Forster G, Kahaly G, Ochs K, et al: Analysis of orbital T cells in thyroid-associated ophthalmopathy, Clin Exp Immunol 112:427–434, 1998.

59. Pappa A, Lightman S, Weetman AP, et al: Analysis of extraocular muscle-infiltrating T cells in thyroid-associated ophthalmopathy (TAO), Clin Exp Immunol 109:362–369, 1997.

60. Aniszewski JP, Valyasevi RW, Bahn RS: Relationship between disease duration and predominant orbital T cell subset in Graves' ophthalmopathy, J Clin Endocrinol Metab 85:776–780, 2000.

61. Kumar S, Coenen M, Scherer P, et al: Evidence for enhanced adipogenesis in the orbits of patients with Graves' ophthalmopathy, J Clin Endocrinol Metab 88:4246–4250, 2003.

62. Bahn RS: Clinical review: pathogenesis of Graves' ophthalmopathy: the cycle of disease, J Clin Endocrinol Metab 88:1939–1946, 2003.

63. Grubech-Loebenstein B, Trieb K, Sztankay A, et al: Retrobulbar T cells from patients with Graves' ophthalmopathy are CD8+ and specifically recognize autologous fibroblasts, J Clin Invest 93:2738–2743, 1994.

64. Otto EA, Kahaly GJ, Wall JR, et al: Orbital tissue-derived T lymphocytes from patients with Graves' ophthalmopathy recognize autologous orbital antigens, J Clin Endocrinol Metab 81:3045–3050, 1996.

65. Smith TJ: Orbital fibroblasts exhibit a novel pattern of responses to proinflammatory cytokines: potential basis for the pathogenesis of thyroid-associated ophthalmopathy, Thyroid 12:197–203, 2002.

66. Smith TJ, Koumas L, Gagnow AM, et al: Orbital fibroblast heterogeneity may determine the clinical presentation of thyroid-associated ophthalmopathy, J Clin Endocrinol Metab 87:385–392, 2002.

67. Koumas L, Smith TJ, Feldon S, et al: Thy-1 expression in human fibroblast subsets defines myofibroblastic or lipofibroblastic phenotypes, J Pathol 163:1291–1300, 2003.

68. Kubota S, Wall J, Hiromatsu Y, et al: The 64-kilodalton eye muscle protein is the flavoprotein subunit of mitochondrial succinate dehydrogenase: the corresponding serum antibodies are good markers of an immune-mediated damage to the eye muscle in patients with Graves' hyperthyroidism, J Clin Endocrinol Metab 83:443–447, 1998.

69. Bernard NF, Nygen TN, Tyutyunikov A, et al: Antibodies against 1D, a recombinant 64-kDa membrane protein, are associated with ophthalmopathy in patients with thyroid autoimmunity, Clin Immunol Immunopathol 70:225–233, 1994.

70. Bahn RS, Gorman CA, Johnson CM, et al: Presence of antibodies in the sera of patients of patients with Graves' disease recognizing a 23 kilodalton fibroblast protein, J Clin Endocrinol Metab 69:622–628, 1989.

71. Mengistu M, Lukes YG, Nagy EV, et al: TSH receptor gene expression in retroocular fibroblasts, J Endocrinol Invest 17:437–441, 1994.

72. Heufelder AE, Dutton CM, Sarkar G, et al: Detection of TSH receptor RNA in cultured fibroblasts from patients with Graves' ophthalmopathy and pretibial dermopathy, Thyroid 3:297–300, 1993.

73. Bahn RS, Heufelder AE, Spitzweg C, et al: Thyrotropin receptor expression in Graves' orbital adipose/connective tissues: potential autoantigen in Graves' ophthalmopathy, J Clin Endocrinol Metab 83:998–1002, 1998.

74. Feliciello A, Fenzi G, Avvedimento EV, et al: Expression of thyrotropin-receptor mRNA in healthy and Graves' disease retro-orbital tissue, Lancet 342:337–338, 1993.

75. Burch HB, Sellitti D, Barnes SG, et al: TSH receptor antisera for the detection of immunoreactive protein species in retroocular fibroblasts obtained from patients with Graves' ophthalmopathy, J Clin Endocrinol Metab 78:1384–1391, 1994.

76. Stadlmayr W, Heufelder AE, Bichlmair AM, et al: TSH receptor transcripts and TSH receptor-like immunoreactivity in orbital and pretibial fibroblasts of patients with Graves' ophthalmopathy and pretibial myxedema, Thyroid 7:3–12, 1997.

77. Perros P, Kendall-Taylor P: Demonstration of thyrotropin binding sites in orbital connective tissue: Possible role in the pathogenesis of thyroid-associated ophthalmopathy, J Endocrinol Invest 17:163–170, 1994.

78. Starkey KJ, Janezic A, Jones G, et al: Adipose thyrotropin receptor expression is elevated in Graves' and thyroid eye disease ex vivo and indicates adipogenesis in progress in vivo, J Mol Endocrinol 30:369–380, 2003.

79. Wakelkamp IM, Bakker O, Baldeschi L, et al: TSH-R expression and cytokine profile in orbital tissue of active vs. inactive Graves' ophthalmopathy patients, Clin Endocrinol 58:280–287, 2003.

80. Many M-C, Costagliola S, Detrait M, et al: Development of an animal model of autoimmune thyroid eye disease, J Immunol 162:4966–4974, 1999.

81. Valyasevi R, Erickson DA, Harteneck DA, et al: Differentiation of human orbital preadipocyte fibroblasts induces expression of functional thyrotropin receptor, J Clin Endocrinol Metab 84:2557–2562, 1999.

82. Erie JC: Ophthalmic history and examination. In Bartley BG, Liesegang TJ, editors: Essentials of Ophthalmology, Philadelphia, 1992, JB Lippincott, pp 3–25.

83. Bartley GB, Waller RR: Graves' ophthalmopathy. In van Heerden JA, editor: Common Problems in Endocrine Surgery, Chicago, 1989, Year Book, pp 25–29.

84. Gorman CA: The measurement of change in Graves' ophthalmopathy, Thyroid 8:539–543, 1998.

85. Anonymous: Classification of eye changes of Graves' disease, Thyroid 2:235–236, 1992.

86. Fells P: Management of dysthyroid eye disease, Br J Ophthalmol 75:245–246, 1991.

87. Neigel JM, Rootman J, Belkin RI, et al: Dysthyroid optic neuropathy: the crowded orbital apex syndrome, Ophthalmology 95:1515–1521, 1988.

88. Bahn RS, Garrity JA, Bartley GB, et al: Diagnostic evaluation of Graves' ophthalmopathy, Endocrinol Metab Clin North Am 17:527–545, 1988.

89. Bartley GB, Gorman CA: Diagnostic criteria for Graves' ophthalmopathy, Am J Ophthalmol 119:792–795, 1995.

90. Bartley GB, Fatourechi V, Kadrmas EF, et al: Clinical features of Graves' ophthalmopathy in an incidence cohort, Am J Ophthalmol 121:284–290, 1996.

91. Feldon SE, Levin L: Graves' ophthalmopathy: V. Etiology of upper eyelid retraction in Graves' ophthalmopathy, Br J Ophthalmol 74:484–485, 1991.

92. Bahn RS, Bartley GB, Gorman CA: Emergency treatment of Graves' ophthalmopathy, Ballieres Clin Endocrinol Metab 6:95–105, 1992.

93. Bogren HG, Franti CE, Wilmarth SS: Normal variations of the position of the eye in the orbit, Ophthalmology 93:1072–1077, 1986.

94. Werner SC: Modification of the classification of the eye changes of Graves' disease: recommendations of the ad hoc committee of the American Thyroid Association, J Clin Endocrinol Metab 44:203–204, 1977.

95. Migliori ME, Gladstone GJ: Determination of the normal range of exophthalmometric values for black and white adults, Am J Ophthalmol 98:438–442, 1984.

96. Amino N, Yuasa T, Yabu Y, et al: Exophthalmos in autoimmune thyroid disease, J Clin Endocrinol Metab 51:1232–1234, 1980.

97. Salvi M, Zhang Z-G, Haegert D, et al: Patients with endocrine ophthalmopathy not associated with overt thyroid disease have multiple thyroid immunological abnormalities, J Clin Endocrinol Metab 70:89–94, 1990.

98. Mourits MPH, Koornneef L, Wiersinga WM, et al: Clinical criteria for the assessment of disease activity in Graves' ophthalmopathy: a novel approach, Br J Ophthalmol 73:639–644, 1989.

99. Waller RR, Jacobson DH: Endocrine ophthalmopathy: Differential diagnosis. In Gorman CA, Campbell RJ, Dyer JA, editors: The Eye and Orbit in Thyroid Disease, New York, 1984, Raven Press, pp 213–220.

100. Bartley GB: The differential diagnosis and classification of eyelid retraction, Ophthalmology 103:168–176, 1996.

101. Gonnering RS: Pseudoretraction of the eyelid in thyroid-associated orbitopathy, Arch Ophthalmol 106:1078–1080, 1988.

102. Werner SC, Coleman DJ, Frazen LA: Ultrasonographic evidence of a consistent orbital involvement in Graves' disease, N Engl J Med 290:1447–1450, 1974.

103. Merlis AL, Schaiberger CL, Adler R: External carotid-cavernous sinus fistula simulating unilateral Graves' ophthalmopathy, J Comput Assist Tomogr 6:1006–1009, 1982.

104. Marino M, Mariotti S, Muratorio A, et al: Mild clinical expression of myasthenia gravis associated with autoimmune thyroid diseases, J Clin Endocrinol Metab 82:438–443, 1997.

105. Bartley GB, Fatourechi V, Kadrmas EF, et al: Long-term follow-up of Graves ophthalmopathy in an incidence cohort, Ophthalmology 103:958–962, 1996.

106. Perros P, Kendall-Taylor P, Crombie AL: Natural history of thyroid associated ophthalmopathy, Clin Endocrinol (Oxf) 42:45–50, 1995.

107. Jacobson DH, Gorman CA: Diagnosis and management of Graves' ophthalmopathy, Med Clin North Am 69:973–988, 1985.

108. Weetman AP, Wiersinga WM: Current management of thyroid-associated ophthalmopathy in Europe: results of an international study, Clin Endocrinol 49:21–28, 1998.

109. Martin B, Jay B: Use of guanethidine eye drops in dysthyroid lid retraction, Proc R Soc Med 62:18–19, 1969.

110. Sisson JC: Stimulation of glucose utilization and glycosaminoglycan production by fibroblasts derived from retrobulbar tissue, Exp Eye Res 12:285–292, 1971.

111. Smith TJ, Bahn RS, Gorman CA: Connective tissue, glycosaminoglycans, and diseases of the thyroid, Endocr Rev 10:366–391, 1989.

112. Smith TJ: Dexamethasone regulation of glycosamino-glycan synthesis in cultured human skin fibroblasts: similar effects of glucocorticoid and thyroid hormone therapy, J Clin Invest 74:2157–2163, 1984.

113. Wiersinga WM: Immunosuppressive treatment of Graves' ophthalmopathy, Trends Endocrinol Metab 1:377–381, 1990.

114. Burman KD: Treatment of autoimmune ophthalmopathy, Endocrinologist 1:102–110, 1991.

115. Marcocci C, Bartalena L, Panicucci M, et al: Orbital cobalt irradiation combined with retrobulbar or systemic corticosteroids for Graves' ophthalmopathy: a comparative study, Clin Endocrinol 27:33–42, 1987.

116. Yamamoto K, Saito K, Takai T, et al: Treatment of Graves' ophthalmopathy by steroid therapy, orbital radiation therapy, plasmapheresis, and thyroxine replacement, Endocrinol Jpn 29:495–501, 1982.

117. Kahaly G, Beyer J: Immunosuppressant therapy of thyroid eye disease, Klin Wochenschr 66:1049–1059, 1988.

118. Kendall-Taylor P, Crombie AL, Perros P: High-dose intravenous methylprednisolone pulse therapy in severe thyroid-associated ophthalmopathy [abstract], Thyroid 2(Suppl 1):29, 1992.

119. Guy JR, Fagien S, Donovan JP, et al: Methylprednisolone pulse therapy in severe dysthyroid optic neuropathy, Ophthalmology 96:1048–1053, 1989.

120. Kahaly GJ, Pitz S, Hommel G, et al: Randomized, single blind trial of intravenous versus oral steroid monotherapy in Graves' orbitopathy, J Clin Endocrinol Metab 90(9):5234–5240, 2005 Sep.

121. Marino M, Morabito E, Brunetto MR, et al: Acute and severe liver damage associated with intravenous glucocorticoid pulse therapy in patients with Graves' ophthalmopathy, Thyroid 2004;14:403–406.

122. Mourits MP, Koornneef L, Wiersinga WM, et al: Clinical criteria for the assessment of disease activity in Graves' ophthalmopathy: a novel approach, Br J Ophthalmol 73:639–644, 1989.

123. Laitt RD, Hoh B, Wakeley C, et al: The value of short tau inversion recovery sequence in magnetic resonance imaging of thyroid eye disease, Br J Radiol 67:244–247, 1994.

124. Hiromatsu Y, Kojima K, Ishisaka N, et al: Role of magnetic resonance imaging in thyroid-associated ophthalmopathy: Its predictive value for therapeutic outcome of immunosuppressive therapy, Thyroid 2:299–305, 1992.

125. Moncayo R, Donnemiller E, Kendler D, et al: Evaluation of immunological mechanisms mediating thyroid-associated ophthalmopathy by radionuclide imaging using the somatostatin analog ^{111}In-octreotide, Thyroid 7:21–29, 1997.

126. Kahaly G, Bockisch A, Hommel G, et al: Indium-111-pentetreotide in Graves' disease, J Nucl Med 39:533–536, 1998.

127. Wiersinga WM: Novel drugs for the therapy of Graves' ophthalmopathy. In Wall JR, How J, editors: Graves' Ophthalmopathy, Cambridge, 1990, Blackwell, pp 111–126.

128. Kahaly G, Schrezenmeir J, Krause U, et al: Cyclosporin and prednisone in treatment of Graves' ophthalmopathy: a controlled, randomized and prospective study, Eur J Clin Invest 16:415–422, 1986.

129. Prummel MF, Mourits MP, Berghout A, et al: Prednisone and cyclosporine in the treatment of severe Graves' ophthalmopathy, N Engl J Med 321:1353–1359, 1989.

130. Dickinson AJ, Vaidya B, Miller M, et al: Kendall-Taylor double-blind, placebo-controlled trial of octreotide long-acting repeatable (LAR) in thyroid-associated ophthalmopathy, J Clin Endocrinol Metab 89:5910–5915, 2004.

131. Wemeau JL, Caron P, Beckers A, et al: Octreotide (long-acting release formulation) treatment in patients with Graves' orbitopathy: clinical results of a four-month, randomized, placebo-controlled, double-blind study, J Clin Endocrinol Metab 90:841–848, 2005.

132. Stan MN, Garrity JA, Bradley EA, et al: Randomized, double-blind, placebo-controlled trial of long-acting release octreotide for treatment of Graves' ophthalmopathy, J Clin Endocrinol Metab 91(12):4817–4824, 2006.

133. Sautter-Bihl M-L: Orbital radiotherapy: recent experience in Europe. In Wall JR, How J, editors: Graves' ophthalmopathy, Cambridge, 1990, Blackwell, pp 145–157.

134. Sautter-Bihl M-L, Heinze HG: Radiotherapy of Graves' ophthalmopathy, Dev Ophthalmol 20:139–154, 1989.

135. Pigeon P, Orgiazzi J, Berthezene F, et al: High voltage orbital radiotherapy and surgical orbital decompression in the management of Graves' ophthalmopathy, Horm Res 26:172–176, 1987.

136. Kriss JP, Peterson IA, Donaldson SS, et al: Supervoltage orbital radiotherapy for progressive Graves' ophthalmopathy: results of a twenty year experience. Acta Endocrinol (Copenh) 121(Suppl 2):154, 1989.

137. Peterson IA, Kriss JP, McDougall IR, et al: Prognostic factors in the radiotherapy of Graves' ophthalmopathy, Int J Radiat Oncol Biol Phys 19:259–264, 1990.

138. Prummel MF, Mourits MP, Blank L, et al: Randomized double-blind trial of prednisone versus radiotherapy in Graves' ophthalmopathy, Lancet 342:949–954, 1993.

139. Bartalena L, Marcocci C, Chiovato L, et al: Orbital cobalt irradiation combined with systemic corticosteroids for Graves' ophthalmopathy: comparison with systemic corticosteroids alone, J Clin Endocrinol Metab 56:1139–1144, 1983.

140. Gorman CA, Garrity JA, Fatourechi V, et al: A prospective, randomized, double-blind, placebo-controlled study of orbital radiotherapy for Graves' ophthalmopathy, Ophthalmology 108:1523–1534, 2001.

141. Prummel MF, Terwee CB, Gerding MN, et al: A randomized controlled trial of orbital radiotherapy versus sham irradiation in patients with mild Graves' ophthalmopathy, J Clin Endocrinol Metab 89(1):15–20, 2004 Jan.

142. Bartalena L, Marcocci C, Gorman CA, et al: Orbital radiotherapy for Graves' ophthalmopathy: useful or useless? Safe or dangerous? J Endocrinol Invest 26:5–16, 2003.

143. Kinyoun JL, Kalina RE, Brower SA, et al: Radiation retinopathy following orbital irradiation for Graves' ophthalmopathy, Arch Ophthalmol 102:1473–1476, 1984.

144. Parsons JT, Fitzgerald CR, Hood CI, et al: The effects of irradiation on the eye and optic nerve, Int J Radiat Oncol Biol Phys 9:609–622, 1983.

145. Salvi M, Vannucchi G, Campi I, et al: Treatment of Graves' disease and associated ophthalmopathy with the anti-CD20 monoclonal antibody rituximab: an open study, Eur J Endocrinol 156:33–40, 2007.

146. El Fassi D, Nielsen CH, Hasselbalch HC, et al: Treatment-resistant severe, active Graves' ophthalmopathy successfully treated with B lymphocyte depletion, Thyroid 16(7):709–710, 2006.

147. El Fassi D, Clemmensen O, Nielsen CH, et al: Evidence of intrathyroidal B-lymphocyte depletion after rituximab therapy in a patient with Graves' disease, J Clin Endocrinol Metab 92:3762–3763, 2007.

148. Lyons CJ, Vickers SF, Lee JP: Botulinum toxin therapy in dysthyroid strabismus, Eye 4:538–540, 1990.

149. Lopatynsky MO, Krohel GB: Bromocriptine therapy for thyroid ophthalmopathy, Am J Ophthalmol 107:680–681, 1989.

150. Harden RM, Chisholm CJS, Cant JS: The effect of metronidazole on thyroid function and exophthalmos in man, Metabolism 16:890–898, 1967.

151. Rogvi-Hansen B, Perrild H, Christensen T, et al: Acupuncture in the treatment of Graves' ophthalmopathy: a blinded randomized study, Acta Endocrinol (Copenh) 124:143–145, 1991.

152. Bartley GB, Fatourechi V, Kadrmas EF, et al: The treatment of Graves' ophthalmopathy in an incidence cohort, Am J Ophthalmol 121:200–206, 1996.

153. Fatourechi V, Garrity JA, Bartley GB, et al: Graves' ophthalmopathy: results of transantral orbital decompression performed primarily for cosmetic indications, Ophthalmology 101:938–942, 1994.

154. Kazim M, Trokel S, Moore S: Treatment of acute Graves' orbitopathy, Ophthalmology 98:1443–1448, 1991.

155. Wilson WB, Manke WF: Orbital decompression in Graves' disease: the predictability of reduction of proptosis, Arch Ophthalmol 109:334–345, 1991.

156. Mourits MPH, Koornneef L, Wiersinga WM, et al: Orbital decompression for Graves' ophthalmopathy by inferomedial, by inferomedial plus lateral, and by coronal approach, Ophthalmology 97:636–641, 1990.

157. DeSanto LW, Gorman CA: Selection of patients and choice of operation for orbital decompression in Graves' ophthalmopathy, Laryngoscope 83:945–959, 1973.

158. DeSanto LW: The total rehabilitation of Graves' ophthalmopathy, Laryngoscope 90:1652–1678, 1980.

159. Gorman CA, DeSanto LW, MacCarty CS, et al: Optic neuropathy of Graves's disease: treatment by transantral or transfrontal orbital decompression, N Engl J Med 290:70–75, 1974.

160. Garrity JA, Fatourechi V, Bergstralh EJ, et al: Results of transantral orbital decompression in 428 patients with severe Graves' ophthalmopathy, Am J Ophthalmol 116:533–547, 1993.

161. Dyer JA: Ocular muscle surgery. In Gorman CA, Campbell RJ, Dyer JA, editors: The Eye and Orbit in Thyroid Disease, New York, 1984, Raven Press, pp 253–262.

162. Bartley GB: The eyelids in Graves' ophthalmopathy. In Bosniak S, editor: Principles and Practice of Ophthalmic Plastic Reconstructive Surgery, Philadelphia, 1997, WB Saunders, pp 514–524.

Chapter 11

AUTONOMOUSLY FUNCTIONING THYROID NODULES AND OTHER CAUSES OF THYROTOXICOSIS

GEORG HENNEMANN

The term *thyrotoxicosis* literally means "poisoning by thyroid hormone." The term includes any situation in a patient who shows clinical and biochemical characteristics of overactivity of thyroid hormone. It involves not only hyperfunction of the thyroid gland, termed *hyperthyroidism*, but also any other condition with elevated thyroid hormone levels in combination with clinical characteristics of overactivity of thyroid hormones. For instance, when thyroid hormones leak from the thyroid gland because of infectious or other damaging processes or are produced outside the thyroid gland in toxic amounts (struma ovarii, thyroid carcinoma metastasis) or ingested in overdose, thyrotoxicosis may ensue. In thyrotoxicosis, free hormone levels are invariably increased. The reverse is not true in that increased free thyroid hormone levels do not always point to thyrotoxicosis. In illness or resistance to thyroid hormones, increased free hormone levels are present while the patients are clinically euthyroid or even sometimes hypothyroid.[1]

The following causes of thyrotoxicosis are distinguished and will be discussed in this chapter:
Graves' disease
Toxic multinodular goiter
Subacute (de Quervain's) thyroiditis
Hashimoto's thyroiditis
Congenital hyperthyroidism
Autonomously functioning thyroid nodules (AFTNs)
Silent or painless thyroiditis
Thyrotoxicosis factitia
Thyrotoxicosis caused by pregnancy and trophoblastic disease
Iodine-induced thyrotoxicosis (IIT)
Hyperthyroidism caused by inappropriate thyroid-stimulating hormone (TSH) secretion
Thyrotoxicosis caused by metastatic thyroid carcinoma
Struma ovarii

Autonomously Functioning Thyroid Nodules

AFTNs are defined as (mostly) single nodules present in the thyroid gland that produce and secrete thyroid hormone independent of stimulation by TSH. On statistical grounds, these nodules are almost always adenoma and seldom carcinoma (see later). For that reason, the term *autonomously functioning adenoma* is often used synonymously. From a functional point of view, three types of AFTN are differentiated: toxic, hot, and warm nodules. Both toxic and hot nodules accumulate more radioactivity on scintiscan than the surrounding (normal) tissue. The patient is thyrotoxic in the first case but euthyroid in the latter. When the nodule is warm, radioactivity in the nodule is similar to that in the surrounding tissue in a euthyroid patient.

EPIDEMIOLOGY AND NATURAL HISTORY

About 5% to 10% of solitary thyroid nodules are toxic. This figure varies from country to country and is higher in Europe.[2,3] In nodules with a diameter of less than 2.5 cm, the proportion that are toxic is only 1.9%, whereas in nodules of 2.5 cm or greater, this figure is 42.6%. In a study of patients 60 years and older with AFTNs, 57% were thyrotoxic. In patients younger than 60 years, thyrotoxicity was noted in only 13%. In patients younger than 40 years, only 19.5% had AFTNs with a diameter of 3 cm or larger, but in older patients, this figure was 45.9%.[2] The proportion of AFTNs that are responsible for the hyperthyroidism of referred patients varies geographically between 1.5% and 44.5% (Table 11-1). About five times more women than men suffer from this disorder.[4] The natural history of the growth of

AFTNs varies. They may stay the same over the years, grow, or shrink. In a group of 159 patients who were observed for 1 to 15 years, an increase in size was seen in 10% and a decrease in 4%.[2] Changes in function of the nodule over the years also occur. In an observation period of 6 years, 10% of patients with AFTNs became toxic, and loss of function due to degeneration was observed in 4%.[2] Development of hyperthyroidism occurred predominantly in nodules greater than 3 cm in diameter,[3] with a minimal volume of 16 mL by ultrasound.[5]

PATHOGENESIS

From a histologic point of view, two types of nodules (Figs. 11-1 and 11-2) may be discerned: a monoclonal and a polyclonal type. Studer and his group developed the concept that even if monoclonal at the molecular level, nodules may become polyclonal from a functional and histologic aspect during evolution. They suggest that individual follicular cells may acquire new qualities that were not present in the mother cells but become inheritable during further replication. Obviously this change supposes some sort of genetic event. This sequence of events may lead to loss of anatomic and functional integrity of the follicular cells. The process might be accelerated by stimulatory factors such as TSH (e.g., in iodine deficiency, by goitrogens) and by local stimulatory and growth factors.[6]

At the genetic level, two types of monoclonal autonomously functioning nodules have been reported. Both are somatic mutations. One involves the TSH receptor (*TSHR*) gene and the other involves the $G_{s\alpha}$ protein gene. Both mutations lead to constitutive activation of the adenylate cyclase system, probably also activation of the inositol phosphates pathways[7] in the follicular cell, and to autonomy of the follicle. Mutations of the TSHR gene, and with a much lower prevalence, the $G_{s\alpha}$ gene, play a major (principal) role in the pathogenesis of AFTN.[8] For those monoclonal toxic adenomas (TA) in which no mutations are found in the TSHR or $G_{s\alpha}$ unit, probably other somatic mutations are involved.[9] In a recent study of 75 hot thyroid nodules, somatic TSH receptor mutations were detected in 57% and $G_{s\alpha}$ mutations in 3% of the nodules.[10] The same group studied females with AFTN, but without mutations in the TSH-R or $G_{s\alpha}$ unit, and

Table 11-1. Frequency of Toxic Adenoma in Various Countries

Location	Period	No. of Toxic Patients	% of Toxic Adenomas
Europe			
Austria	1966-1968	821	44.5
England	1948	107	3.7
Finland	1996	125	18
France			
Paris	1962	24	11.7
Marseilles	1964	537	
Montpellier	1965-1967	240	24
Germany	1965	350	19.7
Greece	1968	686	9.5
Italy	1968	1121	11.4
Switzerland	1967	—	33
General survey	1968	924	27.9*
North America			
Cleveland	1962	2846[†]	1.6
New York	1944	2431[‡]	1.5
Rochester	1912	1627	23.9
Rochester	1954-1965	215	15.8
Southfield, MI	1961-1979	—	2
Australia			
Tasmania	1973[§]	88	17

From Orgiazzi JJ, Mornex R: Hyperthyroidism. In Greer MA (ed): The Thyroid Gland. New York: Raven, 1990, p. 442.

*Patients younger than 50 years.
[†]Graves' disease plus toxic adenoma.
[‡]Thyrotoxicosis submitted to surgery.
[§]Six years after bread iodination.

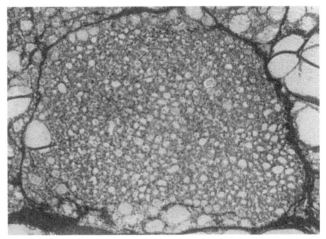

FIGURE 11-1. Uniform nature of cells formed in a nodule by proliferation of only one or a few clones of epithelial cells. (From Studer H, Ramelli F: Simple goiter and its variants: euthyroid and hyperthyroid multinodular goiters. Endocr Rev 3:40, © 1982, The Endocrine Society.)

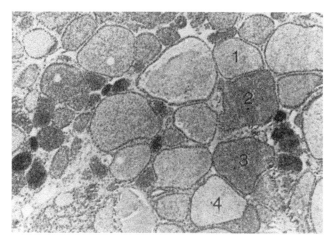

FIGURE 11-2. Autoradiograph of a hot nodule, illustrating areas with different capacity of uptake of radioiodine. (From Studer H, Gerber H, Peter HJ: Multinodular goiter. In DeGroot LJ [ed]: Endocrinology, 2nd ed, vol 1. Philadelphia: WB Saunders, 1989, p 722.)

detected a monoclonal origin in 10 out of 20 of cases when tested for X-chromosome inactivation. This strongly suggests a mutation at other location(s).[10] Although some believe that iodine deficiency can increase mutation rate and functional expression of autonomy[11] in AFTN, others[12] consider the fundamental process of goitrogenesis in (multi)nodular goiter as independent from iodine deficiency but operating through mechanisms that are innate to the hereditary and acquired heterogeneity among the thyrocytes themselves. However, superimposed iodine deficiency may shift clinical expression to younger ages. Van Sande and co-workers[13] hypothesized that as 16 different activating mutations were identified in the TSHR gene, this receptor is in a constrained conformation in its wild-type form. They also report that AFTA have a high level of Na^+/iodide symporter gene expression, a high thyroperoxidase mRNA and protein content, and a low H_2O_2 generation. Inositol uptake was also increased, but inositol phosphates were not increased. TA secreted more thyroid hormone than the quiescent surrounding tissue. Other characteristics of TA were increased cycling of thyrocytes as compared to normal surrounding tissue, little apoptosis, and low expression of early immediate genes.[14] An important study by Fuhrer and co-workers[15] showed that a panel of different activating TSHR mutations caused different functional and morphologic responses in vitro in rat and human primary thyrocytes. Their data suggest that different biologic properties of the TSHR mutants may result in different in vivo phenotypes. Finally, other mutated genes causing AFTN may be located in the AMP cascade.

PATHOLOGY

On macroscopic examination, a solitary toxic nodule is surrounded by normal thyroid tissue that is functionally suppressed. Rarely, a microscopically monotonous picture is seen that consists of uniform follicular cells without signs of malignancy. Usually the picture is heterogeneous with cells of different size, sometimes with signs of fresh and old hemorrhage and calcification. This picture, however, does not exclude a monoclonal origin of the nodule but may be the result of stimulatory local growth factors (see the section entitled "Pathogenesis"). No information is available at present on the exact ratio between primarily monoclonal and polyclonal AFTNs of the thyroid. Sometimes,

autonomously functioning micronodules are present in the surrounding thyroid tissue. This finding is in agreement with the thesis of Studer and co-workers[6] that the true adenoma is one end of a large spectrum of thyroid nodules growing from single thyrocytes or tiny cell families, each replicating with an individual growth rate, whereas the grossly abnormal multinodular goiter is at the other end of the scale.

CLINICAL FEATURES

The signs and symptoms of patients with toxic adenoma are those of thyrotoxicosis, without the specific signs of Graves' disease, such as eye signs, pretibial myxedema, and acropachy. On palpation of the thyroid region, a nodule is found in one of the lobes, usually with a diameter of 3 cm or larger.[2] The thyroid tissue surrounding the nodule and the thyroid lobe on the other side are not usually palpable because of TSH suppression.

LABORATORY DIAGNOSIS

When a single nodule is found in the thyroid and the patient is clinically thyrotoxic, estimation of serum TSH is sufficient for the diagnosis of toxic adenoma. To have an idea about the severity of the thyrotoxicosis, estimation of serum free thyroxine (T_4) is sufficient. If this parameter is normal, serum triiodothyronine (T_3) or free T_3 should be determined because it may be solely elevated in minimal thyrotoxicosis, that is, T_3 toxicosis. If findings on palpation are inconclusive, it is wise to perform a scintiscan of the thyroid. In the case of a toxic nodule, activity is seen in the nodule, with minimal or no activity anywhere else in the thyroid region (Fig. 11-3). The presence of a thyroid carcinoma in an AFTN is rare.[16] Although some authors are of the opinion that the occurrence of carcinoma in an AFTN may be more than coincidental,[17] most thyroidologists believe that such is not the case. The differential diagnosis of a toxic nodule includes relapse of hyperthyroid Graves' disease in remnant thyroid tissue after thyroid surgery or in thyroid dysgenesis. The latter possibility is especially remote. Theoretically, a TSH stimulation test would distinguish between an AFTN and the two other possibilities, but this test is hardly ever necessary in clinical practice. It is of no value to perform fine-needle aspiration cytology of an AFTN, because differentiation between a follicular adenoma and carcinoma is difficult if not impossible with this technique. When a hot nodule is present, that is, prominent uptake in the nodule but less in the surrounding tissue while serum TSH is normal, autonomous function can be tested by performing a T_3 or T_4 suppression test. In the case of autonomous function, uptake in the nodule is still present after the administration of 25 μg T_3 three times daily for 10 days or 125 μg T_4 for 14 days, whereas uptake is suppressed in the surrounding tissue. Sometimes uptake in a single nodule is indistinguishable from uptake in the surrounding tissue, a situation described as a "warm" nodule. This picture may be generated either by normal affinity of the nodular tissue for the isotope or because a nonfunctioning nodule is surrounded by normal thyroid tissue. Thus the possibility of the presence of a carcinoma in a warm nodule is certainly not excluded, which means that it should be evaluated as though it were a cold nodule.

TREATMENT

No treatment of a hot nodule is necessary as long as the patient remains euthyroid. Regular TSH measurement at intervals of a half to 1 year suffices. Most patients remain euthyroid. Occasionally, a hemorrhage in the nodule leads to spontaneous resolution. Treatment of toxic nodules with antithyroid drugs is useless

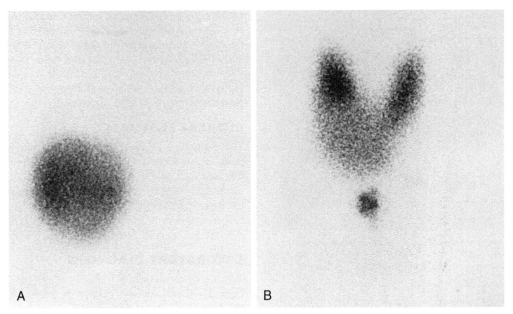

FIGURE 11-3. Thyroid with toxic nodule before **(A)** and after **(B)** treatment with [131]I.

because after discontinuation of medication, relapse invariably occurs. Three modes of treatment of toxic nodules include nodulectomy, administration of radioactive iodine, and percutaneous injection of alcohol into the nodule. Nodulectomy is very effective in rendering the patient euthyroid and has a low surgical complication rate. Surprisingly, permanent hypothyroidism develops in about 5% of patients, perhaps because of coexistent thyroid disease.[2,18] Obviously, the disadvantages of surgery are its operative risks, the residual scar, and its cost, which is high in relation to the other two forms of treatment.

Treatment with radioactive iodine is safe, cheap, and effective. Two reports indicate no risk of posttreatment hypothyroidism 6 months after treatment in a total of 93 patients.[19,20] However, when a longer period of follow-up was taken into account in 23 patients, such as 4 to 16.5 years after treatment, hypothyroidism developed in up to 36%.[21] In another study of 126 patients with autonomously functioning nodules, the percentage of hypothyroidism after a mean period of 10 years was 9.7% when the nodules were hot and 1.5% when toxic.[22] In this and the previous study, no relationship was found between the total dose administered, the size of the nodule, and the development of hypothyroidism. However, if thyroid autoantibodies were present, hypothyroidism occurred in 18% of patients and, when absent, in 1.4%.[22] It is important that when ^{131}I is administered, uptake be present only in the nodule and not in the surrounding tissue or in the other lobe, which could occur after pretreatment with antithyroid drugs. To avoid this complication, pretreatment with T_3 or T_4 might be considered. In some patients, typical Graves' disease has developed months after treatment of a toxic nodule with [131]I. Possibly, antigens released by the ^{131}I therapy induce or exacerbate an autoimmune response.

The third treatment modality is of rather recent date and involves percutaneous alcohol injection into the nodule. Euthyroidism is achieved in 65% to 85% of patients by 12 months after treatment. Injections are repeated 2 to 12 times at weekly intervals. The treatment is usually well tolerated, with few side effects. When nodule volume exceeds 30 mL, results are less favorable.[23,24] All three treatment modalities are acceptable, the choice depending on local circumstances and the patient's preference. Laser photocoagulation of AFTN is the most recent introduced therapy.[25] A recent study showed that its efficacy is comparable to that of ethanol injection, with possibly less ensuing hypothyroidism.[24]

Silent or Painless Thyroiditis

Silent thyroiditis is an autoimmune thyroiditis that usually comes to clinical attention because of symptoms of thyrotoxicosis caused by leakage of thyroid hormone from a painless thyroid gland. The condition often occurs in the postpartum period.

INCIDENCE

The incidence varies geographically. In 1980, this syndrome accounted for 10% of cases of thyrotoxicosis in Japan but only 3% to 4% in New York City.[22,26,27] A random poll showed that silent thyroiditis was uncommon in Argentina, Europe, and the east and west coasts of the United States but occurred more frequently around the Great Lakes and in Canada.[28] Patients are usually between 30 and 60 years old, and the female-to-male ratio is 1.5 to 1. Apart from its association with pregnancy, known then as *postpartum thyroiditis*, the condition is currently rarely diagnosed. Postpartum thyroiditis occurs in 5% to 9% of women in the first year after delivery, especially in those who have circulating autoantibodies against thyroperoxidase.[29]

ETIOLOGY

Silent thyroiditis is an autoimmune lymphocytic thyroiditis, and many patients with this disease have a family history of thyroid disease. Postpartum thyroiditis has been significantly associated with HLA-D3 and HLA-D5.[30] Exposure to iodine, such as in the form of amiodarone or lithium, interleukin (IL)-2, interferon, and etanercept has been suggested as an initiating event.[31-33] Silent thyroiditis is associated with other autoimmune diseases such as rheumatoid arthritis, systemic sclerosis, Graves' disease, primary adrenal insufficiency, systemic lupus erythematosus, idiopathic thrombocytopenic purpura, rubella, and seasonal allergies.[33-38]

PATHOLOGY

Microscopically, follicles are disrupted, and infiltration of lymphocytes and plasma cells occurs. The infiltration may be focal or diffuse, and sometimes formation of lymphoid follicles is seen. Follicular cells may be cuboidal or, when stimulated by TSH in the hypothyroid phase, columnar. Sometimes Hürthle or Askanazy cells are present. These cells are large and oxyphilic and contain many mitochondria. Thyroid tissue obtained during hypothyroidism or the recovery phase shows regenerating follicles with little colloid. Occasionally, persistent lymphocytic infiltration is observed. Extensive fibrosis may ultimately develop. A few multinucleated giant cells are regularly present.[39]

CLINICAL FEATURES

The initial symptoms in 112 patients with 122 episodes of silent thyroiditis have been reviewed.[40] Characteristically, thyroid pain was absent in all cases. The female-to-male ratio was 1.3 : 1. The mean age (±SD) in females and males was 32 ± 8.5 and 24.9 ± 8.2 years, respectively. Recurrences were uncommon. The symptoms are similar to other causes of thyrotoxicosis and varied from mild to severe. Specific signs that are characteristic of Graves' disease, such as eye signs, pretibial myxedema, and acropachy, were absent. The mean duration of the toxic phase in these patients was 3.6 ± 2.0 months. In most reports, the thyroid gland had a firm consistency. In about half the patients, a goiter was present. The course of the disease follows four sequential stages: thyrotoxicosis, euthyroidism, hypothyroidism, and euthyroidism. These stages need not be present in all patients. In one series, 57 of 112 patients became euthyroid, and hypothyroidism did not develop. Clinical hypothyroidism was present in only 32 patients. Hypothyroidism was transient in 24 patients but permanent in 8, who required thyroid hormone substitution. Ultimately, about half of the patients with silent thyroiditis become permanently hypothyroid.[41]

LABORATORY FINDINGS

The acute (first) phase of the disease is characterized by leakage of thyroid hormone and thyroglobulin from the damaged thyroid. This leakage results in elevated serum concentrations of thyroid hormones and thyroglobulin and suppression of serum TSH. Uptake of radioactive iodine by the thyroid is absent in this stage. The C-reactive protein (CRP) and the erythrocyte sedimentation rate (ESR) are mostly, but not always, slightly elevated. The ESR was elevated in 34 of 53 episodes but higher than 40 mm only in 8.[40] This result contrasts with subacute thyroiditis, in which the ESR is invariably much more elevated. T_4 and T_3 start to decline in the first phase and reach normal levels in the second (euthyroid) phase, but TSH remains suppressed. In the third (hypothyroid) phase, thyroid hormone levels are subnormal, and serum TSH starts to rise at the end of this stage. Because of TSH stimulation, the fourth stage is characterized by normalization of serum T_4 and T_3. Serum TSH ultimately normalizes, but normalization can take several months, so temporary subclinical hypothyroidism intervenes. For the mean period of the different phases, see Fig. 11-4.

TREATMENT

The degree of thyrotoxicosis is usually mild in silent thyroiditis, and treatment is not usually necessary. Prescription of α-adrenergic blocking agents may be considered. Antithyroid drugs have a very limited role because the thyrotoxicosis is not the result of increased thyroid hormone synthesis. Propylthio-

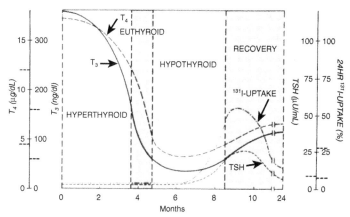

FIGURE 11-4. Schematic representation of the four phases of silent thyroiditis. (From Gegick CG, Harring WB: Painless subacute thyroiditis: a report of two cases. N C Med J 38:387, 1977.)

uracil or ipodate to block peripheral conversion of T_4 to T_3 may be of some value. In more serious cases, prednisone in a dose between 30 and 60 mg/day has a rapid ameliorating effect. The dose should be continued for 1 to 2 weeks and then be slowly tapered.[42] In case of relapsing thyroiditis, prednisone can be reinstituted. It is seldom necessary to perform thyroidectomy. If necessary, radiochemical "thyroidectomy" may be contemplated during remission when sufficient thyroid uptake of radioactive iodine is present for effective treatment, often in the presence of prednisone administration. As was stated, thyrotoxicosis is usually mild, and "definitive" treatment is seldom necessary. After the thyrotoxic phase, temporary hypothyroidism develops in about 40% of patients. If needed, thyroid hormone treatment can be instituted in a dose that allows TSH to remain mildly elevated to promote resumption of thyroid hormone synthesis in the recovery phase. Only a small proportion of patients (see previous discussion) need permanent and full-dose substitution at this stage. Finally, however, permanent hypothyroidism develops in about half of the patients. This result is in contrast to subacute thyroiditis, after which patients almost always become permanently euthyroid. Thus patients who suffered from silent thyroiditis need lifelong follow-up because hypothyroidism may develop years later.[43]

Thyrotoxicosis Factitia

Thyrotoxicosis factitia is primarily a psychiatric disorder. Patients surreptitiously ingest thyroid hormone in excessive amounts. When confronted with the situation, they usually deny doing so. Physicians should be aware of the phenomenon, or the diagnosis might be missed. Patients are usually overtly thyrotoxic but do not show eye signs, except those of sympathetic overactivity, such as eyelid retraction.

Other signs of Graves' disease such as eye signs, pretibial edema, acropachy, and goiter are also absent. Differentiation from Graves' disease is also feasible by color Doppler sonography, which shows absent thyroid vascularity and low-normal peak velocity, whereas these signs are increased in Graves' disease.[44] Because of TSH suppression, the thyroid shrinks and is often not palpable. Thyroid uptake of radioactive iodine is absent. Serum thyroglobulin is low or below detection limits in thyrotoxicosis factitia but elevated in silent thyroiditis. Factitious thyrotoxicosis is not difficult to distinguish from toxic multinodular goiter or toxic adenoma. Differentiation from subacute thyroiditis is easy on clinical grounds, because these patients suffer from frequent severe pain in the thyroid region. Furthermore, the CRP or ESR and serum thyroglobulin concentration are elevated in subacute thyroiditis. The diagnosis of thyrotoxicosis factitia should be considered when laboratory results are contradictory. Psychiatric help is urgently needed for such patients.

Thyrotoxicosis caused by accidental intake of excessive amounts of thyroid hormone has been observed in the "hamburger toxicosis patients." Two epidemics were caused by the inclusion of bovine thyroid in hamburger.[45,46]

Thyrotoxicosis Caused by Pregnancy and Trophoblastic Disease

Human chorionic gonadotropin (hCG) has intrinsic TSH-like activity. In about 2% to 3% of normal pregnancies, gestational transient thyrotoxicosis (GTT) is present because of elevated hCG serum concentrations. Familial gestational hyperthyroidism has recently been described and is caused by a missense mutation in the TSHR that renders it hypersensitive to hCG. Thyrotoxicosis may also be induced by molar pregnancy and by trophoblastic disease in men and women.

TSH-LIKE ACTIVITY OF HUMAN CHORIONIC GONADOTROPIN

The hCG from concentrated human pregnant urine has weak TSH-like activity when tested in a mouse bioassay.[47] The hCG that is purified from molar tissue has intrinsic TSH bioactivity in the same bioassay, though 4000 times less than that of human TSH on a molar basis.[48] However, when produced in sufficient amounts, it may induce clinical hyperthyroidism in humans, as shown in 2 of 20 patients with gestational trophoblastic neoplasia.[49] These patients had extremely high serum (3,220,000 and 6,720,000 IU/L) and urine concentrations of hCG that correlated closely with TSH-like bioactivity. Other patients with moderately

elevated serum hCG levels, between 110,000 and 310,000 IU/L, were euthyroid. When tested on human thyroid cell membranes, 1.0 IU hCG is biologically roughly equivalent to 0.27 μIU hTSH.[50] Both hCG and human luteinizing hormone (HLH) compete with TSH for the TSHR, and hLH also has weak (10 to 100 times higher than hCG) TSH-like activity.[50-52] The β subunit of hCG and hLH share 85% sequence identity in the first 114 amino acids but differ in the carboxyl-terminal peptide because hCG-β contains an extension of 31 amino acids.[53] Carboxypeptidase digestion of hCG, with amino acid residues 142 to 145 cleaved from the β subunit, leads to an increase in its capacity to stimulate adenylate cyclase in human thyroid membranes.[54] A variant of hCG that is lacking the C terminus of the β subunit because of enzymatic cleavage has been identified in pregnancy serum and molar tissue.[55] In studies using human thyroid membranes[56] or a cell line transfected with human TSHR,[57] desialylated forms of hCG exhibited stronger inhibition of TSH-mediated cyclic adenosine monophosphate responses than did native hCG. Both TSH binding and TSH-induced adenylate cyclase stimulation were found to be more effectively inhibited by desialylated variants of hCG than unmodified hCG was.[58] From these and other studies it seems that the biologic effect of hCG is predominantly confined to hCG containing little or no sialic acid. In cultured FRTL-5 cells, hCG has been found to increase iodide uptake, and it also causes a dose-related increment in adenylate cyclase activity and thymidine uptake.[59,60]

GESTATIONAL TRANSIENT THYROTOXICOSIS

GTT occurs in 2% to 3% of pregnant women.[61,62] It is diagnosed mostly between the 8th and the 14th weeks, when hCG levels peak. Fig. 11-5 shows the relationship between hCG and TSH during euthyroid pregnancy. Levels in gestational pregnancy are usually above 75,000 and 100,000 U/L and of sufficient duration to cause hyperthyroidism. About half of patients with GTT have clinical symptoms of hyperthyroidism. Differential diagnosis from Graves' disease is important. GTT is a nonautoimmune type of hyperthyroidism, which means that circulating thyroid autoantibodies and the characteristic symptoms of Graves' disease, such as eye signs, pretibial myxedema, and acropachy, are

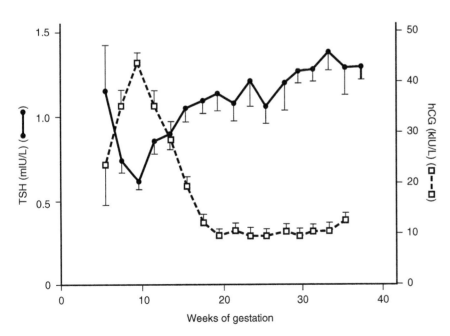

FIGURE II-5. Serum TSH and hCG levels as a function of gestational age. (From Glinoer D et al: J Clin Endocrinol Metab 71:276–287, 1990, with permission.)

absent. Hyperthyroidism disappears spontaneously when serum hCG levels decrease. Treatment with antithyroid drugs is necessary only when hyperthyroidism is severe. In severe cases, hyperemesis is invariably present, and hospital admission is pertinent. In patients with hyperemesis, the β subunit of hCG, but not the α subunit, is elevated in serum.[63] If treatment is necessary in milder cases, administration of β-adrenergic blocking agents is sufficient to suppress symptoms.

FAMILIAL GESTATIONAL HYPERTHYROIDISM

Recently a mother and a daughter were described who suffered from recurrent gestational hyperthyroidism but in whom hCG serum levels were normal during pregnancy. Both patients were heterozygous for a missense mutation, guanine for adenine, at codon 183 in exon 7 in the TSHR gene. This mutation resulted in replacement of a lysine residue by arginine at position 138 of the receptor, which is in the middle of its extracellular N-terminal domain. Because the mutant receptor was about 3.5 times more sensitive to hCG than was the wild type, hyperthyroidism developed in these women during pregnancy. Both women had concomitant hyperemesis as well.[64] No information is as yet available about the frequency of this syndrome.

MOLAR PREGNANCY AND TROPHOBLASTIC DISEASE

Several early reports describe molar pregnancy in combination with hyperthyroidism and disappearance of thyrotoxicosis after removal of a hydatidiform mole.[65-67] Bioassayable serum TSH was decreased in parallel with normalization of thyroid function parameters and a decrease in serum hCG. From the parallelism of thyroid-stimulating and hCG activity, it was suggested that both are caused by the same molecule: hCG.[68] The thyroid stimulator that is extracted from the serum of a patient with hyperthyroidism caused by a mole differed biologically and immunologically from TSH, from hCG found in normal placentas, and from thyroid-stimulating immunoglobulins. It contained less sialic acid and was biologically more active than normal pregnancy hCG.[65,69] In patients with chorionic carcinoma, a similar relationship is present between thyroid-stimulating activity in serum and hCG serum concentrations, the β subunit of human hCG, and quantitation of tumor burden.[70] Choriocarcinoma associated with hyperthyroidism in males is exceedingly rare. About four cases have been reported in the literature.[71] The clinical picture of patients with trophoblastic hyperthyroidism is that of Graves' disease without the specific features of the latter.

Therapeutically, removal of the mole resolves the problem. In the case of choriocarcinoma, total removal of the tumor should be undertaken if possible. If necessary because of the hyperthyroidism, preoperative treatment with β-adrenergic blocking drugs or, in more serious cases, combined with iodide and antithyroid drugs should be initiated. In patients who are not suitable for surgery, antithyroid drug treatment or administration of radioactive iodine in combination with chemotherapy is the best treatment available.

Iodine-Induced Thyrotoxicosis

IIT may be subdivided into different groups: (1) patients from endemic goiter areas, (2) patients with previous nonendemic goiter, (3) patients with previous or with actual Graves' disease, and (4) patients without apparent previous thyroid disease.[72]

One of the best known studies on IIT is that by Connolly and co-workers.[73] They found a steep rise in the incidence of thyrotoxicosis in the late months of 1966 in Tasmania (Australia), an area of iodine deficiency with a high prevalence of goiter. This increase was due to the addition of potassium iodide to bread in early 1966. The increased incidence occurred predominantly in subjects older than 40 years, in whom a rise in incidence from 50 per 100,000 to a maximum of 130 cases per 100,000 was seen in 1967 to 1968. By 1974, the incidence decreased to about the pre-epidemic level. Most thyrotoxic patients had nodular goiter, and few patients had Graves' disease. Later it was recognized that a pre-epidemic increase in the incidence of thyrotoxicosis had been caused by the use of iodophor disinfectants on dairy farms.[74] Despite the continued increase in the iodide supply, the prevalence of IIT decreased after its peak in 1967-1968. It was argued that this increase in thyrotoxicosis starting from 1964, in this area of relative iodine deficiency with a high prevalence of goiter, was due to autonomy in the nodular goiters. For a review of IIT caused by iodine prophylaxis in Tasmania and other countries, see Stanbury and co-workers.[75]

Many substances, such as iodinated drugs, radiographic contrast agents, iodochloroxyquinoline, iodine-containing contrast agents, disinfectants, and iodine-containing drugs, may also cause IIT.[72,76] Precipitation of thyroid storm is rare. Subjects with longstanding goiter are especially susceptible to IIT. In a study of 85 consecutive patients with IIT, a preexisting thyroid disorder was present in at least 20%. Spontaneous reversal to euthyroidism occurred after a mean period of 6 months in 50 of 85 patients. Return to euthyroidism may be preceded by subclinical hypothyroidism.[77] The recently developed nonionic contrast media do not prevent the development of IIT in elderly subjects.[78]

Evidence from human and animal studies suggests that chronic excess iodine intake may modulate thyroid autoimmunity and lead to thyrotoxicosis in genetically susceptible individuals.[79] A necrotic effect of iodide excess has been demonstrated in vivo in various animal species and also in human thyroid follicles in vitro.[80]

The antiarrhythmic drug amiodarone is currently widely used. Because of its high iodine content (37.2%), it has been the cause of IIT in many patients from all parts of the world. Its basic molecular structure has some similarity to that of the iodothyronines. Amiodarone may also interfere with thyroid hormone transport into cells and with pathways of intracellular thyroid hormone metabolism and action.[81] It interferes with 5′-monodeiodination of thyroid hormones, which leads to a decrease in intracellularly derived T_3 from T_4, thus inducing tissue hypothyroidism.[82] Hypothyroidism occurs predominantly in patients with preexisting thyroid autoimmune disease and was recognized in 6% of 467 patients chronically treated with amiodarone.[83] It is being used in many cardiac patients, particularly in France. The reported incidence of IIT caused by amiodarone varies between 0.003% and 11.5%. Estimation of serum total or free T_4 in patients using amiodarone is not specific, because they may be elevated in hyperthyroid, euthyroid, and even hypothyroid patients. The two latter conditions are explained by a decrease in T_4 metabolic clearance by amiodarone because of inhibition of T_4 transport into tissues and subsequent T_4 deiodination. This process results in high T_4 plasma levels and may lead to subnormal tissue T_3 concentrations. To differentiate between these possibilities, determination of serum TSH and T_3 is useful.

Of the two forms of amiodarone-induced thyrotoxicosis, type 1 is due to an iodine-induced increase in thyroid hormone synthesis, and type 2 involves iodine- or amiodarone-induced cytotoxic damage of the thyroid gland, with subsequent leakage of iodothyronines into the circulation. The picture of type 2 on electron microscopy characteristically shows two types of damage: multilamellar lysosomal inclusions and intramitochondrial glycogen inclusions with a morphologic picture of thyrocyte hyperfunction.[84] Thyroid radioactive uptake is usually low to normal in type 1 but low to suppressed in type 2. Serum IL-6 levels are normal to slightly elevated in type 1 and markedly elevated in type 2. Color flow sonography has been shown to differentiate between the two conditions. Type 1 shows normal vascularity (pattern 1) or increased vascularity (pattern 2) with a patchy distribution, whereas type 2 shows no vascularity (pattern 0).[85] Amiodarone-associated IIT type 1 is a serious problem in many instances because of the coexisting heart disease of these patients, and treatment may often be difficult.[86] Administration of a combination of methimazole and potassium perchlorate is reported to be effective in type 1.[87] Treatment of type 2 thyrotoxicosis consists of administration of prednisone starting at a dose of 40 mg/day, for example. Normalization of thyroid hormone levels is achieved in about 1 week.[86] Patients with previous type 2 thyrotoxicosis are at risk for hypothyroidism when given excessive iodine.[88] (For review see Ref. 89.)

Radiographic contrast agents contain between 30% and 50% iodine and may also induce IIT. Patients who have multinodular goiter or live in countries where iodine intake is low are especially at risk.[90] IIT often develops several weeks after the administration of radiographic contrast agents, so follow-up of such patients is advisable. In some instances, prophylactic administration of methimazole might be necessary. In view of the wide use of radiographic contrast agents, the probability of inducing IIT by these substances is probably low, but it might be inversely related to the iodine intake of the population.

Hyperthyroidism Caused by Inappropriate TSH Secretion

These situations are typified by increased production of thyroid hormone with clinical and/or biochemical characteristics of thyrotoxicosis in combination with unsuppressed or even supranormal serum TSH concentrations. This picture may be seen in the presence of a TSH-secreting pituitary tumor or be the result of selective partial pituitary resistance to thyroid hormone.

SELECTIVE PARTIAL TISSUE RESISTANCE OF THE PITUITARY TO THYROID HORMONE

This syndrome is probably part of the spectrum of the syndromes of thyroid hormone resistance, with resistance predominant at the pituitary level. Because only the pituitary is partially resistant to thyroid hormone, the set point of the pituitary, that is, the specific TSH/thyroid hormone ratio needed to ensure normal thyroid gland activation, is set at a higher level of serum thyroid hormone concentration. Because the other body tissues appear to have a sensitivity to thyroid hormone that is at least higher than that of the pituitary but might be even normal, the clinical picture of thyrotoxicosis is present, although without eye symptoms and other characteristics specific for Graves' disease. This syndrome may be inherited in an autosomal-dominant mode.[91-94] Because no pituitary tumor is present, the ratio of TSH α

subunits to total TSH is less than 1, whereas in the case of a TSH-producing pituitary tumor (see following), this ratio is usually above 1.

HYPERTHYROIDISM CAUSED BY A TSH-SECRETING PITUITARY ADENOMA

A TSH-secreting pituitary tumor is a rare condition, although since the use of ultrasensitive TSH measurements, its detection has increased. In a 1993 publication, 2.8% of all pituitary tumors consisted of TSH-producing adenomas.[95] More than 70% of these tumors are macroadenomas.[96] Patients are usually mildly hyperthyroid, and specific symptoms of Graves' disease are lacking. Serum levels of free T_4 and/or free T_3 are elevated, with a normal or increased serum TSH concentration. Visualization of the pituitary by magnetic resonance imaging shows a pituitary tumor. The concentration of TSH α subunits in blood is above normal, as is the ratio of TSH-α/ TSH.[97] Pituitary TSH-secreting adenomas produce normal forms of TSH but secrete them in variable amounts with variable biologic activity, which explains the variable degree of hyperthyroidism in these patients.[98] Treatment consists of surgery and postsurgical pituitary irradiation. About two thirds of patients have normal serum TSH after surgery alone or in combination with irradiation, but only one third of the patients are considered cured.[99] Treatment with somatostatin analogues such as octreotide returns TSH levels to normal in 80% of patients, and tumor size shrinks in 50%. Vision improves in 75%, and euthyroidism returns in almost all patients.[100] Results with long-acting somatostatin analogues have shown them to be effective as well.[100] Somatostatin treatment is also effective in surgical failures.

Thyrotoxicosis Caused by Metastatic Differentiated Thyroid Carcinoma

Thyrotoxicosis resulting from functioning metastasis of differentiated thyroid carcinoma is rare. Recently, 54 cases reported in the literature were analyzed.[101] The age and sex distribution of these patients is no different from that of other patients with differentiated carcinoma but without thyrotoxicosis. About 85% of patients are older than 40 years, and the female-to-male ratio is 3:1. The clinical picture of this type of thyrotoxicosis is no different from other causes of thyrotoxicosis. Iodine uptake and thyroid hormone synthesis by the tumor are generally poor, and excessive hormone production is due to the large mass of metastatic tissue.[102] The inefficient thyroid hormone synthesis is at least partly due to relative iodine deficiency in tumor tissue and the presence of abnormal thyroglobulin.[103] Other deficiencies and abnormalities in the complicated process of thyroid hormone synthesis may, however, be present in carcinomatous tissue. For instance, evidence suggests that expression of the TSH receptor and Na^+/I^- symporter may be absent or low in carcinomatous thyroid tissue.[104] In many cases, clinical symptoms are caused by T_3 toxicosis, with suppressed serum TSH and normal (sometimes even low) serum T_4.[102,103] Recently, increased T_4 to T_3 conversion by deiodinases type I and type II in abundant metastatic mass has been suggested to often produce the T_3 toxicosis in these cases.[105] Uptake of radioactive iodine in metastatic tissue is often absent when the thyroid gland is still present. The metastatic pattern of this type of adenocarcinoma is the same as is usually found in patients with thyroid adenocarcinoma, predominantly in bone, lung, and the mediastinum.

Treatment of metastatic functioning thyroid carcinoma consists of the administration of radioactive iodine. The usual dose ranges between 3700 and 7400 MBq (100 to 200 mCi). Exacerbation of thyrotoxicosis, even precipitating thyroid storm, has been reported.[106] For this reason, radioactive iodine for treatment of a functioning metastatic thyroid carcinoma should be administered with caution and only after adequate preparation of elderly patients with cardiovascular disease. If normal thyroid tissue is still present, it is appropriate to eradicate this tissue either by surgery or by radioactive iodine to ensure more efficient uptake of therapeutic doses of radioactive iodine in the metastatic tissue. Furthermore, it is dangerous to administer the above-mentioned doses of radioiodine in the presence of a normal thyroid gland, because severe radiation thyroiditis may ensue. The combination of Graves' disease and follicular carcinoma may not be a coincidence,[107,108] because recent knowledge suggests an association between Graves' disease and thyroid carcinoma, possibly as a result of longstanding thyroid stimulation by immunoglobulins.[109] In contrast, no significant association between Graves' disease and papillary carcinoma could be detected.[110] Although it has been postulated that thyroid carcinoma in patients with Graves' disease behaves more aggressively,[111] this statement has recently been denied.[112]

Struma Ovarii

Struma ovarii is a rare tumor that occurs in a teratoma or dermoid of the ovary. It constitutes about 1% of all ovarian tumors[113] and may spread to the peritoneum.[114] Often admixed with a carcinoid tumor,[115] it has also been reported to occur in association with multiple endocrine neoplasia type IIA.[116] Ovarian strumal carcinoid tumors have been found to synthesize different peptide hormones, including calcitonin, adrenocorticotropic hormone, somatotropin release–inhibiting factor, neuron-specific enolase, chromogranin, synaptophysin, serotonin, and other peptides.[116,117] Struma ovarii is unilaterally localized in about 90% of patients, and about 80% or more are benign.[118,119] Because differentiation between carcinoid and struma tissue is sometimes difficult, electron microscopic studies in combination with specific immunochemistry are sometimes necessary. Struma ovarii seldom causes hyperthyroidism. In thyrotoxicosis caused by struma ovarii, uptake of radioactive iodine by the thyroid gland is low in the presence of elevated serum thyroid hormones and suppressed TSH. Uptake of radioactive iodine over the ovarian tumor confirms the diagnosis.[120] Although one would suspect that the thyroid gland would be reduced in size in thyrotoxic cases resulting from struma ovarii, in several reports, the thyroid was enlarged.[118-121]

The pathogenesis of hyperthyroidism caused by struma ovarii is not clear. It has been suggested that thyroid-stimulating immunoglobulins stimulate ovarian strumal tissue or that struma ovarii may become autonomous.[122] Treatment of struma ovarii, either with euthyroidism or thyrotoxicosis, should be effected by removal of the ovarian tumor. In the case of coexistent thyrotoxicosis, preparation for surgery should be done by administration of antithyroid drugs, sometimes in combination with β-adrenergic blocking agents. Because of the coexisting teratoma, it is sometimes difficult to determine whether the thyroid tissue in the tumor is benign or malignant. It is not advised that patients with thyrotoxic struma ovarii be treated with radioiodine because of the possibility that the tumor is malignant, which cannot be determined on clinical grounds, and because of the unknown radiation effects on the other ovarian elements.

REFERENCES

1. Docter R, Krenning EP, de Jong M, et al: The sick euthyroid syndrome: changes in thyroid hormone serum parameters and hormone metabolism, Clin Endocrinol (Oxf) 39:499, 1993.
2. Hamburger JI: Evolution of toxicity in solitary nonfunctioning thyroid nodules, J Clin Endocrinol Metab 50:1089, 1980.
3. Bransom CJ, Talbot CH, Henry J, et al: Solitary toxic adenoma of the thyroid gland, Br J Surg 66:590, 1997.
4. Horst W, Rosler H, Schneider C, et al: 306 Cases of toxic adenoma: clinical aspects, findings in radioiodine diagnostics, radiochromatography and histology: Results of 131-I and surgical treatment, J Nucl Med 8:515, 1967.
5. Emrich D, Erlenmaier U, Pohl M, et al: Determination of the autonomously functioning volume of the thyroid, Eur J Nucl Med 20:410, 1993.
6. Studer H, Peter HJ, Gerber H: Natural heterogeneity of thyroid cells: the basis for understanding thyroid function and nodular goiter growth, Endocr Rev 10:125, 1989.
7. O'Sullivan C, Barton CM, Staddon SI, et al: Activation point mutations of the GSP oncogene in human thyroid adenomas, Mol Carcinog 4:345, 1992.
8. Holtzapfel H-P, Bergner B, Wonerof P, et al: Expression of Gas proteins and TSH receptor signaling in hyperfunctioning thyroid nodules with TSH receptor mutations, Eur J Endocrinol 147:109, 2002.
9. Trulzsch B, Krohn K, Wonerow P, et al: Detection of thyroid-stimulating hormone receptor and Gsalpha mutations in 75 toxic thyroid nodules by denaturing gradient gel electrophoresis, J Mol Med 78:684, 2001.
10. Krohn K, Fuhrer D, Holzapfel HP, et al: Clonal origin of toxic thyroid nodules with constitutively activating thyrotropin receptor mutations, J Clin Endocrinol Metab 83:130–134, 1998.
11. Derwahl M: TSH receptor and Gs-alpha gene mutations in the pathogenesis of toxic thyroid adenoma: a note of caution [editorial]. J Clin Endocrinol Metab 81:1783, 1996.
12. Derwahl M, Studer H: Nodular goiter and goiter nodules: where iodine deficiency falls short of explaining the facts, Exp Clin Endocrinol Diabetes 109:250, 2001.
13. Van Sande J, Massart C, Costagliola S, et al: Specific activation of the thyrotropin receptor by trypsin, Mol Cell Endocrinol 119:161, 1996.
14. Deleu S, Allory Y, Radulescu A, et al: Characterization of autonomous thyroid adenoma: metabolism, gene expression, and pathology, Thyroid 10:131, 2000.
15. Fuhrer D, Lewis MD, Alkhafaji F, et al: Biological activity of activating thyroid-stimulating hormone receptor mutants depends on the cellular context, Endocrinology 144:4018, 2003.
16. Sandler MP, Fellmeth B, Salhany KE, et al: Thyroid carcinoma masquerading as a solitary benign hyperfunctioning nodule, Clin Nucl Med 30:410, 1988.
17. Hamburger JI: Solitary autonomously functioning thyroid lesions: diagnosis, clinical features and pathogenetic considerations, Am J Med 58:740, 1975.
18. Eyre-Brook IA, Talbot CH: The treatment of autonomous functioning thyroid nodules, Br J Surg 69:577, 1982.
19. Ratcliffe GE, Cooke S, Fogelman I, et al: Radioiodine treatment of solitary functioning thyroid nodules, Br J Radiol 59:385, 1986.
20. Ross DS, Ridgway EC, Daniels GH: Successful treatment of solitary toxic nodules with relatively low-dose 131I with low prevalence of hypothyroidism, Ann Intern Med 101:488, 1984.
21. Goldstein R, Hart IR: Follow-up of solitary autonomous thyroid nodules treated with 131I, N Engl J Med 309:1473, 1983.
22. Mariotti S, Martino E, Francesconi M, et al: Serum thyroid auto-antibodies as a risk factor for development of hypothyroidism after radioactive iodine therapy for single thyroid "hot" nodule, Acta Endocrinol (Copenh) 113:500, 1986.
23. Lippi F, Ferrari C, Manetti L, et al: Treatment of solitary autonomous thyroid nodules by percutaneous ethanol injection: results of an Italian multicenter study. The Multicenter Study Group, J Clin Endocrinol Metab 81:3261, 1996.
24. Monzani F, Caraccio N, Goletti O, et al: Treatment of hyperfunctioning thyroid nodules with percutaneous ethanol injection: eight years' experience, Exp Clin Endocrinol Diabetes 106(Suppl 4):S54, 1998.
25. Døssing H, Bennedbaek FN, Bonnema SJ, et al: Randomized prospective study comparing a single radioiodine dose and a single laser therapy session in autonomously functioning thyroid nodules, Eur J Endocrinol 157:95, 2007.
26. Tokuda Y, Kasagi K, Lida Y, et al: Sonography of subacute thyroiditis: changes in the findings during the cause of the disease, J Clin Ultrasound 18:21, 1990.
27. Vitug AC, Goldman JM: Silent (painless) thyroiditis: evidence of a geographic variation in frequency, Arch Intern Med 145:437, 1985.
28. Schneeberg NG: Silent thyroiditis, Arch Intern Med 143:2214, 1983.
29. Lazarus JH, Ammari F, Oretti R, et al: Clinical aspects of recurrent postpartum thyroiditis, Br J Gen Pract 47:305, 1997.
30. Farid NR, Hawe BS, Walfish PG: Increased frequency of HLA-D3 and 5 in the syndromes of painless thyroiditis with transient thyrotoxicosis: evidence for an auto immune etiology, Clin Endocrinol 19:669, 1983.
31. Chow CC, Lee S, Shek CC, et al: Lithium-associated transient thyrotoxicosis in four Chinese women with autoimmune thyroiditis, Aust N Z J Psychiatry 27:246, 1993.
32. Sauter MP, Atkins MB, Meir JW, et al: Transient thyrotoxicosis and persistent hypothyroidism during acute autoimmune-thyroiditis after interleukin-2 and inter-

feron-alpha therapy for metastatic carcinoma: a case report, Am J Med 92:441, 1992.

33. Mittra ES, McDougall IR: Recurrent silent thyroiditis: a report of four patients and review of the literature, Thyroid 17:671, 2007.

34. Sakata S, Nagai K, Shibata T, et al: A case of rheumatoid arthritis associated with silent thyroiditis, J Endocrinol Invest 15:377, 1992.

35. Yamamoto M, Fuwa Y, Chimori K, et al: A case of progressive systemic sclerosis (PSS) with silent thyroiditis and anti-bovine thyrotropin antibodies, Endocrinol Jpn 38:265, 1991.

36. Itaka M, Ishii J, Ishikaea N, et al: A case with Graves' disease with false hyperthyrotropinemia who developed silent thyroiditis, Endocrinol Jpn 38:667, 1991.

37. Parker Klien I, Fishman LM, Levey GS: Silent thyrotoxic thyroiditis in association with chronic adrenocortical insufficiency, Arch Intern Med 143:2214, 1983.

38. Magaro M, Zoli A, Altomonte L, et al: The association with silent thyroiditis and active systemic lupus erythematosus, Clin Exp Rheumatol 10:67, 1992.

39. Mizukami Y, Michigishi T, Hashimoto T, et al: Silent thyroiditis: a histologic and immunohistochemical study, Hum Pathol 19:423, 1988.

40. Wolff PD: Transient painless thyroiditis with hyperthyroidism: a variant of lymphocytic thyroiditis? Endocr Rev 1:411, 1980.

41. Gegick CG, Harring WB: Painless subacute thyroiditis: a report of two cases, N C Med J 38:387, 1977.

42. Nicolai TF, Coombs GJ, McKenzie AK, et al: Treatment of lymphocytic thyroiditis with spontaneously resolving hyperthyroidism (silent thyroiditis). Arch Intern Med 142:2281, 1982.

43. Nicolai TF, Coombs GJ, McKenzie AK: Lymphocytic thyroiditis with spontaneously resolving hyperthyroidism and subacute thyroiditis: long-term follow-up, Arch Intern Med 141:1455, 1981.

44. Bogazzi F, Bartalena LA, Vitti P, et al: Color flow Doppler sonography in thyrotoxicosis factitia, J Endocrinol Invest 19:603, 1996.

45. Kinney JS, Hurwitz ES, Fishbein DB, et al: Community outbreak of thyrotoxicosis: epidemiology, immunogenetic characteristics and long-term outcome, Am J Med 84:10, 1988.

46. Hedberg CW, Fishbein DB, Janssen RS, et al: An outbreak of thyrotoxicosis caused by the consumption of bovine thyroid gland in ground beef, N Engl J Med 316:993, 1987.

47. Nisula BC, Ketelslegers J-M: Thyroid-stimulating activity and chorionic gonadotropin, J Clin Invest 54:494, 1974.

48. Kenimer JG, Hershman JM, Higgins HP: The thyrotropin in hydatidiform moles is human chorionic gonadotropin, J Clin Endocrinol Metab 40:482, 1975.

49. Nisula BC, Taliadouros GS: Thyroid function in gestational trophoblastic neoplasia: evidence that the thyrotropic activity of chorion gonadotropin mediates the thyrotoxicosis of choriocarcinoma, Am J Obstet Gynecol 77:138, 1980.

50. Carayon P, Lefort G, Nisula BC: Interaction of human chorionic gonadotropin and human luteinizing hormone with human thyroid membranes, Endocrinology 106:1907, 1980.

51. Williams JF, Davies TF, Catt KJ, et al: Receptor-binding activity of highly purified bovine luteinizing hormone and thyrotropin, and their subunits, Endocrinology 106:1353, 1980.

52. Yoshimura M, Hershman JM, Pang XP, et al: Activation of the thyrotropin (TSH) receptor by human chorionic gonadotropin and luteinizing hormone in Chinese hamster cells expressing human TSH receptors, J Clin Endocrinol Metab 77:1009, 1993.

53. Yoshimura M, Hershman JM: Thyrotropic action of human chorionic gonadotropin, Thyroid 5:425, 1995.

54. Carayon P, Amir S, Nisula B, et al: Effect of carboxypeptidase digestion of the human choriogonadotropin molecule on its thyrotropic activity, Endocrinology 108:1891, 1981.

55. Cole LA, Kardana A: Discordant results in human chorionic gonadotropin assays, Clin Chem 38:263, 1992.

56. Ouchimura H, Nagataki S, Ito K, et al: Inhibition of the thyroid adenylate cyclase response to thyroid-stimulating immunoglobulin G and asialo-chorionic gonadotropin, J Clin Endocrinol Metab 55:347, 1982.

57. Hoerman R, Broecker M, Grossmann M, et al: Interaction of human chorionic gonadotropin (hCG) and asialo-hCG with recombinant human thyrotropin receptor, J Clin Endocrinol Metab 78:933, 1994.

58. Hoerman R, Amir SM, Ingbar SH: Evidence that partially desialylated variants of human chorionic gonadotropin (hCG) are the factors in crude hCG that inhibit the response to thyrotropin in human thyroid membranes, Endocrinology 123:1535, 1988.

59. Davies TF, Platzer M: hCG-induced TSH receptor activation and growth acceleration in FRTL-thyroid cells, Endocrinology 118:2149, 1986.

60. Hershman JM, Lee H-Y, Sugawara M, et al: Human chorionic gonadotropin stimulates iodide uptake, adenylate cyclase, and deoxyribonucleic acid synthesis in cultured rat thyroid cells, J Clin Endocrinol Metab 67:74, 1988.

61. Glinoer D: The regulation of thyroid function in pregnancy: pathways of endocrine adaptation from physiology to pathology, Endocr Rev 18:404, 1997.

62. Glinoer D: Thyroid hyperfunction during pregnancy, Thyroid 8:859, 1998.

63. Goodwin TM, Hershman JM, Cole L: Increased concentration of the free beta-subunit of human chorionic gonadotropin in hyperemesis gravidarum, Acta Obstet Gynecol Scand 73:770, 1994.

64. Rodien P, Bremont C, Rafin Sanson M-L, et al: Familial gestational hyperthyroidism caused by a mutant thyrotropin receptor hypersensitive to human chorionic gonadotropin, N Engl J Med 339:1823, 1998.

65. Hershman JM, Higgins P: Hydatidiform mole: a cause of clinical hyperthyroidism, N Engl J Med 284:573, 1971.

66. Dowling JT, Ingbar SH, Frenkel N: Iodine metabolism in hydatidiform mole and choriocarcinoma, J Clin Endocrinol Metab 20:1, 1960.

67. Kock H, Vessel HV, Stolte L, et al: Thyroid function in molar pregnancy, J Clin Endocrinol Metab 26:1128, 1966.

68. Higgins HP, Hershman JM, Kenimer JG, et al: The thyrotoxicosis of hydatidiform mole, Ann Intern Med 83:307, 1975.

69. Yoshimura M, Pekary AE, Pang XP, et al: Thyrotropic activity of basic isoelectric forms of human chorionic gonadotropin extracted from hydatidiform mole tissues, J Clin Endocrinol Metab 78:862, 1994.

70. Anderson NR, Lockich JJ, McDermott WV Jr, et al: Gestational choriocarcinoma and thyrotoxicosis, Cancer 44:304, 1979.

71. Orgiazzi JJ, Rousset B, Consentino C, et al: Plasma thyrotropic activity in a man with choriocarcinoma, J Clin Endocrinol Metab 39:653, 1974.

72. Fradkin JE, Wolff J: Iodine-induced thyrotoxicosis, Medicine (Baltimore) 62:1, 1983.

73. Connolly RJ, Vidor GI, Stewart JC: Increase in thyrotoxicosis in endemic goitre area after iodination of bread, Lancet 1:500, 1970.

74. Stewart JC, Vidor GI: Thyrotoxicosis induced by iodine contamination of food: a common unrecognized condition? Br Med J 1:372, 1976.

75. Stanbury JB, Ermans AE, Pourdiux P, et al: Iodine-induced hyperthyroidism: occurrence and epidemiology, Thyroid 8:83, 1998.

76. Burman KD, Wartofsky L: Iodine effects on the thyroid gland: biochemical and clinical aspects, Rev Endocr Metab Disord 1:19–25, 2000.

77. Leger AF, Massin JP, Laurent MF, et al: Iodine-induced thyrotoxicosis: analysis of eighty-five consecutive cases, Eur J Clin Invest 14:449, 1984.

78. Martin FIR, Tress BW, Colman P, et al: Iodine-induced hyperthyroidism due to nonionic contrast radiography in the elderly, Am J Med 95:78, 1933.

79. Bournaud C, Orgiazzi JJ: Iodine excess and thyroid autoimmunity, J Endocrinol Invest 26(2 Suppl):49–56, 2003.

80. Many M-C, Mestdagh C, van den Hove M-F, et al: In vitro study of acute toxic effects of high iodide doses on human thyroid follicles, Endocrinology 131:621, 1992.

81. Hennemann G, Docter R, Friesema ECH, et al: Plasma membrane transport of thyroid hormones and its role in thyroid hormone metabolism and bioavailability, Endocr Rev 22:451–476, 2001.

82. Bianco AC, Salvatore D, Gereben B, et al: Biochemistry, cellular and molecular biology, and physiological roles of the iodothyronine selenodeiodinases, Endocr Rev 23:38–89, 2002.

83. Martino E, Aghini-Lombardi F, Bartalena L, et al: Enhanced susceptibility to amiodarone-induced hypothyroidism in patients with thyroid autoimmune disease, Arch Intern Med 154:12, 1994.

84. Cappiello E, Boldorini R, Tosoni A, et al: Ultrastructural evidence of thyroid damage in amiodarone-induced thyrotoxicosis, J Endocrinol Invest 18:862, 1995.

85. Bogazzi F, Bartalena L, Brogioni S, et al: Color flow Doppler sonography differentiates type 1 and type 2 amiodarone-induced thyrotoxicosis, Thyroid 7:541, 1997.

86. Bartalena L, Brogioni S, Grasso L, et al: Treatment of amiodarone-induced thyrotoxicosis, a difficult challenge: Results of a prospective study, J Endocrinol Metab 81:2930, 1996.

87. Reichert LJ, de Rooy HA: Treatment of amiodarone induced hyperthyroidism with potassium perchlorate and methimazole during amiodarone treatment, Br Med J 298:1547, 1989.

88. Roti E, Minelli R, Gardini E, et al: Iodine-induced subclinical hypothyroidism in euthyroid subjects with a previous episode of amiodarone-induced thyrotoxicosis, J Clin Endocrinol Metab 75:1273, 1992.

89 Basaria S, Cooper DS: Amiodarone and the thyroid, Am J Med. 118:706–714, 2005.

90. Martino E, Aghini-Lombardi F, Mariotti S, et al: Amiodarone: a common source of iodine-induced thyrotoxicosis, Horm Res 26:158, 1987.

91. Emerson CH, Utiger RD: Hyperthyroidism and excessive thyrotropin secretion, N Engl J Med 287:328, 1972.

92. Gershengorn MC, Weintraub BD: Thyrotropin-induced hyperthyroidism caused by selective pituitary resistance to thyroid hormone, J Clin Invest 56:633, 1975.

93. Rösler A, Litvin Y, Hage C, et al: Familial hyperthyroidism due to inappropriate thyrotropin secretion successfully treated with triiodothyronine, J Clin Endocrinol Metab 54:76, 1982.

94. Catargi B, Monsaingeon M, Bex-Bachellerie V, et al: A novel thyroid hormone receptor-beta mutation, not anticipated to occur in resistance to thyroid hormone, causes variable phenotypes, Horm Res 57:137, 2002.

95. Mindermann T, Wilson CB: Thyrotropin-producing pituitary adenomas, J Neurosurg 79:521, 1993.

96. Beck-Peccoz P, Brucker-Davis F, Persani L, et al: Thyrotropin-secreting pituitary tumors, Endocr Rev 17:610, 1996.

97. McDermott MT, Ridgway EC: Central hyperthyroidism, Endocrinol Metab Clin North Am 27:187, 1998.

98. Sergi E, Medri G, Papandreou MJ, et al: Polymorphism of thyrotropin and alpha subunit in human pituitary adenomas, J Endocrinol Invest 16:45–55, 1993.

99. Shimon I, Melmed S: Management of pituitary tumors, Ann Intern Med 129:472, 1998.

100. Kienitz T, Quinkler M, Strasburger CJ, et al: Long-term management in five cases of TSH-secreting pituitary adenomas: a single center study and review of the literature, Eur J Endocrinol 157:39–46, 2007.

101. Salvatori M, Saletnich I, Rufini V, et al: Severe thyrotoxicosis due to functioning pulmonary metastasis of well-differentiated cancer, J Nucl Med 39:1202, 1998.

102. Paul SJ, Sisson JC: Thyrotoxicosis caused by thyroid cancer, Endocrinol Metab Clin North Am 19:593, 1990.

103. Nakashima T, Enue K, Shiro-osu A, et al: Predominant T_3 synthesis in the metastatic thyroid carcinoma in a patient with T_3-toxicosis, Metabolism 30:327, 1981.

104. Caillou B, Troalen F, Baudin E, et al: $Na^{+/-}$ symporter distribution in human thyroid tissues: an immunohistochemical study, J Clin Endocrinol Metab 83:4102, 1998.

105. Takano T, Miyauchi A, Ito Y, et al: Thyroxine to triiodothyronine hyperconversion thyrotoxicosis in patients with large metastases of follicular thyroid carcinoma, Thyroid 16:615–618, 2006.

106. Cerletty JM, Listwan WJ: Hyperthyroidism due to functioning metastatic thyroid carcinoma: precipitation of thyroid storm with therapeutic radioactive iodine, JAMA 242:269, 1979.

107. Kasagi K, Takeichi R, Miyamoto S, et al: Metastatic thyroid cancer presenting as thyrotoxicosis: report of three cases, Clin Endocrinol 40:429, 1994.

108. Steffensen FH, Aunsholt NA: Hyperthyroidism associated with metastatic thyroid carcinoma, Clin Endocrinol 41:685, 1994.

109. Mazzaferri EL: Thyroid cancer and Graves' disease [editorial]. J Clin Endocrinol Metab 70:826, 1990.
110. Phitayakorn R, McHenry CR: Incidental thyroid carcinoma in patients with Graves' disease, Am J Surg 195:292, 2008.
111. Belfiore A, Charofalo MR, Giuffrida D: Increased aggressiveness of thyroid cancer in patients with Graves' disease, J Clin Endocrinol Metab 70:830, 1990.
112. Hales IB, McElduff A, Crummer P, et al: Does Graves' disease or thyrotoxicosis affect the prognosis of thyroid cancer? J Clin Endocrinol Metab 75:886, 1992.
113. Ayhan A, Yanik F, Tuncer R, et al: Struma ovarii, Int J Gynaecol Obstet 42:143, 1993.

114. Roth LM, Karseladze AI: Highly differentiated follicular carcinoma arising from struma ovarii: a report of 3 cases, a review of the literature, and a reassessment of so-called peritoneal strumosis, Int J Gynecol Pathol 27:213, 2008.
115. Tamsen A, Mazur MT: Ovarian strumal carcinoid in association with multiple endocrine neoplasia, type IIA, Arch Pathol Lab Med 116:200, 1992.
116. Sakura H, Fujii T, Okamoto K: A study of human calcitonin in an ovarian carcinoid and ovarian cancers, Exp Clin Endocrinol 97:91, 1991.
117. Ozerwenka KF, Schon HJ, Bock P: Immunochemical and ultrastructural studies of an ovarian strumal carcinoid, Wien Klin Wochenschr 102:687, 1990.

118. Kempers RD, Dockerty MB, Hoffman DL, et al: Struma _ovarii-ascitic, hyperthyroid and asymptomatic syndromes, Ann Intern Med 72:883, 1970.
119. Devaney K, Snyder R, Norris HJ, et al: Proliferative and histologically malignant struma ovarii: a clinico-pathologic study of 54 cases, Int J Gynaecol Pathol 12:333, 1993.
120. Pardo-Mindan FJ, Vazquez JJ: Malignant struma ovarii: light and electron microscopic study, Cancer 51:337, 1983.
121. Ross DS: Syndromes of thyrotoxicosis with low radioactive iodine uptake, Endocrinol Metab Clin North Am 27:169, 1998.
122. Bayot MR, Chopra IJ: Coexistence of struma ovarii and Graves' disease, Thyroid 5:469, 1995.

Chapter 12

CHRONIC (HASHIMOTO'S) THYROIDITIS

JOHN H. LAZARUS

Among the inflammatory diseases in the thyroid gland, chronic thyroiditis is the most common disorder. It is also called autoimmune thyroiditis or Hashimoto's thyroiditis. Autoimmune thyroiditis is a lifelong autoimmune disease of the thyroid gland. The enlarged thyroid gland gradually atrophies in association with the development of hypothyroidism in typical patients. The first variety of chronic thyroiditis, struma lymphomatosa, was described by Hakaru Hashimoto in 1912.[1] Hashimoto reported four patients with diffuse goiter and clarified the four histologic characteristics: diffuse lymphocytic infiltration, formation of lymphoid follicles, destruction of epithelial cells, and prolifera-

tion of fibrous tissue. The term Hashimoto's disease or Hashimoto's thyroiditis is sometimes used to refer only to goitrous thyroiditis, but it may usually be considered, in a broad sense, a synonym of chronic thyroiditis or autoimmune thyroiditis, including atrophic and nongoitrous thyroiditis. Although the histopathology was well described, no information on its pathogenesis was available until in 1956, Rose and Witebsky[2] described thyroglobulin antibodies and thyroiditis in rabbits immunized with thyroid extract. In the same year, Roitt, Doniach, and colleagues reported thyroglobulin antibodies in the serum of patients with Hashimoto's thyroiditis.[3] These observations opened a new era in immunopathology and established the value of measuring antibodies in human autoimmune disease. Hashimoto's thyroiditis is one of a number of conditions characterized by the presence of thyroiditis.[4] Salient features of some of these conditions are shown in Table 12-1. Details of suppurative thyroiditis, a bacterial or fungal infection seen in children and young adults, and Riedel's thyroiditis, a rare condition with dense fibrosis, are not shown.

This chapter focuses on Hashimoto's thyroiditis, also known as chronic lymphocytic thyroiditis, chronic autoimmune thyroiditis, and lymphadenoid goiter. In the early stage, patients are euthyroid and have no or a very small goiter. Chronic thyroiditis is subclinical, and the only evidence of autoimmune thyroiditis is the presence of antithyroid antibodies in the serum. Postmortem histologic examination has revealed that positive tests for serum antithyroid antibodies, especially antithyroid microsomal antibodies (now known as thyroid peroxidase antibodies [TPOAb]), in subjects without overt thyroid disease indicate the presence of lymphocytic infiltration into the thyroid.[5] As the disease progresses, patients show a firm, diffuse goiter of small to moderate size and generally are said to have chronic autoimmune thyroiditis. Their thyroid function is variable, ranging from euthyroidism to thyrotoxicosis. A large, firm goiter develops when the disease is more advanced; this type is the classical or goitrous Hashimoto's disease. Further progression of the immune process results eventually in atrophic thyroiditis in association with hypothyroidism. This combination represents the final stage of Hashimoto's disease.

In the general population, the percentages of women and men with serum TPOAb and antithyroglobulin antibodies (TgAb) increase with age, from about 10% in women in reproductive age to as many as 19% or more among elderly women.[6] The

Table 12-1. Thyroiditis Syndromes

Feature	Hashimoto's Thyroiditis	Postpartum Thyroiditis	Sporadic Thyroiditis	Subacute Thyroiditis
Neck pain	No	No	No	Yes++
Age of onset	All ages, peak 30-50 yr	Child-bearing	All ages, peak 30-40 yr	20-60 yr
Sex ratio F:M	8-9:1	—	2:1	5:1
Cause	Autoimmune	Autoimmune	Autoimmune	Unknown
Pathology	Lymphocytic infiltration, germinal centers, fibrosis	Lymphocytic infiltration	Lymphocytic infiltration	Giant cells, granulomas
Thyroid function	Hypo	Hyper/hypo or both	Hyper/hypo or both	Hyper/hypo or both
TPOAb	+++	+++	+++	+/−

Data from Pearce EN, Farwell AP, Braverman LE, et al: Thyroiditis, N Engl J Med 348:2646, 2003.
F, Female; *M,* male; *TPOAb,* thyroid peroxidase antibodies.

prevalence in men is much less—about 5%. Subclinical autoimmune thyroiditis is further evidenced by the fact that thyroid dysfunction develops after delivery in up to 50% of women with positive TPOAb measured in early pregnancy.[7] Therefore, when subclinical autoimmune thyroiditis is included, chronic thyroiditis is a very common disease. One in 10 to 30 women in the general population has autoimmune thyroiditis.

Pathology

In the classic form of Hashimoto's thyroiditis (struma lymphomatosa) with a firm, enlarged thyroid, the normal follicular structure is extensively replaced by lymphocytic and plasma cell infiltrates with the formation of lymphoid germinal centers (Fig. 12-1). Thyroid follicles remain isolated or in small clusters, are small or atrophic, and are empty or contain sparse colloid. Some persistent follicular epithelial cells are transformed into Askanazy cells, which have an eosinophilic granular cytoplasm. These cells are found in many other thyroid diseases and probably represent a damaged state of epithelial cells. Fibrosis of variable extent and lymphocytic infiltration are found in the interstitial tissue.

Autoimmune Abnormalities

INITIATION OF THYROID AUTOIMMUNITY

Similar to other autoimmune diseases, autoimmune thyroiditis can arise from a breakdown of self-tolerance to thyroid antigens. Immunologic self-tolerance is thought to be induced during the perinatal period, when immature lymphocytes are exposed to self-antigens.[8] At this critical point, clonal deletion or induced anergy of autoreactive T cells in the thymus provides self-tolerance to autoantigens. If an abnormality occurs during this period, self-tolerance might not be induced,[8] and autoimmune thyroiditis might develop. An early theory was that a genetically induced organ-specific suppressor T lymphocyte defect could deregulate a thyroid-specific helper T cell population.[9] This view has required redefinition in relation to the role of regulatory T cells in thyroid autoimmunity.[10] Further breakdown in self-tolerance may be induced by altered self-antigen, exposure to environmental antigens that mimic a self-antigen, polyclonal immune activation, or idiotype cross-reaction of self-antigens. These factors may augment low levels of autoimmune thyroiditis. For example, infection, drugs, or other factors might activate autoreactive helper lymphocytes. Locally produced interferon-γ (IFN-γ) may induce major histocompatibility complex (MHC) class II antigen expression on thyroid cell surfaces, which may promote autoimmunity.[11] Environmental factors also play an

Table 12-2. Factors Predisposing to Autimmune Thyroiditis

Genetic	Environmental
HLA	Smoking
CTLA-4	Stress
PTPN22	Iodine and selenium
TG	Drugs (amiodarone, lithium, interleukin-2, interferon-α, HAART, GM-CSF)
	Irradiation, infection
	Pregnancy and post partum

GM-CSF, Granulocyte-macrophage colony-stimulating factor; *HAART,* highly active antiretroviral therapy.

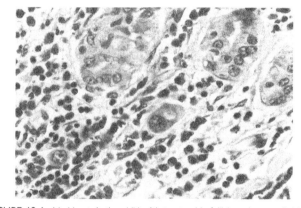

FIGURE 12-1. Hashimoto's thyroiditis. Note atrophic follicles, absent colloid, and infiltrate of lymphocytes, plasma cells, and immunoblasts *(lower left).* (Hematoxylin and eosin [H&E], ×200) (From Livolsi VA. In Falk SA, ed: Thyroid disease: endocrinology, surgery, nuclear medicine and radiotherapy, New York, 1990, Raven Press.)

important role in the pathogenesis of autoimmune thyroiditis. A summary of the genetic and environmental factors that predispose to the condition is shown in Table 12-2. Details are described in subsequent sections.

ENVIRONMENT AND THYROID AUTOIMMUNITY

Three studies all imply that smoking may in fact protect against development of TPO antibodies[12] and inferentially against chronic lymphocytic thyroiditis. The mechanism for these findings is not clear, although it is known that smoking is a definite risk factor for the development of Graves' ophthalmopathy and, to a lesser extent, Graves' disease. Although stress is thought to contribute to the onset of Graves' hyperthyroidism, no good data relate stressful life events to involvement in the origin of Hashimoto's disease. Iodine administration is known to induce thyroiditis in susceptible animals by affecting the antigenicity of thyroglobulin.[13,14] In contrast to iodine, it is a deficiency of selenium that has been noted to cause increased thyroid volume and reduced echogenicity, together with reduction in immune competence.[15]

Amiodarone contains 37% iodine, and many of its effects on the thyroid are iodine mediated; in addition, amiodarone administration results in the appearance of thyroid antibodies in patients who have preexisting thyroid autoimmunity.[16] A similar situation occurs in patients who are receiving lithium therapy.[17] Both of these drugs may have specific immunomodulatory effects, which exacerbate thyroid autoimmunity in Hashimoto's thyroiditis. Interleukin (IL)-2 and Interferon-α (IFN-α) both cause changes in the immune system characterized by alterations in lymphocyte subsets, which may result in autoimmune thyroid disease.[18] Highly active antiretroviral therapy (HAART) and granulocyte-macrophage colony-stimulating factor (GM-CSF) have been noted to be associated with small increases in thyroid autoimmunity in some studies.[19,20] External irradiation, as an accident (e.g., Chernobyl), can result in the expression of autoimmune thyroid disease and the emergence of thyroid antibodies.[21] Although infection (viral or bacterial) is an attractive factor to be considered as a cause of autoimmune thyroid disease, the data related to Hashimoto's thyroiditis are tentative at best.[22,23] The molecular mimicry hypothesis regarding the increased incidence of *Yersinia enterocolitica* noted in patients with Graves' disease has not been confirmed as a causative factor, and this serology is not seen in Hashimoto's disease. The switch in peripheral lymphocyte pattern from Th2 during pregnancy to a Th1 state post partum is associated with the so-called "immune rebound," which is characterized by a rapid rise in titers of thyroid antibodies in women who are known to have these antibodies in early gestation. In about 25% to 30% of these women, permanent autoimmune hypothyroidism occurs. Transient postpartum thyroiditis is seen in the remaining antibody-positive women. Thus pregnancy must be regarded as a specific cause of autoimmune thyroid disease in predisposed women. From the foregoing, it will be appreciated that although environmental factors are important, it is necessary to impose these on the appropriate genetic background to initiate the immune process. This, together with an overview of the immune abnormalities seen in Hashimoto's disease, will be discussed in the following sections.

Genetic Factors

It is widely known that autoimmune thyroid diseases (both Hashimoto's thyroiditis and Graves' disease) occur in families.[24] Fig. 12-2 shows the age at diagnosis in 400 patients with Hashimoto's disease *(panel A)* and shows that those with a positive family history present at a younger age than those who have no family history *(panel B)*. This tendency could be due to genetic predisposition, as well as to environmental influences. Studies of genetic predisposition have revealed that autoimmune thyroid diseases are often associated with particular genetic markers. These markers include histocompatibility lymphocytic antigens, allotypes of immunoglobulin heavy chains, and variations in the T cell receptor (TCR) and the thyroid peroxidase (TPO). More recently, the association of Hashimoto's disease with variants of CTLA-4, PTNP22, and thyroglobulin has been documented.[25] These associations have been examined by linkage analysis, association analysis, and whole genome screening. Findings described in reports are not always consistent with each other, probably because of the subjects chosen and the small sizes of some studies. The main susceptibility genes are shown in Table 12-3.

Recent studies have highlighted the possibility of association of vitamin D receptor gene polymorphisms with increased risk

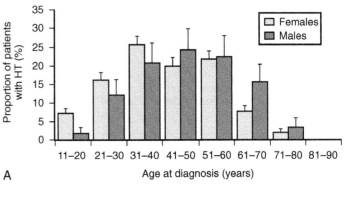

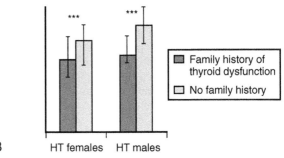

FIGURE 12-2. Age at diagnosis of Hashimoto's thyroiditis **(A)** and median age at diagnosis of those with and without a family history of thyroid dysfunction **(B).** (From Manji N, Carr-Smith JD, Boelaert K, et al: Influences of age, gender, smoking, and family history on autoimmune thyroid disease phenotype, J Clin Endocr Metab 91:4873–4880, 2006.)

Table 12-3. Susceptibility Genes for Hashimoto's Thyroiditis

Gene	Associated Variants	Population Association
HLA-DR	DR3,DR5 (goitrous)	Caucasian
	DR3 and HLA B8 (atrophic)	Caucasian
	DR9 and HLA-Bw46,87	Chinese
HLA-DQ	DQw2 (link dis HLA DR3)	Cauasian
	DQ A0301 (link dis HLA DR4)	Caucasian
	DQ B0201 (link dis HLA DR3)	Caucasian
CTLA-4	A/G49SNP, CT60 SNP	Caucasian, Japanese
	3' UTR AT microsatellite	Koreans, Chinese
PTPN22	R620W SNP	Caucasian
Thyroglobulin	S734A SNP	Caucasian
	T2334C SNP	Japanese
	M1028V, R1999W SNP	

Data from Jacobson EM, Tomer Y: The genetic basis of thyroid autoimmunity, Thyroid 17:949–961, 2007.

Link dis, Linkage disequilibrium; *SNP,* single-nucleotide polymorphism.

for Hashimoto's disease among the Chinese[26] and possibly also in the Croatian population.[27] Other possible candidate susceptibility genes for Hashimoto's include an *IL-6* gene promoter polymorphism[28] and a polymorphism in the *IFN-γ* gene, the latter being associated with severity of the disease.[29] Linkage of specific *TCR* genes to inheritance of Hashimoto's thyroiditis has also been reported. A specific TCR restriction fragment length polymorphism (RFLP) was increased in Hashimoto's thyroiditis, as well as in Graves' disease,[30] and a TaqI RFLP for the *Va* gene of TCR was also increased.[31] TCR Vbeta gene utilization was diminished, but selective expression was not observed in Hashimoto's in contrast to Graves' disease.[32] Inheritance of specific allotypes of the immunoglobulin G (IgG) heavy chain is also seen in autoimmune thyroiditis.[33] The CT60 polymorphism of CTLA-4 maps an important genetic determinant for the risk of Hashimoto's disease across diverse populations[34] and may identify patients with celiac disease who are at risk for Hashimoto's disease and type 1 diabetes.[35] Recently, X chromosome inactivation has been reported to be an important contributor to the increased risk that females may develop Hashimoto's thyroiditis.[36]

Antibodies to Thyroid Antigens

THYROGLOBULIN

Experimental autoimmune thyroiditis with histologic findings similar to those of Hashimoto's thyroiditis can be induced in animals by immunization with human thyroglobulin in an adjuvant. It can also be produced by depleting rats of T cells followed by thyroglobulin (Tg) administration. In both these animal models, strain specificity is vital, indicating the role of MHC class II-encoded susceptibility.[37]

Human Tg has at least 40 antigenic epitopes, but only one or two of these bind human TgAbs.[38] Although the TgAb response in autoimmune thyroid disease (AITD) is typically polyclonal on isoelectric focusing,[39] TgAb from patients with AITD are specific to human Tg and are directed toward a restricted number of epitopes on Tg, unlike rabbit TgAb, which recognizes Tg from other animal species.[40] However, thyroglobulin is not isolated from the immune system in the thyroid follicles but is normally present in the circulation of humans.[14] Thyroglobulin-binding lymphocytes can also be detected in the fetus.[15]

Evidence suggests that TgAb from patients with AITD recognize Tg from normal and AITD thyroids differently, suggesting the presence of antigenic variations between the Tg from healthy and AITD thyroids.[41] TgAb in AITD is mainly IgG (which consists of four subclasses) rather than IgM, which is more likely to be present in healthy individuals.[42] TgAb in AITD states is predominantly of the IgG4 subtype, and the weak complementing fixing property of TgAb is probably due to the predominance of this isotype, which is a poor activator of the complement cascade.[43] This implies that antithyroglobulin antibodies are not directly related to tissue damage in Hashimoto's thyroiditis. The pattern of Tg recognition, as assessed by the use of inhibition of Tg binding by four recombinant TgAb-Fab, showed that the pattern was similar when patients with Hashimoto's disease were compared with patients with Graves' disease.[44]

TgAb are found in patients with AITD but not consistently so, being present in only about 60% of patients.[42] Unlike the thyroid peroxidase antibody (TPOAb), TgAb does not fix complement as stated above, probably because the epitopes on the large molecule are widely spaced and are unable to achieve the cross-linking necessary for complement activation. Further, TgAb is also found in healthy individuals with no evidence of thyroid disease.[45] A role for TgAb in the pathogenesis of AITD therefore remains unproven.

THYROID PEROXIDASE

Thyroid peroxidase (TPO) evokes high-affinity, IgG-class autoantibodies (TPOAb) and TPO-specific T cells that are markers of thyroid infiltration or are implicated in thyroid destruction, respectively.[46] Thyroid peroxidase (TPO), the major antigen in human Hashimoto's disease, was shown to be identical to the previously termed microsomal antigen in the 1980s. TPOAbs in sera from patients with Hashimoto's thyroiditis are predominantly polyclonal. Anti-TPO antibodies can induce complement-dependent cytotoxicity.[47] In fact, antibodies against complement (anti-C1q) are found in patients with Hashimoto's disease, and

they correlate with thyroid-stimulating hormone (TSH) levels. Anti-C1q may be pathogenically involved in destruction in this disease independent of thyroid antibodies.[48] Anti-idiotypic antibodies against TPO antibodies are occasionally found in the sera of patients with autoimmune thyroid disease and might be involved in the regulation of autoimmunity.[49] A study of epitopic recognition patterns of TPOAb in healthy individuals and patients with Hashimoto's thyroiditis has shown that specific immunodominant regions are associated with Hashimoto patients but not with normal controls. Whether the propensity to produce antibodies to certain TPO epitopes is of pathogenetic relevance is not clear.[50] However, TPOAbs can damage thyroid cells as they activate the complement cascade. TPO itself appears to interact with TPO-specific T cells that are implicated in thyroid destruction. TPO antibodies that are transferred passively from mothers with Hashimoto's thyroiditis do not seem to damage the thyroid or to affect thyroid function in the fetus or neonate.[51]

TPOAbs are positive in more than 90% of patients with Hashimoto's thyroiditis, regardless of the presence of hypothyroidism or euthyroidism. The superior diagnostic value of TPOAb rather than TgAb for the confirmation of Hashimoto's thyroiditis has led many hospitals and laboratories to rely solely on TPOAb measurements. This is satisfactory for more than 95% of patients, but in some instances, patients have only TgAb as a marker of thyroid autoimmunity. Currently, the clinical importance of anti-TPO antibodies lies in the diagnosis of thyroid autoimmunity, but T cell–mediated immunity to TPO is an ongoing field of investigation that should improve our understanding of the pathogenesis of Hashimoto's thyroiditis.

THYROID-STIMULATING HORMONE RECEPTOR ANTIBODIES

Thyroid-stimulating hormone (TSH) stimulation-blocking antibody (TSBAb) can inhibit TSH action on thyroid and cause atrophic hypothyroidism in autoimmune thyroiditis.[52] Although the specific epitopes for thyroid-stimulating antibody (TSAb) or TSBAb are still uncertain, the major epitope of TSBAb seems to be found in the C-terminal part of the extracellular domain (around 300 to 400 amino acids),[53] probably in close proximity to that for TSAb.[53] However, in vitro conversion from TSBAb to TSAb after the addition of antihuman IgG antibody suggests that TSAb and TSBAb are not determined solely by their epitopes, and the same TSHR antibody might act as a stimulator or a blocker, depending on the influence of other factors.[54] TSBAb are uncommon as a cause of immune-mediated hypothyroidism, although they have been noted in a few patients with goitrous autoimmune thyroiditis, as well as in patients with atrophic chronic thyroiditis.[52] Regional variations in prevalence have been noted, with the antibody reported more frequently in Japan.

OTHER ANTIBODIES

The Na^+/I^- symporter (NIS), a membrane glycoprotein, mediates iodine uptake into the thyroid follicular cell. Although reports have described antibodies to this moiety in Hashimoto's thyroiditis, evidence that NIS is a major autoantigen now is not generally accepted. For example, anti-NIS antibodies were found to be positive in only 15% of patients with Hashimoto's thyroiditis.[55]

Antibodies to thyroxine (T_4) and triiodothyronine (T_3) sometimes are found in patients with autoimmune or other thyroid diseases. They are seen in 14% and 35%, respectively, of patients with primary hypothyroidism, in most of whom TGAbs are found in high titer.[56] The pathogenetic significance of these antibodies is not known. Probably, they are of little importance as long as the thyroid can produce enough thyroid hormone to sustain adequate serum levels of free hormone. These antibodies interfere with measurements of serum T_4 and T_3, especially in assays of free T_4 and free T_3.[57] Antibovine TSH autoantibodies, occasionally found in Graves' disease, are also reported in Hashimoto's thyroiditis.[58] Their pathogenetic significance is unclear. They are speculated to be anti-idiotypic antibodies to anti-TSH receptor antibodies (TRAbs) in Graves' disease. They may interfere with the measurement of TRAbs and yield unusually high or negative titers. Autoantibodies against several other thyroid components have been reported. Antibodies to colloid antigen-2, distinct from thyroglobulin, have been detected. Antibodies to cell-surface antigen (distinct for TPO) are detected by the patchy immunofluorescent staining of the cell surface or by mixed hemabsorption.

Considerable interest has been expressed in past years in the concept of direct growth-stimulating antibodies or growth-blocking antibodies found in goitrous Hashimoto's thyroiditis and in primary myxedema, respectively.[37] However, contoversy regarding the assay has impeded progress.[59] Following the development of a sensitive bioassay for growth-stimulating antibody, which did report positive findings in goitrous Hashimoto's disease, no studies have explored the use of this assay in greater detail. Autoantibodies against other cellular components, so-called natural antibodies (not always thyroid cell-specific), have also been reported, for example, antibodies to tubulin and calmodulin[60] and the ganglioside asialo-GM1, present in the plasma membrane of human thyroid.[61] Measurement of natural antibodies (to DNA, actin, myoglobin, myosin, trinitrophenyl hapten, and tubulin) has shown that around 50% of a series of Hashimoto's patients are positive for one or more of these antibodies, and this positivity appears to correlate with thyroid antibody activity.[62] Antibodies to other organs related to autoimmune disease (e.g., islet cells, adrenal cortex, gastric mucosa, parathyroid) are found in autoimmune thyroiditis in higher incidence than in the general population.[60] (See section on other autoimmune diseases.)

Cellular Abnormalities

The breakdown of immunologic self-tolerance leads to the presentation of self antigens and the expansion of autoreactive T cells. Consequently, release of inflammatory cytokines and differentiation of B cells producing antibodies occur. The T cells in Hashimoto's disease are of the type 1 helper T cell (Th1) type, characterized by the production of IL-2 and IFN-γ.

It has become clear that regulatory T cells (T-reg) (with CD4+/CD25 surface expression) play an important role in the maintenance of immune tolerance and the prevention of its breakdown. T-reg express FoxP3, a specific gene marker for the inhibition of expression of inflammatory cytokines. Hence, in vivo depletion of this subset exacerbates autimmune disease in the Hashimoto's mouse animal model. The development of transgenic animal models of autoimmune thyroiditis has suggested that T-regs have a role in the progression of Graves' disease to Hashimoto's thyroiditis and subsequent hypothyroidism.[63] In addition to the predominance of the Th1 lymphocyte subset, the B7-1 (CD80) molecule preferentially acts as a co-stimulator for the generation of Th1 cells and has been recognized on thyrocytes in Hashimoto's disease.[64] This phenomenon, together with expression of MHC class II and intercellular adhesion molecule

(ICAM)-1,[65] leads to T cell differentiation from Th0 to Th1 cells and maintenance of thyroid autoimmunity. Thyroid cells in autoimmune thyroid disease also produce several cytokines (e.g., IL-1, IL-6, tumor necrosis factor-β [TNF-β]) that influence lymphocytic responses (vide infra).

In studies of intrathyroid-infiltrating lymphocytic populations, T lymphocytes predominate over B cells and CD8⁺ T lymphocytes are increased in Hashimoto's thyroiditis. Analysis of the gene for the variable region of the a chain (Va gene) of the TCR suggested that the infiltrating T cells are a highly restricted population,[66] raising the possibility of a clonal restriction in this autoimmune disease. However, this has not been confirmed.[67] Several in vitro cytotoxic mechanisms have been demonstrated. Cytotoxic T cells that are specific for thyroid epithelial cells are observed and antibody-mediated cell cytotoxicity activity can be found in the sera of patients with Hashimoto's disease. In addition, complement-dependent cytotoxic antibodies are found in sera from these patients, and natural killer lymphocyte counts correlate inversely with thyroid hormone levels. These factors undoubtedly contribute to thyroid follicular cellular damage. Their importance in the whole destructive cascade has been overshadowed to some extent by the data related to apoptosis of thyroid cells (vide infra).

Cytokines

Cytokines are known to have a wide variety of inflammatory and immunomodulatory effects; therefore, it might be thought that many steps in thyroid autoimmunity are mediated and/or modulated by cytokines.[68]

Characterization of T cells into Th1 and Th2 based on different patterns of cytokine production has aided the understanding of immunologic events in Hashimoto's disease, although the picture in the human is not as clear as in animals. Cytokines associated with Th1 and Th2 are shown in Table 12-4. In general, the pattern of T cell response in autoimmune hypothyroidism is a Th1 pattern. Following activation by autoantigen recognition, thyroid-specific lymphocytes produce IL-2 with induction of T cell proliferation and differentiation. IFN-γ is also produced and natural killer cells activated. Thyroid autoimmunity occurs in humans who received IL-2 or IFN-γ for the treatment of cancer or viral hepatitis.[69,70] A broader range of cytokines then is produced from these activated lymphocytes, resulting in amplification and perpetuation of the immune response. In addition, some cytokines stimulate human lymphocyte antigen (HLA) class II expression on thyroid epithelial cells, which may be important for the amplification and progression of the disease. Data from in vitro effects of cytokines on cultured thyroid cells

Table 12-4. Cytokine Pattern from Th1 and Th2 CD4+ Cells

	Th1	Th2
IL-1	++	++
IL-2	+++	−
IL-4	−	+++
Il-5	−	+++
Il-10	+	+++
IL-13	−	+++
IFN-γ		+++

IFN, Interferon; *IL,* interleukin.

also indicate that some cytokines (e.g., TNF-α, which is mainly produced by monocytes) may be directly cytotoxic to thyroid cells in vivo. The mechanisms of cytokine interaction are not simple. For example, autoantibodies and complement may promote mixed Th1/Th2 cell cytokine response by enhancing the uptake of autoantigens by antigen presenting cells.[71] Another molecule, CTLA-4, whose gene is now a known risk factor for autoimmune thyroid disease, is expressed by activated T and B lymphocytes. Levels of serum CTLA-4 are elevated in autoimmune thyroid disease, and this may play a pathogenetic role in this condition.[72] It should be noted that some cytokines (e.g., IL-1, IL-6) are produced by thyrocytes, as well as by lymphocytes. Thus, interleukins produced by thyrocytes would stimulate intrathyroidal lymphocytes. IL-1 stimulates T cells to release lymphokines and has many other inflammatory effects. IL-1 can induce thyrocyte apoptosis through Fas-Fas ligand interaction (vide infra).

Chemokines

Chemokines are a group of low molecular weight proteins that recruit leukocyte subtypes and other cell types to sites of inflammation. They do this by interacting with G protein–coupled receptors, and they play important roles in initiating and maintaining immunologic responses in Hashimoto's thyroiditis, as well as in other autoimmune endocrine diseases. The main chemokines found in the thyroid in autoimmune thyroid disease are shown in Table 12-5. In human Hashimoto's disease, there is increased expression of CXCL9 and CXCL10, and the serum level of the latter is higher. The role of chemokines is being further investigated with the use of animal models, particularly a transgenic mouse model expressing CCL21. This mouse does not develop hypothyroidism, despite significant lymphoid infiltration.[73] Further work in this area is awaited with interest.

Table 12-5. Chemokines Found in the Thyroid in Autoimmune Thyroid Disease

Type	Name	Receptor
CXC	CXCL1	CXCR1, CXCR2
	CXCL8	CXCR1, CXCR2
	CXCL9	CXCR3
	CXCL10	CXCR3
	CXCL11	CXCR3, CXCR3B, CXCR7
	CXCL12	CXCR4
	CXCL13	CXCR5
	CXCL14	Unknown
CC	CCL2	CCR2
	CCL3	CCR1, CCR5
	CCL4	CCR5
	CCL5	CCR1, CCR3, CCR5
	CCL18	Unknown
	CCL21	CCR7
	CCL22	CCR4
	CCL19	CCR7

Data from Weetman AR: Cellular immune responses in autoimmune thyroid disease, Clin Endocrinol 61:405–413, 2004; Kimura H, Caturegli P: Chemokine orchestration of autoimmune thyroiditis, Thyroid 17:1005–1011, 2007.
C, Cysteine; L, ligand; R, receptor; X, amino acid residue.
CXC have X between two cysteine molecules.

Mechanism for Development of Hypothyroidism

Mounting evidence indicates that destruction of thyroid follicles occurs by the mechanism of apoptosis.[74] Apoptosis or programmed cell death is characterized by progressive digestion of the cell and its genetic material by caspases, which are proteolytic enzymes. Thyroid cells express apoptotic ligands and receptors, for example, TNF, Fas, and TRAIL (tumor necrosis–related apoptosis-inducing ligand). In the normal situation, no cell death occurs, but when the thyroid follicular cells are in contact with infiltrating cytotoxic lymphocytes expressing FasL and Bcl-2, apoptosis develops. Fas is an apoptosis-signaling receptor molecule that is found on the surface of a number of cell types.[75] Interaction of Fas with its ligand regulates a number of physiologic and pathologic processes involved in cell death. Although Fas ligand is expressed in thyrocytes from both normal controls and patients with Hashimoto's thyroiditis, Fas is expressed only in thyrocytes from patients with Hashimoto's thyroiditis.[76] Interleukin-1β, which is abundantly produced by the glands of patients with Hashimoto's thyroiditis, induced Fas expression in normal thyrocytes, and cross-linking of Fas resulted in massive thyrocyte apoptosis. The interaction of the Fas/FasL, which is inhibited in normal thyrocytes, can be activated by proinflammatory cytokines (e.g., IL-1β, IFN-γ, TNF-α), which will arise from Th1 cytokines. Soluble Fas molecules lack the transmembrane domain because of alternative splicing and block Fas-mediated apoptosis. Decreased serum levels of soluble Fas in Hashimoto's disease may also induce destruction of thyroid cells by promoting their apoptosis.[77] Increased serum TSH may inhibit Fas-mediated apoptosis of thyrocytes,[78] and TSBAb may block the inhibitory action of TSH toward Fas-mediated apoptosis, thus inducing thyroid atrophy. Indeed, the expression of FasL on thyrocytes correlated postively with TRAb in Graves' thyrocytes, but no correlation was found with antibody titer in Hashimoto's thyrocytes.[79] However, serum levels of Fas correlate with TPOAb and TSH in Hashimoto's patients,[80] and soluble CD40 correlates with TPOAb.[81] Transgenic expression of FasL on thyroid follicular cells actually prevents autoimmune thyroiditis, possibly through inhibition of lymphocyte infiltation.[82] Mutations of Fas, which induce loss of function, were found in thyroid lymphocytes in 38.1% of patients with Hashimoto's thyroiditis[83] and in 65.4% of patients with malignant lymphoma,[84] which usually develops from Hashimoto's thyroiditis.

The TRAIL molecule is a member of the TNF group that exists in membrane-bound and soluble form. It induces apoptosis through interaction with its receptors via a caspase-dependent pathway. Molecular regulation of apoptosis in the thyroid is unknown, but it is reasonable to suggest that defects in T regulatory cells, referred to in the section on cellular events, are related to the apoptosis. Indeed, the expression of Fas in CD4+ T-reg cells is greater in severe thyroiditis.[85] In summary, Fas/FasL-mediated apoptosis plays an important role in the active stage of the autoimmune process in Hashimoto's thyroiditis and may contribute to the irreversible damage of thyrocytes. Furthermore, soluble CD40 may serve as a marker for these events.

Other mechanisms of cell death in autoimmune thyroiditis include exocytic granules that contain perforin and granzyme B and complement activation. Complement activation may not kill cells but may help to maintain the inflammatory disease by exacerbating the immune process.[86] A schematic overview of the immunopathologic process of the development of thyroid auto-

OVERVIEW OF THE PATHOGENESIS OF AUTOIMMUNE
THYROID DISEASE

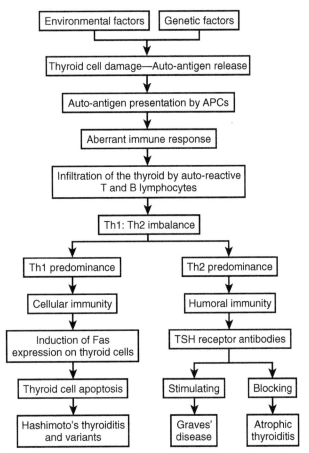

FIGURE 12-3. Development of Hashimoto's thyroiditis and Graves' disease is shown, in addition to the effect of thyroid-stimulating hormone (TSH) receptor blocking antibody. (Adapted from Fontoulakis and Tsatsoulis: on the pathogenesis of autoimmune thyroid disease: a unifying hypothesis, Clin Endocr 60, 397–409, 2004.)

immunity is shown in Fig. 12-3. Inevitably, this is simplistic, and many molecular details still are not clear.

CLINICAL FEATURES

Most patients with Hashimoto's thyroiditis are euthyroid or have subclinical hypothyroidism with goiter and circulating thyroid antibodies. As time passes, overt hypothyroidism will develop at a rate of about 5% per year.[6] The goiter becomes smaller and occasionally atrophies (atrophic thyroiditis). Histologically, fibrosis spreads, and few thyroid follicles remain in this stage of thyroiditis. The patient is usually an asymptomatic female. A goiter may be found incidentally at medical examination, but some patients present with discomfort related to the presence of a goiter. Thyroid enlargement in thyroiditis is usually lobular and irregular. It may be smooth or bosselated. The consistency is often firm and in some cases hard, suggesting a diagnosis of thyroid cancer. In rare cases, thyroid enlargement can encircle the trachea, causing compressive symptoms such as dysphagia, hoaresness, and dysphonia. Very rarely, the goiter is painful, suggesting a diagnosis of subacute thyroiditis. Some patients present with an apparent single thyroid nodule, even in the presence of circulating thyroid antibodies. In this situation, full investigation of the nodule must be performed to exclude malignancy, as the two conditions may coincide. In cases of diagnostic uncertainty, a fine needle biopsy, together with thyroid ultrasound, will clarify the problem. Although most patients will be euthyroid at presentation, some may even be hyperthyroid. Elderly patients are more likely to be found hypothyroid, although the presence of thyroid antibodies does not indicate progression to hypothyroidism at the same rate as in younger patients.[87] As was already mentioned, the presence of circulating thyroid antibodies, particularly TPOAb, is the hallmark of Hashimoto's thyroiditis; however, a minority of patients also have thyroid receptor blocking as well as stimulating immunoglobulins. Hypothyroidism then will be related to the blocking antibodies and the autoimmune process. In some instances, however, a patient may become hyperthyroid because of the stimulating antibodies after many years of replacement of levothyroxine for autoimmune hypothyroidism. Patients with an acute aggravation of thyroid autoimmunity are subject to destruction-induced thyrotoxicosis. These episodes usually are followed by transient hypothyroidism. High iodine ingestion can aggravate autoimmune thyroiditis, thus inducing hypothyroidism.

In children, Hashimoto's disease is less common and titers of antithyroid antibodies are usually lower than in adult patients. Autoimmune thyroid disease is uncommon in children and adolescents, and the prevalence of self-limiting autoimmune thyroiditis is significant.[88] They usually have a small symptomless goiter, and hypothyroidism is uncommon; thyroid dysfunction reverts to normal in up to 50% during follow-up.[89-91]

It is appropriate for patients with subclinical autoimmune thyroiditis to be examined periodically (once or twice a year). At this time, clinical signs of hypothyroidism should be evaluated, in addition to assay of serum T_4 and TSH and thyroid antibodies.

RELATION TO SILENT AND POSTPARTUM THYROIDITIS

Another form of thyroiditis, also believed to be of autoimmune cause, is variably referred to as painless, silent, occult, subacute, subacute nonsuppurative, and atypical (silent) subacute thyroiditis; it is also known as hyperthyroiditis, transient thyrotoxicosis with low thyroidal radioactive iodine uptake (RAIU), and lymphocytic thyroiditis with spontaneously resolving hyperthyroidism. No agreement has been reached on an inclusive name. Features of this disease entity overlap those of De Quervain's thyroiditis and Hashimoto's thyroiditis. The clinical course resembles that of De Quervain's (subacute) thyroiditis, except that no neck or thyroid pain is present and the erythrocyte sedimentation rate is not elevated, at least not to a very high level. Histologically, the condition cannot be differentiated from a milder form of Hashimoto's disease. The clinical features of the condition are firstly characterized by an initial phase of hyperthyroidism due to leakage of intrathyroidal hormones into the circulation after damage to thyroid epithelial cells from inflammation.[92] Thus, thyroid radioactive iodine uptake is low. This transient hyperthyroid phase is followed by hypothyroidism, which may be transient or, in a minority, permanent. A significant percentage of patients with silent thyroiditis have personal or family histories of autoimmune thyroid disease. Most patients have a complete remission, but persistent hypothyroidism develops in some.[93] Recurrence of disease is common in silent thyroiditis but very rare in subacute thyroiditis. It appears that silent thyroiditis is caused by the exacerbation of autoimmune thyroiditis induced by aggravating factors. Thyroiditis frequently recurs, and seasonal allergic rhinitis is reported to be an initiation factor,[94] as well as vigorous massage of the neck.[95]

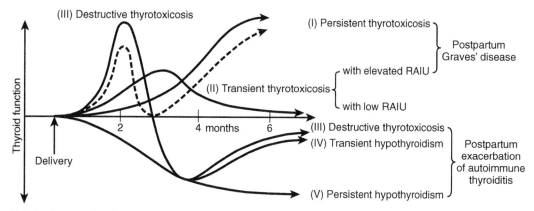

FIGURE 12-4. Thyroid dysfunction occurring after pregnancy. (From Amino N, Tada H, and Hidaka Y: Thyroid disease after pregnancy: postpartum thyroiditis. In Wass JAH, Shalet SM (eds): Oxford textbook of endocrinology and diabetes. Oxford, UK, 2002, Oxford University Press, pp. 527–532.)

The occurrence of lassitude and other symptoms of hypothyroidism related to the postpartum period was first noted in 1948.[96] These complaints were treated successfully with thyroid extract. The syndrome was later confirmed as postpartum thyroiditis (PPT), and the immune nature of the condition has been discussed.[97] Postpartum thyroiditis is essentially silent thyroiditis in the postpartum period. The term postpartum thyroiditis relates to destructive thyroiditis that occurs during the first 12 months postpartum and not to Graves' disease, although the two conditions may be seen concurrently. The origin is related to the change in immune status that follows delivery associated with the development or exacerbation of thyroid dysfunction (Fig. 12-4). PPT with thyroid dysfunction (i.e., postpartum thyroid dysfunction [PPTD]) is characterized by an episode of transient hyperthyroidism followed by transient hypothyroidism. The former presents at about 14 weeks' postpartum and is followed by transient hypothyroidism at a median of 19 weeks. Very occasionally, the hypothyroid state is seen before hyperthyroidism is noted. The thyroid dysfunction that occurs in up to 50% of TPO-antibody positive women ascertained at around 14 weeks' gestation involves 19% with hyperthyroidism alone, 49% with hypothyroidism alone, and the remaining 32% with hyperthyroidism followed by hypothyroidism (i.e., biphasic). Not all women manifest both thyroid states, and the hyperthyroid episode may escape detection as it may be of short duration. PPTD is almost always associated with the presence of antithyroid antibodies, usually anti-TPO antibodies that rise in titer at about 6 weeks' postpartum. Anti-Tg antibody occurs in about 15% and is the sole antibody in less than 5%. However, postpartum thyroid dysfunction has been described in small numbers of women who have not been shown to have circulating thyroid antibodies.[98] Although the clinical manifestations of the hyperthyroid state are not usually severe, lack of energy and irritability are particularly prominent, even in thyroid antibody–positive women who do not develop thyroid dysfunction. In contrast, the symptoms of the hypothyroid phase may be profound. Many classic hypothyroid symptoms occur before the onset of thyroid hormone reduction and persist even when recovery of hormone levels is seen. Postpartum thyroiditis can also occur in women receiving T_4 therapy before pregnancy and after miscarriage. Abundant evidence indicates that postpartum thyroiditis is an immunologically related disease.[98] Biopsy of the thyroid in this syndrome shows lymphocytic infiltration similar to that seen in Hashimoto's thyroiditis.[99]

RELATION TO GRAVES' DISEASE

After treatment, patients with Graves' disease often progress to hypothyroidism,[100] possibly because of the autoimmune tissue destruction described above. Another mechanism for the appearance of hypothyroidism is an increase in TSBAb, which has been found in 11.1% of thyrotoxic patients with Graves' disease who had blocking activity to TSH-induced adenylate cyclase stimulation but no TSAb activity,[101] that is, some patients with Graves' disease have both stimulating and blocking antibodies. When they have predominantly stimulating antibodies, hyperthyroidism develops, and when blocking antibodies become predominant, patients progress to hypothyroidism. The clinical features of patients depend on the balance among stimulating, blocking, and destructive aspects of humoral and cellular immunity. When stimulating factors are predominant, Graves' thyrotoxicosis develops. Predominance of destructive factors, such as antibody dependent cytotoxicity (ADCC), T lymphocyte cytotoxicity, lymphotoxin (TNF), and cytotoxic antibody, may produce Hashimoto's disease or myxedema. Blocking factors such as TSBAb also cause a reduction in thyroid function. Once thyroid cells are destroyed completely, stimulating factors are ineffective. Clinically, it is important to recognize that patients who are receiving levothyroxine for hypothyroidism due to Hashimoto's thyroiditis may develop thyrotoxicosis due to Graves' disease because of the presence of TSAb.[102] This implies of course that viable thyroid tissue is present that has not been completely destroyed by the destructive factors mentioned above.

RELATION TO OTHER AUTOIMMUNE DISEASES

Patients with other autoimmune diseases are often found to be positive for thyroglobulin antibodies; these disorders are thus associated with autoimmune thyroid disease.[4] The incidence is higher than in the general population. Autoimmune thyroid disease is found in association with both organ-specific autoimmune disease (e.g., vitiligo, myasthenia gravis, thrombocytopenic purpura, alopecia, Sjögren's syndrome)[103] and systemic autoimmune disease (e.g., rheumatoid arthritis, systemic lupus erythematosus, progressive systemic sclerosis). An association with other endocrine autoimmune diseases (such as insulin-dependent diabetes mellitus, autoimmune adrenalitis, autoimmune hypoparathyroidism, and autoimmune hypophysitis) is also found in autoimmune thyroiditis (Table 12-6). Such autoimmunity may occur simultaneously in multiple organs (polyendocrine autoimmune disease). During the past decade, it has been

Table 12-6. Risk for Other Autoimmune Diseases in Hashimoto's Thyroiditis

Associated Autoimmune Disease	Relative Risk	95% CI	P Value
Type 1 diabetes mellitus	2.97	1.24-7.11	.028
Rheumatoid arthritis	7.71	5.08-11.72	<.001
Pernicious anemia	31.08	20.23-47.75	<.001
Systemic lupus erythematosus	22.45	7.26-69.36	<.001
Addison's disease	157.13	75.30-327.87	<.001
Celiac disease	20.20	8.45-48.32	<.001
Vitiligo	26.26	15.36-44.91	<.001
Multiple sclerosis	6.22	2.34-16.50	.004
Myasthenia gravis	13.47	1.90-95.42	.072
Ulcerative colitis	3.11	1.17-8.25	.042

Relative risk of diagnosis of other autoimmune diseases in index cases.
Data from Boelaert, Newby, Simmonds, et al: The quantification of other autoimmune diseases in subjects with autoimmune thyroid disease: a large cross-sectional study, Amer J Med, 2009.

realized that celiac disease is more common in patients with Hashimoto's disease than was previously thought. In one recent study, 15% of patients with Hashimoto's disease had positive serology for celiac disease, and, conversely, 21% of patients with celiac disease had positive thyroid antibodies. Screening of patients with Hashimoto's disease for celiac disease and vice versa should be considered.[104] It is important to note that the increased frequency of chronic anemia in patients with autoimmune thyroid disease is due to concomitant autoimmune gastrointestinal disease.[105] On the other hand, the frequency with which patients with autoimmune thyroid disease suffer from another autoimmune disease is low, except for autoimmune gastritis and low B$_{12}$ levels.[106] Antiparietal cell antibodies and/or anti-intrinsic factor antibodies are found in about one third of patients with autoimmune thyroid disease.

Hashimoto's Encephalopathy

Hashimoto's encephalopathy or encephalitis is a rare complication of Hashimoto's thyroiditis. It is a steroid-responsive, relapsing encephalopathy associated with thyroid antibodies. It is more common in females and has been reported in children, adults, and the elderly.[107] Neurologic complications sometimes are associated with thyroid dysfunction, but patients with this encephalopathy are usually euthyroid. It is a treatable, steroid-responsive, progressive or relapsing encephalopathy associated with elevation of thyroid-specific autoantibodies.[108] The condition was first described in 1966[109] and may present as a subacute or acute encephalopathy with seizures and stroke-like episodes, often in association with myoclonus and tremor.[110] Seizures, cognitive decline, and behavioral problems are seen in chidren.[111] It is associated with abnormal electroencephalogram (EEG) and high cerebrospinal fluid proteins without pleocytosis. Some patients have significant residual disability.[112] Antibody to α-enolase has been identified in some patients,[113,114] but this antibody is frequently found in other autoimmune diseases as well. Although this condition may represent an association of an uncommon autoimmune encephalopathy with autoimmune thyroid disease,[115] the finding of TPOAb binding to specific astrocytes is of interest.[116] The autoimmune response to enzymes identified as the IgG autoimmune response in cerebrospinal fluid (CSF) from patients may indicate mechanisms of vascular and or neuronal damage in this autoimmune inflammatory condition.[117]

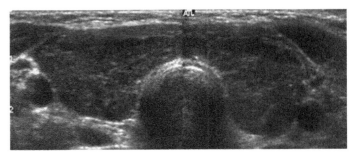

FIGURE 12-5. Ultrasound of patient with Hashimoto's thyroiditis. Note bilateral hypoechogenicity. (Courtesy Dr. Peter Smyth.)

RELATION TO THYROID CANCER

The association between autoimmune thyroiditis and B cell lymphoma is well recognized. Sequence similarity between clonal bands in Hashimoto's thyroiditis and thyroid lymphoma (as determined by polymerase chain reaction [PCR] and sequence determination of immunoglobulin heavy chain gene rearrangements) suggests strongly that primary thyroid lymphoma may evolve from Hashimoto's thyroiditis.[118] It has been generally assumed that differentiated thyroid cancer is not more frequent in patients with Hashimoto's disease, but several reports, including two recent large studies,[119,120] have shown that patients with Hashimoto's disease may be up to three times more likely to have papillary thyroid cancer. Molecular studies have shown that the RET/PTC-RAS-BRAF cascade is expressed more commonly in non-neoplastic follicular cells in thyroiditis, indicating overlapping molecular mechanisms that regulate early tumor development and inflammation in Hashimoto's thyroiditis.[121,122]

DIAGNOSIS

The diagnosis of autoimmune thyroiditis is usually simple to make by clinical observation and serologic tests, especially in overt hypothyroidism. A goiter that may be diffuse or nodular and positive antithyroid antibodies (anti-TPO antibodies and/or antithyroglobulin antibodies) with no evidence of other thyroid disease lead to the diagnosis of goitrous Hashimoto's thyroiditis. Tests of thyroid function (free T$_4$, free T$_3$, and TSH) might not be helpful because thyroiditis is subclinical in about 90% of patients. About 90% of patients with Hashimoto's disease have positive TPOAbs, but no difference is seen in titers and in the prevalence of antibodies between euthyroid and hypothyroid patients. In patients who are found to have thyroid antibodies but no palpable goiter, a thyroid ultrasound will reveal a hypoechoic pattern consistent with Hashimoto's thyroiditis (Fig. 12-5). In patients who have primary hypothyroidism with an atrophic thyroid, the existence of blocking-type anti–thyrotropin receptor (TSHR) antibodies (TSBAbs) can be assessed, although their prevalence is low even in Japan.[123] Histologic examination is confirmative but not necessary for the diagnosis and management of thyroiditis because lymphocytic infiltration into the thyroid is observed in all seropositive patients.[5] Conversely, TPOAb or TgAb is detectable in more than 95% of histologically confirmed cases of Hashimoto's disease. Indeed, detection of the antibodies alone is sufficient for a diagnosis of autoimmune thyroid disease. Antibodies are also found in about 10% of individuals in the general population with no clinical manifestations, and these patients should be considered to have subclinical autoimmune thyroiditis. For the small number of seronegative patients who have overt or latent hypothyroidism, the diagnosis of Hashimoto's thyroiditis is likely and can be confirmed by

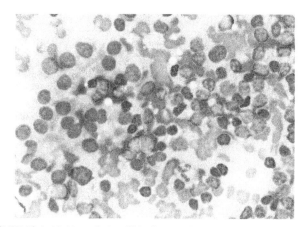

FIGURE 12-6. Hashimoto's thyroiditis: fine needle aspiration biopsy. Note loose clusters of follicular epithelial cells and a range of lymphoid cells. (From Orell SR, Philips J: Monographs in clinical cytology. In Orell SR, ed: The thyroid fine-needle biopsy and cytological diagnosis of thyroid lesions, vol 14, Basel, Switzerland, 1997, Karger, p 68.)

ultrasound examination. Fine needle aspiration biopsy will show cytologic evidence of thyroiditis (Fig. 12-6), but histologic examination is the only way to absolutely prove its existence. Thyroid biopsy will be necessary if the goiter is rapidly increasing and is very hard or fixed, that is, when thyroid tumors are suspected.

During the thyrotoxic phase of acute exacerbation of Hashimoto's thyroiditis, it is necessary to rule out Graves' disease, silent and subacute thyroiditis, and toxic nodular goiter. Graves' thyrotoxicosis lasts for longer than 3 months, but increased thyroid hormone levels in silent thyroiditis usually disappear within 3 months. Patients with Graves' disease have anti-TSHR antibody, and TSH-binding inhibitory immunoglobulin, measured by radioreceptor assay, is positive in about 90% of patients. These antibodies are usually negative in silent thyroiditis, although some exceptions can be found. The serum T_3/T_4 ratio (nanogram per microgram) is a simple indicator of differentiation between the two types of thyrotoxicosis. Eighty percent of patients with Graves' thyrotoxicosis show a ratio of more than 20, but it is less than 20 in those with destructive thyrotoxicosis, including silent thyroiditis. After complete remission of Graves' disease, silent thyroiditis sometimes develops in the same patients. Therefore, the previous history is not useful for differentiation.

NATURAL HISTORY

Most patients with Hashimoto's thyroiditis are euthyroid or have latent hypothyroidism with goiter in their youth. As time passes, some progress to overt hypothyroidism. The goiter becomes smaller and occasionally atrophies. Histologically, fibrosis spreads, and few thyroid follicles remain in this stage of thyroiditis. Thus, elderly patients with Hashimoto's thyroiditis are more likely to be found hypothyroid.

Patients may experience periods of transient hypothyroidism under certain conditions. In some cases of Hashimoto's thyroiditis, the hypothyroidism seems to be reversible.[124] This transient hypothyroidism may occur in the course of Hashimoto's thyroiditis when destruction of the thyroid is slow. Hypothyroidism is often transient when goiter is present and the serum thyroglobulin concentration is high.[125] The thyroid response to TSH after the administration of thyrotropin-releasing hormone can be used to evaluate potential recovery from hypothyroidism in patients undergoing T_4 therapy.[126] In a region where iodine-containing food (such as seaweed) is common, as in Japan, excessive dietary iodine intake (1000 mg/day or more) can cause transient hypothyroidism in patients with subclinical autoimmune thyroiditis. This condition is easily reversible with reduction of iodine intake.[127]

A rare but important complication of Hashimoto's thyroiditis is malignant lymphoma. The tumor arises in patients with Hashimoto's thyroiditis in around 40% to 80% of cases[128]; hence, it has a female preponderance. The patient is usually in the sixth decade or older and presents with a rapidly enlarging neck mass on a background of previously diagnosed autoimmune thyroiditis, often while on levothyroxine treatment. Rapid diagnosis is made by fine needle biopsy and external radiotherapy, and chemotherapy can result in dramatic shrinkage of the tumor with relief of pressure symptoms and remission in most cases.

TREATMENT

No practical way has been found to manipulate the autoimmune abnormality itself. In a study in which euthyroid patients with Hashimoto's thyroiditis were randomly allocated to levothyroxine treatment or simple follow-up, a significant increase in free T_4 and a significant decrease in TSH and antithyroglobulin antibody anti–thyroid peroxidase antibody levels were noted after 15 months in the T_4-treated group. Although no change in cytologic findings was seen, ultrasonography showed a decrease in thyroid volume in L-thyroxine–receiving patients, whereas an increase was detected in patients who were followed without treatment. It seems therefore that thyroid hormone therapy may be beneficial in patients with Hashimoto's thyroiditis, even if they are euthyroid.[129] Recently it was observed that the administration of selenium to patients with Hashimoto's thyroiditis is accompanied by a significant fall in titers of thyroid antibodies compared with a control group.[130] However, no evidence of reversal of the pathology was found. Hypothyroidism in patients with large goiters and high iodine uptake is often transient,[124] especially in patients younger than 30 years. Restriction of high iodine ingestion may be effective in these patients, but surgical resection may be required occasionally. Such patients can be treated successfully with radioiodine, with a size reduction of around 50%.[131] At present, the major approach is to treat the associated hypothyroidism or to attempt to shrink the goiter to release pressure symptoms or simply for cosmetic reasons. T_4 replacement therapy is not always necessary in euthyroid patients with small or moderate goiters. These patients should be examined once a year to detect the later development of hypothyroidism. When hypothyroidism develops, patients should be treated with T_4. The daily replacement dose is 100 to 200 mcg/day (about 2 mcg/kg/day). In patients with long-standing hypothyroidism, replacement therapy should be initiated with a small dose of T_4 and should be built up gradually until a satisfactory maintenance dose is achieved. Hypothyroidism in patients with postpartum thyroiditis is usually transient. In these patients, lifelong T_4 therapy is not necessary. T_3 rather than T_4 therapy may be useful for a short period to quickly relieve hypothyroid symptoms in some cases.

Painful subacute exacerbation of goitrous Hashimoto's disease is rare, and corticosteroid therapy is useful in these cases. About 10% to 20% of patients have recurrent episodes of destructive thyroiditis, but thyroid suppression therapy is not effective for prevention. In rare patients who have frequent recurrences, surgical removal of the gland or ^{131}I therapy has been recommended.

REFERENCES

1. Hashimoto H: Zur Kenntniss der lymphomatösen Veränderung der Schilddrüse (Struma lymphomatosa), Arch Klin Chir 97:219, 1912.
2. Rose NR, Witebsky E: Studies in organ specificity. V. Changes in the thyroid glands of rabbits following activ immunisation with rabbit thyroid extracts, J Immunol 76:417–427, 1956.
3. Roit IM, Doniach D, Campbell PN, et al: Autoantibodies in Hashimoto's disease (lymphadenoid goitre), Lancet ii:820–821, 1956.
4. Pearce EN, Farwell AP, Braverman LE, et al: Thyroiditis, N Engl J Med 348:2646–2655, 2003.
5. Yoshida H, Amino N, Yagawa K, et al: Association of serum antithyroid antibodies with lymphocytic infiltration of the thyroid gland: Studies of seventy autopsied cases, J Clin Endocrinol Metab 46:859, 1978.
6. Vanderpump MPJ: The epidemiology of thyroid disease. In Braverman LE, Utiger RD, editors: Werner & Ingbar's The Thyroid A Fundamental and Clinical Text, ed 9, Philadelphia, 2005, Lippincott Williams & Wilkins, pp 398–406.
7. Lazarus JH: Sporadic and Postpartum thyroiditis. In Braverman LE, Utiger RD, editors: Werner & Ingbar's The Thyroid A Fundamental and Clinical Text, ed 9, Philadelphia, 2005, Lippincott Williams & Wilkins, pp 524–535.
8. Nossal GJ, Pike BL: Evidence for the clonal abortion theory of B-lymphocyte tolerance. 1975, J Immunol 179:5619–5632, 2007.
9. Volpe R, Iitaka M: Evidence for an antigen-specific defect in suppressor T-lymphocytes in autoimmune thyroid disease, Exp Clin Endocrinol 97:133–138, 1991.
10. Quaratino S, Badami E: Regulatory T cells and thyroid autoimmunity. In Wiersinga WM, Drexhage HA, Weetman AP, et al, editors: The Thyroid and Autoimmunity, Stuttgart Verlag, 2007, pp 74–81.
11. Bottazzo GF, Pujol-Borrell R, Hanafusa T, et al: Role of aberrant HLA-DR expression and antigen presentation in induction of endocrine autoimmunity, Lancet 2:1115–1119, 1983.
12. Krassas GE, Wiersinga WM: Smoking and autoimmune thyroid disease: the plot thickens, Eur J Endocrinol 154:777–780, 2006 Jun.
13. Rose NR, Bonita R, Burek CL: Iodine: an environmental trigger of thyroiditis, Autoimmun Rev 1:97–103, 2002.
14. Camargo R, Tomimori E, Neves S, et al: Thyroid and the environment: exposure to excessive nutritional iodine increases the prevalence of thyroid disorders in Sao Paulo, Brazil, Eur J Endocrinol 2008 Jun 27 in press.
15. Bartalena L, Tanda ML, Piantanida A, et al: Environment and thyroid autoimmunity. In Wiersinga WM, Drexhage HA, Weetman AP, et al, editors: The Thyroid and Autoimmunity, Stuttgart, 2007, Verlag, pp 60–73.
16. Martino E, Bartalena L, Bogazzi F, et al: The effects of amiodarone on the thyroid, Endocr Rev 22:240–254, 2001.
17. Lazarus JH: The effects of lithium therapy on thyroid and thyrotropin-releasing hormone, Thyroid 8:909–913, 1998.
18. Sharma RB, Burek CL, Cihakova D, et al: Environmental factors in autoimmune endocrinopathies. In Weetman AP, editor: Autoimmune Diseases in Endocrinology, Totowa, 2008, Humana Press, pp 35–75.
19. Chen F, Day SL, Metcalfe RA, et al: Characteristics of autoimmune thyroid disease occurring as a late complication of immune reconstitution in patients with advanced immunodeficiency virus (HIV) disease, Medicine 84:98–106, 2005.
20. Hoekman K, von Blomberg-von dar F, Wagstaff J, et al: Reversible thyroid dysfunction during treatment with GM-CSF, Lancet 338:541–542, 1991.
21. Eheman CR, Garbe P, Tuttle RM: Autoimmune thyroid disease associated with thyroid irradiation, Thyroid 13:453–464, 2003.
22. Mori K, Munakata Y, Saito T, et al: Intrathyroidal persistence of human parvovirus B19 DNA in a patient with Hashimoto's thyroiditis, J Infect 55:29–31, 2007.
23. Thomas D, Liakos V, Michou V, et al: Detection of herpes virus DNA in post-operative thyroid tissue specimens of patients with autoimmune thyroid disease, Exp Clin Endocrinol Diabetes 116:35–39, 2008.
24. Manji N, Carr-Smith JD, Boelaert K, et al: Influences of age, gender, smoking, and family history on autoimmune thyroid disease phenotype, J Clin Endocrinol Metab 91:4873–4880, 2006.
25. Jacobson EM, Tomer Y: The genetic basis of thyroid autoimmunity, Thyroid 17:949–961, 2007.
26. Lin WY, Wan L, Tsai CH, et al: Vitamin D receptor gene polymorphisms are associated with risk of Hashimoto's thyroiditis Chinese patients in Taiwan, J Clin Lab Anal 20:109–112, 2006.
27. Stefanic M, Papić S, Suver M, et al: Association of vitamin D receptor gene 3'-variants with Hashimoto's thyroiditis in the Croatian population, Int J Immunogenet 35:125–131, 2008.
28. Chen RH, Chang CT, Chen WC, et al: Proinflammatory cytokine gene polymorphisms among Hashimoto's thyroiditis patients, J Clin Lab Anal 20:260–265, 2006.
29. Ito C, Watanabe M, Okuda N, et al: Association between the severity of Hashimoto's disease and the functional +874A/T polymorphism in the interferon-gamma gene, Endocr J 53:473–478, 2006.
30. Ito M, Tanimoto M, Kamura H, et al: Association of HLA antigen and restriction fragment length polymorphism of T cell receptor beta-chain gene with Graves' disease and Hashimoto's thyroiditis, J Clin Endocrinol Metab 69:100–104, 1989.
31. Weetman AP, So AK, Roe C, et al: T-cell receptor alpha chain V region polymorphism linked to primary autoimmune hypothyroidism but not Graves' disease, Hum Immunol 20:167–173, 1987.
32. Zhang J, Zhang M, Wang Y: Infiltrating T-lymphocyte receptor V beta gene family utilization in autoimmune thyroid disease, J Int Med Res 34:585–595, 2006.
33. Tamai H, Uno H, Hirota Y, et al: Immunogenetics of Hashimoto's and Graves' diseases, J Clin Endocrinol Metab 60:62–66, 1985.
34. Kavvoura FK, Akamizu T, Awata TJ, et al: Cytotoxic T-lymphocyte associated antigen 4 gene polymorphisms and autoimmune thyroid disease: a meta-analysis, J Clin Endocrinol Metab 92:3162–3170, 2007.
35. Dallos T, Avbelj M, Barák L, et al: CTLA-4 gene polymorphisms predispose to autoimmune endocrinopathies but not to celiac disease, Neuro Endocrinol Lett 29:334–340, 2008.
36. Yin X, Latif R, Tomer Y, Davies TF: Thyroid epigenetics: X chromosome inactivation in patients with autoimmune thyroid disease, Ann N Y Acad Sci 1110:193–200, 2007.
37. Ludgate M: Animal models of autoimmune disease. In Weetman AP, editor: Autoimmune Diseases in Endocrinology, Totowa, 2008, Humana Press, pp 79–93.
38. Roitt IM, Campbell PN, Doniach D: The nature of the thyroid autoantibodies present in patients with Hashimoto's thyroiditis (lymphadenoid goitre), Biochem J 69:248–256, 1958.
39. Nye L, De Carvalho LP, Roitt IM: An investigation of the clonality of human autoimmune thyroglobulin antibodies and their light chains, Clin Exp Immunol 46:161–170, 1981.
40. Chan CT, Byfield PG, Himsworth RL, et al: Human autoantibodies to thyroglobulin are directed towards a restricted number of human specific epitopes, Clin Exp Immunol 69:516–523, 1987.
41. Kim PS, Dunn AD, Dunn JT: Altered immunoreactivity of thyroglobulin in thyroid disease, J Clin Endocrinol Metab 67:161–168, 1988.
42. McIntosh RS, Asghar MS, Weetman AP: The antibody response in human autoimmune thyroid disease, Clin Sci 92:529–541, 1997.
43. Parkes AB, McLachlan SM, Bird P, et al: The distribution of microsomal and thyroglobulin antibody activity among the IgG subclasses, Clin Exp Immunol 57:239–243, 1984.
44. Latrofa F, Ricci D, Grasso L, et al: Characterization of thyroglobulin epitopes in patients with autoimmune and non-autoimmune thyroid diseases using recombinant human monoclonal thyroglobulin autoantibodies, J Clin Endocrinol Metab 93:591–596, 2007.
45. Guilbert B, Dighiero G, Avrameas S: Naturally occurring antibodies against nine common antigens in human sera. I. Detection, isolation and characterization, J Immunol 128:2779–2787, 1982.
46. McLachlan SM, Rapoport B: Thyroid peroxidase as an autoantigen, Thyroid 17:939–948, 2007.
47. Khoury EL, Hammond L, Bottazzo GF, et al: Presence of the organ-specific "microsomal" autoantigen on the surface of human thyroid cells in culture: Its involvement in complement-mediated cytotoxicity, Clin Exp Immunol 45:316–328, 1981.
48. Potlukova E, Jiskra J, Limanova Z, et al: Autoantibodies against complement C1q correlate with the thyroid function in patients with autoimmune thyroid disease, Clin Exp Immunol 153(1):96–101, 2008 Jul.
49. Tandon N, Jayne DR, McGregor AM, et al: Analysis of anti-idiotypic antibodies against anti-microsomal antibodies in patients with thyroid autoimmunity, J Autoimmun 5:557–570, 1992.
50. Nielsen CH, Brix TH, Gardas A, et al: Epitope recognition patterns of thyroid peroxidase autoantibodies in healthy individuals and patients with Hashimoto's thyroiditis, Clin Endocrinol (Oxf) 2008 in press.
51. Tamaki H, Amino N, Aozasa M, et al: Effective method for prediction of transient hypothyroidism in neonates born to mothers with chronic thyroiditis, Am J Perinatol 6:296–303, 1989.
52. Konishi J, Iida Y, Kasagi K, et al: Primary myxedema with thyrotrophin-binding inhibitor immunoglobulins. Clinical and laboratory findings in 15 patients, Ann Intern Med 103:26–31, 1985.
53. Rees Smith B, Sanders J, Furmaniak J: TSH receptor antibodies, Thyroid 17:923–938, 2008.
54. Amino N, Watanabe Y, Tamaki H, et al: In-vitro conversion of blocking type anti-TSH receptor antibody to the stimulating type by anti-human IgG antibodies, Clin Endocrinol (Oxf) 27:615–624, 1987.
55. Endo T, Kogai T, Nakazato M, et al: Autoantibody against Na+/I-symporter in the sera of patients with autoimmune thyroid disease, Biochem Biophys Res Commun 224:92–95, 1996.
56. Staeheli V, Vallotton MB, Burger A: Detection of human anti-thyroxine and anti-triiodothyronine antibodies in different thyroid conditions, J Clin Endocrinol Metab 41:669–675, 1975.
57. John R, Othman S, Parkes AB, et al: Interference in thyroid function tests in postpartum thyroiditis, Clin Chem 37:1397–1400, 1991.
58. Sakata S, Takuno H, Nagai K, et al: Anti-bovine thyrotropin autoantibodies in patients with Hashimoto's thyroiditis, subacute thyroiditis, and systemic lupus erythematosus, J Endocrinol Invest 14:123–130, 1991.
59. Zakaria M, MacKenzie J: Do thyroid growth-promoting immunoglobulins exist? J Clin Endocrinol Metab 70:308–310, 1990.
60. DeGroot LJ, Quintans J: The causes of autoimmune thyroid disease, Endocr Rev 10:537–562, 1989.
61. Sawada K, Sakurami T, Imura H, et al: Anti-asialo-GM1 antibody in sera from patients with Graves' disease and Hashimoto's thyroiditis, Lancet 2:198, 1980.
62. Jasani B, Parkes AB, Lazarus JH: Natural antibody status in patients with Hashimoto's thyroiditis, J Clin Lab Immunol 51:9–20, 1999.
63. McLachlan SM, Nagayama Y, Pichurin PN, et al: The link between Graves' disease and Hashimoto's thyroiditis: a role for regulatory T cells, Endocrinology 148:5724–5733, 2007.
64. Battifora M, Pesce G, Paolieri F, et al: B7.1 costimulatory molecule is expressed on thyroid follicular cells in Hashimoto's thyroiditis, but not in Graves' disease, J Clin Endocrinol Metab 83:4130–4139, 1998.
65. Weetman AP, Freeman M, Borysiewicz LK, et al: Functional analysis of intercellular adhesion molecule-1-expressing human thyroid cells, Eur J Immunol 20:271–275, 1990.
66. Davies TF, Martin A, Concepcion ES, et al: Evidence of limited variability of antigen receptors on intrathyroidal T cells in autoimmune thyroid disease [see comments], N Engl J Med 325:238–244, 1991.
67. McIntosh RS, Tandon N, Pickerill AP, et al: IL-2 receptor-positive intrathyroidal lymphocytes in Graves' disease. Ananlysis of V alpha transcript microheterogeneity, J Immunol 151:3884–3893, 1993.
68. Nagataki S, Eguchi K: Cytokines and immune regulation in thyroid autoimmunity, Autoimmunity 13:27–34, 1992.
69. Atkins MB, Mier JW, Parkinson DR: Hypothyroidism after treatment with interleukin-2 and lymphokine-

activated killer cells, N Engl J Med 16(318):1557–1563, 1988.

70. Nagayama Y, Ohta K, Tsuruta M, et al: Exacerbation of thyroid autoimmunity by interferon alpha treatment in patients with chronic viral hepatitis: Our studies and review of the literature, Endocr J 41:565–572, 1994.

71. Nielsen CH, Hegedüs L, Rieneck K, et al: Production of interleukin (IL)-5 and IL-10 accompanies T helper cell type 1 (Th1) cytokine responses to a major thyroid self-antigen, thyroglobulin, in health and autoimmune thyroid disease, Clin Exp Immunol 147:287–295, 2007.

72. Saverino D, Brizzolara R, Simone R, et al: Soluble CTLA-4 in autoimmune thyroid diseases: relationship with clinical status and possible role in the immune response dysregulation, Clin Immunol 123:190–198, 2007.

73. Marinkovic T, Garin A, Yokota Y, et al: Interaction of mature CD3+CD4+ T cells with dendritic cells triggers the development of tertiary lymphoid structures in the thyroid, J Clin Invest 116:2622–2632, 2006.

74. Wang SH, Baker JR: The role of apoptosis in thyroid autoimmunity, Thyroid 17:975–979, 2007.

75. Itoh N, Yonehara S, Ishii A, et al: The polypeptide encoded by the cDNA for human cell surface antigen Fas can mediate apoptosis, Cell 66:233–243, 1991.

76. Giordano C, Stassi G, De Maria R, et al: Potential involvement of Fas and its ligand in the pathogenesis of Hashimoto's thyroiditis, Science 275:960–963, 1997.

77. Shimaoka Y, Hidaka Y, Okumura M, et al: Serum concentration of soluble Fas in patients with autoimmune thyroid diseases, Thyroid 8:43–47, 1998.

78. Kawakami A, Eguchi K, Matsuoka N, et al: Thyroid-stimulating hormone inhibits Fas antigen-mediated apoptosis of human thyrocytes in vitro, Endocrinology 137:3163–3169, 1996.

79. Bossowski A, Czarnocka B, Bardadin K, et al: Identification of apoptotic proteins in thyroid gland from patients with Graves' disease and Hashimoto's thyroiditis, Autoimmunity 41:163–173, 2008,

80. Myśliwiec J, Okota M, Nikołajuk A, et al: Soluble Fas, Fas ligand and Bcl-2 in autoimmune thyroid diseases: relation to humoral immune response markers, Adv Med Sci 51:119–122, 2006.

81. Mysliwiec J, Oklota M, Nikolajuk A, et al: Serum CD40/CD40L system in Graves' disease and Hashimoto's thyroiditis related to soluble Fas, FasL and humoral markers of autoimmune response, J Immunol Invest 36:247–257, 2007.

82. Batteux F, Lores P, Bucchini D, et al: Transgenic expression of Fas ligand on thyroid follicular cells prevents autoimmune thyroiditis, J Immunol 164:1681–1688, 2000.

83. Dong Z, Takakuwa T, Takayama H, et al: Fas and Fas ligand gene mutations in Hashimoto's thyroiditis, Lab Invest 82:1611–1616, 2002.

84. Takakuwa T, Dong Z, Takayama H, et al: Frequent mutations of Fas gene in thyroid lymphoma, Cancer Res 61:1382–1385, 2001.

85. Marazuela M, García-López MA, Figueroa-Vega N, et al: Regulatory T cells in human autoimmune thyroid disease, J Clin Endocrinol Metab 91:3639–3646, 2006.

86. Tandon N, Morgan BP, Weetman AP: Expression and function of multiple regulators of complement activation in autoimmune thyroid disease, Immunology 81:643–647, 1994.

87. Lazarus JH, Burr ML, McGregor AM, et al: The prevalence and progression of autimmune thyroid disease in the elderly, Acta Endocrinol 106:199–202, 1984.

88. Weetman AP: The thyroid and autoimmunity in children and adolescents. In Krassas GE, Rivkees SA, Kiess W, editors: Diseases of the Thyroid in Childhood and Adolescence, Basel, 2007, Karger, pp 104–117.

89. Jaruratanasirikul S, Leethanaporn K, Khuntigij P, et al: The clinical course of Hashimoto's thryoiditis in children and adolescents: 6 years longitudinal follow-up, J Pediatr Endocrinol Metab 14:177–184, 2001.

90. Radetti G, Gottardi E, Bona G, et al: The natural history of euthyroid Hashimoto's thyroiditis in children. Study Group for Thyroid Diseases of the Italian Society for Pediatric Endocrinology and Diabetes, J Pediatr 149:827–832, 2006.

91. Wang SY, Tung YC, Tsai WY, et al: Long-term outcome of hormonal status in Taiwanese children with Hashimoto's thyroiditis, Eur J Pediatr 165:481–483, 2006.

92. Woolf PD: Transient painless thyroiditis with hyperthyroidism: a variant of lymphocytic thyroiditis, Endocr Rev 4:411–420, 1980.

93. Nikolai TF, Coombs GJ, McKenzie AK: Lymphocytic thyroiditis with spontaneously resolving hyperthyroidism and subacute thyroiditis: Long-term follow-up, Arch Intern Med 141:1455–1458, 1981.

94. Yamamoto M, Shibuya N, Chen LC, et al: Seasonal recurrence of transient hypothyroidism in a patient with autoimmune thyroiditis, Endocrinol Jpn 35:135–142, 1988.

95. Tachi J, Amino N, Miyai K: Massage therapy on neck: A contributing factor for destructive thyrotoxicosis? Thyroidology 2:25–27, 1990.

96. Roberton HEW: Lassitude, coldness, and hair changes following pregnancy, and their response to treatment with thyroid extract, Brit Med J 2:93–94, 1948.

97. Lazarus JH, Premawardhana LDKE: Postpartum Thyroiditis. In Weetman AP, editor: Contemporary Endocrinology: Autoimmune Diseases in Endocrinology, New Jersey, USA, 2008, Humana Press Inc., pp 177–192.

98. Muller AF, Drexhage HA, Berghout A: Postpartum thyroiditis and autoimmune thyroiditis in women of childbearing age: recent insights and consequences for antenatal and postnatal care, Endocr Rev 22:605–630, 2001.

99. Mizukami Y, Michigishi T, Nonomura A, et al: Postpartum thyroiditis. A clinical, histologic, and immunopathologic study of 15 cases, Am J Clin Pathol 100:200–205, 1993.

100. Wood LC, Ingbar SH: Hypothyroidism as a late sequela in patient with Graves' disease treated with antithyroid agents, J Clin Invest 64:1429–1436, 1979.

101. Macchia E, Concetti R, Carone G, et al: Demonstration of blocking immunoglobulins G, having a heterogeneous behaviour, in sera of patients with Graves' disease: Possible coexistence of different autoantibodies directed to the TSH receptor, Clin Endocrinol 28:147–156, 1988.

102. Gavras I, Thomson J: Late thyrotoxicosis complicating autoimmune thyroiditis, Acta Endocrinol 69:41–46, 1972.

103. Karsh J, Pavlidis N, Weintraub BD, et al: Thyroid disease in Sjogren's syndrome, Arthritis Rheum 23:1326–1329, 1980.

104. Hadithi M, de Boer H, Meijer JW, et al: Coeliac disease in Dutch patients with Hashimoto's thyroiditis and vice versa, World J Gastroenterol 13:1715–1722, 2007.

105. Sibilla R, Santaguida MG, Virili C, et al: Chronic unexplained anaemia in isolated autoimmune thyroid disease or associated with autoimmune related disorders, Clin Endocrinol 68:640–645, 2008.

106. Ness-Abramof R, Nabriski DA, Braverman LE, et al: Prevalence and evaluation of B12 deficiency in patients with autoimmune thyroid disease, Am J Med Sci 33:119–122, 2006.

107. Mocellin R, Walterfang M, Velakoulis D: Hashimoto's encephalopathy: epidemiology, pathogenesis and management, CNS Drugs 21:799–811, 2007.

108. Peschen-Rosin R, Schabet M, Dichgans J: Manifestation of Hashimoto's encephalopathy years before onset of thyroid disease, Eur Neurol 41:79–84, 1999.

109. Brain L, Jellinek EH, Ball K: Hashimoto's disease and encephalopathy, Lancet 2:512–514, 1966.

110. Pozo-Rosich P, Villoslada P, Canton A, et al: Reversible white matter alterations in encephalopathy associated with autoimmune thyroid disease, J Neurol 249:1063–1065, 2002.

111. Gayatri NA, Whitehouse WP: Pilot survey of Hashimoto's encephalopathy in children, Dev Med Child Neurol 47:556–558, 2005.

112. Canton A, de Fabregas O, Tintore M, et al: Encephalopathy associated to autoimmune thyroid disease: A more appropriate term for an underestimated condition? J Neurol Sci 176:65–69, 2000.

113. Ochi H, Horiuchi I, Araki N, et al: Proteomic analysis of human brain identifies fienolase as a nobel autoantigen in Hashimoto's encephalopathy, FEBS Lett 528:197–202, 2002.

114. Yoneda M, Fujii A, Ito A: High prevalence of serum autoantibodies against the amino terminal of alpha-enolase in Hashimoto's encephalopathy, J Neuroimmunol 185:195–200, 2007.

115. Sawka AM, Fatourechi V, Boeve BF, et al: Rarity of encephalopathy associated with autoimmune thyroiditis: A case series from Mayo Clinic from 1950 to 1996, Thyroid 12:393–398, 2002.

116. Blanchin S, Coffin C, Viader F, et al: Anti-thyroperoxidase antibodies from patients with Hashimoto's encephalopathy bind to cerebellar astrocytes, J Neuroimmunol 192:13–20, 2007.

117. Gini B, Laura L, Riccardo C, et al: Novel autoantigens recognised by CSF IgG from Hashimoto's encephalitis revealed by a proteomic approach, J neuroimmunol 196:153–158, 2008.

118. Moshynska OV, Saxena A: Clonal relationship between Hashimoto thyroiditis and thyroid lymphoma, J Clin Pathol 61:438–444, 2008.

119. Cipolla C, Sandonato L, Graceffa G, et al: Hashimoto thyroiditis coexistent with papillary thyroid carcinoma, Am Surg 71:874–878, 2005.

120. Larson SD, Jackson LN, Riall TS, et al: Increased incidence of well-differentiated thyroid cancer associated with Hashimoto thyroiditis and the role of the PI3k/Akt pathway, J Am Coll Surg 204:764–773, 2007.

121. Rhoden KJ, Unger K, Salvatore G, et al: RET/papillary thyroid cancer rearrangement in nonneoplastic thyrocytes: follicular cells of Hashimoto's thyroiditis share low-level recombination events with a subset of papillary carcinoma, J Clin Endocrinol Metab 91:2414–2423, 2006.

122. Kang DY, Kim KH, Kim JM, et al: High prevalence of RET, RAS, and ERK expression in Hashimoto's thyroiditis and in papillary thyroid carcinoma in the Korean population, Thyroid 17:1031–1038, 2007.

123. Tamaki H, Amino N, Kimura M, et al: Low prevalence of thyrotropin receptor antibody in primary hypothyroidism in Japan, J Clin Endocrinol Metab 71:1382–1386, 1990.

124. Yoshinari M, Okamura K, Tokuyama T, et al: Clinical importance of reversibility in primary goitrous hypothyroidism, Br Med J 287:720–722, 1983.

125. Sato K, Okamura K, Ikenoue H, et al: TSH dependent elevation of serum thyroglobulin in reversible primary hypothyroidism, Clin Endocrinol 29:231–237, 1988.

126. Takasu N, Komiya I, Asawa T, et al: Test for recovery from hypothyroidism during thyroxine therapy in Hashimoto's thyroiditis, Lancet 336:1084–1086, 1990.

127. Tajiri J, Higashi K, Morita M, et al: Studies of hypothyroidism in patients with high iodine intake, J Clin Endocrinol Metab 63:412–417, 1986.

128. Wirtzfeld DA, Winston JS, Hicks WL Jr, et al: Clinical presentation and treatment of non-Hodgkin's lymphoma of the thyroid gland, Ann Surg Oncol 8:338–341, 2001.

129. Aksoy DY, Kerimoglu U, Okur H, et al: Effects of prophylactic thyroid hormone replacement in euthyroid Hashimoto's thyroiditis, Endocr J 52:337–343, 2005.

130. Mazokopakis EE, Papadakis JA, Papadomanolaki MG, et al: Effects of 12 months treatment with L-selenomethionine on serum anti-TPO Levels in Patients with Hashimoto's thyroiditis, Thyroid 17:609–612, 2007.

131. Tajiri J: Radioactive iodine therapy for goitrous Hashimoto's thyroiditis, J Clin Endocrinol Metab 91:4497–4500, 2006.

Chapter 13

SUBACUTE AND RIEDEL'S THYROIDITIS

VALÉRIA C. GUIMARÃES

Subacute Thyroiditis

BACKGROUND AND DEFINITION

The term *subacute thyroiditis* (SAT) describes a self-limited inflammatory disorder and the most common cause of thyroid pain, probably of viral origin.[1-5] It was first reported by Mygind[6] in 1895, who described 18 cases of "thyroiditis akuta simplex." The name *De Quervain* traditionally has been associated with this condition, however, probably because he described the pathology of this disorder thoroughly in 1904[7] and again in 1936.[8] SAT occurs in 5% of patients with clinical thyroid disease[9] and frequently follows an upper respiratory tract infection. Its incidence correlates with the peak incidence of enterovirus.[10] Other viruses, such as Epstein-Barr virus and cytomegalovirus, also have been reported, but so far clear evidence for a viral cause is still lacking.[11] There is a strong preponderance of women over men with this condition.[1]

SAT has a multiplicity of synonyms, some reflecting misconceptions regarding the etiology or pathology of the condition. These include De Quervain's thyroiditis, viral thyroiditis, granulomatous thyroiditis, acute or subacute diffuse thyroiditis, acute simple thyroiditis, noninfectious thyroiditis, struma granulomatosa, pseudogranulomatous thyroiditis, giant cell thyroiditis, pseudo–giant cell thyroiditis, migratory "creeping" thyroiditis, and pseudotuberculous thyroiditis. The term *subacute thyroiditis* connotes a temporal quality that might apply to any inflammatory process of intermediate severity and duration. As the term is generally employed, however, it specifically includes only patients showing a pseudogranulomatous pathologic appearance in the thyroid gland (which is virtually specific for the disease) and a characteristic clinical syndrome in which the painful tender goiter also is associated with considerable malaise, fever, and evidence of thyroid dysfunction (described more fully later).[1-5] It generally is distinguishable from a similar disorder, painless or silent thyroiditis, which disturbs thyroid function in a manner similar to SAT but without pain or tenderness and with a different pathologic appearance.

INCIDENCE

Few epidemiologic studies of SAT have been reported.[10,14-22] Compared with other thyroid diseases, SAT is uncommon, occurring at the rate of about 1 case per 5 cases of Graves' disease and 1 case per 15 or 20 cases of Hashimoto's thyroiditis.[19] Although the cause is most likely viral, SAT, similar to all other thyroid conditions, occurs most commonly in women who are 40 to 50 years old. The reported female-to-male ratio is 3 to 6 : 1.[19] it has been noted as a rare cause of hyperthyroidism in pregnancy.[20] It is rare in children and seems to occur in any season of the year,[10,22] with a trend toward more cases in fall and spring.[22] Familial or geographic aggregation of cases is seldom noted. SAT has been reported most commonly from the temperate zone, having been observed in North America, Europe, and Japan. Recently, a few cases were reported in Western Saudi Arabia,[21] although it is rarely reported from many other parts of the world. Associated autoimmune conditions do not seem more common than autoimmune conditions observed in the general population.[22]

Although complete recovery is the rule, recurrence after several years has been reported.[24-27] In one study, four recurrent episodes of SAT occurred in 3 of 222 patients (1.4%). The recurrent episodes were similar to the first episodes of SAT.[27] In a larger study that evaluated data for 3344 patients with SAT between 1970 and 1993, SAT recurred in 48 of 3344 patients (1.4%) (mean 14.5 ± 4.5 years after the first episode). Five patients experienced a third episode (mean 7.6 ± 2.4 years after the second episode).[27] Another cohort study showed a 4% recurrence rate after many years.[22] Theoretically, late recurrence possibly occurs after the disappearance of immunity to the previous viral infection. During an evaluation of subtypes of hypothyroidism over a 4-year period in Denmark, an incidence of subacute thyroiditis of 1.8% was found in a cohort of 685 patients with hypothyroidism.[28]

ETIOLOGY

In 1952, Fraser and Harrison[29] were the first to propose that SAT represents a viral infection of the thyroid gland. Since then, considerable indirect evidence suggests that SAT is most likely the result of a viral infection[30-32] that rarely recurs after a complete recovery, possibly because of immunity to the offending virus.

Clinically, the disease has several characteristics typical of viral infections, including a typical prodrome with myalgias, malaise, and fatigue; absence of leukocytosis; and usually a self-limited course.[1-5] Additionally, clusters of the disease have been reported during outbreaks of viral infection.[1-5,10] It has been described in association with mumps, measles,[1] influenza,[1] the common cold,[1] adenovirus,[1] infectious mononucleosis,[1,12] coxsackievirus,[1] myocarditis,[1] cat-scratch fever,[1] St. Louis encephalitis,[1] hepatitis A,[18] parvovirus B19 infection,[19] and cytomegalovirus infection.[11,13]

In an extensive study reported by Volpé and colleagues,[33] 32 of 71 patients with SAT, who had no evidence of specific viral disease, showed at least fourfold increases in viral antibodies during the thyroid illness. These viral antibodies included antibodies to coxsackievirus, adenovirus, influenza virus, and mumps virus. Coxsackievirus antibodies were found most commonly, and the changes in their titers most closely approximated the course of the disease. In a later study of 10 patients in Singapore, no such antibodies were observed, however.[34] It is possible that the presence of these antibodies may not reflect pathogenic significance, but instead may result from an anamnestic response to the inflammatory thyroid lesion. The thyroid responds with the clinical picture of thyroiditis after invasion by a variety of viruses, and a variety of agents may be causative in the syndrome of SAT.

Certain nonviral infections, such as malaria and Q fever, have been associated with a clinical syndrome that at least simulates SAT.[1] The significance of these observations remains to be determined. In addition, a case of SAT occurring simultaneously with giant cell arteritis has been reported.[35] Several cases of SAT that developed during interferon-α treatment for hepatitis C have been described,[36-38] and more recently, a case of SAT that developed after long-term immunosuppression and lithium therapy following an allogeneic bone marrow transplant was reported.[39]

Several autoimmune phenomena have been described in SAT. Thyroid autoantibodies (antithyroglobulin and antithyroid peroxidase antibodies) have been found in 42% to 64% of patients with SAT.[33] In most of these patients, the antibody titer gradually decreased and remained low or disappeared as the disease faded. Thyroid-stimulating hormone (TSH) receptor antibodies also have been reported in patients with SAT,[40-42] although changes in antibody titer did not correlate with disease activity.[40] Auto-

antibodies to several novel, uncharacterized thyroid antigenic determinants were found in eight of nine patients with SAT tested.[43] These autoantibodies persisted, and their level did not decrease over 39 months after onset of SAT. These antibodies likely arise secondary to the damage caused by viral infection of the thyroid gland because they are typically polyclonal in nature.[43]

There is evidence that T-cell-mediated immunity against thyroid antigens may play a role in the pathogenesis of SAT. During the initial phase of the disease, the gland is infiltrated by T cells, and sensitization of T cells against thyroid antigens has been shown in such patients.[44-46] This sensitization was transitory, however, and likely represented a secondary immune response to the inflammatory release of antigen induced by the viral infection of the gland.[1]

It has been suggested that thyroid-destructive events in the course of SAT may trigger, under a genetic background, thyroid autoimmune disease of various kinds.[47,48] Patients with a previous history of SAT, in about 1% of cases,[2] may develop hypothyroidism as a consequence of previous thyroid damage. The occurrence of Graves' disease after SAT also has been described, although such evidence seems to be extremely rare, with fewer than 20 cases reported in the literature.[49-53]

Infectious agents may induce thyroid autoimmunity by a variety of diverse mechanisms, such as inducing modifications of self-antigens, mimicking self-molecules, inducing polyclonal T-cell activation (e.g., by superantigens), altering the idiotypic network, forming immune complexes, and inducing expression of major histocompatibility complex (MHC) molecules on thyroid epithelial cells. Although indirect data suggesting involvement of the infecting organisms in the pathogenesis of human autoimmune thyroid disease are abundant, only a few studies have employed direct approaches. Such a direct approach would involve isolation or molecular identification of the potentially infecting organisms from the thyroid gland and the subsequent induction of autoimmune thyroid disease in an experimental model.

Although SAT is shown to be associated with thyroid autoimmune phenomena, after recovery all immunologic phenomena should disappear. This is in contrast to the continuing presence of these abnormalities in autoimmune thyroid disease.[54] The transitory immunologic markers observed during the course of SAT seem to be secondary to the release of antigenic material from the thyroid and seem to be a normal, physiologic response to the inflammatory destruction of the gland.[55]

In light of the previous observations, the lack of any direct evidence, and because it is rare for SAT to progress to either Graves' disease or Hashimoto's disease, the corollary is still consistent with the view that antigen-driven events can produce a transient immunologic disturbance, but does not, or is most unlikely to, culminate in chronic autoimmune thyroid disease. It is possible that the illness of SAT might act as a nonspecific stress acting on the immune system to precipitate Graves' disease in a favorable genetic background.[54]

An association between SAT and HLABw35 has been noted in all ethnic groups tested.[56-59] This haplotype seems to confer an unusual susceptibility to SAT, perhaps because it allows one or more viruses to trigger an immune response directed against thyroid tissue.[60] Histocompatibility studies show that 72% of patients with subacute thyroiditis manifest HLA-Bw35.[57-60] Familial occurrence of subacute thyroiditis associated with HLA-B35 has been reported.[61,62] Another HLABw67 was found in 87% of a Japanese population and correlated with a seasonal appearance and a mild course of disease. Thus the susceptibility to subacute thyroiditis is genetically influenced, and it has also been suggested that subacute thyroiditis might occur by transmission of viral infection in genetically predisposed individuals.[13]

CLINICAL FEATURES

Half of patients have a history of an antecedent of upper respiratory infection, followed in days or weeks by the clinical manifestations of SAT itself.[1-5,22,63] SAT begins with a prodrome of generalized myalgias, pharyngitis, low-grade fever, and fatigue. The patient notes pain of varying degrees in the region of the thyroid gland. This pain may involve one lobe, part of a lobe, or the whole thyroid, and it typically radiates from the thyroid gland to the angle of the jaw and to the ear of the affected side. If not bilateral initially, the pain and tenderness often spread to the uninvolved side of the thyroid within days or weeks. It also may radiate to the anterior chest or may be centered only over the thyroid. Moving the head, swallowing, or coughing may aggravate it. Transient vocal cord paresis may occur.[23]

In a few patients, pain is entirely lacking. Although patients without pain often may be categorized as having "silent thyroiditis," surgical thyroidectomy or biopsy has shown the typical granulomatous picture in some of these specimens. Similarly, tenderness may be moderate or severe or, conversely, may be lacking. Some patients notice swelling in the neck. Although the symptoms may be limited to the head and neck, most patients also have systemic symptoms, including malaise, myalgia with or without arthralgia, mild feverishness, and anorexia. These reactions may be minimal or severe, and fever may reach 40°C (104°F).

Symptoms of mild to moderate hyperthyroidism occur in the early phase in most patients.[22] Fifty percent of patients have symptoms of thyrotoxicosis, and the usual symptoms of nervousness, tremulousness, weight loss, heat intolerance, and tachycardia predominate.[1-5,63-66] On physical examination, most patients appear uncomfortable and flushed, with variable fever. The thyroid gland may be only slightly to moderately enlarged, with one lobe larger than the other. The consistency of the involved area is usually firm or hard. With time or treatment, the thyroid tenderness subsides, and the goiter generally disappears within several weeks or months. Signs of mild to moderate hyperthyroidism are present in 50% of cases. About 8% to 16% of patients with this condition are noted to have a preexisting goiter. Cervical lymphadenopathy is rare.

In most patients, SAT lasts 2 to 4 months, although it may last 1 year. When the course is prolonged, the major manifestation is persistent, painful, tender thyroid enlargement, the thyrotoxicosis almost always having subsided earlier. Recurrences after recovery have been reported but are unusual, on the order of 2.3% per year[26] or 4% over 21 years after the first episode.[22]

Sometimes hyperthyroidism may not be apparent clinically but can be detected by biochemical means.[64] This situation is due to a disruptive process within the thyroid gland, with continuous leakage of the colloid into the interstitial spaces, where it is broken down into its component parts, liberating thyroid hormones, thyroglobulin, and other iodoamino acids into the circulation.[26,64-74] Because the thyroid cells during this phase are virtually incapable of producing new thyroid hormone, the colloid that has been stored within the follicles is depleted within 2 to 3 months, resulting in a phase of transient hypothyroidism in patients in whom the process has persisted over the interval.[75] Because disruption of the thyroid parenchyma can continue for

months, hypothyroidism may persist for several weeks. As recovery continues, the follicles regenerate, the colloid is repleted, and normal thyroid function is restored. With recovery, the thyroid is reconstituted, repleted with colloid; thyroid function is restored; and a variable amount of interstitial fibrosis persists.[1-5,64-75] This transient hypothyroidism may be subclinical or overt and occurs in about two thirds of patients.

SAT rarely progresses to permanent hypothyroidism.[1-5,75,76] In these cases, progression may be due to total destruction of the thyroid, with consequent fibrosis. As mentioned before, in rare instances, the disorder may seem to culminate in autoimmune thyroiditis after recovery from SAT.[48,51,53]

DIAGNOSIS

The typical painful SAT usually is obvious when the patient is first seen and should present no difficulties in diagnosis for the endocrinologist.[67,68] In patients who have only a sore throat or ear pain, however, the diagnosis is less obvious, and many patients are initially misdiagnosed with pharyngitis.[64] It is important that the thyroid gland be palpated carefully in patients presenting with upper respiratory infections or complaints of sore neck or throat or earache.

Eventually, patients with Hashimoto's thyroiditis and a few with silent thyroiditis may present with a painful, tender thyroid enlargement that is indistinguishable from SAT.[54] The radioactive iodine uptake is rarely as completely suppressed in Hashimoto's thyroiditis as it is in SAT, and the titers of thyroid autoantibodies are usually high enough to suggest lymphocytic thyroiditis. Acute suppurative thyroiditis initially may mimic SAT, but with time, the findings of fever, more localized tenderness and swelling, and erythema over the involved area of the thyroid should become obvious. A rapidly growing anaplastic carcinoma[77] of the thyroid or hemorrhage into a thyroid nodule can cause thyroid pain and tenderness. In anaplastic carcinomas, the lesion is usually obvious by virtue of its large size, adherence to adjacent structures, lymphadenopathy, and characteristic progressive course. Hemorrhage into a thyroid nodule presents with a localized nature, and the obvious nodule usually leads to the correct diagnosis.

The hallmark of SAT is a markedly elevated erythrocyte sedimentation rate. The serum thyroglobulin and C-reactive protein concentration are similarly elevated.[78] The leukocyte count is normal or slightly elevated. Peripheral blood thyroid hormone concentrations are elevated, with ratios of thyroxine (T_4) to triiodothyronine (T_3) of less than 20, reflecting the proportions of stored hormone within the thyroid,[79] and serum concentrations of thyrotropin are low or undetectable. Serum thyroid peroxidase antibody concentrations are usually normal. The 24-hour radioactive iodine uptake is low (<5%) in the toxic phase of SAT, distinguishing this disease from Graves' disease. Color-flow Doppler ultrasonography also may help to make this distinction; in patients with Graves' disease, the thyroid gland is hypervascular, whereas in patients with painful SAT, the gland is hypoechogenic and has low to normal vascularity.[80]

Fine-needle aspiration biopsy may be useful, but it may show large numbers of histiocytes and be misleading. Occasionally, a large-needle biopsy or a small, open surgical biopsy of the thyroid may be necessary to establish a definite diagnosis.

During the recovery of hypothyroid phases, thyroid test results may be confusing, and a diagnosis of permanent hypothyroidism may be made erroneously unless the history of the earlier stages of the disease is obtained. SAT occasionally presents as a fever of unknown origin with no or minimal thyroid-specific symptoms and has been detected by thallium isotope scanning.

LABORATORY AND IMAGING FINDINGS

Inflammatory Phase

Dynamic changes in thyroid function studies occur with the onset of thyroid inflammation (Fig. 13-1). The destruction of the thyroid follicles results in release and breakdown of the colloid into the interstitial tissue and into the circulation of iodinated materials—protein, proteases, peptides, and amino acids. An increase in serum T_4, T_3, and thyroglobulin and in urinary iodine results.[1-5,64,74]

The increase in serum T_4 and T_3 accounts for the manifestations of hyperthyroidism. In contrast to Graves' disease, in which serum T_3 is usually disproportionately elevated compared with

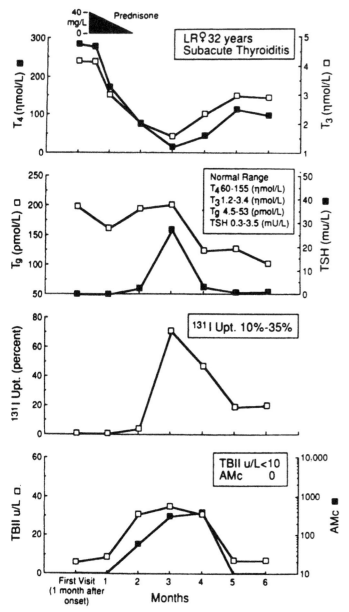

FIGURE 13-1. Salient laboratory features during the course of subacute thyroiditis. *AMc*, Antimicrosomal (antithyroperoxidase) antibody; T_4, thyroxine; T_3, triiodothyronine; *TBII*, thyrotropin-binding inhibitory immunoglobulin; *Tg*, thyroglobulin.

serum T_4, in SAT, the increased serum T_3 is only proportionate to the amount of T_4 released into the circulation. This difference may account for the mildness of the clinical manifestations of hyperthyroidism in SAT because the severity of the clinical manifestations of Graves' disease relates closely to levels of circulating T_3.

In addition, iodoproteins, such as thyroglobulin and iodoalbumin, are discharged from the gland into the circulation.[69] Plasma thyroglobulin may remain elevated long after all other evidence of the inflammatory process has subsided.[71] The decline in plasma T_4 is exponential during the first week, and this phase of hyperthyroidism can continue only until the gland is depleted of its preformed colloid.[73] TSH is usually undetectable in the hyperthyroid phase,[72,73] and the TSH response to thyrotropin-releasing hormone, as expected, is diminished at this time.[81,82]

At the same time, the damage to the thyroid follicular cells results in impaired iodine transport; the 24-hour radioactive iodine uptake is characteristically suppressed to 0% to 1%, revealing a patchy and irregular distribution of the tracer.[1-5,64,69,83,84] Even if only part of the gland is involved, the uptake may be similarly depressed as a result of suppression of pituitary TSH owing to the elevated levels of thyroid hormone.[72,73] Increased perfusion is shown in studies with technetium-99m sestamibi during the acute stage of SAT. This increased uptake in the thyroid region suggests the inflammatory phase of this disease.[85] SAT is one of the hyperthyroid conditions associated with high levels of thyroid hormones but a low radioactive iodine uptake, and such observations are characteristic in the early phase of this disorder. Under these circumstances, only minimal thyroid hormone biosynthesis is sustained, and what is produced leaks out.[69]

Evidently, thyroid cell damage reduces the ability of the gland to respond to TSH so that large doses of TSH generally do not cause a rise in the radioactive iodine uptake except when some parts of the gland are uninvolved.[82] This lack of response to exogenous TSH administration persists during the first weeks of the disease, reflecting continuing thyroid cell impairment and failure of the iodide-concentrating mechanism. Also, the administration of perchlorate or thiocyanate generally does not cause release of excessive amounts of iodine from the gland.[74]

The erythrocyte sedimentation rate is characteristically elevated (often >100 mm/h) in SAT.[1-5,86] If the test is normal or only slightly elevated, the diagnosis of SAT should be suspected. The leukocyte count is normal in about half of patients and elevated in the remainder[1-5,8,86] and has been reported as high as 18 × 10^9/L. The leukocyte counts correlate with serum concentrations of granulocyte colony-stimulating factor.[87] There may be a mild normochromic anemia, and an increase in α_2-globulin frequently is seen as a nonspecific inflammatory response.[88] Alkaline phosphatase and other hepatic enzymes may be elevated in the early phase.[89] It has been suggested that SAT actually represents a multisystem disease also affecting the thyroid gland.[90] There also are increases in serum ferritin,[94] soluble intercellular adhesion molecule-1,[95] selectin,[96] and interleukin-6[97] levels during the inflammatory phase.

Ultrasound examinations show hypoechoic focal areas and can be used for guided fine-needle cytology.[84-103] Magnetic resonance imaging of the thyroid also can help distinguish SAT from Graves' disease during the hyperthyroid phase. The ADC values obtained from the diffusion-weighted images of the patients with Graves' disease are significantly higher than the values of patients with SAT.[104]

Recovery Phase

As the process subsides, the serum T_4, T_3, and thyroglobulin levels decline, but the serum TSH level remains suppressed. The normal concentrations of sex hormone–binding globulin in the hyperthyroid phase probably reflect the short duration of exposure to increased thyroid hormone.[105]

Later, during the recovery phase, the radioiodine uptake becomes elevated with the resumption of the ability of the thyroid gland to concentrate iodide. The serum T_4 concentration may fall below normal; the TSH level may become elevated. Usually, after several weeks or months, all the parameters of thyroid function return to normal. Restoration of iodine stores seems to be much slower and may take more than 1 year after the complete clinical remission.[106,107] Ultimate recovery is the general rule. An occasional patient remains permanently hypothyroid.

Tests of thyroid antibodies are positive in a few cases; these develop several weeks after the onset and tend to decline and disappear thereafter.[33,108] An antibody against an unpurified thyroid antigen persists for years, however, after clinical features have subsided.[43] Also, as mentioned before, antibodies to the TSH receptor, either of the stimulating or of the blocking variety, may appear transiently without relationship to the thyroid functional state.[40-42] In about 2% of patients, SAT may trigger autoreactive B cells to produce TSH receptor antibodies, resulting in TSH antibody–associated dysfunction.[109]

PATHOLOGY

Although it has been reported that SAT may be associated with viral infection, the mechanisms of the destruction and regeneration of thyroid follicles have not been fully elucidated.

Macroscopically, an enlarged thyroid gland is found and is edematous. It may be slightly adherent to adjacent structures, although it can be freed from these without difficulty.

From histologic examination, the process may be diffuse or irregular in its involvement, with various stages of the disease sometimes found within the same specimen.[110] Initially, there is extensive follicular cell destruction, extravasation of colloid, and infiltration of lymphocytes and histiocytes. The lymphocytes and histiocytes tend to congregate around masses of colloid and coalesce into giant cells. With time, there is a variable degree of fibrosis, and areas of follicular regeneration are seen. After recovery, the thyroid appears normal except for minimal residual fibrosis.

The follicular cells sometimes virtually disappear, leaving a fine follicular lining. The initial phase is characterized by the appearance of neutrophils, followed by large mononuclear cells and lymphocytes (Fig. 13-2). The follicles appear much larger than normal, with disruption of the epithelial lining and hyperplasia of the surviving follicular cells. Histiocytes congregate around masses of colloid within the follicles and in the interstitial tissues, producing "giant cells." Because often these giant cells actually consist of masses of colloid surrounded by large numbers of individual histiocytes, they should in such cases be termed *pseudo–giant cells*. True giant cells and granulomas also appear in this disease, however.[111] Marked interstitial edema also is present with lymphocytic infiltration.

The process often is irregularly distributed in either or both lobes.[114] With recovery, the inflammatory reaction recedes, and a variable amount of fibrosis may appear. Areas of follicular regeneration are seen, but there is no caseation, hemorrhage, or calcification. The degree of recovery is generally virtually

complete, aside from the residual fibrosis already mentioned. Only in rare instances is there complete destruction of the thyroid parenchyma leading to permanent hypothyroidism.

Thyroid tissue obtained by fine-needle aspiration biopsy (Fig. 13-3) often shows a mixed and polymorphous inflammatory infiltrate of neutrophils, lymphocytes, and large numbers of histiocytes, which can be misinterpreted. The features of SAT—epithelioid granulomas, multinucleated giant cells, and follicular cells with intravacuolar granules—can be identified.[87,111-113]

An immunohistochemical study of six cases showed the cellular composition of SAT.[115] The giant cells were CD68 positive,

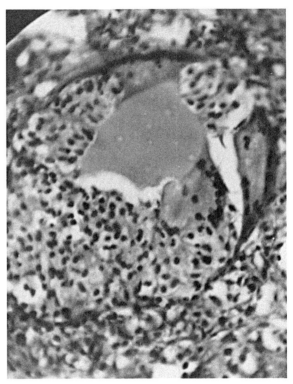

FIGURE 13-2. Pathologic findings in subacute thyroiditis. Note the severe destruction of the thyroid follicle, with the remaining colloid being surrounded by large numbers of histiocytes, giving the appearance of a giant cell (pseudo–giant cell). Marked interstitial edema is noted, with cellular infiltration and considerable destruction of the thyroid parenchyma.

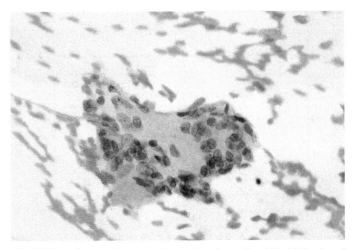

FIGURE 13-3. Fine-needle aspiration findings in subacute thyroiditis. Multinucleated giant cell with lymphocytes.

thyroglobulin negative, and cytokeratin negative. Small lympho-cytes in the granulomas are CD3-positive, CD8-positive, and CD45RO-positive cytotoxic T cells. In the nongranulomatous lesion, the follicles often were infiltrated by CD8-positive T lymphocytes, plasmacytoid monocytes, and histiocytes, resulting in disrupted basement membrane and rupture of the follicles. These findings suggest an intense cellular immune response in SAT. In addition, apoptotic cells are found in regenerating follicular cells in the area of granuloma and rarely found in sites of fibrosis, which might indicate a healing process.[115]

TREATMENT

In some patients, no treatment is required. In mild cases, the relief of symptoms can be achieved with nonsteroidal antiinflam-matory drugs or aspirin (2 to 3 g/day).[1-4] If this therapy fails, as it often does when the symptoms are severe, prednisone or another similar analogue of cortisol is prescribed.[5,116,117] Relief of symptoms occurs often within 24 hours. The basic disease process may not be altered, but the inflammatory response is suppressed, allowing the pathologic process to run its now sub-clinical course.

Treatment with prednisone generally is begun with a single daily dose of 40 mg. Within 8 to 10 days, symptoms markedly decrease, and the dose can be tapered and completely stopped after 4 weeks. The relief of the tenderness in the neck is so dra-matic as to be virtually diagnostic of the problem as being due to SAT. In most instances, exacerbations do not occur, and patients go on to full recovery. Sometimes symptoms flare up again, and the prednisone taper needs to be reversed.[1-5] The recurrence rate of SAT after cessation of prednisone therapy is about 20%, but no difference has been found in routine labora-tory data between recurrent and nonrecurrent groups of patients.[118]

There seems to be no significant difference in the incidence of mild thyroid failure between patients receiving corticosteroid therapy and patients receiving nonsteroidal antiinflammatory drugs. In contrast, long-term hypothyroidism requiring T_4 therapy is significantly more common in the group receiving corticosteroid therapy, as shown in a more recent report.[22] Cor-ticosteroid therapy should be given to improve the symptoms and quality of life without an expectation of reducing long-term thyroid dysfunction.

During the initial phase, the patient may be thyrotoxic and need treatment with β-sympathetic blocking agents, such as propranolol. Sodium iopodate has been employed in the man-agement of the hyperthyroidism of SAT.[120] The treatment was effective in causing normalization of thyroid function, although the inflammatory state persisted for 6 weeks thereafter. There have been reports that the addition of T_4 or T_3 after repeated exacerbations can result in amelioration of the condition and prevent further recurrences.[1-5] Thyroid hormone administration may be useful in situations in which the patient is not already hyperthyroid due to the release of thyroidal contents into the circulation. It is thought that TSH suppression would reduce the thyroid stimulation, which otherwise might prolong the inflam-matory process. Antibiotics are of no value. Thiouracil and TSH have been reported to be beneficial, but such drugs have not found general favor.[4] Because recovery is almost certain, thyroid-ectomy almost never needs to be recommended except in an unusual prolonged course with continuing local distress.[3,4,119]

It is necessary to administer thyroid hormones if the patient enters a phase of hypothyroidism after the acute inflammation. Also, because of the high incidence of transient hypothyroidism,

T_4 therapy should not be considered lifelong if started in the first year. During the recovery process, there may be a marked but transient increase in the 24-hour radioactive iodine uptake, which can reach levels typical of Graves' disease. This increase occurs before reestablishment of normal thyroid function and should not be confused with hyperthyroidism due to Graves' disease.

Riedel's Thyroiditis

BACKGROUND AND DEFINITION

In 1896, Riedel[121-123] described a rare disorder of chronic scleros-ing thyroiditis, occurring especially in women, causing pressure symptoms in the neck, which tends to progress inexorably to complete destruction of the thyroid gland. This disorder is char-acterized pathologically by dense fibrous tissue, which replaces the normal thyroid parenchyma and extends into adjacent tissues, such as muscles, blood vessels, and nerves.[1,3,124,125] Syn-onyms for the term *chronic invasive fibrous thyroiditis* include Riedel's struma, struma fibrosa, ligneous struma, chronic fibrous thyroiditis, and chronic productive thyroiditis. The presence of eosinophils has been shown histologically, suggesting a unique autoimmune response to fibrous tissue. It may include sclerosing mediastinitis, retroperitoneal fibrosis, pseudotumors of the orbit, and sclerosis of the biliary tract.[126]

INCIDENCE

Riedel's thyroiditis is exceedingly rare. Women are four times more likely to be affected than men, and it occurs most commonly between 30 and 50 years of age. In the Mayo Clinic series, it occurred approximately one fiftieth as frequently as Hashimoto's thyroiditis.* The operative incidence over 64 years was 0.06%, and the overall incidence in outpatients was 1.06 per 100,000.[127-130] Only 37 cases were found on review of histol-ogy of 57,000 thyroidectomies.[127] In thyroidectomies performed for all disorders, an incidence between 0.03% and 0.98% was reported from a small group of centers.[126]

ETIOLOGY

Although there has been considerable debate as to whether Riedel's thyroiditis is a primary inflammatory disorder of the thyroid gland, a variant of Hashimoto's thyroiditis, or even end-stage SAT, current evidence suggests that Riedel's thyroid-itis might be a local manifestation of a systemic fibrosing disease.[3,131-133] An autoimmune mechanism is suggested by (1) the presence of mononuclear cell infiltration and vasculitis within the fibrous tissue and the serum antithyroid antibodies present in so many patients[134]; (2) occasional reports of the coexistence of Riedel's thyroiditis with autoimmune disorders such as Addison's disease, type 1 diabetes, pernicious anemia, Graves' disease, and Hashimoto's thyroiditis[136-139]; and (3) the favorable response to glucocorticoid therapy.[140]

The autoantibodies are thought to be reactive to antigens released from destroyed thyroid tissue.[134] The association with other autoimmune diseases is rare and probably coinciden-tal,[134-137] and the response to glucocorticoid therapy may be due to decreased production of cytokines with strong fibrogenic properties.[140]

The absence of other autoantibodies and the presence of a normal serum complement level and a normal lymphocyte sub-

---

*References 1, 3, 124, 125, 127, and 128.

population also are inconsistent with an autoimmune mechanism.[141] When followed for many years, patients with Hashimoto's thyroiditis, a common disease, almost never progress to Riedel's struma, which is a rare entity. The aforementioned evidence does not confirm an autoimmune basis for the disease, and most cases of Riedel's struma are clearly unrelated to such autoimmune disease.

It has been suggested that the key event in this disorder might be proliferation by fibroblasts, in turn induced by cytokine production from B or T lymphocytes or both.[142] Consistent with this suggestion is the finding by Many and associates[142] of histologic modifications similar to modifications observed in Riedel's thyroiditis in nonobese diabetic (NOD) mice during the development of iodine-induced thyroiditis, in the presence of T-helper 2 cytokines favoring autoantibody production. The observations of Heufelder and colleagues[143] of marked tissue eosinophilia and eosinophil degranulation in Riedel's struma have suggested another possibility—that these elements may represent an important fibrogenic stimulus, possibly via the release of eosinophil-derived products. The nature of such products is as yet unknown.

It now is widely believed that Riedel's thyroiditis is more likely to be an isolated or local manifestation of a systemic disease called *idiopathic multifocal fibrosclerosis*. An association between Riedel's thyroiditis and other fibrosing lesions, including mediastinal fibrosis, was first described by Barret[144] in 1958. Since then, many cases of Riedel's thyroiditis in association with retroperitoneal fibrosis,[145-149] mediastinal fibrosis,[145,150-153] sclerosing cholangitis,[154,155] and pseudotumor of the orbit[156,157] have been reported, suggesting they may be variable manifestations of a systemic multifocal fibrosing disorder.

Long-term follow-up of patients with Riedel's thyroiditis (follow-up time 10 years) has shown that one third develop fibrosing disorders of the retroperitoneal space (often leading to ureteral obstruction), chest, or orbits.[138] DeLange and co-workers[131] have cited all of the available literature on this point. Two thirds of patients with Riedel's struma do not develop extracervical fibrosis within the ensuing 10 years, and it is rare for one patient to have extracervical fibrosis in more than one site. Conversely, less than 1% of patients with retroperitoneal fibrosis have Riedel's struma. It is considered likely that these apparently disparate fibrotic lesions may be different manifestations of the same generalized fibrosing disease; however, the thyroid fibrosis seems common, central, and integral to this disease complex, implying an important role for it in the pathogenesis.

The established association of certain drugs with retroperitoneal fibrosis has not been observed with Riedel's struma.[131] Aside from one example of two brothers, children of consanguineous parents, who developed fibrosclerosis in multiple sites (including Riedel's struma in one of the brothers),[142,150] there does not seem to be a genetic predisposition to this condition.

CLINICAL FEATURES

The thyroid gland is normal in size or enlarged, usually symmetrically involved, and extremely hard. Occasionally, involvement may be unilateral. Typically, a lobe of the thyroid and the adjacent skeletal muscle, nerves, blood vessels, trachea, and other tissues are extensively replaced by dense, chronically inflamed fibrous tissue. The mass formed is firm to hard, pale gray, and easily mistaken for cancer on clinical examination or by a surgeon at operation. Diagnostic confusion with sarcoma of the thyroid region has been reported.[158] The involvement of the thyroid in a sense seems to be incidental to the involvement

Table 13-1. Clinical Features: Riedel's versus Hashimoto's Thyroiditis

	Riedel's	Hashimoto's
Age	23-70 yr (mostly >50 yr)	Any age (mostly >20 yr, gradually increasing with age)
Sex (F/M)	2-4:1	4-10:1
Symptoms	Pressure goiter	Often goiter
Thyroid involvement	Unilateral or diffuse	Generally diffuse, occasionally goiter quite large
Thyroid status	Occasionally hypothyroid, rarely hypoparathyroid	Commonly hypothyroid, but may be euthyroid or hyperthyroid
Thyroid antibodies	≤45%	Almost invariably
Follow-up	Often regresses	Usually proceeds to hypothyroidism

of the soft tissue of the neck (Table 13-1). It may occur in a multinodular goiter, mimicking thyroid cancer.[159] Although the etiology is unknown, the disease may develop in the course of subacute thyroiditis.[160]

The disease may remain stable over many years, or it may progress slowly and produce hypothyroidism at a prevalence rate of 25% to 29%.[124,128,130,131,161,162] Dyspnea, dysphagia, hoarseness, and aphonia are caused by the local pressure, and if there is enough pressure on both recurrent laryngeal nerves, there may be stridor. Sensations of suffocation, cough, and heaviness in the neck are common. Pain is unusual, although the sense of pressure may be out of proportion to the size of the goiter.[163-165] The presence or degree of obstruction varies with the extent to which the surrounding structures have been invaded. Occasionally, tetany due to hypoparathyroidism may be observed.[161,162]

Sometimes the disease is asymptomatic and discovered only incidentally. Some patients have only mild and infrequent symptoms, with minimal dysphagia and dyspnea. In severe cases, the entire gland is involved with the fibrotic process, and symptoms are intense; patients present with stridor, severe dyspnea, or attacks of suffocation.

On physical examination, the thyroid gland is rock hard, is densely adherent to adjacent cervical structures (e.g., muscles, blood vessels, and nerves), and may move scarcely on swallowing. It is variable in size, from small to very large.[1,124,125] The lesion may be limited to one lobe, may be present in both, or (as mentioned earlier) may involve the entire gland. It has a harder consistency than carcinoma and is only rarely tender. Although adjacent lymph nodes occasionally are enlarged, when they are present and associated with a hard thyroid mass, a diagnosis of carcinoma is often suspected.[1,124,125]

The clinical importance of Riedel's thyroiditis lies in its ability to result in local obstructive phenomena; in its potential for being confused with carcinoma, especially lymphoma[166] and sarcoma; and in its variable association with fibrosing processes elsewhere in the body.[1,124,125,131,161] The local complications of Riedel's thyroiditis are protean and range from thyroid dysfunction, tracheal and esophageal compression with fibrous mediastinitis,[153] bilateral fibrous parotitis,[167] occlusive vasculitis[148,168] causing an extensive sterile neck abscess,[168] superior vena cava syndrome,[169,170] and cerebral venous sinus thrombosis,[171] obstruction of a ventriculoperitoneal shunt,[172] to pituitary failure.[173] Spontaneous hypoparathyroidism secondary to Riedel's thyroiditis seems to be rare. Only nine previous cases of primary hypoparathyroidism secondary to Riedel's thyroiditis have been reported,[132,174-179] and only two of these showed parathyroid recovery.[162,179] Parathyroid autoantibodies were tested in some cases and were negative. Vascular compromise and progressive ischemia also may contribute to parathyroid dysfunction. The occurrence of cerebral sinus thrombosis suggests that Riedel's thyroiditis may cause venous stasis, vascular damage, and possibly hypercoagulability.[180] Because of fibrotic lesions elsewhere, the examination must include a careful search for compressive signs.

LABORATORY AND IMAGING FINDINGS

Riedel's thyroiditis has no characteristic biochemical findings. Most patients are euthyroid, whereas few are hypothyroid.[125] This difference is probably due to the extent of the nonfunctioning fibrous infiltration of the gland at the time of diagnosis. In the Cleveland Clinic series, 64% of the patients were found to be euthyroid, 32% hypothyroid, and 4% hyperthyroid.[125] Two other large series revealed prevalence rates of hypothyroidism of 25% and 29%.[128,131]

Antithyroid antibodies are present in 67% of reported cases,[129] and a mixed population of B and T cells is present in the thyroid. The occurrence of marked tissue eosinophilia and the extracellular deposition of eosinophil granule major basic protein suggests a role for eosinophils and their products in the development of fibrosis in Riedel's thyroiditis.[143] Fibrosis also may be related to the action of transforming growth factor-$\beta 1$, as seen in murine thyroiditis.[181]

Antinuclear factor was once reported as present.[161] The white blood cell count may be normal or elevated, and the erythrocyte sedimentation rate is usually moderately elevated.[1,124,125] Additionally, fibrosis of the whole gland occasionally can result in hypoparathyroidism, with consequent low serum calcium and high serum phosphorus values.[161,162,182] Thyroid and parathyroid function should be measured in all cases.

On thyroid radionuclide imaging, a heterogeneous pattern of isotope uptake or very low uptake is usually seen, similar to other forms of thyroiditis.[1,124,125] Fluorine-18 fluorodeoxyglucose positron emission tomography images have shown metabolic activity in an abdominal mass and increased glucose metabolism in the thyroid, probably resulting from active inflammation involving lymphocytes, plasma cells, and fibroblast proliferation.[183]

Ultrasonography also can be helpful. On ultrasound, Riedel's thyroiditis is reported to be homogeneously hypoechoic due to fibrosis.[161,184] A thyroid hypodense on computed tomography and hypointense on T1-weighted and T2-weighted magnetic resonance images can suggest Riedel's thyroiditis whether or not invasion to nearby soft tissues is observed. Administration of contrast medium may be helpful in differentiating the normal thyroid parenchyma from the fibrosclerotic mass. Based on current knowledge, no other entity causes diffuse decreased enhancement after gadolinium administration on magnetic resonance imaging or administration of iodinated contrast medium on computed tomography. These radiologic findings may be an important diagnostic tool for Riedel's thyroiditis.[185-187]

Fine-needle aspiration biopsy is usually nondiagnostic in Riedel's thyroiditis because most often only follicular cells are obtained and not the fibrous material characteristic of this type of thyroiditis. In many patients, the diagnosis is established pathologically only by open biopsy or postoperatively.

PATHOLOGY

The gland has been described as woody or very hard. On pathologic examination, the thyroid is replaced by dense fibrosis in which are scattered solitary follicular cells and occasional acini

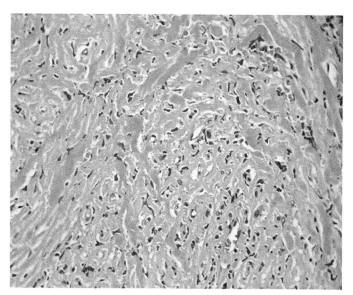

FIGURE 13-4. Pathologic findings of Riedel's thyroiditis. Extensive follicular cell destruction and replacement of thyroid tissue by a dense fibrous tissue and infiltration of lymphocytes.

with small amounts of colloid (Fig. 13-4).[1,124,125,128,130] Extension of the fibrosis beyond the capsule of the thyroid into adjacent structures, such as nerves, blood vessels, and muscles, is a characteristic feature and accounts for the occasional instance in which the parathyroid glands have been obliterated by this fibrosing process. There are no tissue planes, making surgical extirpation virtually impossible (ligneous thyroiditis).[1,124,125] An adenoma may occur in the midst of the fibrous mass. Isolated thyroid amyloidosis has been described in one case of Riedel's struma.[124]

On histologic examination, early lesions show an intense infiltration of lymphocytes, plasma cells, neutrophils, and eosinophils. Subsequently, dense fibrous bands divide the thyroid into progressively smaller lobules. Eventually, dense hyalinized fibrous tissue with a few lymphocytes, plasma cells, and eosinophils replaces the thyroid parenchyma.[128,130] Similar features also are observed in the extracervical fibrosclerotic lesions in the retroperitoneal or mediastinal regions, in the orbit or lacrimal glands, or in cholangitis. An associated arteritis and phlebitis with intimal proliferation, medial destruction, adventitial inflammation, and frequent thrombosis also may occur.[1,124,125,128,130]

DIAGNOSIS AND TREATMENT

Untreated Riedel's thyroiditis is usually slowly progressive, although it may stabilize or regress spontaneously. In some cases, this disease may present a difficult diagnostic challenge, necessitating rapid interventions and a collaborative effort of medical and surgical teams.

The criteria most commonly used to diagnose Riedel's thyroiditis, as reported by Woolner and colleagues[128] and modified further by Schwaegerle and associates,[125] are (1) gross description of a visible fibroinflammatory process involving all or a portion of the thyroid gland, (2) gross or histologic evidence of extension into adjacent structures, (3) absence of granulomatous reaction, and (4) absence of neoplasm.

Although there is no specific therapy for Riedel's thyroiditis, several management strategies are available depending on the clinical features of the disease in the individual patient. Hypothyroidism should be treated with levothyroxine, although it rarely has an effect on goiter size or the progressive spread of fibrosclerosis. In addition, calcium and vitamin D therapy are indicated in cases with associated hypoparathyroidism.[161] Surgical intervention is indicated on two grounds: (1) to exclude malignancy and (2) to relieve tracheal or esophageal compression. In this case, operation should be limited to relief of obstruction, for example, by wedge excision of the thyroid isthmus. Thyroidectomy or neck dissection is not the rule, because the lack of resection planes and the risk of injury to adjacent structures make surgery quite hazardous.[129] Recurrence after surgery also has been reported.[134,135]

Because of the rarity of Riedel's thyroiditis, there have been no extensive clinical trials of the efficacy of medical therapy. Nevertheless, small studies and case reports consistently show a good response to glucocorticoids.[134,162,182,188] These drugs often are used as first-line therapy because of the progressive perithyroidal infiltration and fibrosis with potentially life-threatening destruction of local structures.

In some instances, dramatic responses to glucocorticoids have been described and lasting benefit even after withdrawal.[141,189] In other instances, relapses have occurred when these drugs were stopped.[141,182] The reasons for this variation are unclear, but inflammatory activity and duration of disease may be relevant factors. Glucocorticoids are considered to be more effective when given early in the disease.[182] Initial doses of 100 mg/day of prednisone have been used, but sustained improvement has been reported with lower doses of 15 to 60 mg/day.[166]

In patients who fail to respond to steroid therapy or relapse after withdrawal, tamoxifen therapy should be tried. Tamoxifen, an antiestrogen drug with inhibitory properties for connective tissue proliferation, has been used successfully in the treatment of Riedel's thyroiditis. In one series of four patients with Riedel's thyroiditis who had progressive symptomatic disease despite glucocorticoid therapy and surgery, tamoxifen resulted in subjective and objective improvements.[190] Each of the four patients had a decrease in goiter size of 50% or more, and one had total resolution of the disease. Although not fully understood, tamoxifen's effectiveness in treating disorders such as Riedel's thyroiditis could have been related to the stimulation of transforming growth factor β production. Transforming growth factor β is a known potent growth inhibitor of immature fibroblasts and epithelial cells.[191] Until more effective drugs are found, tamoxifen may be the drug of choice for managing intractable Riedel's thyroiditis. Side effects of tamoxifen include hot flashes and menstrual irregularity. Men report decreased libido.

Immunosuppressive treatment and chemotherapy have been tried in individual cases. Much remains to be learned about the pathophysiology and treatment of Riedel's thyroiditis.

PROGNOSIS

The mortality rate has been reported to range from 6% to 10%, with deaths usually attributed to asphyxia secondary to tracheal compression or laryngospasm.[1,124,125] The mortality rates mentioned are derived from the older literature, however, and may not reflect the (presumably lower) current rates. The course of the lesion may be slowly progressive, may stabilize, or may remit. After surgery, the disease sometimes subsides or takes a benign, self-limiting course. Spontaneous remissions without surgery may occur, and secondary surgery is only rarely required.[1,124,125]

Acknowledgments

The author expresses her gratitude and appreciation to Dr. Inês V. Castro and Dr. Paulo Carneiro for the preparation of Figs. 13-3 and 13-4. The author also thanks Dr. Robert Volpé for permission to use Figs. 13-1 and 13-2.

REFERENCES

1. Volpé R: Subacute and sclerosing thyroiditis. In DeGroot LG, editor: Endocrinology, 3rd ed, Philadelphia, 1995, WB Saunders, pp 742–751.
2. Bastenie PA, Ermans AM: Thyroiditis and thyroid function: clinical, morphological and physiological studies. International Series of Monographs in Pure and Applied Biology. Modern Trends in Physiological Sciences, vol. 36, New York, 1972, Pergamon Press.
3. LiVolsi VA, LoGerfo P, editors: Thyroiditis, Boca Raton, FL, 1981, CRC Press, pp 21–42.
4. Greene JN: Subacute thyroiditis, Am J Med 51:97–108, 1971.
5. Steinberg FU: Subacute granulomatous thyroiditis: a review, Ann Intern Med 52:1014–1025, 1960.
6. Mygind H: Thyroiditis akuta simplex, J Laryngol 91:181–193, 1895.
7. De Quervain F: Die akute nicht eiterige Thyreoiditis und die Beteiligung der Schilddrüse und akuten Intoxikationen und Infectionen überhaupt, Mitt Grenzgebieten Med Chir 2(Suppl):1–165, 1904.
8. De Quervain F, Giordandengo G: Die akute und subakute nicht eiterige thyroiditis, Mitt Grenzgeheiten Med Chir 44:538–590, 1936.
9. Volpe R, Row VV, Ezrin C: Circulating viral and thyroid antibodies in subacute thyroiditis, J Clin Endocrinol Metab 27:1275–1284, 1967.
10. Martino E, Buratti L, Bartalena L, et al: High prevalence of subacute thyroiditis during summer season in Italy, J Endocrinol Invest 10:321–323, 1987.
11. Kawano C, Muroi K, Akioka T, et al: Cytomegalovirus pneumonitis, activated prothrombin time prolongation and subacute thyroiditis after unrelated allogeneic bone marrow transplantation, Bone Marrow Transplant 26:1347–1349, 2000.
12. Volta C, Carano N, Street ME, et al: Atypical subacute thyroiditis caused by Epstein-Barr virus infection in a three-year-old girl, Thyroid 15:1189–1191, 2005.
13. Al Maawali A, Al Yaarubi S, Al Futaisi A: An infant with cytomegalovirus-induced subacute thyroiditis, J Pediatr Endocrinol Metab 21:191–193B, 2008.
14. Dulipsingh L, Ikram Z, Malchoff CD, et al: A cluster of cases of subacute and silent thyroiditis in the northern Connecticut, Greater Hartford area, Conn Med 62:395–397, 1998.
15. Oksa H, Jarvenpaa P, Metsahonkala L, et al: No seasonal distribution in subacute de Quervain's thyroiditis in Finland, J Endocrinol Invest 12:495, 1989.
16. Cordray JP, Nys P, Merceron RE, et al: Frequency of hypothyroidism after de Quervain's thyroiditis and contribution of ultrasonographic thyroid volume measurement [French], Ann Med Interne (Paris) 152:84–88, 2001.
17. de Bruin TW, Riekhoff FP, de Boer JJ: An outbreak of thyrotoxicosis due to atypical subacute thyroiditis, J Clin Endocrinol Metab 70:396–402, 1990.
18. Nordyke RA, Gilbert FI Jr, Lew C: Painful subacute thyroiditis in Hawaii, West J Med 155:61–63, 1991.
19. Nikolai TF: Silent thyroiditis and subacute thyroiditis, In Braverman LE, Utiger R, editors: Werner and Ingbar's The Thyroid: A Fundamental and Clinical Text, ed 6, Philadelphia, 1991, JB Lippincott, pp 720–727.
20. B Hiraiwa T, Kubota S, Imagawa A, et al: B Two cases of subacute thyroiditis presenting in pregnancy, B J Endocrinol Invest 29:924–927, 2006.
21. Qari FA, Maimani AA: Subacute thyroiditis in Western Saudi Arabia, Saudi Med J 26:630–633, 2005.
22. Fatourechi V, Aniszewski J, Fatourechi G, et al: Clinical features and outcome of subacute thyroiditis in an incidence cohort: Olmsted County, Minnesota study, J Clin Endocrinol Metab 88:2100, 2003.
23. B Dedivitis RA, Coelho LS: Vocal fold paralysis in subacute thyroiditis, B Rev Bras Otorrinolaringol 73:138, 2007
24. Tauveron I, Thieblot P, Marcheix JC: Recurrence after 12 years of de Quervain-Crile subacute thyroiditis [French], Rev Med Interne 12:396, 1991.
25. Bauman A, Friedman A: Recurrent subacute thyroiditis: a report of three cases, N Y State J Med 83:987–988, 1983.
26. Iitaka M, Momotani N, Ishii J, et al: Incidence of subacute thyroiditis recurrences after a prolonged latency: 24 year survey, J Clin Endocrinol Metab 81:466–469, 1996.
27. Yamamoto M, Saito S, Sakurada T, et al: Recurrence of subacute thyroiditis over 10 years after the first attack in three cases, Endocrinol Jpn 35:833–839, 1988.
28. Carle A, Laurberg P, Pedersen IB, et al: Epidemiology of subtypes of hypothyroidism in Denmark, Eur J Endocrinol 154:21–28, 2006
29. Fraser R, Harrison RJ: Subacute thyroiditis, Lancet 1:382–386, 1952.
30. Vejlgaard TB, Nielsen OB: Subacute thyroiditis in parvovirus B19 infection, Ugeskr Laeger 156:6039–6040, 1994.
31. Brouqui P, Raoult D, Conte-Devolx B: Coxsackie thyroiditis, Ann Intern Med 114:1063–1064, 1991.
32. Sato M: Virus-like particles in the follicular epithelium of the thyroid from a patient with subacute thyroiditis (de Quervain), Acta Pathol Jpn 25:499–501, 1975.
33. Volpé R, Row VV, Ezrin C: Circulating viral and thyroid antibodies in subacute thyroiditis, J Clin Endocrinol Metab 27:1275–1284, 1967.
34. Yeo PPB, Rauff A, Chan SW, et al: Subacute (de Quervain's) thyroiditis in the tropics. In Stockigt JR, Nagataki S, editors: Thyroid Research VIII, Canberra, 1980, Australian Academy of Science, pp 570–574.

35. Arend SM, Westedt ML: Simultaneous onset of giant cell arteritis and subacute thyroiditis, Ann Rheum Dis 52:839–840, 1993.

36. Falaschi P, Martocchia A, D'Urso R, et al: Subacute thyroiditis during interferon-alpha therapy for chronic hepatitis C, J Endocrinol Invest 20:24–28, 1997.

37. Parana R, Cruz M, Lyra L, et al: Subacute thyroiditis during treatment with combination therapy (interferon plus ribavirin) for hepatitis C virus, J Viral Hepatol 7:393–395, 2000.

38. B Moser C, Furrer J, Ruggieri F: Neck pain and fever after peginterferon alpha-2a, B Schweiz Rundsch Med Pradx 96:205–207, 2007.

39. Obuobie K, Al-Sabah A, Lazarus JH: Subacute thyroiditis in an immunosuppressed patient, J Endocrinol Invest 25:169–171, 2002.

40. Strakosch CR, Joyner D, Wall JR: Thyroid stimulating antibodies in subacute thyroiditis, J Clin Endocrinol Metab 46:345–348, 1978.

41. Wall JR, Strakosch CR, Brandy P, et al: Nature of thyrotropin displacement activity in subacute thyroiditis, J Clin Endocrinol Metab 54:349–353, 1982.

42. Tamai H, Nozaki T, Mukuta T, et al: The incidence of thyroid-stimulating blocking antibodies during the hypothyroid phase in patients with subacute thyroiditis, J Clin Endocrinol Metab 73:245–250, 1991.

43. Weetman AP, Smallridge RC, Nutman TB, et al: Persistent thyroid autoimmunity after subacute thyroiditis, J Lab Clin Immunol 23:1–6, 1987.

44. Wall JR, Fang SL, Ingbar SH, et al: Lymphocyte transformation in response to human thyroid extract in patients with subacute thyroiditis, J Clin Endocrinol Metab 43:587–590, 1976.

45. Totterman TH, Gordin A, Hayry P, et al: Accumulation of thyroid antigen-reactive T lymphocytes in the gland of patients with subacute thyroiditis, Clin Exp Immunol 32:153–158, 1978.

46. Galluzzo A, Giordano C, Andronico F, et al: Leucocyte migration test in subacute thyroiditis: hypothetical role of cell mediated immunity, J Clin Endocrinol Metab 50:1038–1041, 1980.

47. Fukata S, Matsuzuka F, Kobayashi A, et al: Development of Graves' disease after subacute thyroiditis: two unusual cases, Acta Endocrinol (Copenh) 126:495–496, 1992.

48. Bartalena L, Bogazzi F, Pecori F, et al: Graves' disease occurring after subacute thyroiditis: report of a case and review of the literature, Thyroid 6:345–348, 1996.

49. Sheets RF: The sequential occurrence of acute thyroiditis and thyrotoxicosis, JAMA 157:139–140, 1955.

50. Perloff WH: Thyrotoxicosis following acute thyroiditis: a report of 5 cases, J Clin Endocrinol Metab 16:542–546, 1956.

51. Werner SC: Graves' disease following acute (subacute) thyroiditis, Arch Intern Med 139:1313–1315, 1979.

52. Sartani A, Feigl D, Zaidel L, et al: Painless thyroiditis followed by autoimmune disorders of the thyroid: a case report with biopsy, J Endocrinol Invest 3:169–172, 1980.

53. Wartofsky L, Schaaf M: Graves' disease with thyrotoxicosis following subacute thyroiditis, Am J Med 83:761–763, 1987.

54. Volpé R: Autoimmune thyroiditis. In Braverman LE, Utiger R, editors: Werner and Ingbar's The Thyroid: A Fundamental and Clinical Text, ed 6, Philadelphia, 1991, JB Lippincott, pp 921–933.

55. Volpé R: Immunology of the thyroid. In Volpé R, editor: Autoimmune Diseases of the Endocrine System, Boca Raton, FL, 1990, CRC Press, pp 73–240.

56. Bech K, Nerup J, Thomsen M, et al: Subacute thyroiditis de Quervain: a disease associated with HLA-B antigen, Acta Endocrinol 86:504–509, 1977.

57. Nyulassy S, Hnilica P, Buc M, et al: Subacute (de Quervain's) thyroiditis: association with HLA-Bw35 antigen, and abnormalities of the complement system, immunoglobulins and other serum proteins, J Clin Endocrinol Metab 45:270–274, 1977.

58. Tamai H, Goto H, Uno H, et al: HLA in Japanese patients with subacute (de Quervain's) thyroiditis, Tissue Antigens 24:58–59, 1984.

59. Yeo PPB, Chan SH, Aw TC, et al: HLA and Chinese patients with subacute (de Quervain's) thyroiditis, Tissue Antigens 17:249–250, 1981.

60. Ohsako N, Tamai H, Sudo T, et al: Clinical characteristics of subacute thyroiditis classified according to HLA typing, J Clin Endocrinol Metab 80:3653–3656, 1995.

61. Zein EF, Karaa SE, Megarbane A: Familial occurrence of painful subacute thyroiditis associated with human leukocyte antigen-B35, Presse Med 36:808–809, 2007.

62. Hsiao Jy, Hsin SC, Hsieh MC, et al: Subacute thyroiditis following influenza vaccine (Vaxigrip) in a young female, Kaohsiung J Med Sci 22:297–300, 2006.

63. Volpé R, Johnston MW: Subacute thyroiditis: A disease commonly mistaken for pharyngitis, Can Med Assoc J 77:297–307, 1957.

64. Volpé R, Johnston MW, Huber N: Thyroid function in subacute thyroiditis, J Clin Endocrinol Metab 18:65–78, 1958.

65. Alper AT, Hasdemir H, Akyol A, et al: Incessant ventricular tachycardia due to subacute thyroiditis, B Int J Cardiol 116:E22–E24, 2007.

66. Swinburne JL, Kreisman SH: A rare case of subacute thyroiditis causing thyroid storm, Thyroid 17:73–76, 2007.

67. Nishihara E, Ohye H, Amino N, et al: Clinical characteristics of 852 patients with subacute thyroiditis before treatment, Intern Med 47:725–729, 2008.

68. Benbassat CA, Olchovsky D, Tsvetov G, et al: Subacute thyroiditis: clinical characteristics and treatment outcome in fifty-six consecutive patients diagnosed between 1999 and 2005, J Endocrinol Invest 30:631–635, 2007.

69. Ingbar SH, Freinkel N: Thyroid function and metabolism of iodine in patients with subacute thyroiditis, Arch Intern Med 101:339–346, 1958.

70. Dorta T, Beraud T: New investigations on subacute thyroiditis, Helv Med Acta 28:19–41, 1961.

71. Izumi M, Larsen PR: Correlation of sequential change in serum thyroglobulin, triiodothyronine, and thyroxine in patients with Graves' disease and subacute thyroiditis, Metabolism 27:449–460, 1978.

72. Larsen PR: Serum triiodothyronine and thyrotropin during hyperthyroid and recovery phases of subacute non-suppurative thyroiditis, Metabolism 23:467–471, 1974.

73. Weihl AC, Daniels GH, Ridgeway ED, et al: Thyroid function during the early days of subacute thyroiditis, J Clin Endocrinol Metab 44:1107–1114, 1977.

74. Glinoer D, Puttemans N, Van Herle AJ, et al: Sequential study of the impairment of thyroid function in the early stage of subacute thyroiditis, Acta Endocrinol 77:26–39, 1974.

75. Lio S, Pontecorvi A, Caruso M, et al: Transitory subclinical and permanent hypothyroidism in the course of subacute thyroiditis (de Quervain), Acta Endocrinol 106:67–70, 1984.

76. Jay HK: Permanent myxedema: an unusual complication of granulomatous thyroiditis, J Clin Endocrinol Metab 21:1384–1387, 1961.

77. Rosen F, Row VV, Volpé R, et al: Anaplastic carcinoma of thyroid with abnormal circulating iodoprotein: a case simulating subacute thyroiditis, Can Med Assoc J 95:1039–1041, 1966.

78. Pearce EN, Martino E, Bogazzi F, et al: The prevalence of elevated serum C-reactive protein levels in inflammatory and noninflammatory thyroid disease, Thyroid 13:643–648, 2003.

79. Amino N, Yabu Y, Miki T, et al: Serum ratio of triiodothyronine to thyroxine, and thyroxine-binding globulin and calcitonin concentrations in Graves' disease and destruction-induced thyrotoxicosis, J Clin Endocrinol Metab 53:113–116, 1981.

80. Hiromatsu Y, Ishibashi M, Miyake I, et al: Color Doppler ultrasonography in patients with subacute thyroiditis, Thyroid 9:1189–1193, 1999.

81. Demeester-Mirkine N, Brauman H, Corvilain J: Delayed adjustment of the pituitary response in circulating thyroid hormones in a case of subacute thyroiditis, Clin Endocrinol 5:9–14, 1976.

82. Staub JJ: The TRH test in subacute thyroiditis, Lancet 1:868–870, 1975.

83. Lewitus W, Rechnic J, Lubin E: Sequential scanning of the thyroid as an aid to the diagnosis of subacute thyroiditis, Isr J Med Sci 3:847–854, 1967.

84. Hamburger JL, Kadian G, Rossin HW: Subacute thyroiditis—evaluations depicted by serial 131I scintigrams, J Nucl Med 6:560–565, 1965.

85. Hiromatsu Y, Ishibashi M, Nishida H, et al: Technetium-99m sestamibi imaging in patients with subacute thyroiditis, Endocr J 50:239–244, 2003.

86. Nicklaus Muller E, Mullhaupt B, Perschak H: Steroid therapy and course of blood sedimentation rate in de Quervain's thyroiditis, Schweiz Rundsch Med Prax 83:95–100, 1994.

87. Sakane S, Murakami Y, Sasaki M, et al: Serum concentrations of granulocyte colony-stimulating factor (G-CSF) determined by a highly-sensitive chemiluminescent immunoassay during the clinical course of subacute thyroiditis, Endocr J 42:391–396, 1995.

88. Skillern PG, Lewis LA: Fractional plasma protein values in subacute thyroiditis, J Clin Invest 36:780–783, 1957.

89. Kubota S, Matsumoto Y, Amino N, et al: Serial changes in liver function tests in patients with subacute thyroiditis, Thyroid 18: 815, 2008.

90. Hamada S, Yagura T, Ishii H, et al: Subacute thyroiditis as a systemic multisystem disease, In Nagataki S, Torizuka K, editors: The Thyroid 1988. Excerpta Medica International Congress Series 796, Amsterdam, 1988, Elsevier, pp 521–525.

91. Kunz A, Blank W, Braun B: De Quervain's subacute thyroiditis by colour Doppler sonography findings, Ultraschall Med 26:102–106, 2005.

92. Park SY, Kim EK, Kim MJ, et al: Ultrasonographic characteristics of subacute granulomatous thyroiditis, Korean J Radiol 7:229–234, 2006.

93. Omori N, OmoriK, Takano K: Association of the ultrasonographic findings of subacute thyroiditis with thyroid pain and laboratory findings, Endocr J 55:583–588, 2008.

94. Sakata S, Nagai K, Maekawa H, et al: Serum ferritin concentrations in subacute thyroiditis, Metabolism 40:682–688, 1991.

95. Ozata M, Bolu E, Sengul A, et al: Soluble intercellular adhesion molecule-1 concentrations in patients with subacute thyroiditis and in patients with Graves' disease with or without ophthalmopathy, Endocr J 43:517–525, 1996.

96. Hara H, Sugita E, Sato R, et al: Plasma selectin levels in patients with Graves' disease, Endocr J 43:709–713, 1996.

97. Yamada T, Sato A, Aizawa T: Dissociation between serum interleukin 6 rise and other parameters of disease activity in subacute thyroiditis during treatment with corticosteroid, J Clin Endocrinol Metab 81:577–579, 1996.

98. Vulpoi C, Zbranca E, Preda C, et al: Contribution of ultrasonography in the evaluation of subacute thyroiditis, Rev Med Chir Soc Med Nat Iasi 105:749–755, 2001.

99. Lu CP, Chang TC, Wang CY, et al: Serial changes in ultrasound-guided fine needle aspiration cytology in subacute thyroiditis, Acta Cytol 41:238–243, 1997.

100. Bennedbaek FN, Gram J, Hegedus L: The transition of subacute thyroiditis to Graves' disease as evidenced by diagnostic imaging, Thyroid 6:457–459, 1996.

101. Bennedbaek FN, Hegedus L: The value of ultrasonography in the diagnosis and follow-up of subacute thyroiditis, Thyroid 7:45–50, 1997.

102. Benker G, Olbricht TH, Windeck R, et al: The sonographic and functional sequelae of de Quervain's subacute thyroiditis, Acta Endocrinol 117:435–441, 1988.

103. Tokuda Y, Kasagi K, Iida Y, et al: Sonography of subacute thyroiditis: changes in the findings during the course of the disease, J Clin Ultrasound 18:21–26, 1990.

104. Tezuka M, Murata Y, Ishida R, et al: MR imaging of the thyroid: correlation between apparent diffusion coefficient and thyroid gland scintigraphy, J Magn Reson Imaging 17:163–169, 2003.

105. Vierhapper H, Bieglmayer CH, Nowotny P, et al: Normal serum concentrations of sex hormone-binding globulin in patients with hyperthyroidism due to subacute thyroiditis, Thyroid 8:1107–1111, 1998.

106. Fragu P, Rougier P, Schlumberger M, et al: Evolution of thyroid 127I stores measured by x-ray fluorescence in subacute thyroiditis, J Clin Endocrinol Metab 54:162–166, 1982.

107. Rapoport B, Block MB, Hoffer PB, et al: Depletion of thyroid iodine during subacute thyroiditis, J Clin Endocrinol Metab 36:610–611, 1973.

108. Bech K, Feldt-Rasmussen U, Bliddal H, et al: Persistence of autoimmune reactions during recovery of subacute thyroiditis. In Pinchera A, Ingbar SH, McKenzie JM, Fenzi GF, editors: Thyroid Autoimmunity, New York, 1987, Plenum Press, pp 623–625.

109. Itaka M, Momotani N, Hisaoka T, et al: TSH receptor antibody-associated thyroid dysfunction following subacute thyroiditis, Clin Endocrinol 48:445–453, 1998.

110. Volpé R: Subacute and sclerosing thyroiditis. In DeGroot LG, editor: Endocrinology, ed 4, Philadelphia, 1999, WB Saunders, pp 742–751, 1480–1489.

111. Solano JC, Bascunana AG, Perez JS, et al: Fine-needle aspiration of subacute granulomatous thyroiditis (de Quervain's thyroiditis): a clinico-cytologic review of 36 cases, Diagn Cytopathol 16:214–220, 1997.

112. Shabb NS, Salti I: Subacute thyroiditis: fine-needle aspiration cytology of 14 cases presenting with thyroid nodules, Diagn Cytopathol 34:18–23, 2006.

113. Liel Y: The survivor: association of an autonomously functioning thyroid nodule and subacute thyroiditis, Thyroid 17:183–184, 2007.

114. Sari O, Erbas B, Erbas T: Subacute thyroiditis in a single lobe, Clin Nucl Med 26:400–401, 2001.

115. Koga M, Hiromatsu Y, Jimi A, et al: Immunohistochemical analysis of Bcl-2, Bax, and Bak expression in thyroid glands from patients with subacute thyroiditis, J Clin Endocrinol Metab 84:2221–2225, 2002.

116. Singer PA: Thyroiditis: acute, subacute, and chronic, Med Clin North Am 75:61–77, 1991.

117. Volpe R: The management of subacute (de Quervain's) thyroiditis, Thyroid 5:253–255, 1993.

118. Mizukoshi T, Noguchi S, Murakami T, et al: Evaluation of recurrence in 36 subacute thyroiditis patients managed with prednisolone, Intern Med 40:292–295, 2001.

119. Bogazzi F, Dell'Unto E, Tanda ML, et al: Long-term outcome of thyroid function after amiodarone-induced thyrotoxicosis, as compared to subacute thyroiditis, J Endocrinol Invest 29:694–698, 2006.

120. Chopra IJ, Van Herle AJ, Korenman SG, et al: Use of sodium iodate in management of hyperthyroidism in subacute thyroiditis, J Clin Endocrinol Metab 80:2178–2180, 1995.

121. Riedel BM: Ueber Verlauf und Ausgang der chronischer Strumitis, Munch Med Wochenschr 57:1946–1947, 1910.

122. Riedel BM: Vorstellung eines Kranken mit chronischer Strumitis, Verh Ges Chir 26:127–129, 1896.

123. Riedel BM: Die chronische zur Bildung eisenharter Tumoren führende Entzündung der Schilddrüse, Verh Ges Chir 25:101–105, 1896.

124. Bastenie PA: Invasive fibrous thyroiditis (Riedel), In Bastenie PA, Ermans AM, editors: Thyroiditis and Thyroid Function. International Series of Monographs in Pure and Applied Biology, Modern Trends in Physiological Sciences, vol. 36, Oxford, 1972, Pergamon Press, pp 99–108.

125. Schwaegerle SM, Bauer TW, Esselstyn CB: Riedel's thyroiditis, Am J Clin Pathol 90:715–722, 1988.

126. DeCourcey JL: A new theory concerning the etiology of Riedel's struma, Surgery 12:754–762, 1942.

127. Hay ID: Thyroiditis: a clinical update, Mayo Clin Proc 60:836–843, 1985.

128. Woolner LB, McConahey WM, Beahrs O: Invasive fibrous thyroiditis (Riedel's struma), J Clin Endocrinol Metab 17:201–220, 1957.

129. Hay ID, McConahey WM, Carney JA, et al: Invasive fibrous thyroiditis (Riedel's struma) and associated extracervical fibrosclerosis: Bowlby's disease revisited [abstract], Ann Endocrinol 43:29A, 1982.

130. Woolner LB: Thyroiditis: classification and clinicopathologic correlations. In Hazard JB, Smith DE, editors: The Thyroid, Baltimore, 1964, Williams & Wilkins, pp 123–142.

131. DeLange WE, Freling NJM, Molenaar WM, et al: Invasive fibrous thyroiditis (Riedel's struma): a case report with review of the literature, QJM 268:709–717, 1989.

132. Volpé R: Suppurative thyroiditis. In Werner SC, Ingbar SH, editors: The Thyroid: A Fundamental and Clinical Text, ed 4, New York, 1978, Harper & Row, pp 983–985.

133. Degroot LJ, Stanbury JB: The Thyroid and Its Diseases, ed 4, New York, 1975, Wiley & Sons.

134. Zimmermann-Belsing T, Feldt-Rasmussen U: Riedel's thyroiditis: an autoimmune or primary fibrotic disease? J Intern Med 235:271–274, 1994.

135. Lorenz K, Gimm O, Holzhausen HJ, et al: Riedel's thyroiditis: impact and strategy of a challenging surgery, Langenbecks Arch Surg 392:405–412, 2007.

136. Vaidya B, Harris PE, Barrett P, et al: Corticosteroid therapy in Riedel's thyroiditis, Postgrad Med J 73:817, 1997.

137. Drury ME, Sweeney EC, Heffernan SJ: Invasive fibrous thyroiditis, Ir Med J 67:388–390, 1974.

138. Merrington WR: Chronic thyroiditis: a case showing features of both Riedel's and Hashimoto's thyroiditis, Br J Surg 35:423–426, 1948.

139. Rose E, Rayster HP: Invasive fibrous thyroiditis (Riedel's struma), JAMA 176:224–226, 1961.

140. Bendtzen K: Clinical significance of cytokines: Natural and therapeutic regulation, Semin Clin Immunol 8:5–18, 1991.

141. Katsikas D, Shorthouse AJ, Taylor S: Riedel's thyroiditis, Br J Surg 63:929–931, 1976.

142. Many MC, Carpentier S, Eggermont J, et al: Towards an experimental model for Riedel's fibrous thyroiditis [abstract], J Endocrinol Invest 4(Suppl):92, 1998.

143. Heufelder AE, Goellner JR, Bahn RS, et al: Tissue eosinophilia and eosinophil degranulation in Riedel's invasive fibrous thyroiditis, J Clin Endocrinol Metab 81:977–984, 1996.

144. Barret NR: Idiopathic mediastinal fibrosis, Br J Surg 46:207–218, 1958.

145. Rao CR, Ferguson GC, Kyle VN: Retroperitoneal fibrosis associated with Riedel's struma, Can Med Assoc J 108:1019–1021, 1973.

146. Turner-Warwich R, Nabarro JD, Doniach D: Riedel's thyroiditis and retroperitoneal fibrosis, Proc R Soc Med 59:596–598, 1966.

147. Gleeson MH, Taylor S, Dowling RH: Multifocal fibrosclerosis, Proc R Soc Med 63:1309–1311, 1970.

148. Meijer S, Hoitsma HF, Scholtmeijer R: Idiopathic retroperitoneal fibrosis in multifocal fibrosclerosis, Eur Urol 2:258–260, 1976.

149. Nielson HK: Multifocal idiopathic fibrosclerosis: two cases with simultaneous occurrence of retroperitoneal fibrosis and Riedel's thyroiditis, Acta Med Scand 208:119–123, 1980.

150. Comings DS, Skubi KB, Van Eyes J, et al: Familial multifocal fibrosclerosis, Ann Intern Med 66:884–892, 1967.

151. Husband P, Knudsen A: Idiopathic cervical and retroperitoneal fibrosis: report of a case treated with steroids, Postgrad Med J 52:788–793, 1976.

152. Raphael HA, Beahrs OH, Woolner LB, et al: Riedel's struma associated with fibrous mediastinitis: report of a case, Mayo Clin Proc 41:375–382, 1966.

153. Wold LE, Weiland LH: Tumefactive fibro-inflammatory lesions of the head and neck, Am J Surg Pathol 7:477–482, 1983.

154. Hache L, Utz DC, Woolner LB: Idiopathic fibrous retroperitonitis, Surg Gynecol Obstet 115:737–744, 1962.

155. Bartholemew LG, Cain JC, Woolner LB, et al: Sclerosing cholangitis: its possible association with Riedel's struma and fibrous retroperitonitis, N Engl J Med 269:8–12, 1963.

156. Andersen SR, Seedorf HH, Halberg P: Thyroiditis with myxedema and orbital pseudotumor, Acta Ophthalmol (Rbh) 41:120–125, 1963.

157. Arnott EJ, Greaves DP: Orbital involvement in Riedel's thyroiditis, Br J Ophthalmol 49:1–5, 1965.

158. Torres-Montaner A, Beltran M, Romero de la Osa A, et al: Sarcoma of the thyroid region mimicking Riedel's thyroiditis, J Clin Pathol 54:570–572, 2001.

159. Annaert M, Thijs M, Sciot R, et al: Riedel's thyroiditis occurring in a multinodular goiter, mimicking thyroid cancer, J Clin Endocrinol Metab 92:2005–2006, 2007.

160. Cho MH, Kim CS, Park JS, et al: Riedel's thyroiditis in a patient with recurrent subacute thyroiditis: a case report and review of the literature, Endocr J 54:559–562, 2007.

161. Best TB, Munro RE, Burwell S, et al: Riedel's thyroiditis associated with Hashimoto's thyroiditis, hypoparathyroidism, and retroperitoneal fibrosis, J Endocrinol Invest 14:767–772, 1991.

162. Chopra D, Wool MS, Crosson A, et al: Riedel's struma associated with subacute thyroiditis, hypothyroidism and hypoparathyroidism, J Clin Endocrinol Metab 46:869–871, 1978.

163. Heufelder AE, Hay ID, Carney JA, et al: Coexistence of Graves' disease and Riedel's (invasive fibrous) thyroiditis: further evidence of a link between Riedel's thyroiditis and organ-specific autoimmunity, Clin Invest 72:788–793, 1994.

164. Heufelder AE, Hay ID: Further evidence for autoimmune mechanisms in the pathogenesis of Riedel's invasive thyroiditis, J Intern Med 238:85–86, 1995.

165. Shaw AFB, Smith RP: Riedel's chronic thyroiditis: with a report of six cases and a contribution to the pathology, Br J Surg 13:93–108, 1925.

166. Vigouroux C, Escourolle H, Mosnier-Pudar H, et al: Riedel's thyroiditis and lymphoma: Diagnostic difficulties, Presse Med 25:28–30, 1996.

167. Hines RC, Scheuermann HA, Royster HP, et al: Invasive fibrous (Riedel's) thyroiditis with bilateral fibrous parotitis, JAMA 213:869–871, 1970.

168. Geissler B, Wagner T, Dorn R, et al: Extensive sterile abscess in an invasive fibrous thyroiditis (Riedel's thyroiditis) caused by an occlusive vasculitis, J Endocrinol Invest 24:111–115, 2001.

169. Abet D, Francisci MP, Sevestre H, et al: Superior vena cava syndrome and Riedel's thyroiditis: Report of a case: Review of the literature, J Mal Vasc 16:298–300, 1991.

170. Yasmeen T, Khan S, Gonsh F, et al: Riedel's thyroiditis: report of a case complicated by spontaneous hypoparathyroidism, recurrent laryngeal nerve injury, and Horner's syndrome, J Clin Endocrinol Metab 87:3543–3547, 2002.

171. Vaidya B, Coulthard A, Goonetilleke A, et al: Cerebral venous sinus thrombosis: a late sequel of invasive fibrous thyroiditis, Thyroid 8:787–790, 1998.

172. Natt N, Heufelder AE, Hay ID, et al: Extracervical fibrosclerosis causing obstruction of a ventriculo-peritoneal shunt in a patient with hydrocephalus and invasive fibrous thyroiditis (Riedel's struma), Clin Endocrinol (Oxf) 47:107–111, 1997.

173. Kelly WF, Mashiter K, Taylor S, et al: Riedel's thyroiditis leading to severe but reversible pituitary failure, Postgrad Med J 55:194–198, 1979.

174. Lo JC, Loh KC, Rubin AL, et al: Riedel's thyroiditis presenting with hypothyroidism and hypoparathyroidism: dramatic response to glucocorticoid and thyroxine therapy, Clin Endocrinol (Oxf) 48:815–818, 1998.

175. Crile C Jr: Thyroiditis, Ann Surg 127:640–654, 1948.

176. Austoni M, Conte N, Zaccaria M, et al: Tiroidite di Riedel associata a ipoparatiroidismo, Folia Endocrinol 25(Suppl 6):495–501, 1972.

177. Marin F, Araujo R, Paramo C, et al: Riedel's thyroiditis associated with hypothyroidism and hypoparathyroidism, Postgrad Med J 268:709–717, 1989.

178. McRorie ER, Chalmers J, Campbell IW: Riedel's thyroiditis complicated by hypoparathyroidism and hypothyroidism, Scott Med J 38:27–28, 1993.

179. Casoli P, Tumiati B: Hypoparathyroidism secondary to Riedel's thyroiditis: A case report and review of the literature, Ann Ital Med Int 14:54–57, 1999.

180. Vaiydya B, Coulthard A, Goonetilleke A, et al: Cerebral venous sinus thrombosis: a late sequel of invasive fibrous thyroiditis, Thyroid 8:787–790, 1998.

181. Chen K, Wei Y, Sharp GC, et al: Characterization of thyroid fibrosis in a murine model of granulomatous experimental autoimmune thyroiditis, J Leukoc Biol 68:828–835, 2000.

182. Thomson JA, Jackson IMD, Duguid WP: The effect of steroid therapy on Riedel's thyroiditis, Scott Med J 13:13–16, 1968.

183. Drieskens O, Blockmans D, Van den Bruel A, et al: Riedel's thyroiditis and retroperitoneal fibrosis in multifocal fibrosclerosis: positron emission tomographic findings, Clin Nucl Med 27:413–415, 2002.

184. Perez Fontan FJ, Cordido Carballido F, Pombo Felipe F, et al: Riedel thyroiditis: US, CT, and MR evaluation, J Comput Assist Tomogr 17:324–325, 1993.

185. Ozgen A, Cila A: Riedel's thyroiditis in multifocal fibrosclerosis: CT and MR imaging findings, Am J Neuroradiol 21:320–321, 2000.
186. Takahashi N, Okamoto K, Sakai K, et al: MR Findings with dynamic evaluation in Riedel's thyroiditis, Clin Imaging 26:89–91, 2002.
187. Papi G, Corrado S, Cesinaro AM, et al: Riedel's thyroiditis: clinical, pathological and imaging features, Int J Clin Pract 56:65–67, 2002.

188. Rodriguez I, Ayala E, Caballero C, et al: Solitary fibrous tumor of the thyroid gland: report of seven cases, Am J Surg Pathol 25:1424–1428, 2001.
189. Owen K, Lane H, Jones MK: Multifocal fibrosclerosis: a case of thyroiditis and bilateral lacrimal gland involvement, Thyroid 1187–1190, 2001.

190. Few J, Thompson NW, Angelos P, et al: Riedel's thyroiditis: treatment with tamoxifen, Surgery 120:993–999, 1996.
191. Arteaga CL, Tandon AK, Von Hoff DD, et al: Transforming growth factor β: potential autocrine growth inhibitor of estrogen receptor-negative human breast cancer cell, Cancer Res 48:3808–3904, 1988.

Chapter 14

HYPOTHYROIDISM AND MYXEDEMA COMA

WILMAR M. WIERSINGA

Hypothyroidism is a syndrome characterized by the clinical and biochemical manifestations of thyroid hormone deficiency in the target tissues of thyroid hormone. Strictly speaking, hypothyroidism denotes deficient thyroid gland production of thyroid hormone. This deficiency may be caused by an abnormality in the thyroid gland itself (primary hypothyroidism) or by insufficient thyroid-stimulating hormone (TSH) stimulation of the thyroid gland resulting from an abnormality in the pituitary or hypothalamus (secondary and tertiary, or central, hypothyroidism). Most patients with thyroid hormone deficiency have primary hypothyroidism. Symptoms and signs of thyroid hormone deficiency in a few patients are caused by loss-of-function mutations in genes involved in thyroid hormone signaling in target tissues. The term **hypothyroidism** may be used in a broader sense to indicate deficient thyroid hormone action in target tissues, regardless of its cause.

The first step in the spontaneous development of primary hypothyroidism is a slight decrease in thyroid secretion of thyroxine (T_4), which causes increased release of TSH. The decreased T_4 secretion results in a modest decrease in the serum concentration of free thyroxine (FT_4), which still remains within the normal reference range, but serum TSH increases to values above the upper normal limit because of the exquisite sensitivity of the pituitary thyrotroph for circulating thyroid hormone (giving rise to the log-linear relationship between serum TSH and FT_4). The condition is known as subclinical hypothyroidism. The increase in TSH induces preferential thyroid secretion of triiodothyronine (T_3) by stimulating the synthesis of T_3 more than T_4 and by increasing thyroidal 5′-monodeiodination of T_4 into T_3.[1,2] The fractional conversion rate of T_4 to T_3 in extrathyroidal tissues (notably the brain) increases. These mechanisms result in a relative overproduction of T_3 compared with T_4 and serve—in view of the greater biological potency of T_3 than T_4—to restrict the impact of thyroid hormone deficiency in peripheral tissues. This preferential T_3 production explains why in subclinical hypothyroidism the serum concentration of T_3 sometimes exceeds the upper normal limit. Progression of thyroid disease causes a greater decline in thyroidal

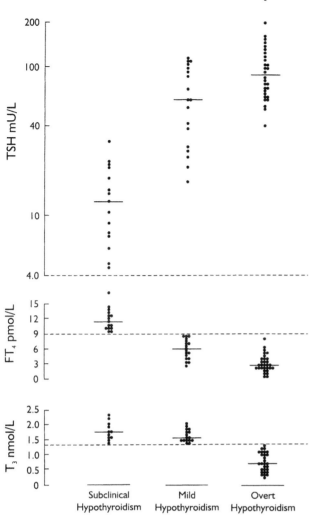

FIGURE 14-1. Individual and median values of thyroid function tests in various grades of primary hypothyroidism. Interrupted horizontal lines indicate upper (thyroid-stimulating hormone [TSH]) and lower (free thyroxine [FT$_4$] and triiodothyronine [T$_3$]) limits of the normal reference range. Progression from grade I to III can be observed in the transition from the euthyroid to the severely hypothyroid state and vice versa on treatment of hypothyroidism.

Grade I	Subclinical hypothyroidism	TSH slightly elevated	FT$_4$ normal	T$_3$ normal or slightly elevated
Grade II	Mild hypothyroidism	TSH moderately high	FT$_4$ low	T$_3$ normal
Grade III	Overt hypothyroidism	TSH very high	FT$_4$ low	T$_3$ low

Table 14-1. Prevalence and Incidence of Primary Hypothyroidism in Adults as Established in the Whickham Survey

		Women	**Men**
Prevalence	Hypothyroidism	18/1000	1/1000
	Unsuspected	3/1000	0/1000
	Known	15/1000	1/1000
	Subclinical hypothyroidism	75/1000	28/1000
Incidence	Hypothyroidism	4.1/1000/yr	0.6/1000/yr

Data from Tunbridge et al[4] and Vanderpump et al.[5]

secretion of T$_4$ and results in serum FT$_4$ levels below the normal reference range and a further rise in serum TSH; serum T$_3$ remains within normal limits because of maintenance of T$_3$ production. Finally, when serum T$_4$ has decreased even further, serum T$_3$ values fall into the subnormal range. Hypothyroidism is a graded phenomenon (Fig. 14-1) that ranges from subclinical hypothyroidism to myxedema coma, the most severe manifestation of the syndrome.

History

Hypothyroidism as a clinical syndrome was described in 1874 by Gull under the name of **myxedema** in view of the swollen skin **(edema)** and its excessive content of mucin **(myx-).** In 1883, Semon noted striking similarities between patients with myxedema and patients who had undergone total thyroidectomy. The Clinical Society of London nominated a committee to investigate this matter. In 1888, the committee reported in what has become a classic paper[3] that cretinism, myxedema, and post-thyroidectomy changes all were due to loss of thyroid function. In 1891, Murray reported cure of myxedema by hypodermic injections of sheep thyroid extract. Simply eating ground or dried animal thyroid tissue proved equally effective. The active principle of thyroid extract was isolated by Kendall on Christmas Day, 1914, and was named **thyroxine.** Harrington elucidated the precise constitution of thyroxine in 1926 and was able to synthesize it. Desiccated thyroid remained the usual treatment for hypothyroidism, however, because thyroxine was more expensive and less efficacious owing to poor absorption of the free acid. As of the 1960s, levothyroxine sodium surplanted gradually desiccated thyroid as the preferred treatment modality for hypothyroidism.

Epidemiology

Primary hypothyroidism is a common disease worldwide, especially in iodine-deficient areas. It also is a prevalent disease in iodine-replete regions. The most extensive epidemiologic data have been obtained from a population-based study of subjects 18 years old and older in Whickham County in northeast England (Table 14-1).[4,5] The initial survey was done between 1972 and 1974, with a follow-up 20 years later. The data seem representative of other countries inasmuch as similar figures have been reported from Sweden, Japan, and the United States.[6] Most striking are the high prevalence (especially of subclinical hypothyroidism), the marked female preponderance, and the increasing occurrence with advancing age. The mean age at diagnosis of hypothyroidism in women is 60 years. Most cases are due to chronic autoimmune thyroiditis (incidence of 3.5 per 1000 women per year), followed by destructive treatment for thyrotoxicosis (incidence of 0.6 per 1000 women per year). The probability of spontaneous hypothyroidism developing in women at a particular time increases with age: from 1.4 per 1000 per year at ages 20 to 25, to 14 per 1000 per year at 75 to 80 years. Risk factors for progression to overt hypothyroidism include the presence of thyroid autoantibodies and an already elevated TSH (Table 14-2). The risk correlates directly with the serum concentration of thyroid peroxidase autoantibodies and with the extent of the TSH increase. The probability that hypothyroidism will develop increases even at TSH levels in the high-normal range of 2 to 5 mU/L, independent of age or antibody status.[5,7]

Table 14-2. Percentage of Women Acquiring Spontaneous Primary Hypothyroidism During 20 Years of Follow-up in the Whickham Survey

| Initial Serum TSH | Initial Thyroid Autoantibodies | |
	Negative	Positive
Normal	4%	27%
Elevated	33%	55%

Data from Vanderpump et al[5] and Wang and Crapo.[6]
TSH, Thyroid-stimulating hormone.

Table 14-3. Causes of Hypothyroidism

Central (Hypothalamic/Pituitary) Hypothyroidism

Loss of functional tissue
  Tumors (pituitary adenoma, craniopharyngioma, meningioma, dysgerminoma, glioma, metastases)
  Trauma (surgery, irradiation, head injury)
  Vascular (ischemic necrosis, hemorrhage, stalk interruption, aneurysm of internal carotid artery)
  Infections (abscess, tuberculosis, syphilis, toxoplasmosis)
  Infiltrative (sarcoidosis, histiocytosis, hemochromatosis)
  Chronic lymphocytic hypophysitis
  Congenital (pituitary hypoplasia, septo-optic dysplasia, basal encephalocele)
Functional defects in TSH biosynthesis and release
  Mutations in genes encoding for TRH receptor, TSHβ, or pituitary transcription factors POUIFI, PROPI, LHX3, HESXI
  Drugs: dopamine, glucocorticoids, levothyroxine withdrawal, bexarotene

Primary (Thyroidal) Hypothyroidism

Loss of functional thyroid tissue
  Chronic autoimmune thyroiditis
  Reversible autoimmune hypothyroidism (silent and postpartum thyroiditis, cytokine-induced thyroiditis)
  Surgery and irradiation (^{131}I or external irradiation)
  Infiltrative and infectious diseases, subacute thyroiditis
  Thyroid dysgenesis
Functional defects in thyroid hormone biosynthesis and release
  Congenital defects in thyroid hormone biosynthesis
  Iodine deficiency and iodine excess
  Drugs: antithyroid agents, lithium, natural and synthetic goitrogenic chemicals, tyrosine kinase inhibitors

Peripheral (Extrathyroidal) Hypothyroidism

Mutations in genes encoding for MCT8, SECISBP2, or TRβ
Consumptive hypothyroidism

MCT8, Monocarboxylate transporter 8; *SECISBP2,* selenocysteine insertion sequence-binding protein 2; *TRH,* thyrotropin-releasing hormone; *TSH,* thyroid-stimulating hormone; *TRβ,* thyroid hormone receptor β.

Pathogenesis

The various causes of hypothyroidism can be classified according to their site of interference (in the hypothalamus-pituitary, in the thyroid gland, or in the peripheral target tissues) and their nature (organic lesions resulting in loss of functional tissue, or functional disturbances resulting in deficient hormone biosynthesis and release) (Table 14-3). Most cases of hypothyroidism are acquired and permanent; congenital hypothyroidism and transient forms of hypothyroidism are in the minority.

CENTRAL HYPOTHYROIDISM

Reduced T_4 secretion in central hypothyroidism is due to insufficient stimulation of the thyroid gland by TSH, which is caused by lesions in the pituitary (secondary hypothyroidism) or the hypothalamus (tertiary hypothyroidism resulting from deficient thyrotropin-releasing hormone [TRH] release). The term **central hypothyroidism** is preferred because lesions sometimes involve both sites, which prevents clear-cut distinction. Although an absent TSH response to exogenous TRH would suggest a pituitary cause, and a delayed response would suggest a hypothalamic cause,[8] the TSH profiles after TRH are not well correlated to the anatomic site of the lesion. Basal serum TSH values in central hypothyroidism can be low, normal, or even slightly elevated (up to 10 mU/L).[9,10] The apparent paradox of central hypothyroidism in the presence of a normal or increased serum TSH concentration is explained by the reduced biological activity of TSH in these patients related to abnormal sialylation of TSH. Central hypothyroidism also is associated with a decreased nocturnal TSH surge (because of loss of the usual nocturnal increase in TSH pulse amplitude, but not TSH pulse frequency), which might hamper further maintenance of normal thyroid function.[11,12]

The prevalence of central hypothyroidism in the general population is unknown; a rough estimate is 0.005%. The sex distribution is about equal, and central hypothyroidism occurs with peaks in childhood and in adults 30 to 60 years old.[13] Congenital cases are due to pituitary hypoplasia, midline defects such as septo-optic dysplasia (TSH deficiency in 20%), Rathke's pouch cysts, or rare loss-of-function mutations in genes encoding for TRH receptors, the TSH-β subunit, or pituitary transcription factors. Childhood cases are caused most often by craniopharyngioma (TSH deficiency in 53%) or cranial irradiation for brain tumors (TSH deficiency in 6%).[14] Adult cases most frequently are due to pituitary macroadenomas (hypothyroidism in 10% to 25%) and pituitary surgery or irradiation. TSH deficiency caused by loss of functional tissue usually becomes manifest after the development of growth hormone and gonadotropin deficiency.[13] TSH deficiency sometimes may disappear after selective adenomectomy.[15] Cranial radiotherapy for brain tumors causes hypothyroidism in 65%, depending on the radiation dose; the onset varies between 1 and 26 years after irradiation.[16]

Radiotherapy for pituitary tumors is followed by hypothyroidism in at least 15% (55% when combined with surgery).[17] Less common causes include traumatic brain injury and subarachnoid hemorrhage,[18] ischemic necrosis from postpartum hemorrhage (Sheehan's syndrome) and severe shock, pituitary apoplexy (hemorrhage in a pituitary adenoma), infiltrative diseases, and lymphocytic hypophysitis.[19] Lymphocytic hypophysitis most likely is an autoimmune disease that occurs predominantly in women during pregnancy and the postpartum period and is characterized by a pituitary mass and hypopituitarism.[19] Despite the many known causes of central hypothyroidism, idiopathic cases are still encountered.

In critically ill patients receiving dopamine, serum TSH and the T_4 production rate decrease by 60% and 56%, respectively, as a result of direct inhibition of pituitary TSH.[20] Transient functional inhibition of TSH release is observed after withdrawal of long-term levothyroxine suppressive therapy, which may last 6 weeks.[21] Glucocorticoid excess dampens pulsatile TSH release, which rarely results in decreased serum FT_4.[22] Octreotide therapy does not cause hypothyroidism despite its inhibition of TSH secretion. High doses of bexarotene, a specific retinoid X receptor agonist used in the treatment of cutaneous T cell lymphoma, cause central hypothyroidism by strongly inhibiting TSH secretion.[23]

CHRONIC AUTOIMMUNE THYROIDITIS

Hypothyroidism secondary to chronic autoimmune thyroiditis is caused mainly by destruction of thyrocytes. The goitrous variant (hypothyroid Hashimoto's goiter) is characterized by massive lymphocytic infiltration of the thyroid with the formation of germinal centers, oxyphilic changes in thyrocytes called Hürthle or Askanazy cells, and some fibrosis. In the atrophic variant (atrophic myxedema), fibrosis is the predominant feature, along with lymphocytic infiltration. The less common goitrous variant is characterized by a diffuse goiter of firm "rubbery" consistency; the histology remained essentially unaltered after 20 years, and the goiter did not regress despite T_4 treatment in 43% of cases.[24] Many patients with chronic autoimmune thyroiditis are euthyroid, and a few have an initial transient hyperthyroid stage (labeled as **Hashitoxicosis**). **Hashimoto's disease** is used by many authors as an umbrella term to indicate autoimmune-mediated destruction of thyrocytes, frequently but not always resulting in hypothyroidism, as opposed to Graves' disease, in which TSH receptor–stimulating antibodies usually result in hyperthyroidism. The two disease entities overlap and can be viewed as opposite ends of a continuous spectrum of thyroid autoimmunity. Destruction of thyrocytes and development of hypothyroidism in Hashimoto's disease are mediated by cytotoxic T cells and cytokines (especially interferon-γ and tumor necrosis factor) released by infiltrating T cells and macrophages. Humoral immunity appears less important in this respect, but (a subset of) thyroid peroxidase (TPO) antibodies may contribute via antibody-dependent, cell-mediated cytotoxicity, complement-mediated cytotoxicity, and inhibition of TPO enzymatic activity. TSH receptor–blocking antibodies enhance thyroid atrophy and hypothyroidism, possibly also by inducing apoptosis; their prevalence is low except in Japanese patients.[25]

Genetic and environmental factors enhance the susceptibility of individuals to develop the disease and may determine the direction of the evolving autoimmune reaction. Autoimmune thyroid disease runs in families (80% of patients have a positive family history) and is four to ten times more common in women. Autoimmune hypothyroidism in whites is weakly associated with HLA-DR and CTLA4 polymorphisms; other, still unidentified genes probably are involved. Iodine intake has been identified as an environmental factor because the prevalence of autoimmune hypothyroidism is higher in iodine-replete than in iodine-deficient areas,[26] and the incidence increases after supplemental iodine is introduced. Smoking decreases the risk for developing TPO antibodies and hypothyroidism.[27]

REVERSIBLE AUTOIMMUNE HYPOTHYROIDISM

Chronic Autoimmune Thyroiditis

Autoimmune hypothyroidism may revert spontaneously into euthyroidism in connection with the disappearance of TSH receptor–blocking antibodies.[28] The presence of a goiter and high thyroidal radioiodine uptake increase the likelihood of spontaneous recovery.[29] The incidence of spontaneous recovery is about 5%,[30] but in Japan—in the face of a high ambient iodine intake—iodide restriction alone restores euthyroidism in one third of patients.[29] Autoimmune hypothyroidism, however, is permanent in most patients. Peculiar cases of alternating hypothyroidism and hyperthyroidism are explained by changes in coexisting TSH receptor–blocking and TSH receptor–stimulating antibodies.[31]

Silent and Postpartum Thyroiditis

Silent or painless thyroiditis and postpartum thyroiditis are variant forms of chronic autoimmune thyroiditis. Thyroid histology shows lymphocytic infiltration with no germinal centers or fibrosis. The autoimmune attack is intense (resulting mainly in T cell–mediated destructive thyroiditis) but transient, which

explains the characteristic pattern of transient thyrotoxicosis followed by transient hypothyroidism in the recovery stage. Each stage lasts 2 to 8 weeks. Most patients remain asymptomatic and revert spontaneously to euthyroidism. Occurrence is common in the first year after delivery: The incidence of postpartum thyroiditis is 4% to 6% and 25% in patients with type 1 diabetes mellitus.[32-34] Several patterns are recognized: Thyrotoxicosis alone occurs in 38%, thyrotoxicosis followed by hypothyroidism occurs in 26%, and hypothyroidism alone occurs in 36%. TPO antibodies in serum of 100 kU/L or greater at 12 weeks' gestation predict to a certain extent postpartum thyroiditis (positive predictive value 0.50, negative predictive value 0.98).[33] Thyroid antibody titers decrease in the second and third trimesters and increase postpartum. Women with postpartum thyroiditis are at risk for recurrent postpartum thyroiditis after delivery (about 40%) and for permanent hypothyroidism (20% to 30% after 5 years) related to higher antibody titers and absence of a thyrotoxic phase.

Cytokine-Induced Thyroiditis

Treatment for malignant tumors or for hepatitis C or B with interleukin-2 or interferon-α is causally related to the de novo occurrence of TPO antibodies and the development of thyroid dysfunction.[35,36] Typical features are similar to features of silent and postpartum thyroiditis and include sudden onset, biphasic pattern of thyrotoxicosis followed by hypothyroidism (although hypothyroidism alone is most frequent), and spontaneous resolution after discontinuation of treatment. The incidence is about 6%; risk factors include female sex and preexisting TPO antibodies.[36]

POSTOPERATIVE AND POSTIRRADIATION HYPOTHYROIDISM

Surgery

Total thyroidectomy results in overt hypothyroidism within 1 month. Subtotal thyroidectomy for Graves' hyperthyroidism is followed by hypothyroidism in 40% after 10 years[37]; risk factors include a small thyroid remnant, lymphocytic infiltration, and subsequent exposure to iodine. Most patients become hypothyroid in the first year after surgery; thereafter, the cumulative incidence of hypothyroidism increases by only 1% to 2% per year. Immediate postoperative hypothyroidism does not always indicate permanent hypothyroidism; it may resolve spontaneously by 6 months. Subtotal thyroidectomy for (toxic) nodular goiter carries a much lower risk (about 15%) for postoperative hypothyroidism.

Radioactive Iodine

Radioactive iodine (^{131}I) treatment for Graves' hyperthyroidism results in a cumulative incidence of hypothyroidism of 70% after 10 years,[37] depending on the dose of ^{131}I administered. Most cases occur in the first year (spontaneous return to euthyroidism is observed in some patients); thereafter, the annual incidence of hypothyroidism is 0.5% to 2%, also related to persisting chronic autoimmune thyroiditis. Hypothyroidism after ^{131}I treatment for toxic nodular goiter is less common (6% to 13%).[38] ^{131}I treatment for nontoxic goiter to reduce goiter size carries a cumulative risk of 58% for the development of hypothyroidism in 8 years, the risk being related to the (relatively high) dose of ^{131}I and the presence of TPO antibodies.[39] Hypothyroidism caused by ionizing radiation has been reported in subjects exposed to atomic or hydrogen bomb explosions.

External Irradiation

External radiotherapy of the neck for Hodgkin's or non-Hodgkin's lymphoma causes hypothyroidism in 25% to 50% of patients; the risk is related to the radiation dose, the use of iodine-containing contrast agents before radiotherapy, and the duration of follow-up.[40] The risk is decreased when the thyroid is shielded during mantle field irradiation. External radiotherapy for head and neck cancer has an actuarial risk of 40% for the development of subclinical hypothyroidism and 15% for overt hypothyroidism 3 years after treatment.[41] Another study with a median follow-up of 4.4 years reports a 5-year incidence rate of 48%, with a median time of 1.4 years (range, 0.3 to 7.2 years) to the onset of elevated TSH values.[42] Total body irradiation with subsequent bone marrow transplantation for acute leukemia or aplastic anemia is associated with (mainly subclinical) hypothyroidism in about 25% and usually occurs after 1 year; it is transient in half of patients.[43]

INFILTRATIVE AND INFECTIOUS DISEASES

A rare cause of hypothyroidism is thyroidal infiltration by systemic disease.[44] Hypothyroidism is observed in the course of invasive fibrous thyroiditis of Riedel's (30% to 40%), cystinosis (86% in adults), progressive systemic sclerosis, and amyloidosis. Infections of the thyroid gland are rare and are associated with preexisting thyroid disease and immunocompromising conditions. Occasionally, damage to the thyroid causes hypothyroidism. In contrast, hypothyroidism in the recovery phase of subacute thyroiditis of de Quervain (related to previous viral infections) is a common event.

CONGENITAL HYPOTHYROIDISM

Congenital hypothyroidism can be permanent (incidence 1 in 3100 newborns) or transient. Causes include loss of functional thyroid tissue (thyroid dysgenesis), functional defects in thyroid hormone biosynthesis (related to loss-of-function mutations in genes encoding for the TSH receptor, Na^+/I^- symporter, thyroglobulin, TPO, dual oxidase 2, or dehalogenase 1), and thyroid hormone resistance (mutated TRβ).

IODINE DEFICIENCY AND IODINE EXCESS

Hypothyroidism can be caused by iodine deficiency or iodine excess. Inorganic iodide in excess of daily doses of 500 to 1000 μg inhibits organification of iodide, known as the **Wolff-Chaikoff effect**. Usually, the thyroid gland escapes the Wolff-Chaikoff effect after several weeks because autoregulatory mechanisms inhibit thyroid iodide transport, and the intrathyroidal iodine concentration consequently falls below the level required for inhibition of organification. Failure to escape results in hypothyroidism, which occurs in the presence of underlying thyroid disease, such as chronic autoimmune thyroiditis, previous subacute or postpartum thyroiditis, and ^{131}I or surgical therapy.[45] Iodide-induced hypothyroidism may be due to inorganic iodide or organic iodine compounds that are deiodinated in vivo. Sources of iodine excess include an iodine-rich diet (e.g., in Japan with high consumption of seaweed[29]) and iodine-containing medications, such as potassium iodide, vitamins, kelp, topical antiseptics, radiographic contrast agents, and amiodarone.[45] The incidence of amiodarone-induced hypothyroidism in areas with high environmental iodine intake is higher than in areas with low iodine intake (22% and 5%)[46]; cases occur predominantly in the first 18 months of amiodarone

treatment, especially in women with preexisting thyroid antibodies.[47]

DRUG-INDUCED HYPOTHYROIDISM

Drugs that cause hypothyroidism through interference with thyroid hormone production or release in the thyroid gland[48] include thiouracils and imidazoles (used as treatment for thyrotoxicosis), lithium, cytokines (see Reversible Autoimmune Hypothyroidism), iodine (see Iodine Deficiency and Iodine Excess), and a variety of environmental and industrial goitrogenic chemicals. Examples of the latter group include naturally occurring goitrogens, such as flavonoids and resorcinol (present in watersheds of the coal-rich and shale-rich regions of Colombia and Kentucky), and industrial pollution with polychlorinated biphenyls. Lithium inhibits thyroidal iodide transport and release of T_4 and T_3. Long-term lithium treatment results in goiter in 50%, subclinical hypothyroidism in about 20%, and hypothyroidism in about 20%; goiter and hypothyroidism usually occur in the first 2 years of treatment, especially in patients with preexisting thyroid antibodies. Tyrosine kinase inhibitors like sunitinib induce hypothyroidism in about 50%; the responsible mechanism is incompletely understood.[49,50]

CONSUMPTIVE HYPOTHYROIDISM

Hepatic and cutaneous hemangiomas often express high levels of type 3 iodothyronine-5-deiodinase (D_3), which catalyzes the conversion of T_4 and T_3 into biologically inactive rT_3 and $3,3'-T_2$. In infants with large hemangiomas, hypothyroidism can occur as the result of D_3-induced degradation of thyroid hormone at rates that exceed the synthetic capacity of the thyroid gland.[51,52] Removal of the tumor restores euthyroidism.

Clinical Features

Systemic manifestations vary considerably, depending on the cause, duration, and severity of the hypothyroid state. The characteristic clinical finding is slowing of physical and mental activity and many organ functions. The characteristic pathologic finding is accumulation of hyaluronic acid and other glycosaminoglycans in interstitial tissue, which is related to loss of the inhibitory effects of thyroid hormone on the synthesis of hyaluronate, fibronectin, and collagen by fibroblasts.[53] The hydrophilic properties of glycosaminoglycans lead to a peculiar mucinous nonpitting edema (myxedema) that is most obvious in the dermis but can be present in many organs.

ENERGY AND NUTRIENT METABOLISM

Thyroid hormone deficiency causes slowing of a wide variety of metabolic processes, which results in decreased resting energy expenditure, oxygen consumption, and use of substrates. Reduced thermogenesis is related to the characteristic cold intolerance of hypothyroid patients. The decline in metabolic rate and substrate use contributes to decreased appetite and food intake. Body weight increases on average by 10% because of an increase in body fat and retention of water and salt.

Serum leptin in some but not all studies is slightly low, returning to normal levels after treatment.[54,55] Whether thyroid hormone regulates leptin secretion independent of body mass index and body fat remains controversial.[56,57] The other adipocytokines have normal (adiponectin) or slightly low (resistin) serum concentrations.[55] Hypothyroidism delays glucose absorption from the intestine. Insulin secretion in response to oral glucose is appropriate for the slightly flattened oral glucose tolerance curve. Hepatic gluconeogenesis and glucose use usually remain normal, and blood glucose levels are maintained within normal limits. The occurrence of hypoglycemia in hypothyroid patients should alert the physician to concomitant diseases (e.g., hypopituitarism). The development of hypothyroidism in patients with insulin-dependent diabetes mellitus may require lowering of the insulin dose to counteract the decreased rate of insulin degradation.

Synthesis and degradation of proteins are reduced in hypothyroidism; one of the obvious consequences during childhood is impaired growth. Biosynthesis of fatty acids and lipolysis also are reduced. An increase in total cholesterol in serum occurs, largely as the result of an increase in low-density lipoprotein (LDL)-cholesterol (explained by decreased expression of the T_3-responsive liver LDL receptor, which is involved in LDL clearance), combined with an increase in apolipoprotein B, lipoprotein (a), and possible triglycerides.[58] An increase in the oxidizability of LDL particles occurs,[59] along with a decrease in the metabolism of serum remnant-like particles reflecting chylomicrons and very low-density lipoprotein (VLDL) remnants.[60] HDL2 but not HDL3 is increased modestly with higher apoprotein AI but not AII. The changes in serum lipids result in an atherogenic lipid profile that is reversible upon treatment.

SKIN AND APPENDAGES

Skin changes are prevalent among hypothyroid patients. The skin is dry, pale, thick, and rough with scales, and it feels cold. Dryness is related to decreased function of sebaceous and sweat glands. Pallor is related to decreased skin blood flow and anemia. Yellowish discoloration of the skin may be present, especially on the palms and soles, because of the deposition of carotene, which is converted to a lesser extent to vitamin A. The thick rough skin with scales is caused by mucinous swelling of the dermis and hyperkeratosis of the stratum corneum in the epidermis. The nonpitting swelling is most marked in the extremities and the face and gives rise to the so-called myxedema face (Fig. 14-2). This classic appearance of primary hypothyroidism is seen less often nowadays, probably because of earlier diagnosis achieved by widespread use of the TSH assay. The hair becomes dull, coarse, and brittle. Hair loss occurs in 50%; it usually is diffuse and involves the scalp, beard, and genital hair and less often the eyebrows. Nail deformities also are common: The nails become thin and brittle, have grooves, and grow more slowly.

NERVOUS SYSTEM

Thyroid hormones are essential for normal brain development; congenital hypothyroidism, if left untreated, results in mental retardation and neurologic abnormalities. In adult hypothyroid patients, a generalized decrease in regional cerebral blood flow and in cerebral glucose metabolism has been shown.[61] Studies using phosphorus 32 nuclear magnetic resonance spectroscopy of the frontal lobe of adult hypothyroid patients reported reversible alterations in phosphate metabolism.[62] The low-voltage electroencephalogram, prolonged central motor conduction time, and reduced visual and somatosensory-evoked potential amplitude with longer latency in adult hypothyroid patients are reversible with T_4 treatment. These findings indicate that the adult human brain is a thyroid hormone–responsive organ and provide a biological basis for the prevalent neurobehavioral symptoms and cognitive impairment associated with adult hypothyroidism.[61,63,64]

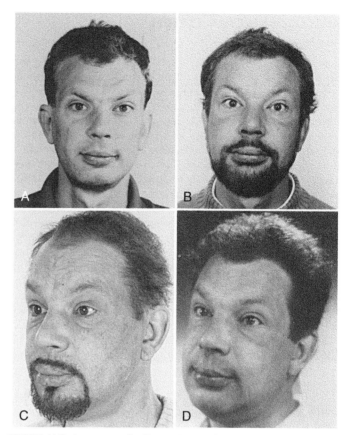

FIGURE 14-2. Appearance of a 47-year-old man 12 years **(A),** 5 years **(B),** and 3 years **(C)** before hypothyroidism secondary to atrophic myxedema **(D)** was diagnosed. Note the typical myxedema face characterized by puffy nonpitting swelling of the skin and coarse facial features. (Reproduced with permission of the patient.)

Typically, a hypothyroid patient is slow in movement and thought, is less alert, and is less able to concentrate and memorize. Speech becomes slow and often hoarse. Hearing can be impaired. The patient sleeps longer and may fall asleep during the daytime. Hypothyroidism is listed as one of the rare but treatable causes of dementia.[65] Patients may accept the limitations in physical and mental activity as part of the unavoidable aging process, but many become anxious or depressed. Rarely, severe anxiety and agitation occur, a condition known as **myxedematous madness.** Depression develops in more than 40%, most likely related to reduced synthesis and turnover of brain 5-hydroxytryptamine; central 5-hydroxytryptamine activity is reduced in hypothyroid patients.[66]

Thyroid hormone deficiency may give rise to several reversible neurologic syndromes. Cerebellar ataxia may occur, especially in elderly people, and is associated with an unsteady gait and intention tremor. More common (30%) is the carpal tunnel syndrome, which is linked to entrapment of the median nerve by thickening of the connective tissue of tendon sheaths.[67,68] Complaints of paresthesias occur in 64%, and signs of sensorimotor axonal neuropathy are observed in 42%.[67] Hashimoto's encephalopathy is a vaguely defined condition in which otherwise unexplained clinical manifestations of central nervous system dysfunction are linked to the presence of TPO antibodies; serum TSH can be normal or slightly elevated.[69] The condition responds to glucocorticoids, but the relationship to thyroid autoimmunity is currently uncertain.

MUSCULOSKELETAL SYSTEM

Muscles

Muscle symptoms are prevalent in hypothyroid patients and include myalgia, weakness, stiffness, cramps, and easy fatigability.[67,68,70] The biochemical substrate of these complaints is provided in part by an increase in the inorganic phosphate-to-adenosine triphosphate (ATP) ratio in resting muscle and by an important decrease in phosphocreatine in working hypothyroid muscle with a greater decrease in intracellular pH than in controls.[71] Impairment of mitochondrial oxidative metabolism also has been shown in subclinical hypothyroidism.[72] Transition from white fast type II to red slow type I muscle fibers is involved in the change in muscle bioenergetics, which is probably multifactorial. The histopathology varies; most common is type II fiber atrophy, but fiber hypertrophy may be present along with interstitial edema and sarcoplasmic degeneration.[70] Rarely, chronic hypothyroid myopathy results in increased volume of muscles (notably in the tongue and extremities), which may cause entrapment syndromes.[73] Serum creatine kinase (MM fraction derived from skeletal muscle) is often elevated and correlates with the severity of hypothyroidism. The decreased rate of muscle contractility in hypothyroidism is evident from slow deep tendon reflexes. The half-relaxation time of the Achilles reflex is prolonged in many hypothyroid patients, but substantial overlap is seen in euthyroid subjects.

Joints

Arthralgia and joint stiffness are common complaints. Synovial effusions (usually of the knee) are rare.

Bones

Hypothyroidism leads to decreased bone formation and bone resorption, but bone mineral density is comparable with that of matched controls. Urinary excretion of hydroxyproline and serum alkaline phosphatase and osteocalcin levels can be decreased; serum calcium is usually normal.

CARDIOVASCULAR SYSTEM

Changes in cardiovascular dynamics in hypothyroidism include an increase (of 50% to 60%) in peripheral vascular resistance and a decrease (of 30% to 50%) in cardiac output.[74,75] Aortic stiffness is increased.[76] As a result, mean blood pressure is largely unaltered, although systolic pressure may decrease and diastolic pressure may increase. The increase in systemic vascular resistance is due to endothelial dysfunction and impaired vascular smooth muscle relaxation. The decrease in cardiac output is due to a decrease in stroke volume and heart rate. The pre-ejection time and isovolumetric contraction time are prolonged, and the ventricular relaxation rate during diastole is slower.[75] The mechanism of reduced cardiac contractility with subnormal systolic and diastolic performance is multifactorial. Changes in T3-dependent myocardial gene expression are involved, especially in genes that code for calcium regulatory proteins.[77] Blood volume is decreased. Edema may develop through albumin extravasation as a result of increased capillary permeability; it may give rise to pericardial, pleural, or peritoneal effusions.

Cardiovascular symptoms of hypothyroid patients include dyspnea and decreased exercise tolerance; the hemodynamic response to exercise usually is preserved. Physical examination may reveal a slow pulse rate, diastolic hypertension (in 20%), weak heart sounds, occasionally cardiac enlargement (caused by pericardial effusion or, rarely, by T4-reversible cardiomyopathy[77]), and peripheral nonpitting or pitting edema (rarely caused by heart failure except when cardiac disease is preexisting). The electrocardiogram may show bradycardia, low-voltage conduction disturbances, and nonspecific ST-T changes. Symptomatic ischemic heart disease with anginal complaints occurs in about 3%; the reduced need for oxygen in view of the hypometabolic state might give some protection.[78] The atherogenic profile of serum lipids and the hyperhomocysteinemia[79] in hypothyroidism suggest a greater prevalence of coronary atherosclerosis in these patients.[80]

RESPIRATORY SYSTEM

Respiratory symptoms of hypothyroidism include shortness of breath and sleep apnea. Shortness of breath can be caused by the cardiac effects of thyroid hormone deficiency, by weakness of respiratory muscles, by pleural effusion, or by impaired pulmonary function. In most nonobese hypothyroid patients, pulmonary function is nearly normal. Reduced ventilatory drive is observed in 34%; the depressed response to hypercapnia or hypoxia usually is restored rapidly on T4 treatment.[81] Severe obstructive sleep apnea occurs in 7.7%,[82] in part as a result of increased size of the tongue and pharyngeal muscles with a slow and sustained muscle contraction; the contribution of reduced ventilatory drive to sleep apnea is less marked but can be substantial in obese patients.

UROGENITAL SYSTEM

Kidneys and Fluid Metabolism

Renal plasma flow and glomerular filtration rate are reduced in hypothyroidism in accordance with the changes in cardiovascular hemodynamics. Serum creatinine is increased by 10% to 20%, and hyponatremia sometimes occurs.[79,83] Hyponatremia is associated with increased total body water and sodium content in hypothyroidism, which is a result of the increased vascular permeability and extravascular accumulation of hydrophilic glycosaminoglycans. Free water clearance in hypothyroidism is diminished, regardless of the presence of hyponatremia. Plasma arginine vasopressin frequently is increased in hypothyroid patients; arginine vasopressin levels increase normally in response to hypertonic saline, but they are not suppressed normally after water ingestion. The syndrome of inappropriate antidiuresis in hypothyroidism is not fully understood,[84] but a purely renal vasopressin-independent mechanism seems to be involved,[85] presumably related to increased expression of aquaporin water channels in the kidney.[86] The significance of low serum atrial natriuretic peptide concentrations in hypothyroidism is unclear.[72]

REPRODUCTIVE SYSTEM

Juvenile hypothyroidism results in delayed sexual maturation; it seldom results in precocious puberty (explained by spillover of the action of TRH on gonadotropes and the action of TSH on follicle-stimulating hormone receptors[87,88]). In adult hypothyroid men, semen analysis is usually normal; erectile dysfunction is common but fully reversible.[89] Serum sex hormone–binding globulin, free testosterone, follicle-stimulating hormone, and luteinizing hormone levels most often are normal. In adult hypothyroid women, pulsatile gonadotropin release in the follicular phase is normal,[90] but the ovulatory surge may not occur. Irregular—often anovulatory—cycles occur in 23% (three times as often as in the general population); oligomenorrhea and menorrhagia are most common.[91] Some patients are seen initially with the galactorrhea-amenorrhea syndrome, which is due to hyperprolactinemia induced by thyroid hormone deficiency. Despite restricted fertility, conception may occur with a successful pregnancy outcome. Pregnancy-induced hypertension is two to three times more common in hypothyroid women. The prevalence of an elevated TSH among pregnant women is about 2%.[92] The IQs of children born to affected mothers are 7 points lower than the IQs of controls.[93] The spontaneous abortion rate is higher in hypothyroid mothers who do not receive adequate levothyroxine treatment than in mothers who do.[94]

GASTROINTESTINAL SYSTEM

Hypothyroidism causes a decrease in electrical and motor activity of the esophagus, stomach, small intestine, and colon. Gastric emptying and intestinal transit times are prolonged.[95] The decreased motility explains the common complaint of constipation, which may range from mild to severe (rarely with paralytic ileus and intestinal pseudo-obstruction). Small intestinal bacterial overgrowth is common,[96] but intestinal absorption is mostly normal. Malabsorption may be due to pernicious anemia or celiac disease, both of which frequently are associated with autoimmune hypothyroidism. About 25% of patients with chronic autoimmune thyroiditis have parietal cell antibodies; some patients have achlorhydria and vitamin B_{12} malabsorption. Myxedematous ascites is rare.

Slightly abnormal liver function test results are common[97] but usually fully reversible (except when caused by associated autoimmune liver disease). Hypotonia of the gallbladder may occur.

HEMATOPOIETIC SYSTEM

Erythrocytes

Anemia occurs in about 30% and usually is mild and normocytic normochromic. It develops as a normal response to the decreased oxygen requirement and results in a decrease in erythropoietin and erythropoiesis with slight bone marrow hypoplasia. Because of the concomitant decrease in plasma volume, the anemia is less marked than it otherwise would be. The anemia disappears slowly with T_4 treatment. Microcytic hypochromic anemia is seen in 2% to 15% and most often is due to iron deficiency caused by excessive menstrual bleeding or by reduced iron absorption in the case of hypochlorhydria; both conditions are common in hypothyroid women. Macrocytic hyperchromic anemia indicates vitamin B_{12} or folic acid deficiency and is caused by the hypothyroid state itself or by pernicious anemia associated with chronic autoimmune thyroiditis.

Leukocytes and Thrombocytes

Granulocyte, lymphocyte, and platelet counts usually are normal in hypothyroidism. Leukopenia might indicate associated vitamin B_{12} or folic acid deficiency. Mean platelet volume can be decreased.

Hemostasis

Hypothyroid patients may have bleeding symptoms, such as easy bruising, menorrhagia, or prolonged bleeding after tooth extraction. Hypothyroidism is associated with a hypocoagulable state: Bleeding time in vivo and clotting time in vitro are prolonged. Coagulation tests reveal low or normal factor VIII activity and decreased von Willebrand factor antigen and activity.[98,99] Desmopressin rapidly reduces these abnormalities[100] and may be valuable for the acute treatment of bleeding or as cover for surgery. Usually the clinical relevance of these abnormalities is limited, as illustrated by no excess blood loss or bleeding complications during and after surgery in a large series of hypothyroid patients.[101]

ENDOCRINE SYSTEM

Pituitary

The decrease in growth hormone secretion in hypothyroidism is related to an increase in hypothalamic somatostatinergic tone[102] and results in low insulin-like growth factor (IGF-1) serum concentrations. It may cause dramatic growth retardation in hypothyroid children. Serum IGF-2, IGF-binding protein-1 (IGFBP-1), and IGFBP-3 are also decreased, whereas IGFBP-2 is increased; these changes are reversed with T_4 treatment.[103]

Moderate hyperprolactinemia occurs in 8% of hypothyroid patients, especially in young women, but is not related to the severity of thyroid hormone deficiency.[104] It may cause galactorrhea and amenorrhea, particularly in long-standing hypothyroidism. Increased expression of hypothalamic TRH due to diminished negative feedback exerted by T_3 might explain the (reversible) hyperprolactinemia in hypothyroidism.

Hypothyroidism in the presence of a pituitary mass does not always indicate central hypothyroidism. The hypersecretion of TSH in primary hypothyroidism is accompanied by hyperplasia and hypertrophy of pituitary thyrotrophs. Rarely, this alteration may cause a distinct pituitary macroadenoma in severely hypothyroid patients with high TSH levels (even with impaired vision) that shrinks after thyroid hormone therapy.[105]

Parathyroid

Thyroid hormone deficiency reduces the activity of osteoclasts and osteoblasts (only the latter possess nuclear T_3 receptors), which results in a slow rate of bone resorption and formation in the bone structural unit. Because of decreased bone resorption, serum calcium levels are decreased slightly, followed by an increase in parathyroid hormone and 1,25-dihydroxyvitamin D and an increase in intestinal calcium absorption. Calcium losses in urine and feces are decreased.

Adrenal Cortex

Metabolic clearance and, to a lesser extent, production of cortisol are decreased in hypothyroidism[106]; serum cortisol and 24-hour urinary cortisol remain within normal limits. The adrenal response to exogenous adrenocorticotropic hormone and the pituitary response to hypoglycemia or metyrapone usually are maintained or slightly decreased. Some patients with chronic autoimmune thyroiditis have associated autoimmune adrenalitis. Hypocortisolemia by itself may cause slightly elevated TSH levels that return to normal with glucocorticoid replacement, illustrating the negative feedback of cortisol on TSH secretion.[107]

Hypothyroidism decreases angiotensinogen production in the liver and serum angiotensin-converting enzyme and plasma renin activity. Serum aldosterone remains normal: The decrease in clearance is neutralized by a decrease in secretion.[74] The effects of these changes in the renin-angiotensin-aldosterone system are minimal and are not responsible for the hypertension in hypothyroid patients.

Sympathoadrenal System

Serum norepinephrine concentrations are increased in hypothyroid patients because of an increased production rate; epinephrine production is not affected. The increased central sympathetic output seems to be compensatory for the reduced response to catecholamines in target tissues such as the heart.[108] Mechanisms involved include a reduced number of β-adrenergic receptors and postreceptor defects, which contributes to impaired lipolysis, glycogenolysis, and gluconeogenesis.

Diagnosis

Two phases can be distinguished in the diagnosis of hypothyroidism. First, it should be ascertained whether a thyroid hormone deficiency exists (syndromal diagnosis). Thereafter, the cause of the demonstrated thyroid hormone deficiency should be looked for (nosologic diagnosis). Diagnosis of the hypothyroid syndrome starts with the history and physical examination and ends—in the case of sufficient clinical suspicion—with an assay of TSH and FT$_4$ in serum. One of the rationales for clinical examination is to increase the pretest likelihood of hypothyroidism so that fewer patients need hormone tests; because of the higher prevalence of hypothyroidism in the remaining patients, the diagnostic accuracy of hormone tests increases. The rationale for a nosologic diagnosis is to look for cases of potentially reversible hypothyroidism and increase awareness of the possible existence of other conditions associated with a specific cause.

SYNDROMAL DIAGNOSIS

Clinical Assessment

Statistical methods based on the frequency of symptoms and signs in patients and controls have been applied to the clinical diagnosis of hypothyroidism. The Billewicz score consists of points given in a weighted manner for the presence or absence of 17 symptoms and signs.[109] Application of this score to patients suspected of having hypothyroidism increases the pretest probability of hypothyroidism by 15% to 19%.[110] A simpler score is derived by awarding 1 point each for the presence of 12 symptoms and signs (Table 14-4)[111]; because of a high frequency in euthyroid controls, cold intolerance and pulse rate had predictive values less than 70% and were excluded from the score. The score was higher in older than in younger control women; cor-

rection for age is done by adding 1 point for women younger than age 55. The positive predictive value for hypothyroidism is 96.9% with a score of 6 or more points; the negative predictive value for exclusion of hypothyroidism is 94.2% with a score of 2 points or less. Sixty-two percent of all overt hypothyroid and 24% of subclinical hypothyroid patients are classified as clinically hypothyroid by this new score; the corresponding figures with the Billewicz score are 42% and 6%. Receiver operating curves of both scores, however, are similar.

The clinical diagnosis of hypothyroidism can be easy but also difficult because of the nonspecific nature of the symptoms and signs and the marked diversity of findings.[112] It is incompletely understood why the clinical manifestations of thyroid hormone deficiency vary considerably among patients. Chilliness, paresthesias, weight gain, and muscle cramps occur less frequently in elderly patients, who also have fewer clinical signs than younger patients.[113] Smokers have more severe manifestations of hypothyroidism.[114]

Biochemical Assessment

The ideal diagnostic test for hypothyroidism would be one that accurately measures the effect of thyroid hormone deficiency on target tissues. Peripheral tissue function tests, such as serum cholesterol and creatine kinase, lack sufficient sensitivity and specificity to be of much use. Serum TSH is the best assay for detection of hypothyroidism. By using the flow diagram presented in Fig. 14-3, the following results can be obtained:

1. **TSH normal.** Euthyroidism is almost certain, and no additional tests are necessary. The only exception is central hypothyroidism; usually, clinical examination offers sufficient clues to suspect hypothalamic/pituitary disease because isolated TSH deficiency is rare.
2. **TSH elevated, FT$_4$ decreased.** Primary hypothyroidism is almost always present. In a few cases, TSH values of 5 to 15 mU/L are associated with central hypothyroidism.
3. **TSH elevated, FT$_4$ normal.** The results indicate subclinical hypothyroidism and sometimes nonthyroidal illness.
4. **TSH elevated, FT$_4$ increased.** This peculiar combination of test results indicates one of the rare patients with thyroid

Table 14-4. Accuracy of 12 Symptoms and Signs in the Diagnosis of Primary Hypothyroidism

Symptoms and Signs	Sensitivity, %	Specificity, %	Positive Predictive Value, %	Negative Predictive Value, %	Score if Present
Symptoms					
Hearing impairment	22	98	90	53	1
Diminished sweating	54	86	80	65	1
Constipation	48	85	76	62	1
Paresthesia	52	83	75	63	1
Hoarseness	34	88	73	57	1
Weight increase	54	78	71	63	1
Dry skin	76	64	68	73	1
Physical Signs					
Slow movements	36	99	97	61	1
Periorbital puffiness	60	96	94	71	1
Delayed ankle reflex	77	94	92	80	1
Coarse skin	60	81	76	67	1
Cold skin	50	80	71	62	1
Sum of all symptoms and signs if present*					12†

From Zulewski H, Müller B, Exer P, et al: Estimation of tissue hypothyroidism by a new clinical score: evaluation of patients with various grades of hypothyroidism and controls. J Clin Endocrinol Metab 82:771–776, 1997. Copyright © 1997, The Endocrine Society.
*Add 1 point for women younger than 55 years.
†Hypothyroid, ≥6 points; intermediate, 3 to 5 points; euthyroid, ≤2 points.

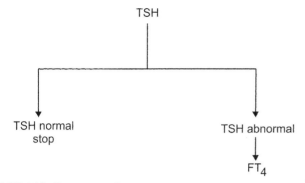

FIGURE 14-3. Flow diagram for the biochemical diagnosis of hypothyroidism. *FT₄,* Free thyroxine; *TSH,* thyroid-stimulating hormone.

hormone resistance or thyrotoxicosis caused by a TSH-producing adenoma.

5. **TSH decreased, FT₄ decreased.** These results are compatible with central hypothyroidism, hypothyroidism after recent therapy for thyrotoxicosis, or nonthyroidal illness.
6. **TSH decreased, FT₄ increased or normal.** Hypothyroidism is excluded. The results indicate overt thyrotoxicosis, subclinical hyperthyroidism, or rarely, nonthyroidal illness.

NOSOLOGIC DIAGNOSIS

The history and physical examination usually provide important clues to the cause of the hypothyroidism. Symptoms and signs of hypopituitarism and pituitary mass effects suggest the presence of central hypothyroidism. Physical examination may reveal a goiter, but many, if not most, hypothyroid patients have no palpable thyroid gland. Goitrous hypothyroidism occurs in goitrous Hashimoto's disease (with the characteristic firm rubbery consistency), in postpartum and subacute thyroiditis, in iodine deficiency, in iodine excess (small firm goiter), and in drug-induced cases. The most useful laboratory test is the assay of TPO antibodies indicating chronic autoimmune thyroiditis. Thyroid scans usually show low, inhomogeneous uptake of the radioisotope.

Clues for potentially reversible hypothyroidism can be obtained from the history (recent delivery? exposure to iodine excess? use of antithyroid drugs? recent thyroid surgery or ¹³¹I therapy?). In patients with chronic autoimmune thyroiditis, the presence of a goiter, preserved thyroidal radioiodine uptake, and homogeneous distribution of the tracer increase the likelihood of reversible hypothyroidism.[29]

Recovery of hypothyroidism by elimination of its cause is possible in cases secondary to (antithyroid) drugs or iodine excess. Spontaneous recovery from hypothyroidism in the natural course of the disease is the rule in subacute thyroiditis; it is common in postpartum thyroiditis, occurs less frequently in hypothyroidism that develops in the first 6 months after surgery or ¹³¹I therapy for thyrotoxicosis, and is exceptional (5%) in chronic autoimmune thyroiditis.

Treatment

Most hypothyroid patients need lifelong replacement therapy with T₄. In the few patients with a high likelihood of reversible hypothyroidism, one may refrain from treatment or, if symptoms and signs are severe, prescribe T₄ for a few months. The goal of treatment is restoration of the euthyroid state in all tissues. Gradual disappearance of the systemic manifestations of hypothyroidism can be expected several weeks to months after initiation of therapy; symptoms and signs related to the skin, appendages, and nervous system resolve slowly. Treatment of hypothyroid patients is gratifying because the symptoms and signs are usually fully reversible.

REPLACEMENT WITH THYROXINE

T₄ is prescribed as levothyroxine sodium, which comes in tablets of different strength. The sodium salt increases the gastrointestinal absorption of levothyroxine, which is greater in the fasting (80%) than in the fed state (60%).[115] Absorption of T₄ seems to be greater in the evening at 22.00 hours than in the morning at 06.30 hours before breakfast.[116] Generic and brand name levothyroxine preparations are most often bioequivalent,[117] but altered bioavailability from changes in the formulation of preparations has been reported.[118] About 25% of the exogenous T₄ is converted into T₃ and provides 80% of the circulating T₃ pool.[115] The half-life of serum T₄ is approximately 7 days, which allows a single daily dose of levothyroxine sodium. Omission of an occasional tablet has little or no clinical relevance.

The initial daily dose of levothyroxine sodium depends on the severity and the duration of the hypothyroid state, the age of the patient, and the coexistence of cardiac disease. In the case of mild hypothyroidism, short duration of hypothyroidism, young age, and no heart disease, one may opt to start with a full replacement dose (on average 1.6 μg/kg/d, but with large interindividual variation).[119] In the case of more severe or long-standing hypothyroidism, older age, and especially the presence of ischemic heart disease, it is prudent to start with a low dose (25 to 50 μg daily). Too high a starting dose under these circumstances may be poorly tolerated by the patient, who is accustomed to a low metabolic rate, which is now reversed. The patient may experience agitation, palpitations, and worsening or development of anginal complaints because of the increased need for oxygen. Individualization of the initial dose is recommended, and the same holds true for the rate at which the initial dose is increased until the full replacement dose has been reached. In high-risk cases, the daily levothyroxine sodium dose can be increased by 25 to 50 μg every 4 weeks, and it takes 3 to 6 months before the euthyroid state is restored. The mean replacement dose of levothyroxine sodium is 125 μg daily, in line with the daily production rate of 100 μg of thyroxine in normal subjects; it varies, however, between 50 and 200 μg (Fig. 14-4). The final dose required is a function of body weight (especially lean body mass) and initial TSH value,[120] but it is not always predictable. The dose should be titrated against serum TSH and FT₄ concentrations. These assays should be done no earlier than 4 to 6 weeks after a change in T₄ dose, when a new steady state has been established. One aims for TSH values in the low normal range, which results in FT₄ values that are significantly higher than values in controls (see Fig. 14-4) and often slightly above the upper normal limit.[115] The high T₄ levels under these circumstances serve to maintain serum T₃ (predominantly derived from 5'-deiodination of T₄) in the midnormal range. In patients with central hypothyroidism, one should rely primarily on normalization of serum FT₄, which frequently suppresses serum TSH to less than 0.1 mU/L.[121]

Some patients feel better with a slightly higher dose of levothyroxine sodium and consequently suppressed TSH. This dose can be accepted as long as serum T₃ is still within the normal range and serum TSH is (arbitrarily) not lower than 0.2 mU/L.

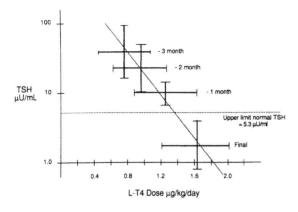

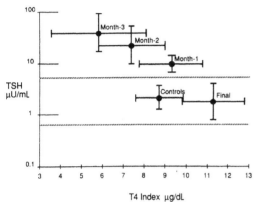

FIGURE 14-4. Dosage titration of levothyroxine (L-T4) *(top panel)* and the free thyroxine (T4) index *(bottom panel)* as a function of serum thyroid-stimulating hormone (TSH). Values are expressed by month, counting backward from the final dose. The bars represent 1 standard deviation from the mean. (Reprinted from Fish LH, Schwartz HL, Cavanaugh J, et al: Replacement dose, metabolism, and bioavailability of levothyroxine in the treatment of hypothyroidism: role of triiodothyronine in pituitary feedback in humans. N Engl J Med 316:764–770, 1987. Copyright © 1987, Massachusetts Medical Society. All rights reserved.)

Table 14-5. Conditions Requiring Adjustment of the Replacement Dose of Thyroxine for Hypothyroidism

Increased Dose Requirement

Decreased intestinal absorption of T_4
  Malabsorption (e.g., celiac disease) and short-bowel syndrome[127]
  Dietary fiber supplements[128]
  Drugs: bile acid sequestering agents (colestipol, cholestyramine[129]),
    α-sucralfate,[130] aluminum hydroxide,[131] ferrous sulfate,[132] raloxifene,[133]
    calcium carbonate[134]
Increased need for T_4
  Weight gain
  Estrogens[135]
  Pregnancy[136]
Increased clearance of T_4
  Phenobarbital, phenytoin, carbamazepine, rifampicin[137]
Precise mechanism unknown
  Amiodarone,[138] sertraline,[139] chloroquine[140]
Noncompliance[141]

Decreased Dose Requirement

Decreased need for T_4
  Weight loss
  Androgens[142]
Decreased clearance of T_4
  Old age[143]

decreases the bioavailability of T_4 and necessitates a higher dose in patients with high intake of dietary fiber (whole-wheat bread, granola, bran).[128] T_4 and T_3 conjugates are excreted in bile and partially deconjugated in the intestine, with the release of small amounts of T_4 and T_3 for reabsorption. Interference with this enterohepatic circulation of thyroid hormone by bile acid–sequestering agents may cause a slight increase in TSH in levothyroxine-treated patients, but not in normal subjects.[129] Other drugs, such as sucralfate,[130] aluminum hydroxide,[131] ferrous sulfate,[132] raloxifene,[133] and calcium carbonate,[134] also decrease the absorption of T_4. Serum T_4 is often above normal in many levothyroxine-treated patients with normal TSH. The effect of these drug interactions is modest and largely can be avoided by taking levothyroxine sodium and the other drug several hours apart.

Considerable weight gain may increase the need for T_4. Estrogen therapy[135] and pregnancy[136] also require additional thyroid hormone in most hypothyroid patients, probably because of increased serum concentrations of T_4-binding globulin. Levothyroxine requirements increase by about 50% in most pregnant women during the first half of pregnancy and plateau by week 16; median onset of TSH increase occurs at 8 weeks' gestation.[136] It is prudent to anticipate these events, and assessment of thyroid function in each trimester is recommended. After delivery, the dose used before pregnancy can be reinstituted.

Several antiepileptic and tuberculostatic drugs increase the clearance of T_4 by stimulating the mixed-function oxygenases responsible for hepatic drug oxidation.[137] Serum TSH increases in levothyroxine-treated hypothyroid patients when amiodarone is administered,[138] possibly as a result of the inhibition of T_4 conversion into T_3. The mechanism by which other drugs, such as sertraline[139] and chloroquine,[140] increase T_4 requirements is unknown. The most common reason for persistently elevated TSH values despite apparently adequate replacement doses is poor compliance of the patient with intake of levothyroxine tablets. Noncompliance is a challenge to the treating physician who seeks to solve this difficult management problem; in the process, it is important to not lose the patient's confidence. One

TSH values of 0.1 mU/L or less carry a risk for atrial fibrillation[122] and bone loss[123] (especially in postmenopausal women). Long-term levothyroxine therapy at TSH-suppressive doses increases the risk for ischemic heart disease in patients younger than age 65 years.[124] No or just a slight excess of fractures has been observed in patients maintained with levothyroxine even if TSH is suppressed.[125,126]

Lifelong treatment with levothyroxine sodium, when properly monitored, seems to be free of complications. Long-term morbidity and mortality are normal. Cutaneous allergy to the dye used to color the tablets is rarely observed.

FACTORS REQUIRING DOSE ADJUSTMENT

When euthyroidism has been restored by the full replacement dose of levothyroxine, this usually suffices to check the patient's thyroid state once a year. The main reason for the annual follow-up visit is to enhance compliance with lifelong levothyroxine sodium treatment. Some patients need adjustment of the levothyroxine sodium dose for reasons outlined in Table 14-5.

Increased Dose Requirement

T_4 is absorbed mainly from the small intestine, which explains the higher dose requirements in malabsorption and short-bowel syndromes.[127] Nonspecific absorption of T_4 by dietary fibers option is to administer levothyroxine under supervision once weekly.[141] A slightly larger dose than seven times the normal daily dose may be required; a single weekly dose of 1000 μg of levothyroxine sodium given orally seems to be effective and well tolerated.

Decreased Dose Requirement

Considerable weight loss may decrease the need for levothyroxine. In women receiving long-term levothyroxine replacement therapy, administration of androgens for breast cancer may result—via a decrease in serum T_4-binding globulin—in thyrotoxicosis within 4 weeks; the levothyroxine dose has to be reduced by 25% to 50%.[142] Production and metabolic clearance rates of T_4 are slightly decreased in old age; the net result is no change in the serum FT_4 concentration. The levothyroxine replacement dose decreases in elderly people by about 25% in association with the decrease in lean body mass with age.[143]

OTHER THYROID HORMONE PREPARATIONS

Animal Thyroid Extract

Extracts of animal thyroid glands (primarily cattle) were the first thyroid hormone preparations available. Desiccated thyroid, although effective, is no longer used in view of the lack of precise standardization and the availability of synthetic levothyroxine. After ingestion of desiccated thyroid, elevated serum concentrations of T_3 can occur in the postabsorptive period and cause transient thyrotoxic symptoms, such as palpitations. These effects do not occur after a dose of levothyroxine, which is converted gradually into T_3.

Liothyronine Sodium

After oral liothyronine administration, serum T_3 concentrations reach elevated values within hours, with a decline to basal levels in the next couple of hours. The half-life of liothyronine is approximately 1 day. Liothyronine preparations can be useful in the management of patients with thyroid cancer or myxedema coma.

Combination of Levothyroxine and Liothyronine

Synthetic levothyroxine and liothyronine have been combined in a single tablet in a ratio of 4:1. New interest in this kind of formula has been inspired by animal studies showing that the euthyroid state of thyroidectomized rats could be restored in all tissues only by the combination of levothyroxine and liothyronine and not by levothyroxine alone,[144] and likewise by human studies reporting impaired psychological well-being and neurocognitive functioning of hypothyroid patients despite adequate treatment with thyroxine.[145,146] However, a meta-analysis of 11 randomized clinical trials found no differences in the effectiveness of T_4 and T_3 combination therapy versus T_4 monotherapy in terms of bodily pain, depression, anxiety, fatigue, and quality of life.[147]

INTERFERENCE WITH COEXISTENT CONDITIONS

Cortisol Deficiency

Treatment for hypothyroidism in patients with glucocorticoid deficiency may provoke adrenal insufficiency because the adrenal is incapable of meeting the increasing demand for cortisol caused by the increased metabolic rate. Glucocorticoids should be given before levothyroxine therapy is started.

Ischemic Heart Disease

Levothyroxine increases the need for oxygen in the myocardium. Worsening or de novo development of anginal complaints should call for tempering of the levothyroxine dose or institution of antianginal drugs. Alternatively, coronary artery bypass surgery or angioplasty is a safe procedure, even when euthyroidism has not yet been restored.[101,148]

Surgery

Surgery in hypothyroid patients is associated with increased risk for several minor perioperative complications.[101] A higher incidence of heart failure and gastrointestinal and neuropsychiatric complications has been reported. Patients have fever less frequently with infection.

Drugs

The metabolism of many drugs is slowed in hypothyroidism, which results in higher sensitivity to a loading dose and a lower maintenance dose. Hypothyroid patients can experience marked respiratory depression after a single small dose of morphine. Restoration of the euthyroid state may require dose adjustments, for example, an increase in the dose of digoxin or insulin. Treatment for adult growth hormone deficiency with recombinant human growth hormone decreases serum FT_4, sometimes into the hypothyroid range.[149]

Myxedema Coma

Myxedema coma is a rare, life-threatening clinical condition in patients with long-standing, severe untreated hypothyroidism. The term is largely a misnomer because most patients are not comatose. Rather, the entity represents a form of decompensated hypothyroidism in which a precipitating event leads to functional disorders of the cardiovascular and central nervous systems, which, if not recognized and reversed, frequently have a fatal outcome.[150]

PATHOGENESIS

A normal body core temperature is preserved in compensated hypothyroidism because of neurovascular adaptations, including chronic peripheral vasoconstriction, mild diastolic hypertension, and diminished blood volume. The hypothyroid heart also compensates by performing more work at a given amount of oxygen through better coupling of ATP to contractile events. These adaptations to thyroid hormone deficiency maintain homeostasis, albeit at a precarious balance. A further reduction in blood volume (e.g., secondary to gastrointestinal bleeding or the use of diuretics) may disrupt this precarious balance, which homeostatic mechanisms are no longer able to restore. Likewise, the already compromised ventilatory drive may progress to respiratory failure by intercurrent pulmonary infection. Impairment in central nervous system function can be provoked further by stroke, the use of sedatives, and hyponatremia (a common phenomenon in severe hypothyroidism).

DIAGNOSIS

The three key diagnostic features of myxedema coma are as follows:

1. **Altered mental status:** from disorientation and lethargy to psychosis and coma

2. **Defective thermoregulation:** hypothermia or the absence of fever despite infectious disease
3. **Precipitating event:** cold exposure, infection, drugs (diuretics, sedatives, tranquilizers), trauma, stroke, heart failure, gastrointestinal bleeding

Most cases of myxedema coma occur in elderly women in winter. Early recognition is crucial, but in many cases the condition is diagnosed late, often after inadequate response to treatment for the precipitating event. The presence of cool pale skin and the absence of mild diastolic hypertension are warning signs of impending myxedema coma. Serum FT_4 is low; serum TSH is usually high but sometimes is elevated only slightly because of the effect of intercurrent nonthyroidal illness. Serum creatine phosphokinase most often is extremely elevated.

TREATMENT

Rapid institution of thyroid hormone replacement therapy and supportive measures (Table 14-6) is essential for a successful outcome; the prognosis remains poor, however, with a mortality of at least 20%. Patients should be monitored closely for vital signs.

No consensus has been reached regarding the most appropriate dose, route of administration, and form (liothyronine or levothyroxine) of thyroid hormone replacement. Too high a dose may provoke cardiac ischemia and arrhythmias. Oral administration may be less efficacious because of reduced gastrointestinal absorption. T_3 abruptly increases metabolism, which carries a risk for cardiac complications, but T_4 may be converted less well into T_3 because of nonthyroidal illness. The severity of the patient's condition might be considered, but clinical experience indicates that too conservative an approach worsens the outcome. Current recommendations include a starting dose of 300 to 500 µg of levothyroxine given intravenously, followed by 50 to 100 µg of levothyroxine intravenously daily until oral medication can be taken. If no improvement is seen within 24 to 48 hours, liothyronine might be given (e.g., 10 µg given intravenously every 4 hours or 25 µg given intravenously every 8 hours).

Hypothermia is treated just with blankets; active rewarming is dangerous because the peripheral vasodilation induced may provoke vascular collapse. Mechanical respiratory assistance is indicated at the first signs of respiratory failure, and one should not delay endotracheal intubation. Hypoxia is worsened by anemia, a common finding in hypothyroidism. In case of hypotension, transfusion of whole blood may restore blood volume and oxygen-carrying capacity. Digoxin and diuretics should be used cautiously for congestive heart failure. Hypoglycemia might indicate hypopituitarism or primary adrenal insufficiency; however, also in the absence of hypoglycemia or hypocortisolemia, all patients should receive intravenous hydrocortisone

(100 to 200 mg daily in divided doses) in view of the blunted cortisol response to stress in severe hypothyroidism. Finally, one should try to identify precipitating factors and eliminate them if possible. Infection (pneumonia or urosepsis) is present in 35% but is not easily detected because fever, tachycardia, and leukocytosis are usually absent. A differential count of leukocytes and cultures should be ordered, and broad-spectrum antibiotics are indicated even if the suspicion of infection is modest.

Subclinical Hypothyroidism and Screening

Subclinical hypothyroidism is defined as an elevated serum TSH concentration in the presence of normal serum FT_4 and T_3. It is a prevalent condition (see Table 14-1) that occurs most often in women and elderly people.[4] The causes can be endogenous (chronic autoimmune thyroiditis, subacute thyroiditis, postpartum thyroiditis) or exogenous (^{131}I therapy, thyroidectomy, antithyroid drugs).

The natural course of subclinical hypothyroidism secondary to chronic autoimmune thyroiditis is reasonably well known.[5] Spontaneous return to normal TSH values occurs in 5% to 6%. Progression to overt hypothyroidism is a common event, especially if thyroid antibodies are present (see Table 14-2); the annual incidence is about 5%.

SYSTEMIC MANIFESTATIONS

The term **subclinical hypothyroidism** suggests the absence of symptoms and signs of thyroid hormone deficiency, but clinical experience tells otherwise. Nonspecific complaints (fatigue and weight gain), depressive feelings, and mild cognitive disturbances (poor ability to concentrate, poor memory) can be present. Subjects score higher on a clinical scale for hypothyroidism (Fig. 14-5).[111] Peripheral tissue function tests frequently indicate a limited degree of thyroid hormone deficiency; examples include prolongation of the Achilles tendon reflex relaxation time, prolongation of systolic time intervals, a decrease in cardiac

Table 14-6. Characteristics and Treatment of Myxedema Coma

Hypothyroxinemia	Large doses of intravenous levothyroxine
Hypothermia	Blankets, no active rewarming
Hypoventilation	Mechanical ventilation
Hypotension	Cautious volume expansion with crystalloid or whole blood
Hyponatremia	Mild fluid restoration
Hypoglycemia	Glucose administration
Hypocortisolemia	Glucocorticoid administration
Precipitating event	Identification and elimination by specific treatment

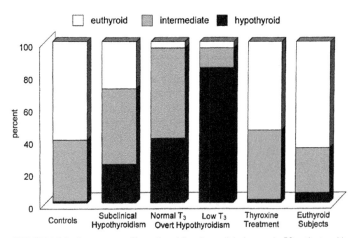

FIGURE 14-5. Assessment of hypothyroidism by a clinical score in 50 patients with overt hypothyroidism, 80 age-matched controls, 93 patients with subclinical hypothyroidism, 67 hypothyroid patients treated with thyroxine, and an additional 109 euthyroid subjects. T_3, triiodothyronine. (From Zulewski H, Müller B, Exer P, et al: Estimation of tissue hypothyroidism by a new clinical score: evaluation of patients with various grades of hypothyroidism and controls. J Clin Endocrinol Metab 82:771–776, 1997. Copyright © 1997, The Endocrine Society.)

contractility, impairment of muscle energy metabolism, and an increase in LDL cholesterol.[151]

TREATMENT

Treatment for subclinical hypothyroidism is still debated. A Cochrane analysis of randomized clinical trials found that levothyroxine therapy had no effect on survival, cardiovascular morbidity, symptoms, or quality of life, although lipid profiles and left ventricular function improved.[152] Nevertheless, meta-analyses of population-based studies demonstrate a higher prevalence and incidence of ischemic heart disease and mortality, at least in women and subjects younger than 65 years.[153,154] In view of this, thyroxine therapy might be considered in subjects younger than 65 years if TSH is >10 mU/L and/or TPO antibodies are present. In case TSH is <10 mU/L and TPO antibodies are absent, thyroxine therapy still might be warranted in individuals with a high background for cardiovascular risk, symptoms, pregnancy, and infertility.[151] When in doubt because of nonspecific complaints, a trial of T_4 treatment for at least 3 months can be considered.

SET POINT

Subclinical hypothyroidism seems to be a misnomer, but how some subjects with subclinical thyroid dysfunction experience clinical symptoms and signs, whereas other subjects are really asymptomatic despite similar serum FT_4 concentrations, remains an unanswered question. Repeated measurements of thyroid function in the same individual over time show a narrow fluctuation around the mean value. Apparently, each individual is characterized by a fixed relationship between serum TSH and FT_4 concentrations; this point can be considered the working point of the pituitary-thyroid axis of that individual. From longitudinal observations in subjects in whom abnormal thyroid function develops, it can be deduced that an intraindividual log-linear relationship exists between TSH and FT_4, as depicted by a straight line[115]; the working point moves along this line, upward in the case of hypothyroidism (Fig. 14-6). The position of the working point of an individual determines the changes in thyroid function test results that are maximally allowed within the conventional reference range before they are labeled abnormal. In the example depicted in Fig. 14-6, the subject with subclinical hypothyroidism and a serum FT_4 of 12 mol/L might have an original working point at 18 mol/L (indicating a decrease in serum FT_4 by 33%) or at 15 mol/L (indicating a decrease in

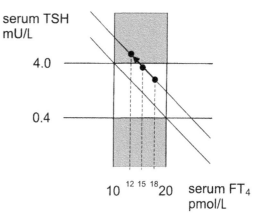

FIGURE 14-6. The log-linear relationship between thyroid-stimulating hormone (TSH) and free thyroxine (FT_4) of a particular individual is depicted by a straight line; the working point of that individual moves upward along this line if hypothyroidism develops. Variation between individuals is given by the different location of the working point on the same or parallel lines. The upper hatched area represents subclinical hypothyroidism, and the central area encompasses the normal range of TSH and FT_4. For further explanation, see the text.

serum FT_4 by 20%). It is conceivable that symptoms and signs are present in the former but not in the latter situation.

SCREENING

In view of the high prevalence of thyroid disease in the general population, the question arises of whether a screening program for adults is justified.[6] A simple, inexpensive, and accurate screening test is available: the sensitive TSH assay. The disease to be screened (hypothyroidism and thyrotoxicosis) has a high prevalence and can be treated effectively. The burden of disease is limited, however, and it has not been proved that clinical outcome is improved by early diagnosis and treatment in the asymptomatic stage. Nevertheless, a computer-derived decision model concludes that it is cost effective to screen persons in the general community for mild hypothyroidism with a serum TSH combined with a serum cholesterol every 5 years after the age of 35 years.[155] Screening of elderly women is especially cost effective. For the time being, case finding is a suitable alternative, that is, determination of serum TSH in patients (especially pregnant women and older women) who consult the physician because of unrelated problems. A high degree of suspicion of thyroid function disorder is warranted in patients with nonspecific complaints.

REFERENCES

1. Ishii H, Inada M, Tanaka K, et al: Induction of outer and inner ring monodeiodinases in human thyroid gland by thyrotropin, J Clin Endocrinol Metab 57:500–505, 1983.
2. Lum SM, Nicoloff JT, Spencer CA, et al: Peripheral tissue mechanism for maintenance of serum triiodothyronine values in a thyroxine-deficient state in man, J Clin Invest 73:570–575, 1984.
3. Ord WM: Report of a committee of the Clinical Society of London nominated December 14, 1883 to investigate the subject of myxoedema, Trans Clin Soc Lond 8:15, 1888.
4. Tunbridge WMG, Evered DC, Hall R, et al: The spectrum of thyroid disease in the community: the Whickham survey, Clin Endocrinol 7:481–493, 1977.
5. Vanderpump MPJ, Tunbridge WMG, French JM, et al: The incidence of thyroid disorders in the community:

A twenty-year follow-up of the Whickham survey, Clin Endocrinol 43:55–68, 1995.
6. Wang C, Crapo LM: The epidemiology of thyroid disease and implication for screening, Endocrinol Metab Clin North Am 26:189–218, 1997.
7. Strieder TGA, Tijssen JGP, Wenzel BE, et al: Prediction of progression to overt hypo- or hyperthyroidism in female relatives of patients with autoimmune thyroid disease using the Thyroid Events Amsterdam (THEA) score, Arch Int Med 168:1–7, 2008.
8. Faglia G: The clinical impact of the thyrotropin-releasing hormone test, Thyroid 8:903–908, 1998.
9. Horimoto M, Nishikawa M, Ishihara T, et al: Bioactivity of thyrotropin (TSH) in patients with central hypothyroidism: comparison between in vivo 3,5,3'-triiodothyronine response to TSH and in vitro bioactivity of TSH, J Clin Endocrinol Metab 80:1124–1128, 1995.

10. Persani L, Ferretti E, Borgato S, et al: Circulating thyrotropin bioactivity in sporadic central hypothyroidism, J Clin Endocrinol Metab 85:3631–3635, 2000.
11. Samuels MH, Lillehei K, Kleinschmidt-Demasters BK, et al: Patterns of pulsatile glycoprotein secretion in central hypothyroidism and hypogonadism, J Clin Endocrinol Metab 70:391–395, 1990.
12. Adriaanse R, Brabant G, Endert E, et al: Pulsatile TSH release in patients with untreated pituitary disease, J Clin Endocrinol Metab 77:205–209, 1993.
13. Vance ML: Hypopituitarism, N Engl J Med 330:1651–1662, 1994.
14. Schmiegelow M, Feldt-Rasmussen U, Rasmussen AK, et al: A population-based study of thyroid function after radiotherapy and chemotherapy for a childhood brain tumor, J Clin Endocrinol Metab 88:136–140, 2003.

15. Arafah BM: Reversible hypopituitarism in patients with large non-functioning pituitary adenomas, J Clin Endocrinol Metab 62:1173–1179, 1986.

16. Constine LS, Woolf PD, Cann D, et al: Hypothalamic-pituitary dysfunction after radiation for brain tumors, N Engl J Med 328:87–94, 1993.

17. Snijder PJ, Fowble BF, Schatz NJ, et al: Hypopituitarism following radiation therapy of pituitary adenomas, Am J Med 81:457–462, 1986.

18. Schneider HJ, Kreitschmann-Andermahr I, Ghigo E, et al: Hypothalamopituitary dysfunction following traumatic brain injury and aneurysmal subarachnoid hemorrhage: a systematic review, JAMA 298:1429–1438, 2007.

19. Bellastella A, Bizzarro A, Coronella C, et al: Lymphocytic hypophysitis: a rare or underestimated disease? Eur J Endocrinol 149:363–376, 2003.

20. Kaptein EM, Spencer CA, Kamile MB, et al: Prolonged dopamine administration and thyroid hormone economy in normal and critically ill subjects, J Clin Endocrinol Metab 51:387–393, 1980.

21. Vagenakis AG, Braverman LE, Azizi F, et al: Recovery of pituitary thyrotropic function after withdrawal of prolonged thyroid suppression therapy, N Engl J Med 293:681–684, 1975.

22. Adriaanse R, Brabant G, Endert E, et al: Pulsatile thyrotropin secretion in patients with Cushing's syndrome, Metabolism 43:782–786, 1994.

23. Sherman SI, Gopal J, Haugen BR, et al: Central hypothyroidism associated with retinoid X receptor-selective ligands, N Engl J Med 340:1075–1079, 1999.

24. Hayashi Y, Tamai H, Fukata S, et al: A long-term clinical, immunological, and histological follow-up study of patients with goitrous chronic lymphocytic thyroiditis, J Clin Endocrinol Metab 61:1172–1178, 1985.

25. Arikawa K, Ichikawa Y, Yoshida T, et al: Blocking type antithyrotropin receptor antibody in patients with nongoitrous hypothyroidism: its incidence and characteristics of action, J Clin Endocrinol Metab 60:953–959, 1985.

26. Laurberg P, Pedersen KM, Hreidarsson A, et al: Iodine intake and the pattern of thyroid disorders: a comparative epidemiological study of thyroid abnormalities in the elderly in Iceland and in Jutland, Denmark, J Clin Endocrinol Metab 83:765–769, 1998.

27. Asvold BO, Bjøro T, Nilsen TI, et al: Tobacco smoking and thyroid function: a population-based study, Arch Int Med 167:1428–1432, 2007.

28. Takasu N, Yamada T, Takasu M, et al: Disappearance of thyrotropin-blocking antibodies and spontaneous recovery from hypothyroidism in autoimmune thyroiditis, N Engl J Med 326:513–518, 1992.

29. Kasagi K, Iwata M, Misaki T, et al: Effect of iodine restriction on thyroid function in patients with primary hypothyroidism, Thyroid 13:561–567, 2003.

30. Nikolai TF: Recovery of thyroid function in primary hypothyroidism, Am J Med Sci 297:18–21, 1989.

31. Kraiem Z, Baron E, Kahana L, et al: Changes in stimulating and blocking TSH receptor antibodies in a patient undergoing three cycles of transition from hypo- to hyperthyroidism and back to hypothyroidism, Clin Endocrinol 36:211–216, 1992.

32. Gerstein HC: How common is postpartum thyroiditis? A methodologic overview of the literature, Arch Intern Med 150:1397–1400, 1990.

33. Kuypens JL, Pop VJ, Vader HL, et al: Prediction of postpartum thyroid dysfunction: can it be improved? Eur J Endocrinol 139:36–43, 1998.

34. Alvarez-Marfany M, Roman SH, Drexler AJ, et al: Long-term prospective study of postpartum thyroid function in women with insulin dependent diabetes mellitus, J Clin Endocrinol Metab 79:10–16, 1994.

35. Vialettes B, Guillerand MA, Viens P, et al: Incidence rate and risk factors for thyroid dysfunction during recombinant interleukin-2 therapy in advanced malignancies, Acta Endocrinol 129:31–38, 1993.

36. Prummel MF, Laurberg P: Interferon-α and autoimmune thyroid disease, Thyroid 13:547–551, 2003.

37. Nofal MN, Beierwaltes WH, Patno ME: Treatment of hyperthyroidism with sodium iodide I-131, a 16-year experience, JAMA 197:605–610, 1966.

38. Huysmans DA, Corstens FH, Kloppenborg PW: Long-term follow-up in toxic solitary autonomous thyroid nodules treated with radioactive iodine, J Nucl Med 32:27–30, 1991.

39. Le Moli R, Wesche MFT, Tiel-van Buul MMC, et al: Determinants of long-term outcome of radioiodine therapy of sporadic non-toxic goitre, Clin Endocrinol 50:783–789, 1999.

40. Smith RE, Adler RA, Clark P, et al: Thyroid function after mantle irradiation in Hodgkin's disease, JAMA 245:46–49, 1981.

41. Tell R, Sjödin H, Lundell G, et al: Hypothyroidism after external radiotherapy for head and neck cancer, Int J Radiat Oncol Biol Phys 39:303–308, 1997.

42. Mercado G, Adelstein DJ, Saxton JP, et al: Hypothyroidism: A frequent event after radiotherapy and after radiotherapy with chemotherapy for patients with head and neck carcinoma, Cancer 92:2892–2897, 2001.

43. Katsanis E, Shapiro RS, Robison LL, et al: Thyroid dysfunction following bone marrow transplantation: long-term follow-up of 80 pediatric patients, Bone Marrow Transplant 5:335–340, 1990.

44. Pearce EN, Farwell AP, Braverman LE: Thyroiditis, New Engl J Med 348:2646–2655, 2003.

45. Braverman LE: Iodine and the thyroid: 33 years of study, Thyroid 4:351–356, 1994.

46. Martino E, Safran M, Aghini-Lombardi F, et al: Environmental iodine intake and thyroid dysfunction during chronic amiodarone therapy, Ann Intern Med 101:28–34, 1984.

47. Trip MD, Wiersinga WM, Plomp TA: Incidence, predictability, and pathogenesis of amiodarone-induced thyrotoxicosis and hypothyroidism, Am J Med 91:507–511, 1991.

48. Surks MI, Sievert R: Drugs and thyroid function, N Engl J Med 333:1688–1694, 1995.

49. Desai J, Yassa L, Marqusee E, et al: Hypothyroidism after sunitinib treatment for patients with gastrointestinal stromal tumours, Ann Int Med 145:660–664, 2006.

50. Mannavola D, Coco P, Vannucchi G, et al: A novel tyrosine-kinase selective inhibitor, sunitinib, induces transient hypothyroidism by blocking iodine uptake, J Clin Endocrinol Metab 92:3531–3534, 2007.

51. Huang SA, Tu HM, Harney JW, et al: Severe hypothyroidism caused by type 3 iodothyronine deiodinase in infantile hemangiomas, N Engl J Med 343:185–189, 2000.

52. Huang SA, Fish SA, Dorfman DM, et al: A 21-year-old woman with consumptive hypothyroidism due to a vascular tumor expressing type 3 iodothyronine deiodinase, J Clin Endocrinol Metab 87:4457–4461, 2002.

53. Smith TJ, Bahn RS, Gorman CA: Connective tissue, glycosaminoglycans, and diseases of the thyroid, Endocr Rev 10:366–391, 1989.

54. Diekman MJ, Romijn JA, Endert E, et al: Thyroid hormones modulate serum leptin levels: observations in thyrotoxic and hypothyroid women, Thyroid 8:1081–1086, 1998.

55. Iglesias P, Alvarez Fidalgo P, Codoceo R, et al: Serum concentrations of adipocytokines in patients with hyperthyroidism and hypothyroidism before and after control of thyroid function, Clin Endocrinol 59:621–629, 2003.

56. Hsieh CJ, Wang PW, Wong ST, et al: Serum leptin concentrations of patients with sequential thyroid function changes, Clin Endocrinol 57:29–34, 2002.

57. Brackhik M, Marcisz C, Giebel S, et al: Serum leptin and ghrelin levels in premenopausal women with stable body mass index during treatment of thyroid dysfunction, Thyroid 18:545–550, 2008.

58. Pearce EN: Hypothyroidism and dyslipidemia: modern concepts and approaches, Curr Cardiol Rep 6:451–456, 2004.

59. Diekman T, Demacker PNM, Kastelein JJP, et al: Increased oxidizability of low-density lipoproteins in hypothyroidism, J Clin Endocrinol Metab 83:1752–1755, 1998.

60. Ito M, Takamutsu J, Matsuo T, et al: Serum concentrations of remnant-like particles in hypothyroid patients before and after thyroxine replacement, Clin Endocrinol 58:621–626, 2003.

61. Constant EL, De Volder AG, Ivanocin A, et al: Cerebral blood flow and glucose metabolism in hypothyroidism: a positron emission tomography study, J Clin Endocrinol Metab 86:3864–3870, 2001.

62. Smith CD, Ain KB: Brain metabolism in hypothyroidism studied with ^{31}P magnetic-resonance spectroscopy, Lancet 345:619–620, 1995.

63. Dugbartey AT: Neurocognitive aspects of hypothyroidism, Arch Intern Med 158:1413–1418, 1998.

64. Burmeister LA, Ganguli M, Dodge HH, et al: Hypothyroidism and cognition: Preliminary evidence for a specific defect in memory, Thyroid 11:1177–1185, 2001.

65. Knopman DS, Petersen RC, Cha RH: Incidence and causes of nondegenerative nonvascular dementia: a population-based study, Arch Neurol 63:218–221, 2006.

66. Cleare AJ, McGregor A, O'Keane V: Neuroendocrine evidence for an association between hypothyroidism, reduced central 5-HT activity and depression, Clin Endocrinol 43:713–719, 1995.

67. Duyff RF, Van den Bosch J, Laman DM, et al: Neuromuscular findings in thyroid dysfunction: a prospective clinical and electrodiagnostic study, J Neurol Neurosurg Psychiatry 68:750–755, 2000.

68. Cakir M, Samanci N, Balci N, et al: Musculoskeletal manifestations in patients with thyroid disease, Clin Endocrinol 59:162–167, 2003.

69. Chong JY, Rowland LP, Utiger RD: Hashimoto encephalopathy: syndrome or myth? Arch Neurol 60:164–171, 2003.

70. Madariaga M: Polymyositis-like syndrome in hypothyroidism: review of cases reported over the past twenty-five years, Thyroid 12:331–336, 2002.

71. Kaminsky P, Robin-Lherbier B, Brunotte F, et al: Energetic metabolism in hypothyroid skeletal muscle, as studied by phosphorus magnetic resonance spectroscopy, J Clin Endocrinol Metab 74:124–129, 1992.

72. Monzani F, Caraccio N, Siciliano G, et al: Clinical and biochemical features of muscle dysfunction in subclinical hypothyroidism, J Clin Endocrinol Metab 82:3315–3318, 1997.

73. Hsu I-H, Thadhani RI, Daniels GH: Acute compartment syndrome in a hypothyroid patient, Thyroid 5:305–308, 1995.

74. Diekman MJM, Harms MPM, Endert E, et al: Endocrine factors related to changes in total peripheral vascular resistance after treatment of thyrotoxic and hypothyroid patients, Eur J Endocrinol 144:339–346, 2001.

75. Klein I, Danzi S: Thyroid disease and the heart, Circulation 116:1725–1735, 2007.

76. Obuobie K, Smith J, Evans LM, et al: Increased central arterial stiffness in hypothyroidism, J Clin Endocrinol Metab 87:4662–4666, 2002.

77. Ladenson PW, Sherman SI, Baughman KL, et al: Reversible alterations in myocardial gene expression in a young man with dilated cardiomyopathy and hypothyroidism, Proc Natl Acad Sci U S A 89:5251–5255, 1992.

78. Bengel FM, Nekolla SG, Ibrahim T, et al: Effect of thyroid hormones on cardiac function, geometry, and oxidative metabolism assessed noninvasively by positron emission tomography and magnetic resonance imaging, J Clin Endocrinol Metab 85:1822–1827, 2000.

79. Diekman MJM, van der Put NM, Blom HJ, et al: Determinants of changes in plasma homocysteine in hyperthyroidism and hypothyroidism, Clin Endocrinol 54:197–204, 2001.

80. Cappola AR, Ladenson PW: Hypothyroidism and atherosclerosis, J Clin Endocrinol Metab 88:2438–2444, 2003.

81. Ladenson PW, Goldenheim PD, Ridgway EC: Prediction and reversal of blunted ventilatory responsiveness in patients with hypothyroidism, Am J Med 84:877–883, 1988.

82. Pelttari L, Rauhala E, Polo O, et al: Upper airway obstruction in hypothyroidism, J Intern Med 236:177–181, 1994.

83. Hollander JG den, Wulkan RW, Mantel MJ, et al: Correlation between severity of thyroid dysfunction and renal function, Clin Endocrinol 62:423–427, 2005.

84. Hanna FWF, Scanlon MF: Hyponatraemia, hypothyroidism and role of arginine-vasopressin, Lancet 350:755–756, 1997.

85. Sahun M, Villabona C, Rosel P, et al: Hypothyroidism is associated with plasma hypo-osmolality and impaired water excretion that is vasopressin-independent, J Endocrinol 168:435–445, 2001.

86. Yeum CH, Kim SW, Kim NH, et al: Increased expression of aquaporin water channels in hypothyroid rat kidney, Pharmacol Res 46:85–88, 2002.

87. Bruder JM, Samuels MH, Bremner WJ, et al: Hypothyroidism-induced macroorchidism: Use of a gonad-

otropin-releasing hormone agonist to understand its mechanism and augment adult stature, J Clin Endocrinol Metab 80:11–16, 1995.

88. Anasti JN, Flack MR, Froehlich J, et al: A potential novel mechanism for precocious puberty in juvenile hypothyroidism, J Clin Endocrinol Metab 80:276–279, 1995.

89. Krassas GE, Tziomalos K, Papadopoulou F, et al: Erectile dysfunction in patients with hyper- and hypothyroidism: how common and should we treat? J Clin Endocrinol Metab 93:1815–1819, 2008.

90. Samuels MH, Veldhuis JD, Henry P, et al: Pathophysiology of pulsatile and copulsatile release of thyroid-stimulating hormone, luteinizing hormone, follicle-stimulating hormone, and alpha-subunit, J Clin Endocrinol Metab 71:425–432, 1990.

91. Krassas GE, Pontikides N, Kaltsas FL, et al: Disturbances of menstruation in hypothyroidism, Clin Endocrinol 50:655–659, 1999.

92. Smallridge RC, Ladenson PW: Hypothyroidism in pregnancy: consequences to neonatal health, J Clin Endocrinol Metab 86:2349–2353, 2001.

93. Haddow JE, Palomaki GE, Allan WC, et al: Maternal thyroid deficiency during pregnancy and subsequent neuropsychological development of the child, N Engl J Med 341:549–555, 1999.

94. Abalovich M, Gutierrez S, Alcaraz G: Overt and subclinical hypothyroidism complicating pregnancy, Thyroid 12:63–68, 2002.

95. Rahman Q, Haboubi NY, Hudson PR, et al: The effect of thyroxine on small intestinal motility in the elderly, Clin Endocrinol 35:443–446, 1991.

96. Lauritano EC, Bilotta AL, Gabrielli M, et al: Association between hypothyroidism and small intestinal bacterial overgrowth, J Clin Endocrinol Metab 92:4180–4184, 2007.

97. Saha B, Maity C: Alterations of serum enzymes in primary hypothyroidism, Clin Chem Lab Med 40:609–611, 2002.

98. Squizzato A, Romualdi, Büller HR, et al: Clinical review: thyroid dysfunction and effects on coagulation and fibrinolysis: a systematic review, J Clin Endocrinol Metab 92:2415–2420, 2007.

99. Manfredi E, Zaane B van, Gerdes VE: Hypothyroidism and acquired von Willebrand's syndrome: a systematic review, Haemophilia 14:423–433, 2008.

100. Erfurth EM, Ericsson U-BC, Egervalh K, et al: Effect of acute desmopressin and of long-term thyroxine replacement on haemostasis in hypothyroidism, Clin Endocrinol 42:373–378, 1995.

101. Ladenson PW, Levin AA, Ridgway EC, et al: Complications of surgery in hypothyroid patients, Am J Med 77:261–266, 1984.

102. Valcavi R, Valente F, Dieguez C, et al: Evidence against depletion of the growth hormone (GH)-releasable pool in human primary hypothyroidism: studies with GH-releasing hormone, pyridostigmine, and arginine, J Clin Endocrinol Metab 77:616–620, 1993.

103. Miell JP, Zini M, Quin JD, et al: Reversible effects of cessation and recommencement of thyroxine treatment on insulin-like growth factors (IGFs) and IGF-binding proteins in patients with total thyroidectomy, J Clin Endocrinol Metab 79:1507–1512, 1994.

104. Raber W, Gesol A, Nowotny P, et al: Hyperprolactinaemia in hypothyroidism: clinical significance and impact of TSH normalization, Clin Endocrinol 58:185–191, 2003.

105. Sarlis NJ, Brucker-Davis F, Doppman JL, et al: MRI-demonstrated regression of a pituitary mass in a case of primary hypothyroidism after a week of acute thyroid hormone therapy, J Clin Endocrinol Metab 82:808–811, 1997.

106. Iranmanesh A, Lizarralde G, Johnson ML, et al: Dynamics of 24-hour endogenous cortisol secretion and clearance in primary hypothyroidism assessed before and after partial thyroid hormone replacement, J Clin Endocrinol Metab 70:155–161, 1990.

107. Topliss DJ, White EL, Stockigt JR: Significance of thyrotropin excess in untreated primary adrenal insufficiency, J Clin Endocrinol Metab 50:52–56, 1980.

108. Silva JE: Intermediary metabolism and the sympathoadrenal system in hypothyroidism. In Braverman LE, Utiger RD, editors: The thyroid: a Fundamental and Clinical Text, ed 9, Philadelphia, 2005, Lippincott Williams & Wilkins, pp 817–823.

109. Billewicz WL, Chapman RS, Crooks J, et al: Statistical methods applied to the diagnosis of hypothyroidism, QJM 38:255–266, 1969.

110. Seshadri MS, Samuel BU, Kanagasabapathy AS, et al: Clinical scoring system for hypothyroidism: is it useful? J Gen Intern Med 4:490–492, 1989.

111. Zulewski H, Müller B, Exer P, et al: Estimation of tissue hypothyroidism by a new clinical score: evaluation of patients with various grades of hypothyroidism and controls, J Clin Endocrinol Metab 82:771–776, 1997.

112. Tachman ML, Guthrie GP: Hypothyroidism: diversity of presentation, Endocr Rev 5:456–465, 1984.

113. Doucet J, Trivalle C, Chassagne P, et al: Does age play a role in clinical presentation of hypothyroidism? J Am Geriatr Soc 42:984–986, 1994.

114. Müller B, Zulewski H, Huber P, et al: Impaired action of thyroid hormone associated with smoking in women with hypothyroidism, N Engl J Med 333:964–969, 1995.

115. Fish LH, Schwartz HL, Cavanaugh J, et al: Replacement dose, metabolism, and bioavailability of levothyroxine in the treatment of hypothyroidism: role of triiodothyronine in pituitary feedback in humans, N Engl J Med 316:764–770, 1987.

116. Bolk N, Visser TJ, Kalsbeek A, et al: Effect of evening vs morning thyroxine ingestion on serum thyroid hormone profiles in hypothyroid patients, Clin Endocrinol 66:43–48, 2007.

117. Dong BJ, Hauck WW, Gambertoglio JG, et al: Bioequivalence of generic and brand-name levothyroxine products in the treatment of hypothyroidism, JAMA 227:1205–1213, 1997.

118. Olveira G, Almaraz MC, Soriguer F, et al: Altered bioavailability due to changes in the formulation of a commercial preparation of levothyroxine in patients with differentiated carcinoma, Clin Endocrinol 46:707–711, 1997.

119. Roos A, Linn-Rasker SP, Domburg RT van, et al: The starting dose of levothyroxine in primary hypothyroidism treatment: a prospective, randomized, double-blind trial. Arch Intern Med 165:1714–1720, 2005.

120. Kabadi UM, Jackson T: Serum thyrotropin in primary hypothyroidism: a possible predictor of optimal daily levothyroxine dose, Arch Intern Med 155:1046–1048, 1995.

121. Shimon I, Cohen O, Lubetsky A, et al: Thyrotropin suppression by thyroid hormone replacement is correlated with thyroxine level normalization in central hypothyroidism, Thyroid 12:823–827, 2002.

122. Sawin CT, Geller A, Wolf PA, et al: Low serum thyrotropin concentrations as a risk factor for atrial fibrillation in older persons, N Engl J Med 331:1249–1252, 1994.

123. Uzzan B, Campos J, Cucherat M, et al: Effects on bone mass of long term treatment with thyroid hormones: a meta-analysis, J Clin Endocrinol Metab 81:4278–4289, 1996.

124. Leese GP, Jung RT, Guthrie C, et al: Morbidity in patients on L-thyroxine: a comparison of those with a normal TSH to those with a suppressed TSH, Clin Endocrinol 37:500–503, 1992.

125. Vestergaard P, Weeke J, Hoeck HC, et al: Fractures in patients with primary idiopathic hypothyroidism, Thyroid 10:335–340, 2000.

126. Sheppard MC, Holder R, Franklyn J: Levothyroxine treatment and occurrence of fracture of the hip, Arch Intern Med 162:338–343, 2002.

127. d'Estève-Bonetti L, Bennet AP, Malet D, et al: Gluten-induced enteropathy (coeliac disease) revealed by resistance to treatment with levothyroxine and alfacalcidol in a 68-year old patient: a case report, Thyroid 12:633–636, 2002.

128. Liel Y, Harman-Boehm I, Shany S: Evidence for a clinically important adverse effect of fiber-enriched diet on the availability of levothyroxine in adult hypothyroid patients, J Clin Endocrinol Metab 81:857–859, 1996.

129. Harmon SM, Seifert CF: Levothyroxine-cholestyramine interaction reemphasized, Ann Intern Med 115:658–659, 1991.

130. Havrankova J, Lahaie R: Levothyroxine binding by sucralfate [erratum appears in Ann Intern Med 118:398, 1993], Ann Intern Med 147:445–446, 1992.

131. Sperber AD, Liel Y: Evidence for interference with the intestinal absorption of levothyroxine sodium by aluminium hydroxide, Arch Intern Med 152:183–184, 1992.

132. Campbell NRC, Hasinoff BB, Stalts H, et al: Ferrous sulfate reduces thyroxine efficacy in patients with hypothyroidism, Ann Intern Med 117:1010–1013, 1992.

133. Siraj ES, Gupta MK, Reddy SS: Raloxifene causes malabsorption of levothyroxine, Arch Intern Med 163:1367–1370, 2003.

134. Singh N, Singh PN, Hershman JM: Effects of calcium carbonate on the absorption of levothyroxine, JAMA 283:2822–2825, 2000.

135. Arafah BM: Increased need for thyroxine in women with hypothyroidism during estrogen therapy, N Engl J Med 344:1743–1749, 2001.

136. Alexander EK, Marqusee E, Lawrence J, et al: Timing and magnitude of increases in levothyroxine requirements dusring pregnancy in women with hypothyroidism, New Engl J Med 351:241–249, 2004.

137. Isley WL: Effect of rifampin therapy on thyroid function tests in a hypothyroid patient on replacement L-thyroxine, Ann Intern Med 107:517–518, 1987.

138. Figge J, Dluhy RG: Amiodarone-induced elevation of thyroid stimulating hormone in patients receiving levothyroxine for primary hypothyroidism, Ann Intern Med 113:553–555, 1990.

139. McCowen KC, Garber JR, Spark R: Elevated serum thyrotropin in thyroxine-treated patients with hypothyroidism given sertraline, N Engl J Med 337:1010–1011, 1997.

140. Munera Y, Hugues FC, Le Jeunne C, et al: Interaction of thyroxine sodium with antimalarial drugs, Br Med J 314:1593, 1997.

141. Grebe SKG, Cooke RR, Ford HC, et al: Treatment of hypothyroidism with once weekly thyroxine, J Clin Endocrinol Metab 82:870–875, 1997.

142. Arafah BM: Decreased levothyroxine requirement in women with hypothyroidism during androgen therapy for breast cancer, Ann Intern Med 121:247–251, 1994.

143. Griffin JE: Hypothyroidism in the elderly, Am J Med Sci 299:334–345, 1990.

144. Escobar-Morreale HF, Escobar del Ray F, Obregon MJ, et al: Only the combined treatment with thyroxine and triiodothyronine ensures euthyroidism in all tissues of the thyroidectomized rat, Endocrinology 137:2490–2502, 1996.

145. Saravanan P, Chau W-F, Roberts N, et al: Psychological well-being in patients on 'adequate' doses of L-thyroxine: results of a large, controlled community-based questionnaire study, Clin Endocrinol 57:577–585, 2002.

146. Wekking EM, Appelhof BC, Fliers E, et al: Cognitive functioning and well-being in euthyroid patients on thyroxine replacement therapy for primary hypothyroidism, Eur J Endocrinol 153:747–753, 2005.

147. Grozinsky-Glasberg S, Fraser A, Nahskoni E, et al: Thyroxine-triiodothyronine combination therapy versus thyroxine monotherapy for clinical hypothyroidism: meta-analysis of randomized controlled trials, J Clin Endocrinol Metab 91:2592–2599, 2006.

148. Sherman SI, Ladenson PW: Percutaneous transluminal coronary angioplasty in hypothyroidism, Am J Med 90:367–370, 1991.

149. Porretti S, Giavoli C, Ronchi C, et al: Recombinant human GH replacement therapy and thyroid function in a large group of adult GH-deficient patients: when does L-T4 therapy become mandatory? J Clin Endocrinol Metab 87:2042–2045, 2002.

150. Wartofsky L: Myxedema coma, Endocrinol Metab Clin North Am 35:687–698, 2006.

151. Biondi B, Cooper DS: The clinical significance of subclinical thyroid dysfunction, Endocr Rev 29:76–131, 2008.

152. Villar HC, Saconato H, Valente O, et al: Thyroid hormone replacement in subclinical hypothyroidism, Cochrane Database Syst Rev 18:CD003419, 2007.

153. Ochs N, Auer R, Bauer DC, et al: Meta-analysis: subclinical thyroid dysfunction and the risk for coronary heart disease and mortality, Ann Intern Med 148:832–845, 2008.

154. Razvi S, Shakoor A, Vanderpump M, et al: The influence of age on the relationship between subclinical hypothyroidism and ischaemic heart disease: a meta-analysis, J Clin Endocrinol Metab 93:2998–3007, 2008.

155. Danese MD, Powe NR, Sawin CT, et al: Screening for mild thyroid failure at the periodic health examination: a decision and cost-effectiveness analysis, JAMA 276:285–292, 1996.

Chapter 15

NONTHYROIDAL ILLNESS SYNDROME: A Form of Hypothyroidism

LESLIE J. DE GROOT

Serum thyroid hormone levels drop during starvation and illness. In mild illness, this involves only a decrease in serum triiodothyronine (T$_3$) levels. However, as the severity of the illness increases, there is a drop in both serum T$_3$ and thyroxine (T$_4$). This decrease of serum thyroid hormone levels is seen in starvation, sepsis, surgery, myocardial infarction, bypass, bone marrow transplantation, and in fact probably any severe illness.[1-9] The condition has been called the *euthyroid sick syndrome* (ESS). An alternative designation, which does not presume the metabolic status of the patient, is *nonthyroidal illness syndrome*, or NTIS.

Low T$_3$ States

Starvation, and more precisely carbohydrate deprivation, appears to rapidly inhibit deiodination of T$_4$ to T$_3$ by type 1 iodothyronine deiodinase in the liver, thus inhibiting generation of T$_3$ and preventing metabolism of reverse T$_3$ (rT$_3$).[10] Consequently there is a drop in serum T$_3$ and elevation of reverse T$_3$. Since starvation induces a decrease in basal metabolic rate,[11] it has been argued, teleologically, that this decrease in thyroid hormone represents an adaptive response by the body to spare calories and protein by inducing some degree of hypothyroidism. Patients who have only a drop in serum T$_3$, representing the mildest form of the NTIS, do not show clinical signs of hypothyroidism. Nor has it been shown that this decrease in serum T$_3$ (in the absence of a drop in T$_4$) has an adverse physiologic effect on the body or that it is associated with increased mortality.

Nonthyroidal Illness Syndrome With Low Serum T$_4$

As the severity of illness, and often associated starvation, progresses, there is the gradual development of a more complex syndrome associated with low T$_3$ *and* usually low T$_4$ levels. Generally thyroid-stimulating hormone (TSH) levels are low or normal despite the low serum hormone levels, and rT$_3$ levels are normal or elevated. A large proportion of patients in an intensive care unit setting have various degrees of severity of NTIS with low T$_3$ and T$_4$. Plikat et al. found that 23% of patients admitted to an ICU during a 2-year period had low free T$_3$, low free T$_4$, and low or normal TSH, and that these findings gave a greatly increased risk of death.[12] Girvent et al. note that NTIS is highly prevalent in elderly patients with acute surgical problems and is associated with poor nutrition, higher sympathetic response, and worse postoperative outcome.[13] Surprisingly, during the past 3 decades, many endocrinologists have assumed that NTIS is a beneficial physiologic response,[14-17] but actual evidence for this view is unavailable.

A marked decrease in serum T$_3$ and T$_4$ in NTIS is associated with a high probability of death. NTIS was found in a group of 20 patients with severe trauma, among whom 5 died, and the drop in T$_3$ correlated with the Apache II score.[18] NTIS found in patients undergoing bone marrow transplantation was associated with a high probability of fatal outcome.[19] NTIS was typical in elderly patients undergoing acute surgery and was associated with a worse prognosis.[20] All of 45 non-dopamine-treated children with meningococcal septicemia had low T_3, T_4, and thyroxine-binding globulin (TBG), without elevated TSH. When serum T_4 levels drop below 4 g/dL, the probability of death is about 50%, and with serum T_4 levels below 2 g/dL, the probability of death reaches 80%.[21-23] Obviously such associations do not prove that hypothyroidism is the cause of these complications or deaths, but the fact of hypothyroidism must at least raise the consideration of treatment.

Physiologic Interpretations of NTIS

Several conceptual explanations of NTIS can be followed through the literature:

1. The abnormalities represent test artifacts, and assays would indicate euthyroidism if proper tests were employed.
2. The serum thyroid hormone abnormalities are due to inhibitors of T_4 binding to proteins, and the tests do not appropriately reflect free hormone levels. Proponents of this concept may or may not take the position that a binding inhibitor is present throughout body tissues, rather than simply in serum, and that the binding inhibitor may also inhibit uptake of hormone by cells or prevent binding to nuclear T_3 receptors and thus inhibit action of hormone.
3. In NTIS, T_3 levels in the pituitary are normal because of enhanced local deiodination. Thus the pituitary is actually euthyroid, while the rest of the body is hypothyroid. This presupposes enhanced intrapituitary $T_4 > T_3$ deiodination as the cause.
4. Serum hormone levels are artifactually low, the patients are biochemically euthyroid, and this is (teleologically) a beneficial physiologic response which should not be altered by treatment.

5. Serum hormone levels are in fact low, and the patients are biochemically hypothyroid, but this is (teleologically) a beneficial physiologic response and should not be altered by treatment.
6. Lastly, NTIS is in part a form of secondary hypothyroidism, the patient's serum and tissue hormone levels are truly low, tissue hypothyroidism is present, this is probably disadvantageous to the patient, and therapy should be initiated if serum thyroxine levels are depressed below the danger level of 4 µg/dL.

SERUM HORMONE LEVELS AND TISSUE HORMONE SUPPLIES IN NTIS

Serum T_3 and Free T_3

With few exceptions, reports on NTIS indicate that serum T_3 and free T_3 levels are low.[24-30] Chopra and co-workers reported that free T_3 levels were low (Fig. 15-1),[31] or in a second report, often normal.[32] However, it is important to note that in the second report, the patients with "NTIS" actually had average serum T_4 levels that were *above* the normal mean and did not have significant NTIS. Sapin et al. compared free T_3 levels found in patients with NTIS by direct dialysis, microchromatography, analogue, two-step immune extraction, and a labeled antibody RIA method.[30] Results were significantly below normal by five of the methods and low in the most severe cases by one method. Faber et al. evaluated thyroid hormone levels in 34 seriously ill patients, most of whom had low T_4 and free T_4 index values, and found generally normal free T_3 and free T_4 using an ultrafiltration technique.[33] A point to consider is that some ultrafiltration techniques fail to exclude thyroid hormone–binding proteins from the filtrate and give spuriously high free hormone values.[34]

Serum rT_3 may be reduced, normal, or elevated and is not a reliable indicator of abnormal thyroid hormone supply. While it may be expected that rT_3 should always be elevated, this is not true, and often it is within the normal range. Peeters et al.[35] found in patients with NTIS, serum TSH, T_4, T_3, and the T_3/rT_3 ratio were lower, whereas serum rT_3 was higher than in normal sub-

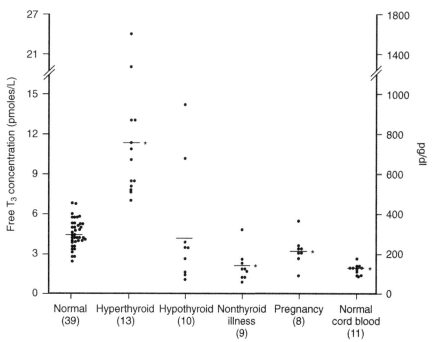

FIGURE 15-1. Free T_3 concentrations in different groups of patients, as reported by Chopra et al.[31] In this report, patients with NTIS have significantly lowered free T_3 levels than normal subjects. *NTIS,* Nonthyroidal illness syndrome; T_3, triiodothyronine.

*cf normal, p<0.05

jects ($P < 0.0001$). Liver D1 is down-regulated, and D3 (which is not evident in liver and skeletal muscle of healthy individuals) is induced, particularly in disease states associated with poor tissue perfusion. The level of rT_3 reflects the action of several enzymes and presumably, as well, tissue metabolic function. Induction of D3 would tend to increase rT_3. Degradation of rT_3 is reduced by decreased function of the same D1 enzyme that generates T_3. Moreover, formation of rT_3 is limited by the low level of substrate (T_4) in serum and in tissues and perhaps by inhibition of T_4 entry into cells. Personal experience treating patients with NTIS (unpublished) shows that when T_4 is given and repletes serum hormone levels, generation of rT_3 rapidly increases, and levels often become significantly elevated.

Serum T_4

Serum T_4 levels are reduced in NTIS in proportion to the severity and, probably, length of the illness.[24-35] In acute, short-term trauma such as cardiac bypass[36] or in short-term starvation,[37] there is no drop in serum T_4. However, with increasing severity of trauma, illness, or infection, there is a drop in T_4, which may become extreme. As indicated, serum T_4 levels below 4 µg/dL are associated with a marked increased risk of death (up to 50%), and once T_4 is below 2, prognosis becomes extremely guarded. In neonates, low total T_4 and TSH are associated with a greater risk of death and severe intraventricular hemorrhage. It is suggested that thyroid hormone supplementation might be a potential benefit in infants with the lowest T_4 values.[27]

Total serum T_4 is reduced in part because of a reduction in TBG. One reason for this reduction appears to be because of cleavage of TBG. Schussler's group recognized a rapid drop in TBG to 60% of baseline within 12 hours after bypass surgery, and their data suggest that this is due to cleavage of TBG by protease, which causes TBG to lose its T_4-binding activity.[38] Further studies by this group demonstrated the presence of a cleaved form of TBG present in serum of patients with sepsis.[39]

The impact of meningococcal sepsis on peripheral thyroid hormone metabolism and binding proteins was studied in 69 children with meningococcal sepsis. All children had decreased total T_3 and total T_3/rT_3 ratios without elevated TSH. Lower total T_4 levels were related to increased turnover of TBG by elastase. Lowered TBG is a partial explanation for lower total T_4 and T_3 in NTIS.[40]

Serum Free Thyroxine

A major problem in understanding NTIS is in analyzing data on the level of free T_4. Free T_4 is believed by most workers to represent hormone availability to tissues, although it is in fact intracellular T_3 that binds to the receptors. The results of free T_4 assays in NTIS are definitely method dependent. They may be influenced by a variety of variables, including (alleged) inhibitors present in serum or the effect of agents such as drugs, metabolites, or free fatty acids in the serum or assay. Assays which include an estimate of TBG capacity to estimate free hormone typically return low values for calculated free thyroxine in NTIS. Methods using T_3 analogs in the assay also give levels that are depressed. The free T_4 level determined by dialysis varies widely, as does T_4 measured by ultrafiltration[25-29]; the majority of reports are of normal or low values but in some samples, elevated values.[25,26,41-43]

In theory, methods utilizing equilibrium dialysis may allow dilution of dialyzable inhibitors. Compounds such as 3-carboxy-4-methyl-5-propyl-2-furan-propanoic acid, indoxyl sulfate, and hippuric acid, can accumulate in severe renal failure.[44] However, these compounds probably do not interfere with serum hormone

assays. Free fatty acids, if elevated to 2 to 5 mmol/L, can displace T_4 binding to TBG and elevate free T_4. Free fatty acids almost never reach such levels in vivo.[45,46] However, even small quantities of heparin (0.08 units/kg given IV, or 5000 units given SC), commonly given to patients in an ICU, can lead to in vitro generation of free fatty acids during extended serum dialysis for "free T_4" assay and falsely augment apparent free hormone levels.[47] This is probably a widespread and serious problem, which explains many instances of apparently elevated free T_4 levels in patients with acute illness.

Results obtained using ultrafiltration also are variable. Wang et al.[48] found that in patients with NTIS, free T_4 measured by ultrafiltration was uniformly low (average of 11.7 ng/L), but when measured by equilibrium dialysis, free T_4 was near normal, at 18 ng/L. By ultrafiltration, free T_3 was also (not surprisingly) found to be low and similar to free T_3 by radioimmune assay. Chopra[32] found levels below the normal mean, ±2 SD, when measured by dialysis; 6 of 9 were low when measured by ultrafiltration, and 7 of 9 were low when measured by standard resin-uptake-corrected free T_4. The means of the NTIS patients in this study were clearly below the mean of normals.

Thus, although free T_4 is low in most assays that involve a correction for TBG levels, there is still some question as to the true free T_4 in patients with NTIS. It is of interest that this problem does not carry over to estimates of free T_3, which are depressed in most studies. There might be two reasons for this difference. Firstly, the depression of total T_3 is proportionately greater than of total T_4. Secondly, factors which affect thyroid hormone binding are more apt to alter T_4 assays than T_3, since T_4 is normally more tightly bound to TBG than is T_3.

IS THERE EVIDENCE FOR SUBSTANCES IN SERUM WHICH CAN AFFECT T_4 BINDING TO PROTEINS?

Mendel et al.[49] carefully review the studies that have claimed the presence of dialyzable inhibitors of binding and point out that many of these studies must be viewed with caution.[44,45,50-53] Numerous artifacts are present in both dialysis assays and ultrafiltration assays. They also point out that while the low free T_4 by resin uptake assays found in NTIS generally do not agree with the clinical status of the patient, it is equally true that clinical assessment generally does not fit with the high free T_4 results found by some equilibrium dialysis assays in NTIS.

An argument that completely refutes the importance of factors in serum inhibiting binding of thyroid hormone is provided in the clinical study of Brent and Hershman (Fig. 15-2).[54] These researchers gave 1.5 µg of T_4 per kg body weight daily to 12 of 24 patients with severe NTIS and followed serum hormone levels over 14 days. T_4 levels returned to the normal range within 3 days of therapy. Thus the thyroxine pool was easily replenished, and T_4 levels reached normal values. Not surprisingly, because of reduced T_4>T_3 deiodination, T_3 levels did not return to the normal range until the end of the study period in the few patients who survived. However, the ability of intravenous thyroxine in replacement doses to promptly restore the plasma pool to normal clearly shows that neither a loss of serum TBG nor an inhibitor of binding could be the main cause of low serum T_4 in this group of severely ill patients.

TSH LEVELS

Serum TSH in NTIS is typically normal or reduced and may be markedly low, although usually not less than 0.05 µU/mL.[16,24,25,28,29,31,55] However, to use usual endocrinology logic, these TSH levels are almost always inappropriately low for the observed serum T_4 and T_3. Third-generation assays with sensitivity down to 0.001 U/mL may allow differentiation of patients with hyperthyroidism from those with NTIS, although there can be overlap in these very disparate conditions.[56] Serum TSH in patients with NTIS may have reduced biological activity, perhaps because of reduced thyrotropin-releasing hormone (TRH) secretion and reduced glycosylation. Some patients are found with a TSH level above normal, and elevation of TSH above normal commonly occurs transiently if patients recover from NTIS (Fig. 15-3).[16,29,54] This elevation of TSH strongly suggests that the patients are recovering from a hypothyroid state, during which the ability of the pituitary to respond had been temporarily inhibited.

Responsiveness of the pituitary to TRH during NTIS is variable: many patients respond less than normal,[57] and others respond normally.[58] "Normal" responsiveness in the presence of *low* TSH may suggest that there is a hypothalamic abnormality as a cause of the low TSH and low T_4. There is also a diminution or loss of the diurnal rhythm of TSH,[59] and in some studies, there is evidence for reduction of TSH glycosylation, with lower TSH bioactivity.[60] A logical alternative explanation is that the low TSH is in fact the proximate cause of the low thyroid hormone levels. Hypothalamic function is impaired in patients with NTIS and, because of low TRH, results in low TSH and thus low output of thyroid hormones by the thyroid.

There is other evidence of diminished hypothalamic function in patients with serious illness. Serum testosterone drops rapidly, as do follicle-stimulating hormone (FSH) and luteinizing hormone (LH).[61,62] Typically serum cortisol is elevated as part of a stress response, but this is not always the case. Some patients develop hypotension in association with apparent transient central hypoadrenalism, have low or normal serum ACTH, and cortisol levels under 20 μg/dL. The patients respond dramatically to cortisol replacement and may manifest normal adrenal function at a later time if they recover.

Centrally mediated hyposomatotropism, hypothyroidism, and pronounced hypoandrogenism were observed in a study of patients in the catabolic state of critical illness. In these patients, pulsatile LH secretion and mean LH secretions are very low, even in the presence of extremely low circulating total testosterone and low estradiol. Pulsatile growth hormone (GH) and TSH secretion are also, as is known, suppressed. Interleukin 1 β (IL-1β) levels are normal, whereas IL-6 and tumor necrosis factor α (TNF-α) are elevated. Exogenous IV gonadotropin-releasing hormone (GnRH) partially return serum testosterone levels toward normal but do not completely overcome hypoandrogenism, suggesting that combined deficiency of GH, GnRH, and TSH secretagogues may be important in this low androgen syndrome.[63]

THYROID HORMONE TURNOVER

Kaptein et al.[64,65] studied a group of patients who were critically ill, all of whom had total T_4 below 4 μg/dL, low fT_4 index, low normal free T_4 by dialysis, and TSH which was normal or slightly elevated. In these patients, the mean T_4 by dialysis was significantly below the normal mean. There was on average a 35% decrease in thyroxine disposal per day (Table 15-1). The T_4 production rate in NTIS was significantly below the mean of 17 normal subjects (p < 0.005). In a similar study of T_3 kinetics,[65] free T_3 was found to be 50% of normal serum values. The production rate of T_3 was reduced by 83% (Table 15-2). These two studies document a dramatic reduction in provision of T_4 and T_3

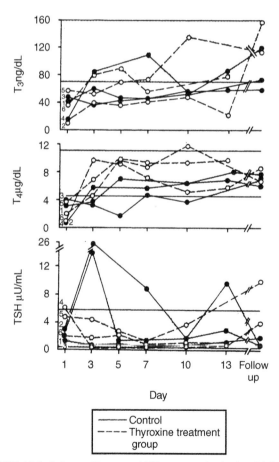

FIGURE 15-2. Patients with severe NTIS were randomized and left untreated *(control, solid lines)* or given IV T_4 *(thyroxine-treated group, dashed lines)* over 2 weeks.[54] Serum T_3, T_4, and TSH concentrations are shown for the survivors of the control *(filled circles)* and T_4-treated groups *(open circles)* during the study period and at the time of follow-up. *NTIS,* Nonthyroidal illness syndrome; *IV,* intravenous; T_3, triiodothyronine; T_4, thyroxine; *TSH,* thyroid-stimulating hormone.

Table 15-1. T_4 Kinetics in the Low T_4 State of Nonthyroidal Illness[64]

Case Number	TT$_4$ (μg/dL)	FT$_4$ (ng/dL)	PR (μg/d/m^2)
Normal Subjects (n = 19)			
Mean	7.1	2.21	50.3
±SE	0.4	0.13	3.4
Sick Patients			
1	2.7	2.05	32.4
2	3.0	1.23	51.1
3	1.2	0.48	39.0
4	1.4	1.04	23.7
5	1.3	0.75	22.2
6	3.0	1.35	34.6
7	1.9	1.33	36.6
8	2.0	1.88	25.3
9*	0.4	0.28	10.0
10*	1.5	1.50	13.7
11*	1.6	1.70	18.4
Mean	1.8	1.24	27.9
±SE	0.2	0.17	3.7
P	<0.001	<0.001	<0.001

FT$_4$, Free thyroxine; *PR,* production rate; *TT$_4$,* total thyroxine.
*Patients receiving dopamine.
All P values are for unpaired t tests.

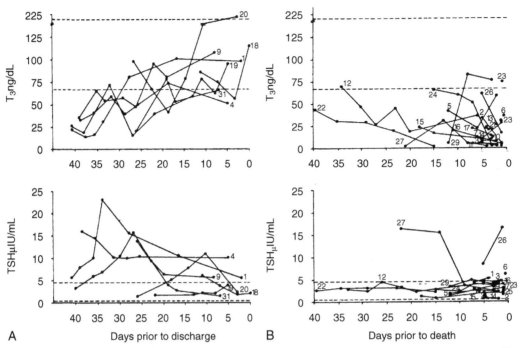

FIGURE 15-3. T_3 and TSH concentrations are shown in patients with nonthyroidal illness who were eventually discharged from hospital *(left panels)*.[29] The *broken line* indicates ±2 SD of the mean value in the normal subjects. The *right panel* displays T_3 and TSH concentrations in patients with NTIS who died. Subjects are indicated by numbers. Note the elevated TSH in some patients who recovered and the generally dropping T_3 and low TSH levels in patients who died.[29] *NTIS,* Nonthyroidal illness syndrome; *SD,* standard deviation; T_3, triiodothyronine; *TSH,* thyroid-stimulating hormone.

Table 15-2. T_3 Kinetics in the Low-T_4 State of Nonthyroidal Illness[65]

Case Number	TT₃ (ng/dL)	FT₃ (pg/dL)	PR (μg/d/m2)
Normal Subjects (n = 12)			
Mean	162	503	23.47
±SE	5	46	2.12
Sick Patients			
3	30	272	6.18
5	42	247	5.67
6	25	151	5.41
7	34	266	8.39
12*	45	282	6.07
Mean	35	244	6.34
±SE	4	24	0.53
P	<0.001	<0.001	<0.005

FT₃, Free triiodothyronine; *PR,* production rate; *TT₃,* total triiodothyronine.
*Patient receiving dopamine.

to peripheral tissues, which would logically indicate that the effects of hormone lack (hypothyroidism) should be present. A third study reported dramatically reduced total T_4 and T_3 turnover, with normal thyroidal secretion of T_3 in patients with NTIS due to uremia.[66] However, this was a calculated rather than directly measured value, was highly variable, and does not negate the extreme reduction in T_3 supply due to diminished T_4>T_3 conversion in peripheral organs.

T₄ ENTRY INTO CELLS AND GENERATION OF T₃

Using deiodination of T_4 as an index of cellular transport of T_4 into rat hepatocytes, Lim et al.[67] and Vos et al.[68] found that serum from patients with NTIS inhibited T_4 uptake. Sera from critically ill NTIS patients caused reduced T_4 uptake compared to control

sera in one study, and the authors considered elevated nonesterified fatty acids (NEFA) and bilirubin and reduced albumin to play a role. Serum from patients with mild NTIS did not cause impaired deiodination of T_4 and T_3.[69] Inhibition of uptake of T_4 into hepatocytes caused by sera of patients with NTIS also was observed by Sarne and Refetoff.[70] There is a diminution in the "reducing equivalents" available for the deiodination of T_4 to T_3 in liver, and presumably elsewhere, thus lowering transport and the function of the type 1 iodothyronine deiodinase.[71] In animals, and probably in man, there is also a drop in the level of type 1 iodothyronine deiodinase enzyme, apparently due to hypothyroidism, since it can be reversed by giving T_3. Recently a study was performed on blood, liver, and skeletal-muscle biopsies of patients immediately after death in intensive care unit settings. Liver T_4 deiodinase 1 was found to be down-regulated, and deiodinase 3 was induced in liver and muscle, especially in situations associated with poor tissue perfusion. These changes contribute to the low generation of T_3 and its increased metabolism in NTIS, thus lowering the intracellular T_3 levels.[35]

In theory, reduced cellular uptake would cause tissue hypothyroidism, reduced T_3 generation and serum T_3 levels, and elevated serum T_4, which is not observed. It is likely that reduced hormone supply in NTIS is caused by multiple factors, and that reduced cell uptake is one of the factors. T_4 is converted to T_3, although at a reduced rate. In addition, T_4 is rapidly converted to rT_3 by an intracellular process, suggesting that entry into cells is not seriously impaired, but the pathways of intracellular deiodination are abnormal.

THYROID HORMONE IN TISSUES

There are few significant data on thyroid hormone in tissues of patients with NTIS.[72] In one study, there was of a dramatically reduced level of T_3 in tissues (Table 15-3). While most samples

Table 15-3. Tissue T_3 Concentrations in Nonthyroidal Illness Syndrome (nmol of T_3/kg of Wet Weight)[72]

Tissue	Control Group			NTI Group	
	Mean	SD	P	Mean	SD
Cerebral cortex	2.2	0.9	<.05	1.2	1.1
Hypothalamus	3.9	2.2	<.01	1.4	1.2
Anterior pituitary	6.8	2.5	<.005	3.7	1.1
Liver	3.7	2.3	<.01	0.9	0.9
Kidney	12.9	4.3	<.001	3.7	2.8
Lung	1.8	0.8	<.01	0.8	0.5
Skeletal muscle	2.3	1.2	NS	>10.9	
Heart	4.5	1.5	NS	>16.3	

NS, Not significantly different; *NTI*, nonthyroidal illness; T_3, triiodothyronine.*Patients receiving dopamine.

had very low levels of T_3 compared to normal tissues, some patients with NTIS showed sporadically and inexplicably high levels of T_3 in certain tissues, especially skeletal muscle and heart.

Peeters et al.[73] investigated 79 patients who died after intensive care, some of whom received thyroid hormone treatment. Tissue iodothyronine levels were positively correlated with serum levels, indicating that the decrease in serum T_3 during illness is associated with decreased levels of tissue T_3. Higher serum T_3 levels in patients who received thyroid hormone treatment were accompanied by higher levels of liver and muscle T_3, with evidence for tissue-specific regulation. Tissue rT_3 and the T_3/rT_3 ratio were correlated with tissue deiodinase activities. Monocarboxylate transporter 8 expression was not related to the ratio of the serum over tissue concentration of the different iodothyronines.[73]

Information on expression of TRs in human tissues during illness is limited. Increased expression of the messenger ribonucleic acid (mRNA) for thyroid hormone receptors $\alpha 1$, $\alpha 2$, and $\beta 1$ has been reported in cardiac tissue of patients with dilated cardiomyopathy; $\alpha 1$ and $\alpha 2$ isoforms also had increased expression in ischemic heart disease.[74] Rodriguez-Perez et al. studied subcutaneous fat and skeletal muscle in patients with septic shock.[75] In muscle, mRNA for TR$\beta 1$ and RXR gamma was reduced, and mRNA for RXR alpha was increased, compared to normals. In adipose tissue, MCT8, TR$\beta 1$, TR$\alpha 1$, and RXR gamma mRNAs were lower. The authors conclude that in these patients, tissue responses were oriented toward decreased hormone levels and decreased hormone action. In animals, starvation and illness are associated with a reduction in thyroid hormone receptor levels. In experimental studies in mice, LPS induces NTIS, and this is associated with an early decrease in binding of the RXR/TR dimer to DNA due to limiting amounts of RXR, and later an up to 50% decrease in levels of RXR and TR protein.[76-77]

ARE PATIENTS WITH NTIS CLINICALLY HYPOTHYROID?

It is straightforward that the clinical parameters of severe hypothyroidism are absent in patients with NTIS. However, these patients usually present with a serious illness and are diagnostically challenging in view of their complicated state. Many are febrile, have extensive edema, have sepsis or pneumonia, may have hypermetabolism associated with burns, have severe cardiac or pulmonary disease, and in general have features that could easily mask evidence of hypothyroidism. Further, the common clinical picture of hypothyroidism does not develop within 2 to 3 weeks of complete thyroid hormone deprivation, but rather requires a much longer period for expression. General laboratory tests are also suspect. Thus starvation or disease-induced altera-

tions in cholesterol, liver enzymes, TBG, creatine kinase, and even basal metabolic rate generally rule out the use of these associated markers for evidence of hypothyroidism. Angiotensin-converting enzyme levels are low,[78] as seen in hypothyroidism, while high-affinity testosterone-binding globulin (TeBG) and osteocalcin levels are not altered.[79] Antithrombin III levels are reduced in a septic rat model of NTIS. T_3 supplementation returned the sepsis-induced decrease in antithrombin III levels toward normal.[80]

Mechanism of Thyroid Hormone Suppression in NTIS

It is probable that the cause of NTIS is multifactorial and may differ in different groups of patients. Specifically, the changes in liver disease and renal disease are probably somewhat different from those occurring in other forms of illness. Certainly one important cause of the drop in serum T_3 is a decreased generation of T_3 by type 1 iodothyronine deiodinase.[81] If reduced entry of T_4 into cells was a primary event and the major problem, then serum T_4 levels would become elevated rather than suppressed. Some studies have suggested that individuals with NTIS may have selenium deficiency, and this may contribute to a malfunction of the selenium-dependent iodothyronine deiodinase.[82] However, supplements of 500 µg of selenium given to patients in a surgical ICU during the first 5 days after serious injury caused only modest changes in thyroid hormones. The data did not suggest a major role for selenium deficiency in this condition.[83]

The overall degradation of thyroid hormone, both thyroxine and T_3, is radically diminished in the NTIS syndrome in the presence of low hormone serum levels. The reduced degradation cannot *produce* the lowering of serum hormone levels; a primary reduction in degradation would increase serum hormone. The change in degradation must be secondary to the low hormone supply. Schussler and co-workers have observed a sharp drop in TBG levels during cardiac bypass surgery, which their studies indicate is due to some selective consumption of TBG. It is possible that this occurs because of activation of serine protease inhibitors (serpins) at sites of inflammation, which cleave the TBG into an inactive form.[38]

Considerable evidence suggests that an alteration in hypothalamic and pituitary function causes the low production of T_4, which in turn causes the low production of T_3. In rats, starvation reduces hypothalamic mRNA for TRH, reduces portal serum TRH, and lowers pituitary TSH content.[84] A recent study documents low TRH mRNA in hypothalamic paraventricular nuclei[85] in NTIS patients (Fig. 15-4). Responses to administered TRH vary in different reports, being suppressed or even augmented.[57,58] Administration of TRH has been suggested as an effective means of restoring serum hormone levels to normal in individuals with NTIS. A recent report of great significance by Van den Berghe and co-workers proves that administration of TRH to patients with severe NTIS leads directly to increased TSH levels, increased T_4 levels, and increased T_3 levels.[86] This data is strong support (albeit not proof) for the role of diminished hypothalamic function as an important factor causing NTIS.

Quite possibly the production of TRH, and responses to TRH, are reduced by cytokines (to be discussed later) or by glucocorticoids.[87] The diurnal variation in glucocorticoid levels at least in part controls the normal diurnal variation in TSH levels, perhaps by affecting pituitary responsiveness to TRH.[88] High levels of

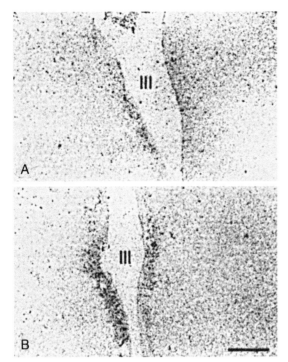

FIGURE 15-4. In situ hybridization study demonstrating mRNA for TRH in the periventricular nuclei of **A,** a subject who died with NTIS and **B,** a subject who died accidentally. In patients with NTIS, mRNA for TRH is significantly reduced.[85] *mRNA*, Messenger ribonucleic acid; *NTIS*, nonthyroidal illness syndrome; *TRH*, thyrotropin-releasing hormone.

glucocorticoids in Cushing's disease suppress TSH and cause a modest reduction in serum hormone levels.[89] High levels of glucocorticoids are known to suppress pituitary response to TRH in man.[87] Stress-induced elevation of glucocorticoids in animals causes suppression of TSH and serum T_4 and T_3 hormone levels.[90] Thus stress-induced glucocorticoid elevation may be one factor affecting TRH and TSH production.

Why should pituitary production of TSH be diminished in the presence of low serum thyroid hormone levels? A possibility is that there is augmented intrapituitary conversion of T_4 to T_3, thus allowing the pituitary to remain "euthyroid" while the rest of the body is actually hypothyroid. There is experimental support for this idea in a uremic rat model of NTIS.[91] Another suggestion is that some other metabolite of thyroxine may be involved in control of pituitary responsiveness. For example, possibly triiodoacetic acid (triac) or tetraiodoacetic acid (tetrac) generated by metabolism of thyroxine could control pituitary responsiveness,[92] but there is no experimental proof of this idea, and even if true, it would mean that the pituitary was normal but the rest of the body hypothyroid. As suggested earlier, elevated serum cortisol levels could play a role. The most obvious possibility is that low TSH stems from diminished TRH production, as previously described. It must also be remembered that the defect in pituitary function is not restricted to TSH, but that LH and FSH are also suppressed in seriously ill patients, and testosterone is reduced, in contrast to the generally augmented glucocorticoid response. Quite possibly these changes are the effect on the hypothalamus of neural integration of multiple factors including stress, starvation, glucocorticoids, and cytokines.

Van den Berghe has proposed that the changes in endocrine function seen during severe illness have a biphasic course. Possibly the initial suppression of T_3 levels represents a genetically engineered adaptive response of the organism, allowing reduced metabolic rate and conservation of energy and protein stores for a longer period of time, while the animal or man goes through a period of starvation. However, the circumstances surrounding severe illness, and the resuscitative efforts applied in an intensive care unit over 1 or more weeks, presumably have not resulted in some genetically induced metabolic response, since survival under such extreme organ failure is a very recent phenomenon. This second phase of the syndrome, with associated suppression of thyroid hormone and other pituitary hormones and a variety of other changes, represents in this construction a maladaptive response. Patients in this situation tend to have elevated insulin levels, nitrogen wasting, retention of fats if calories are made available, and a variety of other metabolic abnormalities that include neuropathy and cardiomyopathy. These authors consider that provision of multiple hormonal support, including thyroid hormone, growth hormone, and androgens, may be beneficial.[93-96]

CYTOKINES IN NTIS

In a series of septic patients studied shortly after admission to an ICU, total T_4, free T_4, total T_3, and TSH were depressed, and IL-1β, soluble interleukin-2 receptor (sIL-2R), IL-6, and TNF-α were elevated.[97] The hypothalamo-pituitary-adrenal axis was activated as expected. The data suggest central suppression of TSH as the cause of the problem, but the relation to cytokines is unclear, as seen in the following reports. Hermus et al.[98] showed that continuous infusion of IL-1 in rats causes suppression of TSH, T_3, and free T_4. Higher doses of IL-1 were accompanied by a febrile reaction and suppression of food intake, which presumably played some role in the altered thyroid hormone economy. IL-1 did not reproduce the diminution in hepatic 5′-deiodinase activity believed to be so characteristic of NTIS. IL-1 is also known to impair thyroid hormone synthesis by human thyrocytes and is enhanced in many diseases associated with NTIS.[99] van der Poll et al.[100] studied the effect of IL-1 receptor blockade in human volunteers to determine if it could alter the NTIS induced by endotoxin. Blockade of IL-1 activity was achieved by infusing recombinant human IL-1 receptor antagonist, but this did not prevent the drop in T_4, free T_4, T_3, and TSH or the rise in rT_3 caused by endotoxin. This is evidence against an important role for IL-1.

Interferon γ

Interferon-γ (IFN-γ) 100 μg/m^2 administered subcutaneously to normal volunteers did not alter TNF-α levels, caused a small elevation of IL-6 levels, and thus did not support a role for IFN-γ in the pathogenesis of the euthyroid sick syndrome in humans.[101]

Tumor Necrosis Factor

TNF is another proinflammatory cytokine that is thought to be involved in many of the illnesses associated with NTIS.[102,103] Infusion of recombinant TNF in man by van der Poll et al.[104] produced a decrease in serum T_3 and TSH and an increase in rT_3. Free T_4 was transiently elevated in association with a significant rise in FFA levels. These studies suggest that TNF could be involved when recombinant IL-6 given to humans activates the hypothalamic pituitary axis; as noted previously, this could secondarily suppress TSH production. However, Chopra et al.[102] did not find TNF to be closely correlated with hormone changes in NTIS. van der Poll et al.[103,104] gave human subjects endotoxin, which caused lowering of T_4, free T_4, T_3, and TSH. TNF blockade by a recombinant TNF receptor-IgG fusion protein did not alter the response, indicating that TNF did not cause the changes in hormone economy induced by administration of endotoxin. Nagaya et al.[105] have proposed a mechanism through which TNF could reduce serum T_3. TNF-α was found during in vitro studies to activate nuclear factor κB (NF-κB), which in turn inhibits the T_3-induced expression of 5′-DI, which would lower T_3 generation in liver.

Interleukin 6

Serum IL-6 is often elevated in NTIS,[106] and its level is inversely related to T_3 levels.[107] Stouthard et al.[108] gave recombinant human IL-6 chronically to human volunteers. Short-term infusion of IL-6 caused a suppression of TSH, but daily injections over 42 days caused only a modest decrease in T_3 and a transient increase in rT_3 and free T_4 concentrations. IL-6 could be involved in the NTIS syndrome, although the mechanism was not defined. In an animal model of NTIS studied by Wiersinga and collaborators,[109] antibody blockade of IL-6 failed to prevent the induced changes in thyroid hormone economy typical of NTIS. Boelen et al. studied the levels of IFN, IL-8, and IL-10 in patients with NTIS and found no evidence that they had a pathogenic role.[110] Short-term administration of recombinant IFN-γ to normal subjects caused a minimal elevation of IL-6, no alteration in TNF, and did not significantly alter thyroid hormone levels.[111] Michalaki et al. observed that serum T_3 drops early after abdominal surgery as an early manifestation of the NTIS syndrome, prior to an increase in serum IL-6 or TNF-α, suggesting that these changes in cytokines do not induce the drop in T_3.[112]

The potential interaction between cytokines and the hypothalamic-pituitary-thyroid axis is certainly complicated, and cytokines themselves operate in a network. For example, IL-1 and TNF can stimulate secretion of IL-6. Activation of TNF and IL-1 production is associated with the occurrence of cytokine inhibitors in serum, which are actually fragments of the cytokine receptor or actual receptor antagonists. Soluble TNF receptor and IL-1 RA are receptor antagonists, which can inhibit the function of the free cytokines. These molecules are increased in many infectious, inflammatory, and neoplastic conditions. Boelen et al.[113] found evidence that the NTIS is "an acute phase response" generated by activation of a cytokine network. Soluble TNF, soluble TNF receptor, soluble IL-2 receptor antagonist, and IL-6 all inversely correlated with serum T_3 levels.

While the studies noted fail to pinpoint one cytokine as the crucial mediator, we can be convinced that striking changes in cytokines co-occur during NTIS and probably play a pathogenic role by mechanisms yet undefined.

OTHER FACTORS ALTERING SERUM T_4 SUPPLY

Altered CNS Metabolism

In healthy men going through two 4.5 hour long sessions of induced hypoglycemia, TSH, fT_3 and fT_4 are significantly reduced.[114] Perinatal asphyxia, recognized by low Apgar scores, is associated with a depression of TSH, T_4, and T_3, and the reductions are greatest in infants with hypoxic/ischemic encephalopathy. In this study, 6 of 11 infants with $fT_4 < 2$ng/dL died. These data suggest, not surprisingly, that reduced substrate or O_2 supply to the CNS could induce hypothalamic/pituitary dysfunction.[114,115]

Glucagon

Administration of glucagon to dogs caused a significant fall in serum T_3, suggesting that stress-induced hyperglucagonemia

may be a contributor to the NTIS syndrome by altering intracellular metabolism of T_4.[116]

Dopamine

Dopamine given in support of renal function and cardiac function must play a role in many patients who develop low hormone levels while in an intensive care unit setting. Dopamine inhibits TSH secretion directly, depresses further the already abnormal thyroid hormone production, and induces significant worsening of the low hormone levels. Withdrawal of dopamine infusion is followed by a prompt dramatic elevation of TSH, a rise in T_4 and T_3, and an increase of the T_3/rT_3 ratio. All of these changes suggested to Van den Berghe et al.[117] that dopamine makes some patients with NTIS hypothyroid, inducing a condition of iatrogenic hypothyroidism, and that treatment (presumably by administering thyroid hormone), "should be evaluated."

Leptin

Leptin plays a key role in control of thyroid hormone levels during starvation in animals. During starvation, leptin levels drop. With this there is diminished stimulation of TRH, thus diminished secretion of TSH, and lowered thyroid hormone levels. Administration of leptin appears to work via the arcuate nucleus of the hypothalamus to induce production of pro-opiomelanocortin (POMC), and thus α-melanocyte-stimulating hormone (αMSH), and reduce Agouti-related protein (AgRP). Normally αMSH stimulates the melanocortin 4 receptor (MC4R), whereas AgRP suppresses it. Presumably through these actions, a lack of leptin during starvation leads to diminished stimulation of the MC4R receptor on the TRH neurons in ventricular nuclear centers and thus diminished TRH secretion. Administration of leptin partially reverses this sequence.[118] These actions appear to be part of an energy-conserving scheme related to thyroid changes during starvation and are associated with leptin-induced increase in appetite, decreased energy expenditure, and modified neuroendocrine function. Naturally the relevance of this to human physiology is as yet unclear, but the data strongly suggest that leptin is involved in the down-regulation of thyroid function during acute starvation.[119-120] In clinical trials, stimulation of growth hormone secretion by GH secretagogues leads to increased insulin and leptin levels in severely ill ICU patients. To date, studies of leptin levels in patients with NTIS have indicated they are normal or elevated, not low.[86,121]

Atrial Natriuretic Peptides

Atrial natriuretic peptides, including amino acids 1 to 30, amino acids 31 to 67 (known as *vessel dilator*), 79 to 98 (kaliuretic hormone), and 99 to 126 (atrial natriuretic hormone), derived from the ANH prohormone, significantly decreased circulating concentrations of total T_4, free T_4, and free T_3, when given to healthy humans for 60 minutes. A reciprocal increase in TSH lasted for 2 or 3 hours after cessation of the administration of these hormones, suggesting that the effect was a direct inhibition of thyroid hormone release from the thyroid gland rather than an action of the hormones upon the hypothalamus or pituitary. No data are available on these factors in NTIS[122] (Table 15-4).

Diagnosis

Typically the endocrinologist is presented with a severely ill patient in whom there is no prior history suggestive of pituitary disease, in whom clinical findings of hypothyroidism are either absent or

Table 15-4. Summary of Observations in Nonthyroidal Illness Syndrome

1. Hypothalamic mRNA for TRH is reduced, and cytokines may be responsible.
2. TSH levels are inappropriately low for serum hormone levels, presumably because of reduced secretion.
3. TRH injection causes an elevation of TSH, T_4, and T_3, reversing many aspects of the syndrome and suggesting low TRH secretion may be a primary problem.
4. Measured serum levels of apparent free T_4 and T_3 may be low or normal, but no assay can be certified to be free of artifact.
5. Inhibitors of T_4, and T_3, binding to serum proteins and possibly receptors, have been postulated but remain of unproven significance.
6. T_4 and T_3 production rates have been clearly demonstrated to be markedly reduced.
7. Based on scant data, levels of hormone in most tissues are greatly reduced in proportion to decreased blood hormone levels.
8. Serum hormone was (in the one study available) restored by administration of physiologic doses of hormone.
9. Replacement hormone therapy has not been shown to be disadvantageous, and in some studies it appears to be beneficial.
10. Major abnormalities are also present in GH, LH, T, and insulin physiology.

masked by other disorders, with a T_4 and FTI (by an index method) that are low, a low or normal TSH, and, if measured, a low T_3. If T_4 is below 4 µg/dL in this setting, the diagnosis of NTIS, associated with a potentially fatal outcome, may be assumed; rT_3 may be normal or elevated and is not diagnostic. An elevated TSH suggests the presence of prior hypothyroidism, which should be treated. Finding positive antithyroid antibody titers supports the diagnosis of primary hypothyroidism but does not prove it.

Serum cortisol should be measured. Transient, apparently central, hypoadrenalism may occur in severe illness.[123-125] Cortisol should be above 20 µg/dL, and commonly is above 30. If below 20, ACTH should be drawn, and the patient should be given supportive cortisol therapy. Serum cortisol should certainly be determined if thyroid hormone is to be given. Since CBG may be reduced, it is advisable to measure serum free cortisol if possible. It is useful to determine FSH in postmenopausal women as a sign of pituitary function, but this is less clearly valuable in men. If there is a reason to consider hypopituitarism, a CAT scan of the pituitary is appropriate, or at least a skull film.

Use of aspirin, dilantin, and carbamazepine should be noted, since they can lower T_4 and FTI as measured by several "index" methods. Dopamine used in the setting of severe illness can induce clear-cut hypothyroidism. Hyperthyroidism is the typical cause of suppression of TSH below 0.1 µU/mL, but it is rarely difficult to exclude this diagnosis in the setting of severely depressed T_4 and T_3.

Is Thyroid Hormone Treatment of NTIS Advantageous or Disadvantageous?

Two valuable studies are available on replacement therapy using thyroid hormone in patients with NTIS. In the study by Brent and Hershman,[54] replacement with 1.5 µg T_4 IV per kilogram body weight daily, in 12 patients, promptly returned serum T_4 levels to normal (thereby proving that a binding defect was not the cause of the low T_4) but did not normalize T_3 levels over a period of 2 to 3 weeks. However, in both the treated and control group, mortality was 80%.[54] Clearly this excellent small study,

which used for primary therapy what would now be considered the wrong hormone, failed to show either an advantageous or disadvantageous effect. It is possible that the failure to show a positive effect was due to the failure of T_3 levels to be restored to normal. In a study of severely burned patients given 200 µg T_3 daily, again there was no evidence of a beneficial or disadvantageous effect.[126] Mortality was not so great, as in the Brent and Hershman study, but it is entirely possible that the high levels of T_3 provided worsened the hypermetabolism known to be present in burn patients and could have, at these levels, been disadvantageous.

An important study by Acker et al. certainly advises caution regarding T_4 therapy in patients with acute renal failure. Numerous studies in animals have documented a beneficial effect of T_4 therapy in experimental acute renal failure.[127] In a randomized, controlled prospective study of patients with acute renal failure (ARF), treated patients received 150 µg of thyroxine a total of four times intravenously over 2 days.[128] The single difference recognized in the subsequent laboratory data was a suppression of TSH. T_4 treatment had no effect on any measure of ARF severity. Among other questions, it is not clear that serum T_3 levels were ever altered. However, mortality was higher in the thyroxine group (43% versus 13%) than in the control group. It is of interest that, as the authors state, "the observed mortality in the controls in this study was less than that typically seen in our institution in ARF and ICU patients, whereas the 43% mortality noted in the thyroid group better approximates both our experience and that reported in the literature for ICU patients." It will be difficult to replicate this study (although this reader believes it should be replicated). But it is uncertain whether the small dose of thyroxine administered over 2 days actually is related to the mortality, considering that the mortality in the treated group was that usually observed, whereas the control happened to have a much lower mortality.[128] The same group has also studied the effect of thyroid hormone treatment on posttransplant acute tubular necrosis. T_3 treatment during the posttransplant period did not alter outcome in a beneficial or derogatory manner.[129]

Studies from animals are often quoted in the literature as an argument against treatment of NTIS or for the therapy. A study of sepsis induced in animals showed no difference in mortality, but some animals treated with thyroid hormone died earlier than did those that were untreated.[130] Chopra et al. induced NTIS in rats by injection of turpentine oil. The reduction in T_4, T_3, free T_4 index, and TSH were associated with no clear evidence of tissue hypothyroidism, and urinary nitrogen excretion was normal. Thyroid hormone replacement with T_4 or T_3 did not significantly alter enzyme activities or urinary nitrogen excretion.[131] Healthy pigs were subjected to 20 minutes of regional myocardial ischemia by Hsu and collaborators,[132] and this was associated with a drop in T_3, free T_3, and elevated rT_3. Some animals were treated with 0.2 µg T_3 per kilogram for five doses over 2 hours. While myocardial infarction size was not altered, the pigs treated with T_3 showed a more rapid improvement in cardiac index. Oxygen consumption did not alter. It should be noted that the T_3 levels fell back to normal levels within 4 hours of the last T_3 dose, suggesting that more prolonged therapy might have been beneficial. Katzeff et al.[133] studied a model of NTIS induced by caloric restriction in young rats. In these animals, T_3 was reduced, and there was a decrease in LV relaxation time, SERCA2 mRNA, and αMHC mRNA. All changes were reversed to normal values by supplementation with T_3, suggesting that the low-T_3 syndrome was related to the pathologic cardiac changes. Sepsis and multisystem organ failure are often associated with disseminated intravascular coagulation and consumption of coag inhibitors such as antithrombin III. Chapital studied a model of sepsis in rats and showed that T_3 supplementation reduced the decrease in antithrombin III levels, which presumably would reflect a beneficial effect.[134] Dogs subjected to hemorrhagic shock recovered more cardiovascular function when given T_3 intravenously than did untreated animals.[135] Neurologic outcome after anoxia is improved in dogs by T_3 treatment.[136]

Short-term studies on T_3 replacement of patients in shock, in patients with respiratory disease, in subjects who are brain dead and potential organ donors, and in patients undergoing coronary artery bypass grafts all suggest modest cardiovascular benefits from the administration of T_3. One study reports benefit by replacing T_3 to elevate the depressed T_3 levels in premature infants.[137] Other studies found no apparent effects. Children treated with T_3 postoperatively when they have undergone cardiac surgery also require less cardiac support. T_3 administration (one dose of approximately 6 μg IV) did not alter cardiac performance in brain-dead transplant donors.[138-139] Coronary artery bypass, as studied by Klemperer and collaborators,[36] was associated with a drop in serum T_3; IV administration of T_3 elevated T_3 above normal, augmented cardiac output, and reduced the need for pressor support but had no other effect. In this study, however, the patients had a very favorable prognosis and minimal NTIS, so the study primarily shows that administration of T_3 had no adverse effect under these circumstances. In a study reported several years ago, T_3 administration to critically ill neonates with severe respiratory distress appeared to improve survival. Infants of less than 37 weeks gestational age or weighing less than 220 grams were given prophylactic doses of thyroxine and T_3 daily and had a lower mortality rate than untreated infants.[137] Use of thyroid hormone replacement in children after cardiac surgery has been extensively reviewed by Haas et al., with the conclusion that it is a desirable treatment option, especially in high-risk patients.[140] Goarin et al. studied the effect of T_3 administration in brain-dead organ donors and found that although it returned T_3 levels to normal, it did not improve hemodynamic status or myocardial function.[141] Pingitore et al. gave T_3 by IV infusion for 3 days to patients with chronic heart failure. Heart rate, plasma norepinephrine (down 52%), natriuretic peptide, and aldosterone (down 23%) were all significantly diminished, and ventricular performance improved, without side effects.[142] In a randomized study of patients for 24 hours after coronary bypass, correction of the usual drop in serum T_3 by IV T_3 infusion had no beneficial or deleterious effect on cardiac parameters.[143] Of interest, it also did not affect leucine flux or urinary nitrogen excretion, contrary to the usual assumption that a drop in serum T_3 should spare body protein. The general outcome of these studies is that they weakly support the use of T_3, and none of the studies found evidence of damage caused by treatment.[144-150]

In summary, it can be stated that there is no clear evidence that thyroxine or triiodothyronine treatment of NTIS in animals or man is disadvantageous, and no certain proof that it is advantageous. However, what evidence there is suggests it may be beneficial. The argument has been raised that administration of thyroid hormone in NTIS would prevent the elevation in TSH commonly seen in recovering patients. This seems rather specious. More objectively, the elevation of TSH is another suggestion that the few patients who survive the ordeal were originally hypothyroid and left untreated. Lastly, it is unlikely that administration of replacement hormone during NTIS would be harmful,

even if all of the evidence presented suggesting hypothyroidism was erroneous, and the patients were in fact euthyroid.

IF THYROID HORMONE REPLACEMENT IS GIVEN, WHAT SHOULD IT BE?

Clearly the high mortality rate in patients with T_4 under 4 μg/dL suggests that this is a target group in whom thyroid hormone administration should be considered. In this group of patients, there appears to be no obvious contraindication to replacement therapy, with the possible exception of people who have cardiac decompensation or arrhythmias. Even here, the evidence is uncertain. There is no clear evidence that administration of replacement doses of T_3 to patients with low cardiac output is disadvantageous, and in fact current studies using intravenous T_3 in these patients indicate it is well tolerated and may be beneficial.[151] Arrhythmias obviously also raise a question, but again, there is no evidence that replacement of thyroid hormone to a normal level would cause trouble in control of arrhythmias. Low free T_3 levels are reported to be associated with an increased incidence of fibrillation after cardiac surgery in elderly patients.[152] Thus even in this group of patients, it is reasonable to suggest therapy. It should also be noted that among patients with NTIS, there will certainly be patients who are clearly hypothyroid—based on known disease, treatment with dopamine, or elevated TSH—who need replacement therapy by any standard.

If therapy is to be given, it cannot be thyroxine alone, since this would fail to promptly elevate T_3 levels.[54] Treatment should include oral, or if this is impractical, intravenous T_3, and probably should be at the replacement level of approximately 50 μg/day given in divided doses. It may be appropriate to give slightly higher doses, such as 75 μg/day for 3 to 4 days to increase the body pool more rapidly, followed by replacement doses as described. Coincidentally, it is appropriate to start replacement with T_4. Serum levels of T_4 and T_3 should be followed at frequent intervals (every 48 hours) and dosages adjusted to achieve a serum T_3 level at least low normal (70 to 100 ng/dL) prior to the next scheduled dose. If treatment is successful, T_3 administration can gradually be reduced, and thyroxine administration can be increased to replacement levels as deiodination increases. Because of the marked diminution in T_4 to T_3 deiodination, and shunting of T_4 toward rT_3, replacement with T_4 may initially only lead to elevation of rT_3 and have very little effect upon T_3 levels, or physiologic action. In this situation, continued administration of T_3 would be preferred.

ADDITIONAL SUPPORTIVE HORMONAL THERAPY TO CONSIDER

Although this discussion concentrates on the potential value of treating patients with NTIS with replacement thyroid hormone, several important recent studies expand the concept to other areas, including treatment of the associated hyperglycemia, relative adrenal insufficiency, use of beta blockers in burn patients, and possible use of GHRH and testosterone. Van den Berghe and co-workers have suggested that the acute and prolonged critical illness responses are entirely different neuroendocrine conditions. In protracted severe illness, patients are kept alive with conditions that previously caused death. However, this process has unmasked a variety of nonspecific wasting syndromes that include protein loss, accumulation of fat stores, hyperglycemia and insulin resistance, hypoproteinemia, hypercalcemia, potassium depletion, and hypertriglyceridemia. In prolonged illness, cortisol values are elevated, although ACTH levels are low, indicating that other mechanisms are driving the steroid response.

Growth hormone secretory pulses are reduced, and the mean concentration is low in prolonged critical illness. FSH and LH are reduced, and testosterone levels are reduced. These authors maintain that the reduced neuroendocrine drive, present in the chronic phase of illness in an intensive care setting, is unlikely to be an evolutionary preserved beneficial process. They suggest that the administration of hypothalamic physiotropic releasing peptides may be a safer strategy than the administration of peripherally active hormones.[93]

Conclusions

This review has presented the arguments for administration of replacement T_3 and T_4 hormone in patients with NTIS. However, it is impossible to be certain at this time that it is either beneficial to replace hormone or whether this could be harmful. Only a prospective study will be adequate to prove this point, and probably this would need to involve hundreds of patients. One cannot envisage that replacement of thyroxin or T_3 can "cure" patients with NTIS. The probable effect, if any is achieved, will be a modest increment in overall physiologic function and a decrease in mortality. Perhaps this would be 5%, 10%, or 20%. If effective, thyroid hormone replacement will be one of many beneficial treatments given the patient, rather than a single magic bullet which would reverse all the metabolic changes going wrong in these severely ill patients. Ongoing studies document the beneficial effects of hormone replacement in these acutely and severely ill patients. Possibly therapy will ultimately involve replacement of peripheral hormones, or may instead be via growth hormone–releasing peptide (GHRP), TRH, GnRH, insulin, adrenal steroids, and leptin.

REFERENCES

1. McIver B, Gorman CA: Euthyroid sick syndrome: An overview, Thyroid 7:125–132, 1997.
2. DeGroot LJ: "Non-thyroidal illness syndrome" is functional central hypothyroidism, and if severe, hormone replacement is appropriate in light of present knowledge, J Endocrinol Invest 26:1163–1170, 2003.
3. Stathatos N, Wartofsky L: The euthyroid sick syndrome: is there a physiologic rationale for thyroid hormone treatment? J Endocrinol Invest 26:1174–1179, 2003.
4. Hennemann G, Docter R, Krenning EP: Causes and effects of the low T_3 syndrome during caloric deprivation and non-thyroidal illness: an overview, Acta Med Kaust 15:42–45, 1988.
5. Phillips RH, Valente WA, Caplan ES, et al: Circulating thyroid hormone changes in acute trauma: prognostic implications for clinical outcome, J Trauma 24:116–119, 1984.
6. Vardarli I, Schmidt R, Wdowinski JM, et al: The hypothalamo-hypophyseal-thyroid axis, plasma protein concentrations and the hypophyseogonadal axis in low T_3 syndrome following acute myocardial infarct, Klin Wochenschrift 65:129–133, 1987.
7. Eber B, Schumacher M, Langsteger W, et al: Changes in thyroid hormone parameters after acute myocardial infarction, Cardiology 86:152–156, 1995.
8. Holland FW, Brown PS, Weintraub BD, et al: Cardiopulmonary bypass and thyroid function: a "euthyroid sick syndrome." Ann Thorac Surg 52:46–50, 1991.
9. Vexiau P, Perez-Castiglioni P, Socie G, et al: The "euthyroid sick syndrome": Incidence, risk factors and prognostic value soon after allogeneic bone marrow transplantation, Br J Hematol 85:778–782, 1993.
10. Harris ARC, Fang SL, Vagenakis AG, et al: Effect of starvation, nutriment replacement, and hypothyroidism on in vitro hepatic T_4 to T_3 conversion in the rat, Metabolism 27:1680–1690, 1978.
11. Welle SL, Campbell RG: Decrease in resting metabolic rate during rapid weight loss is reversed by low-dose thyroid hormone treatment, Metabolism 35:289–291, 1986.
12. Plikat K, Langgartner J, Buettner R, et al: Frequency and outcome of patients with nonthyroidal illness syndrome in a medical intensive care unit, Metabolism 56(2):239–244, 2007 Feb.
13. Girvent M, Maestro S, Hernandez R, et al: Euthyroid sick syndrome, associated endocrine abnormalities, and outcome in elderly patients undergoing emergency operation, Surgery 123:560–567, 1998.
14. Wartofsky L, Burman KD: Alterations in thyroid function in patients with systemic illnesses: the "Euthyroid Sick Syndrome", Endocrine Rev 3:164–217, 1982.
15. Kaptein EM: Clinical relevance of thyroid hormone alterations in nonthyroidal illness, Thyroid International 4:22–25, 1997.
16. Docter R, Krenning EP, de Jong M, et al: The sick euthyroid syndrome: changes in thyroid hormone serum parameters and hormone metabolism, Clin Endocrinol 39:499–518, 1993.

17. Chopra IJ, Huang TS, Boado R, et al: Evidence against benefit from replacement doses of thyroid hormones in nonthyroidal illness: studies using turpentine oil–injected rat, J Endocrinol Invest 10:559–564, 1987.
18. Schilling JU, Zimmermann T, Albrecht S, et al: Low T_3 syndrome in multiple trauma patients – a phenomenon or important pathogenetic factor? Medizinische Klinik 3:66–69, 1999.
19. Schulte C, Reinhardt W, Beelen D, et al: Low T_3-syndrome and nutritional status as prognostic factors in patients undergoing bone marrow transplantation, Bone Marrow Transplantation 22:1171–1178, 1998.
20. Girvent M, Maestro S, Hernandez R, et al: Euthyroid sick syndrome, associated endocrine abnormalities, and outcome in elderly patients undergoing emergency operation, Surgery 123:560–567, 1998.
21. Maldonado LS, Murata GH, Hershman JM, et al: Do thyroid function tests independently predict survival in the critically ill? Thyroid 2:119, 1992.
22. Vaughan GM, Mason AD, McManus WF, et al: Alterations of mental status and thyroid hormones after thermal injury, J Clin Endocrinol Metab 60:1221, 1985.
23. De Marinis L, Mancini A, Masala R, et al: Evaluation of pituitary-thyroid axis response to acute myocardial infarction, J Endocrinol Invest 8:507, 1985.
24. Surks MI, Hupart KH, Pan C, et al: Normal free thyroxine in critical nonthyroidal illnesses measured by ultrafiltration of undiluted serum and equilibrium dialysis, J Clin Endocrinol Metab 67:1031–1039, 1988.
25. Melmed S, Geola FL, Reed AW, et al: A comparison of methods for assessing thyroid function in nonthyroidal illness, J Clin Endocrinol Metab 54:300–306, 1982.
26. Kaptein EM, MacIntyre SS, Weiner JM, et al: Free thyroxine estimates in nonthyroidal illness: comparison of eight methods, J Clin Endocrinol Metab 52:1073–1077, 1981.
27. Kantor M, et al: Admission thyroid evaluation in very-low-birth-weight infants: association with death and severe intraventricular hemorrhage, Thyroid 13:965, 2003.
28. Chopra IJ, Solomon DH, Hepner GW, et al: Misleadingly low free thyroxine index and usefulness of reverse triiodothyronine measurement in nonthyroidal illnesses, Ann Int Med 90:905–912, 1979.
29. Bacci V, Schussler GC, Kaplan TB: The relationship between serum triiodothyronine and thyrotropin during systemic illness, J Clin Endocrinol Metab 54:1229–1235, 1982.
30. Sapin R, Schlienger JL, Kaltenbach G, et al: Determination of free triiodothyronine by six different methods in patients with nonthyroidal illness and in patients treated with amiodarone, Ann Clin Biochem 32:314–324, 1995.
31. Chopra IJ, Taing P, Mikus L: Direct determination of free triiodothyronine (T_3) in undiluted serum by equilibrium dialysis/radioimmunoassay, Thyroid 6:255–259, 1996.
32. Chopra IJ: Simultaneous measurement of free thyroxine and free 3,5,3'-triiodothyronine in undiluted serum

by direct equilibrium dialysis/radioimmunoassay: evidence that free triiodothyronine and free thyroxine are normal in many patients with the low triiodothyronine syndrome, 1998.
33. Faber J, Kirkegaard C, Rasmussen B, et al: Pituitary-thyroid axis in critical illness, J Clin Endocrinol Metab 65(2):315–320, 1987 Aug.
34. Fritz KS, Wilcox RB, Nelson JC: Quantifying spurious free T_4 results attributable to thyroxine-binding proteins in serum dialysates and ultrafiltrates, Clin Chem 53(5):985–988, 2007 May.
35. Peeters RP, Wouters PJ, Kaptein E, et al: Reduced activation and increased inactivation of thyroid hormone in tissues of critically ill patients, J Clin Endocrinol Metab 88(7):3202–3211, 2003 Jul.
36. Klemperer JD, Klein I, Gomez M, et al: Thyroid hormone treatment after coronary-artery bypass surgery, N Engl J Med 333:1522–1527, 1995.
37. Osburne RC, Myers EA, Rodbard D, et al: Adaptation to hypocaloric feeding: physiologic significance of the fall in T_3, Metabolism 32:9–13, 1983.
38. Afandi B, Schussler GC, Arafeh A-H, et al: Selective consumption of thyroxine-binding globulin during cardiac bypass surgery, Metabolism 49:270–274, 2000.
39. Jirasakuldech B, Schussler GC, Yap MG, et al: A characteristic serpin cleavage product of thyroxine-binding globulin appears in sepsis sera, J Clin Endocrinol Metab 85:3996–3999, 2000.
40. den Brinker M, Joosten KF, Visser TJ, et al: Euthyroid sick syndrome in meningococcal sepsis: the impact of peripheral thyroid hormone metabolism and binding proteins, J Clin Endocrinol Metab 90(10):5613–5620, 2005.
41. Uchimura H, Nagataki S, Tabuchi T, et al: Measurements of free thyroxine: comparison of percent of free thyroxine in diluted and undiluted sera, J Clin Endocrinol Metab 42:561–566, 1976.
42. Nelson JC, Weiss RM: The effect of serum dilution on free thyroxine concentration in the low T_4 syndrome of nonthyroidal illness, J Clin Endocrinol Metab 61:239–246, 1985.
43. Wang R, Nelson JC, Weiss RM, et al: Accuracy of free thyroxine measurements across natural ranges of thyroxine binding to serum proteins, Thyroid 10:31–39, 2000.
44. Kaptein EM: Thyroid hormone metabolism and thyroid diseases in chronic renal failure, Endocrine Rev 17:45–63, 1996.
45. Liewendahl K, Helenius T, Naveri H, et al: Fatty acid–induced increase in serum dialyzable free thyroxine after physical exercise: implication for nonthyroidal illness, J Clin Endocrinol Metab 74:1361–1365, 1992.
46. Mendel CM, Frost PH, Cavalieri RR: Effect of free fatty acids on the concentration of free thyroxine in human serum: the role of albumin, J Clin Endocrinol Metab 63:1394–1399, 1986.
47. Jaume JC, Mendel CM, Frost PH, et al: Extremely low doses of heparin release lipase activity into the plasma and can thereby cause artifactual elevations in the

serum-free thyroxine concentration as measured by equilibrium dialysis, Thyroid 6:79–83, 1996.

48. Wang Y-S, Hershman JM, Pekary AE: Improved ultrafiltration method for simultaneous measurement of free thyroxine and free triiodothyronine in serum, Clin Chem 31:517–522, 1985.

49. Mendel CM, Laufhton CW, McMahon FA, et al: Inability to detect an inhibitor of thyroxine-serum protein binding in sera from patients with nonthyroidal illness, Metabolism 40:491–502, 1991.

50. Chopra IJ, Huang T-S, Beredo A, et al: Evidence for an inhibitor of extrathyroidal conversion of thyroxine to 3,5,3'-triiodothyronine in sera of patients with nonthyroidal illnesses, J Clin Endocrinol Metab 60:666, 1985.

51. Wang R, Nelson JC, Wilcox RB: Salsalate administration—a potential pharmacological model of the sick euthyroid syndrome, J Clin Endocrinol Metab 83:3095–3099, 1998.

52. Csako G, Zweig MH, Benson C, et al: On the albumin-dependence of the measurement of free thyroxine. II. Patients with nonthyroidal illness, Clin Chem 33:87–92, 1987.

53. Chopra IJ, Chua Teco GN, Mead JF, et al: Relationship between serum free fatty acids and thyroid hormone binding inhibitor in nonthyroid illnesses, J Clin Endocrinol Metab 60:980–984, 1985.

54. Brent GA, Hershman JM: Thyroxine therapy in patients with severe nonthyroidal illnesses and lower serum thyroxine concentration, J Clin Endocrinol Metab 63:1–8, 1986.

55. Chopra IJ: Nonthyroidal illness syndrome or euthyroid sick syndrome? Endocrine Pract 2:45–52, 1996.

56. Franklyn JA, Black EG, Betteridge J, et al: Comparison of second and third generation methods for measurement of serum thyrotropin in patients with overt hyperthyroidism, patients receiving thyroxine therapy, and those with nonthyroidal illness, J Clin Endocrinol Metab 78:1368–1371, 1994.

57. Vierhapper H, Laggner A, Waldhausl W, et al: Impaired secretion of TSH in critically ill patients with "low T4-syndrome". Acta Endocrinol 101:542–549, 1982.

58. Faber J, Kirkegaard C, Rasmussen B, et al: Pituitary-thyroid axis in critical illness, J Clin Endocrinol Metab 65:315–320, 1987.

59. Arem R, Deppe S: Fatal nonthyroidal illness may impair nocturnal thyrotropin levels, Am J Med 88:258–262, 1990.

60. Lee H-Y, Suhl J, Pekary AE, et al: Secretion of thyrotropin with reduced concanavalin-A-binding activity in patients with severe nonthyroid illness, J Clin Endocrinol Metab 65:942, 1987.

61. Spratt DI, Bigos ST, Beitins I, et al: Both hyper- and hypogonadotropic hypogonadism occur transiently in acute illness: bio- and immunoactive gonadotropins, J Clin Endocrinol Metab 75:1562–1570, 1992.

62. Spratt DI, Cox P, Orav J, et al: Reproductive axis suppression in acute illness is related to disease severity, J Clin Endocrinol Metab 76:1548–1554, 1993.

63. Van den Berghe G, Weekers F, Baxter RC, et al: Five-day pulsatile gonadotropin-releasing hormone administration unveils combined hypothalamic-pituitary-gonadal defects underlying profound hypoandrogenism in men with prolonged critical illness, J Clin Endocrinol Metab 86:3217–3226, 2001.

64. Kaptein EM, Grieb DA, Spencer CA, et al: Thyroxine metabolism in the low thyroxine state of critical nonthyroidal illnesses, J Clin Endocrinol Metab 53:764–771, 1981.

65. Kaptein EM, Robinson WJ, Grieb DA, et al: Peripheral serum thyroxine, triiodothyronine and reverse triiodothyronine kinetics in the low thyroxine state of acute nonthyroidal illnesses. A noncompartmental analysis, J Clin Invest 69:526–535, 1982.

66. Lim VS, Fang VS, Katz AI, et al: Thyroid dysfunction in chronic renal failure. A study of the pituitary-thyroid axis and peripheral turnover, Kinetics of thyroxine and triiodothyronine, J Clin Invest 60(3):522–534, 1997.

67. Lim C-F, Docter R, Visser TJ, et al: Inhibition of thyroxine transport into cultured rat hepatocytes by serum of nonuremic critically ill patients: effects of bilirubin and nonesterified fatty acids, J Clin Endocrinol Metab 76:1165–1172, 1993.

68. Vos RA, de Jong M, Bernard BF, et al: Impaired thyroxine and 3,5,3'-triiodothyronine handling by rat hepatocytes in the presence of serum of patients with nonthyroidal illness, J Clin Endocrinol Metab 80:2364–2370, 1995.

69. Lim C-F, Docter R, Krenning EP, et al: Transport of thyroxine into cultured hepatocytes: effects of mild nonthyroidal illness and calorie restriction in obese subjects, Clinical Endocrinol 40:79–85, 1994.

70. Sarne DH, Refetoff S: Measurement of thyroxine uptake from serum by cultured human hepatocytes as an index of thyroid status: reduced thyroxine uptake from serum of patients with nonthyroidal illness, J Clin Endocrinol Metab 61:1046–1052, 1985.

71. Krenning D, et al: Decreased transport of thyroxine (T4), 3, 3', 5-triiodothyronine (T3) and 3,3',5'-triiodothyronine (rT3) into rat hepatocytes in primary culture due to a decrease of cellular ATP content and various drugs, FEBS Lett 140:229–233, 1982.

72. Arem R, Wiener GJ, Kaplan SG, et al: Reduced tissue thyroid hormone levels in fatal illness, Metabolism 42:1102–1108, 1993.

73. Peeters RP, van der Geyten S, Wouters PJ, et al: Tissue thyroid hormone levels in critical illness, J Clin Endocrinol Metab 90(12):6498–6507. Epub 2005 Sep 20, 2005.

74. d'Amati G, di Gioia CRT, Mentuccia D, et al: Increased expression of thyroid hormone receptor isoforms in end-stage human congestive heart failure, J Clin Endocrinol Metab 86:2080–2084, 2001.

75. Rodriguez-Perez A, Palos-Paz F, Kaptein E, et al: Identification of molecular mechanisms related to nonthyroidal illness syndrome in skeletal muscle and adipose tissue from patients with septic shock, Clin Endocrinol (Oxf) 68(5):821–827, 2008.

76. Sanchez B, Jolin T: Triiodothyronine-receptor complex in rat brain: effects of thyroidectomy, fasting, food restriction, and diabetes, Endocrinology 129:361–367, 1991.

77. Beigneux A, et al: Sick euthyroid syndrome is associated with decreased TR expression and DNA binding in mouse liver, Am J Physiol Endocrinol Metab 284:E228–E236, 2003.

78. Brent GA, Hershman JM, Reed AW, et al: Serum angiotensin converting enzyme in severe nonthyroidal illness associated with low serum thyroxine concentration, Ann Intern Med 100:680–683, 1986.

79. Seppel T, Becker A, Lippert F, et al: Serum sex hormone-binding globulin and osteocalcin in systemic nonthyroidal illness associated with low thyroid hormone concentrations, J Clin Endocrinol Metab 81:1663–1665, 1996.

80. Chapital AD, Hendrick SR, Lloyd L, et al: The effects of triiodothyronine augmentation on antithrombin III levels in sepsis, Am Surg 67(3):253–255, 2001 Mar.

81. Kaplan MM: Subcellular alterations causing reduced hepatic thyroxine-5'-monodeiodinase activity in fasted rats, Endocrinology 104:58–64, 1979.

82. Berger MM, Lemarchand-Beraud T, Cavadini C, et al: Relations between the selenium status and the low T3 syndrome after major trauma, Intensive Care Med 22:575–581, 1996.

83. Berger MM, Reymond MJ, Shenkin A, et al: Influence of selenium supplements on the post-traumatic alterations of the thyroid axis: a placebo-controlled trial, Intensive Care Med 27:91–100, 2001.

84. Blake NG, Eckland JA, Foster OJF, et al: Inhibition of hypothalamic thyrotropin-releasing hormone messenger ribonucleic acid during food deprivation, Endocrinology 129:2714–2718, 1991.

85. Fliers E, Guldenaar SEF, Wiersinga WM, et al: Decreased hypothalamic thyrotropin-releasing hormone gene expression in patients with nonthyroidal illness, J Clin Endocrinol Metab 82:4032–4036, 1997.

86. Van den Berghe G, De Zegher F, Baxter RC, et al: Neuroendocrinology of prolonged critical illness: effects of exogenous thyrotropin-releasing hormone and its combination with growth hormone secretagogues, J Clin Endocrinol Metab 83:309–319, 1998.

87. Nicoloff JT, Fisher DA, Appleman MD Jr: The role of glucocorticoids in the regulation of thyroid function in man, J Clin Invest 49:1922, 1970.

88. Brabant G, Brabant A, Ranft U: Circadian and pulsatile thyrotropin secretion in euthyroid man under the influence of thyroid hormone and glucocorticoid administration, J Clin Endocrinol Metab 65:83, 1987.

89. Benker G, Raida M, Olbricht T, et al: TSH secretion in Cushing's syndrome: relation to glucocorticoid excess, diabetes, goiter, and the "sick euthyroid syndrome", Clin Endocrinol 33:777–786, 1990.

90. Bianco AC, Nunes MT, Hell NS, et al: The role of glucocorticoids in the stress-induced reduction of extrathyroidal 3,5,3'-triiodothyronine generation in rats, Endocrinology 120:1033–1038, 1987.

91. Lim VS, Passo C, Murata Y, et al: Reduced triiodothyronine content in liver but not pituitary of the uremic rat model: demonstration of changes compatible with thyroid hormone deficiency in liver only, Endocrinology 114:280–286, 1984.

92. Beale E, Srivastava P, Liang H, et al: Triiodothyroacetic acid (T3AC): is it an intracellular autocrine acting form of thyroid hormone? Abstract No. OR1–1 presented at the 79th Annual Meeting of the Endocrine Society, Minneapolis, MN, 1997.

93. Van den Berghe G, de Zegher F, Bouillon R: Acute and prolonged critical illness as different neuroendocrine paradigms, J Clin Endocrinol Metab 83:1827–1834, 1998.

94. Van den Berghe G, et al: Intensive insulin therapy in critically ill patients, N Engl J Med 345:1359–1367, 2001.

95. Van den Berghe G, Schoonheydt K, Becx P, et al: Insulin therapy protects the central and peripheral nervous system of intensive care patients, Neurology 64(8):1348–1353, 2005 Apr 26.

96. Weekers F, Giulietti AP, Michalaki M, et al: Metabolic, endocrine, and immune effects of stress hyperglycemia in a rabbit model of prolonged critical illness, Endocrinology 144(12):5329–5338, 2003 Dec. Epub 2003 Aug 28.

97. Mönig H, Arendt T, Meyer M, et al: Activation of the hypothalamo-pituitary-adrenal axis in response to septic or non-septic diseases—implications for the euthyroid sick syndrome, Intensive Care Med 25:1402–1406, 1999.

98. Hermus RM, Sweep CG, van der Meer MJ, et al: Continuous infusion of interleukin-1 beta induces a nonthyroidal illness syndrome in the rat, Endocrinology 131:2139–2146, 1992.

99. Cannon JG, Tompkins RG, Gelfand JA, et al: Circulating interleukin-1 and tumor necrosis factor in septic shock and experimental endotoxin fever, J Infect Dis 161:79–84, 1990.

100. van der Poll T, Van Zee KJ, Endert E, et al: Interleukin-1 receptor blockade does not affect endotoxin-induced changes in plasma thyroid hormone and thyrotropin concentrations in man, J Clin Endocrinol Metab 80:1341–1346, 1995.

101. de Metz J, Romijn JA, Endert E, et al: Administration of interferon-γ in healthy subjects does not modulate thyroid hormone metabolism, Thyroid 10:87–91, 2000.

102. Chopra IJ, Sakane S, Chua Teco GN: A study of the serum concentration of tumor necrosis factor—in thyroidal and nonthyroidal illnesses, J Clin Endocrinol Metab 72:1113–1116, 1991.

103. van der Poll T, Endert E, Coyle SM, et al: Neutralization of TNF does not influence endotoxin-induced changes in thyroid hormone metabolism in humans, Am J Physiol 276:R357–R362, 1999.

104. van der Poll T, Romijn JA, Wiersinga WM, et al: Tumor necrosis factor: a putative mediator of the sick euthyroid syndrome in man, J Clin Endocrinol Metab 71:1567–1572, 1990.

105. Nagaya T, Fujieda M, Otsuka G, et al: A potential role of activated NF-kappa B in the pathogenesis of euthyroid sick syndrome, J Clin Invest 106(3):393–402, 2000.

106. Bartalena L, Brogioni S, Grasso L, et al: Relationship of the increased serum interleukin-6 concentration to changes of thyroid function in nonthyroidal illness, J Endocrinol Invest 17:269–274, 1994.

107. Boelen A, Platvoet-ter Schiphorst MC, Wiersinga WM: Association between serum interleukin-6 and serum 3,5,3'-triiodothyronine in nonthyroidal illness, J Clin Endocrinol Metab 77:1695–1699, 1993.

108. Stouthard JML, van der Poll T, Endert E, et al: Effects of acute and chronic interleukin 6 administration on thyroid hormone metabolism in humans, J Clin Endocrinol Metab 79:1342–1346, 1994.

109. Boelen A, Platvoet-ter Schiphorst MC, Wiersinga WM: Immunoneutralization of interleukin 1, tumor necrosis factor, interleukin-6 or interferon does not prevent the LPS-induced sick euthyroid syndrome in mice, J Endocrinol 153:115–122, 1997.

110. Boelen A, Platvoet-ter Schiphorst MC, Wiersinga WM: Relationship between serum 3,5,3'-triiodothyronine and serum interleukin 8, interleukin 10 or interferon gamma in patients with nonthyroidal illness, J Endocrinol Invest 19:480–483, 1996.

111. De Metz J, Romijn JA, Endert E, et al: Administration of Interferon-γ in healthy subjects does not modulate thyroid hormone metabolism, Thyroid 10:87–91, 2000.

112. Michalaki M, Vagenakis AG, Makri M, et al: Dissociation of the early decline in serum T₃ concentration and serum IL-6 rise and TNFα in nonthyroidal illnss syndrome induced by abdominal surgery, J Clin Endocrinol Metab 86:4198–4205, 2001.

113. Boelen A, Platvoet-ter Schiphorst MC, Wiersinga WM: Soluble cytokine receptors and the low 3,5,3'-triiodothyronine syndrome in patients with nonthyroidal disease, J Clin Endocrinol Metab 80:971–976, 1995.

114. Schultes B, et al: Acute and prolonged effects of insulin-induced hypoglycemia on the pituitary-thyroid axis in humans, Metabolism 51:1370–1374, 2002.

115. Pereira D, Procianoy R: Effect of perinatal asphyxia on thyroid-stimulating hormone and thyroid hormone levels, Acta Pediatr 92:339–345, 2003.

116. Custro N, Scafidi V, Costanzo G, et al: Role of high blood glucagon in the reduction of serum levels of triiodothyronine in severe nonthyroid diseases, Minerva Endocrinol 14:221–226, 1989.

117. Van den Berghe G, de Zegher F, Lauwers P: Dopamine and the sick euthyroid syndrome in critical illness, Clin Endocrinol 41:731–737, 1994.

118. Legradi G, Emerson CH, Ahima RS, et al: Leptin prevents fasting-induced suppression of prothyrotropin-releasing hormone messenger ribonucleic acid in neurons of the hypothalamic paraventricular nucleus, Endocrinology 138:2569–2576, 1997.

119. Legradi G, Emerson CH, Ahima RS, et al: Arcuate nucleus ablation prevents fasting-induced suppression of proTRH mRNA in the hypothalamic paraventricular nucleus, Neuroendocrinology 68:89–97, 1998.

120. Flier JS, Harris M, Hollenberg AN: Leptin, nutrition, and the thyroid: the why, the wherefore, and the wiring, J Clin Invest 105:859–861, 2000.

121. Bornstein SR, et al: Leptin levels are elevated despite low thyroid hormone levels in the "euthyroid sick" syndrome, J Clin Endocrinol Metab 82(12):4278–4279, 1997.

122. Vesely DL, San Miguel GI, Hassan I, et al: Atrial natriuretic hormone, vessel dilator, long-acting natriuretic hormone, and kaliuretic hormone decrease the circulating concentrations of total and free T₄ and free T₃ with reciprocal increase in TSH, J Clin Endocrinol Metab 86:5438–5442, 2001.

123. Kidess AI, Caplan RH, Reynertson RH, et al: Transient corticotropin deficiency in critical illness, Mayo Clin Proc 68:435–441, 1993.

124. Merry WH, Caplan RH, Wickus GG, et al: Acute adrenal failure due to transient corticotropin deficiency in postoperative patients, Surgery 116:1095–1100, 1994.

125. Lambert SWJ, Bruining HA, DeLong FH: Corticosteroid therapy in severe illness, N Engl J Med 337:1285–1292, 1997.

126. Becker RA, Vaughan GM, Ziegler MG, et al: Hypermetabolic low triiodothyronine syndrome of burn injury, Critical Care Med 10:870–875, 1982.

127. Siegel N, et al: Beneficial effect of thyroxine on recovery from toxic acute renal failure, Kidney Int 25:906–911, 1984.

128. Acker CG, Singh AR, Flick RP, et al: A trial of thyroxine in acute renal failure, Kidney Int 57:293–298, 2000.

129. Acker CG, Flick R, Shapiro R, et al: Thyroid hormone in the treatment of post-transplant acute tubular necrosis (ATN), Am J Transplant 2:57–61, 2002.

130. Little JS: Effect of thyroid hormone on survival after bacterial infection, Endocrinology 117:1431–1435, 1985.

131. Chopra IJ, Huang TS, Boado R, et al: Evidence against benefit from replacement doses of thyroid hormones in nonthyroidal illness: studies using turpentine oil-injected rat, J Endocrinol Invest 10:559, 1987.

132. Hsu R-B, Huang T-S, Chen Y-S, et al: Effect of triiodothyronine administration in experimental myocardial injury, J Endocrinol Invest 18:702–709, 1995.

133. Katzeff HL, Powell SR, Ojamaa K: Alterations in cardiac contractility and gene expression during low T₃ syndrome: prevention with T₃, Amer J Physiol 273:E951–E956, 1997.

134. Chapital AD, Hendrick SR, Lloyd L, et al: The effects of triiodothyronine augmentation on antithrombin III levels in sepsis, Am Surg 67:253–255, 2001.

135. Shigematsu H, Shatney CH: The effect of triiodothyronine and reverse triiodothyronine on canine hemorrhagic shock, Nippon Geka Gakkai Zasshi 89:1587–1593, 1988.

136. Facktor MA, Mayor GH, Nachreiner RF, et al: Thyroid hormone loss and replacement during resuscitation from cardiac arrest in dogs, Resuscitation 26:141–162, 1993.

137. Schoenberger W, Grimm W, Emmrich P, et al: Thyroid administration lowers mortality in premature infants, Lancet 2:1181, 1979.

138. Novitzky D, Cooper D, Reichart B: Hemodynamic and metabolic responses to hormonal therapy in brain-dead potential organ donors, Transplantation 43:852–855, 1987.

139. Novitzky D, et al: Improved cardiac allograft function following triiodothyronine therapy to both donor and recipient, Transplantation 49:311–316, 1990.

140. Haas NA, Camphausen CK, Kececioglu D: Clinical review: thyroid hormone replacement in children after cardiac surgery: is it worth a try? Crit Care 10(3):213, 2006.

141. Goarin JP, Cohen S, Riou B, et al: The effects of triiodothyronine on hemodynamic status and cardiac function in potential heart donors, Anesth Analg 83:41–47, 1996.

142. Pingitore A, Galli E, Barison A, et al: Acute effects of triiodothyronine (T₃) replacement therapy in patients with chronic heart failure and low-T₃ syndrome: a randomized, placebo-controlled study, J Clin Endocrinol Metab 93(4):1351–1358, 2008.

143. Spratt DI, Frohnauer M, Cyr-Alves H, et al: Physiological effects of nonthyroidal illness syndrome in patients after cardiac surgery, Am J Physiol Endocrinol Metab 293(1):E310–E315, 2007.

144. Hesch R, et al: Treatment of dopamine-dependent shock with triiodothyronine, Endocr Res Commun 8:299–301, 1981.

145. Meyer T, et al: Treatment of dopamine-dependent shock with triiodothyronine: preliminary results, Dtsch Med Wochenschr 104:1711–1714, 1979.

146. Dulchavsky S, et al: Beneficial effects of thyroid hormone administration on metabolic and hemodynamic function in hemorrhagic shock, FASEB J 4:A952, 1990.

147. Dulchavsky S, et al: T₃ preserves respiratory function in sepsis, J Trauma 31:753–759, 1991.

148. Dulchavsky S, Hendrick S, Dutta S: Pulmonary biophysical effects of triiodothyronine (T₃) augmentation during sepsis-induced hypothyroidism, Trauma 35:104–109, 1993.

149. Klemperer J, et al: Thyroid hormone treatment after coronary-artery bypass surgery, N Engl J Med 333:1522–1527, 1995.

150. Bennett-Guerro E, et al: Duke T₃ Study Group, Cardiovascular effects of intravenous triiodothyronine in patients undergoing coronary artery bypass graft surgery. A randomized, double-blind, placebo-controlled trial, J Am Med Assoc 275:687–692, 1996.

151. Hamilton MA, Stevenson LW: Thyroid hormone abnormalities in heart failure: possibilities for therapy, Thyroid 6:527–529, 1996.

152. Kokkonen L, Majahalme S, Kööbi T, et al: Atrial fibrillation in elderly patients after cardiac surgery: postoperative hemodynamics and low postoperative serum triiodothyronine, J Cardiothorac Vasc Anesth 19(2):182–187, 2005 Apr.

Chapter 16

MULTINODULAR GOITER

LASZLO HEGEDÜS, RALF PASCHKE, KNUT KROHN, and STEEN J. BONNEMA

Basic Aspects

DEFINITION AND CLINICAL MANIFESTATION

Benign nodular thyroid disease is a heterogeneous thyroid disorder that is highly prevalent in iodine-deficient areas. On a very general basis, it can be divided into solitary nodular and multinodular thyroid disease. Histologically, benign thyroid nodules are distinguished (1) as encapsulated lesions (true adenomas) or adenomatous nodules that lack a capsule, and (2) by morphologic criteria according to the World Health Organization (WHO) classification.[1] On functional grounds, nodules are classified as cold, normal, or hot, depending on whether they show decreased, normal, or increased uptake on scintiscan. Approximately 50% to 85% of all nodules are cold, up to 40% are scintigraphically indifferent, and about 10% are hot,[2,3] although the prevalence will vary geographically with the iodine supply and with the clinical setting.

Classification of thyroid nodules on the basis of results from clonality studies implies that most thyroid nodules are "true"

thyroid tumors compared with polyclonal hyperplastic nodules. Traditionally, only thyroid adenomas are considered true tumors, on the basis of an exclusive histologic definition—the presence of a capsule and a growth pattern that are different from the surrounding normal parenchyma in an otherwise normal thyroid gland. Strict histologic criteria for an adenoma and its differentiation from hyperplastic thyroid nodules or adenomatous nodules (without a capsule) are, however, difficult to obtain in the frequent presence of goiter or thyroiditis. The biological basis for separating hyperplastic thyroid nodules from true tumors, therefore, should also depend on their clonality.[4] Because many thyroid nodules without a capsule (adenomatous nodules) are monoclonal, a mixed functional and molecular definition of true thyroid tumors, as outlined in Fig. 16-1, appears objective and consistent. In contrast to solitary nodular thyroid disease, which has a more uniform clinical, pathologic, and molecular picture, multinodular nontoxic goiter (MNG) and multinodular toxic goiter (MNTG) make up a mixed group of nodular entities. Thus a combination of hyper-, hypo-, or normally functioning thyroid lesions usually is found within the same thyroid gland. The overall balance of functional properties of individual thyroid nodules within a multinodular goiter ultimately determines the functional status in the individual patient, which may be seen as euthyroidism (normal thyroid-stimulating hormone [TSH] and free thyroid hormone levels), subclinical hyperthyroidism (low or suppressed TSH and normal free thyroid hormone levels), or overt hyperthyroidism (suppressed TSH and elevated free thyroid hormone levels). The term MNG is applied in the first scenario, and MNTG refers to the latter situations. It is important to emphasize that this functional characterization is not stationary, but patients with MNTG usually have a history of long-standing MNG.[5] In general, development of MNG proceeds in two phases: global activation of thyroid epithelial cell proliferation (e.g., as the result of iodine deficiency or other goitrogenic stimuli) leading to goiter, and a focal increase in thyroid epithelial cell proliferation causing thyroid nodules. So far, the most common stimulus for local proliferation is a somatic mutation, as detailed in the following section.

ENVIRONMENT VERSUS HEREDITY

Until recently, nontoxic goiter was regarded mainly as a consequence of iodine deficiency. However, a number of goitrogens[6-8] and cigarette smoking are important environmental risk factors in the origin of nontoxic goiter. The impact of smoking, most likely mediated by thiocyanate, which competitively inhibits the iodide transport into the thyroid, has been extensively studied.[6,9] Additional etiologically important factors consist of gender,[10,11]

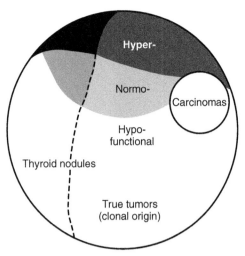

FIGURE 16-1. Classification of thyroid nodules on the basis of results from clonality studies. Such studies imply that most thyroid nodules are "true" thyroid tumors compared with polyclonal hyperplastic nodules. Traditionally, only thyroid adenomas are considered true tumors. This is based solely on a histologic definition—the presence of a capsule and a growth pattern that is different from the surrounding normal parenchyma in an otherwise normal thyroid gland.

age,[12] and increased body mass index (BMI).[13] The effect of a certain goitrogen is influenced by the degree of iodine sufficiency and therefore varies regionally and interindividually. However, it is most likely that interactions between environmental factors and individual genetic determinants ultimately determine the onset of the goiter.[10] Nontoxic goiter appearing early in life, often clustering in families, suggests strong genetic susceptibility, whereas environmental determinants are more likely to have additive or triggering effects. However, in an individual, it may be impossible to evaluate the relative contribution of genetic predisposition and a multitude of potential environmental factors.

In contrast to sporadic goiters, caused by spontaneous recessive genomic variations, most cases of familial goiter present an autosomal dominant pattern of inheritance, indicating predominant genetic defects.[14-16] Gene-gene interactions or various polygenic mechanisms (i.e., synergistic effects of several variants or polymorphisms) could increase the complexity of the pathogenesis of nontoxic goiter and offer an explanation for its genetic heterogeneity. A strong genetic predisposition is indicated by family and twin studies. Thus, children of parents with goiter have a significantly higher risk for developing goiter compared with children of nongoitrous parents.[17] The high incidence in females and the higher concordance in monozygotic than in dizygotic twins also suggest a genetic predisposition.[10] Moreover, preliminary evidence reveals a positive family history for thyroid disease in those who have postoperative relapse of goiter, which can occur from months to years after surgery.[18,19]

The development of nontoxic goiter is most likely a continuous process that starts with thyroid hyperplasia. Therefore, defects in genes that play an important role in thyroid physiology and thyroid hormone synthesis could predispose to the development of goiter, especially in cases of borderline or overt iodine deficiency. Such defects could lead to dyshormonogenesis as an immediate response, thereby indirectly explaining the nodular transformation of the thyroid as a late consequence of dyshor-

monogenesis, as a form of maladaptation.[12] Genes that encode the proteins involved in thyroid hormone synthesis, such as the thyroglobulin gene (*TG* gene), the thyroid peroxidase gene (*TPO* gene), the sodium-iodide symporter gene (*SLC5A5*), the Pendred syndrome gene (*SLC26A4*), the TSH receptor gene (*TSH-R* gene), the iodotyrosine deiodinase gene (*DEHAL1*), and the thyroid oxidase 2 gene (*THOX2*), are convincing candidate genes in familial euthyroid goiter. Originally, several mutations in these genes were identified in patients with congenital hypothyroidism. However, in cases of less severe functional impairment that can still be compensated, the contribution of variants of these genes in the development of nontoxic goiter is possible. Moreover, in case of mutations in the *TG* gene,[20,21] *SLC26A4*,[22,23] and *SLC5A5*,[24,25] patients with nontoxic goiter have also been identified.

LINKAGE STUDIES

To identify novel susceptibility loci, as well as to account for the coinheritance of different genomic regions, and to further improve the understanding of the genetic mechanisms that contribute to the development of nontoxic familial goiter, linkage analyses have been performed. A genome-wide linkage analysis has identified a candidate locus, MNG1 on chromosome 14q31, in a large Canadian family with 18 affected individuals.[15] This locus was confirmed in a German family with recurrent euthyroid goiters.[26] A dominant pattern of inheritance with high penetrance was assumed in both investigations. Moreover, a region on 14q31 between MNG1 and the *TSH-R* gene was identified as a potential positional candidate region[26] for nontoxic goiter. However, in the earlier study by Bignell et al.,[15] the *TSH-R* gene was clearly excluded. Furthermore, an X-linked autosomal dominant pattern and linkage to a second locus MNG2 (Xp22) was identified in an Italian pedigree with nontoxic familial goiter.[27] To identify additional candidate regions, the first extended genome-wide linkage analysis was performed to detect susceptibility loci in 18 Danish, German, and Slovakian euthyroid goiter families.[14] Assuming genetic heterogeneity and a dominant pattern of inheritance, four novel candidate loci on chromosomes 2q, 3p, 7q, and 8p were identified. An individual contribution was attributable to four families for the 3p locus and to one family for each of the other loci, respectively. On the basis of previously identified candidate regions and established environmental factors, nontoxic goiter can be defined as a complex disease (Fig. 16-2). However, for the first time, a more prevalent putative locus, present in 20% of the families investigated, was identified.[14]

The candidate region on 3p[14] suggests a dominant pattern of inheritance for goiter. However, whereas linkage studies are suitable for the detection of candidate genes with a strong effect, it is possible to miss weak genetic defects of first-line candidate gene variants or of novel genes by linkage studies. Moreover, it is conceivable that the sum of several weak genetic variations in different genomic regions could lead to goiter predisposition. Therefore, the widely accepted risk factors such as iodine deficiency, smoking, old age, and female gender are likely to interact with and/or trigger the genetic susceptibility. In the future, loci identified by linkage analysis and/or association studies could reveal important genetic risk factors for familial nontoxic goiter. Further narrowing down the candidate regions and performing association studies with SNP markers in additional families and especially in case control association studies is necessary to identify the specific candidate genes for hereditary nontoxic goiter.

GENOME SCREEN IN FAMILIES WITH EUTHYROID GOITERS

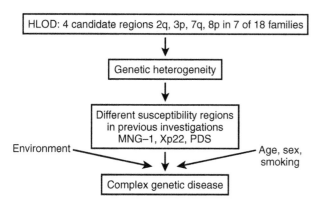

FIGURE 16-2. The identification of different susceptibility loci together with established environmental risk factors suggests that nontoxic goiter should be characterized as a complex disease. HLOD is the calculation of LOD score (logarithm of odds score) with respect to genetic heterogeneity.

MUTAGENESIS AS THE CAUSE OF NODULAR TRANSFORMATION LEADING TO MULTINODULAR GOITER

Most goiters become nodular with time. From animal models of hyperplasia caused by iodine depletion,[28] we have learned that besides an increase in functional activity, a tremendous increase in thyroid cell number occurs. These two events very likely orchestrate a burst of mutation events. It is known that thyroid hormone synthesis goes along with increased H_2O_2 production and free radical formation,[29] which may damage genomic DNA and cause mutations. Together with a higher spontaneous mutation rate, a higher replication rate often will prevent mutation repair and increase the mutation load of the thyroid, thereby also randomly affecting genes crucial for thyrocyte physiology. Mutations that confer a growth advantage (e.g., TSH-R or $G_s\alpha$ protein mutations) very likely initiate focal growth. Hence, autonomously functioning thyroid nodules (AFTNs) are likely to develop from small cell clones that contain advantageous mutations, as shown for the TSH-R in "hot" microscopic regions of euthyroid goiters.[30]

Epidemiologic studies, animal models, and molecular/genetic data outline a general theory of nodular transformation. Based on the identification of somatic mutations and the predominant clonal origin of AFTNs and cold thyroid nodules (CTNs), the following sequence of events could lead to thyroid nodular transformation that occurs in three steps, as outlined in Fig. 16-3.[17] First, iodine deficiency, nutritional goitrogens, or autoimmunity may cause diffuse thyroid hyperplasia. Then, at this stage of thyroid hyperplasia, increased proliferation together with possible DNA damage due to H_2O_2 action causes a higher mutation load (i.e., a higher number of cells bearing mutations). Some of these spontaneous mutations confer constitutive activation of the cyclic adenosine monophosphate (cAMP) cascade (e.g., TSH-R and $G_s\alpha$ mutations), which stimulates growth and function. Finally, in a proliferating thyroid, growth factor expression (e.g., insulin-like growth factor 1 [IGF-1], transforming growth factor β [TGF-β], or epidermal growth factor [EGF]) is increased. As a result of growth factor co-stimulation, most cells divide and form small clones. After increased growth factor expression ceases, small clones with activating mutations further proliferate if they can achieve self-stimulation. They thus can form small foci, which may develop into thyroid nodules. This mechanism may

explain AFTNs by advantageous mutations that initiate growth and function of the affected thyroid cells, as well as CTNs by mutations that stimulate proliferation only (e.g., *ras* mutations, other mutations in the RAS/RAF/MEK/ERK/MAP cascade). Moreover, nodular transformation of thyroid tissue due to TSH-secreting pituitary adenomas[31] and nodular transformation of thyroid tissue in Graves' disease[32] and in goiters of patients with acromegaly[33] could follow a similar mechanism, because thyroid pathology in these patients is characterized by early thyroid hyperplasia.

As an alternative to the increase in cell mass, and as illustrated by those individuals who do not develop a goiter when exposed to iodine deficiency, the thyroid might also adapt to iodine deficiency without extended hyperplasia.[34] Although the mechanism that allows this adaptation is poorly understood, data from a mouse model suggest an increase of mRNA expression of TSH-R, sodium iodine symporter (NIS), and TPO in response to iodine deficiency, which might be a sign of increased iodine turnover in the thyroid cell in iodine deficiency.[35] Moreover, expansion of the thyroid microvasculature, caused by upregulation of vascular endothelial growth factor and other proangiogenic factors, is an additional mechanism that might help the thyroid to adapt to iodine deficiency.[36]

OXIDATIVE STRESS AS THE DOWNSIDE OF THYROID HORMONE SYNTHESIS

Because of the slow proliferation rate of thyroid epithelial cells, a long period (tens of years) between initiation of the tumor and appearance of MNG would seem likely. Therefore, the prevalence of thyroid tumors is a paradox that can be explained only by a high frequency of tumor initiation and/or enhanced thyroid epithelial cell proliferation. The origin of tumor formation in the thyroid therefore could be a natural or induced high mutation rate and aberrant growth stimulation in the thyroid gland. The latter very likely involves endogenous growth factors and/or exogenous goitrogenic substances.

Proliferation is very important for the manifestation of mutagenesis, and DNA replication during cell division leads to mispairing of damaged nucleotides, causing fixation of spontaneous mutations into the genome and a certain mutation load of dividing cells. Hence, compared with highly proliferating and therefore tumor-prone tissues—such as the colon, endometrium, skin, prostate, or breast—proliferation of the thyroid is rather low. If mutations occurred in the thyroid at a similar rate as in other tissues, the tumor incidence ought to be much lower than it actually is.

The main function of the thyroid gland is to synthesize the thyroid hormones L-3,5,3′,5′-tetraiodothyronine (T_4) and L-3,5,3′-triiodothyronine (T_3). To do so, the thyroid gland takes up iodine from food and incorporates it into thyroglobulin (Tg)—the precursor of the thyroid hormones. Iodination of tyrosyl residues on Tg requires high concentrations of H_2O_2 and oxidized iodine, which are generated by the enzymes thyroid oxidase 1 (THOX1), thyroid oxidase 2 (THOX2), and TPO.

Besides being a substrate in the hormone synthesis, H_2O_2 could be a major source of free radicals and reactive oxygen species (ROS). Because these molecules can cause substantial damage to a cell and impair normal function, thyroid epithelial cells are likely to have a potent defense mechanism to counterbalance potential damage mediated by free radicals. It has been shown that antioxidant enzymes, such as glutathione peroxidases (GPXs) or TPO, are upregulated during thyroid hormone synthesis.[37] GPX3 has been suggested to directly interfere with

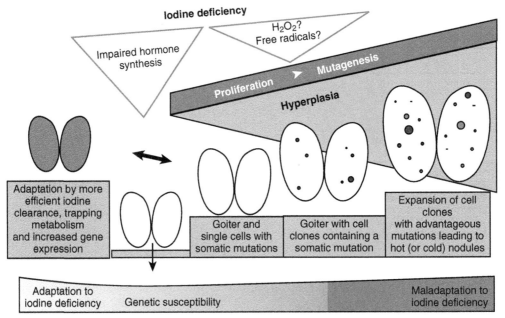

FIGURE 16-3. Hypothesis for thyroid nodular transformation. The starting point for the development of the multinodular nontoxic goiter (MNG) is hyperplasia induced by goitrogenic stimuli (e.g., iodine deficiency). Iodine deficiency increases mutagenesis directly (production of H_2O_2/free radicals) or indirectly (proliferation and increased number of cell divisions). Subsequently, hyperplasia forms cell clones. Some of them contain somatic mutations of the *TSH-R*, leading to autonomously functioning thyroid nodules (*filled circles*), or they contain mutations that lead to dedifferentiation and therefore cold thyroid nodules or cold adenomas (*open circles*).

thyroid hormone synthesis by affecting the concentration of H_2O_2.[38] If antioxidant defense is not effective enough, excessive damage (e.g., peroxidation) should be detectable in lipids, DNA, and proteins of thyroid epithelial cells.

In thyrocytes, H_2O_2-mediated cytotoxicity appears to be dose dependent, requiring only low concentrations to result in thyroid cell apoptosis rather than necrosis, which could function as a barrier for tumorigenesis.[39] Furthermore, findings in the thyroid glands of male Wistar rats suggest that the predominant cytotoxic response to oxidative stress might differ depending on the functional state of the gland.[39] Moreover, ample evidence for excessive oxidative DNA damage has been found in the thyroid gland.[40] Does this affect the spontaneous mutation rate (SMR) in the thyroid at large? It is most interesting to note that a strikingly high SMR was found in the thyroid gland of mice[41]: with an 8- to 10-fold higher number compared with liver, the thyroid stands out from many other tissues. Indeed, the SMR in mouse thyroid glands without any experimental mutagenic challenge shows values that usually are found only in other organs (e.g., liver) of animals treated with mutagens like ethyl nitrosourea or benzo[a]pyrene.[42] The above data point to a connection between thyroid hormone metabolism, oxidative DNA damage, and SMR in the normal thyroid gland that may represent the basis for frequent tumorigenesis.

On top of this generally high mutation rate in the normal thyroid gland, environmental and lifestyle factors may add to the pool of DNA damage and increase mutagenesis and tumor initiation. Tobacco smoke, as previously mentioned,[9] because it is one of the prime suspects in thiocyanate-induced blocking of iodine transport into the thyrocyte, could lead to intracellular iodine deficiency.

As outlined in the aforementioned, H_2O_2-mediated ROS generation is very likely to be an important starting point for thyroid tumor development (Fig. 16-4). Because iodine and H_2O_2 act as co-substrates in thyroid hormone synthesis, changes in iodine concentration are very likely to affect the H_2O_2 concentration. In fact, generation of H_2O_2 is inhibited by iodide in vivo and in vitro.[43] H_2O_2 generation—which is mandatory for the organification of iodine—is, moreover, stimulated by TSH (in contrast to many other aspects of thyroid hormone synthesis, it is unclarified whether cAMP is the second messenger in H_2O_2 generation), which increases the expression of genes important for thyroid hormone synthesis (e.g., *NIS, TPO*).[29] Low iodine levels and markers of increased thyroid functionality suggest activation of H_2O_2 generation, which could result in DNA damage and somatic mutations.[44] Consequently, low iodine and high H_2O_2 levels should activate antioxidative defenses, which should be detectable in the cellular regulation of enzymes involved in the defense against oxidative stress.

Indeed, a higher expression of mRNA for superoxide dismutase 3 (SOD3)—the extracellular SOD isoform that preferentially acts in the lumen, where H_2O_2 is generated—is detected during experimental iodine deficiency in mice.[35] Moreover, oxidative stress and antioxidant defenses are enhanced in hyperplastic and involuting glands.[45]

Differential expression of additional antioxidant enzymes[40] underlines the importance of the antioxidant defense in the iodine-deficient thyroid gland. Moreover, glutathione peroxidases are selenium proteins. It therefore is very likely that selenium deficiency could impair the antioxidant defense and exacerbate oxidative stress (see Fig. 16-4). An increased oxidative burden in the thyroid gland through iodine deficiency is also suggested by results of the comet assay with repair-enzyme protocols to detect oxidative DNA damage.[35] As a consequence, early molecular conditions for nodular and tumor transformation in the thyroid gland consist of a sequence of molecular events that include oxidative stress and DNA damage as the triggers for somatic mutations. The oxidative burden is already detectable in the normal thyroid gland and is very likely to be linked to hormone synthesis and H_2O_2 production. Additionally, environmental conditions (e.g., iodine deficiency) have the potential to aggravate this situation. In general, any external factor (e.g.,

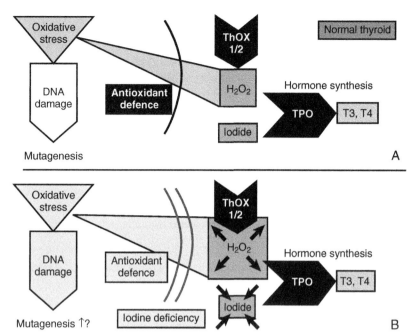

FIGURE 16-4. Mechanisms that might cause mutagenesis in the thyroid gland. The figure shows the key molecules involved in those parts of thyroid hormone synthesis which—in conditions of iodine and most likely also selenium deficiency—lead to oxidative stress, DNA damage, and possibly mutagenesis. *ROS,* Reactive oxygen species; *THOX,* thyroid oxidase; *TPO,* thyroid peroxidase. **A,** In the normal thyroid gland, the enzymes THOX1 and THOX2 generate H_2O_2, and TPO transfers oxidized iodine to tyrosyl residues of thyroglobulin, the precursor for T_3 and T_4 synthesis. H_2O_2 is, however, a source of ROS, which—with other oxidative stress—can cause DNA damage. Normally, antioxidant defense could prevent oxidative stress and DNA damage. Selenoproteins like glutathione peroxidase 3 are part of the defense. **B,** Conditions of iodine deficiency increase levels of H_2O_2 and might increase the amount of oxidative stress and DNA damage. Additional selenium deficiency decreases selenoproteins and thereby could weaken antioxidative defense, which exacerbates oxidative stress and DNA damage.

smoking) that increases oxidative stress, causes DNA damage, or increases the SMR might aggravate the risk for tumor genesis. Also, any factor that increases proliferation (e.g., goitrogens) in all likelihood shortens the time to development of a detectable thyroid tumor.

HOT THYROID NODULES

Somatic point mutations that constitutively activate the TSH-R were first identified by Parma and coworkers in hyperfunctioning thyroid adenomas.[46] However, in different studies, the prevalence of *TSH-R* and $G_s\alpha$ mutations in autonomously functioning thyroid nodules has been reported to vary from 8% to 82% and from 8% to 75%, respectively.[46-49] Available studies differ in the extent of mutation detection and in screening methods. A comparison with respect to the obvious differences between studies has been done elsewhere.[50,51] A comprehensive study using the more sensitive denaturing gradient gel electrophoresis[52,53] revealed a frequency of 57% *TSH-R* mutations and 3% $G_s\alpha$ mutations in 75 consecutive, autonomously functioning thyroid nodules.[54] These results raise the question of the molecular origin of *TSH-R* and $G_s\alpha$ mutation-negative nodules. A possible answer is given by clonal analysis of these AFTNs, which demonstrates a predominant clonal origin of thyroid nodules and implies a neoplastic process driven by genetic alteration.

In addition to the intracellular signaling network that is connected to the TSH-R, the extracellular action of different growth factors enhances the complexity of the signal flux into the thyroid cell. Growth factors like IGF-1, EGF, TGF-β, and fibroblast growth factor (FGF) stimulate growth and dedifferentiation of thyroid epithelial cells.[55] Studies focused on insulin and IGF show a permissive effect of insulin and IGF-1 on TSH signaling[56,57] as well as a cooperative interaction of TSH and insulin/IGF-1.[58] Other studies suggest inactivation of TGF-β signaling in AFTNs due to constitutively activated TSH-R (e.g., resulting from *TSH-R* mutations).[59] This assumption is supported by the finding of decreased expression of TGF-β_1 mRNA after TSH stimulation of thyrocytes.[60] Because TGF-β_1 has been shown to inhibit iodine uptake, iodine organification, and thyroglobulin expression,[61] as well as cell proliferation in different cell culture systems,[62,63] these findings suggest that inactivation of TGF-β signaling is a major prerequisite for increased proliferation in AFTNs.[64] Signal modulation of the TSH-R that would define the cause of AFTNs and the clinical phenotype therefore could take part at a number of stages and very likely involve genetic/epigenetic, gender-related, and environmental factors.

COLD THYROID NODULES

The term "cold" indicates reduced uptake on scintiscan. Because a histologic diagnosis typically is employed to exclude thyroid malignancy, many investigations of thyroid nodules refer only to the histologic diagnosis of thyroid adenoma. This histologic entity should not be confounded with the scintigraphically characterized entity "cold nodule," which, like AFTNs or "warm nodules," can appear histologically as thyroid adenomas or adenomatous nodules according to the WHO classification.[1] In contrast, focal hyperplasia is not very well explained on the molecular level and has been discussed in detail elsewhere as the cause of thyroid tumors.[65,66] A monoclonal origin has been detected for most cold thyroid nodules, which implies nodular development from a single mutated thyroid cell.[67]

With reference to their functional status (i.e., reduced iodine uptake), failure in the iodide transport system and failure of the organic binding of iodide were detected as functional aberrations of cold thyroid nodules long before the molecular components of iodine metabolism were known. Subsequently, decreased expression of the Na^+/I^- symporter (NIS) in thyroid carcinomas and benign cold thyroid nodules were suggested as the molecular mechanisms underlying the failure of iodide transport (reviewed in references 68 and 69). However, a defective cell membrane targeting the NIS protein is a more likely molecular mechanism accounting for the failure of iodine uptake in CTNs.[68,70] The ultimate cause of this defect is currently unknown.

Compared with iodine transport, the organic binding of iodine is a multistep process with a number of protein components that still awaits final characterization.[71] mRNA expression of enzymatic components (e.g., TPO, flavoproteins) and the substrate of iodination (i.e., Tg) have been quantified in CTNs without significant differences compared with normal follicular tissue.[72,73] TPO, Tg, and thyroid-specific oxidases (THOX) have been successfully screened for molecular defects, especially in congenital hypothyroidism.[74]

Although CTNs could be regarded as a form of focal hypothyroidism, somatic mutations in enzymes that catalyze organic binding of iodine would need to exert a growth advantage on the affected cell to cause the development of a thyroid nodule. At least in the case of inactivating mutations in the *TPO* or *THOX* genes, growth advantage could result from a lack of enzyme activity, which would reduce not only thyroid hormone synthesis but also follicular iodide trapping in organic iodo compounds. Because these compounds have been shown to inhibit thyroid epithelial cell proliferation,[75] reduced synthesis could have a proliferative effect. Therefore, somatic *TPO* or *THOX* mutations could be a molecular cause of CTN. However, mutations in the *TPO* gene have not been detected.[76] A study of 40 cold thyroid adenomas and adenomatous nodules detected *ras* mutations in only a single case.[67] Moreover, in the same set of CTNs, no point mutations in the mutational hot spots of the *BRAF* gene were detected.[77] This is in line with the lack of *BRAF* mutations in benign follicular adenomas in other studies.[78,79] So far, only one study has detected a single *BRAF* mutation in a set of 51 follicular adenomas.[80] Moreover, the gene expression for approximately 10,000 full-length genes was compared between CTNs and their corresponding normal surrounding tissue.[81] Increased expression of histone mRNAs and of cell cycle–associated genes like cyclin D1, cyclin H/cyclin-dependent kinase (CDK) 7, and cyclin B most likely reflects a molecular setup for increased proliferation in CTNs.[82] In accordance with the low prevalence of *ras* mutations in CTNs,[67] reduced expression of *ras*-MAPK (mitogen-activated protein kinase) cascade–associated genes was found, which might suggest minor importance of this signaling cascade. Furthermore, gene rearrangements unique to thyroid adenomas have recently been the focus (reviewed in reference 83). These studies led to the identification of the thyroid adenoma–associated gene (THADA) that encodes a death receptor–interacting protein.[84] Although also reported for thyroid follicular carcinoma,[85] the finding of loss of heterozygosity (LOH) at the TPO locus is characteristic for some CTNs (about 15%) but rather points to defects in a gene near *TPO* on the short arm of chromosome 2. Although the frequency of each of these DNA aberrations is rather low, together these chromosomal changes need to be considered in further elucidation of the molecular origin of CTNs.

Clinical Aspects

OCCURRENCE

Epidemiologic studies of multinodular goiter are hampered by problems such as selection criteria (age and gender), influence of environmental factors (e.g., iodine intake, smoking habits), evaluation of size and morphology (palpation, ultrasound, or scintigraphy), and determination of thyroid function, and whether subjects with subclinical hyperthyroidism are categorized as euthyroid or hyperthyroid. Only thyroid nodules of at least 10 mm can be identified reliably by palpation.[86] With the use of ultrasound, nodules as small as 2 mm are readily detected. It therefore is not surprising that the prevalence of nodules is increased several-fold if sonographic examination is applied, because 70% of thyroid nodules disclosed by sonography are smaller than 10 mm in diameter.[86,87]

Most studies have focused on middle-aged women and the elderly, whereas only a few have documented the prevalence of multinodular thyroid disease in a cross-sectional investigation of the adult population in a community. Longitudinal studies covering many years are necessary to give valid figures on incidence, etiologic risk factors, and the natural history. Such studies that take the above-mentioned problems into consideration are not available. These limitations therefore should be borne in mind when the available data are considered.[87] Iodine deficiency is still the most frequent single cause of multinodular endemic goiter worldwide. Considerable regional variation exists even in nonendemic goiter areas. In the Whickham survey, 16% of the cohort had simple goiter.[88] In men, the prevalence declined with age from 7% in those younger than 25 years to 4% in those older than 65 years. Among women, the frequency declined from 31% in those younger than 45 years to 12% in those older than 75 years. This finding fits the observation that lean body mass, known to decline with age, is the major determinant of thyroid size.[87] Illustrating the influence of iodine intake on the epidemiology of sporadic goiter, 31 of 423 (7.3%) 68-year-olds had goiter in Jutland, Denmark (low iodine intake area), versus 2 of 100 (2%) in Reykjavik, Iceland (high iodine intake area).[89]

A cross-sectional study of the community in Whickham found a prevalence of hyperthyroidism of 25 per 1000 women and 2 per 1000 men in an adult population.[88] Others have reported similar figures.[88] The yearly incidence of hyperthyroidism (all types) varies between 0.1 and 0.2 per 1000 men and between 0.3 and 1.3 per 1000 women. As with nontoxic goiter, iodine intake is of paramount importance. In Denmark, a country with a borderline sufficient iodine intake, multinodular toxic goiter accounts for 50% of patients with hyperthyroidism, whereas Iceland, with a high iodine intake, has a lower proportion of multinodular goiter (6%) and a greater number of cases of Graves' disease.[89]

NATURAL HISTORY

The natural history of multinodular goiter, with respect to goiter growth and function, varies and is difficult to predict in a given patient. The spontaneous growth rate in selected populations has been estimated to be up to 20% yearly[90] but usually is much lower. No specific parameter exists that can predict the growth potential of multinodular goiter, which can be accurately assessed by serial yearly measurements of the size of the goiter and individual nodules by ultrasonography.[91]

Painful nodules are usually the result of hemorrhage into a nodule or a cyst in the goiter. The diagnosis is readily made by ultrasonographic examination and fine-needle aspiration biopsy. Such a growing painful nodule may represent thyroid malignancy and should be investigated accordingly. Multinodular goiter is not usually associated with a significantly increased risk for the development of thyroid malignancy. The risk of malignancy in thyroid nodules occurring within a multinodular goiter has not been completely clarified, but most authors find a similar frequency in uninodular and multinodular goiters.[92]

Patients with nontoxic multinodular goiter can become hyperthyroid or, less commonly, hypothyroid. Hyperthyroidism in such patients often develops insidiously, in contrast to that of Graves' disease. It often begins with a prolonged period of subclinical hyperthyroidism characterized by low serum TSH and normal serum free T_4 and triiodothyronine (T_3) concentrations.[87] This hyperthyroid state is the consequence of goiter growth and an associated increase in the mass of autonomously hormone-producing thyroid cells. Hyperthyroidism can also be the result of an increase in iodine intake from iodine-containing drugs such as disinfectants and amiodarone or from radiographic contrast agents, which, in a goiter with increased autonomous iodine metabolism, leads to the production of excessive amounts of thyroid hormone. Little is known of the incidence and the time frame for this progression from the nodular nontoxic goiter toward the nodular toxic goiter. In a large population-based cross-sectional study in an iodine-deficient area, nodular autonomy increased with age and reached 15% in elderly people.[93] It appears from a few longitudinal studies[87] that within 5 years, hyperthyroidism will emerge in approximately 10% of patients with a nodular goiter. In a few cases, autonomy of some of the thyroid nodules may return.

Development of hypothyroidism in a patient with multinodular nontoxic goiter is rarer. This observation is difficult to explain, but the situation is probably caused by coexisting autoimmune thyroiditis.

DIAGNOSIS

Clinical Examination

Pertinent clinical signs and symptoms are given in Table 16-1, and diagnostic aspects are summarized in Table 16-2. For most, the thyroid gland does not become palpable until the volume has doubled. A visibly diffusely enlarged goiter has often reached a volume of 30 to 40 mL. Detection of nodules depends on their size, morphology, and location within the thyroid parenchyma, the anatomy of the patient's neck, and the training of the physician. Among patients who present with a palpable nodule,

approximately half have more than one lesion by sonographic examination.[86] Sonography detects approximately five times as many nodules as thyroid palpation, and twice as many when only nodules larger than 2 cm are considered.[86,87] Awareness, however, may depend on localization, speed of growth, and the possible pain or discomfort related to hemorrhage into a nodule (see Table 16-2).

Inspection and palpation of the neck, preferably done with the patient swallowing gulps of water and with the head tilted slightly backward, may disclose anything from a single nodule in an otherwise normal nonpalpable thyroid to a large compressive multinodular gland extending retroclavicularly or into the mediastinum. However, clinical examination is associated with considerable interobserver and intraobserver variation regarding size and morphology of the thyroid.[94]

Although clinical diagnosis of nodular goiter usually is considered to be straightforward, differential diagnostic considerations include goitrous autoimmune thyroiditis, thyroid cancer, and, rarely, long-standing Graves' disease, in which the gland may become firm and irregular. It should be borne in mind that physical examination of the thyroid includes examination of the neck, as well as the regional lymph nodes and the trachea, but also that glands harboring malignancy are in many cases indistinguishable from those that are not.

Laboratory Investigations

Because the transition from nontoxic to toxic goiter is part of the natural history of this disease,[87] and because detection of borderline but clinically relevant hyperthyroidism requires laboratory tests, annual screening with a sensitive TSH assay is recommended. The possibility of hyperthyroidism must be considered in any goitrous patient with otherwise unexplained illness. This point is particularly true for patients with cardiac failure or arrhythmia. Subnormal serum TSH values should lead to a determination of free T_4 and free T_3. Even in the presence of normal serum thyroid hormone levels, suppressed serum TSH should lead to treatment, especially in the elderly.[95]

Thyroglobulin in serum is positively correlated with thyroid size, but this marker is too inaccurate at the individual level to have any independent value in the diagnosis of goiter.

Calcitonin, a marker of medullary thyroid cancer (MTC) when elevated in serum, can aid in the early detection of sporadic cases of this disease. Routine determination in nodular thyroid disease has been suggested. Large-scale studies demonstrate a prevalence of MTC in the range of 0.4% to 1.37%.[87,96] Studies vary with regard to the diagnostic setup and the fraction of patients with histologic verification. Basal or stimulated calcitonin levels were generally more sensitive than fine-needle aspiration biopsy (FNAB) in detecting MTC, and the routine use of serum calcitonin is recommended by most authors of these studies.[87,96] However, a clear conclusion is not easy to draw from the existing data. Cost-benefit must be taken into consideration, and a high false-positive rate will result in many unnecessary thyroidectomies. It is also evident from international surveys[97-100] that no consensus has been reached on this issue. More than 30% of European clinicians measure basal serum calcitonin routinely,[97,99] whereas only very few in North America use this strategy except in cases of a family history of thyroid cancer.[98,100]

Antithyroid antibodies (TPO and TG antibodies) in serum in our opinion should be determined routinely in the workup of these patients. This recommendation is based mainly on the fact that Hashimoto's thyroiditis may be mistaken for simple multinodular goiter, and that these antibodies may be recognized as

Table 16-1. Clinical Signs and Symptoms of Multinodular Goiter

- Slowly growing nodular anterior neck mass
- Tracheal deviation or compression, upper airway obstruction, dyspnea
- Occasional cough and dysphagia, globulus
- Sudden pain or enlargement secondary to hemorrhage
- Superior vena cava obstruction syndrome
- Pemberton's sign: obstruction of the thoracic inlet by the arms extended over the head
- Enlargement during pregnancy
- Gradually developing hyperthyroidism
- Iodide-induced thyrotoxicosis
- Recurrent nerve palsy (rare)
- Phrenic nerve palsy (rare)
- Horner's syndrome (rare)

Table 16-2. Diagnosis of Multinodular Goiter

- Multinodularity on examination
- Asymmetry, tracheal deviation
- No adenopathy
- Thyroid-stimulating hormone normal or decreased, free thyroxine and free triiodothyronine normal or increased, thyroglobulin elevated
- Calcitonin normal
- Thyroid antibodies negative in approximately 90%
- Scintigraphy with hot and cold areas
- Ultrasound finding of nodularity (nonhomogeneity); cysts and calcifications are common
- Computed tomography and magnetic resonance imaging demonstrating a nonhomogeneous mass
- Lung function testing may demonstrate impaired inspiratory capacity
- Benign cytology by fine-needle aspiration of dominant nodules

markers of increased risk for ^{131}I-induced hypothyroidism, as well as Graves' disease, in patients with toxic[101] and nontoxic multinodular goiter.[102]

[131]*I uptake* determination aids in the diagnosis of iodine contamination, ensures that uptake is adequate, and allows calculation of the ^{131}I dose before ^{131}I therapy is provided. However, it is used routinely in the workup of such patients only by a minority of clinicians.[99,100]

Diagnostic Imaging

Although not adequately investigated, it has been stated repeatedly that imaging rarely provides information that is decisive for clinical management in individual cases. Although simple and cheap, neck palpation is notoriously imprecise with regard to thyroid gland morphology and size determination.[94] For this purpose, several imaging methods are available: sonography, scintigraphy, computed tomography (CT) scan, magnetic resonance (MR) imaging, and perhaps positron emission tomography (PET). Of these, sonography clearly has first priority among clinicians.[97-100]

Scintigraphy has little place in the anatomo-topographic evaluation of the nodular goiter, but it aids in verification of the clinical diagnosis and allows determination of the relative mass of hyperfunctioning (hot) and nonfunctioning (cold) thyroid areas. If a clinically dominant nodule is cold on scintigraphy, it should be treated as a solitary cold nodule—the risk for malignancy being the same.[87,92] Nodules with high uptake by scintigraphy almost never harbor clinically significant malignancy, although exceptions have been reported.[99m]Tc used as tracer may result in false-positive uptake in 3% to 8% of thyroid nodules,[87] and iodine isotopes are devoid of this problem. Nevertheless, comparative studies have been unable to demonstrate any clinically significant differences between the two tracers.[87] Tracers like [201]Thallium and ^{99m}Tc-MIBI have an increased uptake in differentiated malignant thyroid nodules, but sensitivity and specificity do not support their general use.[103,104] Many disregard thyroid scintigraphy in the initial evaluation of patients with nontoxic nodular goiter.[87,99,100] Nevertheless, more than two thirds of ETA members[97,99] routinely use scintigraphy, and less than 25% of ATA members prefer such a strategy.[98,100] Indisputable indications for scintigraphy in the setting of a nodular goiter include hyperthyroidism (to visualize hot nodules suitable for ^{131}I therapy) and identification of a follicular neoplasm with FNAB, because warm nodules with great certainty are benign.[87]

Ultrasound, which is used often in Europe[97,99] and less so in the United States,[98,100] allows determination of total thyroid volume and individual nodule size and evaluation of regional lymph nodes, regional blood flow, nodule vascularity, and elasticity.[87,105] It aids in the performance of accurate biopsies[91] and is of great help in therapeutic procedures such as cyst puncture and alcohol and laser sclerosis of solid or cystic nodules.[91,106-108] In the vast majority of patients, ultrasound can neither confirm nor exclude malignancy.[91] For an objective determination of thyroid size, whether before therapy, such as in the dose calculation of ^{131}I, or for follow-up post therapy, it is the technique of choice,[91] although it is less useful with very large goiters.[87]

Computed tomography and *magnetic resonance imaging* are generally of little value except for evaluation of a retroclavicular or intrathoracic goiter, and for evaluation and follow-up of malignant thyroid disease. MR is thought to be more precise than CT in the anatomo-topographic evaluation of the substernal goiter.[87] However, whether CT or MR is preferred probably depends on cost and availability.

In the differentiation between malignant and benign thyroid lesions, [18F]-2-deoxy-2-fluoro-D-glucose *positron emission tomography* (FDG-PET) may be a potentially useful tool in the evaluation of thyroid nodules with indeterminate cytologic findings. Because this method has a very low false-negative rate for the detection of malignant lesions, a number of unnecessary thyroidectomies may be avoided.[109] Noteworthy, thyroid nodules detected incidentally by FDG-PET harbor cancer in 25% to 50% of cases.[110]

Many patients with goiter appear to have upper airway obstruction due to tracheal compression. Most often, the inspiratory component of the respiration is compromised, but this is often overlooked during a routine examination because respiratory symptoms usually are absent.[87] *Routine radiography* of the trachea has no place in patients with a compressive goiter, because this method is too insensitive for detection of a clinically significant tracheal obstruction.[87] Determination of the smallest cross-sectional tracheal area by MR imaging or CT seems more useful in this setting.[87] Thus, a *flow volume loop* rather than tracheal imaging should be used for the evaluation of respiratory capacity in the patient with a goiter, in particular if the goiter is very large; however, this strategy is rarely used by clinicians.[99,100]

Fine-Needle Aspiration Biopsy (FNAB)

The possibility of thyroid malignancy should be considered in all patients with multinodular goiters, and the use of ultrasonography guidance has been shown to enhance the diagnostic efficacy of FNAB.[92] If the initial FNAB is nondiagnostic owing to limited cellularity, a repeated test is advocated.[111] FNAB cannot rule out malignancy but probably can reduce the risk of overlooking malignancy to below 1% and, in the worst case, could lead to delays in making the correct diagnosis. If malignancy is clinically suspected, a benign cytology should be disregarded naturally and the patient offered surgery. In subjects referred for evaluation of symptomatic multinodular nontoxic goiter and offered surgery, the incidence of carcinoma is 1% to 4%.[87] This figure includes small papillary carcinomas of dubious clinical significance. In unselected patients with multinodular goiter, the prevalence of clinically important malignancy is probably less than 1%. It is important to note that hyperthyroidism does not exclude the possible presence of malignancy,[87] although the risk seems inversely correlated with falling serum TSH levels.[112]

The examination should focus on the dominant nodule ("index nodule") or nodules or on those that have a different consistency from other nodules within the gland.[87] It has been recommended that nodules measuring less than 10 mm, detected incidentally, do not require an FNAB.[113] However, Papini et al.[114] demonstrated thyroid malignancy in 6% of nonpalpable lesions of 8 to 15 mm in size in multinodular goiters (9% in solitary thyroid nodules). The risk was similar in nodules smaller or greater than 10 mm. Whether carcinomas found in nodules other than the index nodule constitute clinically significant cancers or just incidental microcarcinomas remains an unsolved issue, leaving the clinician with no clearcut guidelines for management. Sonographic features may guide the clinician to include FNAB in nodules other than the index nodule. If scintigraphy is performed, we recommend FNAB in up to two nodules, provided they are scintigraphically cold.[87]

In our opinion, neither diagnostic imaging nor FNAB is necessary in most patients with nodular thyroid disease if the preferred treatment is surgery. However, if a nonsurgical treatment is considered, we support the liberal use of diagnostic imaging and FNAB.[87]

Treatment

Nodular thyroid disease is very common, but most of these goiters do not cause significant symptoms and are best left untreated. Treatment may be indicated in cases of
1. Large goiter or progressive growth of the entire gland or individual nodules
2. Signs of cervical compression
3. Overt or subclinical hyperthyroidism
4. Marked neck disfigurement
5. Cosmetic complaints
6. Suspicion of thyroid cancer

In a number of clinical situations, a discrepancy is seen between clinical findings and complaints of patients. In this context, the decision whether to treat can be more difficult.

No ideal treatment is available for goiter, and no consensus has been reached.[87,99,100,115] This is reflected by the fact that a third of clinicians would refrain from treatment when facing a patient with moderate discomfort due to a multinodular nontoxic goiter of 50 to 80 g in which malignancy has been ruled out.[99,100] Comparative studies of available options are sparse. It is important to note that no study has evaluated health-related quality of life using a disease-specific questionnaire.[116] Thus, treatment is not only a matter of goiter reduction. Patient satisfaction, the risks for hypothyroidism and goiter recurrence, and the fear of overlooking a thyroid cancer are all important issues that should be taken into account. It follows that the optimal treatment for toxic and nontoxic multinodular goiter is controversial, and at present the treatment choice must be based on individual factors.

The nontoxic and the toxic multinodular goiter should be regarded as the same disease but at different evolutionary stages. Because many of the data regarding surgery and ^{131}I therapy apply to both conditions, the treatment options are discussed in concert. Tables 16-3 and 16-4 list effects and side effects of the various treatment options.

ANTITHYROID DRUGS

Antithyroid drugs are indicated if the nodular goiter is complicated by coexisting hyperthyroidism. These drugs normalize thyroid function, but remission is very rare and lifelong treatment should be anticipated. Also, further goiter growth may be seen, possibly as a result of using these drugs. Antithyroid drugs are indicated before thyroid surgery to lower the operative risk and can be stopped during the immediate postoperative period.[117] To reduce the risk for exacerbation of hyperthyroidism, it has been recommended to render the patient euthyroid with antithyroid drugs prior to ^{131}I treatment. Usually, the antithyroid drug is discontinued at least 4 days before and is resumed no sooner than 3 days afterward.[117] A meta-analysis, based mainly on studies of Graves' disease, found that the use of methimazole and propylthiouracil in conjunction with ^{131}I therapy results in a decreased remission rate.[118] Whether this applies also to toxic multinodular goiter patients is unknown. One study has shown attenuation of goiter reduction if methimazole is resumed after ^{131}I therapy despite a neutral effect on thyroid function.[119]

IODINE SUPPLEMENTATION

Iodine supplementation for treatment of goiter is used by some clinicians, particularly in Europe.[99] In a placebo-controlled trial, the median volume of diffuse goiters was reduced from 29 to 18 mL, but thyroid dysfunction and antibodies appeared in 10% of patients.[120] The efficacy of iodine supplementation, once a nodular goiter has developed, has only very scarcely been evaluated. In nodular goiter, iodine is no better than L-T4 suppression therapy for goiter reduction in comparative trials. But the major hindrance involving the use of iodine is the fact that a sudden increase of intake may induce thyrotoxicosis in predisposed individuals.[87]

THYROID HORMONE TREATMENT

Thyroid hormone therapy for suppression of pituitary TSH secretion has been much used in the patient with nontoxic multinodular goiter.[99,100] Although L-T4 suppressive therapy is effective in reducing the volume of diffuse nontoxic goiters by up to 30%,[121] few controlled studies have examined nontoxic multinodular goiter[90,122] by employing sonography for objective size monitoring. In one study,[90] 58% of patients had a significant (>13%) decrease in thyroid volume, but regrowth was seen after discontinuation of therapy. Wesche et al.[122] in a randomized trial found a median reduction of goiter volume in the ^{131}I-treated group of 38% and 44% after 1 and 2 years, respectively; corresponding values in the L-T4–treated group were 7% and 1%, respectively, and these were nonsignificant.

L-T4 dose is often targeted toward a partially suppressed serum TSH level.[99,100] The consequence is subclinical hyperthyroidism that adversely affects the skeleton and the cardiovascular system.[95] Because lifelong therapy probably is needed to avoid goiter recurrence, and because the natural history of the disease involves progression toward hyperthyroidism due to autonomous function of the thyroid nodules,[87] L-T4 treatment in fact is not feasible in most patients.[123] Based on the aforementioned, L-T4 treatment should be abandoned on this indication.[87,124,125]

SURGERY

The goal of surgery is removal of all thyroid tissue with a nodular appearance, usually by a unilateral hemithyroidectomy and subtotal resection of the contralateral lobe. A bilateral subtotal resection cannot be recommended. Only extremely rarely is a thoracic approach necessary. Further resection is not usually recommended if final pathologic evaluation incidentally reveals a unilateral cancer that is smaller than 1 cm. This not uncommon finding accounts for most cancers found in surgical series, a majority of which are of little if any clinical significance.[126] Macroscopically normal perinodular tissue often harbors microscopic growth foci, which explains the relatively high risk for recurrence in these patients.[127] In the case of a toxic nodular goiter, thyroid function is normalized more rapidly after surgery than after ^{131}I therapy on the assumption that antithyroid drugs are not used postoperatively.[87]

Surgery leads to rapid decompression, resulting in improved respiratory function if affected presurgically.[128] Not all patients are surgical candidates, but among those undergoing surgery, the surgical mortality rate is less than 1% in experienced centers. Disadvantages include the general risks and side effects of a surgical procedure. Specific risks include transient (6%) or permanent (2%) vocal cord paralysis, transient (6%) or permanent (5%) hypoparathyroidism, and postoperative bleeding (1%).[129] Others have reported lower figures.[130] Complications are related

Table 16-3. Treatment Options for Patients With Nontoxic Multinodular Goiter

Treatment	Advantages	Disadvantages	Comments
Surgery	Significant goiter reduction Rapid decompression of vital structures Allows pathologic examination	Not all patients eligible Postoperative hemorrhage (1%) Recurrent laryngeal nerve injury (1%-2%) Hypoparathyroidism (0.5%-5%) Hypothyroidism* and goiter recurrence* Postoperative tracheomalacia (rare) Risk rates are slightly increased in cases of large goiter, intrathoracic extension, or reoperation	Standard therapy for large goiters or when rapid decompression is required Total thyroidectomy should be considered to avoid goiter recurrence
Thyroxine	Outpatient Low cost May prevent new nodule formation	Low efficacy Mainly impact on the perinodular volume Treatment should be lifelong and aimed at TSH suppression, which induces side effects caused by subclinical hyperthyroidism and inadvertent effects on bone and the heart	Its role on the wane owing to adverse effects and lack of efficacy Not recommended by the authors
Radioiodine	Halving of thyroid volume within 1 year Improves inspiratory capacity over long term Most often outpatient Can be repeated successfully Few subjective side effects	Gradual reduction of the goiter Decreasing effect with increasing size Small risk of acute goiter enlargement Risk of thyroiditis: 3% Risk of transition into Graves' disease: 5% One-year risk of hypothyroidism: 15%-20% Small risk of radiation-induced ophthalmopathy Treatment needs to be repeated in some Risk of radiation-induced malignancy unsettled	Has replaced surgery as the standard therapy in some European countries Should be contemplated instead of reoperation and in those who decline or are not fit for surgery, also in case of a very large goiter (high-dose radioiodine) For data in relation to rhTSH-stimulated therapy, please see the text

rhTSH, Recombinant human thyroid-stimulating hormone; TSH, thyroid-stimulating hormone.
*The percentage of patients affected depends on the extent of surgery.

Table 16-4. Treatment Options for Patients With Toxic Multinodular Goiter

Treatment	Advantages	Disadvantages	Comments
Surgery	Significant goiter reduction Rapid achievement of euthyroidism Allows pathologic examination	Not all patients eligible Surgical mortality and morbidity a little higher than in nontoxic goiter Persistence or recurrence of hyperthyroidism* Hypothyroidism*	Standard therapy for a large goiter or when rapid decompression is required Treatment of choice if radioiodine is not feasible
Antithyroid drugs	Easiest treatment option	Lifelong treatment needed Very little chance of remission Adverse effects in approximately 5% Continuous goiter growth	Major indications are before thyroid surgery and before and after radioiodine, particularly in elderly patients and those with concurrent health problems. Long-term treatment recommended only when surgery or radioiodine cannot be used
Radioiodine	Effective in rendering patients euthyroid and in reducing thyroid volume Most often outpatient Few subjective side effects	Only gradual reversal of hyperthyroidism Gradual reduction of the goiter Small risk for acute goiter enlargement Risk for thyroiditis: 3% Risk for transition into Graves' disease: 5% Five-year risk for hypothyroidism: 15% Small risk for radiation-induced ophthalmopathy Treatment needs to be repeated in some.	Standard therapy unless the goiter is very large (>100 mL) High-dose radioiodine (inpatient treatment) may be an option in those with a very large goiter not fit for or who decline surgery

*The percentage of patients affected depends on the extent of surgery.

to increasing goiter size and extent of the resection.[130,131] Novel techniques may reduce the operation time, the postoperative pain, and the length of the hospital stay.[132,133] Postoperative tracheomalacia, necessitating intubation, may ensue in approximately 5% of patients operated for large goiters.[87] A matter of concern is the apparently high prevalence (7% to 17%) of thyroid carcinomas in substernal goiters,[87,134] but this seemingly high frequency probably is influenced by selection bias.

The long-term risk for hypothyroidism after subtotal resection of multinodular goiters is insufficiently described but is approximately 10% to 20%, as reported for toxic multinodular goiters,[87] and is related to the extent of the resection. Recurrence of the nontoxic multinodular goiter is seen in 15% to 40% of patients on long-term follow-up.[87] Postoperative use of L-T4 is preferred by many clinicians[99,100] to avoid recurrence; however, based on results from randomized trials,[87] the use of L-T4 generally cannot be recommended,[87] nor can the use of iodine.[135] A reoperation for recurrent goiter results in a threefold to 10-fold increase in risk for permanent vocal cord paralysis or hypoparathyroidism.[130,131] [131]I therapy seems to be a favorable alternative in these cases. Goiter recurrence can be completely avoided, if a total thyroidectomy is carried out initially, in some centers with the same low rate of complications as was reported with subtotal thyroidectomy.[136]

RADIOIODINE THERAPY

[131]I treatment is considered safe and appropriate in nearly all types of hyperthyroidism, especially that occurring in elderly patients.[117] Generally, ^{131}I is thought to carry a lower rate of complications and a lower cost than surgery.[117] This fact has led a number of centers to offer ^{131}I as the first choice of therapy for most patients. In contrast to surgery, which cures nearly all patients and normalizes hyperthyroidism within a few days,[137] only 50% become euthyroid within 3 months of ^{131}I therapy, given that antithyroid drugs are not administered.[101] Twenty to 40% need additional ^{131}I therapy, and even up to five treatment sessions will not cure all patients.[101] In contrast, persistence of hyperthyroidism after surgery is rare.[137]

Besides being able to cure hyperthyroidism, it has long been recognized that use of ^{131}I results in shrinkage of the thyroid gland. During the past 25 years, ^{131}I therapy for symptomatic multinodular nontoxic goiter therefore has been introduced in a number of mainly European centers as a nonsurgical alternative to L-T4 therapy.[87,99] Thyroid volume reduction is of the same magnitude in toxic and nontoxic multinodular goiters, that is, approximately 40% after 1 year[101,122,138-140] and 50% to 60% after 2 years, without further reduction.[101,138] Sixty percent of this decrease is seen within 3 months of initiation of therapy.[101,138] In addition to relief of compressive symptoms, ^{131}I therapy results in less tracheal compression, which improves pulmonary function, particularly the inspiratory component.[139,140] Because of the often large goiters, normalization of thyroid volume, as is seen in diffuse toxic and nontoxic goiters, can rarely be achieved,[87] but symptoms in most cases are considerably improved, and patient satisfaction is high.[140,141] If a secondary increase in thyroid volume is seen, this should raise the suspicion of malignancy. Generally, ^{131}I doses of 100 μCi (3.7 MBq) per gram of thyroid tissue corrected for 100% 24 hour ^{131}I uptake have been given.[101,122,138-140] However, whether such dose adjustment is worthwhile has been questioned,[117,142] and fixed doses are given in a number of centers.[117] Treatment can be repeated if further goiter reduction is required in a euthyroid patient.[87,138]

Radiation thyroiditis, seen in 3% within the first months of ^{131}I therapy,[102] is easily treated with salicylates or corticosteroids. Another complication is a Graves'-like autoimmune hyperthyroidism, which is seen in 5%. Rare cases of ^{131}I-induced Graves' ophthalmopathy have also been reported.[87] Pretreatment presence of anti-TPO antibodies confers a significantly increased risk for this complication,[87] which most likely is triggered by ^{131}I-related release of thyroid antigens and is associated with the appearance of TSH receptor antibodies typically 3 to 6 months after ^{131}I therapy. It also can be seen after surgical manipulation of the thyroid or after subacute thyroiditis.[87] The condition is often self-limiting but may necessitate therapy.

Although early goiter enlargement caused by radiation therapy may be seen, on average ^{131}I therapy is not followed by any significant acute thyroid enlargement.[139,143] The risk for permanent hypothyroidism after ^{131}I therapy in multinodular goiters ranges from 14% to 58% within 5 to 8 years.[87,101,138] It occurs more commonly in patients with a small goiter and when anti-TPO antibodies are present.[87] [131]I therapy, given for Graves' disease for decades, until recently was not thought to be followed by any clinically significant increased risk for cancer death.[144,145] However, a recent study questions these findings.[146] Data regarding ^{131}I therapy in multinodular goiter are sparse, and in the case of nontoxic goiter, nonexistent. In the study by Ron et al.,[144] 1089 patients were treated for a toxic nodular goiter, and these individuals had a 31% increase in overall cancer mortality,

nearly exclusively attributable to thyroid malignancy. However, a similar pattern was seen in patients with the same disease but not treated with [131]I. Hence, the disclosure of a thyroid cancer in a nodular goiter after ^{131}I therapy raises the question, whether malignancy in a nodule was overlooked at the time of therapy.

In some European countries, ^{131}I therapy has replaced surgery as the treatment of choice in most patients.[87,99] However, the optimum treatment remains to be established, ideally through comparative randomized trials, including data on effects, side effects, costs, and patient satisfaction.

The efficacy of ^{131}I therapy in multinodular goiter is hampered by irregular ^{131}I uptake in the gland, and the relative goiter reduction is inversely correlated with initial goiter size.[139] A high dietary iodine intake diminishes efficacy. However, recombinant human TSH (rhTSH) has the potential of increasing the 24-hour ^{131}I uptake more than fourfold,[147-149] and the effect is inversely correlated to the initial thyroid ^{131}I uptake.[147-149] Moreover, pretreatment with rhTSH causes a more homogeneous distribution of ^{131}I within the nodular gland.[150] These properties of rhTSH are ideal in the context of ^{131}I therapy for multinodular goiter. Indeed, several studies, including two randomized, double-blinded trials,[151,152] have confirmed that rhTSH, in doses from 0.1 mg to 0.9 mg and administered 24 hours before ^{131}I therapy, improves goiter reduction by 35% to 55% within a year, when compared with conventional ^{131}I therapy (Fig. 16-5). The impact of rhTSH pre-stimulation is most pronounced in patients with a low baseline thyroid ^{131}I uptake.[149,151,152] rhTSH-augmented ^{131}I therapy also results in reduced tracheal compression and enhancement of the inspiratory reserve, as shown in a randomized trial.[153] We have speculated that the effects of rhTSH might be mediated through factors beyond the increase in thyroid iodine uptake.[151,152]

As an alternative to aiming at increased thyroid irradiation and goiter shrinkage, rhTSH allows a reduction in ^{131}I activity while still retaining a mean goiter reduction of approximately 40% within the first 12 months.[154] With this approach, extrathyroidal irradiation is diminished,[155] which may render ^{131}I therapy more attractive in young patients.

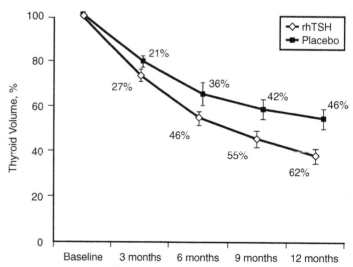

FIGURE 16-5. Effect of ^{131}I therapy on nontoxic multinodular goiter comparing patients randomized to pretreatment with 0.3 mg recombinant human thyrotropin or placebo 24 hours before therapy is given. The y-axis represents the mean change (%) in thyroid volume. The between-group difference at 12 months was highly significant (P = .005). (Data from Nielsen et al., Arch Intern Med 2006; 166:1476-1482.)

rhTSH per se, in doses from 0.3 mg to 0.9 mg, results in a transient 25% to 35% enlargement of the thyroid gland[156,157]; this may be potentially dangerous in patients with goiter. However, rhTSH-augmented ^{131}I therapy is generally well tolerated, particularly when a dose of 0.1 mg or lower is used. With a higher rhTSH dose, the patient may experience cervical pain and a temporary rise in thyroid hormones within the first week after ^{131}I therapy.[149,151,152,158,159] In parallel with improved goiter reduction, a higher frequency of hypothyroidism is encountered after rhTSH-augmented ^{131}I therapy is provided.[151,152,159] When safety aspects have been further evaluated, rhTSH-augmented ^{131}I therapy may well become a routine option in many patients with symptomatic multinodular goiter who decline surgery.

PERCUTANEOUS INTERVENTIONAL THERAPY

Percutaneous ethanol injection therapy (PEIT) has been used for longer than a decade in solitary hot, toxic, and even cold thyroid nodules.[87,108] The most convincing effect is seen in solitary thyroid cysts.[108] Theoretically, PEIT can be used in multinodular goiter. Drawbacks are related to pain, risk for recurrent laryngeal nerve damage, and the possibility of extrathyroidal fibrosis complicating subsequent surgery. Interstitial laser photocoagulation was introduced recently and seems to have the same effect as PEIT with possibly fewer side effects.[107] No controlled studies in multinodular goiter have examined either technique.

Acknowledgments

The work of L.H. and S.B. has been generously supported by the Agnes and Knut Mørks Foundation, the A.P. Møller Relief Foundation, and the Novo Nordisk Foundation. Research by R.P and K.K. was funded by D.F., Thyssen Stiftung, Krebshilfe, and Wilhelm Sander Stiftung.

REFERENCES

1. Hedinger C, Williams ED, Sobin LH: The WHO histological classification of thyroid tumors: a commentary on the second edition, Cancer 63:908–911, 1989.
2. Belfiore A, La Rosa GL, La Porta GA, et al: Cancer risk in patients with cold thyroid nodules: relevance of iodine intake, sex, age, and multinodularity, Am J Med 93:363–369, 1992.
3. Knudsen N, Perrild H, Christiansen E, et al: Thyroid structure and size and two-year follow-up of solitary cold thyroid nodules in an unselected population with borderline iodine deficiency, Eur J Endocrinol 142:224–230, 2000.
4. Chan JKC, Hirokawa M, Evans H, et al: Follicular adenoma. In DeLellis RA, Lloyd RV, Heitz PU, et al, editors: WHO Classification of Tumours. Pathology and Genetics of Tumours of Endocrine Organs, Lyon, 2004, IARC Press, pp 98–103.
5. Berghout A, Wiersinga WM, Smits NJ, et al: Interrelationships between age, thyroid volume, thyroid nodularity, and thyroid function in patients with sporadic nontoxic goiter, Am J Med 89:602–608, 1990.
6. Knudsen N, Laurberg P, Perrild H, et al: Risk factors for goiter and thyroid nodules, Thyroid 12:879–888, 2002.
7. Pisarikova B, Herzig I, Riha J: [Inorganic anions with a potential goitrogenic effect in drinking water supply for humans and animals], Vet Med (Praha) 41:33–39, 1996.
8. Scanelli G: [Lithium thyrotoxicosis, Report of a case and review of the literature], Recenti Prog Med 93:100–103, 2002.
9. Brix TH, Hansen PS, Kyvik KO, et al: Cigarette smoking and risk of clinically overt thyroid disease: a population-based twin case-control study, Arch Intern Med 160:661–666, 2000.
10. Brix TH, Kyvik KO, Hegedüs L: Major role of genes in the etiology of simple goiter in females: a population-based twin study, J Clin Endocrinol Metab 84:3071–3075, 1999.
11. Knudsen N, Bulow I, Laurberg P, et al: Parity is associated with increased thyroid volume solely among smokers in an area with moderate to mild iodine deficiency, Eur J Endocrinol 146:39–43, 2002.
12. Krohn K, Fuhrer D, Bayer Y, et al: Molecular pathogenesis of euthyroid and toxic multinodular goiter, Endocr Rev 26:504–524, 2005.
13. Hansen PS, Brix TH, Bennedbæk FN, et al: Genetic and environmental causes of individual differences in thyroid size: a study of healthy Danish twins, J Clin Endocrinol Metab 89:2071–2077, 2004.
14. Bayer Y, Neumann S, Meyer B, et al: Genome-wide linkage analysis reveals evidence for four new susceptibility loci for familial euthyroid goiter, J Clin Endocrinol Metab 89:4044–4052, 2004.
15. Bignell GR, Canzian F, Shayeghi M, et al: Familial nontoxic multinodular thyroid goiter locus maps to chromosome 14q but does not account for familial nonmedullary thyroid cancer, Am J Hum Genet 61:1123–1130, 1997.
16. Neumann S, Bayer Y, Reske A, et al: Further indications for genetic heterogeneity of euthyroid familial goiter, J Mol Med 81:736–745, 2003.
17. Brix TH, Hegedüs L: Genetic and environmental factors in the aetiology of simple goitre, Ann Med 32:153–156, 2000.
18. Geerdsen JP, Hee P: Nontoxic goitre. I. Surgical complications and longterm prognosis, Acta Chir Scand 148:221–224, 1982.
19. Piraneo S, Vitri P, Galimberti A, et al: Ultrasonographic surveillance after surgery for euthyroid goitre in patients treated or not with thyroxine, Eur J Surg 163:21–26, 1997.
20. Corral J, Martin C, Perez R, et al: Thyroglobulin gene point mutation associated with non-endemic simple goitre, Lancet 341:462–464, 1993.
21. Gonzalez-Sarmiento R, Corral J, Mories MT, et al: Monoallelic deletion in the 5′ region of the thyroglobulin gene as a cause of sporadic nonendemic simple goiter, Thyroid 11:789–793, 2001.
22. Everett LA, Glaser B, Beck JC, et al: Pendred syndrome is caused by mutations in a putative sulphate transporter gene (PDS), Nat Genet 17:411–422, 1997.
23. Masmoudi S, Charfedine I, Hmani M, et al: Pendred syndrome: phenotypic variability in two families carrying the same PDS missense mutation, Am J Med Genet 90:38–44, 2000.
24. Fujiwara H, Tatsumi K, Miki K, et al: Recurrent T354P mutation of the Na+/I⁻ symporter in patients with iodide transport defect, J Clin Endocrinol Metab 83:2940–2943, 1998.
25. Matsuda A, Kosugi S: A homozygous missense mutation of the sodium /iodide symporter gene causing iodide transport defect, J Clin Endocrinol Metab 82:3966–3971, 1997.
26. Neumann S, Willgerodt H, Ackermann F, et al: Linkage of familial euthyroid goiter to the multinodular goiter-1 locus and exclusion of the candidate genes thyroglobulin, thyroperoxidase, and Na+/I− symporter, J Clin Endocrinol Metab 84:3750–3756, 1999.
27. Capon F, Tacconelli A, Giardina E, et al: Mapping a dominant form of multinodular goiter to chromosome Xp22, Am J Hum Genet 67:1004–1007, 2000.
28. Many MC, Denef JF, Hamudi S, et al: Effects of iodide and thyroxine on iodine-deficient mouse thyroid: a morphological and functional study, J Endocrinol 110:203–210, 1986.
29. Raspe E, Dumont JE: Tonic modulation of dog thyrocyte H2O2 generation and I− uptake by thyrotropin through the cyclic adenosine 3′,5′-monophosphate cascade, Endocrinology 136:965–973, 1995.
30. Krohn K, Wohlgemuth S, Gerber H, et al: Hot microscopic areas of iodine deficient euthyroid goiters contain constitutively activating TSH receptor mutations, J Pathology 192:37–42, 2000.
31. Abs R, Stevenaert A, Beckers A: Autonomously functioning thyroid nodules in a patient with a thyrotropin-secreting pituitary adenoma: possible cause–effect relationship, Eur J Endocrinol 131:355–358, 1994.
32. Studer H, Huber G, Derwahl M, et al: [The transformation of Basedow's struma into nodular goiter: a reason for recurrence of hyperthyroidism], Schweiz Med Wochenschr 119:203–208, 1989.
33. Cheung NW, Boyages SC: The thyroid gland in acromegaly: an ultrasonographic study, Clin Endocrinol (Oxf) 46:545–549, 1997.
34. Dumont JE, Ermans AM, Maenhaut C, et al: Large goitre as a maladaptation to iodine deficiency, Clin Endocrinol (Oxf) 43:1–10, 1995.
35. Maier J, van Steeg H, van Oostrom C, et al: Iodine deficiency activates antioxidant genes and causes DNA damage in the thyroid gland of rats and mice, Biochim Biophys Acta 1773:990–999, 2007.
36. Gerard AC, Poncin S, Caetano B, et al: Iodine deficiency induces a thyroid stimulating hormone-independent early phase of microvascular reshaping in the thyroid, Am J Pathol 172:748–760, 2008.
37. Howie AF, Arthur JR, Nicol F, et al: Identification of a 57-kilodalton selenoprotein in human thyrocytes as thioredoxin reductase and evidence that its expression is regulated through the calcium-phosphoinositol signaling pathway, J Clin Endocrinol Metab 83:2052–2058, 1998.
38. Howie AF, Walker SW, Akesson B, et al: Thyroidal extracellular glutathione peroxidase: a potential regulator of thyroid-hormone synthesis, Biochem J 308:713–717, 1995.
39. Demelash A, Karlsson JO, Nilsson M, et al: Selenium has a protective role in caspase-3-dependent apoptosis induced by H2O2 in primary cultured pig thyrocytes, Eur J Endocrinol 150:841–849, 2004.
40. Krohn K, Maier J, Paschke R: Mechanisms of disease: hydrogen peroxide, DNA damage and mutagenesis in the development of thyroid tumors, Nat Clin Pract Endocrinol Metab 3:713–720, 2007.
41. Maier J, van Steeg H, van Oostrom C, et al: Deoxyribonucleic acid damage and spontaneous mutagenesis in the thyroid gland of rats and mice, Endocrinology 147:3391–3397, 2006.
42. van Steeg H, Mullenders LH, Vijg J: Mutagenesis and carcinogenesis in nucleotide excision repair-deficient XPA knock out mice, Mutat Res 450:167–180, 2000.

43. Cardoso LC, Martins DC, Figueiredo MD, et al: Ca(2+)/nicotinamide adenine dinucleotide phosphate-dependent H(2)O(2) generation is inhibited by iodide in human thyroids, J Clin Endocrinol Metab 86:4339–4343, 2001.
44. Cooke MS, Evans MD, Dizdaroglu M, et al: Oxidative DNA damage: mechanisms, mutation, and disease, FASEB Journal 17:1195–1214, 2003.
45. Poncin S, Gerard AC, Boucquey M, et al: Oxidative stress in the thyroid gland: from harmlessness to hazard depending on the iodine content, Endocrinology 149:424–433, 2008.
46. Parma J, Duprez L, Van Sande J, et al: Somatic mutations in the thyrotropin receptor gene cause hyperfunctioning thyroid adenomas, Nature 365:649–651, 1993.
47. Führer D, Holzapfel HP, Wonerow P, et al: Somatic mutations in the thyrotropin receptor gene and not in the Gs alpha protein gene in 31 toxic thyroid nodules, J Clin Endocrinol Metab 82:3885–3891, 1997.
48. Georgopoulos NA, Sykiotis GP, Sgourou A, et al: Autonomously functioning thyroid nodules in a former iodine-deficient area commonly harbor gain-of-function mutations in the thyrotropin signaling pathway, Eur J Endocrinol 149:287–292, 2003.
49. Gozu HI, Bircan R, Krohn K, et al: Similar prevalence of somatic TSH receptor and Gs alpha mutations in toxic thyroid nodules in geographical regions with different iodine supply in Turkey, Eur J Endocrinol 155:535–545, 2006.
50. Vassart G: Activating mutations of the TSH receptor, Thyroid 14:86–87, 2004.
51. Krohn K, Paschke R: Progress in understanding the etiology of thyroid autonomy, J Clin Endocrinol Metab 86:3336–3345, 2001.
52. Garcia-Delgado M, Gonzalez-Navarro CJ, Napal MC, et al: Higher sensitivity of denaturing gradient gel electrophoresis than sequencing in the detection of mutations in DNA from tumor samples, Biotechniques 24:72, 74, 76, 1998.
53. Trulzsch B, Krohn K, Wonerow P, et al: DGGE is more sensitive for the detection of somatic point mutations than direct sequencing, Biotechniques 27:266–268, 1999.
54. Trülzsch B, Krohn K, Wonerow P, et al: Detection of thyroid-stimulating hormone receptor and Gs alpha mutations in 75 toxic thyroid nodules by denaturing gradient gel electrophoresis, J Mol Med 78:684–691, 2001.
55. Van Sande J, Parma J, Tonacchera M, et al: Somatic and germline mutations of the TSH receptor gene in thyroid diseases, J Clin Endocrinol Metab 80:2577–2585, 1995.
56. Dugrillon A, Bechtner G, Uedelhoven WM, et al: Evidence that an iodolactone mediates the inhibitory effect of iodide on thyroid cell proliferation but not on adenosine 3′,5′-monophosphate formation, Endocrinology 127:337–343, 1990.
57. Roger PP, Servais P, Dumont JE: Stimulation by thyrotropin and cyclic AMP of the proliferation of quiescent canine thyroid cells cultured in a defined medium containing insulin, FEBS Lett 157:323–329, 1983.
58. Eggo MC, Bachrach LK, Burrow GN: Interaction of TSH, insulin and insulin-like growth factors in regulating thyroid growth and function, Growth Factors 2:99–109, 1990.
59. Eszlinger M, Krohn K, Frenzel R, et al: Gene expression analysis reveals evidence for inactivation of the TGF-beta signaling cascade in autonomously functioning thyroid nodules, Oncogene 23:795–804, 2004.
60. Gärtner R, Schopohl D, Schaefer S, et al: Regulation of transforming growth factor beta 1 messenger ribonucleic acid expression in porcine thyroid follicles in vitro by growth factors, iodine, or delta-iodolactone, Thyroid 7:633–640, 1997.
61. Taton M, Lamy F, Roger PP, et al: General inhibition by transforming growth factor beta 1 of thyrotropin and cAMP responses in human thyroid cells in primary culture, Mol Cell Endocrinol 95:13–21, 1993.
62. Depoortere F, Pirson I, Bartek J, et al: Transforming growth factor beta(1) selectively inhibits the cyclic AMP-dependent proliferation of primary thyroid epithelial cells by preventing the association of cyclin D3-cdk4 with nuclear p27(kip1). Mol Biol Cell 11:1061–1076, 2000.
63. Grubeck-Loebenstein B, Buchan G, Sadeghi R, et al: Transforming growth factor beta regulates thyroid growth. Role in the pathogenesis of nontoxic goiter, J Clin Invest 83:764–770, 1989.
64. Krohn K, Emmrich P, Ott N, et al: Increased thyroid epithelial cell proliferation in toxic thyroid nodules, Thyroid 9:241–246, 1999.
65. Derwahl M, Studer H: Nodular goiter and goiter nodules: Where iodine deficiency falls short of explaining the facts, Exp Clin Endocrinol Diabetes 109:250–260, 2001.
66. Studer H, Peter HJ, Gerber H: Natural heterogeneity of thyroid cells: the basis for understanding thyroid function and nodular goiter growth, Endocr Rev 10:125–135, 1989.
67. Krohn K, Reske A, Ackermann F, et al: Ras mutations are rare in solitary cold and toxic thyroid nodules, Clin Endocrinol 55:241–248, 2001.
68. Dohan O, Baloch Z, Banrevi Z, et al: Rapid communication: predominant intracellular overexpression of the Na(+)/I(−) symporter (NIS) in a large sampling of thyroid cancer cases, J Clin Endocrinol Metab 86:2697–2700, 2001.
69. Dohan O, De la Vieja A, Paroder V, et al: The sodium/iodide Symporter (NIS): characterization, regulation, and medical significance, Endocr Rev 24:48–77, 2003.
70. Tonacchera M, Viacava P, Agretti P, et al: Benign nonfunctioning thyroid adenomas are characterized by a defective targeting to cell membrane or a reduced expression of the sodium iodide symporter protein, J Clin Endocrinol Metab 87:352–357, 2002.
71. Dunn JT, Dunn AD: Update on intrathyroidal iodine metabolism, Thyroid 11:407–414, 2001.
72. Lazar V, Bidart JM, Caillou B, et al: Expression of the Na+/I− symporter gene in human thyroid tumors: a comparison study with other thyroid-specific genes, J Clin Endocrinol Metab 84:3228–3234, 1999.
73. Caillou B, Dupuy C, Lacroix L, et al: Expression of reduced nicotinamide adenine dinucleotide phosphate oxidase (ThoX, LNOX, Duox) genes and proteins in human thyroid tissues, J Clin Endocrinol Metab 86:3351–3358, 2001.
74. De Vijlder JJ: Primary congenital hypothyroidism: defects in iodine pathways, Eur J Endocrinol 149:247–256, 2003.
75. Pisarev MA, Krawiec L, Juvenal GJ, et al: Studies on the goiter inhibiting action of iodolactones, Eur J Pharmacol 258:33–37, 1994.
76. Krohn K, Paschke R: Loss of heterozygosity at the thyroid peroxidase gene locus in solitary cold thyroid nodules, Thyroid 11:741–747, 2001.
77. Krohn K, Paschke R: BRAF mutations are not an alternative explanation for the molecular etiology of ras mutation negative cold thyroid nodules, Thyroid 14:359–361, 2004.
78. Xing M, Vasko V, Tallini G, et al: BRAF T1796A transversion mutation in various thyroid neoplasms, J Clin Endocrinol Metab 89:1365–1368, 2004.
79. Puxeddu E, Moretti S, Elisei R, et al: BRAF(V599E) mutation is the leading genetic event in adult sporadic papillary thyroid carcinomas, J Clin Endocrinol Metab 89:2414–2420, 2004.
80. Soares P, Trovisco V, Rocha AS, et al: BRAF mutations and RET/PTC rearrangements are alternative events in the etiopathogenesis of PTC, Oncogene 22:4578–4580, 2003.
81. Eszlinger M, Krohn K, Berger K, et al: Gene expression analysis reveals evidence for increased expression of cell cycle-associated genes and Gq-protein-protein kinase C signaling in cold thyroid nodules, J Clin Endocrinol Metab 90:1163–1170, 2005.
82. Krohn K, Stricker I, Emmrich P, et al: Cold thyroid nodules show a marked increase of proliferation markers, Thyroid 13:569–576, 2003.
83. Bol S, Belge G, Thode B, et al: Structural abnormalities of chromosome 2 in benign thyroid tumors. Three new cases and review of the literature, Cancer Genet Cytogenet 114:75–77, 1999.
84. Rippe V, Drieschner N, Meiboom M, et al: Identification of a gene rearranged by 2p21 aberrations in thyroid adenomas, Oncogene 22:6111–6114, 2003.
85. Ward LS, Brenta G, Medvedovic M, et al: Studies of allelic loss in thyroid tumors reveal major differences in chromosomal instability between papillary and follicular carcinomas, J Clin Endocrinol Metab 83:525–530, 1998.
86. Tan GH, Gharib H, Reading CC: Solitary thyroid nodule. Comparison between palpation and ultrasonography, Arch Intern Med 155:2418–2423, 1995.
87. Hegedüs L, Bonnema SJ, Bennedbæk FN: Management of simple nodular goiter: current status and future perspectives, Endocr Rev 24:102–132, 2003.
88. Vanderpump MP, Tunbridge WM, French JM, et al: The incidence of thyroid disorders in the community: a twenty-year follow-up of the Whickham Survey, Clin Endocrinol (Oxf) 43:55–68, 1995.
89. Laurberg P, Pedersen KM, Vestergaard H, et al: High incidence of multinodular toxic goitre in the elderly population in a low iodine intake area vs. high incidence of Graves' disease in the young in a high iodine intake area: comparative surveys of thyrotoxicosis epidemiology in East-Jutland Denmark and Iceland, J Intern Med 229:415–420, 1991.
90. Berghout A, Wiersinga WM, Drexhage HA, et al: Comparison of placebo with L-thyroxine alone or with carbimazole for treatment of sporadic non-toxic goitre, Lancet 336:193–197, 1990.
91. Hegedüs L: Thyroid Ultrasound, Endocrinol Metab Clin North Am 30:339–360, 2001.
92. Tollin SR, Mery GM, Jelveh N, et al: The use of fine-needle aspiration biopsy under ultrasound guidance to assess the risk of malignancy in patients with a multinodular goiter, Thyroid 10:235–241, 2000.
93. Aghini-Lombardi F, Antonangeli L, Martino E, et al: The spectrum of thyroid disorders in an iodine-deficient community: the Pescopagano survey, J Clin Endocrinol Metab 84:561–566, 1999.
94. Jarløv AE, Nygaard B, Hegedüs L, et al: Observer variation in the clinical and laboratory evaluation of patients with thyroid dysfunction and goiter, Thyroid 8:393–398, 1998.
95. Surks MI, Ortiz E, Daniels GH, et al: Subclinical thyroid disease: scientific review and guidelines for diagnosis and management, JAMA 291:228–238, 2004.
96. Elisei R, Bottici V, Luchetti F, et al: Impact of routine measurement of serum calcitonin on the diagnosis and outcome of medullary thyroid cancer: experience in 10,864 patients with nodular thyroid disorders, J Clin Endocrinol Metab 89:163–168, 2004.
97. Bennedbæk FN, Perrild H, Hegedüs L: Diagnosis and treatment of the solitary thyroid nodule. Results of a European survey, Clin Endocrinol (Oxf) 50:357–363, 1999.
98. Bennedbæk FN, Hegedüs L: Management of the solitary thyroid nodule: results of a North American survey, J Clin Endocrinol Metab 85:2493–2498, 2000.
99. Bonnema SJ, Bennedbæk FN, Wiersinga WM, et al: Management of the nontoxic multinodular goitre: a European questionnaire study, Clin Endocrinol (Oxf) 53:5–12, 2000.
100. Bonnema SJ, Bennedbæk FN, Ladenson PW, et al: Management of the nontoxic multinodular goiter: a North American survey, J Clin Endocrinol Metab 87:112–117, 2002.
101. Nygaard B, Hegedüs L, Ulriksen P, et al: Radioiodine therapy for multinodular toxic goiter, Arch Intern Med 159:1364–1368, 1999.
102. Nygaard B, Knudsen JH, Hegedüs L, et al: Thyrotropin receptor antibodies and Graves' disease, a side-effect of ^{131}I treatment in patients with nontoxic goiter, J Clin Endocrinol Metab 82:2926–2930, 1997.
103. Okumura Y, Takeda Y, Sato S, et al: Comparison of differential diagnostic capabilities of ^{201}Tl scintigraphy and fine-needle aspiration of thyroid nodules, J Nucl Med 40:1971–1977, 1999.
104. Demirel K, Kapucu O, Yucel C, et al: A comparison of radionuclide thyroid angiography, (99m)Tc-MIBI scintigraphy and power Doppler ultrasonography in the differential diagnosis of solitary cold thyroid nodules, Eur J Nucl Med Mol Imaging 30:642–650, 2003.
105. Rago T, Santini F, Scutari M, et al: Elastography: new developments in ultrasound for predicting malignancy in thyroid nodules, J Clin Endocrinol Metab 92:2917–2922, 2007.
106. Bennedbæk FN, Karstrup S, Hegedüs L: Percutaneous ethanol injection therapy in the treatment of thyroid and parathyroid diseases, Eur J Endocrinol 136:240–250, 1997.
107. Døssing H, Bennedbæk FN, Hegedüs L: Effect of ultrasound-guided interstitial laser photocoagulation on benign solitary solid cold thyroid nodules—a randomised study, Eur J Endocrinol 152:341–345, 2005.

108. Bennedbæk FN, Hegedüs L: Treatment of recurrent thyroid cysts with ethanol: a randomized double-blind controlled trial, J Clin Endocrinol Metab 88:5773–5777, 2003.

109. Sebastianes FM, Cerci JJ, Zanoni PH, et al: Role of 18F-fluorodeoxyglucose positron emission tomography in preoperative assessment of cytologically indeterminate thyroid nodules, J Clin Endocrinol Metab 92:4485–4488, 2007.

110. Kang KW, Kim SK, Kang HS, et al: Prevalence and risk of cancer of focal thyroid incidentaloma identified by 18F-fluorodeoxyglucose positron emission tomography for metastasis evaluation and cancer screening in healthy subjects, J Clin Endocrinol Metab 88:4100–4104, 2003.

111. Baloch Z, Livolsi VA, Jain P, et al: Role of repeat fine-needle aspiration biopsy (FNAB) in the management of thyroid nodules, Diagn Cytopathol 29:203–206, 2003.

112. Haymart MR, Repplinger DJ, Leverson GE, et al: Higher serum thyroid stimulating hormone level in thyroid nodule patients is associated with greater risks of differentiated thyroid cancer and advanced tumor stage, J Clin Endocrinol Metab 93:809–814, 2008.

113. Tan GH, Gharib H: Thyroid incidentalomas: management approaches to nonpalpable nodules discovered incidentally on thyroid imaging, Ann Intern Med 126:226–231, 1997.

114. Papini E, Guglielmi R, Bianchini A, et al: Risk of malignancy in nonpalpable thyroid nodules: predictive value of ultrasound and color-Doppler features, J Clin Endocrinol Metab 87:1941–1946, 2002.

115. Bhagat MC, Dhaliwal SS, Bonnema SJ, et al: Differences between endocrine surgeons and endocrinologists in the management of non-toxic multinodular goitre, Br J Surg 90:1103–1112, 2003.

116. Watt T, Grønvold M, Rasmussen AK, et al: Quality of life in patients with benign thyroid disorders. A review, Eur J Endocrinol 154:501–510, 2006.

117. Weetman AP: Radioiodine treatment for benign thyroid diseases, Clin Endocrinol (Oxf) 66:757–764, 2007.

118. Walter MA, Briel M, Christ-Crain M, et al: Effects of antithyroid drugs on radioiodine treatment: systematic review and meta-analysis of randomised controlled trials, BMJ 334:514, 2007.

119. Bonnema SJ, Bennedbæk FN, Gram J, et al: Resumption of methimazole after 131I therapy of hyperthyroid diseases: effect on thyroid function and volume evaluated by a randomized clinical trial, Eur J Endocrinol 149:485–492, 2003.

120. Kahaly G, Dienes HP, Beyer J, et al: Randomized, double blind, placebo-controlled trial of low dose iodide in endemic goiter, J Clin Endocrinol Metab 82:4049–4053, 1997.

121. Perrild H, Hansen JM, Hegedüs L, et al: Triiodothyronine and thyroxine treatment of diffuse non-toxic goitre evaluated by ultrasonic scanning, Acta Endocrinol (Copenh) 100:382–387, 1982.

122. Wesche MF, Tiel-Van Buul MM, Lips P, et al: A randomized trial comparing levothyroxine with radioactive iodine in the treatment of sporadic nontoxic goiter, J Clin Endocrinol Metab 86:998–1005, 2001.

123. Fast S, Bonnema SJ, Hegedüs L: The majority of Danish non-toxic goitre patients are ineligible for Levothyroxine suppressive therapy, Clin Endocrinol (Oxf) 69:653–658, 2008.

124. Hegedüs L: The thyroid nodule, N Engl J Med 351:1764–1771, 2004.

125. Cooper DS, Doherty GM, Haugen BR, et al: Management guidelines for patients with thyroid nodules and differentiated thyroid cancer, Thyroid 16:109–142, 2006.

126. Ito Y, Uruno T, Nakano K, et al: An observation trial without surgical treatment in patients with papillary microcarcinoma of the thyroid, Thyroid 13:381–387, 2003.

127. Hegedüs L, Nygaard B, Hansen JM: Is routine thyroxine treatment to hinder postoperative recurrence of non-toxic goiter justified? J Clin Endocrinol Metab 84:756–760, 1999.

128. Pradeep PV, Tiwari P, Mishra A, et al: Pulmonary function profile in patients with benign goiters without symptoms of respiratory compromise and the early effect of thyroidectomy, J Postgrad Med 54:98–101, 2008.

129. Erickson D, Gharib H, Li H, et al: Treatment of patients with toxic multinodular goiter, Thyroid 8:277–282, 1998.

130. al Suliman NN, Ryttov NF, Qvist N, et al: Experience in a specialist thyroid surgery unit: a demographic study, surgical complications, and outcome, Eur J Surg 163:13–20, 1997.

131. Thomusch O, Machens A, Sekulla C, et al: Multivariate analysis of risk factors for postoperative complications in benign goiter surgery: prospective multicenter study in Germany, World J Surg 24:1335–1341, 2000.

132. Morrissey AT, Chau J, Yunker WK, et al: Comparison of drain versus no drain thyroidectomy: randomized prospective clinical trial, J Otolaryngol 37:43–47, 2008.

133. Youssef T, Mahdy T, Farid M, et al: Thyroid surgery: Use of the LigaSure Vessel Sealing System versus conventional knot tying, Int J Surg 2008 May 23 [Epub ahead of print].

134. Torre G, Borgonovo G, Amato A, et al: Surgical management of substernal goiter: analysis of 237 patients, Am Surg 61:826–831, 1995.

135. Feldkamp J, Seppel T, Becker A, et al: Iodide or L-thyroxine to prevent recurrent goiter in an iodine-deficient area: prospective sonographic study, World J Surg 21:10–14, 1997.

136. Pappalardo G, Guadalaxara A, Frattaroli FM, et al: Total compared with subtotal thyroidectomy in benign nodular disease: personal series and review of published reports, Eur J Surg 164:501–506, 1998.

137. Porterfield JR Jr, Thompson GB, Farley DR, et al: Evidence-based management of toxic multinodular goiter (Plummer's disease), World J Surg 32:1278–1284, 2008.

138. Nygaard B, Hegedüs L, Gervil M, et al: Radioiodine treatment of multinodular non-toxic goitre, Br Med J 307:828–832, 1993.

139. Bonnema SJ, Bertelsen H, Mortensen J, et al: The feasibility of high dose iodine 131 treatment as an alternative to surgery in patients with a very large goiter: effect on thyroid function and size and pulmonary function, J Clin Endocrinol Metab 84:3636–3641, 1999.

140. Huysmans DA, Hermus AR, Corstens FH, et al: Large, compressive goiters treated with radioiodine, Ann Intern Med 121:757–762, 1994.

141. Bonnema SJ, Nielsen VE, Hegedüs L: Long-term effects of radioiodine on thyroid function, size and patient satisfaction in non-toxic diffuse goitre, Eur J Endocrinol 150:439–445, 2004.

142. Jarløv AE, Hegedüs L, Kristensen LØ, et al: Is calculation of the dose in radioiodine therapy of hyperthyroidism worth while? Clin Endocrinol (Oxf) 43:325–329, 1995.

143. Nygaard B, Faber J, Hegedüs L: Acute changes in thyroid volume and function following 131I therapy of multinodular goitre, Clin Endocrinol (Oxf) 41:715–718, 1994.

144. Ron E, Doody MM, Becker DV, et al: Cancer mortality following treatment for adult hyperthyroidism. Cooperative Thyrotoxicosis Therapy Follow-up Study Group, JAMA 280:347–355, 1998.

145. Franklyn JA, Maisonneuve P, Sheppard M, et al: Cancer incidence and mortality after radioiodine treatment for hyperthyroidism: a population-based cohort study, Lancet 353:2111–2115, 1999.

146. Metso S, Auvinen A, Huhtala H, et al: Increased cancer incidence after radioiodine treatment for hyperthyroidism, Cancer 109:1972–1979, 2007.

147. Huysmans DA, Nieuwlaat WA, Erdtsieck RJ, et al: Administration of a single low dose of recombinant human thyrotropin significantly enhances thyroid radioiodide uptake in nontoxic nodular goiter, J Clin Endocrinol Metab 85:3592–3596, 2000.

148. Nielsen VE, Bonnema SJ, Boel-Jørgensen H, et al: Recombinant human thyrotropin markedly changes the 131I kinetics during 131I therapy of patients with nodular goiter: an evaluation by a randomized double-blinded trial, J Clin Endocrinol Metab 90:79–83, 2005.

149. Albino CC, Mesa CO Jr, Olandoski M, et al: Recombinant human thyrotropin as adjuvant in the treatment of multinodular goiters with radioiodine, J Clin Endocrinol Metab 90:2775–2780, 2005.

150. Nieuwlaat WA, Hermus AR, Sivro-Prndelj F, et al: Pretreatment with recombinant human TSH changes the regional distribution of radioiodine on thyroid scintigrams of nodular goiters, J Clin Endocrinol Metab 86:5330–5336, 2001.

151. Bonnema SJ, Nielsen VE, Boel-Jørgensen H, et al: Improvement of goiter volume reduction after 0.3 mg recombinant human thyrotropin-stimulated radioiodine therapy in patients with a very large goiter: a double-blinded, randomized trial, J Clin Endocrinol Metab 92:3424–3428, 2007.

152. Nielsen VE, Bonnema SJ, Boel-Jørgensen H, et al: Stimulation with 0.3-mg recombinant human thyrotropin prior to iodine 131 therapy to improve the size reduction of benign nontoxic nodular goiter: a prospective randomized double-blind trial, Arch Intern Med 166:1476–1482, 2006.

153. Bonnema SJ, Nielsen VE, Boel-Jørgensen H, et al: Recombinant human thyrotropin stimulated radioiodine therapy of large nodular goiters facilitates tracheal decompression and improves inspiration, J Clin Endocrinol Metab 93:3981–3984, 2008.

154. Nieuwlaat WA, Huysmans DA, Van Den Bosch HC, et al: Pretreatment with a single, low dose of recombinant human thyrotropin allows dose reduction of radioiodine therapy in patients with nodular goiter, J Clin Endocrinol Metab 88:3121–3129, 2003.

155. Nieuwlaat WA, Hermus AR, Ross HA, et al: Dosimetry of radioiodine therapy in patients with nodular goiter after pretreatment with a single, low dose of recombinant human thyroid-stimulating hormone, J Nucl Med 45:626–633, 2004.

156. Nielsen VE, Bonnema SJ, Hegedüs L: Transient goiter enlargement after administration of 0.3 mg of recombinant human thyrotropin in patients with benign nontoxic nodular goiter: a randomized, double-blind, crossover trial, J Clin Endocrinol Metab 91:1317–1322, 2006.

157. Nielsen VE, Bonnema SJ, Hegedüs L: Effects of 0.9 mg recombinant human thyrotropin on thyroid size and function in normal subjects: a randomized, double-blind, cross-over trial, J Clin Endocrinol Metab 89:2242–2247, 2004.

158. Cohen O, Ilany J, Hoffman C, et al: Low-dose recombinant human thyrotropin-aided radioiodine treatment of large, multinodular goiters in elderly patients, Eur J Endocrinol 154:243–252, 2006.

159. Silva MN, Rubio IG, Romao R, et al: Administration of a single dose of recombinant human thyrotrophin enhances the efficacy of radioiodine treatment of large compressive multinodular goitres, Clin Endocrinol (Oxf) 60:300–308, 2004.

Chapter 17

IODINE DEFICIENCY DISORDERS

GERALDO MEDEIROS-NETO and MEYER KNOBEL

Iodine deficiency is the world's most common endocrine problem, the easiest of the major nutritional deficiencies to correct, and the most preventable cause of mental retardation in many underdeveloped countries.[1,2] Given these facts, it is remarkable that iodine deficiency continues to be a major public health problem. It is best known for causing endemic goiter, but its manifestations and consequences reach much deeper into human pathology (Table 17-1). Goiter, although frequently the most obvious feature, is much less important than the adverse effects of iodine deficiency on normal development, particularly normal development of the brain.[3,4] To emphasize the more severe consequences, this health problem is now described as *iodine deficiency disorders* (IDD) instead of endemic goiter.

For many years, it has been recognized that a close and inverse relationship usually, if not always, exists between iodine in the soil and water and the appearance of endemic goiter and allied diseases. Nevertheless, it cannot be said as of this writing that the cause of iodine deficiency disorders has been completely determined in all cases, or even in any case, because nutritional, constitutional, genetic, or immunologic factors may be additive in the sum total of causes that lead to the appearance of these diseases. Therefore, iodine deficiency is a necessary cause, although it may not always be a sufficient cause. The role of iodine deficiency as the main etiologic factor in endemic goiter and cretinism has been extensively confirmed by the success of iodine prophylaxis programs in several countries, although iodine deficiency has persisted despite readily available means of supplementation, such as iodized salt and iodized oil.[1]

Iodine Supply

Iodine is found in relative abundance in marine plants and animals, in the thyroid gland of vertebrates, in deposits of organic origin, in certain natural mineral water, in sedimentary phosphate rock, and in association with certain mineral deposits. Most of the iodine ingested by humans comes from food of animal and plant origin. This iodine, in turn, is derived from the soil. Only a relatively small fraction is derived from drinking water. A most important factor in the depletion of iodine has been glaciation, which removes old soil and scrapes bare the virgin rocks, which have iodine concentrations far lower than those of the covering soil. This situation is found in regions that remained longest under Quaternary glaciers and lost their iodine when the ice thawed.[5]

Optimal Iodine Intake

Iodine is an essential component of the thyroid hormones thyroxine (T_4) and triiodothyronine (T_3) and contributes 65% and 59% of their respective molecular weights. To meet the demand

Table 17-1. Spectrum of Iodine Deficiency Disorders

Fetus

Abortions
Stillbirths
Congenital anomalies
Increased perinatal mortality
Neurologic cretinism: mental deficiency, deaf-mutism, spastic diplegia,
 deafness
Myxedematous cretinism: dwarfism, mental deficiency, epiphyseal dysplasia
Psychomotor defects

Neonate

Neonatal goiter
Neonatal hypothyroidism

Child and Adolescent

Goitrous juvenile hypothyroidism
Impaired mental function
Retarded physical development

Adult

Goiter with its complications
Hypothyroidism
Impaired mental function
Iodine-induced hyperthyroidism
Spontaneous hyperthyroidism in the elderly

Adapted from Hetzel BS, Dunn JT, Stanbury JB (eds): The Prevention and Control of Iodine Deficiency Disorders. Amsterdam: Elsevier, 1987.

for adequate hormone, the thyroid has developed an elaborate mechanism for concentrating iodine from the circulation and converting it into hormone, which it then stores and releases into the circulation as needed. The recommended intake of iodine is at least 90 μg/day for children aged 0 to 5 years, 120 μg/day for children aged 6 to 10 years, 150 μg/day for adolescents older than 12 years and adults, and 250 μg/day for pregnant or lactating women.[1,6] About 90% of iodine is eventually excreted in urine. The median urinary iodine concentration in casual samples, expressed as micrograms per liter or deciliter, is currently the most practical biochemical laboratory marker of community iodine nutrition.[7] Recommendations by the International Council for the Control of Iodine Deficiency Disorders, the World Health Organization, and the United Nations International Children's Emergency Fund set 100 μg/L as the minimal urinary iodine concentration for iodine sufficiency.[6] Daily iodine intake for population estimates can be extrapolated from urinary iodine concentration using estimates of mean 24-hour urine volume and assuming an average iodine bioavailability of 92% using the formula: urinary iodine (μg/L) × 0.0235 × body weight (kg) = daily iodine intake.[8,9] This figure roughly corresponds to a daily intake of 150 μg iodine. A report on iodine nutrition in the United States indicated adequate iodine intake for the overall U.S. population,[10] but the median concentration decreased more than 50% between 1971 and 1974 (320 ± 6.0 μg/L) and 1988 and 1994 (145 ± 3.0 μg/L). Low urinary iodine concentrations (50 μg/L) were found in 11.7% of the 1988-1994 population, a 4.5-fold increase over the proportion in the 1971-1974 study. Possible reasons for this decline included changes in national food consumption patterns (lower salt intake) and food industry practices. A more recent evaluation found a median urine iodine of 153 μg/L (men) and 124 μg/L (women) and did not vary with increasing age, indicating that the U.S. adult population is iodine sufficient.[11]

IODINE NUTRITION DURING PREGNANCY AND LACTATION

Iodine is particularly critical for pregnant women.[6] During pregnancy, several physiologic changes take place in maternal thyroid economy which together lead to an increase in thyroid hormone production of approximately 50% above the preconception baseline hormone production. To achieve the necessary increment in thyroid hormone production, the iodine intake needs to be increased during early pregnancy.[2] Also early in pregnancy, there is an increase in renal glomerular filtration leading to increased plasma iodide clearance. Women should have an adequate iodine intake, corresponding to 150 μg/day, to ensure that intrathyroidal iodine stores are replenished before they became pregnant. A recent guideline[12] reached the consensus that iodine nutrition during pregnancy and breastfeeding should range between 200 and 300 μg/day, with an average of 250 μg/day. The prevalence of postpartum thyroiditis does not seem to be related to the iodine intake status of a population.[13] Accordingly in a case-control study,[14] there was a difference in iodine excretion in the immediate postpartum period between 73 women who developed postpartum thyroiditis and 135 women who did not. With regard to the effect of changes in iodine intake on the occurrence of postpartum thyroiditis, the data are conflicting. On the one hand, there are data indicating that increased iodine intake can influence the severity of thyroid dysfunction in postpartum thyroiditis. In Sweden, an iodine-sufficient area, 20 women who were thyroid peroxidase (TPO) positive in early pregnancy were treated with iodine (0.15 mg/d) for 40 weeks postpartum. In those women who developed thyroid dysfunction, thyroid-stimulating hormone (TSH) levels were higher, and T4 levels were lower, compared with the group who received no medication.[15] On the other hand, in Denmark, in an area with mild to moderate iodine insufficiency, a placebo-controlled, randomized, double-blind trial was accomplished to verify the impact of iodine supplementation (0.15 mg/d) during pregnancy and the postpartum period in 72 TPO antibody–positive women.[16,17] It was concluded that iodine supplementation did not induce or worsen postpartum thyroiditis.[17]

The most reasonable conclusion is that there is no proven further benefit in providing pregnant women with more than 300 μg/day. In most countries with a well-established salt iodination program, pregnancies are not at risk of having iodine deficiency. In case of situations in which ingestion of iodized salt should be restricted, preparations of potassium iodide may be used as oral supplements associated or not to multivitamin tablets. In areas with no iodide supplementation and difficult socioeconomic conditions, it is recommended to administer orally iodized oil as early in gestation as possible (400 mg of iodine given orally will cover thyroid needs for 1 year). The best single parameter to evaluate the adequacy of iodine nutrition is urine iodine, which should range between 150 and 250 μg/L. These values may vary during pregnancy,[18] and iodine supplementation may be needed in late pregnancy. Accordingly, it was shown that prolonged iodized salt significantly improves maternal thyroid economy and reduces the risk of maternal thyroid insufficiency during gestation, probably because of nearly restoring intrathyroidal iodine stores.[19]

With regard to iodine nutrition during breastfeeding, thyroid hormone production and urinary iodine excretion return to normal, but iodine is efficiently concentrated by the mammary gland. Since breast milk provides approximately 100 μg/day of iodine to the infant, it is recommended that the breastfeeding mother should continue to take 250 μg per day of iodine.[6]

Prevalence

It is much easier to list the iodine-sufficient countries than those with different degrees of iodine deficiency. In the beginning of the 1990s, it was estimated that 29% of the global population lived in areas of iodine deficiency. Historically, the occurrence of thyroid disease in Europe has been dominated by iodine deficiency with some geographical variation. Severe iodine deficiency with endemic cretinism and goiter in the major part of the population was primarily found in the Alps and in other mountainous regions, but milder forms of iodine deficiency were present in regions of nearly every European country. As reviewed previously by Delange,[20] iodine deficiency has been eradicated in some European countries for many years, but other countries have lagged behind, especially in prevention of mild to moderate iodine deficiency. Owing to keen efforts by dedicated, hard-working people, the situation has improved in recent years. The number of European countries affected by iodine deficiency is steadily decreasing, and the efforts and results in the fight to prevent and control iodine deficiency have markedly progressed. During the 10 years between 1994 and 2004, the number of European countries which were considered iodine sufficient went from only 5 to 21.[21]

In 2007, WHO estimated that nearly 2 billion individuals had an insufficient intake of iodine, including a third of all school-aged children (Table 17-2).[22] The lowest prevalence of iodine deficiency is in the Americas (10.6%), where the proportion of households consuming iodized salt is the highest in the world (about 90%). The highest prevalence of iodine deficiency is in Europe (52%), where the household coverage with iodized salt is the lowest (about 25%), and many countries have weak or nonexistent control programs for iodine-deficiency disorders.

Iodine deficiency remains a public health problem in 47 countries (Fig. 17-1). However, progress has been made since 2003; 12 countries have progressed to optimum iodine status, and the percentage of school-aged children at risk of iodine deficiency has decreased by 5%.[5] However, iodine intake is more than adequate or even excessive in 34 countries, increased from 27 in 2003. In Australia and the United States, two countries that were previously iodine sufficient, iodine intake is falling. Australia is now mildly iodine deficient, and in the United States, the median urinary iodine is 145 μg/L, as mentioned, which is still adequate but half the median value of 311 μg/L noted in 1970. These changes emphasize the importance of regular monitoring of iodine status in countries to detect both low and excessive intakes of iodine.

Table 17-2. Proportion of Population and Number of Individuals in the General Population (All Age Groups) With Insufficient Iodine Intake*

WHO Regions	Inadequate Iodine Nutrition (Urinary Iodine <100 μg/L)		
	% General Population (Million)	% School-Age Children 6-12 Years (Million)	% Households With Access to Iodized Salt
Africa	41.5 (312.9)	40.8 (57.7)	66.6
Americas	11.0 (98.6)	10.6 (11.6)	86.8
Eastern Mediterranean	30.0 (503.6)	48.8 (43.3)	47.3
Europe	52.0 (459.7)	52.4 (38.7)	49.2
South Asia	47.2 (259.3)	30.3 (73.1)	61.0
Western Pacific	21.2 (374.7)	22.7 (41.6)	89.5
Total worldwide	30.6 (1900.9)	31.5 (263.7)	70.0

Adapted from WHO/ICCIDD/UNICEF: Assessment of the Iodine Deficiency Disorders and Monitoring Their Elimination, 3rd edition. Geneva: WHO, 2007; and Zimmermann MB, Jooste PL, Pandav CS: Iodine-deficiency disorders. Lancet 372:1251–1262, 2008.
*By WHO regions during the period between 1994 and 2006 and proportion of households using iodized salt.

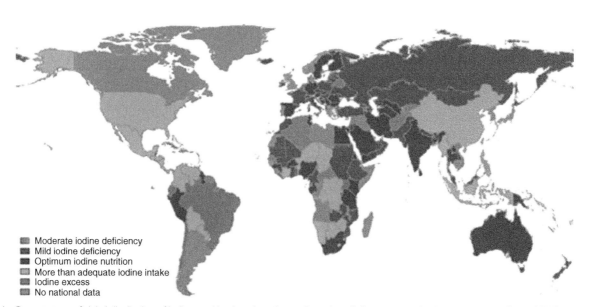

- Moderate iodine deficiency
- Mild iodine deficiency
- Optimum iodine nutrition
- More than adequate iodine intake
- Iodine excess
- No national data

FIGURE 17-1. Current status of global distribution of iodine nutrition based on the median urinary iodine concentration by country, according to WHO database on iodine deficiency. (Data from de Benoist B, McLean E, Andersson M: Iodine deficiency in 2007: Global progress since 2003, Food Nutr Bull 29:195–202, 2008.)

Recent reports on goiter and iodine deficiency in Europe[20] have indicated, however, that goiter persists in adults (but is seldom seen in children) in Bulgaria, Czechoslovakia, the Netherlands, Belgium, and Switzerland.[21] According to a relatively recent study, the iodine status of the Swiss population is currently adequate.[23] Substantial areas of high goiter prevalence persist in Austria, Hungary, Romania, Poland, the constituent countries of the former Yugoslavia (Slovenia, Croatia, Bosnia and Herzegovina, Macedonia, Serbia, Montenegro), and western Russia. In other countries (southwestern Germany, Greece, Italy, Portugal, Spain, and Turkey), iodine prophylaxis is not mandatory, and goiter and even endemic cretinism continue to be major problems, either nationally or regionally (goiter prevalence rates of 18% to 22%).

Iodine deficiency has been a public health problem in most Latin American countries. Iodine status has been reassessed over the last 15 years, and programs have been implemented for the control of IDD. Great progress has been made, particularly in the aggressive push for iodized salt use. But problems remain, such as weak governmental support and lack of effective monitoring of salt iodization in some countries, threatening the effective and sustained elimination of IDD in the region. Data on the present situation, however, are incomplete because regular monitoring is carried out in only a few countries. Moreover, different methods were used to measure iodine in urine and salt, and goiter was evaluated only by palpation. Using the ThyroMobil model, which has proven to be a convenient and efficient model for standardized and rapid evaluation for urinary iodine and goiter prevalence in Europe, 163 sites in 13 countries were visited to assess randomly selected schoolchildren of both genders, 6 to 12 years of age. The median urinary iodine concentration (8208 samples) varied from 72 to 540 µg/L. The Guatemala median was below the recommended range of 100 to 200 µg/L; Bolivia, Nicaragua, El Salvador, Mexico, and Argentina were at 100 to 200 µg/L; and Peru, Honduras, Paraguay, Venezuela, Brazil, Ecuador, and Chile were higher than 200 µg/L, including three (Brazil, Ecuador, Chile) greater than 300 µg/L. Urinary iodine concentration correlated with the iodine content of salt in all countries. Median values of thyroid volume were within the normal range for age in all countries, but the goiter prevalence varied markedly from 3.1% in Bolivia to 25.0% in Nicaragua because of scatter.[24,25]

In the sub-Himalayan area of Pakistan, the overall prevalence of goiter is 39.7%, and endemic cretinism is common.[26] In India, despite intensive efforts to promote iodized salt, only about half the population is covered, and coverage is especially poor in low socioeconomic populations. Iodized salt is unavailable in many rural markets, or salt sold as iodized is poorly or incompletely iodized or both.[27] The Himalayas of India, Nepal, Bhutan, and southern China, as well as the mountains extending into northern Burma, Thailand, Laos, and Vietnam, have long been known as goitrous areas.

It is estimated that 30 million Chinese have goiter, and possibly 200,000 suffer from the consequences of endemic cretinism.[28] Accordingly, new cases of cretinism have been recently detected in isolated regions of Western China.[29] An intensive program of salt iodination and administration of iodized oil (orally and intramuscularly), however, has reduced the prevalence of goiter and iodine deficiency in China. A 1995 national survey among children aged 8 to 12 years showed a total goiter rate of 20.4%. A 1997 national survey of children in the same age group reported a total goiter rate of 10.9% and a median urinary iodine level of 300.2 µg/L. According to the surveillance

results of 2002, the coverage of iodized salt had reached 95.2%, and the coverage of qualified iodized salt had reached 88.8%. With the implementation of the new standards for edible salt, the quality of iodized salt improved, and in 2002, the median urinary iodine among children 8 to 10 years of age was 241.2 µg/L. Furthermore, the study confirmed that the goiter rate among children in the 8-to-10 age group was continuing to decline over time, from 20.4% in 1995 down to 5.8% by 2002, so IDD can presently be considered as extensively eliminated in this country[30] The Philippines and Indonesia are severely iodine deficient.[31] Worse conditions persist in the remote regions of African countries.[32] In sub-Saharan Africa, 64% of households use iodized salt, but coverage varies widely from country to country.[33] In countries such as Sudan, Mauritania, Guinea-Bissau, and the Gambia, coverage is less than 10%, whereas in Burundi, Kenya, Nigeria, Tunisia, Uganda, and Zimbabwe, it is more than 90%. Further, iodine status varies from iodine deficiency in countries such as Ethiopia, Sierra Leone, and Angola to iodine excess in Democratic Republic of the Congo, Uganda, and Kenya.[34,35] However, many countries have outstanding programs—Nigeria, for example, which has been recognized as the first African country to successfully eliminate iodine deficiency.[36] In South Africa, coverage of adequately iodized household salt (i.e., iodized at >15 mg/kg) was 62.4% of households 2 years after the introduction of compulsory iodization at a level of 40 to 60 mg/kg. A total of 7.3% of households used noniodized agricultural salt and salt obtained directly from producers. The iodine concentration in salt was lower in rural areas than in urban and periurban areas. The consequences of using undeiodized or noniodized salt were most likely to be experienced in the country's three northern provinces, among people in the low socioeconomic categories, and in rural households[37] (Fig. 17-2).

As assessed by measurements of urinary iodine, many countries have achieved the elimination of iodine deficiency—for example, Algeria, Kenya, Cameroon, Tanzania (Africa); Iran, Lebanon, Tunisia (Eastern Mediterranean); Bhutan, China, Indonesia, India, Thailand (Asia); Venezuela, Peru, Ecuador (Latin America); and Switzerland, Austria, Great Britain, Finland, Norway, Sweden, Poland, Macedonia, Croatia, the Czech Republic, Slovakia, and Bulgaria in Europe.[5] However, in spite of the tremendous improvement of the implementation of programs of iodized salt, 35.2% of the general population in the world still had a urinary iodine below 100 µg per liter in 2003,[22] and the percentage of the world population affected by goiter did not appreciably change between 1990 (12%)[40] and 1999 (13%).[41]

Etiology

Absolute and chronic iodine deficiency is the main cause of endemic goiter and allied disorders. It is entirely possible that in certain limited situations other etiologic factors such as genetic predisposition in highly inbred and isolated groups and the presence of effective goitrogens in unusual dietary situations (Table 17-3). The arguments supporting iodine deficiency as the cause of endemic goiter are: (1) an association between low iodine content in the food and water and the appearance of the disease in the population; (2) a reduction in goiter incidence that occurs when iodine is added to the diet; and (3) demonstration that the metabolism of iodine and thyroid changes in patients with endemic goiter are similar to those produced in animals subjected to a low-iodine diet.

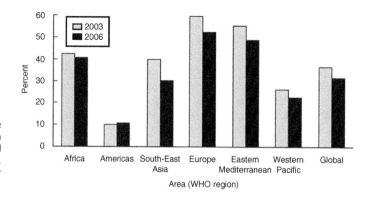

FIGURE 17-2. Change in the prevalence of individuals with an insufficient iodine intake between 2003 and 2006. Insufficient iodine intake in school-aged children has decreased by 5%, the largest decreases occurring in Southeast Asia and Europe. The Americas remained stable. (Data from de Benoist B, McLean E, Andersson M: Iodine deficiency in 2007: Global progress since 2003, Food Nutr Bull 29:195–202, 2008.)

Table 17-3. Natural Goitrogens Associated With Endemic Goiter

Goitrogens	Agent	Action
Millet, soy	Flavonoids	Impair thyroperoxidase activity
Cassava, sweet potato, sorghum	Cyanogenic glucosides metabolized to thiocyanates	Inhibit iodine thyroidal uptake
Babassu coconut, mandioca	Flavonoids	Inhibit thyroperoxidase
Cruciferous vegetables: cabbage, cauliflower, broccoli, turnips	Glucosinolates	Impair iodine thyroidal uptake
Seaweed (kelp)	Iodine excess	Inhibits release of thyroidal hormones
Malnutrition	Vitamin A deficiency	Increases TSH stimulation
	Iron deficiency	Reduces heme-dependent thyroperoxidase thyroidal activity
	Selenium deficiency	Accumulates peroxides and causes deiodinase deficiency; impairs thyroid hormone synthesis

Adapted from Zimmermann MB, Jooste PL, Pandav CS: Iodine-deficiency disorders, Lancet 372:1251–1262, 2008.

Natural goitrogens (see Table 17-3) may be considered significant determinants of the prevalence of endemic goiter, either in iodine-deficient areas or in localities where iodine intake is abundant, as in the coal-rich Appalachian area of eastern Kentucky.[42] Goitrogenic effects may be related to the consumption of certain foodstuffs (cassava, millet, babassu coconut, piñon, vegetables from the genus *Brassica*, and soybean).[44] The goitrogenic factor in cassava is related to the hydrocyanic acid liberated from the cyanogenetic glucoside (linamarin) and endogenously changed to thiocyanate, which competitively inhibits trapping and promotes the efflux of intrathyroidal iodine.[43] Pearl millet is one of the most important food crops in the semiarid tropics (large portions of Africa and Asia). Millet porridge is rich in C-glucosylflavones and also contains thiocyanate. Both are additive in their antithyroid effects. In Darfur province of western Sudan, the goiter prevalence in schoolchildren was linked to the level of consumption of millet.[44] Babassu coconut is largely consumed in northern Brazil, and studies have demonstrated the possible presence of flavonoids in the edible part of the nut.[45] Thus in areas where millet and babassu coconut are a major component of the diet, their ingestion may contribute to the

genesis of goiter. Furthermore, flavonoids, besides being potent inhibitors of thyroid peroxidase, also interact with thyroid hormone at the peripheral level.[46] Turnips, like cabbage, cauliflower, and broccoli, contain glucosinolates whose metabolites compete with iodine for thyroidal uptake.[44] Soy-containing foods and dietary supplements are widely consumed for putative health benefits (e.g., cancer chemoprevention, beneficial effects on serum lipids associated with cardiovascular health, reduction of osteoporosis, relief of menopausal symptoms), but studies of soy isoflavones in experimental animals suggest possible adverse effects as well, like enhancement of reproductive organ cancer, modulation of endocrine function, and antithyroid effects (due to flavonoids which impair thyroid peroxidase activity).[47] Antithyroid effects may also be extended by increasing the loss of T_4 from the blood via bile into the gut and may cause goiter when iodine intake is limited.[48]

Excess consumption of iodine-rich kelp (dry seaweed, 80 to 200 mg iodine per day) has caused sporadic and even endemic goiter in humans. In this case, goiter is common in some families and more frequent in girls at puberty, which suggests possible influences of additional genetic and hormonal factors. The organification of iodine and, consequently, the synthesis of T_4 and T_3 were lower than normal, and iodine-rich colloid goiter was observed in patients from the goiter-endemic coast of Hokkaido, Japan, after thyroidectomy.[49]

Generalized malnutrition (protein-calorie deprivation) has been recognized as an additive factor in the prevalence of endemic goiter in afflicted populations. On the basis of epidemiologic data recorded in 5- to 14-year-old South African children, it was recently shown that vitamin A supplements are effective in treating vitamin A deficiency in areas of mild ID. It also has an additional benefit: through suppression of the pituitary *TSHβ* gene, vitamin A supplements can decrease TSH thyroid hyperstimulation and thereby reduce the risk of goiter.[50] Vitamin A deficiency was also reported to impair thyroglobulin (TG) synthesis and thyroidal iodine uptake.[51]

Another stimulator of follicular cell growth that acts synergistically with endogenous TSH is the anti-GAL antibody.[52] This human polyclonal antibody was found to mimic the in vitro TSH effects of stimulation of cyclic adenosine monophosphate synthesis, ^{125}I uptake, and cellular proliferation of cultured porcine thyrocytes. Anti-GAL antibodies were found to be higher in goitrous individuals and positively correlated with the size of goiter. Whether these antibodies contribute to the pathogenesis of the disease needs further clarification.

Besides iodine, several minerals and trace elements such as iron, selenium, and zinc are essential for normal thyroid hormone metabolism. Iron deficiency impairs thyroid hormone synthesis by reducing activity of heme-dependent thyroid peroxidase. Iron-deficiency anemia blunts and iron supplementation improves the efficacy of iodine supplementation.[53] In several regions of the world, people are exposed to inadequate selenium supply because the selenium content of surface soil has been depleted by erosion and glacial washout, similar to iodine. In spite of that, it was shown that selenium did not significantly influence thyroid volume in borderline iodine sufficiency, because the iodine status was most likely the more important determinant.[54]

Zinc status also affects thyroid function. Research established a relationship between zinc deficiency and thyroid hormone levels. Zinc is required for the proper function of $1,5'$-deiodinase, the enzyme required for the conversion of thyroxine to triiodothyronine.[55] In animal studies, severely zinc-deficient rats had flattened epithelial cells, colloid accumulation, and lower T_3 concentration; marked alterations of follicle cellular architecture, including signs of apoptosis, were found.[56] In a zinc deletion–repletion study carried out in humans, TSH, total T_4, and free T_4 tended to decrease during the depletion phase and returned to control levels after zinc repletion.[57]

In addition to the aforementioned natural goitrogens, exposure to environmental chemicals may have deleterious thyroid-system effects in humans during development, especially in the nervous system, and also may adversely impact thyroid hormone metabolism (Table 17-4). The effects of some chemicals may be profound: the antithyroperoxidase (anti-TPO) activity of resorcinol is 26 times the activity of propylthiouracil. Many halogenated compounds compete with natural hormones for binding to protein carriers (transthyretin and to a lesser degree thyroxine-binding globulin), although the clinical consequences are unclear. Polychlorinated biphenyls (PCBs) may have a possible effect on thyroid hormone–regulated genes.[58] Disulfides from coal processes[44] and from sedimentary rock drained by water into deep wells are believed to be the cause of the incomplete reduction of endemic goiter after the use of iodized salt in Colombia.[59] Perchlorate is a competitive inhibitor of the sodium/iodine symporter, decreasing the active transport of iodine into the thyroid.

There has been concern that naturally occurring perchlorate and industrial contamination of water supplies with perchlorate might pose a health hazard by inducing or aggravating underlying thyroid dysfunction. So far, available evidence has demonstrated that long-term, large but intermittent exposure to perchlorate does not adversely affect thyroid function, despite a lowering of the thyroid radioactive iodide uptake (RAIU).[60] Tobacco smoking is a major source of thiocyanate in humans, which inhibits the function of the iodide transporter in the lactating mammary gland. Smoking during the period of breastfeeding dose-dependently reduces breast milk iodine content to about half and, consequently, exposes the infant to increased risk of iodine deficiency.[61] In brief, it seems that most goitrogens do not have a major clinical effect unless there is coexisting iodine deficiency.

Pathophysiology

Goiter was regarded as an obligatory response to prolonged and severe iodine deficiency, and an increase in thyroid iodine clearance was shown to be the basic mechanism of iodine conservation (for a review of iodine deficiency disorders, see ref. 63). Subsequently, a shift in thyroid hormone synthesis in favor of T_3 indicated an additional mechanism. These concepts have improved our understanding of how humans cope with low iodine intake, as well as the effects that both lack of iodine and adaptation mechanisms have on thyroid physiology. Thus, adaptation to iodine deficiency involves a number of biochemical and physiologic adjustments that ultimately result in maintenance of the intracellular concentration of T_3 within normal limits. These mechanisms are listed in Table 17-5.

INCREASE IN THYROID CLEARANCE OF PLASMA INORGANIC IODINE

An increase in thyroid clearance of plasma inorganic iodine is the fundamental adaptive mechanism by which the thyroid gland maintains a constant concentration of accumulated iodine in the

Table 17-4. Environmental Chemicals With Potential Thyroid-System Deleterious Effects in Humans

Environmental Agents	Class	Mechanism	Effects on Thyroid Hormones
Perchlorate, chlorate, bromate, disulfides from coal processes, smoking	Iodine transport	Competition/block of NIS	Decreased thyroidal synthesis of T_3 and T_4
Methimazole, propylthiourea, amitrole, mancozeb, benzophenone 2,1-methyl-3-propyl-imidazole-2-thione	Synthesis inhibitors	Inhibition of TPO	Decreased thyroidal synthesis of T_3 and T_4
Hydroxyl-PCBs, EMD 49209; pentachlorophenol	Transport disruption	Altered binding to serum transport proteins	Unknown
Acetochlor, phenobarbital, 3-methylcolanthrene, PCBs, 1-methyl-3-propyl-imidazole-2-thione	Enhanced hepatic catabolism	Up-regulation of glucosyltransferases or sulfotransferases (via CAR/PRX or AhR)	Increased biliary elimination of T_3 and T_4
TCPOBOP, pregnenolone-16α-carbonitrile, TCDD, rifampicin, phenobarbital, oltipraz	Enhanced cellular transport	Up-regulation of OATPs or MCT transporters via CAR/PXR or AhR	Increased biliary elimination of T_3 and T_4
Hydroxylated PCBs, triclosan, pentachlorophenol	Sulfotransferases	Inhibition of sulfotransferases	Decreased sulfation of THs
FD&C Red dye #3, propylthiouracil, PCBs, octyl-methoxycinnamate	Deiodinases	Inhibition or up-regulation of deiodinases	Decreased peripheral synthesis of T_3
Tetrabromobisphenol A, bisphenol A, hydroxyPCBs	TR agonists and antagonists	Direct or indirect alterations in TR-TRE binding	Altered activation of TH-dependent gene transcription

Adapted from Crofton KM: Thyroid disrupting chemicals: Mechanisms and mixtures, Int J Androl 31:209–223, 2008.
AhR, Aryl hydrocarbon receptor; *CAR*, constitutive androstane receptor; *EMD49209*, 3-methyl-4′,6-dihydroxy-3′,5′-diiodo-flavone; *FD&C red dye #3*, 2′,4′,5′,7′-tetraiodofluorescein disodium salt, commonly called *erythrosine*, a dye agent that imparts a watermelon red color, listed for use in food, drugs, and cosmetics (FD&C); *MCT*, monocarboxylate transporter; *NIS*, sodium iodide symporter; *OATP*, organic anion-transporting polypeptide; *PCBs*, polychlorinated biphenyls; *PXR*, pregnane-X receptor; *TCDD*, 2,3,7,8 tetrachlorodibenzo-p-dioxin; *TCPOBOP*, 1,4-bis-[2-(3,5-dichloropyridyloxy)]benzene; *TH*, thyroid hormone; *TPO*, thyroid peroxidase; *TR*, nuclear thyroid receptor; *TRE*, T_3 response element.

Table 17-5. Mechanisms Involved in the Adaptation to Iodine Deficiency

Increased thyroid clearance of plasma inorganic iodine
Hyperplasia of the thyroid and morphologic abnormalities
Changes in iodine stores and thyroglobulin synthesis
Modifications of the iodoamino acid content of the gland
Enrichment of thyroid secretion in T_3
Enhanced peripheral conversion of T_4 to T_3 in some tissues
Increased thyroid-stimulating hormone production

T_3, Triiodothyronine; T_4, thyroxine.

presence of chronic iodine deficiency. A clear inverse relationship between the plasma inorganic iodine concentration and thyroid clearance was found by several authors. The relationship is such that the product of thyroid clearance and iodine concentration is constant within the observed range of serum iodine concentrations. This product represents absolute iodine uptake, which is the mass of iodine available to the gland per unit of time. Despite the elevated clearance, absolute iodine uptake tends to be lower in iodine-deficient areas, thus indicating that the compensatory mechanism is neither perfect nor complete. An inability to fully compensate for the low plasma inorganic iodine with an appropriate increase in thyroid clearance probably accounts for the fall in iodine concentration in endemic goiter. The increased iodine trapping reflects TSH stimulation, as well as an intrinsic autoregulatory mechanism dependent on the intrathyroidal iodine concentration.

HYPERPLASIA OF THE THYROID

Although thyroid clearance may be increased without a demonstrable goiter, the anatomic accompaniment of functional activity is an increase in gland mass. Another interesting point is that iodine-concentrating ability is not uniformly distributed among follicular cells, even in normal glands. A certain level of TSH-dependent, autonomous iodine trapping is a feature of normal thyroid follicles, and the generation of new follicles from mother cells with an inherently high capacity for iodine trapping could well explain the heterogeneity in iodine metabolism among the follicles of glands affected by endemic goiter.[64] Partial autonomy of iodine trapping could also account for the persistently high uptake after the administration of iodine supplements. Deficiency of cytosolic superoxide dismutase in endemic goitrous tissue has been claimed to cause more prolonged exposure to oxygen free radicals and contribute to the degenerative changes found in these tissues.[65]

As long as adaptation to iodine is effective, increased thyroid volume may be considered as a mechanism to store iodine during periods of increased supply to provide for less favorable periods. However, this adaptive mechanism has its limits.[66] The capacity to synthesize thyroid hormones is not proportional to the increase of volume, and particularly in voluminous goiter, the thyroid function becomes insufficient.

CHANGES IN IODINE STORES AND THYROGLOBULIN SYNTHESIS

A constant finding reported in endemic goiter is a drastic reduction in iodine concentration, expressed in iodine per gram of tissue. The amount of organic iodine in a thyroid affected by endemic goiter may range from 1.0 to 2.5 mg, in contrast with values of 10 mg obtained in normal control glands. Concomitantly, thyroid iodine turns over much faster, as shown by an increase in the rate of release of ^{131}I from the gland. The presence

of two compartments of organic iodine in an iodine-deficient gland has been postulated: a slow- and a fast-releasing compartment, with different sizes. The fast-release pattern is seen in children and adolescents with small, diffuse goiters and is associated with a rapid rise in plasma-bound ^{131}I. Most adult goitrous patients have a slow-release pattern, with normal or low protein-bound ^{131}I and a prolonged biological half-life of thyroid ^{131}I. Such observations suggest that intrathyroidal iodine in these longstanding multinodular glands is turning over at a subnormal rate. Slow secretion of the tracer is apparently due to dilution in a large endogenous pool of stable iodine, largely as monoiodotyrosine (MIT) and diiodotyrosine (DIT), which are present to an excessive degree in the poorly iodinated TG.

MODIFICATION OF THE IODOAMINO ACID CONTENT OF THE GLAND

Experimental studies in the rat show that thyroid hyperplasia induced by iodine deficiency is associated with an altered pattern of iodine distribution within the gland.[67] An increase in labeled MIT and a decrease in the concentration of DIT, as well as a progressive increase in the ratio of T_3 to T_4, are the main changes in the thyroid gland occurring during prolonged iodine deficiency and are directly related to the degree of iodine depletion of the gland. These alterations caused by iodine deficiency appear to be associated with a structural change in TG. Experimental studies have shown a greater degree of heterogeneity in the TG molecule. Its altered sedimentation peak, significantly lower than 19 S, indicates failure of TG maturation. In large human goiters, as the concentration of iodine is reduced, the MIT/DIT ratio increases, and the fraction of tracer found in the form of T_4 and T_3 is markedly reduced. Possibly, many of the iodotyrosyl groups do not have the spatial configuration that favors the normal coupling process, and therefore only a small fraction of the iodine accumulated is actually incorporated into the normal pathway of hormone synthesis and secretion. A significant amount of iodine seems to be wasted by incorporation into iodocompounds that are clearly different from TG, that are resistant to hydrolysis, and that have a very long half-life and low molecular weight. These iodocompounds are at least in part fragments of TG.

PREFERENTIAL SECRETION OF TRIIODOTHYRONINE

The enhanced synthesis and release of T_3 at the expense of T_4 constitute an additional adaptive mechanism entirely different from those described above. T_3 contains one iodine atom less than T_4 does, and its biological activity is greater. Therefore, increasing the T_3/T_4 ratio of the hormones actually secreted by the thyroid makes the secretion biologically more active, although it contains less iodine. Data on thyroidal and extrathyroidal iodine kinetics obtained from experimental models and in humans with goiter have suggested preferential T_3 release. Coupling of MIT and DIT seems to be favored over that of two DIT molecules and is directly related to the decreasing levels of TG iodination. A low level of TG iodination and intense TSH stimulation are necessary conditions for increasing T_3 biosynthesis and release.

ENHANCED PERIPHERAL CONVERSION OF THYROXINE TO TRIIODOTHYRONINE

A compensatory increase in the peripheral conversion of T_4 to T_3 can occur in those with chronic iodine deficiency. It has been demonstrated in iodine-deficient animals that a striking increase in the conversion of T_4 to T_3 is observed in the cerebral cortex, whereas the liver shows a change in the opposite direction.[68] Thus tissues highly dependent on T_4 for their intracellular content of T_3, such as the brain, undergo a significant increase in conversion of T_4 to T_3 in the presence of chronic deficiency of iodine, and this adaptation may prevent harmful consequences on brain development in the early stages of life. Brain growth is characterized by two periods of maximal growth velocity. The first one occurs during the first and second trimesters between the third and fifth months of gestation. This phase corresponds to neuronal multiplication, migration, and organization. The second phase takes place from the third trimester onwards up to the second and third years postnatally. It corresponds to glial cell multiplication, migration, and myelination. The first phase occurs before fetal thyroid has reached its functional capacity. During this phase, the supply of thyroid hormones to the growing fetus is almost exclusively of maternal origin, whereas during the second phase, the supply of thyroid hormones to the fetus is essentially of fetal origin (Fig. 17-3).[69] An important recent issue regarding thyroid function and regulation in the fetus is the concept that thyroid hormones are transferred from mother to fetus both before and probably after the onset of fetal thyroid function.[70] Thyroid hormones, especially T_4, are already available to embryonic and fetal tissues before the onset of fetal thyroid function, which occurs in humans at mid-gestation (about 22 weeks). Thus the T_4 and T_3 found in early human fetuses up to mid-gestation are likely to be entirely or mostly of maternal origin. This transfer decreases but persists during later gestation. Iodine deficiency in the fetus is the result of iodine deficiency in the mother, and an insufficient supply of thyroid hormones to the developing brain may result in mental retardation.

INCREASED THYROTROPIN PRODUCTION

In iodine deficiency, as in other thyroid conditions with a limited glandular reserve, subjects with normal serum T_3 and low T_4 levels may have elevated levels of serum TSH even though they are clinically euthyroid. A clear-cut increase in the mean level of serum TSH was found in subjects living in areas where the iodine supply was reduced, and no difference was evident between individuals with and without goiter.[71] Also, it has been demonstrated that serum TSH levels correlate much better with serum T_4 than with serum T_3. When T_4 is low, the pituitary seems to be hypothyroid, whereas most other tissues are not metabolically affected, provided that the serum T_3 level is normal or elevated. The most elevated TSH values have been observed in newborns and young adults living in areas with severe endemic goiter, whereas in longstanding multinodular goiter, the increased thyroid mass and the presence of autonomous areas may bring serum TSH levels toward the normal range. An increased sensitivity of endemic goiter tissue to TSH has been proposed as an additional factor for continuous goiter growth. Both thyroid peroxidase activity and 5'-deiodinase (5'DI) activity are elevated in the presence of normal serum TSH, and this increased activity has been claimed to be related to increased tissue sensitivity to TSH. In an attempt to further delineate the role of TSH in the pathogenesis of goiter, various investigators have administered thyrotropin-releasing hormone (TRH) to goitrous patients. The exaggerated and sustained TSH response to TRH observed in most studies indicates an increase in pituitary TSH reserve and

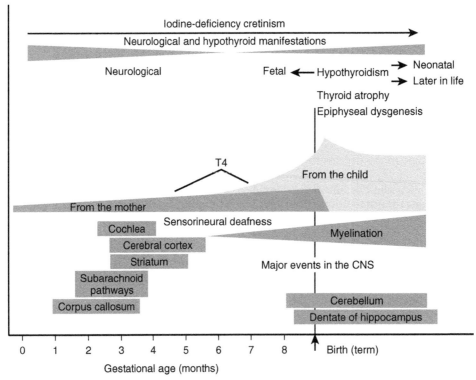

FIGURE 17-3. Proposed time course of the neurodevelopmental events and neurologic alterations associated with iodine deficiency during fetal and neonatal life. Prenatal maternal hypothyroxinemia secondary to severe iodine deficiency results in fetal neurodevelopmental damage. In addition, continuing postnatal thyroid hormone deficiency acts to determine the severity and is responsible for the varied clinical manifestations of postnatal hypothyroidism. (Data from Berbel P, Obregón MJ, Bernal J et al: Iodine supplementation during pregnancy: A public health challenge, Trends Endocrinol Metab 18:338–343, 2007.)

less than optimal T_4-induced TSH suppression at the pituitary level. This finding further documents the role in the pituitary of intracellular T_3 generated from T_4 in suppressing TSH (see Fig. 17-2).

ASSOCIATED PATHOLOGY

In most regions of the globe in which selenium deficiency is endemic, iodine deficiency is also endemic, but the converse is not true. Selenium deficiency is more severe in China and Tibet[72] than in central Africa[73] and could affect many organs, including the thyroid gland. The essential selenium is involved in thyroid hormone synthesis, metabolism, and action.[74] Selenium is an integral component of two important enzymes: glutathione peroxidase and iodothyronine deiodinase. The former catalyzes the breakdown of hydrogen peroxide, thereby protecting against oxidative damage. The later catalyzes the deiodination of T_4 to T_3. Selenium and iodine are thus linked biochemically because both are involved in thyroid hormone production. Selenium deficiency impairs the function of 5′ DI, a selenocysteine-containing protein which plays a major role in T_4 deiodination in peripheral tissues.

Clinical and Laboratory Diagnosis

The clinical picture of endemic goiter is identical to that of sporadic or simple goiter, the difference being only epidemiologic. Classically, infants and children up to school age have only diffuse enlargement of the thyroid gland. Further thyroid growth is often observed until puberty (mostly in girls) and constitutes what is commonly called *diffuse colloid goiter*. After adolescence, the gland becomes more nodular and grows in size as the adult ages. A few patients (less than 15% of the adult goitrous population) may exhibit very large multinodular glands, with the total mass estimated to be over 150 g. Age and gender influence the prevalence of goiter, females being more often affected than males.

The presence of endemic goiter does not cause any other recognized changes in the body unless the patient is hypothyroid, which is unusual. Goitrous individuals in areas of endemic goiter seem to feel perfectly good, are able to perform hard work, and show no signs of intellectual or physical impairment. A few patients with very large goiters may show symptoms of tracheal compression, with dyspnea or other symptoms caused by compression of the jugular veins. The intensity of the symptoms and signs resulting from compression on structures surrounding the goiter is not necessarily dependent on goiter size. Large, pendulous goiters can be seen in patients who do not have any other complaint. On the other hand, relatively small goiters enclosed in the upper thoracic region can generate signs of tracheal obstruction.

A frequent complication in large multinodular goiters is hemorrhage or infarction of a thyroid nodule, often accompanied by an inflammatory reaction and an abrupt rise in serum TG concentration. Hyperthyroidism, often caused by an autonomously functioning adenoma, is frequently observed if patients have access to even a small iodine load.[75] Thyroiditis, a rare complication, is often subacute and sometimes focal. The pathologic features of endemic goiter do not materially differ from those of simple nodular goiter. Follicular and anaplastic carcinomas and especially sarcomas are more frequent in regions of endemic goiter. The prevalence of these tumor types means that highly aggressive thyroid cancer prevails in countries with endemic goiter, whereas relatively benign forms (papillary carcinomas)

are less frequently recognized.[76] The prognosis of thyroid cancer in regions of endemic goiter is worse than in goiter-free areas because most patients are first seen with a tumor stage in which no cure by surgery can be expected. Highly aggressive, prognostically poor types of thyroid malignancy preponderate in patients with endemic goiter. Iodine supplementation results in a relative decrease in these tumor types and hence forms of thyroid cancer with a better prognosis.

As a whole, the following tests are advised for assessment of iodine nutrition in populations: urinary iodine concentration, goiter rate, serum TSH, thyroid hormones, and serum TG. These indicators are complementary in that urine iodine concentration is a sensitive indicator of recent iodine intake (days), and TG shows an intermediate response (weeks to months), whereas changes in the goiter rate show long-term iodine nutrition (months to years).[5]

Serum thyroid hormone levels are a further index of the effects of iodine deficiency. Thyroid hormone concentrations are generally poor indicators of iodine status. In iodine-deficient populations, serum T_3 and TSH rise or remain unchanged, and serum T_4 usually falls. However, these changes are often within the normal range, and the overlap with iodine-sufficient populations is large enough to make thyroid hormone concentrations an insensitive measure of iodine nutrition. However, TSH is a sensitive indicator of iodine status in the newborn period. Elevated serum TSH, but for exceptional pathologic situations, indicates an insufficiency in the saturation of the T_3 receptor in the brain, whatever the level of serum thyroid hormones. Therefore, elevated serum TSH constitutes an indicator of the potential risk of iodine deficiency on brain development. Serum T_4 and T_3 are less specific indicators of iodine deficiency because they are modified usually only in conditions of at least moderate iodine deficiency.[41] In moderate and severe iodine deficiency, serum T_4 is low, but T_3 is variable or occasionally high due to preferential T_3 secretion by the thyroid. Elevated serum T_3 despite low serum T_4 is considered a protective mechanism for most parts of the body, except the brain, where T_3 is produced locally and not derived from the circulating T_3.

Serum T_3 levels in inhabitants of regions where goiter is endemic are typically normal or moderately elevated at a time when serum T_4 and free T_4 are low normal or low. Elevated serum T_3 levels provide an explanation for the apparent paradox of clinical euthyroidism despite subnormal T_4 levels. Serum TSH is elevated in goitrous patients with low T_4 and correlates better with serum T_4 than with serum T_3 levels. The serum T_3/T_4 ratio is commonly used to express the adaptive processes that were described earlier. Euthyroid subjects living in areas where iodine is abundant have a mean ratio of 15:1, whereas in areas of endemic goiter, mean T_3/T_4 ratios are higher. Treatment with iodized oil causes a progressive fall in this ratio. Serum reverse T_3 (rT_3) tends to follow the direction of serum T_4, but in the serum of pregnant women from areas of endemic goiter, rT_3 is significantly higher than rT_3 levels in nonpregnant subjects from the same region. An increased binding capacity of thyroxine-binding globulin is observed and may be related to the elevated serum T_3 concentrations. This increased capacity could play an important role in the maintenance of a normal level of free T_3.

Serum TG, which represents a sensitive marker of thyroid abnormalities and iodine deficiency in epidemiologic studies, is often elevated in patients with endemic goiter.[77,78] Increased serum TG concentrations in endemic goiter could be partly related to the reduced concentration of iodine in goitrous tissue and the intrathyroidal metabolic changes secondary to persistent and chronic iodine deficiency. In areas of endemic goiter, serum TG increases owing to greater thyroid mass and TSH stimulation. Serum TG is well correlated with the severity of iodine deficiency as measured by urinary iodine.[77] Whole blood from finger pricks spotted on filter paper cards can be used to measure serum TSH and serum TG as indicators of thyroid hyperstimulation and the consequence of the state of hyperstimulation, respectively.[79]

EVALUATION OF THE IODINE STATUS IN IODINE DEFICIENCY

In addition to the determination of serum levels of TSH, thyroid hormones, and TG, the following indicators of iodine status are evaluated in an iodine-deficient population: (1) the urinary iodine concentration and (2) the estimation of thyroid size.[41]

According to WHO recommendations, quantification of urinary iodine concentration expressed as μg of iodine per volume (μg I/L, pg I/dL or μg I/dL) is accepted as a good marker of the dietary iodine intake. Therefore, it is the index of choice for evaluating the degree of iodine deficiency and for measuring the improvement in iodine status after iodine prophylaxis. Iodine intake for metabolic studies is best determined from a 24-hour urine sample, but logistics make it impractical to use such measurements for epidemiologic studies. Collections of 24-hour urine are difficult to obtain and are not necessary. Relating urinary iodine to creatinine is also not practical, because urinary creatinine decomposes after 3 days without refrigeration. Furthermore, the creatinine level varies depending on age, sex, muscle mass, diseases, pH conditions, and nutritional status of the population. For these reasons and to avoid errors introduced in the performance of different creatinine assays, the WHO has recommended for epidemiologic studies the evaluation of iodine concentrations in casual spot samples, provided a sufficient number of specimens is collected. Because the frequency distribution of urinary iodine is usually skewed towards elevated values, the median is considered instead of the mean. It is appropriate to mention that the concentration of iodine in a spot or casual urine sample cannot be used to diagnose iodine deficiency in an individual. The urinary iodine concentration may vary up to threefold in an individual during a day.[80] This means that it is necessary to collect repeated urine samples from an individual over a period of time and estimate the median or average, in order to evaluate their iodine status. Also, the urinary iodine (UI) concentration (μg/L) is not interchangeable with 24-hour UI excretion (μg/24 h). The two values are interchangeable only if the volume of urine passed in 24 hours is one liter. The average volume of urine passed by an adult is approximately 1.5 L/24 h. Therefore, the median UI excretion given as μg/24 h will be 50% higher than the median iodine excretion given as μg/L.[81]

Several methods of determination of urinary iodine have been reported, and almost all depend on the Sandell-Kolthoff reaction, in which iodide catalyzes the reduction of yellow ceric ammonium sulfate to the colorless cerous form in the presence of arsenious acid; the rate of color disappearance is proportional to the amount of iodide.[82] An optimal urinary iodine concentration is 100 to 200 μg/L, corresponding approximately to a daily intake of 150 to 300 μg for adults.

The prevalence of goiter is an index of longstanding iodine deficiency and, therefore, is less sensitive than urinary iodine in the evaluation of a recent change in the status of iodine intake. Traditionally, neck palpation can detect the enlarged thyroid of moderate or severe iodine deficiency but is less reliable in mild deficiency. Recently, thyroid ultrasonography has introduced a more precise and accurate means for quantitative estimate of

thyroid volume. Norms have been established for the thyroid volume of iodine-sufficient children related to age, gender, and body mass. The total goiter rate is related to the severity of iodine deficiency as follows: no iodine deficiency, 0% to 4.9%; mild deficiency, 5.0% to 19.9%; moderate deficiency, 20.0% to 29.9% and severe deficiency, more than 30%.[41] Furthermore, a thyroid is considered as goitrous when its volume is above the 97th percentile established for sex, age, and body surface area in iodine-replete populations.[83] In areas of endemic goiter, although the thyroid size predictably decreases in response to increases in iodine intake, thyroid size might not return to normal for months or years after correction of iodine deficiency. During this transition period, the goiter rate is difficult to interpret, because it indicates both a population's history of iodine nutrition and its present status. Moreover, palpation of goiter in regions of mild iodine deficiency has poor sensitivity and specificity; in such areas, measurement of thyroid volume by ultrasound is preferable for the classification of goiter.[84]

Principles of Treatment

In areas of iodine deficiency, goiter prevalence may be very high, and multinodularity develops frequently, especially in goiters of longstanding.

Treatment of endemic goiter can be carried out by oral administration of L-thyroxine (100 to 200 mcg/day) for a prolonged period. This putative suppressive therapy induces, through a decrease in TSH and the TSH response to TRH, functional atrophy of the goiter. Results are often satisfactory in relatively small colloid goiters but less effective in large multinodular glands. Triac (triiodothyroacetic acid) is used in the treatment of thyroid gland hypertrophy in nontoxic goiter for its suppressive effect on pituitary-thyroid function. In agreement, a study by Brenta and colleagues demonstrated that Triac is effective as a goiter-shrinkage agent.[85] These authors reported that when compared to L-thyroxine, the action appeared to be more important in reduction of goiter size, although it did not attain a significant level. In addition, it was associated with a relative advantage concerning a significantly lower incidence of adverse events. Therefore, Triac could be an alternative for the treatment of nontoxic diffuse goiter and nodular goiter.

Iodine administration is equally effective when introduced as adjunctive therapy with L-thyroxine or intramuscularly as iodized oil. The increased thyroidal secretion of thyroid hormones suppresses pituitary TSH, and more than half of the treated population experiences a remarkable reduction in goiter size. Surgery should be considered when the goiter is very large, when more than a third of the normal width of the tracheal lumen is affected, and when malignancy is suspected. In patients who have previously had thyroid surgery, the possibility of shrinking the gland with radioiodine should be considered.

Administration of ^{131}I in euthyroid or hyperthyroid multinodular goiter, to both decrease the size and to treat thyrotoxicosis, has become more popular over the years because of its efficacy and safety.[86] Even in the case of large goiters causing substantial tracheal compression with concomitant airflow obstruction, treatment with radioactive iodine can be very effective. Also, ^{131}I treatment can be used in patients in whom surgery is not an option because of increased risk. The goal is to reduce thyroid size, which can be achieved only by relatively large doses of the isotope. However, in patients with longstanding, large, nodular goiter after iodide supplementation whose RAIU is low or normal, RAIU can be enhanced. Recently, recombinant human thyrotropin has been used to stimulate RAIU in patients with nodular goiter,[87] allowing approximately 50% to 60% reduction of the therapeutic dose and causing a more homogeneous glandular distribution of radioiodine without compromising the efficacy of thyroid volume reduction. A rather high percentage (32%) of patients will become hypothyroid after treatment, as also noted in subjects treated with radioiodine for Graves' disease. Although controversial, prophylactic L-thyroxine treatment in these patients could be instituted to hinder recurrence of the goiter and persistence of hypothyroidism.[87]

In patients affected by endemic nontoxic goiter, iodine alone or in combination with L-T_4 has been proposed as an efficient alternative therapeutic tool to treatment with L-T_4 alone.[88] Among the advantages derived from this combination is the possibility of using lower doses of L-T_4 with less TSH suppression than that attained in the course of L-T_4 monotherapy.

Endemic Cretinism

Endemic cretinism is now largely a disease in remote, underdeveloped areas of the Third World (Fig. 17-4). It occurs when iodine intake is below a critical level of 25 μg/day and may affect up to 10% of populations living in conditions of severe iodine deficiency.[63] The disorder is found in India, Indonesia, China, Oceania (Papua New Guinea), Africa (Congo Kinshasa), and South America (Ecuador, Peru, Bolivia). In all these locations, with the exception of Congo Kinshasa, neurologic features are predominant. *Endemic cretinism* may be defined as irreversible changes in mental development in individuals born in an area of endemic goiter; such individuals exhibit a combination of some of the following characteristics not explained by other causes: (1) a predominantly neurologic syndrome consisting of defects of hearing and speech associated or not with characteristic disorders of stance and gait of varying degree, (2) stunted growth, (3) mental deficiency, and (4) hypothyroidism. In its fully developed form, mental deficiency, deaf-mutism, and motor spastic diplegia are associated with or without goiter. This condition is referred to as the *neurologic form* of endemic cretinism, in contrast to the *myxedematous form* (see Fig. 17-3). The typical myxedematous cretin has a lesser degree of mental retardation, severe hypothyroidism, and nonpalpable thyroid. It should be made clear, however, that the two types of endemic cretinism represent polar opposites of a wide spectrum of clinical abnormalities. Although the myxedematous type is more common in Congo Kinshasa, the condition may be found in the Himalayas, Western China, Sicily (Italy), and South America (Bolivia and Peru).

In central Africa (Congo Kinshasa), the intensity of cretinism was found to be proportional to the degree of hypothyroidism; the severity was also shown to correlate with selenium deficiency.[89] According to experimental results, it was suggested that in central Africa (Congo Kinshasa) thyroid destruction might originate from the interaction of three factors: iodine and selenium deficiencies (by increasing H_2O_2 accumulation), selenium deficiency (by decreasing cell defense and promoting fibrosis), and SCN overload (by triggering follicular cell necrosis), explaining the thyroid atrophy characteristic of the myxedematous form of cretinism. Furthermore, a hypothesis was put forth that defective glutathione peroxidase caused by selenium deficiency results in a lack of protection against peroxidative damage induced by high levels of H_2O_2 in the thyroid cell.[90] Glutathione peroxidase activity was found to be decreased in selenium-deficient areas in Congo Kinshasa and the Central African Republic (formerly Ubangi-Shari), and the enzyme activity in cretins was half the level in normal subjects. The same observation on serum glutathione peroxidase activity was recently made in a selenium-deficient population in the Lhasa district in central Tibet.[91] Selenium supplementation for 2 months corrected the enzyme levels in both normal subjects and endemic cretins.[92] However, this treatment also produced decreases in serum T_4 and T_3 and an increase in TSH. In view of these findings, it is advisable to provide iodine supplementation before administration of selenium in populations deficient in both these elements.

An interesting unifying hypothesis was proposed[93] to explain the clinical picture of endemic cretinism. The authors suggested that the clinical expression of endemic cretinism is determined by the sum of two pathophysiologic events. The first event is fetal hypothyroidism secondary to severe iodine deficiency, which occurs in all cretins and represents the prenatal action of thyroid hormone insufficiency on brain development, transmitted from mother to fetus, resulting in the neurologic abnormalities of the disorder. The second event is the persistence of postnatal hypothyroidism effects on both somatic and brain development from continuing iodine lack and other mechanisms causing thyroid failure, which entails the development of myxedematous cretinism.

DEAF-MUTISM AND ENDEMIC CRETINISM

An endemic cretin is frequently partially or completely deaf. Lesions can be produced experimentally in the organ of Corti in the chick by injecting an antithyroid drug into the yolk sac. Also, antithyroid drug (propylthiouracil) administered to pregnant mice or to pups after birth causes abnormalities in the tectorial membrane of the organ of Corti and results in deafness. These

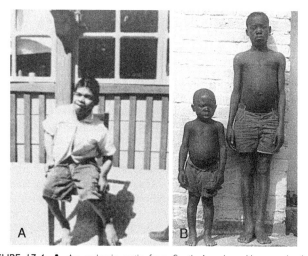

FIGURE 17-4. **A,** An endemic cretin from South America with a predominant neurologic pattern comprising deaf-mutism, spastic diplegia, goiter, and mental retardation. Although thyroid hormone levels are usually normal, an exaggerated and sustained thyroid-stimulating hormone response to thyrotropin-releasing hormone is observed frequently and suggests a low thyroid reserve. **B,** Two boys of the same age in Congo Kinshasa (formerly Zaire, central Africa). The boy on the left has an endemic myxedematous type of cretinism with severe thyroid insufficiency and dwarfism. Thyroid atrophy commonly is found later in life in myxedematous cretins and has been attributed to environmental agents or blocking autoantibodies or both. These two physiognomic forms of the syndrome represent polar opposites of a wide spectrum of clinical abnormalities which varies from one geographic area to another, with mixed characteristics.

experiments strongly suggest that intrauterine hypothyroidism somehow damages the developing auditory system and causes deafness and other neurologic defects. This has been confirmed by auditory brainstem evoked-potential studies which showed no cochlear or brainstem responses even at the highest sound frequencies, indicating a cochlear lesion. In accordance, Halpern[94] has consistently found profound congenital petrous temporal bone changes and underdeveloped cochleas (incomplete turns, fragmented and enlarged vestibular aqueduct) in the majority of both neurologic and hypothyroid adult cretins. These findings are suggestive of a premature arrest of the auditory system. Its absence in sporadic congenital hypothyroidism may be a result of the protective action of thyroid hormone passing to the fetus from the mother.

DIAGNOSIS OF ENDEMIC CRETINISM

Differentiation between sporadic congenital hypothyroidism and endemic cretinism is important both clinically and etiologically. The former is a result of hypothyroidism caused by developmental anomalies or metabolic defects, whereas the latter is associated with severe iodine deficiency in the maternal-fetal unit. Thus the common form of endemic cretinism during childhood or in adults, unlike untreated sporadic congenital hypothyroidism, is often not associated with severe clinical hypothyroidism. The three characteristic features of neurologic endemic cretinism in its fully developed form are extremely severe mental deficiency together with squint, deaf-mutism, and motor spasticity, with disorders of the arms and legs of a characteristic nature. As it would be expected with a deficiency disease, there is a wide range in the severity of the clinical features in the population affected. Mental deficiency is characterized by a marked impairment of the capacity for abstract thought, but vision is unaffected. Autonomic, vegetative, personal, and social functions and memory appear to be relatively well preserved except in the most severe cases.

Deafness is the striking feature. This may be complete in as many as 50% of cretins. As described previously, early damage to the developing auditory system has been confirmed by auditory brainstem evoked-potential studies which showed no cochlear or brainstem responses even at the highest sound frequencies. Such findings suggest a cochlear lesion. In subjects with reduced hearing, a high-tone defect is apparent. Deafness is sometimes absent in subjects with other signs of cretinism. All totally deaf cretins studied were mute, and many with some hearing had no intelligible speech.

The motor disorder shows a characteristic proximal rigidity of both lower and upper extremities and the trunk. There is a corresponding proximal spasticity with markedly exaggerated deep tendon reflexes at the knees, adductors, and biceps. Spastic involvement of the feet and hands is unusual or, if present, is much milder than that of the proximal limbs. Function of the hands and feet is characteristically preserved so that most cretins can walk. This observation is very useful in differentiating cretinism from other forms of cerebral palsy commonly encountered in endemic areas, such as cerebral palsy from birth injury or meningitis.

In addition to frank cretinism, a larger proportion of the population (estimated to be three to five times as great) suffers from some degree of mental retardation and coordination defect. The typical myxedematous cretin has a less severe degree of mental retardation than the neurologic cretin. Affected individuals have had all the features of extremely severe hypothyroidism present since early life, as in unrecognized sporadic congenital hypothyroidism: severe growth retardation; incomplete maturation of the features, including the naso-orbital configuration; atrophy of the mandibles; puffy features; myxedematous, thickened, and dry skin; dry and rare hair, eyelashes, and eyebrows; and much-delayed sexual maturation. Contrasting with the general population and with neurologic cretinism, goiter is usually absent, and the thyroid is often not even palpable, suggesting thyroid atrophy. This diagnosis is confirmed by thyroid scans that show the thyroid in a normal location but of small volume with a very heterogeneous and patchy distribution of the tracer. Thyroidal uptake of radioiodine is much lower than in the general population. The serum levels of T_4 and T_3 are extremely low, often undetectable, and TSH is dramatically high. Markedly enlarged sella turcicae have been demonstrated, suggesting pituitary adenomas. Myxedematous cretinism used to be particularly common in Congo Kinshasa.

NEONATAL HYPOTHYROIDISM IN IODINE-DEFICIENT AREAS

A serious consequence of chronic iodine deficiency is a higher incidence of neonatal hypothyroidism. In India and Congo Kinshasa, it has been reported that this condition is 200- to 500-fold more frequent than in countries with adequate iodine intake.[5] In iodine-deficient areas of India, as many as 4% of newborn babies have a cord blood serum T_4 level below 2 µg/dL, and in Congo Kinshasa, low T_4 concentrations have been observed in up to 10%.[95] Further deterioration in thyroid function occurred in Congo Kinshasan children between 2 and 4 years of age, followed by a pronounced prevalence of hypothyroidism between 5 and 7 years of age. This pattern is linked to persistent iodine deficiency accompanied by an increased thiocyanate load originating from very high consumption of cassava.[96]

Experimental work has confirmed that severe iodine deficiency affects brain development by reducing both maternal and fetal thyroid function. When sheep or marmosets are maintained on a severely iodine-deficient diet for 6 to 12 months before pregnancy and also during pregnancy, reduced brain weight and low DNA content of the fetal cerebral cortex occur as early as day 70 of gestation.[97]

Similarly, the number of spines on the shafts of pyramidal neurons from the visual cortex of iodine-deficient rats is lower than in animals supplemented with iodine.[98] This finding supports the concept that thyroid hormone affects brain maturation through specific effects on the rate of cell differentiation and gene expression.[99,100] The primary action of thyroid hormone on gene expression is mediated through interaction of the T_3 receptors with responsive elements located in gene regulatory regions. Some of the genes known to be responsive to thyroid hormones in the brain contain T_3-responsive elements (TREs), and in some cases the action of T_3 has been shown to be at the transcriptional level in vitro. Genes containing TREs in their promoter or intronic regions include those encoding myelin basic protein (MBP), the Purkinje cell–specific gene (PCP2), which encodes a G protein nucleotide exchange factor, the calmodulin-binding and protein kinase C (PKC) substrate neurogranin (RC3), prostaglandin D2 synthetase, the transcription factor hairless, the neuronal cell–adhesion molecule (NCAM), and the early response gene NGFI-A.[100] The severe neurologic damage found in endemic cretinism is probably due to thyroid hormone deficiency early in pregnancy (first trimester), and it might have become irreversible by birth, at which time thyroid hormones reverse the hypothyroidism, if present, but not the neurologic deficits. Both forms of the syndrome can be prevented by correction of the severe

Table 17-6. WHO-Recommended Iodine Supplementation*

Age Groups	Oral Dose (a)[†] (mg Iodine) 3 months	6 months	12 months	Intramuscular Dose (b)[‡] (mg Iodine) >1 year
Pregnant women	50-100	100-300	300-480	480
Women of reproductive age (15-49 years)	100-200	200-480	400-960	480
Lactating women[§]	—	—	—	480
Infants & children				
0-1 years	20-40	50-100	100-300	240
1-5 years	40-100	100-300	300-480	480
6-15 years	100-200	200-480	400-960	480
Males 16-45 years	100-200	200-480	400-960	480

Adapted from references 1, 63, and 136.

*Doses, frequency, and duration of effectiveness of administering oral and intramuscular iodine supplementation using an iodized oil preparation in the prevention of the disorders induced by iodine deficiency.

[†](a) Lipiodol (capsule): 1 capsule (0.4 mL) contains about 200 mg iodine; Oriodol (capsule): 1 capsule (0.57 mL) contains about 300 mg iodine.

[‡](b) Lipiodol (ultra fluid)/Ethiodol: 1 mL contains about 480 mg iodine.

[§]Data unavailable for lactating women.

iodine deficiency before pregnancy by iodized oil injections. When given in the first trimester, however, iodized oil does not prevent the syndrome of endemic cretinism, which suggests that the effects of maternal iodine deficiency arise very early. Thus, elemental iodine, apart from its hormonal role, may be essential for normal neural tube development, but the mechanism responsible for this action is unknown.

Prophylaxis and Treatment of Iodine-Deficiency Disorders

Prevention of endemic goiter and cretinism by the addition of iodine supplements to the daily diet has been accepted and widely used since the beginning of the 20th century. The main resources for mass correction of iodine deficiency are iodized salt and iodized oil.

IODIZED SALT

Iodized salt is considered the most appropriate measure for iodine supplementation.[101] There are two forms of iodine which can be used to iodize salt: iodide and iodate, usually as the potassium salt. Iodate is less soluble and more stable than iodide and is therefore preferred for tropical moist conditions. Both are generally referred to as "iodized salt."

The sources of most common salt are solar evaporation of sea water and salt mines. Sea salt, as usually produced, does not contain enough iodine to meet minimal human needs because the average iodine content of ocean salts is approximately 2 ppm. Human salt consumption (5 to 15 g/day) varies widely among cultures and with climatic conditions. Thus the level of iodination of salt may be varied to conform to regional conditions (1:25,000 to 1:100,000). It is accepted that 30 ppm (30 mg of potassium iodate per kilogram of salt) is the lowest level that will ensure the provision of 100 µg of iodine per day. Many local problems confound the program of iodination of salt for the many millions of people at risk. Inadequate iodinate of the salt, difficulties in importing potassium iodate, problems of transportation and coordination of distribution efforts, and the consumption of poorly iodinated "cattle" salt by the rural population are the main problems that have obstructed effective iodination prophylaxis. Successful salt iodination programs have been implemented in many countries and are highly dependent on continuous surveillance of the iodized salt produced and consumed.[102]

IODIZED OIL

Intramuscular injection or oral administration of the iodized ethyl esters of fatty acids of poppy seed (Lipiodol, Ethiodol, Oriodol), rape seed (Brassiodol), walnut, and soybean oil (475 to 540 mg iodine per milliliter) has been used for the prevention of endemic goiter and cretinism.[134-137] Intramuscular doses have varied from 0.5 to 1.0 mL in infants and young children to 0.5 to 2.0 mL for adults (Table 17-6). The physiology and pharmacology of iodized oil in goiter prophylaxis have been extensively reviewed.[137] Intramuscular administration of iodized oil was started in Papua New Guinea and extended to South America, the former Zaire (now Congo Kinshasa), Nepal, Sudan, Indonesia, India, and China. Oral administration of iodized soybean oil was extensively studied in various countries and also reported to be effective in a mass population program to control endemic goiter.[138]

The use of iodized oil, also in children, has proved to be effective not only in reducing the frequency of endemic goiter but also in reducing the size of established goiters and in preventing the major neuromotor, physical, and mental deficits that are found in association with endemic goiter and endemic cretinism.[139] Iodized oil provides effective, safe, and economically sound prophylaxis against endemic goiter and related disabilities in situations in which salt iodination is not feasible for economic or political reasons.

Iodine Excess

Universal salt iodization (USI) is a highly beneficial measure in the fight against iodine deficiency. During USI programs, occasionally population groups or individuals turn up to have or to acquire excessive iodine intake. Such inappropriate iodine intake occurs in a sporadic or endemic setting. The former situation, often self-limited, is caused by iodine-containing drugs, radiographic contrast media, or occasional intake of seaweed. Endemic circumstances of iodine excess needing work-ups to establish and correct causes are: deliberate high legal salt iodine standard to compensate for possible losses in storage, unintentional overi-

Table 17-7. Tolerable Upper Intake Level for Iodine by Age Group

Age Group	European Commission/ Scientific Committee on Food, 2002 (µg/day)	U.S. Institute of Medicine, 2001 (µg/day)
1-3 yr	200	200
4-6 yr	250	300
7-10 yr	300	300
11-14 yr	450	300
15-17 yr	500	900
Adult	600	1100
Pregnant women	600	1100

Adapted from Zimmermann MB: Iodine requirements and the risks and benefits of correcting iodine deficiency in populations, J Trace Elem Med Biol 22:81–92, 2008.

odination of salt, and high salt intake or usual eating of food naturally rich in iodine (i.e., seaweed consumed in coastal areas in Japan).

TOXIC EFFECTS OF EXCESS INTAKE

Most people who are iodine sufficient are remarkably tolerant to high dietary intakes of iodine. Iodine intakes of up to 1000 µg per day are well tolerated by most adults, since the thyroid is able to adjust to a wide range of intakes and regulates the synthesis and release of thyroid hormones. In children, chronic intakes of 500 µg per day or more are associated with increased thyroid volume, which is an early sign of thyroid dysfunction.[103] European and U.S. expert committees have recommended tolerable upper intakes for iodine (Table 17-7) but caution that individuals with chronic iodine deficiency might respond adversely to intakes lower than these.[9]

Both a chronic shortage and an acute increase in iodine intake of a population carry an augmented risk of thyroid disease, but the consequences are more severe in iodine deficiency than iodine excess. The most serious and common complication of salt iodization is the development of iodine-induced hyperthyroidism, which affects mainly older people with nodular goiters. Other possibilities are the aggravation or even the induction of autoimmune thyroiditis, goiter, and a change in the pattern of thyroid cancer.[104]

IODINE-INDUCED HYPERTHYROIDISM

An increase in the incidence of iodine-induced hyperthyroidism (IIH) has been reported after the institution of iodized salt programs in Europe and South America and after the introduction of iodized bread in Denmark and Tasmania.[105,106] IIH was more frequently seen in patients older than 40 years and was closely associated with increasing weight and nodularity of the goiter and with the existence of nonhomogeneity on thyroid scans.[107] These large multinodular goiters, adapted to chronic iodine deficiency, have autonomous areas particularly susceptible to small loads of iodine and produce excessive amounts of T_3 or T_4.

A mild and transient form of hyperthyroidism characterized by a blunted TSH response to TRH is frequently observed in endemic goiter patients moving to urban areas, where iodized salt is commonly used.[108,109]

An outbreak of IIH was reported in Africa, particularly in two African countries after the introduction of salt with a higher level of iodination.[110] In a severely iodine-deficient area of Kivu in Zaire (now Congo Kinshasa),[111] 25% of 200 unselected adult subjects with visible goiter had an undetectable serum level of thyrotropin (TSH). In half of the TSH-suppressed patients, serum thyroid hormones reached the level of overt hyperthyroidism. High serum thyroid hormone levels remained unchanged at a 1-year interval, which suggests that the hyperthyroidism was not temporary. The urinary iodide concentrations of these patients did not differ from the levels observed in euthyroid patients, 240 µg/L. In most of these patients, the clinical picture was not characteristic of hyperthyroidism.

In Zimbabwe, all cases of hyperthyroidism detected by laboratory tests in the main hospital of Harare from 1991 to 1995 were reviewed.[112] Since 1993, a threefold increase was demonstrated after the consumption of salt iodinated at a level of 30 to 90 ppm. Fatal outcomes occurred mainly from cardiac complications. The median concentration of urinary iodide in the population was 280 µg/L.

In a recent report from China, the cumulative 5-year incidence of overt hyperthyroidism, overt hyperthyroidism caused by Graves' disease, and subclinical hyperthyroidism was similar in subjects in three different communities in which iodine intake was low, more than adequate and excessive. After 5 years, 72% of the patients were euthyroid (without medication). This study may indicate that IIH is of short duration with a tendency to a normal thyroid function in relation to time, and that there is no relationship between iodine intake and hyperthyroidism, at least in people with a rather broad range of iodine intake.[113]

The reason for the development of IIH after iodine supplementation appears to be that iodine deficiency increases thyrocyte proliferation and mutation rates (due to mutational events in thyroid cells) that lead to autonomy of function.[114] When the mass of cells with such mutations becomes sufficient and the iodine supply is increased, the subject may become hyperthyroid. These changes may occur in localized foci within the gland or in the process of nodule formation. IIH may also occur with an increase in iodine intake in those whose hyperthyroidism (Graves' disease) is not expressed because of iodine deficiency. The risks of IIH are principally to the elderly, who may have heart disease, and to those who live in regions with limited access to medical care. The same situation is also found in endemic goiter areas when iodized oil injections are introduced.[115] This hyperthyroidism is often transient, and hormone production will eventually decrease in 6 to 12 months without a need for therapy unless cardiovascular disease and related complications are present.

Diagnosis of Iodine-Induced Hyperthyroidism

IIH is an occasional consequence of the correction of iodine deficiency, occurring most frequently in older subjects with multinodular goiter. This complication is usually mild and self-limited, but may be serious and occasionally lethal. The most important clinical manifestations are cardiovascular.

Clinical diagnosis of IIH is often subtle. The features may develop slowly over time and be mistakenly attributed to aging or chronic illness. The appearance of clinical features compatible with hyperthyroidism, especially in the presence of a goiter and a recent increase of iodine intake, should prompt the physician to pursue the diagnosis further. The appropriate laboratory tests are the same as for hyperthyroidism from other causes. The most valuable is the serum TSH by a sensitive assay (i.e., one that measures to 0.1 µU/mL or below); a depressed value favors a diagnosis of hyperthyroidism. Another supportive laboratory result is elevation in free thyroxine. Urinary iodine determinations are rarely helpful in diagnosing the individual patient with IIH because they define only iodine nutrition and not the level of thyroid function.

Treatment of Iodine-Induced Hyperthyroidism

Therapy for IIH varies with the underlying pathology and the amounts of iodine involved. The patient with nodular goiter who has become hyperthyroid with increasing dietary iodine is treated by one of the conventional measures for hyperthyroidism: antithyroid drugs, radioactive iodine, or surgery.

Hyperthyroidism associated with pharmacologic amounts of iodine is more complicated to treat. The large iodine load depresses iodine uptake by the thyroid and makes ^{131}I treatment less feasible. Amiodarone can cause thyrotoxicosis both from excess iodine and also from thyroid inflammation induced by the drug itself. The usual treatment is antithyroid drugs, with or without perchlorate, for the IIH and corticosteroids for thyroid inflammation. In patients resistant to drugs, thyroidectomy may be necessary, but euthyroidism must be achieved with antithyroid drugs during the perioperative period, or thyroid storm may ensue.

Correction of the hyperthyroidism is the best treatment for the cardiac manifestations of IIH. It has been shown that angina will resolve in approximately 50% of those who develop it. Atrial fibrillation spontaneously reverts to sinus rhythm in approximately 60% of patients within 6 months of becoming euthyroid. β-Adrenergic blocking agents, such as propranolol, are effective in controlling the ventricular rate in either atrial fibrillation or sinus rhythm and are the drugs of choice for treatment of this problem. Atrial thromboembolism has ranged from 8% to as high as 40% in patients with thyrotoxicosis and atrial fibrillation. The risk warrants the strong consideration of anticoagulant therapy until euthyroidism is restored, because the majority of these emboli are cerebrovascular.[116]

IODINE EXCESS AND CHRONIC AUTOIMMUNE THYROID DISEASE

It is recognized that excessive dietary iodine may increase the risk of thyroiditis, hyperthyroidism, hypothyroidism, and goiter.[117] In healthy adults, short-term iodine intakes of 500 to 1500 μg/day have mild inhibitory effects on thyroid function. According to experimental conditions, excessive iodine intake can precipitate spontaneous thyroiditis in genetically predisposed beagles, rats, or chickens.[118] The mechanism involved in iodine-induced thyroiditis in animal models could be that elevated dietary iodine triggers thyroid autoimmune reactivity by increasing the antigenicity of more highly iodinated forms of TG or by inducing damage of the thyroid and cell injury by free radicals.[102] However, it was shown that the frequency of thyroid autoantibodies and hypothyroidism was higher in iodine-replete populations than in iodine-deficient populations. Pearce et al.[119] found that during prolonged excess iodine exposure there were marked increases in serum total iodine concentrations, the prevalence of goiter, elevated serum TSH values, and elevated serum thyroid peroxidase antibody values increased. The occurrence of all abnormalities decreased after removal of excess iodine from the drinking water system.

In a study conducted in China, the researchers examined the effect of regional differences in iodine intake on the incidence of thyroid disease in 3018 subjects during a 5-year follow-up study. They came from three regions with different levels of iodine intake (median urinary iodine 84, 243, and 651 μg/L, respectively). It has been found that the cumulative incidence of subclinical hypothyroidism and autoimmune thyroiditis was higher in subjects with median urinary iodine concentration more than 243 μg/L.[120] Subjects who were TPOAb and TGAb positive at baseline developed thyroid autoimmunity more frequently than seronegative individuals. High iodine intake was a risk factor for developing hypothyroidism in antibody-positive subjects. They conclude that a constant exposure to excessive iodine intake increased the incidence of hypothyroidism and positive TgAb.[121] Studies conducted in Greece before and after introduction of iodized salt in iodine-deficient mountainous areas confirmed a higher prevalence of Hashimoto's thyroiditis (by fine-needle aspiration smears) from 5.9% at baseline to 13.9% after 8 years of iodine sufficiency.[118] In Sao Paulo (Brazil) after 5 years of excessive iodine intake (iodine concentration in salt: 40 to 100 ppm), the urinary iodine excretion was greater than 300 μg/L in 45.6% of the population. The prevalence of chronic autoimmune thyroiditis increased to 16.9% of the included subjects and was higher (21.5%) in women.[122]

In contrast with these observations, thyroid antibodies did not appear in 43 goitrous patients living in areas of chronic iodine deficiency followed up during 60 months after an injection of iodized oil.[123] Similarly, the daily administration of iodine during pregnancy to 38 women living in an iodine-deficient area was not followed by the occurrence of thyroid autoantibodies from 2 to 21 days after delivery.[124] Laurberg et al.,[125] studying the importance of the population iodine intake level for the prevalence rate of various thyroid abnormalities in elderly subjects, compared random samples of subjects from Jutland, Denmark, with low iodine intake (median urinary iodine of 38 μg/L) and from Iceland, with longstanding relatively high iodine intake (median urinary iodine of 150 μg/L). These authors reported that the frequency of thyroid autoantibodies were in general more common in Jutland. The population with the highest prevalence of autoantibodies had a high occurrence of goiter and thyroid hyperfunction. Similarly, Aghini-Lombardi et al.[126] reported that in a community of Southern Italy with mild iodine deficiency (median urinary iodide of 55 μg/L), the detection of low titers of autoantibodies was relatively frequent (12.6%) but that only 3.5% also had the thyroid echographic pattern of diffuse hypoechogenicity consistent with diffuse autoimmune thyroiditis, a prevalence that is no different from that observed in iodine-sufficient areas. Overall, the prevalence of thyroid antibodies in children in relation to iodine intake is not well established, although an equal prevalence of TPO antibodies in iodine-replete and moderately iodine-deficient patients was demonstrated.[127] At variance with this last data, Weetman[128] suggests that the effect of dietary iodine on thyroid autoimmunity seems at best modest.

IODINE AND THYROID CANCER

Enhanced secretion of TSH has been linked with increased risk of thyroid carcinoma, especially in subjects living in iodine-deficient areas. There is a tendency for higher incidence rates of thyroid cancers detected at autopsy from endemic goiter areas, although the relationship of thyroid cancer and endemic goiter has been debated without agreement being reached on many aspects, including causal relationship.[76]

The proposed mechanisms implicating growth factors associating low iodine intake to thyroid carcinogenesis can be summarized as follows:

- Increased TSH stimulation: low T_4 synthesis associated to higher TSH secretion will promote follicular cell proliferation.
- Thyroid cell responsiveness to TSH is increased in iodine-deficient thyroid cells (increased Ca^{++} and cAMP pathways).

- Increased thyroid-cell EGF-induced proliferation: decreased intracellular organified iodine intermediate (iodolactone or 2-iodohexadecanal) will result in EGF-induced cell proliferation.
- Decreased TGF-β production: thyroid cell proliferation is inhibited by TGF-β. Iodine deficiency will result in a decrease of negative growth regulation.
- Increased angiogenesis may promote tumor growth.

Iodine supplementation is accompanied by a change in the epidemiologic pattern of thyroid cancer, with an increased prevalence of occult papillary cancer discovered at autopsy.[76] For example, follicular carcinoma is the predominant histologic variety in Africa, which has prevailed over the decades owing to persisting iodine deficiency. On the other hand, reports suggest a relative rise in papillary tumors, implying in improved iodination.[129] Accordingly, the prognosis has significantly improved because of a shift towards differentiated forms of thyroid cancer that are diagnosed at earlier stages.[130] Moreover, careful monitoring of the incidence of thyroid cancer in Switzerland following iodine supplementation showed that this incidence continuously decreased.[131] Slowinska-Klencka et al.[132] compared the cytologic diagnoses in 3572 patients to the results of postoperative histopathologic examinations in Poland between 1985 and 1990, when iodine deficiency was progressively corrected. The frequency of neoplastic lesions significantly decreased throughout the examined period, and the ratio of papillary/follicular carcinoma increased, as did the occurrence of cytologically diagnosed chronic thyroiditis. Overall, it appears that the correction in iodine supply reduces the risk of and morbidity from thyroid cancer. It can probably be set forth that correction of iodine deficiency far exceeds its risks.[133]

Overall, the literature data indicate that:
- Nutritional iodine intake and incidence of cancer remains a controversial issue.
- There is weak evidence that low iodine intake would increase the temporal incidence of thyroid malignancy in a given population.
- High iodine intake, however, is also associated with an increased incidence of thyroid cancer (other environmental factors may be present).

With regard to iodine prophylaxis and variations in thyroid cancer incidence, the data indicate[76] that:
- After iodine prophylaxis, a clear relationship has been demonstrated between increased iodine nutrition and elevation of the PTC/FTC ratio.
- This has occurred even in modest increases in iodine urinary excretion.
- A decrease in prevalence of anaplastic thyroid cancer was also observed in most areas.

In conclusion, available evidence from animal experiments, epidemiologic studies, and from the introduction of iodine prophylaxis has demonstrated a relationship between iodine intake and the types of thyroid carcinoma, while no clear evidence exists for a relationship between the overall cancer incidence and iodine intake. All the studies are in general hampered by difficulty in comparing populations, since many factors have to be considered other than iodine intake, such as ethnicity, other dietary factors (e.g., selenium), histologic examination, and radiation. Knowledge of all these factors has an influence also on the diagnostic work-up and management of patients in each population.

REFERENCES

1. WHO, ICCIDD, UNICEF: Assessment of the iodine deficiency disorders and monitoring their elimination, 3rd edition, Geneva, 2007, WHO.
2. DeLange F, Hetzel B: The iodine deficiency disorders. In DeGroot LE, Hannemann G, editors: The thyroid and its diseases. Available at: http://www.thyroidmanager.org/ (accessed on August, 2008).
3. Morreale de Escobar G, Obregon MJ, Escobar del Rey F: Role of thyroid hormone during early brain development, Eur J Endocrinol 151(Suppl 3):U25–37, 2004.
4. Bernal J: Thyroid hormones and brain development, Vitam Horm 71:95–122, 2005.
5. Zimmermann MB, Jooste PL, Pandav CS: Iodine-deficiency disorders, Lancet 372:1251–1262, 2008.
6. WHO Secretariat, Andersson M, de Benoist B, et al: Prevention and control of iodine deficiency in pregnant and lactating women and in children less than 2 years old: conclusions and recommendations of the Technical Consultation, Public Health Nutr 10:1606–1611, 2007.
7. Dunn JT, Crutschfield HE, Gutekunst R, et al: Two simple methods for measuring iodine in urine, Thyroid 3:119–123, 1993.
8. Delange F: Iodine requirements during pregnancy, lactation and the neonatal period and indicators of optimal iodine nutrition, Public Health Nutr 10:1571–1580, 2007.
9. Zimmermann MB: Iodine requirements and the risks and benefits of correcting iodine deficiency in populations, J Trace Elem Med Biol 22:81–92, 2008.
10. Hollowell JG, Staehling NW, Hannon WH, et al: Iodine nutrition in the United States: trends and public health implications. Iodine excretion data from National Health and Nutrition Examination Surveys I and III (1971–1974 and 1988–1994), J Clin Endocrinol Metab 83:3401–3408, 1998.
11. Haddow JE, McClain MR, Palomaki GE, et al: Urine iodine measurements, creatinine adjustment and thyroid deficiency in an adult USA population, J Clin Endocr Metab 92:1019–1022, 2007.
12. Abalovich M, Amino N, Barbour LA, et al: Management of thyroid dysfunction during pregnancy and postpartum: an Endocrine Society Clinical Practice Guideline, J Clin Endocrinol Metab 92(Suppl 8):S1–47, 2007.
13. Muller AF, Drexhage HA, Berghout A: Postpartum thyroiditis and autoimmune thyroiditis in women of child-bearing age: recent insights and consequences for antenatal and postnatal care, Endocr Rev 22:605–630, 2001.
14. Othman S, Phillips DI, Lazarus JH, et al: Iodine metabolism in postpartum thyroiditis, Thyroid 2:107–111, 1992.
15. Kampe O, Jansson R, Karlsson FA: Effects of L-thyroxine and iodide on the development of autoimmune postpartum thyroiditis, J Clin Endocrinol Metab 70:1014–1018, 1990.
16. Nøhr SB, Jorgensen A, Pedersen KM, et al: Postpartum thyroid dysfunction in pregnant thyroid peroxidase antibody-positive women living in an area with mild to moderate iodine deficiency: is iodine supplementation safe? J Clin Endocrinol Metab 85:3191–3198, 2000.
17. Laurberg P, Nohr SB, Pedersen KM, et al: Thyroid disorders in mild iodine deficiency, Thyroid 10:951–963, 2000.
18. Stilwell G, Reynolds PJ, Paramesvaran V, et al: The influence of gestational stage on urinary iodine excretion in pregnancy, J Clin Endocr Metab 93:1737–1742, 2008.
19. Moleti M, Lo Presti VP, Campolo MC, et al: Iodine prophylaxis using iodized salt and risk of maternal thyroid failure in conditions of mild iodine deficiency, J Clin Endocrinol Metab 93:2616–2621, 2008.
20. Delange F: Iodine deficiency in Europe and its consequences: an update, Eur J Nucl Med 29(Suppl 2):S404–S416, 2002.
21. Andersson M, de Benoist B, Darnton-Hill I, et al: Iodine deficiency in Europe: a continuing public health problem, Geneva, 2007, World Health Organization.
22. de Benoist B, McLean E, Andersson M: Iodine deficiency in 2007: global progress since 2003, Food Nutr Bull 29:195–202, 2008.
23. Hess SY, Zimmermann MB, Torresani T, et al: Monitoring the adequacy of salt iodization in Switzerland: a national study of schoolchildren and pregnant women, Eur J Clin Nutr 55:162–166, 2001.
24. Rossi AC, Tomimori E, Camargo R, et al: Searching for iodine deficiency disorders in schoolchildren from Brazil: the ThyroMobil project, Thyroid 11:661–663, 2001.
25. Pretell EA, Delange F, Hostalek U, et al: Iodine nutrition improves in Latin America, Thyroid 14:590–599, 2004.
26. Subraman P: Goiter and iodine deficiency disorders control through universal iodination of salt in India, IDD Newsletter 3:12–16, 1997.
27. Ategbo E, Sankar R, Schultink W: Pushing in the right direction: steady progress in control of IDD in India, IDD Newsletter 21:1–4, 2005.
28. Teng XC, Hu FN, Teng WP, et al: The study of thyroid diseases in a community not using iodized salt, Chin J Prev Medicine 136:176–179, 2002.
29. Chen ZP: New cretins discovered in Southern Xinjiang, China, IDD Newsletter 23:18, 2007.
30. Zhao J, van der Haar F: Progress in salt iodization and improved iodine nutrition in China, 1995–99, Food Nutr Bull 25:337–343, 2004.
31. Delange F, Bürgi H, Chen ZP, et al: World status of monitoring of iodine deficiency disorders control programs, Thyroid 12:915–924, 2002.
32. Okosieme OE: Impact of iodination on thyroid pathology in Africa, J R Soc Med 99:396–401, 2006.
33. UNICEF: The state of world children 2007. www.unicef.org/nutrition/files/SOWC06_Table 2.pdf (accessed on August, 2008).

34. Aguayo VM, Scott S, Ross J, et al: Sierra Leone: investing in nutrition to reduce poverty: a call for action, Public Health Nutr 6:653–657, 2003.
35. Abuye C, Berhane Y: The goiter rate, its association with reproductive failure, and the knowledge of iodine deficiency disorders (IDD) among women in Ethiopia: cross-section community based study, BMC Public Health 7:316, 2007.
36. Egbuta J, Onyezili F, Vanormelingen K: Impact evaluation of efforts to eliminate iodine deficiency disorders in Nigeria, Public Health Nutr 6:169–173, 2003.
37. Jooste PL, Weight MJ, Lombard CJ: Iodine concentration in household salt in South Africa, Bull World Health Organ 79:534–540, 2001.
38. WHO: WHO global database on iodine deficiency. http://www.who.int/whosis/database (acessed on July, 2008).
39. de Benoist B, Anderson M, Takkouche B, et al: Prevalence of iodine deficiency worldwide, Lancet 362:1859–1860, 2003.
40. WHO, UNICEF, ICCIDD: Indicators for assessing Iodine Deficiency Disorders and their control through salt iodization, Geneva: 1994, WHO publ, WHO/NUT/94.6:1–55.
41. WHO, UNICEF, ICCIDD: Assessment of the Iodine Deficiency Disorders and monitoring their elimination, Geneva: 2001, WHO publ, WHO/NHD/01.1:1–107.
42. Gaitan E, Cooksey RC, Legan J, et al: Antithyroid and goitrogenic effects of coal-water extracts from iodine-sufficient goiter areas, Thyroid 3:49–53, 1993.
43. Ngudi DD, Kuo YH, Lambein F: Cassava cyanogens and free amino acids in raw and cooked leaves, Food Chem Toxicol 41:1193–1197, 2003.
44. Vanderpas J: Nutritional epidemiology and thyroid hormone metabolism, Annu Rev Nutr 26:293–322, 2006.
45. Gaitan E, Cooksey RC, Legan J, et al: Antithyroid effects in vivo and in vitro of babassu and mandioca: a staple food in goiter areas of Brazil, Eur J Endocrinol 131:138–144, 1994.
46. Schröder-van der Elst JP, Smit JW, Romijn HA, et al: Dietary flavonoids and iodine metabolism, Biofactors 19:171–176, 2003.
47. Doerge DR, Chang HC: Inactivation of thyroid peroxidase by soy isoflavones, in vitro and in vivo, J Chromatogr B Analyt Technol Biomed Life Sci 777:269–279, 2002.
48. Bell DS, Ovalle F: Use of soy protein supplement and resultant need for increased dose of levothyroxine, Endocr Pract 7:193–194, 2001.
49. Suzuki H, Higuchi T, Sawa K, et al: Endemic coast goiter in Hokkaido, Japan, Acta Endocrinol 50:161–176, 1965.
50. Zimmermann MB, Jooste PL, Mabapa NS, et al: Vitamin A supplementation in iodine-deficient African children decreases thyrotropin stimulation of the thyroid and reduces the goiter rate, Am J Clin Nutr 86:1040–1044, 2007.
51. Ingenbleek Y: Vitamin A deficiency impairs the normal mannosylation, conformation and iodination of the thyroglobulin: a new etiological approach to endemic goiter, Experientia Suppl 44:264–297, 1983.
52. Knobel M, Umezawa ES, Cardia MS, et al: Elevated anti-galactosyl antibody titers in endemic goiter, Thyroid 9:493–498, 1999.
53. Zimmermann MB: The influence of iron status on iodine utilization and thyroid function, Annu Rev Nutr 26:367–389, 2006.
54. Brauer VF, Schweizer U, Köhrle J, et al: Selenium and goiter prevalence in borderline iodine sufficiency, Eur J Endocrinol 155:807–812, 2006.
55. Kralik A, Eder K, Kirchgessner M: Influence of zinc and selenium deficiency on parameters relating to thyroid hormone metabolism, Horm Metab Res 28:223–226, 1996.
56. Ruz M, Codoceo J, Galgani J, et al: Single and multiple selenium-zinc-iodine deficiencies affect rat thyroid metabolism and ultrastructure, J Nutr 129:174–180, 1999.
57. Wada L, King JC: Effect of low zinc intakes on basal metabolic rate, thyroid hormones and protein utilization in adult men, J Nutr 116:1045–1053, 1986.
58. Brucker-Davis F: Environmental disrupters of thyroid hormone action. In Henry HL, Norman AN, editors: Encyclopedia of Hormones, New York, 2003, Elsevier-Academic Press, pp 535–537.
59. Lindsay RH, Hill JB, Gaitan E, et al: Antithyroid effects of coal-derived pollutants, J Toxicol Environ Health 37:467–481, 1992.
60. Braverman LE: Clinical studies of exposure to perchlorate in the United States, Thyroid 17:819–822, 2007.
61. Laurberg P, Nøhr SB, Pedersen KM, et al: Iodine nutrition in breast-fed infants is impaired by maternal smoking, J Clin Endocrinol Metab 89:181–187, 2004.
62. Crofton KM: Thyroid disrupting chemicals: mechanisms and mixtures, Int J Androl 31:209–223, 2008.
63. Delange F: The disorders induced by iodine deficiency, Thyroid 4:107–128, 1994.
64. Knobel M, Bisi H, Peres CA, et al: Correlated functional and morphological aspects in human multinodular simple goiter tissues, Endocr Pathol 4:205–214, 1993.
65. Sugawara M, Kita T, Lee ED, et al: Deficiency of superoxide dismutase in endemic goiter tissue, J Clin Endocrinol Metab 67:1156–1161, 1988.
66. Dumont JE, Ermans AM, Maenhaut C, et al: Large goiter as a maladaptation to iodine deficiency, Clin Endocrinol (Oxf) 43:1–10, 1995.
67. Stübner D, Gärtner R, Greil W, et al: Hypertrophy and hyperplasia during goiter growth and involution in rats: separate bioeffects of TSH and iodine, Acta Endocrinol (Copenh) 116:537–548, 1987.
68. Obregon MJ, Escobar del Rey F, Morreale de Escobar G: The effects of iodine deficiency on thyroid hormone deiodination, Thyroid 15:917–929, 2005.
69. Berbel P, Obregón MJ, Bernal J, et al: Iodine supplementation during pregnancy: a public health challenge, Trends Endocrinol Metab 18:338–343, 2007.
70. Morreale de Escobar G, Obregon MJ, Escobar del Rey F: Is neuropsychological development related to maternal hypothyroidism or to maternal hypothyroxinemia? J Clin Endocrinol Metab 85:3975–3987, 2000.
71. Dumont JE, Ermans AM, Maenhaut C, et al: Large goiter as a maladaptation to iodine deficiency, Clin Endocrinol (Oxf) 43:1–10, 1995.
72. Xia Y, Hill KE, Byrne DW, et al: Effectiveness of selenium supplements in a low-selenium area of China, Am J Clin Nutr 81:829–834, 2005.
73. Chanoine JP: Selenium and thyroid function in infants, children and adolescents, Biofactors 19:137–143, 2003.
74. Schmutzler C, Mentrup B, Schomburg L, et al: Selenoproteins of the thyroid gland: expression, localization and possible function of glutathione peroxidase 3, Biol Chem 388:1053–1059, 2007.
75. Lima N, Medeiros-Neto GA: Transient thyrotoxicosis in endemic goiter patients following exposure to a normal iodine intake, Clin Endocrinol (Oxf) 21:631–637, 1984.
76. Knobel M, Medeiros-Neto G: Relevance of iodine intake as a reputed predisposing factor for thyroid cancer, Arq Bras Endocrinol Metabol 51:701–712, 2007.
77. Knudsen N, Bulow I, Jorgensen T, et al: Serum Tg: a sensitive marker of thyroid abnormalities and iodine deficiency in epidemiological studies, J Clin Endocrinol Metab 86:3599–3603, 2001.
78. van den Briel T, West CE, Hautvast JG, et al: Serum thyroglobulin and urinary iodine concentration are the most appropriate indicators of iodine status and thyroid function under conditions of increasing iodine supply in school children in Benin, J Nutr 131:2701–2706, 2001.
79. Zimmermann MB, de Benoist B, Corigliano S, et al: Assessment of iodine status using dried blood spot thyroglobulin: development of reference material and establishment of an international reference range in iodine-sufficient children, J Clin Endocrinol Metab 91: 4881–4887, 2006.
80. Als C, Helbling A, Peter K, et al: Urinary iodine concentration follows a circadian rhythm: a study with 3023 spot urine samples in adults and children, J Clin Endocrinol Metab 85:1367–1369, 2000.
81. Laurberg P, Andersen S, Bjarnadóttir RI, et al: Evaluating iodine deficiency in pregnant women and young infants—complex physiology with a risk of misinterpretation, Public Health Nutr 10:1547–1552, 2007.
82. Baloch Z, Carayon P, Conte-Devolx B, et al: Guidelines Committee, National Academy of Clinical Biochemistry: Laboratory medicine practice guidelines. Laboratory support for the diagnosis and monitoring of thyroid disease, Thyroid 13:3–126, 2003.
83. Zimmermann MB, Hess SY, Molinari L, et al: New reference values for thyroid volume by ultrasound in iodine-sufficient schoolchildren: a World Health Organization/Nutrition for Health and Development Iodine Deficiency Study Group report, Am J Clin Nutr 79:231–237, 2004.
84. Zimmermann M, Saad A, Hess S, et al: Thyroid ultrasound compared with World Health Organization 1960 and 1994 palpation criteria for determination of goiter prevalence in regions of mild and severe iodine deficiency, Eur J Endocrinol 143: 727–731, 2000.
85. Brenta G, Schnitman M, Fretes O, et al: Comparative efficacy and side effects of the treatment of euthyroid goiter with levo-thyroxine or triiodothyroacetic acid, J Clin Endocrinol Metab 88:5287–5292, 2003.
86. Weetman AP: Radioiodine treatment for benign thyroid diseases, Clin Endocrinol (Oxf) 66:757–764, 2007.
87. Medeiros-Neto G, Marui S, Knobel M: An outline concerning the potential use of recombinant human thyrotropin for improving radioiodine therapy of multinodular goiter, Endocrine 33:109–117, 2008.
88. Carella C, Mazziotti G, Rotondi M, et al: Iodized salt improves the effectiveness of L-thyroxine therapy after surgery for nontoxic goiter: a prospective and randomized study, Clin Endocrinol (Oxf) 57:507–513, 2002.
89. Köhrle J, Jakob F, Contempré B, et al: Selenium, the thyroid, and the endocrine system, Endocr Rev 26:944–984, 2005.
90. Contempre B, de Escobar GM, Denef JF, et al: Thiocyanate induces cell necrosis and fibrosis in selenium- and iodine-deficient rat thyroids: a potential experimental model for myxedematous endemic cretinism in central Africa, Endocrinology 145:994–1002, 2004.
91. Li S, Wei H, Zheng Q: Elimination of iodine-deficiency disorders in Tibet, Lancet 371:1980–1981, 2008.
92. Contempre B, Dumont J, Bebe N, et al: Effect of selenium supplementation in hypothyroid subjects of an iodine and selenium deficient area: the possible danger of indiscriminate supplementation of iodine-deficient subjects with selenium, J Clin Endocrinol Metab 73:213–215, 1991.
93. Boyages SC, Halpern JP: Endemic cretinism: toward a unifying hypothesis. Thyroid 3:59–71, 1993.
94. Halpern JP: Studies of hearing abnormality in endemic cretinism in Qinghai Province, PRC. In Stanbury JB, editor: The Damaged Brain of Iodine Deficiency: Cognitive Behavioral, Neuromotor and Educative Aspects, New York, 1994, Cognizant Communication, pp 273–277.
95. Geelhoed GW: Metabolic maladaptation: individual and social consequences of medical intervention in correcting endemic hypothyroidism, Nutrition 15:908–932, 1999.
96. Teles FF: Chronic poisoning by hydrogen cyanide in cassava and its prevention in Africa and Latin America, Food Nutr Bull 23:407–412, 2002.
97. de Escobar GM, Obregón MJ, del Rey FE: Iodine deficiency and brain development in the first half of pregnancy, Public Health Nutr 10:1554–1570, 2007.
98. Pedraza PE, Obregon MJ, Escobar-Morreale HF, et al: Mechanisms of adaptation to iodine deficiency in rats: thyroid status is tissue specific. Its relevance for man, Endocrinology 147(5):2098–2108, 2006.
99. Kilby MD: Thyroid hormones and fetal brain development, Clin Endocrinol (Oxf) 59:280–281, 2003.
100. Bernal J, Guadano-Ferraz A, Morte B: Perspectives in the study of thyroid hormone action on brain development and function, Thyroid 13:1005–1012, 2003.
101. Dunn JT: Iodine should be routinely added to complementary foods, J Nutr 133:3008S–3010S, 2003.
102. Delange F, Lecomte P: Iodine supplementation: benefits outweigh risks, Drug Safety 22:89–95, 2000.
103. Knobel M, Medeiros-Neto G: Pediatric Aspects of Thyroid Function and Iodine. In Krassas GE, Rivkees SA, Kiess W, editors: Diseases of the Thyroid in Childhood and Adolescence. Pediatr Adolesc Med, vol 11, Basel, 2007, Karger, pp 56–79.
104. Lauberg P, Bullow Pedersen I, Knudsen N, et al: Environmental iodine intake affects the type of nonmalignant thyroid disease, Thyroid 11:457–469, 2001.
105. Rasmussen LB, Ovesen L, Christensen T, et al: Iodine content in bread and salt in Denmark after iodization and the influence on iodine intake, Int J Food Sci Nutr 58:231–239, 2007.

106. Seal JA, Doyle Z, Burgess JR, et al: Iodine status of Tasmanians following voluntary fortification of bread with iodine, Med J Aust 186(2):69–71, 2007.
107. Delange F, de Benoist B, Alnwick D: Risks of iodine-induced hyperthyroidism after correction of iodine deficiency by iodized salt, Thyroid 9:545–556, 1999.
108. Corvilain B, van Sande J, Dumont JE, et al: Autonomy in endemic goiter, Thyroid 8:107–113, 1998.
109. Gołkowski F, Buziak-Bereza M, Trofimiuk M, et al: Increased prevalence of hyperthyroidism as an early and transient side-effect of implementing iodine prophylaxis, Public Health Nutr 10:799–802, 2007.
110. Okosieme OE: Impact of iodination on thyroid pathology in Africa, J R Soc Med 99:396–401, 2006.
111. Bourdoux P, Ermans AM, Mukalay A, et al: Iodine-induced thyrotoxicosis in Kivu, Zaire, Lancet 347:552–553, 1996.
112. Todd CH, Allain T, Gomo ZA, et al: Increase in thyrotoxicosis associated with iodine supplements in Zimbabwe, Lancet 346:1563–1565, 1995.
113. Yang F, Shan Z, Teng X, et al: Chronic iodine excess does not increase the incidence of hyperthyroidism: a prospective study community base epidemiological survey in China, Eur J Endocrinol 156:403–408, 2007.
114. Corvilain B, van Sande J, Dumont JE, et al: Autonomy in endemic goiter, Thyroid 8:107–113, 1998.
115. Martins MC, Lima N, Knobel M, et al: Natural course of iodine-induced thyrotoxicosis (Jod-Basedow) in endemic goiter area: a 5-year follow-up, J Endocrinol Invest 12:239–244, 1989.
116. Dunn JT, Semigran MJ, Delange F: The prevention and management of iodine-induced hyperthyroidism and its cardiac features, Thyroid 8;101–106, 1998.
117. Zimmermann MB, Ito Y, Hess SY, et al: High thyroid volume in children with excess dietary iodine intakes, Am J Clin Nutr 81:840–844, 2005.
118. Papanastasiou L, Vatalas IA, Koutras DA, et al: Thyroid autoimmunity in the current iodine environment, Thyroid 17:729–739, 2007.
119. Pearce EN, Gerber AR, Gootnick DB, et al: Effects of chronic iodine excess in a cohort of long-term American workers in West Africa, J Clin Endocrinol Metab 87:5499–5502, 2002.
120. Teng W, Shan Z, Teng X, et al: Effect of iodine intake on thyroid diseases in China, N Engl J Med 354:2783–2793, 2006.
121. Li Y, Teng D, Shan Z, et al: Anti-thyroperoxidase and anti-thyroglobulin antibodies in a 5-year follow-up survey of populations with different iodine intakes, J Clin Endocr Metab 93:1751–1757, 2008.
122. Camargo RYA, Tomimori E, Neves SC, et al: Thyroid and environment: exposure to excessive nutritional iodine increases the prevalence of thyroid disorders in Sao Paulo, Brazil, Eur J Endocr 159:293–299, 2008.
123. Knobel M, Medeiros-Neto G: Iodized oil treatment for endemic goiter does not induce the surge of positive serum concentrations of antithyroglobulin or antimicrosomal autoantibodies, J Endocrinol Invest 9:321–324, 1986.
124. Liesenkötter KP, Göpel W, Bogner U, et al: Earliest prevention of endemic goiter by iodine supplementation during pregnancy, Eur J Endocrinol 134:443–448, 1996.
125. Laurberg P, Pedersen KM, Hreidarsson A, et al: Iodine intake and the pattern of thyroid disorders: a comparative epidemiological study of thyroid abnormalities in the elderly in Iceland and in Jutland, Denmark, J Clin Endocrinol Metab 83:765–769, 1998.
126. Aghini-Lombardi F, Antonangeli L, Martino E, et al: The spectrum of thyroid disorders in an iodine-deficient community: the Pescopagano survey, J Clin Endocrinol Metab 84:561–566, 1999.
127. Kabelitz M, Liesenkötter KP, Stach B, et al: The prevalence of anti-thyroid peroxidase antibodies and autoimmune thyroiditis in children and adolescents in an iodine replete area, Eur J Endocrinol 148:301–307, 2003.
128. Weetman AP: The thyroid and autoimmunity in children and adolescence. In Krassas GE, Rivkees SA, Kiess W, editors: Diseases of the Thyroid in Childhood and Adolescence, vol 11, Basel, 2007, Karger, pp 104–117.
129. Okosieme OE: Impact of iodination on thyroid pathology in Africa, J R Soc Med 99:396–401, 2006.
130. Bacher-Stier C, Riccabona G, Totsch M, et al: Incidence and clinical characteristics of thyroid carcinoma after iodine prophylaxis in an endemic goiter country, Thyroid 7:733–741, 1997.
131. Franceschi S: Iodine intake and thyroid carcinoma: a potential risk factor, Exp Clin Endocrinol Diabetes 106(Suppl 3):S38–S44, 1998.
132. Slowinska-Klencka D, Klencki M, Sporny S, et al: Fine-needle aspiration biopsy of the thyroid in an area of endemic goiter: influence of restored sufficient iodine supplementation on the clinical significance of cytological results, Eur J Endocrinol 146:19–26, 2002.
133. Braverman LE: Adequate iodine intake: the good far outweighs the bad, Eur J Endocrinol 139:14–15, 1998.
134. Benmiloud M, Chaouki ML, Gutekunst R, et al: Oral iodized oil for correcting iodine deficiency: optimal dosing and outcome indicator selection, J Clin Endocrinol Metab 79:20–24, 1994.
135. Untoro J, Schultink W, West CE, et al: Efficacy of oral iodized peanut oil is greater than that of iodized poppy seed oil among Indonesian schoolchildren, Am J Clin Nutr 84:1208–1214, 2006.
136. Zimmermann MB, Connolly K, Bozo M, et al: Iodine supplementation improves cognition in iodine-deficient schoolchildren in Albania: a randomized, controlled, double-blind study, Am J Clin Nutr 83:108–114, 2006.
137. Wolff J: Physiology and pharmacology of iodized oil in goiter prophylaxis, Medicine 80:20–36, 2001.
138. Tonglet R, Bourdoux P, Minga T, et al: Efficacy of low oral doses of iodized oil in the control of iodine deficiency in Zaire, N Engl J Med 326:236–241, 1992.
139. Zimmermann M, Adou P, Torresani T, et al: Low-dose oral iodized oil for control of iodine deficiency in children, Br J Nutr 84:139–141, 2000.

Chapter 18

THYROID NEOPLASIA

FURIO PACINI, STEFANIA MARCHISOTTA, and LESLIE J. DE GROOT

Thyroid cancer is statistically a minor health problem that accounts for less than 1% of all human malignancies and for 0.4% of all cancer deaths and kills only 8 in 1 million people per year in the United States. Its clinical importance, however, is much greater, because up to 4% of the population harbor clinically detectable thyroid nodules that must raise the possible diagnosis of thyroid cancer. Even higher is the prevalence of small thyroid nodules discovered incidentally at neck ultrasound performed for other diseases. This discussion evaluates the problem of the thyroid nodule and, subsequently, the management of diagnosed thyroid cancer.

Thyroid Nodules

INCIDENCE AND PREVALENCE OF NODULES

Thyroid nodules are the most common endocrine lesions, particularly in countries where dietary iodine intake is low. The main problem posed by the discovery of a thyroid nodule is the distinction between its benign or malignant nature and, consequently, its appropriate treatment.

In the past 20 years, the problem has been solved largely by the introduction into clinical practice of fine-needle aspiration cytology (FNAC), which has allowed diagnosis of the nature of thyroid nodules with great sensitivity and specificity. FNAC has resulted in a significant reduction in the number of nodules sent to the surgeon and, if surgery is needed, in better planning of the surgery to be performed.

In countries where iodine deficiency has been corrected by iodine prophylaxis, palpable thyroid nodules are present in about 4% to 5% of the general population.[1-8] Early data on prevalence came from the population sampled in Framingham, Massachusetts,[1] where 4% were found to have a palpable thyroid nodule (or nodules). Half the lesions were considered multinodular, and half were solitary. New nodules appeared, with an incidence of 1 per 1000 per year.[2] A study from Connecticut indicated a prevalence of only 2% of clinically nodular glands in an adult population.[6] Of all thyroid glands that on surgical resection prove to contain solitary nodules, 70% to 80% prove to be benign adenomas, and about 10% to 30% are malignant growths.[3,4]

In autopsy series, the incidence of thyroid nodules in apparently normal thyroid glands is also very high. In a report from the Mayo Clinic[5] on 1000 consecutive autopsies in individuals with clinically normal thyroid glands, an age-related increase in thyroid weight and nodularity was noted. Fifty percent had one or more nodules, and 12% had a solitary nodule. The prevalence of thyroid carcinoma was 2.1%. If we also consider nonpalpable nodules, which are discovered more and more commonly during ultrasound exploration for nonthyroidal diseases (e.g., carotid exploration, hypercalcemia, cervical adenopathies [Table 18-1]), the prevalence of thyroid nodules can be as high as 20% to 30% in unselected populations and even higher in older age groups.[6,9-11]

A higher prevalence of thyroid nodules is usually reported in countries affected by moderate or severe iodine deficiency, where diffuse goiter is common and evolves over time to multinodular goiter. The problem of whether thyroid cancer is more common in this environment is still debated. In a prospective study performed by Belfiore and colleagues in an iodine-deficient area of Sicily (Italy), the prevalence of thyroid nodules was higher with

Table 18-1. Prevalence of Nonpalpable Thyroid Nodules Detected on Ultrasound

Series	Purpose of Examination	Prevalence, %
Harlocker et al.	Hyperparathyroidism	46
Stark et al.	Hyperparathyroidism	40
Carroll et al.	Carotid examination	13
Ezzat et al.	Prospective	67
Brander et al.	Prospective	27
Woestyn et al.	Prospective	19
Tomimori et al.	Prospective	17

Data from Tan GH, Gharib H: Thyroid incidentalomas: management approaches to nonpalpable nodules discovered incidentally on thyroid imaging, Ann Intern Med 126:226, 1997.

respect to a control area with sufficient iodine intake.[12] The number of thyroid cancers was not increased when expressed as a percentage of the nodules, but absolute numbers were higher because of the higher prevalence of thyroid nodules.

Most thyroid nodules are benign, particularly in multinodular goiters, although great variation is observed between clinical and surgical series. The incidence of thyroid carcinoma is around 3% to 4% of all thyroid nodules, and its mortality accounts for only 0.4% of all cancer deaths. It is the cancer with the largest increase year by year among all human cancers, particularly papillary microcarcinomas, which probably are due to screening effect at neck ultrasound.[13-16] Although it is difficult to know the real malignant potential of these small tumors, it has been demonstrated that the incidence of malignancy among incidental micronodules is the same as that of clinical thyroid nodules.[12] All findings above justify a conservative therapeutic approach, whenever possible, because surgical treatment of all clinical or incidental thyroid nodules, without any selection, would expose an extraordinary number of people to surgical treatment. Furthermore, given that only a few of them will have thyroid carcinoma, and that many of them, especially if operated on by inexperienced surgeons, will have surgical complications, and that the financial cost will be high, one must realize that surgical treatment of thyroid nodules must be rigorously based on a rational diagnostic protocol.

NATURE AND PATHOLOGY OF NODULES

Thyroid nodules are not a unique disease but are the clinical manifestation of several different thyroid diseases. They may be single or multiple and may be found in the context of a normal gland or a diffuse goiter. In multinodular goiter, one of the nodules may become clinically dominant in terms of growth, dimension, and functional character. A clinical-pathologic classification of thyroid nodules is presented in Table 18-2.

Benign Neoplasia

Most adenomas are follicular and have a histologic appearance characteristic of thyroid tissue. Adenomas usually exhibit a uniform orderly architecture and few mitoses and show no lymphatic or blood vessel invasion. They are characteristically enveloped by a discrete fibrous capsule or a thin zone of compressed surrounding thyroid tissue. Fetal and embryonal adenomas show a progressively reduced "adult" structure. Whether papillary adenoma is a real entity is debatable; most observers believe that all papillary tumors should be considered carcinomas. Others believe that some papillary tumors are benign adenomas. It is our impression that papillary tumors are best thought of as carcinomas, although the degree of invasive potential may be very

Table 18-2. Clinical and Pathologic Classification of Thyroid Nodules

Non-neoplastic nodules
  Hyperplastic
    Spontaneous
    Thyroid hemiagenesis
    Compensatory after partial thyroidectomy
  Inflammatory
    Acute bacterial thyroiditis
    Subacute thyroiditis
    Hashimoto's thyroiditis
Benign neoplasia
  Nonfunctioning
    Adenoma
    Cyst
    Thyroglossal cyst
  Functioning
    Toxic (or pretoxic) adenoma
Malignant neoplasia
  Primary carcinomas
    Papillary
    Follicular
    Anaplastic
    Medullary
  Lymphomas
  Thyroid metastasis from other primaries
Nonthyroidal lesions
  Cystic hygroma
  Aneurysm
  Parathyroid adenoma or cyst

slight in some instances. The same confusion extends to Hürthle cell adenomas. Many pathologists consider all these tumors low-grade carcinomas in view of their common late recurrence. For this reason, the nondefinitive term Hürthle cell tumor is commonly used. Hürthle cell tumors are found on electron microscopy to be packed with mitochondria, which accounts for their special eosinophilic staining quality.

On gross inspection, nearly half of all single nodules have a gelatinous appearance, are composed of large colloid-filled follicles, and are not completely surrounded by a well-defined fibrous capsule. In our classification, these nodules are listed as colloid variants of follicular adenomas. Many pathologists report them as colloid nodules and suggest that each is a focal process perhaps related to multinodular goiter rather than a true adenoma. These tumors are not usually surrounded by a capsule of compressed normal tissue and often show degeneration of parenchyma, hemosiderosis, and colloid phagocytosis. The histologic pattern of various benign tumors of the thyroid is shown in Fig. 18-1.

The first distinction to be made among benign nodules is between functioning ("hot" on thyroid scan) and nonfunctioning ("cold") nodules. Whereas a "hot" nodule is almost synonymous with a benign nodule, a "cold" nodule is not synonymous with a malignant nodule, because only a minority will turn out to be thyroid carcinomas. Cold nodules can be solid or cystic (around 10% to 20% of the total). However, mixed, solid-cystic forms are also common and should be considered solid in terms of frequency of malignancy. As a general rule, thyroid carcinoma is more common among solid, single, cold nodules.

Thyroid adenomas are usually monoclonal "new growths"[17] that are formed in response to the same sort of stimuli that produce carcinomas. Heredity does not appear to play a major role in their appearance. One clue to their origin is that they are four times more common in women than in men, although no definitive relationship of estrogen to cell growth has been

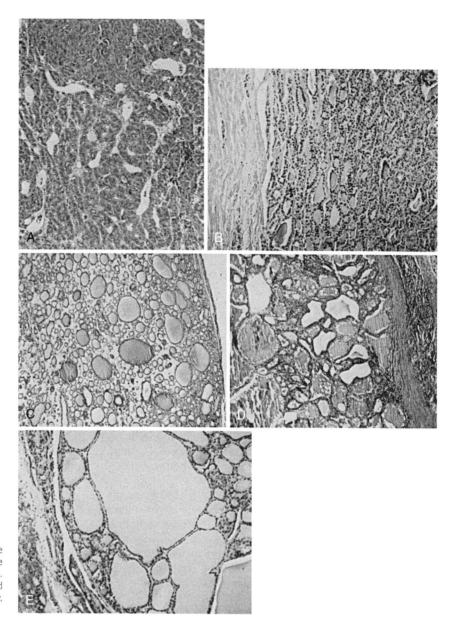

FIGURE 18-1. Histologic pattern of various benign tumors of the thyroid. **A,** Embryonal adenoma. **B,** Fetal adenoma. Note the sharp margin, capsule, and tiny follicles. **C,** Follicular adenoma. **D,** Hyperplastic variant of follicular adenoma. **E,** Colloid-filled variant. (Courtesy Dr. Francis Straus, Department of Pathology, University of Chicago.)

demonstrated. Thyroid radiation, chronic thyroid-stimulating hormone (TSH) stimulation, and oncogenes (see following) are believed to be related to the origin of these lesions; these are discussed in the following section on thyroid cancer.[18] Of specific interest in relation to benign nodules is the observation by Parma and colleagues that activating mutations of the TSH receptor are the specific cause of most hyperfunctioning adenomas[19] and the common involvement of *ras* gene mutations found in follicular adenomas.[19] In view of the frequent discovery of *ras* gene mutation in follicular (and also papillary) thyroid carcinomas, the question is whether a *ras* mutated follicular adenoma should be considered as a pre-neoplastic lesion that should always be treated surgically.

Non-Neoplastic Nodules

These lesions are not true nodules but represent focal areas of glandular hyperplasia that arise spontaneously or, more commonly, as a consequence of previous partial thyroidectomies. Also, thyroid hemiagenesis may rarely be manifested as hyper-plasia of the existing lobe and mimic a thyroid nodule. Nodule(s) associated with Hashimoto's thyroiditis are the expression of lymphocytic infiltration and fibrosis. Nodules seen during the initial phase of subacute thyroiditis are a result of the inflammatory process that gives origin to typical granulomas.

Micronodules

Micronodules are nodules 1 cm or less in diameter. With the routine use of neck ultrasound, the discovery of micronodules is increasing, and nearly 50% of women older than 60 years have such nodularities. One view is that micronodules in general are not clinically relevant and, in the absence of other clinically suspicious findings, do not require investigation or treatment. The usual advice is to repeat thyroid ultrasound at regular intervals and reconsider therapy if growth is seen. However, in light of evidence that the frequency of malignancy is the same in micronodules or macronodules,[12] an alternative view is that the former should be evaluated by FNAC under ultrasound guidance.

COURSE AND SYMPTOMS

Adenomas grow slowly, remain dormant for years, must reach a size of 0.5 to 1 cm before they can be palpated, and are typically asymptomatic. Thus, they often are discovered accidentally by the patient or the physician, and they rarely produce local symptoms.

About 70% of thyroid nodules or adenomas are hypofunctional in terms of accumulation of radioactive iodide and are "cold" on isotope scans. About 20% may be borderline in function and on isotope scan appear to have uptake similar to that of the remainder of the thyroid. One in 10 (or less) is hyperfunctional; these nodules concentrate iodide avidly, may suppress function of the normal gland, and may even produce thyrotoxicosis. This process, which typically occurs when the functioning nodule has grown large enough in diameter, is seen most often in older patients. Activating TSH receptor mutations have been found by Parma and coworkers to be the cause of most hyperfunctional adenomas[19] and are common in "hot" nodules in patients with multinodular goiter.[20,21] These mutations involve the extracellular loops of the transmembrane domain and the transmembrane segments, and in transfection studies, they have been proved to induce constitutive activation of the TSH receptor. Mutations of the stimulatory guanosine triphosphate–binding protein subunit are also present in some patients with hyperfunctioning thyroid adenomas.[22] Hot nodules are almost invariably associated with low or suppressed serum TSH levels. The finding of subnormal serum TSH at the first patient evaluation is the hallmark of hyperfunctioning nodules and is the test of choice that should dictate the need for thyroid scanning. When serum TSH is normal, there is no need to perform routine thyroid scan.

Usually, a benign nodule, once formed, seems to be committed to this "lifestyle" indefinitely. However, pathologic evidence suggests that true follicular adenomas (or Hürthle cell adenomas) can transform into invasive carcinoma. Sequential change from hyperplasia to adenoma formation to invasive carcinoma has been found in patients with congenital goitrous hypothyroidism, and it can be produced experimentally in animals.

Interesting studies have described the metabolic function of nodules. Cold nodules are typically unable to transport iodide into the thyroid as a result of a specific deletion of some element of the transport mechanism.[23] They are not able to maintain a concentration gradient for iodide between the thyroid cell and serum, although peroxidase function in the tissue may be intact.[24,25] In such adenomas, thyrotropin is able to bind to the cell membrane and activate adenyl cyclase, but subsequent metabolic steps are lacking. Other "cold nodules" have been shown to lack peroxidase enzyme.[26] These studies suggest that adenoma formation is associated with genetic mutational events that cause loss or dysfunction of specific enzymes in the iodide metabolic pathway. Recent cloning of the Na^+/I^- symporter (NIS) gene,[27] the gene responsible for iodine uptake by the follicular cell, has confirmed this hypothesis, demonstrating that cold nodules in multinodular goiters and follicular adenomas have reduced NIS messenger RNA (mRNA) and protein expression, thus opening a new field of research for the development of novel therapeutic strategies based on gene manipulation.

CLINICAL EVALUATION AND MANAGEMENT OF NODULES

The aim of clinical evaluation is to detect nodules that should be referred to a surgeon. Among benign lesions, the aim is to

Table 18-3. Clinical Features Suggesting Malignancy of a Thyroid Nodule

History
  External irradiation during childhood
  Familial history of medullary cancer
  Age <20 or >60 yr
  Male sex
Thyroid nodule
  Rapidly growing (especially during L-thyroxine therapy)
  Firm or hard or painful
  Fixed to soft tissue
  Local symptoms
Suspicious finding at thyroid ultrasounds (microcalcifications, hypoechogenicity, irregular margins or no halo, solid intranodule vascularity, more tall than wide)
Other
  Lymphadenopathy
  Dysphagia, hoarseness

differentiate between adenomas (functioning or nonfunctioning), cysts, and nodules in the context of an underlying benign thyroid disease. This differential diagnosis is extremely important decisions regarding the most appropriate therapy. Similarly important in benign lesions is the detection of clinical symptoms or signs (e.g., compression of the trachea or the esophagus, a recurrent nerve deficit) that per se could suggest a need for surgical therapy. The clinical and laboratory features associated with a high risk for cancer are listed in Table 18-3.

Factors that must be considered when a decision on management is reached include history of the lesion; age, sex, and family history of the patient; physical characteristics of the gland; the presence of local symptoms; laboratory evaluation results; and ultrasonographic features.

Personal History

The age of the patient is an important consideration because the ratio of malignant to benign nodules is higher in youth and lower in older age. In a study involving nonirradiated children with cold thyroid nodules, a twofold increased risk for thyroid cancer, regardless of sex,[28] was found when compared with the rate for similar adults.[2] In adult men, nodules are less common, and a greater proportion are malignant.

Rarely, the family history may be helpful in decision making regarding surgery. Patients with the heritable multiple endocrine neoplasia (MEN) syndrome, type 1, may have thyroid adenomas, parathyroid adenomas, islet cell tumors, and adrenal tumors, whereas patients with MEN type 2 may have pheochromocytomas, medullary thyroid carcinomas, hyperparathyroidism, and mucosal neuromas.[29-31] Familial medullary cancer (without MEN) is also possible. Furthermore, we have noted that 6% to 12% of patients with differentiated thyroid carcinoma have one or (less frequently) more family members with a history of malignant (nonmedullary) thyroid neoplasm, most often papillary.[32] Familial papillary thyroid tumors occur in Cowden's disease, Gardner's syndrome, and familial polyposis coli[33] but most of the time are not associated with other manifestations (nonsyndromic). Recently, it has been reported that isolated familial papillary thyroid cancer displays the feature of "genetic anticipation," that is, the tendency for a familial cancer to present at an earlier age and with a more aggressive phenotype in subsequent generations compared with the first generation.[32] As is discussed in the following sections, a history of prior irradiation to the head or neck during infancy or childhood is strongly associated with the subsequent occurrence of carcinoma.[34] A history of such radiation exposure and the presence of a palpable nodule or nodules must raise the possibility of thyroid cancer, which requires a cytologic diagnosis.

The epidemic of childhood papillary thyroid cancer observed in Belarus and Ukraine after the Chernobyl nuclear accident[35] is believed to be the result of contamination from radioactive fallout, mainly iodine isotopes, which were released in huge amounts into the atmosphere. Several studies have reported no increase in the risk for thyroid cancer after diagnostic or therapeutic exposure to ^{131}I. However, the possibility that many naturally occurring thyroid carcinomas may be caused by fallout radiation after nuclear tests, other radiation sources, or natural background radiation must be seriously considered.

The history of the neck lump itself is important. Recent onset, growth, hoarseness, pain, regional nodes, symptoms of brachial plexus irritation, and local tenderness all suggest malignancy but of course do not prove it. The usual cause of sudden swelling and tenderness in a nodule is hemorrhage into a benign lesion. Although the presence of a nodule for many years suggests a benign process, some cancers grow slowly. In our series, the average time from recognition of a nodule to the diagnosis of cancer was 3 years.

Coexisting benign thyroid disease is important in the evaluation of cancer risk associated with a thyroid nodule. A history of residence in an endemic goiter zone during the first decades of life is relevant and must raise the possibility of multinodular goiter as the true diagnosis. Hashimoto's thyroiditis is often associated with discrete nodules, which are an expression of the autoimmune process. The frequency of thyroid carcinoma is not increased in patients with Hashimoto's thyroiditis; however, Hashimoto's thyroiditis is a common preexisting condition in patients in whom thyroid lymphoma develops.[36] Higher risk for differentiated thyroid cancer has been noted in patients with Graves' disease and cold thyroid nodules,[36-39] and increased aggressiveness of such Graves' disease–associated thyroid cancer has been proposed.[40] In the experience of the authors and of other groups,[41,42] the response to traditional therapy and the final outcome of patients with thyroid cancer and Graves' disease are not different with respect to thyroid cancer patients without Graves' disease.

Physical Examination Findings

In the era of thyroid ultrasound, evaluation of the thyroid gland has been enormously facilitated; however, accurate palpation of the thyroid gland and the cervical node chains is still of paramount importance in the evaluation of thyroid nodular pathology. It gives an idea of the number and size of the nodule(s), their consistency and motility, and the status of the rest of the thyroid gland, as well as the presence and the importance of lymph node involvement.

The adenoma typically is felt as a discrete lump in an otherwise normal gland, and it moves with the thyroid. Enlarged lymph nodes should be carefully sought, particularly in the area above the isthmus, in the cervical chains, and in the supraclavicular areas. Their presence suggests malignant disease unless a good alternative diagnosis (e.g., recent oropharyngeal sepsis, viral infection) is apparent. Fixation of the nodule to strap muscles or to the trachea is alarming. Characteristically, a benign thyroid adenoma is part of the thyroid and moves with deglutition, but it can be moved in relation to the strap muscles and within the gland substance to some extent. Pain, tenderness, or sudden swelling of the nodule usually indicates hemorrhage into the nodule but can also indicate invasive malignancy. Hoarseness

may arise from pressure or from infiltration of a recurrent laryngeal nerve by a neoplasm. Obviously, the presence of a firm, fixed lesion associated with pain, hoarseness, or any one of these features should signal some degree of alarm. It is worth noting that these signs are not specific for the diagnosis of malignancy. In a study that correlated suspicious clinical features with the histologic diagnosis, the authors reported benign disease in 29% of patients with palpable cervical adenopathy, in 50% of patients with hard nodules, in 29% of patients with apparent nodule fixation, and in 17% of patients with true vocal cord paralysis.[43] The converse situation, the absence of such characteristics, suggests but does not prove benignity. Fluctuance within the lesion suggests the presence of a cyst that is usually benign.

The presence of a diffusely multinodular gland, ascertained on the basis of palpation, ultrasound, or scanning, generally is interpreted as a sign of safety. Multinodular goiters coming to surgery have a significant prevalence of carcinoma (4% to 17%), but this finding is believed to be caused largely by selection of patients for surgery, and is not believed to be typical of multinodular goiter in the general population.[44] If one area within a multinodular goiter seems different from the remainder of the gland on the basis of palpation or function, or has demonstrated rapid growth, or if two discrete nodules are found in a gland that is otherwise normal, one should consider malignant change rather than a benign multinodular goiter.

Occasionally, in addition to a nodule, the gland exhibits the diffuse enlargement and firm consistency of chronic thyroiditis, a palpable pyramidal lobe, and antibody test results that may be positive. These findings strongly suggest thyroiditis but do not disclose the nature of the nodule, which must be evaluated independently. It should be remembered that 14% to 20%[45,46] of thyroid cancer specimens contain diffuse or focal thyroiditis.

Thyroid Function Tests

Unless a toxic adenoma is present, the patient is usually euthyroid, and this impression is supported by normal values for serum-free thyroxine (FT_4), free triiodothyronine (FT_3), and TSH. Low thyroid hormones or elevated TSH results should raise the question of thyroiditis. Several centers advocate measurement of serum antithyroid autoantibodies (antithyroglobulin [anti-Tg] and antithyroperoxidase [anti-TPO]) in every new patient in search of an underlying autoimmune thyroid disease. The serum Tg concentration may be elevated, as in all other goitrous conditions. Its increase is related mainly to the size of the nodule, rather than to its nature and to the size of the thyroid gland.[47] Thus, serum Tg measurement is not a valuable tool in the differential diagnosis. On the contrary, elevation of circulating calcitonin levels in a patient with a thyroid nodule is almost always diagnostic of medullary thyroid cancer. Several prospective studies have shown that routine measurement of circulating calcitonin in thyroid nodules allows the preoperative diagnosis of medullary thyroid carcinoma with better accuracy than is seen with FNAC[48-51] (Table 18-4). A large retrospective study involving more than 10,000 patients seen at a single institution has recently confirmed that on calcitonin screening, the incidence of medullary thyroid carcinoma (MTC) is 1 in 250 unselected thyroid nodules—higher than was previously believed. In addition, the study demonstrated that such screening offers the possibility of finding MTCs before they have metastasized, thus increasing the chance for definitive cure. Comparison with an historical group of patients with MTC diagnosed before the screening showed a significantly better long-term outcome for MTC detected by calcitonin screening.[52] According to these

Table 18-4. Medullary Thyroid Cancer Diagnosed by Routine Measurement of Serum Calcitonin and by Fine-Needle Aspiration Cytology in Nodular Thyroid Diseases

Authors	Patients	MTC Detected by CT	MTC Detected by FNAC
Pacini, 1994	1385	8 (0.57%)	2 (0.14%)
Rieu, 1995	469	4 (0.85%)	1 (0.21%)
Vierhapper, 1997	1062	13 (1.22%)	—
Niccoli, 1977	1167	12 (1.02%)	3 (0.25%)
Elisei, 2004	10,864	44 (0.4%)	20 (0.18%)
Costante, 2007	5817	15 (0.25%)	6 (0.1%)

CT, Computed tomography; *FNAC,* fine-needle aspiration cytology; *MTC,* medullary thyroid carcinoma.

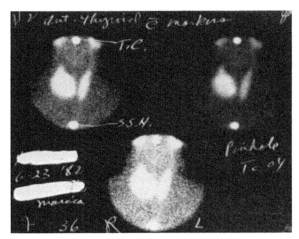

FIGURE 18-2. Scintillation scan view of a functioning nodule in a 36-year-old woman. At surgery, the nodule proved to be a mixed papillary-follicular neoplasm.

authors, measurement of serum calcitonin should be included in the diagnostic evaluation of thyroid nodules at the first visit of the patient; this has been incorporated into the European Thyroid Association guidelines,[53] but not the American Thyroid Association guidelines.[54a] Cost-effectiveness, one of the major issues in screening for thyroid nodules, has been calculated recently, and the result favored calcitonin screening.[55] Calcitonin assay is, of course, mandatory in the presence of a suggestive family history or coincident features of the MEN2 syndromes.

Routine measurement of serum calcium is advocated by several centers. The aim is not directly related to the diagnosis of thyroid nodules, but rather to detection of undiagnosed parathyroid adenomas.

Imaging

Thyroid Ultrasound

Thyroid ultrasound is becoming more and more popular in the first-line evaluation of thyroid nodules. Good technique demonstrates nodules, if they are larger than 3 mm; indicates cystic areas; and may reveal a capsule around the nodule and the size of the lobes. It often displays multiple nodules when only one is noted clinically, and it allows the discovery of suspicious lymph nodes in the neck. This technique is more sensitive than thyroid scan, is noninvasive, involves less time, allows serial examination, and usually is less expensive. From 3% to 20% of lesions are found to be totally or partially cystic. Purely cystic lesions are reported to have a lower incidence of malignancy than do solid tumors (3% vs. 10%), and diagnosis of a cyst raises the possibility of aspiration therapy.[56] Some specific features (e.g., hypoechoic, solid, irregular halo, microcalcifications, shape) are indicative, although not diagnostic, of malignant nodules. The study of blood flow by Doppler ultrasonography may provide indicative information, and, very recently, a new technique called "elastographic ultrasound" was applied to the differential diagnosis with great specificity and sensitivity.[57,58]

Isotope Scans and Other Imaging Techniques

Isotope scintiscans provide only functional information regarding activity of the nodules; their use has been much reduced since neck ultrasound was introduced,[59,60] because the same functional information is revealed by measurement of serum TSH levels. In cases of multinodular goiter, scintiscan is still useful in distinguishing the nodules to be submitted to FNAC (the cold one). Nodules that are hyperfunctional and that produce hyperthyroidism are rarely malignant, and those that accumulate iodide in concentrations equal to the surrounding normal thyroid tissue are usually but not always benign[61,62] (Fig.

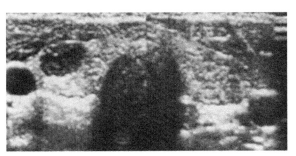

FIGURE 18-3. Sagittal echo scan of a palpable 2 cm single nodule showing a lesion in the R lobe. On aspiration, 2 mL of brownish colloid was obtained. The few cells present showed Hürthle cell changes.

18-2). Cold nodules are typically benign, but when viewed the other way, most thyroid cancers are seen as inactive areas on thyroid scan. In practice, except for the specific case of a toxic nodule, scans are probably of little help in the differential diagnosis, and the tendency to omit scanning from diagnostic maneuvers is growing. Scintiscans can confirm the diagnosis of multinodular goiter and can show the presence of diffuse disease (e.g., Hashimoto's thyroiditis) in some patients when nodularity is suspected.

Other scanning techniques have not found a place in routine preoperative evaluation (Fig. 18-3). Computed tomography (CT) is expensive but occasionally useful, especially in unusually large substernal glands. Magnetic resonance imaging (MRI) is rarely necessary but is useful for identifying abnormal nodes. Fluorine-18-fluoro-deoxyglucose (FDG)–positron emission tomography (PET) is generating great interest in general oncology but has no particular role in the diagnosis of thyroid nodules, even if sporadic reports of positive uptake in malignant nodules have been published.[63,64]

Chest radiograph and soft tissue x-ray films of the neck are useful for ascertaining the presence of compression signs (e.g., indentation or deviation of the trachea), which are particularly common when the tumor is larger than 3 or 4 cm in diameter. Fine, stippled calcifications through the tumor (psammoma bodies) are virtually pathognomonic of papillary cancer. Patchy or "signet ring" calcification occurs in old cysts and degenerating adenomas and has no such connotation. The presence of such signs is very well detected by thyroid ultrasound.

Fine-Needle Aspiration Cytology

Although all the above mentioned procedures may provide some indication, only the results of FNAC can give a definitive answer regarding the nature of a thyroid nodule. FNAC has now been widely adopted after initial favorable reports by Walfish and colleagues[65] and Gershengorn and colleagues.[66] It has replaced the core needle biopsy previously used to provide a histologic diagnosis.[67] In expert hands, adequate specimens can be obtained in more than 90% of patients, with a diagnostic sensitivity and specificity near or superior to 95%. Willems and Lowhagen, in reviewing a collected series of nearly 4000 surgically proven fine-needle aspiration (FNA) studies, found that 11.8% were considered malignant lesions.[68] False-negative diagnoses of cancer were made in 6.6% to 27.5%, and false-positive diagnoses in only 0% to 2%. Currently, the results of FNAC are viewed as the "gold standard" for diagnosis in most cases, and they play a crucial role in the selection of patients for surgery.[69-71] Gharib and coworkers analyzed data on 10,000 FNA procedures and found it to be the preferred first step in diagnosis.[72] Diagnostic accuracy was nearly 98%, with fewer than 2% false positives and false negatives. Miller and colleagues compared FNA, large-needle aspiration, and cutting needle biopsy.[73] They found that FNAC examination was able to detect almost all carcinomas, but they believe that cutting needle biopsy is a useful additional procedure, especially with larger (more than 2 to 3 cm) nodules.

FNAC should always be performed with ultrasound guidance, especially in smaller (or less discrete) or partially cystic nodules. It is demonstrated that, with respect to pre-FNAC years, various centers using the results of FNAC for therapeutic decisions have observed a 35% to 75% reduction in the number of patients sent to surgery; a twofold to threefold increase in the percentage of cancers found at surgery; and a variable, but constant, reduction in the cost of thyroid nodule management.

FNAC is performed with a 22 to 25 gauge needle. Specimen adequacy requires a minimum of two slides (from separate aspirates) showing at least six to eight cell clusters.[74] The method is simple, inexpensive, and very well tolerated and, if necessary, may be repeated several times. Complications are very rare and consist mainly of hematomas. In several large series, it has been found that around 70% (range, 53% to 90%) of aspirates are classified as benign; 4.0% (1% to 10%) as malignant or suspicious for malignancy; 10% (5% to 23%) as indeterminate, mainly represented by "follicular neoplasia"; and 17% (15% to 20%) as inadequate for diagnosis.[75-78] When the sample obtained is of good quality (i.e., high cellularity), the cytologic diagnosis of thyroid carcinoma, especially in the case of a papillary histotype, is highly reliable, and false-negative or false-positive results are very rare. Medullary thyroid carcinoma is diagnosed easily by cytology in classic cases, but sometimes the cellular pattern is atypical and can be interpreted as follicular and even papillary proliferation. Problems may arise in the case of thyroid lymphoma, because the smear may be composed of follicular cells mixed with lymphocytes, which can mimic chronic lymphocytic thyroiditis or may be confused with anaplastic carcinoma. Cytology of cystic nodules shows the presence of colloid, necrotic material, macrophages, and rare epithelial cells. In most cases, these lesions are benign, but the possibility of cystadenocarcinoma must be considered. The cytologic diagnosis of follicular or Hürthle cell neoplasia is particularly challenging. A variety of techniques have been applied to improve the accuracy of interpretation of FNA cytology in this setting, including staining with antibodies to thyroid peroxidase (TPO) and the search for *MUC1*

gene expression and telomerase activity, as well as galectin-3 expression.[79-85] However, none of these potential markers has been entered into clinical practice because of conflicting results or low sensitivity.

The major limitation of FNAC is the inadequacy of specimens, even after repeat attempts. The rate of inadequacy is variable among different centers, with a realistic estimation of between 15% and 25%.[75-76] Inadequacy raises the question of therapy for the nodule with nondiagnostic FNAC. Some authors recommend surgical treatment for all these nodules, whereas others select for surgery only those suspicious by other clinical or laboratory features. Even if only the most suspicious nodules with inadequate FNAC are selected for surgery, the yield of malignancy at histology is relatively low and ranges from 8% to 19%.[74,86,87] In any case, patients should be carefully monitored by repeat FNAC and referred to a surgeon in the event that a nodule increases in size.

An additional indication for FNAC is the diagnostic evaluation of cervical nodes, both at initial evaluation and when a diagnosis of thyroid cancer has already been established. In the case of lymph nodes suspected of being of thyroid metastatic origin, FNAC may be integrated with the measurement of Tg in the liquid recovered when the needle used for the aspiration is washed. As is shown in Fig. 18-4, in the case of a metastatic lesion from differentiated thyroid carcinoma, this technique demonstrates the presence of high levels of Tg.[88,89]

In conclusion, FNAC should be performed on any thyroid nodule. In the case of multinodular goiter, FNAC should be performed on as many nodules as possible. The largest nodule is not necessarily the one associated with malignancy; thus, FNA should be performed under the guidance of sonographic features rather than on the basis of size.[12] In dubious cases, FNAC may be repeated immediately or over the years, if the final decision is to not operate on the patient. It is worth mentioning that the preoperative diagnosis of thyroid carcinoma is useful not only for selecting patients to be operated on, but also for planning in advance the most appropriate surgical procedure.

Diagnostic Protocol

A possible practical diagnostic approach to patients with thyroid nodules is schematically represented in Fig. 18-5.

Serum thyroid hormone and TSH measurement and thyroid ultrasound are performed as first-line exploration. Determination of antithyroid antibodies is calcitonin are also helpful.

If TSH is suppressed or low, a thyroid scan is performed to confirm the presence of an autonomously functioning nodule; the subsequent approach will depend on the presence of clinical or subclinical thyrotoxicosis and on the size of the nodule. If the nodule is cold and cystic, FNAC will be performed both as a therapeutic technique (evacuation) and as a diagnostic tool to detect the small percentage of cystic adenocarcinomas. If the nodule is cold and totally or partially solid, the therapeutic decision will depend on the results of FNAC.

THERAPY

A complete diagnostic evaluation, as previously outlined, is a prerequisite to determining the appropriate choice of treatment for thyroid nodules. The problem involves whether the nodule requires any therapy, and, if so, whether it is manageable by medical or surgical therapy.

Surgical Therapy

We favor selecting the malignant nodules for surgery, and we suggest medical therapy or follow-up for the others. However,

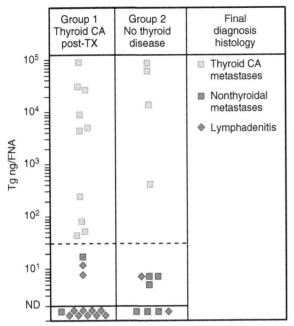

FIGURE 18-4. Concentration of thyroglobulin (Tg) in fine-needle aspirates of neck masses from patients with (group 1) or without (group 2) known thyroid cancer, according to the final diagnosis at histology. (From Pacini F, Fugazzola L, Lippi F, et al: Detection of thyroglobulin in fine needle aspirates of nonthyroidal neck masses: a clue to the diagnosis of metastatic thyroid cancer, J Clin Endocrinol Metab 74:1401, ©1992, The Endocrine Society.)

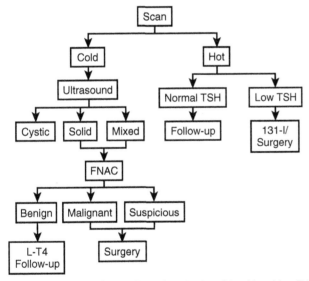

FIGURE 18-5. Flow chart for the diagnostic evaluation of thyroid nodules. *FNAC*, Fine-needle aspiration cytology; *L-T₄*, levothyroxine; *TSH*, thyroid-stimulating hormone. Currently, isotope scanning is omitted unless there is evidence for excess thyroid hormone production.

surgical treatment should also be suggested for some benign lesions, either single or associated with multinodular goiter, when they are large enough to produce symptoms and signs of discomfort or aesthetic concern. Another surgical indication is for questionable nodules, including those characterized by follicular proliferation on FNAC.

If surgery is selected, we believe that it is crucial to work in conjunction with a surgeon who has frequent and continuous experience in thyroid surgery to obtain good results. This is not to say that resection of a thyroid lobe for a nodule is a difficult

procedure; however, if more extensive surgery is required, and especially if total or near-total thyroidectomy and lymph node resection are indicated, it is imperative that the surgeon have the proper knowledge and experience to reduce the possibility of damage to recurrent laryngeal nerves and parathyroid glands.

Surgery for Nodules With FNAC Indicative of Malignancy

When the malignant nature of a nodule has been established by FNAC, the recommended surgical procedure should be total (or near-total) thyroidectomy regardless of the size of the nodule, without the need for frozen section examination, which has a rate of false-negative results in excess of false-positive results for FNAC (near zero). This procedure decreases the risk for local recurrence and is performed with almost no morbidity under expert hands. Moreover, it facilitates postsurgical radioiodine ablation and adequate follow-up.[90-92] Surgery should be preceded by careful staging of the disease in the neck. This is accomplished by thyroid and neck ultrasound. Any suspicious lymph node must be submitted to confirmatory FNAC to alert the surgeon of the presence of metastatic disease. If positive nodes are seen, the surgeon should perform the most appropriate dissection of lymph node chains (central compartment, homolateral modified neck dissection, or bilateral). The need for routine dissection of the central node compartment in the absence of suspicious ultrasonographic findings is debated. Recent European and American guidelines[53,54a] suggest that the central neck should be explored and all nodes removed by the surgeon in cases of papillary and Hürthle cell thyroid cancer, but not follicular thyroid cancer. However, the benefits of prophylactic "en bloc" central node dissection in the absence of preoperative or intraoperative evidence of nodal disease are controversial. No evidence suggests that it improves recurrence or mortality rates, but it does permit accurate staging of the disease that may guide subsequent treatment and follow-up.

This approach, which emphasizes more extensive nodal surgery and less use of ^{131}I, represents an interesting return to concepts in vogue and discarded five decades ago. Bonnet et al.[54b] reported a series of 115 patients with papillary tumors of 1 to 2 cm and no preoperatively recognized cervical nodes, whose surgery arbitrarily included en bloc dissection of midcervical (level VI) nodes and lateral (level III and IV) nodes, and sometimes level II and V nodes. Patients probably had more advanced tumors than are seen in average cases, in that 29% were invasive and 37% multifocal. This extensive nodal surgery changed therapy in 11%, in whom no nodes were found, and who therefore received no [131]I. Complications included hypoparathyroidism and vocal cord paralysis (0.9% each). Certainly this "prophylactic" node dissection may preclude discovery of nodes at a later date, thus preventing a small number of patients from being exposed to 30 mCi of [131]I. Whether this is a fair trade for the certain increase in side effects that would follow application of the approach in general practice remains very uncertain, and this approach cannot be recommended at present.

Surgery for Nodules With Indeterminate or Suspicious FNAC

Among solitary thyroid nodules with an indeterminate ("suspicious," "follicular neoplasm," or Hürthle cell neoplasm) biopsy, the risk for malignancy is approximately 20%.[93-95] For solitary nodules that are repeatedly nondiagnostic on biopsy, the risk for malignancy is unknown but is probably closer to 5% to 10%.[96] In these cases, the surgical procedure should be discussed with the patient. For those who prefer a more limited surgical procedure, thyroid lobectomy associated with frozen section examination is the recommended initial surgical approach.

Because of increased risk for malignancy, total thyroidectomy is indicated in patients with large tumors (>4 cm) when marked atypia is seen on biopsy, when the biopsy reading is "suspicious for papillary carcinoma," in patients with a family history of thyroid carcinoma, in patients with a history of radiation exposure,[97-99] in patients with bilateral nodular disease, and in those who prefer to undergo bilateral thyroidectomy to avoid the possibility of requiring a future surgery.

Surgery for Differentiated Thyroid Cancer Detected at Final Histology Without Total Thyroidectomy Performed

If a patient is referred after less than near-total thyroidectomy, completion thyroidectomy should be proposed in the case of a large tumor, multifocality, extrathyroidal extension, and/or vascular invasion or evidence of local or distant metastases, previous history of radiation exposure, or unfavorable histology.[96,101] In cases of primary tumors between 10 and 20 mm in diameter that have been diagnosed at postoperative definitive histopathology, the indication for completion thyroidectomy should be discussed with the patient on the basis of the risks and benefits of reoperative surgery, including the potential risk for surgical morbidity. Depending on the size of the thyroid remnant, an effective alternative to completion thyroidectomy when the risk for persistent disease is low may be radioiodine ablation of residual thyroid tissue.[102]

Whenever surgery is performed for nodules with no suspicion of malignancy, the usual procedure is lobectomy, which is relatively harmless and has an incidence of complications approaching zero. Usually, patients are discharged within 2 to 3 days. Complications are more common when more extensive dissection is done, as will be discussed subsequently. The thyroid specimen itself, any abnormal areas in the gland, and any abnormal appearing lymph nodes should be examined immediately by frozen section. Differentiating benign from malignant thyroid lesions is admittedly difficult, especially with frozen sections, but experienced pathologists can make the distinction with a high degree of reliability. Occasionally, follicular lesions are believed by the pathologist to be benign at surgery, but permanent sections reveal changes that indicate malignancy. Reoperation with near-total thyroidectomy is probably desirable in these patients, because up to one third can be expected to have residual tumor in the contralateral lobe.[103] To avoid these second operations, we recommend lobectomy and contralateral subtotal resection for very cellular follicular lesions as the initial procedure. Occasionally, a small papillary or follicular cancer is found in the pathologic specimen after the operation has concluded. If this cancer is less than 1 cm and has a well-demarcated single focus, and the patient is younger than 45 years, nothing further need be done therapeutically, but follow-up by periodic thyroid ultrasound is recommended. After surgery, all patients are maintained on replacement levothyroxine therapy in the hope of preventing recurrence of other nodules. Serum TSH should be maintained in the low-normal range.

Medical Therapy

Benign Solid Cold Nodule

Appropriate management of these nodules is strongly debated. A meta-analysis[104] has indicated that about 25% respond to thyroxine treatment with a decrease in size, whereas the remainder remain unchanged, at least over several months. Some physi-

cians believe that once malignancy has been ruled out, medical therapy is indicated for solid cold nodules with normal or subnormal thyroid function, especially when associated with thyroid enlargement. The drug of choice is levothyroxine. Some physicians advocate a dose sufficient to suppress pituitary TSH secretion as demonstrated by a serum TSH level less than 0.1 µU/mL. The rationale for this therapy is the unequivocal observation that TSH is, to some extent, a growth factor not only for the normal thyroid but also for thyroid nodules. Experimental and clinical evidence has shown that even mild iodine deficiency elicits subminimal increases in TSH levels, which leads first to glandular hyperplasia and later to multinodular goiter. On the other hand, the functional heterogeneity and the variable degree of mitogenicity of follicular cells upon stimulation by TSH offer an explanation for the appearance of a nodule without diffuse goiter. When the nodule and/or the goiter is of recent origin, suppression of TSH stimulation by levothyroxine is often sufficient to eliminate the nodule, or at least to reduce its size and that of the thyroid gland. In long-standing cases, both the nodules and the goiter are seldom cured, but a significant reduction in size and arrest of the progression are likely to occur.

Once instituted, levothyroxine therapy must go on for years to be effective.[106] Age is very important in the selection of patients to be treated. Treatment is indicated in young patients and in adults up to about 45 to 50 years of age. In older patients, the opportunity to initiate suppressive therapy must be considered on an individual basis after other underlying diseases such as heart problems are excluded. However, if a patient is already receiving levothyroxine treatment and shows good compliance and no side effects, treatment can be continued after age 50 years and even after age 60 years with the daily dosage slightly decreased.

An alternative approach is to aim for a TSH of 0.3 to 1 µU/mL, because this level will have some suppressive effect, perhaps will inhibit the growth of nodules over subsequent years, and is free of the minimal risk for mild thyrotoxicosis.

At the other end of the spectrum of opinion are physicians who believe that thyroxine therapy is useless and who simply offer continued observation without treatment.

Another aspect to be considered is functional thyroid status. Before instituting levothyroxine therapy, to avoid iatrogenic thyrotoxicosis, one must be certain that the patient is perfectly euthyroid, and that serum TSH, measured with an ultrasensitive assay, is not already suppressed, as so often can happen in multinodular goiters with areas of functional autonomy.

The last important aspect is the dose to be given. The usual suppressive dose is between 1.5 and 2 µg/kg/day, administered in the morning. The dose is checked after 3 to 4 months by measuring FT_3, which should stay in the normal range, and TSH, which should be in the range selected, with an FT_4 value usually in the upper limit of the normal range. If results show that TSH is not suppressed, or that the patient has been overtreated, an appropriate dosage modification will be made, with another hormonal control determined 3 to 4 months later and then yearly.

Once the few precautions described above are observed, levothyroxine treatment is generally useful and safe. Our own experience and data from the literature indicate that significant shrinkage is obtained in 15% to 50% of the nodules, and that many others do not progress. Side effects on the heart and bone, described by some authors, are not observed when careful avoidance of subclinical thyrotoxicosis is maintained.[107]

When clinical signs of hyperthyroidism suddenly develop during levothyroxine therapy, one must suspect the occurrence of functional autonomy of the nodule(s), and levothyroxine treatment must be withdrawn immediately. An indication for referring the patient to a surgeon is an increase in size of the nodule during levothyroxine therapy. Such a situation is not unusual and, although regarded as suspicious, does not constitute definite evidence of malignancy.

Autonomously Functioning Thyroid Nodule

The incidence of cancer in an autonomously functioning thyroid nodule (AFTN) (hot nodule) is so low that the therapeutic approach is dictated mainly by the presence of thyrotoxicosis and/or the size of the nodule. Sometimes hot nodules are found in the presence of detectable TSH, with the extranodular uptake being reduced but not suppressed. Many AFTNs are associated with subclinical thyrotoxicosis, the only abnormality being a low or undetectable serum TSH. Overt thyrotoxicosis is present in the remaining cases. AFTNs tend to occur in young adults, and they are usually smaller than 3 cm.

AFTNs of small dimension (<3 cm), without thyrotoxicosis, can be left untreated and observed. About 20% to 30% of the nodules, and a greater percentage when they are larger than 3 cm, evolve to thyrotoxicosis, sometimes decades after discovery. In the case of thyrotoxicosis, three therapeutic options are available: (1) surgery, (2) radioiodine, and (3) ethanol injection. Radioiodine is a very effective therapy and is the treatment of choice in many patients with AFTNs. Euthyroidism and a variable degree of tumor shrinkage are always attained after ^{131}I treatment, but a hard nodule usually persists for life. No agreement has been reached on the best activity of ^{131}I to be administered. In our experience, standard doses of 15 mCi usually are sufficient to abolish the function of the nodule, although they induce late hypothyroidism in about 20% of patients.[108] Surgery is an acceptable alternative therapy and is indicated for large nodules (>3 cm) and for patients who refuse to be treated with radioiodine. Surgery consists of total lobectomy and, in the case of thyrotoxicosis, must be performed after normal thyroid function has been restored by adequate preparation with antithyroid drugs (methimazole or propylthiouracil). The development of hypothyroidism after treatment is unusual after surgery and occurs in about 10% of cases after radioiodine therapy. Replacement therapy probably is indicated, also in patients who remain euthyroid, to avoid late compensatory hyperplasia of the remaining lobe.

A third therapeutic option for the treatment of AFTN has been proposed by Italian authors and consists of percutaneous intranodular ethanol injection (PEI).[109,110] The mechanism of action of ethanol is based on induction of cellular dehydration, followed by coagulative necrosis and vascular thrombosis and occlusion. The technique, when performed by well-trained staff, is effective and safe. Transient local pain is the most common side effect. PEI may be considered a possible alternative to surgery and radioiodine in selected cases (i.e., small nodules easily accessible to palpation). This method has now been used for several years, and so far evaluation has not revealed long-term complications. Recently, the indication for PEI therapy has been extended successfully by an Italian group to the treatment of large AFTN in conjunction with radioiodine therapy.[111,112]

Thyroid Cysts

Thyroid cysts are managed easily by aspiration, but recurrence of the cyst is very common. Suppressive therapy with levothyroxine may reduce the risk for relapse, especially if aspiration is performed after a few months of levothyroxine treatment, but the risk for relapse remains significantly high. An emerging alternative therapy is cyst sclerotherapy by ethanol injection into the nodule after complete aspiration of the cystic fluid.[113] The technique appears to be effective and safe: It might become the treatment of choice for thyroid cysts. When the above mentioned therapy fails to avoid cyst recurrence, or when the size of the nodule is too large, surgery is necessary.

A small proportion (about 3%) of cystic nodules diagnosed as thyroid cysts do not originate from the follicular epithelium but rather from the parathyroids. These cysts may be suspected from the color of the cystic fluid, which usually, but not always, is transparent like water. The final diagnosis is achieved easily by a finding of high concentrations of parathyroid hormone and low or undetectable concentrations of Tg in the fluid aspirate.[114] Most of the time, calcemia is normal. The differential diagnosis between thyroid and parathyroid cysts has important therapeutic implications in that parathyroid cysts do not tend to recur after FNA and of course do not respond to levothyroxine treatment.

Thyroid Carcinoma

EPIDEMIOLOGY

Thyroid cancer accounts for less than 1% of all cases of malignant neoplasia. It is rare in children and increases in frequency with age; it is among the five most common cancers in the second, third, and fourth decades of life. Differentiated thyroid cancers are two to four times as common in females as in males; however, the female preponderance decreases in prepubertal and postmenopausal ages, which suggests that sex hormones might play some role in the pathogenesis. In the United States over the past two decades, thyroid cancer has had one of the largest increases in incidence among all human cancers.[115] It occurs primarily as small papillary tumors (microcarcinoma), suggesting that the increase is due mainly to ascertainment bias after neck ultrasonography was introduced into clinical practice. As proof of this idea, the rate of death from thyroid cancer is stable, confirming that the increase is the result of subclinical, indolent tumors.[16]

In the past, the estimated incidence of thyroid nodules was about 1 per 1000 persons per year, and that of thyroid carcinoma in various part of the world ranged from 0.5 to 10 cases per 100,000 persons per year. Thus, 0.5% to 10% of patients with thyroid nodules had thyroid cancer.[116] It is not certain that carcinoma occurs with increased frequency in areas of endemic goiter, although a clear increase has been seen in the relative proportions of follicular and anaplastic neoplasms. Studies by Sampson and coworkers[117] and by Fukunaga and Yatani[118] indicate that a high prevalence (up to 5.7%) of unsuspected microcarcinoma may exist in adults. These lesions most often are smaller than 0.5 cm in greatest dimension, are papillary in nature, and are believed to behave in a relatively benign manner. They are detected effectively only by a pathologist. Recognition of such "minimal thyroid cancers" does not demand the same therapeutic response as does the discovery of a larger tumor, although small tumors can certainly metastasize and are occasionally fatal. Studies from the Mayo Clinic suggest that the incidence of thyroid cancer is about 36 per million cases per year but increases to 60 per million if small, occult tumors are included in the statistics.[119] A significant proportion of thyroid cancers are not diagnosed during life and are not the cause of death of the patient. The prevalence of neoplasm at autopsy is highly variable, depending on the population selected and the care of the survey. Prevalence ranges from 0.1% to 2.7%.[120,121] Two studies of consecutive autopsies of patients dying in hospitals found that 2.7% of thyroids harbored unsuspected thyroid cancer, and that an equivalent percentage had metastatic carcinoma in the gland.[121,122] Accurate pathologic examination of resected multinodular goiters, so common in areas of iodine deficiency, is able to detect many occult tumors, which again might be of no relevance from the clinical point of view. All these data provide evidence for leisurely growth of most thyroid tumors.

When compared with other malignancies, thyroid cancer is probably the most curable cancer, with very high long-term survival rates, at least in the well-differentiated histotypes. However, some patients are at high risk for recurrent disease or even death. Most patients can be identified at the time of diagnosis with the use of well-defined prognostic indicators.

PATHOLOGY

Histologic diagnosis of malignancy is usually very simple, but in some tumors it is difficult. Pathologic examination of thyroid tumors is organized to differentiate between benign and malignant lesions; to define pathologic prognostic factors among variants of papillary and follicular carcinoma; and to detect large cell anaplastic cancer, medullary cancer, and rare forms of thyroid cancer. A schematic classification and definition of thyroid tumors is presented in Table 18-5.

Papillary and follicular carcinomas are the two most common entities, usually referred to as differentiated thyroid cancer. The diagnosis of papillary carcinoma is based on the presence of typical features, including nuclear inclusions. The diagnosis of follicular carcinoma is based on the presence of follicular differentiation without the features typical of papillary cancer.[123]

Table 18-5. Classification and Definition of Thyroid Tumors

Epithelial Thyroid Tumors	Definition
Benign	
Follicular adenoma	A benign encapsulated tumor with evidence of follicular cell differentiation
Malignant	
Papillary carcinoma	A malignant epithelial tumor with evidence of follicular differentiation, alterations in papillary and follicular structure, and characteristic nuclear changes
Follicular carcinoma	A malignant epithelial tumor showing follicular cell differentiation without the diagnostic features of papillary carcinoma
Undifferentiated carcinoma	A highly malignant tumor composed in part or wholly of undifferentiated cells
Medullary carcinoma	A malignant tumor showing evidence of C cell differentiation
Malignant Nonepithelial Tumors	
Sarcoma	A malignant tumor lacking all evidence of epithelial differentiation and showing definite evidence of specific sarcomatous differentiation
Hemangioendothelioma	A highly malignant tumor with extensive necrosis or hemorrhage and a vascular-like cleft lined by cells displaying features of endothelial cells
Malignant lymphoma	A malignant tumor with positive staining for leukocyte common antigen or similar antigens
Secondary tumors	Pathologic features depend on the primary tumor

Modified from Hedinger C, Williams ED, Sobin LH: Histologic typing of thyroid tumors, vol II. In International histological classification of tumors, ed 2, Berlin, 1988, Springer-Verlag.

Immunostaining for Tg is almost always positive in both papillary and follicular tumors and may serve to confirm the thyroid origin of a metastasis.

Papillary Thyroid Carcinoma: Classic Type

According to their size and extension, papillary carcinomas may be classified as microcarcinomas, carcinomas limited to the thyroid gland, and carcinomas extending outside the thyroid.

Microcarcinomas are tumors smaller than 1 cm in diameter; they are also called "occult." They may have the features of a classic small papillary carcinoma, or they may appear as unencapsulated sclerotic nodules of a few millimeters, infiltrating the surrounding thyroid. Microcarcinomas are found in 5% to 35% at autopsy, depending on the geographic area and the method used,[5,124] but they are very rare in childhood. As a result of general improvements in diagnostic techniques, the number of microcarcinomas selected for surgery is increasing. Their prognosis is very good.[125,126]

Larger, clinically detectable tumors represent nearly 70% of all papillary cancers. They appear as firm nonencapsulated or partly encapsulated tumors.[123,127] A few papillary cancers may be partly necrotic or cystic. Papillary cancer is often multicentric in one lobe and bilateral, with a frequency varying between 20% and 80% in different series.[128-130]

Microscopically, papillary carcinomas contain papillary areas with a focal distribution or with a diffuse pattern. The papillae consist of a stromal-vascular axis lined by characteristic cells. The presence of true papillae is a peculiar feature of papillary thyroid cancer, and these papillae must be differentiated from the pseudopapillae and the macropapillae seen in Graves' disease, in benign nodules, or in goiter with hypothyroidism.

Other aspects may be associated with the papillae. Follicles filled with colloid or a trabecular or lobular aspect, squamous metaplasia, and psammoma bodies are other distinguishing features present in 40% to 50% of tumors. Also typical of papillary lesions are areas of sclerosis found in the central portion of the tumor or at the periphery.

Nuclei are characteristic. They are larger than those found in normal follicular cells when superimposed on one another, are pale and transparent at the center, and contain hypodense chromatin and prominent nuclear membranes. The shape is irregular and may be "fissured" like "coffee grains." Large, circular, well-delimited intranuclear inclusions, an expression of cytoplasmic invagination, are present.[131] In the absence of other features of the tumor, the diagnosis of papillary cancer is based on typical features of the nuclei.[123]

Scattered lymphocytes are often found at the invasive periphery of the tumor. More rarely, a true lymphocyte infiltrate resembling chronic lymphocytic thyroiditis is seen within the tumor; this is associated with a favorable prognosis.[132]

Commonly and early in the disease, papillary carcinoma invades lymphatic vessels. Invasion progresses from the perithyroid chains to more distant chains. Nodes along the recurrent nerve most often are involved. Lymphatic spread within the thyroid is probably the reason for the high frequency of multifocality of the tumor.[128,129] Venous invasion and distant metastases (most often to the lung and bone) are rare and account for 5% to 7% of cases.[133]

Variants of Papillary Thyroid Carcinoma

The more frequent variant of papillary thyroid cancer is the follicular variant. It is grossly encapsulated[134,135] and shows a diffuse pattern of follicular growth with colloid-containing follicles. The papillary nature of this tumor can be recognized by the findings of clear nuclei, psammoma bodies, desmoplastic reaction, and lymphocytic infiltration. Lung metastases are common and respond well to conventional treatment. The prognosis is similar to that of the classic variants. They often are found in young subjects, and 21% of the post-Chernobyl childhood thyroid cancers in Belarus were classified as follicular variants.[136]

The rare diffuse sclerosing variant is found most often in children and young adults.[137] Its characteristics are those of diffuse thyroid enlargement as seen in goiter, but with both lobes replaced by a very firm and calcified tumor. At microscopy, this form is almost always multicentric. Tumor papillae are associated with squamous metaplasia without keratinization and abundant psammoma bodies. Extensive lymphocytic infiltration of the gland is often found, and lymph node metastases are present in 100% of cases. Also, distant metastases are common. The prognosis is less favorable than for classic papillary cancer, although the response to treatment may be excellent.

In the tall cell variant[138] and the columnar cell variant,[139] the tumor is usually large and extends outside the thyroid gland. These tumors have a papillary pattern, and the cells are tall and have a granular, eosinophilic cytoplasm. Vascular invasion is commonly seen, and the tumors are typical of older patients. A poor prognosis has been reported with this variant.

The encapsulated variant is characterized by a capsule similar to an adenoma but focally invaded. Microscopically, the typical cytologic and nuclear features of papillary tumor and psammoma bodies are found. This variant represents 8% to 13% of cases.[140]

In subjects affected by polyposis coli, papillary thyroid cancer has typical features: common multifocality with classic papillary aspects associated with solid areas and elongated cells.

Follicular Thyroid Carcinoma

At variance with the papillary histotype, follicular carcinoma usually is seen as a solitary, more or less encapsulated nodule in the thyroid. Depending on the degree of invasiveness, the tumor is classified as minimally invasive (encapsulated) or widely invasive.[123] The distinction has great prognostic impact because the prognosis is more severe when more extensive vascular invasion is present.[141]

Minimally invasive carcinomas represent more than 50% of cases. The diagnosis of malignancy is based totally on the demonstration of unequivocal vascular invasion and/or invasion of the full thickness of the capsule. Examination of multiple blocks, including the periphery of the nodule, is often necessary to exclude or confirm the presence of invasion. Cytologically, they cannot be distinguished from benign adenomas. Thus, FNAC is of no help in the differential diagnosis between benign and malignant lesions. Frozen section can lead to misdiagnosis and is not recommended by some experts in the field.

Widely invasive tumors present few diagnostic problems. They show widespread infiltration of blood vessels and surrounding thyroid tissue. The capsule, when present, is infiltrated in several areas and is grossly disrupted.

In minimally and widely invasive follicular carcinoma, the morphology is variable and ranges from well differentiated with well-formed follicles full of colloid to poorly differentiated with a solid, cellular growth pattern.

Follicular cancer invades blood vessels but rarely invades lymphatics. Metastases are spread hematogenously to the lungs, bones, and, less commonly, the brain and liver.[133] Metastases are very common with the widely invasive variant, less common with the minimally invasive variant.

Variants of Follicular Carcinoma

Clear cell tumor is a rare variant, with architectural and clinical features similar to those of the usual follicular carcinomas. The cells are clear because of the formation of intracytoplasmic vesicles, glycogen or fat accumulation, or intracellular Tg deposition. These tumors must be distinguished from clear cell adenoma, from parathyroid adenoma or carcinoma, and particularly from metastatic clear cell renal carcinoma.

The oxyphilic cell type (or Hürthle cell type) is composed of cells derived from the follicular epithelium and characterized by large size with abundant granular, eosinophilic cytoplasm; large nuclei; and prominent nucleoli. The granular appearance of the cytoplasm is conferred by the large number of mitochondria inside the cell. Hürthle cell tumors can also be of papillary lineage, as shown by the presence of *RET/PTC* mutations.

Because Hürthle cells can be found in papillary carcinomas and in a number of benign conditions (e.g., nodular goiter, hyperthyroidism, Hashimoto's thyroiditis, benign nodules), the same criteria for malignancy mentioned for follicular tumors (i.e., invasion) apply to oxyphilic cell tumors. As with follicular carcinoma, macroscopically the oxyphilic variant is seen as a solitary thyroid nodule with complete or partial encapsulation. In several series, the prognosis for this variant has been reported as less favorable than for the follicular cell type.[142]

Insular carcinoma is also a rare variant.[143] It is a poorly differentiated, invasive follicular cancer with a solid aspect and follicular differentiation represented by small vesicles with very little colloid. The cells are very homogeneous in shape and smaller and more dense than in typical follicular cancer. The general picture may resemble that of carcinoid tumors. Metastases, very common, are found in lymph nodes and in distant organs. The prognosis is poor.

Other Tumors

Anaplastic cancer originates from the follicular epithelium, but its high degree of undifferentiation does not allow the recognition of any feature of the thyroid gland. It represents 5% to 15% of all thyroid cancers and is one of the most aggressive human cancers. Local extension at diagnosis and distant metastases are almost the rule.

Medullary tumors derive from the calcitonin-secreting parafollicular C cells of the thyroid. They occur as solid masses of spindle or rounded cells with large nuclei, much fibrosis, and deposits of amyloid. In the familial syndromes MEN2A and MEN2B, C cell hyperplasia precedes the cancer and typically is present in the gland. Immunochemical staining for calcitonin is useful for differentiating medullary thyroid tumors from other histologic types, especially when the origin of metastatic adenocarcinoma is being considered.

Other rare tumors include primary thyroid lymphoma or tumor arising from other cell types.

CAUSES
Oncogenes

The most interesting new concept in tumor causes relates to the role played by oncogenes and tumor suppressor genes. Recent advances in molecular biology have resulted in significant improvement in our understanding of the pathogenesis of thyroid carcinoma.[144] Gene rearrangements involving the *RET* and *TRK* proto-oncogenes have been demonstrated as causative events specific for a subset of the papillary histotype. Oncogenic activa-

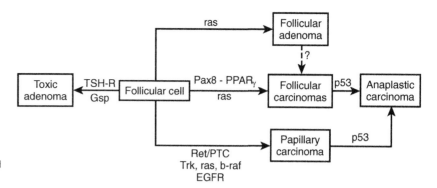

FIGURE 18-6. Proposed model of molecular events in thyroid tumorigenesis. *TSHR,* Thyroid-stimulating hormone receptor.

tion of these genes is accomplished by fusion of their tyrosine kinase domain with the N-terminal promoter sequences of other genes in the same or other chromosomes. *TRK* oncogenes are created by rearrangement of the *NTK1* gene, which encodes a receptor for nerve growth factor and is linked to at least three different activating genes.[142] In the case of *RET* rearrangements, the resulting chimeric oncogenes have been called *PTC,* an acronym for papillary thyroid carcinoma.[145,146] Several chimeric forms have been identified, the most common being *RET/PTC* 1, 2, and 3. Although strictly associated with papillary thyroid carcinoma, *RET/PTC* is found in less than half of cases unassociated with irradiation.[146-149] In papillary thyroid carcinomas occurring after irradiation, the frequency of *RET/PTC* activation is between 60% and 80%, either in Belarus children heavily exposed to radiation after the Chernobyl nuclear disaster[150-153] or in patients who received external radiation treatment during childhood.[154] Worthy of note, these radiation-induced tumors are often of the solid variant of papillary cancer, and the oncogene involved is mainly *RET/PTC* 3, particularly in the youngest subjects. In spontaneous tumors or in classic papillary variants of radiation-induced cancers, *RET/PTC* 1 is the predominant rearrangement.[155] Based on this finding, one can speculate that *RET/PTC* 3 is linked specifically to radiation and to solid papillary tumors arising in young patients (most Belarus cancers were diagnosed in children) with or without the cooperation of radiation. This second hypothesis is supported by data showing a significant correlation between high rates of *RET/PTC* activation and lower age at diagnosis in Italian patients not exposed to radiation.[156]

Recently, another oncogene, *BRAF,* has been associated specifically with *PTC* with a frequency even higher (around 40%) than that of *RET/PTC* rearrangements.[157] Apparently, the activation of *BRAF* and *RET/PTC* does not occur in the same tumor. Mutated forms of the *H-ras, K-ras,* and *N-ras* oncogenes are found in differentiated thyroid cancer; however, in this case, the mutations are not restricted specifically to malignant lesions, because the same mutations have been found in benign thyroid nodules.[158] It is conceivable that mutations of the *ras* gene family may represent early events in thyroid tumorigenesis. Activating mutations of the genes encoding the thyrotropin receptor and the α subunit of the G_s protein, similar to those found in toxic adenomas and probably of irrelevant pathogenic importance, have been reported in a few hyperfunctioning follicular carcinomas.[159] Inactivating mutations of the *p53* tumor suppressor gene are rare in patients with differentiated thyroid carcinoma but common in those with undifferentiated thyroid carcinoma.[150,160]

Expression of C-myc and C-fos is stimulated in normal thyroid tissue by TSH and occurs in adenomas and carcinomas,[161]

perhaps as a consequence of the neoplastic phenotype. The tumor suppressor gene at the 11q13 locus is lost in some follicular adenomas and carcinomas.[162] Farid and coworkers found that the *RB tumor suppressor* gene is also mutated or deleted in a high proportion of thyroid tumors.[163]

As far as follicular neoplasms are concerned, a specific oncogene originating by mutation of a gene with tumor suppressor function, *PAX8/PPARγ,* has been associated with the malignant phenotype with high frequency.[164] Recently activating mutations of the *epidermal growth factor receptor (EGFR)* gene have been identified in a subset of patients with papillary thyroid cancer. This observation suggests that EGFR-tyrosine-kinase inhibitors may be used in the treatment of a subset of patients with PTC.[165]

Based on the gene defects discovered in the different types of thyroid carcinoma, a hypothetical model of the sequential changes involved in tumorigenesis of follicular thyroid cells is offered in Fig. 18-6.

Regarding differentiated thyroid cancer, it is known that cancer tissues often lose their ability to concentrate and to organify iodide; this is why neoplastic tissue often is cold on scintiscan. At the molecular level, a possible explanation for this finding comes from experiments that suggest that the NIS gene (coding for a basolateral membrane protein that actively transports the iodide into the thyroid follicular cells) is less expressed in tumor than in normal thyroid tissue.[166] It is agreed that NIS protein expression correlates with radioactive iodine (^{131}I) uptaking activity, suggesting that NIS protein levels may predict the therapeutic efficacy of radioiodide therapy for thyroid cancer. However, to be effective, the NIS protein must maintain its physiologic polarization on the plasma membrane. In a recent study, loss of polarization with cytoplasmic localization of NIS has been reported in tumor tissues lacking radioiodine uptake. Posttranscriptional events may cause this defect in membrane targeting localization of the NIS protein. Such alterations might explain reduced iodide uptake in cases of thyroid cancer with normal NIS mRNA expression levels.

Ionizing Radiation

External irradiation of the neck during childhood increases the risk for papillary thyroid carcinoma.[34,45,167-170] The latency period between exposure and diagnosis is usually 5 years, is maximal at about 20 years, remains high for about 20 years, and then decreases gradually. A linear dose response relationship is found between external irradiation and thyroid cancer, starting with radiation doses as low as 10 cGy and up to 1500 cGy. Beyond this point, the risk for thyroid cancer decreases, probably because of thyroid cell killing. A major risk factor is young age at the time of irradiation; after the age of 15 or 20 years, the

Table 18-6. Thyroid Cancer in Belarus Before and After the Chernobyl Accident

Age, Yr	1974-1985	1986-1998	Fold Increase
3-14	8	600	75.0
15-18	13	132	10.1
19-29	117	438	3.7
>29	1254	4279	3.4
All	1392	5449	3.9

risk is much reduced. In children exposed to a dose of 1 Gy (100 rad) to the thyroid, excess risk for thyroid cancer is 7.7-fold.[167]

Diagnostic or therapeutic administration of ^{131}I to adults does not seem to be associated with an increased risk for thyroid cancer.[168-170] However, the increased incidence of papillary thyroid cancer in children in the Marshall Islands after atomic bomb testing and, more recently, in Belarus and Ukraine after the Chernobyl nuclear reactor accident[35,171-174] indicates a direct carcinogenic effect of radioactive isotopes, both ^{131}I and/or short-lived isotopes, on the thyroid gland. At variance with the cancers observed after external irradiation, the post-Chernobyl cancers diagnosed in Belarus and Ukrainian children and young adults (Table 18-6) developed after a very short mean latency period (6.5 years on average) from exposure to diagnosis.[171] Whether these discrepancies are caused by different radiation doses to the thyroid; by the very young age of the patients, when the growing thyroid is particularly sensitive to radiation; or by a combination of these and other environmental factors(iodine deficiency) is still a matter of discussion.

Other Factors

In countries where iodine intake is adequate, differentiated thyroid cancers account for more than 80% of all thyroid carcinomas, with the papillary histotype being the more common form (60% to 80%). In areas with nutritional iodine deficiency, a relative increase in follicular and anaplastic cancer with respect to papillary tumors is the rule, but no definitive demonstration of an increased prevalence of thyroid cancer has been made in such countries.[168,170] Chronic stimulation by slightly elevated TSH levels may be the underlying mechanism for thyroid hyperplasia and, possibly, carcinomatous degeneration in iodine-deficient countries. In thyroid hyperplasia in humans, whether induced by congenital metabolic defects or by other causes, the resultant elevation in TSH levels can lead to carcinomatous degeneration if the hypothyroidism is unrecognized and remains untreated for decades.[175]

Abnormalities in TSH receptors have been sought in tumor cells. It appears that differentiated tumors have normal receptors, presumably explaining their TSH-dependent growth, whereas anaplastic cancers lack high-affinity receptors and thus respond poorly to TSH.[176] The thyroid-stimulating immunoglobulins present in the sera of patients who have coincident autoimmune thyroid disease may cause tumor growth, and they occasionally appear to make tumors behave more aggressively, but usually concurrence of Graves' disease does not worsen the prognosis.[33] Although no evidence indicates that thyroid-stimulating immunoglobulins cause malignancy, it is of interest that up to 6% of thyroid glands removed because of Graves' disease harbor a carcinoma.[38,177] It has been reported that positive associations exist between Hashimoto's thyroiditis (or multinodular goiter) and thyroid cancer.

Genetic factors influencing the development of thyroid cancer have been reported, including chromosome instability in patients with medullary thyroid carcinoma.[178] An increased incidence of HLA-DR1 in differentiated thyroid carcinoma was reported by one group[179] but was not found by others.[180] We recently detected an association of HLA-DR7 with differentiated follicular thyroid cancer in patients without a previous history of head and neck irradiation, but not in those with radiation-associated thyroid cancer.[181]

Thyroid carcinomas are present in several familial syndromes, including Cowden's disease (hamartomas, multinodular goiters, and thyroid, breast, colon, and lung cancer),[182] familial adenomatous polyposis,[183,184] Gardner's syndrome,[185] and familial chemodectomas.[186] The incidence of thyroid cancer is estimated to be increased 100-fold above baseline in patients with intestinal polyposis.[183,184] However, familial differentiated thyroid cancer in the context of these syndromes is very rare. A large majority of familial cancers (almost always papillary) occur as isolated, nonsyndromic, papillary thyroid cancer, in which no candidate predisposing oncogene has been detected. This form of familial cancer has been reported in 3% to 10% of patients in different series.[33,187] Recently, an epidemiologic study demonstrated that these pedigrees exhibit the phenomenon of "genetic anticipation," consisting of the appearance of thyroid carcinoma at an earlier age with increased aggressiveness in the second and subsequent generations.[32] In the same families, a germline alteration has been demonstrated, consisting of short telomeres and increased telomerase activity, leading to genomic instability and possibly predisposing to the risk for thyroid carcinoma.[188]

DIAGNOSIS, CLINICAL FEATURES, AND COURSE

In past decades, the feature of differentiated (papillary and follicular) and commonly of medullary thyroid carcinoma was the discovery, often fortuitous, of an asymptomatic thyroid nodule. Recently, the most frequent presentation of thyroid carcinoma has been a positive biopsy of a nodule discovered at neck ultrasound performed for nonthyroidal diseases or for benign thyroid disorders.[16,189,190] Sometimes, particularly in children, one or more metastatic lymph nodes may be the first sign of the disease. More rarely, distant metastases in the lung or the bone from follicular carcinoma may be the initial symptom. Hoarseness, dysphagia, and dyspnea are seldom hallmarks of the tumor; these findings are suggestive of advanced stages of the disease. At physical examination, the nodule, usually single, is firm; is movable during swelling; and often is not distinguishable from a benign lesion. Carcinoma should be suspected when the nodule is single in an otherwise normal thyroid; when it is found in children or adolescents, in males, or in association with ipsilateral enlarged lymph nodes; and, particularly, when a history of previous exposure to external radiation is present. Whatever the manifestation, the final diagnosis of malignancy must rely on the results of FNAC, which should be performed on any palpable nodule. Provided that an adequate specimen is obtained, three cytologic results are possible: benign, malignant, or indeterminate (or suspicious). False-negative and false-positive results are rare. Other diagnostic procedures are seldom useful in the diagnostic evaluation of thyroid nodules, with the exception of measurement of serum calcitonin, whose increase may be pathognomonic of medullary thyroid cancer.[48,191] Measurement of thyroid hormones and TSH may help in revealing the small proportion of "hot," almost invariably benign, nodules. Positive thyroid autoantibodies suggest the presence of an underlying autoimmune disease, which reduces but does not extinguish the possibility of an association with thyroid malignancy. Thyroid ultrasonography, although not able to differentiate benign and

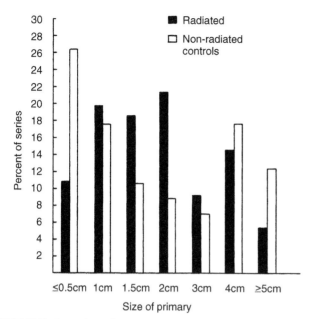

FIGURE 18-7. Comparison of the distribution of the size of primary tumors among 100 non–radiation-associated thyroid malignancies and an equal number of radiation-associated tumors. All were differentiated thyroid carcinomas. The distribution of sizes was not statistically different, although the radiation-associated tumors were slightly larger on average in this comparison than were tumors lacking association with prior x-ray treatment.

malignant lesions, is useful for assessing the number and size of the nodule(s) and the structure of the extranodular thyroid, and for guiding the aspiration of poorly palpable nodules.

Papillary carcinomas occur at any age. They are found in children and increase in frequency to highest incidence in the third and fourth decades.[192] Papillary carcinomas remain in the thyroid gland for a long time, and multicentric lesions are present in half of patients. One third are found initially to have nodal metastases, about 10% have extrathyroidal invasion, and 7.5% have distant metastases.[42,193] These tumors may exist for decades without producing serious symptoms or causing death.[194] They tend to metastasize to cervical lymph nodes and, ultimately, to the lungs. It is an especially benign process in young adults and rarely causes death in persons younger than 40 years. In older patients, the disease is more invasive and behaves in some instances like undifferentiated carcinoma.[195] Positive cervical nodes do not seem to carry an adverse risk in young individuals, but they do imply a worse prognosis in patients older than 40 years (Fig. 18-7). Pulmonary metastasis may be manifested as large "snowballs" or may give a diffuse mottling appearance on chest radiography. Almost all papillary cancer metastases have some ability to take up ^{131}I when first diagnosed. Occasionally, these lesions produce large amounts of thyroid hormone. Obstructive pulmonary disease, arteriovenous shunting, hypoxia, and cyanosis tend to develop gradually in patients with extensive pulmonary metastases. As noted previously, the primary lesions are commonly found to have areas with both papillary and follicular patterns, and the metastatic deposits may be of either variety. Lesions with mixed papillary and follicular elements in the primary tumor behave more or less like papillary cancers, but in our experience, they tend to be more malignant, with greater incidences of recurrence, invasion, and death than are seen in lesions with a purely papillary histology. The mortality from papillary cancer is 8% to 20%, mainly among older patients who have fixed or invasive cervical lesions or distant metastases

at the time of diagnosis[125] (Fig. 18-8). About half of patients who die of this disease succumb because of local invasion.

Papillary carcinoma tends to be aggressive in preteenagers. Children have lymph node or pulmonary metastases more often than adults do,[196] and the tumor causes death in 10% or more of patients. Treatment is essentially as outlined for adults, but long-term follow-up is stressed because of the continued occurrence of relapse.

Follicular cancers occur in an older age group, with peak incidence in the fifth decade of life. They are manifested commonly as a slowly growing thyroid mass, with extrathyroidal invasion in 25%, involvement of local nodes in 5% to 10%, and distant metastases in 10% to 20%. The histologic pattern ranges from almost normal appearing thyroid tissue to rather anaplastic looking sheets of cells. Direct invasion of strap muscles and the trachea is characteristic, and resectability depends on this feature. These lesions tend to metastasize to the lungs and bone. Bone metastases are usually osteolytic. Commonly, lesions retain the ability to accumulate radioactive iodide and thus are theoretically susceptible to ^{131}I treatment. The results, which are not so satisfactory, are discussed below. Follicular cancers are more lethal than papillary tumors, and mortality over the 10 to 15 years following diagnosis is 10% to 50%, again primarily in patients with fixed or invasive disease or distant metastases at the time of initial diagnosis.[125]

Hürthle cell carcinomas behave much as other follicular tumors do.[141] They have a pronounced tendency to recur in the neck many years after the original resection and to cause death by local invasion. Hürthle cell carcinomas often accumulate ^{131}I poorly and may not be amenable to this therapy.

Medullary thyroid cancer was first described as a unique tumor of the thyroid characterized by sheets of cells with large nuclei, fibrosis, multicentricity, and extensive amyloid deposits, with an unexpectedly benign course.[128] These tumors account for 4% to 10% of thyroid cancers and now are known to be derived from the C cells, or parafollicular cells, which are of ultimobranchial origin.[197] About 70% occur alone, and 30% occur as part of MEN2A in association with pheochromocytoma, parathyroid adenoma, and cutaneous lichen amyloidosis; or as part of MEN2B in association with unilateral or bilateral pheochromocytomas, mucosal neuromas, neurofibromas, café-au-lait spots, and possibly Gardner's syndrome.[29,198] Hyperplasia of the C cells precedes the development of cancer.[198] Medullary tumors secrete calcitonin and carcinoembryonic antigen, which allows their diagnosis, and in addition can produce serotonin, prostaglandins, adrenocorticotropic hormone, histaminase, and other peptides.[199-201] Calcitonin is produced in excess, but patients typically are eucalcemic. In sporadic cases, the diagnosis can be achieved by measuring calcitonin levels in the basal condition[48] or after a provocative stimulus with calcium infusion or pentagastrin stimulation.[202,203] In familial cases, the discovery that germline point mutations of the *ret* proto-oncogene are specific causative events in almost 100% of affected kindreds[204] has allowed the development of genetic screening tests for the early diagnosis and preventive treatment of familial medullary thyroid cancer.[205] Tumors follow a course almost like that of follicular cancer and often can be controlled by surgery.

Undifferentiated tumors occur with various configurations, and this has given rise to terms such as giant cell carcinoma, carcinosarcoma, and epidermoid carcinoma. They behave much as invasive tumors elsewhere: They tend to cause local invasion and compression of structures in the neck, and they metastasize to the lymph nodes and lungs. Perhaps no more than 10% are

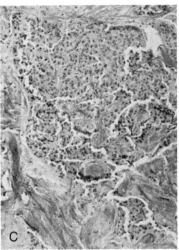
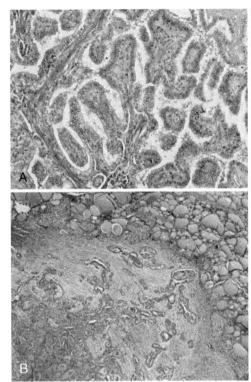

FIGURE 18-8. **A,** Histologic pattern of malignant tumors of the thyroid-papillary carcinoma. Note the tall cells and the fibrovascular core of the papillae. **B,** Follicular adenocarcinoma showing fair preservation of architecture, active colloid resorption, and vesicular nuclei. **C,** Medullary carcinoma with sheets of large cells, fibrosis, and amyloid visible by Congo red staining. (Courtesy Dr. Francis Straus, Department of Pathology, University of Chicago.)

resectable when first discovered; the remainder are rapidly and uniformly lethal within 6 months to 1 year. A variety of evidence suggests that some anaplastic cancers originate from long-existing differentiated thyroid cancer.[206] A subgroup of tumors previously classified as anaplastic, with characteristic islands of cells, have been designated as the insular variants of follicular carcinoma. These tumors are less aggressive than the usual anaplastic cancer; because they often collect therapeutically useful quantities of ^{131}I, their recognition is important.[207]

Lymphomas may originate in the thyroid gland. In 30% to 80% of cases, the thyroid gland is extensively involved with Hashimoto's thyroiditis, and hypothyroidism may be present as well. It appears probable that lymphomas arise from the lymphocytes associated with thyroiditis. Lymphomas are typically of the diffuse, large cell variety. The clinical picture is usually that of a rapidly enlarging neck mass producing symptoms from pressure on contiguous structures in an adult. The lesion spreads to adjacent lymph node clusters, enlarges rapidly, and is often painful. Confusion with thyroiditis or small cell carcinoma is common on biopsy unless appropriate tumor cell markers are identified. Although the incidence is low, Hashimoto's disease is definitely a risk factor for lymphoma.

Metastatic carcinomas occur in a significant proportion of patients dying of other malignancies. These come from melanomas; breast tumors; pulmonary carcinomas; gastric, pancreatic, and intestinal carcinomas; lymphomas; cervical carcinomas; and renal cancers. It sometimes is difficult to differentiate these lesions from primary thyroid cancer. Rarely, thyroidectomy is needed for this purpose.

PROGNOSTIC FACTORS AND SELECTION OF THERAPY

Most patients, particularly those with differentiated histotypes, have high cure rates after initial treatment, but some are at risk for recurrence or death. Univariate analysis of the risk for recur-

rence or death has considered several potential prognostic factors that are based on epidemiologic, biological, clinical, pathologic, and, more recently, molecular features of the tumor, as listed in Table 18-7. Recently, point mutations of *BRAF* have been associated in independent series with an adverse prognosis and more aggressive behavior, including frequent loss of iodine uptake.[208] Factors more commonly associated with an adverse prognosis are reported in Table 18-8.

Age and Sex

In the papillary and follicular histotypes, the risk for recurrence and cancer-related death increases linearly with age at diagnosis.[42,125,127,209-216] In older patients, clinical relapse occurs more rapidly after initial treatment, and the interval between detection of recurrence and death is shorter.[211] Older patients tend to have more locally aggressive tumors and a higher incidence of distant metastases at diagnosis and more aggressive histologic variants. Their metastases often lack ^{131}I uptake. On the other hand, children and adolescents have an excellent long-term prognosis and a very low mortality rate, even when affected by metastatic disease.[196,217-219] Male sex has been reported as an independent risk factor in some series[42,211,215,220] but not in others. Its importance as a prognostic factor is always less than that of age.

Associated Autoimmune Phenomena

With the exception of one report,[40] no major differences have been found in several series of patients with differentiated thyroid cancer with or without Graves' disease with regard to clinical features and response to therapy[37,39,41,177,221-223] or tumor-related mortality.[224] On the contrary, the association of Hashimoto's thyroiditis[225] or lymphocytic infiltration[132] with papillary thyroid cancer seems to confer a better prognosis. In a series from Italy,[226] circulating thyroid autoantibodies were found in 23% of patients with differentiated thyroid cancer. No difference in final outcome was found between antibody-positive and antibody-negative

Table 18-7. Prognostic Factors for Differentiated Thyroid Carcinoma

Patient-related factors
  Age
  Sex
  Autoimmune thyroid diseases
Histopathologic factors
  Tumor histotype and its variants
  Tumor grade and DNA ploidy
  Tumor burden
    Primary tumor
    Multicentric tumor
    Extrathyroidal invasion
    Lymph node metastases
    Distant metastases
Molecular factors
  Oncogenes, antioncogenes, and oncogene-encoded proteins
Treatment-related factors
  Extent of primary surgery
  [131]I ablation of thyroid residue
Tumor markers
  Serum thyroglobulin
Prognostic scoring systems
  EORTC
  Institute Gustave-Roussy
  TNM
  AMES
  Clinical class
  AGES-MACIS
  Ohio State University

AGES, Age, grade (Broders'), tumor extent, size of primary; *AMES*, age, distant metastases, extent and size of primary tumor; *EORTC*, European Organization for Research on Treatment of Cancer; *MACIS*, distant metastases, age, completeness of surgery, invasion of extrathyroidal tissue, size; *TNM*, primary tumor, lymph node status, distant metastases.

Table 18-8. Factors Associated With Adverse Prognosis

Older age
Distant metastases
Less well-differentiated histologic variant
  Follicular, widely invasive, tall cells, columnar cells, oxyphilic cells, Hürthle cells, insular
Large tumor size
Extrathyroidal invasion
Multicentricity
Lymph node metastases
High tumor grade and DNA aploidy
Male sex
BRAF(V600E) mutation

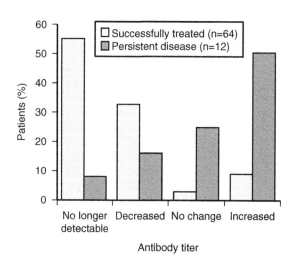

FIGURE 18-9. Changes in antithyroid autoantibody titers in relation to tumor outcome in differentiated thyroid cancer. (Data from Pacini F, Mariotti S, Formica N, et al: Thyroid autoantibodies in thyroid cancer: incidence and relationship with tumour outcome, Acta Endocrinol [Copenh] 119:373, 1988.)

patients. The disappearance of circulating antibodies was correlated with effective treatment of the disease, whereas their persistence was associated with stable or progressive disease (Fig. 18-9), suggesting that complete removal of thyroid autoantigens after effective treatment is followed by disappearance of the corresponding autoantibodies.[227]

Histopathologic Factors

A poor prognosis has been reported with the tall cell variant,[138,228] the columnar cell variant,[229] and the oxyphilic variant[230,231] of papillary thyroid cancer. A good prognosis is found with the encapsulated[140,232,233] and follicular variants.[127,134,139] An intermediate prognosis has been reported for the diffuse sclerosing variant.[137,234]

Widely invasive follicular cancers have a less favorable prognosis than do minimally invasive tumors. Other follicular variants (e.g., the Hürthle cell, insular, and trabecular variants) are often associated with a poor prognosis.[211,235,236]

Tumor Grade and DNA Ploidy

Tumor grade was a significant prognostic factor both by univariate analysis and by multivariate analysis in papillary thyroid carcinoma studied at the Mayo Clinic[225] and in three European series.[210,237,238]

In the report by Joensuu and colleagues, DNA aneuploidy was an adverse factor in univariate analysis but was not an independent prognostic factor.[239] In the Mayo Clinic series, abnormal DNA content was associated with higher cancer mortality in high-risk tumors.[42]

Size of the Primary Tumor and Multicentricity

Microcarcinomas (or minimal or occult) have an excellent prognosis in terms of survival and relapse-free survival, whatever the extent of the primary surgical treatment. Several series have reported a progressive increase in risk for recurrence and tumor-specific mortality with increasing size of the primary tumor.* Tumor size seems to be more predictive in papillary than in follicular tumors.

Multicentricity, whether an expression of intrathyroidal metastases or of multiple primary tumoral foci,[232] has been associated with significantly higher rates of lymph node metastasis,[232,242,243] locally persistent disease and distant metastases,[232] and 30-year mortality.[240]

Extrathyroidal Invasion

Extrathyroidal invasion is present in 5% to 10% of papillary tumors and in 3% to 5% of follicular tumors; it exposes the patient to higher rates of local recurrence and distant metastases, as well as to a higher percentage of tumor-related death.† Invasion limited to the thyroid capsule, without infiltration of soft tissues, carries the same adverse prognosis that is seen with overt extrathyroidal invasion.[221]

Lymph Node Metastases

Lymph node metastases are present in 37% to 65% in different series of papillary carcinoma‡ and much less often (nearly 17%)

*References 42, 193, 216, 235, 240, and 241.
†References 42, 193, 210, 232, 240, 244, and 245.
‡References 42, 125, 127, 193, 235, 246, and 247.

in the follicular histotype.[248] Local node involvement is found with microcarcinomas and with large tumors and may be bilateral in cases of bilateral tumor. Some authors have shown that regional lymph node metastases are associated with higher rates of tumor recurrence and cancer-specific mortality,* whereas others have found that cumulative survival is not significantly affected.[42,133,229,252] In the series of Ohio State University,[240] the presence of lymph node metastases was an important independent prognostic factor that predicted cancer death. Bilateral cervical and mediastinal nodes were particularly likely to be associated with cancer death. In the series of the Department of Endocrinology in Pisa, of 304 patients with lymph node metastases, 253 (83.2%) were cured after surgery and ^{131}I therapy, 37 (12.1%) had persistent progressive disease, and 14 (4.6%) died of their disease during a mean follow-up period of 12 years. Taken together, these data indicate that lymph node metastases are a potential cause of death and underscore the importance of early and thorough treatment.

Distant Metastases

Distant metastases at diagnosis confer the poorest prognosis in patients with papillary, follicular, or medullary thyroid carcinoma. Tumor-specific mortality of patients with distant metastases ranges from 36% to 47% at 5 years and reaches approximately 70% at 15 years.[42,236,253-255] Univariate analysis has shown the following factors to be associated with better prognosis in the case of distant metastases: young age, well-differentiated histotype, localization in the lung rather than in bone, small size, and the presence of ^{131}I uptake. However, multivariate analysis has shown that the extent of metastatic involvement rather than the site (lung or bone) has prognostic value.[236,256,257] The best outcome is found with micronodular metastases visible with radioiodine whole body scanning (WBS) but not visible with standard radiographs.[133,196,236,253,256-259]

Oncogenes, Antioncogenes, and Oncogene-Encoded Proteins

The presence of gene alterations or of oncogene-encoded proteins has been correlated with prognosis. Loss of expression of thyroid-specific differentiation genes (e.g., the *TSH receptor, Tg,* and *TPO* genes) is associated with poor outcomes of poorly differentiated or undifferentiated tumors.[260] Somatic mutations of the *p53* oncogene or hyperexpression of its encoded protein is found exclusively in poorly differentiated and anaplastic tumors.[160,261] Point mutations of the *ras* gene and overexpression of p21 protein have been found in papillary thyroid carcinoma and have been correlated with poor survival rates.[262] Likewise, c-myc expression has been correlated with more aggressive thyroid carcinomas.[263]

In a retrospective study comparing patients with papillary thyroid cancer with or without *RET/PTC* rearrangements, no difference was noted in their outcomes.[264] On the contrary, point mutations of *BRAF* have been associated with an adverse prognosis and more aggressive behavior, including frequent loss of iodine uptake.[208] Somatic *RET* proto-oncogene mutations, found in 50% of cases of sporadic medullary thyroid carcinoma, have been associated with metastatic progression and worse outcomes than those of tumors not carrying the mutation.[265,266]

The above findings represent only the beginning of a new way to look into tumor biology and indicate that exploration of oncogenes and oncogene products may yield new insights with regard to the prognosis for thyroid tumors.

---

*References 193, 211, 220, 240, 245, and 249-251.

Extent of Primary Surgery

Total (or near-total) thyroidectomy is associated with fewer cancer recurrences and tumor-related deaths.[267-270] In the Mayo Clinic series, the extent of surgery significantly affected the risk for local recurrence.[125] Data from the University of Chicago revealed that when compared with lobectomy or bilateral subtotal resection, near-total thyroidectomy decreased the risk for death in papillary tumors larger than 1 cm and decreased the risk for recurrence among all patients.[193] A much higher frequency of recurrent cancer in the form of lung metastasis has been reported with subtotal thyroidectomy.[271] In another series, patients with tumors 1.5 cm or larger, multicentric tumors, local invasion, or cervical metastases had significantly fewer recurrences after total (11.3%) than after subtotal (22.0%) thyroidectomy.[272] Similar results have been observed in the series of the Institute of Endocrinology in Pisa.

[131]I Ablation of Thyroid Residue

Postsurgical radioiodine ablation of the thyroid residue may destroy microscopic neoplastic foci and may reduce the risk for relapse. Whereas some authors have found no significant effect of ^{131}I ablation on the rate of recurrence or tumor-related death,[42,210] others have shown beneficial effects in terms of both recurrence and long-term survival,[193,235] at least in patients with tumors larger than 1.5 cm. However, no randomized study is available, and retrospective studies suffer from the comparison of groups of patients (ablated vs. not ablated) not always accurately matched with regard to other important clinicopathologic factors. Ablation increases the sensitivity of subsequent ^{131}I WBS and the specificity of serum Tg determination, and it provides reassurance to the patient when these tests are negative on subsequent examination.

Serum Thyroglobulin Measurement

Serum Tg measured after initial treatment gives valuable predictive information on subsequent disease evolution. After surgical treatment has been provided, and when ^{131}I imaging is negative, the finding of undetectable serum Tg in the absence of thyroid hormone administration is an excellent indicator of definitive cure.[273-275] On the contrary, persistence of elevated serum Tg concentrations requires extensive clinical evaluation, including WBS after the administration of therapeutic doses of ^{131}I and imaging studies, to detect the site of Tg production and to plan the most appropriate treatment.[236,276]

Prognostic Scoring Systems

Prognostic scoring systems based on multiple regression analysis of prognostic factors are intended to distinguish between low-risk patients to be treated with less aggressive protocols and high-risk patients to be treated with the most aggressive therapy.

Several scoring systems are available (Table 18-9). The EORTC (European Organization for the Research and Treatment of Cancer) system considers age at diagnosis, sex, principal histotype, extrathyroidal invasion, and distant metastases.[277,278] The Institut Gustave-Roussy system is based on age at diagnosis and histotype.[211] The TNM system (by the International Union Against Cancer) is based on the extent of the primary tumor (T), lymph node status (N), the presence of distant metastases (M), and, since the last version, age (younger or older than 45 years) and capsule (encapsulated or nonencapsulated).[279,280] AMES, an acronym for age, distant metastases, and extent and size of the primary tumor,[281] was subsequently modified to DAMES by adding DNA ploidy.[282] AGES includes age, grade (by Broders'

Table 18-9. Variables Considered in Different Prognostic Scoring Systems for Differentiated Thyroid Cancer

Variable	EORTC	TNM	AMES	AGES	MACIS	Clinical Class	Ohio Un	IGR
Age	Yes	Yes	Yes	Yes	Yes			Yes
Sex	Yes							
Histology	Yes							Yes
Extrathyroid invasion	Yes	Yes	Yes	Yes	Yes	Yes	Yes	
Extent of primary tumor	Yes	Yes	Yes	Yes	Yes	Yes		
Lymph node metastases	Yes				Yes	Yes		
Distant metastases	Yes	Yes	Yes	Yes	Yes	Yes	Yes	
Tumor capsule	Yes							
Histologic grade				Yes				
Completeness of surgery					Yes			

IGR, Institut Gustave-Roussy; other acronyms as listed in Table 18-7.

classification), tumor extent (local invasion and distant metastases), and size of the primary tumor.[42] In 1993, AGES was revised to MACIS, which includes distant metastases, age, completeness of surgery, invasion of extrathyroidal tissues, and size.[224] The Ohio State University system considers tumor size, the presence or absence of cervical metastases, multiple tumors, local tumor invasion, and distant metastases.[240] Clinical Class, a very simple and effective staging system developed at the University of Chicago,[193] consists of four classes that depend on the extent of tumor tissue: Class I includes patients with single or multiple intrathyroidal foci; class II patients have lymph node metastases; in class III are patients whose tumors (or unresectable lymph nodes) have invaded outside the thyroid gland; and class IV patients have distant metastases. This classification is primarily anatomic but correlates well with prognosis.

INITIAL TREATMENT FOR THYROID CANCER

In differentiated thyroid cancer, each prognostic system defines low- and high-risk patients. We find that the distinction between low- and high-risk groups is clearly reflected in the simple Clinical Class staging just described. High-risk patients are mainly those with invasive or metastatic disease. However, in most instances, it is impossible to stage cancer correctly at the time of surgery because final pathologic review, node status, and results of ^{131}I scanning are unavailable. Some "low-risk" tumors unfortunately behave as though they were "high risk," and this difference cannot be predicted.[283] Complications of surgery are minimal in the hands of an experienced surgeon.[193,284] Thyroxine replacement probably is indicated in every patient who has had thyroid cancer, regardless of the extent of surgery. Radiation exposure from ^{131}I scanning and ablation is equal to that of one CT scan and is probably inconsequential. More complete thyroid surgery (at least a lobectomy plus contralateral subtotal thyroidectomy or near-total thyroidectomy) improves the overall prognosis, even for low-risk patients with tumors larger than 1 cm in clinical classes I and II.[126,193] Ablation with ^{131}I decreases recurrence and may[126,193,285] or may not[42] decrease deaths, but it clearly improves the value of postablation WBS and makes serial Tg measurements useful. Further study is needed to prove the value of routine postoperative ^{131}I ablation.[286] For these reasons, we believe that the patient's best interest is served in most cases by more complete surgery, postoperative ^{131}I ablation, T[4] replacement, and careful follow-up, as described in the following.

Class I Differentiated (Papillary and Follicular) Carcinoma

The minimal surgical procedure for thyroid carcinoma should be total (or near-total) thyroidectomy, whenever the diagnosis

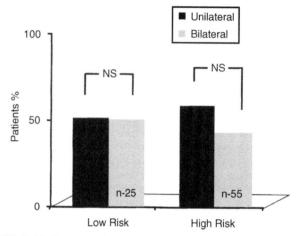

FIGURE 18-10. Percentage of contralateral tumor involvement in low- and high-risk patients who underwent completion thyroidectomy for differentiated thyroid cancer.

has been made before surgery at FNAC. Less extended procedures (lobectomy and subtotal thyroidectomy) may be considered in cases of papillary thyroid cancer discovered accidentally at final histology after surgery for benign disorders, provided that the tumor was small (<1 to 1.5 cm), unifocal, and intrathyroidal, and had favorable histology. The value of total or near-total thyroidectomy for low-risk patients has been confirmed by the results of second "completion" thyroidectomy performed in the centers of the two authors of this chapter. The percentage of patients with detectable tumor in the reoperative specimens was 31% at the University of Chicago[103] and 44% at the University of Pisa.[130] In the last series, no difference in the rate of second tumors was found between patients defined as low risk or high risk at the time of the first operation (Fig. 18-10). In any surgical procedure, recurrent laryngeal nerves and parathyroid glands should be identified carefully, and portions of the thyroid (especially the posterior capsule on the contralateral side) may be left behind, if necessary, to prevent damage.

In lesions that are found to be multicentric on the basis of observations by the surgeon or the pathologist, greater effort is made to perform total thyroidectomy, as long as it can be done without compromise of the parathyroid glands. After surgery, residual thyroid tissue is ablated by ^{131}I administration in most cases, especially in patients who have multicentric foci or a history of irradiation. All patients are given suppressive therapy with thyroid hormone.

Our own experience[193] and long-term follow-up of 576 cases of papillary thyroid cancer by Mazzaferri and Young[268,285] appear to support this approach. Patients with near-total thyroidectomy and postoperative ablation had a significantly improved prognosis, especially when follow-up extended over 10 to 15 years. Massin and coworkers found that "complete thyroidectomy" and ^{131}I ablation gave the lowest incidence of late metastatic recurrence,[271] as did Samaan and colleagues,[126] who found that ^{131}I treatment was the most important influence on recurrence and survival.

Most series reporting on the results of total or near-total thyroidectomy indicate that hypoparathyroidism occurs in 1% to 15% of patients, and recurrent unilateral nerve damage occurs in 2% to 5%, but fortunately, bilateral nerve injury is rare.[287] It is because of these complications and the apparently satisfactory results attained with lobectomy that some investigators prefer the simpler procedure. On the other hand, 20% to 80% of stage I thyroid cancers are multicentric.[128,288] It is clear that not all these foci are of clinical importance, but the recurrence rate of cancer in the contralateral lobe after unilateral lobectomy is at least 6%, and some patients with recurrence eventually die of their lesion.[271,289,290] Because of known multicentricity, the ability of our collaborating surgeons to avoid hypoparathyroidism, and the associated improved prognosis,[193] we prefer the more extensive resection. Surgeons who are especially skilled in performing thyroidectomies can hold the incidence of hypoparathyroidism to about 1% and have an equally low incidence of recurrent nerve damage.

In past years, more radical procedures, including prophylactic radical neck dissection, were advocated for thyroid carcinomas. Forty-six percent of patients with presumed stage I disease were found, in fact, to have lymph node involvement when specimens were studied thoroughly after prophylactic neck dissection.[291] Apparently, however, these lymph node metastases, when not clinically detectable, in some way are controlled by the body's defense mechanisms and rarely lead to death of the patient. Thus, recent opinion is controversial regarding prophylactic central node dissection but is definitively in agreement against radical or en bloc neck dissection.

Because follicular lesions tend to be more directly invasive and lethal than papillary lesions,[141] many surgeons pursue a more aggressive operative approach with stage I follicular cancer than with papillary cancer and perform routine near-total thyroidectomy in patients with the former lesion.[292] Postoperative ^{131}I thyroid ablation and continuous thyroid hormone administration are considered essential.[293]

Up to 20% of low-grade follicular neoplasms are misdiagnosed on operative frozen section as benign, with the diagnosis achieved 1 to 3 days later after review of permanent sections. If the lesion is smaller than 1 cm, unicentric, and intrathyroidal, and the patient is younger than 45 years, no further surgery is required, and, as indicated before, some physicians accept lobectomy as a definitive procedure. In general, in patients with lesions larger than 1 cm who are older than 45 years or with multifocality, we prefer reoperation to achieve near-total thyroidectomy, along with subsequent ^{131}I therapy. As was already mentioned, in an analysis of patients who have undergone a second operation, we found that in 31% of operations at the University of Chicago[103] and in 44% of those performed at the University of Pisa,[130] residual cancer was recovered on the remaining lobe.[67] This problem is best avoided by performing at least a lobectomy plus contralateral subtotal thyroidectomy if any question about the benignity of the "adenoma" is still unanswered at the time of surgery.

The use of radioactive iodide, as described above, can be questioned, because the ablative dosage exposes these patients, who often are young, to 10 to 15 rad of whole body radiation.

Although the genetic and carcinogenic risks of this radiation dosage cannot be ignored completely, they are minimally different from the average background whole body radiation exposure that individuals normally receive by age 30 years, and most likely do not represent a significant hazard. In addition, the recent introduction of thyroid ablation aided by a recombinant human TSH (rhTSH) preparation may result in lower radiation doses to the whole body, thereby preserving the quality of life.[294,295]

Class II Differentiated Carcinoma

Less disagreement surrounds the management of class II disease. The usual procedure is a near-total or total thyroidectomy.[271,296] Small portions of the gland may be left in situ (for later radioiodide ablation), if necessary, to preserve recurrent laryngeal nerves or viability of the parathyroid glands. A modified neck dissection is performed to remove involved nodes. An attempt is made to retain the jugular vein and sternocleidomastoid muscles, and an en bloc resection is not attempted, except occasionally in patients with metastatic follicular cancer. If both sides of the neck are involved, resections usually are staged, because otherwise the incidence of tracheal edema requiring tracheotomy is significant. Radical neck dissection with removal of the jugular vein and sternocleidomastoid muscle is not favored, because the disease usually can be managed by the less mutilating procedure, and uninvolved nodes that become apparent at a later date generally can be resected successfully. Patients are given ^{131}I to ablate residual thyroid tissue after surgery and for treatment of functioning metastases found on scanning.

Class III Differentiated Carcinoma

Patients with class III disease should receive a near-total or total thyroidectomy, appropriate lymph node dissection, and resection of all possibly invading neoplasm. The tendency at present is to avoid mutilating surgery in patients younger than 45 years in an effort to resect all cancerous tissue, because less extensive surgery,[131]I treatment, and suppressive thyroid hormone therapy usually lead to prolonged survival or cure, even if complete excision of the tumor is impossible.[297] [131]I therapy is given as discussed in the following section. External irradiation may be useful in preventing recurrence.[298] However, because most cases appear to be controlled by surgery and ^{131}I, and because definitive experience with supplemental prophylactic irradiation is not always available, the usual course is to withhold irradiation until recurrence is seen in younger patients, but to advise prophylactic treatment in patients older than 45 to 50 years who have known residual disease after surgery and radioactive iodine (RAI) treatment.

Class IV Differentiated Disease

Patients with a thyroid mass and solitary metastasis to the lung or bone probably should have thyroidectomy and excision of the single metastasis, because cure or prolonged survival may be obtained. If multiple metastases are present, thyroidectomy is probably the quickest way to achieve hypothyroidism, so that uptake of radioactive iodide in the metastases and possible therapies can be evaluated.

Hürthle Cell Carcinoma

It is clear that Hürthle cell tumors range in invasiveness from zero to an aggressively locally invading lesion or a tumor with rapidly growing pulmonary metastases. These variations result in a wide range of opinion on therapy. We advocate treatment as described for follicular cancer, of which these are a subgroup.

Postoperative ^{131}I ablation is carried out, although its value may be restricted because many Hürthle cell tumors fail to accumulate [131]I. Invasive tumors (class III) should be treated with mantle irradiation. [131]I treatment is attempted for class III or IV tumors, but it usually is not possible despite the presence of functioning metastases as proved by elevated Tg levels.

Lymphoma

Staging should include neck, chest, and abdominal CT scans and bone marrow biopsy. If the disease appears to be limited to the thyroid gland and contiguous lymph nodes, thyroidectomy is advised, although occasionally only biopsy is possible. Patients with intrathyroidal lymphoma or disease limited to the neck and upper part of the mediastinum have been treated conventionally by mantle irradiation to about 45 Gy over a 3 to 4 week period.[299] Because the overall survival rate at 5 years has been about 50%,[299-301] patients increasingly are being treated primarily by chemotherapy followed by radiotherapy. Patients with more extensive disease and those who relapse are given chemotherapy.

Undifferentiated Thyroid Carcinoma

Undifferentiated thyroid carcinoma is among the most aggressive malignant tumors in humans. Management of this type of cancer is cause for major concern because its poor prognosis is not ameliorated by surgery, chemotherapy, or radiotherapy. As soon as a diagnosis of undifferentiated thyroid cancer has been made, total thyroidectomy should be attempted. Unfortunately, infiltration of the soft tissues of the neck, almost invariably present at surgery, makes radical surgery impossible. External radiotherapy is used after surgery to control local disease, but this treatment is generally unsatisfactory.[302] Several chemotherapeutic protocols, including single (doxorubicin) and combination (doxorubicin plus cisplatin) drugs, have been totally disappointing.[303,304] The combination of radiotherapy and chemotherapy has been used with very modest advantage.[305-307] With any form of treatment, mean survival ranges between 3 and 12 months after diagnosis,[305-308] although individual survival exceeding 2 to 3 years has been reported.[309]

Because radical surgery, as mentioned earlier, is rarely feasible, a novel approach is to use hyperfractionated radiotherapy in combination with chemotherapy as initial treatment, with surgery left as a second step.[310] The idea is to control and reduce the primary tumor with medical therapy, thus giving the surgeon a better chance to perform a radical thyroidectomy. Further radiotherapy and chemotherapy may be added after surgery to stabilize the results of treatment. With this integrated therapeutic approach, complete local control has been obtained in 5 of 16 patients, and 3 patients survived longer than 20 months in one study.[311] Other schemes based on the same combination of radiotherapy and chemotherapy have been used with similar results.[312,313]

The discovery of point mutations of the *p53* tumor suppressor gene specifically associated with undifferentiated thyroid carcinoma[160,314] has opened a new field of research aimed at the development of more effective treatment strategies at the molecular level. Recent studies using tyrosine kinase inhibitors are discussed in the following sections.

RADIOIODINE ABLATION OF POSTSURGICAL THYROID REMNANTS

The rationale for postsurgical radioiodine thyroid ablation is based on the following considerations. Destroying any residual thyroid cell will facilitate subsequent follow-up based on serum Tg measurement and diagnostic radioiodine WBS; furthermore, ^{131}I may destroy microscopic foci of multicentric papillary carcinoma, thus decreasing subsequent tumor recurrence. The indication for thyroid ablation should be based on risk stratification and evidence-based benefit for patients. Recent guidelines[53,54] suggest that for unifocal micropapillary carcinomas (<1 cm) with favorable histology and no extrathyroidal extension, the long-term prognosis is already so good that it cannot be improved by thyroid ablation. In this category of patients, no evidence of any benefit by thyroid ablation is evident, and thus it should not be recommended. In all other patients at intermediate or high risk for relapse, thyroid ablation is associated with a decrease in rate of relapse and with an increase in survival rate.

Traditionally, postoperative ^{131}I therapy was performed 4 to 6 weeks after surgery without thyroid hormone administration in the interim, or later, after replacement therapy was discontinued. Recently, thyroid ablation after rhTSH stimulation instead of T_4 withdrawal entered clinical practice, after preliminary clinical trials had demonstrated similar rates of successful thyroid ablation compared with thyroid hormone withdrawal and significant expense, with preservation of quality of life and reduced total body radiation.[315,316] It is possible to prepare patients by using a reduced T_4 dose protocol, as described later (see ^{131}I whole body scans), which adequately stimulates the thyroid and prevents symptomatic hypothyroidism. When an rhTSH preparation is used, thyroid ablation is effective with fixed doses of 50 to 100 mCi of radioiodine.[295] Lower rates of ablation have been observed in some reports, when 30 mCi doses were used,[317] but equivalent effectiveness has been found in other studies,[317a] and very significant reductions in radiation exposure, expense, and patient inconvenience are gained when the lower dose is used. Although use of a 100 mCi ablation dose is widespread, because it was used in the initial trial of rhTSH, many studies show that it is not superior in effectiveness to lower doses, compels hospitalization, and provides significantly larger whole body radiation. Post-therapy WBS is performed 5 to 10 days after treatment. Among patients who have undergone total or near-total thyroidectomy, total ablation is achieved in nearly 80% after 30 or 100 mCi doses[318] after thyroid hormone withdrawal, and in the same percentage after 50 or 100 mCi after use of an rhTSH preparation. Execution of a diagnostic ^{131}I WBS with a 1 to 2 mCi tracer dose before ablation is naturally less informative than the post-therapy scan with the larger dose, and has been abandoned in many centers. The diagnostic scan occasionally, although infrequently, does provide evidence of unrecognized neck nodes, metastatic disease suggesting an altered dose of ^{131}I, or lack of neck uptake due to level of completeness of surgery or sometimes to iodine contamination.

DIAGNOSTIC AND THERAPEUTIC FOLLOW-UP AFTER SURGERY AND THYROID ABLATION

It is well known that a great majority of local recurrences or distant metastases develop or are detected in the first 2 to 3 years after diagnosis. However, in a minority of cases, distant metastases may develop in late follow-up—even as late as 20 years after initial treatment[133]; this suggests that follow-up of differentiated thyroid cancer should go on throughout the patient's life.

Five percent to 20% of patients with differentiated thyroid cancer have local or regional recurrence, which usually is caused by persistent or recurrent disease in thyroid remnants or lymph nodes after incomplete initial treatment, or may be the expression of aggressive tumors. Local or regional disease may be detected easily by palpation, ultrasonography, or CT scan. WBS performed after diagnostic or therapeutic doses of ^{131}I is most important in revealing disease.

According to several large series, the frequency of distant metastases in differentiated thyroid carcinoma ranges between 10% and 18% of cases.[133,253,271,319-322] Sometimes, distant metastases, particularly in bone, may be the initial symptom of the disease, but usually (in two thirds of cases), they are discovered at the time of the primary diagnosis or soon after thyroidectomy, when the first ^{131}I WBS is performed.[133] However, distant metastases may develop later in the course of follow-up—even as late as 20 years after initial treatment.[133]

The lungs are the most common site of distant metastases, followed by the bones. The combination of lung and bone disease is found in about one third of patients with distant metastases. Other less common localizations may occur to the brain, the liver, and the skin, all of which are more likely to occur in association with lung or bone metastases. The pattern of metastatic lung involvement may vary from one or more macronodules (>1 cm in diameter) to a diffuse micronodular spread.[133,319,320] The latter usually is not detected by chest radiography and sometimes not even by CT scanning, but it can be diagnosed easily with ^{131}I WBS. Commonly, especially in papillary tumors, enlarged lymph nodes in the mediastinum may be present.[258,271] Bone metastases are associated mainly with the follicular histotype and tend to occur in older patients. The vertebrae, pelvis, and ribs are the sites more often affected, but occasionally any skeletal segment may be affected. Single lesions are present in one third of patients. Most metastases are detectable by both WBS and radiography, but a minority (about 25%) are visible only by WBS.[133,323] This latter group is the one most likely to respond to ^{131}I therapy.

Diagnostic and therapeutic strategies for monitoring patients with differentiated thyroid carcinoma are well established and very effective in detecting and treating most patients who are not cured after initial treatment. Basically, after total thyroidectomy and radioiodine ablation of thyroid residue, powerful tools are available to raise suspicions of local or distant metastases and to localize them: These include serum Tg measurement, neck ultrasound, and ^{131}I WBS. However, a substantial proportion of patients may have local or distant disease that does not concentrate radioiodine and thus is not apparent on diagnostic ^{131}I WBS. In these patients, imaging should include CT scan and PET scan. On the other hand, radioiodine therapy and reoperation are very effective modalities of treatment for metastatic patients with well-differentiated carcinoma.

Diagnostic Procedures

Clinical, Ultrasonographic, and Radiographic Examination

Clinical examination with accurate palpation of the thyroid bed and lymph node chains of the neck is performed every 6 to 12 months in any patient being monitored for thyroid carcinoma.

Ultrasonography of the neck has gained increasing importance and should be complementary to the clinical examination. In expert hands, ultrasonography is able to recognize metastatic lymph nodes smaller than 5 mm. Small, thin, oval lymph nodes detected by palpation or by ultrasound may be a normal finding in the neck and should not create unnecessary concern. If lymph node metastases are suspected, ultrasonographically guided FNA for cytology and for Tg measurement should be performed.[88]

Routine chest and bone radiographs are of little diagnostic value in the early discovery of distant metastases to the lungs or bones, particularly in patients who have undetectable levels of serum Tg. These tests are useful in patients with known metastatic disease, for monitoring the evolution of lesions, and in patients with negative ^{131}I WBS but elevated serum Tg levels suggestive of metastases that do not take up radioiodine. In this setting, PET with FDG has been indicated recently as a new, promising tool for the localization of unknown sources of serum Tg.[324-326] The method is based on enhanced glucose metabolism, observed as a nonspecific feature of neoplastic cells, including poorly differentiated thyroid tumors. FDG uptake can be seen when the patient is on L-thyroxine therapy, although it was found to be higher when the patient is hypothyroid.[327] In a recent meta-analysis of data from a multicentric study in patients with Hürthle cell tumors, PET results were informative in detecting metastatic foci in almost all cases, with a sensitivity of 92%, a specificity of 80%, a positive predictive value of 92%, and a negative predictive value of 80%.[328] The usefulness of FDG-PET has been investigated in patients with well-differentiated thyroid cancer with negative ^{131}I scan and elevated serum Tg levels. In two recent studies,[329,330] FDG-PET correctly detected metastatic disease in 94.6% of patients, influencing the therapeutic strategy in many cases. Taken together, these data indicate that FDG-PET is a promising imaging technique for the localization of residual or metastatic tumor in patients with poorly differentiated thyroid cancer and in those with well-differentiated thyroid cancer deprived of iodine uptake. However, FDG-PET is commonly negative in patients with low positive TG levels (5 to 15 ng/mL) who have negative isotope and CT scans.

Serum Thyroglobulin Measurement

Tg, the principal iodoprotein of the thyroid gland, is produced and released into the circulation by normal and neoplastic follicular cells, but not by other cell systems in the body. Thus, serum Tg measurement can be used in clinical practice as a specific and sensitive tumor marker of differentiated thyroid cancer.[331] After total thyroid ablation, undetectable serum Tg levels are found in patients free of disease, whereas detectable and often elevated serum Tg concentrations are found in patients with persistent or recurrent disease.[274,332,333] Two important factors must be considered when a serum Tg value is interpreted: (1) the level of serum TSH; and (2) the presence of circulating anti-Tg autoantibodies. Tg production by neoplastic cells is, at least in part, under TSH control. As a consequence, serum Tg concentrations are lowered, even to undetectable levels, during TSH suppression by thyroid hormone administration, and they are increased after withdrawal of therapy.[273,305,334] Serum Tg results may be altered artifactually by circulating anti-Tg antibodies, which are present in about 15% of patients.[226] Antibodies interfere with the Tg assay by producing false-positive or false-negative results, depending on the assay used.[335] Thus, serum anti-Tg antibodies should be measured any time serum Tg is measured. After thyroid ablation and in the absence of tumor, serum Tg should be theoretically undetectable, but in clinical practice, stimulated serum Tg levels less than 2 ng/mL (or less than 1), when measured in a sensitive assay that uses the World Health Organization standard, are considered as evidence of no residual disease.

As a rule, patients with undetectable TSH-stimulated serum Tg levels may be considered free of disease.[274,332,333] On the contrary, in patients with distant metastases, serum Tg concentrations are elevated when measured after TSH stimulation, and are reduced but still detectable during levothyroxine treatment. In the case of lymph node metastases, serum Tg may be low or undetectable during levothyroxine therapy but may become elevated after TSH stimulation.[274,319] Comparison of the results of serum Tg measurement versus ^{131}I WBS shows good agreement between these two techniques.[336,337] Detectable serum Tg levels usually are associated with positive WBS and indicate the presence of residual or metastatic disease. Undetectable serum Tg levels are found in patients with a negative scan and indicate that the patient is in complete remission. However, as is shown in Fig. 18-11, serum Tg assay is superior to WBS in predicting the presence of metastases in a significant proportion of patients (about 13%) who have increased serum Tg levels but negative basal WBS, as demonstrated by the presence in these patients of abnormal foci of ^{131}I uptake after administration of therapeutic doses of [131]I.[276,338-340] A representative example of this possibility is shown in Fig. 18-12.

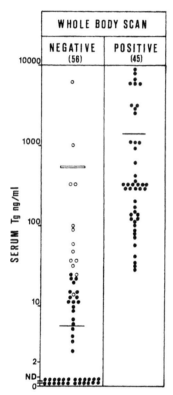

FIGURE 18-11. Relationship between serum thyroglobulin (Tg) and ^{131}I uptake at whole body scanning in patients with differentiated thyroid cancer (after total thyroidectomy). *Open symbols* in the left column indicate patients with proven nonfunctioning metastases. (Data from Pacini F, Pinchera A, Giani C, et al: Serum thyroglobulin concentrations and 131-I whole body scans in the diagnosis of metastases from differentiated thyroid carcinoma [after thyroidectomy], Clin Endocrinol [Oxf] 13:107, 1980.)

[131]I Whole Body Scan

Many metastatic well-differentiated thyroid cancers retain the ability to concentrate iodine, which is the rationale for the traditional diagnostic and therapeutic use of ^{131}I in metastatic thyroid cancer. Radioiodine uptake by metastatic tissue is dependent on TSH stimulation, thus requiring (until recently) a state of hypothyroidism. For this reason, total thyroidectomy and ablation of postsurgical thyroid remnants are the fundamental prerequisites for radioactive imaging. The other important point is withdrawal of levothyroxine therapy for a period long enough to induce high serum levels of endogenous TSH.[341,342] The minimum level of serum TSH required for adequate incorporation of ^{131}I in neoplastic tissues is around 30 µU/mL, a level usually achieved after 20 days without levothyroxine and 2 weeks without L-triiodothyronine. Unfortunately, this period of hypothyroidism may be very uncomfortable for many patients.

Alternatively, moderate hypothyroidism can be induced by reducing the patient's daily dose by 50%. In patients who have previously been ablated, and who are not receiving excessive doses of thyroxine, TSH will be raised to an average value of 50 µU/mL after 6 weeks. In practice, it is useful to measure serum TSH in the fifth week, and if it is above 20 µU/mL, satisfactory elevation (>30 µU/mL) will be anticipated in the sixth week at the time of the scan. It may take a longer period to elevate the TSH to a satisfactory level if patients have an on-treatment TSH value less than 0.1 µU/mL.

Another requirement for effective ^{131}I uptake is that the patient cannot be contaminated by recent ingestion of stable iodine, which would prevent the uptake of radioactive iodine by the metastases. A serum TSH that is not sufficiently high and contamination by iodine are the most common causes of false-negative ^{131}I WBS; therefore, it is necessary to check the serum TSH concentration before ^{131}I WBS and ^{131}I therapy, and to measure urinary iodine excretion if uptake is low.

Some 48 to 72 hours after the administration of ^{131}I, WBS is performed by rectilinear scan or a gamma camera. [131]I doses of 2 mCi generally are used as tracer; higher doses are not indicated because of the possibility that they will produce a sublethal radiation effect in the metastatic cells (i.e., stunning effect) that prevents uptake of the therapeutic dose of ^{131}I to be administered after a few days.[343]

If no abnormal ^{131}I uptake is found, despite elevation of serum Tg while not receiving levothyroxine, a therapeutic dose of [131]I (100 mCi) can be administered, and a post-therapy scan obtained 5 to 7 days later. This procedure will allow the identification of

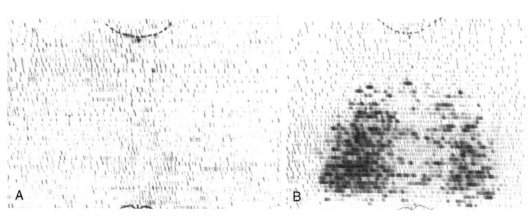

FIGURE 18-12. Representative example of a patient with negative diagnostic whole body scanning **(A)** that becomes positive for diffuse lung metastases on the post-therapy (100 mCi of ^{131}I) scan **(B)**.

small foci of ^{131}I in more than 80% of those patients with a negative basal scan and elevated serum Tg concentrations.[276,338,339] The question of whether such a procedure may have therapeutic effect is controversial. Evidence in favor of a therapeutic effect comes from a comparison between patients treated or untreated for positive Tg and negative WBS.[340] In the treated group, most patients with post-therapy evidence of lung disease were cured after one or more courses of radioiodine. However, this study stressed the important finding that in the untreated group, a large proportion of patients achieved normalization of serum Tg concentrations despite receiving no treatment. In our opinion, the most acceptable protocol in this setting is to give one course of empirical radioiodine treatment for every case of negative scan and positive Tg in the serum as a diagnostic procedure. Further treatments are advocated only in the presence of lung disease seen on the post-therapy scan. In cases of lymph node metastases, surgery is a better option, and no treatment is advocated when the post-therapy scan is negative. In this case, the search for metastases should include other imaging techniques such as CT, MRI of the neck and lung, bone scintigraphy, liver echography, and PET scan.

Whenever a metastasis has been localized by WBS, a complete radiologic assessment should be obtained. In bone metastases, the aim is to assess whether the location is accessible to radical surgical therapy, which, in the case of a single location, may be curative.[323,344] In cases of lung metastases, it is extremely important to establish the presence of one or more macronodular lesions or multiple micronodules not visible on plain chest film but only on CT scan. This point is of relevant prognostic utility because diffuse lung metastases not detectable by radiography but able to take up radioiodine (such as those commonly encountered in children) are highly responsive to ^{131}I treatment.[217,318]

Clinical, biochemical, and scintigraphic evaluations and radioiodine therapy, if needed, should be performed every 6 to 12 months in patients with persistent disease. Patients considered disease free (i.e., negative scan and undetectable serum Tg without levothyroxine therapy) on two occasions may be monitored annually with a clinical examination and serum TSH and Tg measurements. Any other tests are unnecessary as long as serum Tg remains undetectable. In this circumstance, the dose of L-thyroxine may be shifted from suppressive to replacement, with acceptance of a TSH level in the low-normal range. If serum Tg becomes detectable during levothyroxine therapy, ^{131}I WBS should be planned immediately.

Use of Recombinant Human TSH in the Diagnostic Evaluation of Differentiated Thyroid Cancer

A major advance in the management of differentiated thyroid cancer has been the development of human TSH made by recombinant techniques (i.e., recombinant human TSH [rhTSH]). Administration of this drug is an effective alternative to thyroid hormone withdrawal for monitoring patients treated with total thyroidectomy and thyroid ablation.

The idea to use exogenous TSH stimulation, instead of endogenous stimulation, dates many years back, when injection of bovine TSH was used to stimulate patients with thyroid cancer. The results were disappointing: The degree of stimulation was inadequate; side effects were common; and, most of all, immunity against TSH did occur.[345] After cloning of the human TSH gene,[346] hyperexpression of its encoded protein was induced in eukaryotic cells by recombinant techniques, thus allowing the recovery of large amounts of highly purified rhTSH (Thyrogen, Genzyme Therapeutics). The drug alters for the better the post-

operative management of patients with thyroid carcinoma. In clinical trials, the drug has proved very effective.[347,348] In patients with suppressed TSH levels (<0.1 μU/mL), two daily 0.9 mg injections stimulate thyroidal ^{131}I uptake and Tg secretion to a degree equal to 2 to 3 weeks of hormone withdrawal. The results of WBS performed after rhTSH and after levothyroxine withdrawal have shown very good but not perfect concordance between the two techniques. Side effects are minimal, and no anti-TSH antibody formation has been detected, at least in the short term. Thus, it is possible to stimulate ^{131}I uptake and Tg secretion without induction of hypothyroidism, which makes ^{131}I WBS and Tg testing more acceptable to patients and doctors.

Several independent works have confirmed the efficacy of rhTSH based on follow-up in clinical practice. Robbins and colleagues[349] compared two groups of patients with differentiated thyroid cancer (DTC) undergoing follow-up for DTC after thyroxine (L-T$_4$) withdrawal (161 patients) and after rhTSH (128 patients). The authors found that the results of diagnostic WBS and of stimulated serum Tg obtained with the two methods had the same positive and negative predictive value in the detection of residual disease. Based on these findings, it is proposed that follow-up of patients with DTC may be based on periodic serum Tg measurement and ^{131}I uptake after stimulation with rhTSH, with the aim of selecting patients with persistent disease to be given the more appropriate treatment. Pacini and colleagues,[350] in a prospective study of 72 patients with undetectable basal serum Tg concentration, found that the rhTSH-stimulated peak serum Tg was able to detect 100% of metastatic patients. These authors also reported that the diagnostic WBS was not informative in the 41 patients with undetectable rhTSH-stimulated serum Tg and in 8 of the 31 patients who converted from undetectable to detectable after rhTSH. The conclusion of these authors was that in patients with undetectable basal levels of serum Tg, rhTSH-stimulated Tg measurement represents an informative test to distinguish disease-free patients (those not requiring WBS) from diseased patients (those requiring additional diagnostic and/or therapeutic procedures). Similar results have been reported by Mazzaferri and Kloos in 107 patients.[351] Also in this series, the diagnostic yield of the WBS was very low compared with information derived by the rhTSH-stimulated serum Tg measurement. Of 107 patients who were clinically free of disease, 10% had persistent tumor that was identified only with an rhTSH-stimulated serum Tg level greater than 2 ng/mL.

The notion that serum Tg measurement is more sensitive than diagnostic WBS in detecting residual disease is not limited to the setting of patients stimulated by exogenous rhTSH. When endogenous TSH stimulation has been used, the utility of the routine use of diagnostic WBS has been questioned. Two large retrospective series[352,353] of patients undergoing routine diagnostic follow-up after L-T$_4$ withdrawal have shown that when serum Tg is undetectable, the diagnostic WBS is always negative or may show marginal residual uptake in the thyroid bed, thus not adding any relevant information. After more than 10 years of follow-up, most of these patients were free of disease, and local recurrence (metastatic lymph nodes) was detected (usually by neck ultrasound) in as few as 0.6% of patients. Even when serum Tg is detectable, a significant proportion of patients (around 20%) may have false-negative WBS. In most of these patients, residual disease may be visualized on the post-therapy scan performed after administration of high doses of [131]I (100 to 150 mCi). The low clinical yield of diagnostic WBS compared with that of serum Tg measurement has been confirmed recently in a large retrospective study at the University of Pisa, which tested more than

300 patients after rhTSH stimulation.[354] In this study, the results of rhTSH-stimulated Tg, combined with the results of neck ultrasonography, had the highest diagnostic accuracy (nearly 100%) in detecting patients with residual disease. With the exception of one patient with a single bone metastasis taking up radioiodine but not producing Tg, diagnostic WBS was not helpful in detecting metastatic disease. At variance with this result, a similar study carried out at the Memorial Sloan-Kettering Cancer Center in New York found that rhTSH-WBS was superior to rhTSH-stimulated Tg in a significant proportion of metastatic patients.[355] The apparent reason for this discrepancy may be related to the different study population, composed mostly of low-risk patients in the Pisa study and of very high-risk patients in the New York series.

As reported in a recent editorial by Wartofsky[356] and in a paper by Mazzaferri and colleagues,[357] altogether the available evidence is sufficient to propose diagnostic follow-up of patients with DTC based mainly on the use of rhTSH-stimulated serum Tg and post-therapy scan when ^{131}I treatment is indicated. Such an attitude will preserve the patient's quality of life by preventing hypothyroidism and will save many unnecessary diagnostic WBSs, reducing the need for imaging and ^{131}I WBS for a minority of patients with strong suspicion of residual disease. A tentative flow chart for the use of rhTSH in differentiated thyroid cancer is presented in Fig. 18-13.

As after L-T$_4$ withdrawal, patients with circulating anti-Tg antibodies may have falsely depressed serum Tg levels when stimulated with rhTSH. These patients may benefit only from the information derived from ^{131}I WBS and from other common imaging techniques, including neck ultrasound.

Finally, it may be noted that long-term prospective comparisons of these methods are not yet available. "Traditionalists" may wish to continue using 2 mCi ^{131}I scans prior to ablation in order to know distribution and amount of actual radioiodine uptake testing (RAIU), and may wish to have both scan and Tg data at the time of further treatment in the belief that it is useful to know the extent and localization of RAIU before large amounts of isotope are given. Both tests may be useful at least in the first few years of follow-up.

TREATMENT

Local and Regional Recurrences

After primary surgery, recurrences in the neck may develop in the thyroid bed and in surrounding soft tissues or in the regional lymph nodes. They carry an unfavorable prognosis, and most patients dying of differentiated thyroid cancer are included in this group.[252,358,359] The prognosis is better when recurrent cancer is diagnosed by ^{131}I scintigraphy rather than clinically, and when the tumor is able to concentrate iodine.[133,358,360] Any clinically detectable local recurrence should be treated by surgery if possible, although radical reoperation involving central dissection is difficult and risks complications to the parathyroid glands and recurrent laryngeal nerve.

Recurrent disease in the lateral cervical nodes is easier to treat surgically because the operative field has not been dissected previously. The preferred surgical procedure is a modified radical neck dissection. When lymph nodes concentrate iodine, treatment with ^{131}I is a partially effective adjunct to reoperation. Two or three therapeutic courses of ^{131}I are effective in treating more than 60% of patients.[133] If nodal disease persists after ^{131}I, reoperation with the use of an intraoperative isotope probe[361] may be considered.

Local recurrences that cannot be excised completely and that do not take up ^{131}I can benefit from external radiotherapy.[362]

Treatment for Distant Metastases

Effective treatment for distant metastases depends largely on the size, location, and number of metastatic lesions, and their ability to take up radioiodine. Micronodular diffuse lung metastases and, to a lesser extent, small metastatic bone foci revealed by WBS in the absence of radiographic changes have the greatest chance of cure. This observation is particularly true in children, who often have a diffuse pattern of metastatic pulmonary spread and do exceptionally well with radioiodine therapy.[133,196,217] Macronodules in the lung and large bone metastases carry a poor prognosis. Loss of radioiodine uptake is also a prognostic indicator of poor outcome. Taken together, these findings emphasize the concept that early recognition and early treatment of distant metastases are of paramount importance to the final outcome.

Surgical Treatment

The decision to treat distant metastases by surgery depends on their location, spread, ability to concentrate radioiodine, and radiologic pattern.

Lung metastases are typically treatable by radioiodine therapy, with the choice of surgical therapy left to a minority of selected cases. Patients eligible for surgery are those with a single macronodular lesion or more than one in the same lobe, with or without mediastinal lymph node involvement, particularly when they are devoid of radioiodine uptake. Too few patients have undergone surgery for lung metastases to allow a statistical conclusion to be made on their outcomes. However, some appear to achieve long-term remission and, in less advanced cases (one single pulmonary nodule), even definitive cure.[363]

The surgical approach to bone metastases is gaining support because of their relative insensitivity to radioiodine

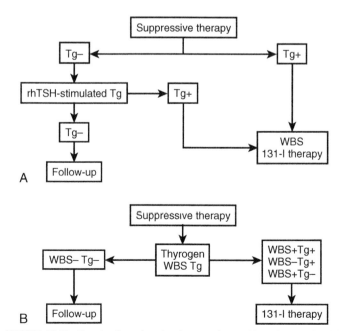

FIGURE 18-13. Tentative flow chart for the use of recombinant human thyroid-stimulating hormone (rhTSH) in the diagnostic follow-up of differentiated thyroid cancer after thyroidectomy. **A,** This panel applies to centers that will base their decision mainly on thyroglobulin (Tg) evaluation. **B,** This panel applies to those using the combination of Tg and whole body scanning (WBS).

therapy.[323,344,363,364] The intent of bone surgery may be palliative or curative. Palliation is required for pathologic fractures or to ameliorate neurologic symptoms resulting from spinal cord compression by vertebral metastases. Curative surgery is possible in single, localized metastases. For large metastases not radically resectable, surgery may be of help in reducing tumor mass to allow more effective action of radioiodine therapy.

Brain metastases are extremely rare and range from 0.15% to 1.3% in different series[364-368]; they carry a very poor prognosis. Although brain metastases usually demonstrate ^{131}I uptake, the therapy of choice, whenever feasible, is surgery, because of severe neurologic symptoms.

Radioiodine Treatment

The role and the indications for ^{131}I therapy in the management of distant metastases from differentiated thyroid carcinoma are well established. Results are reproducible in large series of patients and indicate complete response in 35% to 45% of patients.[133,318-321] Lung metastases, particularly when micronodular, respond better than do bone metastases. The poor prognosis of patients with bone metastases usually is linked to the bulkiness of the lesions and the presence of tumor cells that do not concentrate [131]I.[323,360] In adult patients, the treatment dose is usually 100 to 200 mCi, repeated every 6 to 8 months. Lower doses (empirically 1 mCi/kg body weight) should be used in children with lung metastases, particularly of the diffuse type, to avoid the risk for radiation-induced pulmonary fibrosis.[217,369]

An alternative method is to adjust the dosage of ^{131}I to a maximally tolerable level based on dosimetric analysis of a tracer dose. With this method, doses of 200 to 500 mCi sometimes are given. Because it is cumbersome, expensive, and of unproven benefit, the protocol currently is used in only a few institutions.

In a review of 118 patients with distant metastases treated with ^{131}I therapy,[133] 43 patients (36.4%) were cured (defined as negative WBS and undetectable serum Tg while not receiving levothyroxine), 28 (23.7%) died of their disease, and the others had persistent disease. Metastases from papillary tumors exhibited better response than did those from follicular tumors. The risk for dying was higher if lung metastases were macronodular and detectable by chest radiography, if bone metastases were multiple, and if both lung and bone metastases were present. The mean cumulative dose of ^{131}I used in cured patients was 233 mCi, delivered in 2.2 treatment courses over a 3.4 year period. Loss of radioiodine uptake was seen in 5.2% of patients after a mean cumulative dose of 161 mCi. Six patients with single bone metastases and one with a macronodular lung metastasis were given surgical therapy. In the series of the Institut Gustave Roussy in Paris, the authors followed more than 400 patients with distant metastases and found that overall survival after treatment was associated with the size of the metastases, their location, and their ability to take up radioiodine. Better response was observed in radioiodine avid, micronodular lung metastases, and the worst outcome was found with large bone metastases.[370]

As was previously mentioned, some patients (15% to 20%) have elevated serum Tg levels and no uptake detectable by diagnostic WBS.[336,337] The site of metastatic involvement in such patients, usually the lung or mediastinal lymph nodes, may be detected by WBS performed 5 to 7 days after the administration of high doses of [131]I (100 mCi).[234,296,297] This procedure is also of possible therapeutic value. A few days after administration of ^{131}I therapy, a transient increase in serum Tg concentration occurs and can be explained by release into the circulation of stored Tg by radiation-damaged tumor cells. Furthermore, progressive normalization of WBS and serum Tg levels over years[276,338,339] and normalization of chest CT scans in patients with radiographic evidence of micronodular lung metastases[338] have been observed in patients periodically treated with this treatment modality. This treatment does expose patients to significant radiation, and as of this time, there is no proof that it alters outcome or prolongs life.

Side effects after the administration of therapeutic ^{131}I doses usually are very mild, and most are reversible in a few days. They consist mainly of gastrointestinal symptoms, nausea and occasionally vomiting, and acute sialoadenitis. In patients given more than 100 mCi, dry mouth often develops, and salivary obstruction or loss of saliva leading to dental problems may occur. More serious complications affect the blood and bone marrow. An increased risk for leukemia on the order of 5 cases per 1000 treated patients has been documented by several published series, especially in patients who received more than 600 mCi total dosage.[318] The risk increases with increasing cumulative doses, with reduction of the interval between treatments, and with administration of total whole body radiation doses per treatment greater than 2 Gy.[371] Pancytopenia has been reported in 4.4% of patients treated with mean ^{131}I doses of 536 mCi.[372] In the same study, anemia was found in about 25% of patients, and thrombocytopenia was found in one third.

Another rare complication of radioiodine therapy is radiation-induced pulmonary fibrosis, which may develop in patients repeatedly treated for lung metastases, particularly of the diffuse type. Children seem to be particularly prone to this complication. In adults, generally no more than 60 to 70 mCi should be deposited in the lungs during treatment.

Finally, transient and permanent testicular damage limited to the germinal epithelium has been reported in men, as has transient ovarian failure in women, after treatment with high levels of [131]I.[373,374] ^{131}I-induced genetic damage in the offspring of patients treated with ^{131}I has not been documented in recent series addressing this issue.[375,376] The only anomaly reported was an increased frequency of miscarriage in women treated with ^{131}I during the year before conception.

Levothyroxine Suppressive Therapy

Both the function and the growth of metastatic thyroid cells are under TSH control. It is a common observation that bone or lung metastases increase in size and take up radioiodine during a period of levothyroxine withdrawal, whereas reduction in size and depressed uptake are observed with levothyroxine administration. Serum Tg, a marker of cell function, increases dramatically during hypothyroidism, whereas it returns to low levels during hormone therapy. Suppression of endogenous TSH to low or undetectable levels is a true antineoplastic therapy and should never be omitted in patients with active disease.

The drug of choice is levothyroxine, and the effective dosage is between 1.6 and 2.2 μg/kg body weight. A higher dosage is usually required in children. In every patient, an attempt should be made to use the smallest dose necessary to suppress TSH secretion. Adequacy of therapy is monitored by measurement of serum TSH. Serum TSH theoretically should be undetectable with an ultrasensitive assay, but levels less than 0.1 μU/mL are probably acceptable. FT$_3$ should be in the normal range to avoid iatrogenic thyrotoxicosis. When these guidelines are followed, levothyroxine suppressive therapy is safe and largely devoid of long-term side effects on the heart or bone.[107]

Table 18-10. Possible Indications for Radiation Therapy

Tumor	Stage	Treatment
Papillary or follicular	Invasive, patient younger than 45 yr	Possibly 4000 rad at 2 to 3 cm depth to thyroid bed after RAI treatment; value uncertain in this instance
	Invasive or possible residual, patient older than 45 yr	5000 rad* to the thyroid bed after RAI treatment
	Recurrent, patient of any age	5000 rad* to the thyroid bed after RAI treatment
	Isolated lesion in bone	5000-6000 rad, as required for symptoms after RAI treatment
Medullary	Stage III	4000-5000 rad† to the thyroid bed
	Abnormal or increasing thyrocalcitonin	5000 rad† to the mantle
	Recurrent tumor, isolated metastasis	5000-6000 rad* to the area 5000-6000 rad for symptoms
Lymphoma	All	5000 rad† to the thyroid and mantle
Anaplastic	All	4500-5500 rad† to the thyroid and mantle

RAI, Radioactive iodine. Treatment (15-20 MV Electrons or ^{60}Co).
Note: Spinal cord dosage does not exceed 3000* or 3500† rad.

A shift from suppressive therapy to replacement therapy is appropriate in patients who have well-documented stable and complete remission, as assessed by a negative ^{131}I WBS and undetectable stimulated serum Tg in the absence of anti-Tg antibodies and negative neck ultrasound.

Radiation Therapy

Radiation therapy is appropriate for any class III differentiated tumor not responding to ^{131}I therapy or hormone suppression, for class III Hürthle cell tumors and follicular cancers in older patients, for any expanding class IV lesion, for painful osseous metastases, and for lymphomas and undifferentiated tumors.[377] Unfortunately, no adequate studies are available to assess the value of prophylactic radiation after resection of class III tumors. Prophylactic mantle radiotherapy may be useful in patients with medullary thyroid cancer who have residual hypercalcitoninemia after surgery in the absence of detectable lesions (Table 18-10), but the value of this treatment is debated.[378]

Chemotherapy

A variety of traditional chemotherapeutic approaches have been attempted with minimal success. The overall response rate of thyroid cancer to various chemotherapeutic agents, including the alkylating agents 5-fluorouracil and methotrexate, is estimated to be 10% to 15%, which is comparable with that for other solid tumors.[379] Bleomycin and especially doxorubicin (Adriamycin) have been reported to provide a higher percentage of remission (20% to 33%).[313,379-384] However, response to these chemotherapeutic agents is partial and of short duration, with limitation imposed by toxicity of the medication. Chemotherapeutic agents given in combination appear to be slightly more effective than doxorubicin alone.[313,379-384] Chemotherapy in differentiated thyroid carcinoma, preferably doxorubicin, is warranted in class III and IV lesions after other modalities of therapy have been exhausted and tumor growth is certain (Table 18-11). Recently, an Italian study reported an improvement in the rate of success when an administered chemotherapy scheme was based on the use of epirubicin and cis-platinum, administered while the

Table 18-11. Reported but Largely Unsuccessful Chemotherapy Protocols for Thyroid Carcinoma (see text)

Primary tumor
  Progressive differentiated thyroid cancer, symptomatic medullary cancer, anaplastic cancer; two programs have been proposed:
    Doxorubicin (Adriamycin) + cis-diamminedichloroplatinum + VP-16
    Doxorubicin (Adriamycin) + cis-diamminedichloroplatinum
Secondary therapy for failure of primary treatment
  Differentiated cancer: bleomycin + cyclophosphamide
  Medullary cancer: fluorouracil + streptozocin
  Anaplastic cancer: bleomycin + hydroxyurea

patient was under endogenous or exogenous TSH stimulation.[385] The rationale for this protocol is based on the assumption that tumor cells may be more prone to be killed if they are in a state of active replication, as can be obtained by stimulating them with TSH, rather than in a quiescent state, as may be observed during suppression of circulating TSH. As was already mentioned, chemotherapy may be used in combination with external irradiation for the treatment of anaplastic thyroid carcinoma after surgery.

Novel Therapeutic Strategies for Poorly Differentiated Thyroid Cancer

A small but significant proportion of patients with thyroid cancer do not respond to any of the above mentioned treatment modalities and eventually die of thyroid cancer. New therapeutic strategies are needed for these patients. Several research strategies are being implemented, and some new therapeutic approaches have already been entered into clinical trials.

One idea has been to reinduce a pattern of well differentiation in poorly differentiated or undifferentiated tumors, the so-called "redifferentiation therapy." Poorly differentiated tumors are characterized by loss of expression of differentiation genes specific for the thyroid gland, such as the *TSH receptor* gene, the *thyroglobulin* gene, or the *NIS* gene. The last is the gene responsible for iodine uptake, and its expression is often lower in thyroid cancer cells as compared with normal follicular cells[386]; it is completely abolished in tumors no longer responsive to radioiodine therapy. Reinducing expression of the *NIS* gene would again render the tumors sensitive to the effects of radioiodine. Retinoids are biologically active metabolites of vitamin A, with growth-inhibiting and differentiation-inducing properties. They have been used for treatment and chemoprevention of several human cancers (e.g., acute promyelocytic leukemia) and recently were proposed as a potential agent of redifferentiation in thyroid cancer. In vitro, treatment for follicular thyroid carcinoma cell lines with retinoic acid (RA) exerted significant antiproliferative effects,[387] elicited an increase in NIS mRNA expression and iodine uptake,[388,389] and, by decreasing extracellular matrix degradation, had beneficial effects on metastatic behavior.[390] In vivo, 13-cis-retinoic acid (Roacutan) has been used in several limited series of poorly differentiated thyroid cancer with the aim of reinducing iodine uptake, at doses of 1.0 to 1.5 mg/kg body weight for 2 to 6 weeks. Reinduction of ^{131}I uptake was observed in 5 of 12, 8 of 20, and 4 of 10 patients in three different series.[391-393] Taken together, results of the in vitro and in vivo studies may be interpreted as evidence of redifferentiation deserving of continued clinical evaluation.

Another futuristic approach is gene therapy, whose essence is the introduction of DNA into target cells. Although cancer is a multigenic disease, with more than one gene being dysfunctional, several oncogenes have been unequivocally associated with thyroid carcinoma and may become the target for gene therapy. Several approaches to thyroid cancer have been specifically proposed.[394]

Reintroduction of the p53 Tumor Suppressor Gene

In tumors lacking a functional *p53* gene (as in most cases of undifferentiated thyroid carcinoma), there may be one way to proceed. *p53* is a tumor suppressor gene that normally is devoted to arresting the cell cycle to allow repair of DNA damage or to induce apoptosis. When *p53* is mutated, this mechanism is not working, and cells with genomic alterations are free to survive and propagate. Reintroduction of *p53* into thyroid carcinoma cell lines with *p53* mutations converted the cells to a more differentiated phenotype. Expression of thyroid-specific genes was stimulated, modulation by TSH was restored, tumorigenic potential was reduced, and proliferation was inhibited.[395-399] So far, treatment of patients by this approach has been tested in a few patients with advanced lung carcinoma[400] but never in those with thyroid carcinoma.

Suicide gene therapy is an approach in which gene transfer is used to introduce into the tumor cells a vector coding for a "sensitizing enzyme" that is able to activate a chemotherapeutic agent (pro-drug) only in the cells in which the sensitizing enzyme is expressed. Several pro-drug/sensitizing enzyme systems for thyroid carcinoma have been tested in vitro.[401]

Immunotherapy

Immune response against cancer antigens is somehow impaired in oncologic patients through a number of mechanisms. The use of immunostimulatory agents that enable the host to enhance anticancer immunity is a promising strategy for cancer therapy. Experimental studies in vitro and in animal models by Zhang and colleagues[402-404] have confirmed the feasibility of this approach in MTC. They used a replication-defective adenovirus to transduce MTC cell lines with the murine interleukin-2 (IL-2) gene under the control of the human cytomegalovirus promoter. After infection, the murine (and human) MTC cell line secreted large amounts of IL-2. When these cells were injected into syngeneic animals, IL-2–positive tumor cells showed markedly reduced tumor growth. Furthermore, these authors were able to show that immunity against MTC cells was long-lasting, and that the adenovirus vector used was safe in other organs.

Targeted Therapy

Although the above mentioned strategies are far from the stage of entering clinical practice, the new approach of targeted therapy seems to be more promising. Outstanding progress over the past 20 years in the genetics of thyroid cancer has led to the discovery of oncogenes that have a pathogenic role in follicular and medullary thyroid cancer (MTC) initiation and progression. Most act through the RTK/RAS/RAF/MAPK pathway or the phosphatidylinositol 3-kinase (PI3K)/Akt pathway, and all of them confer constitutive activation to transformed cells.

New Agents Inhibiting Tyrosine Kinases

As in several other human malignancies, knowledge of molecular alterations has prompted the search for new agents able to inhibit the function of specific oncoproteins, with the aim of shutting down uncontrolled growth of neoplastic cells and, hopefully, producing less toxicity in normal cells, so-called "targeted therapy." In thyroid cancer, the logical approach has been to develop molecules that block the RTK/MAPK and the PI3K/AKT pathways, that is, those activated by *RET/PTC, RAS,* and *BRAF* mutations. The effects of some experimental drugs are not restricted to a single protein, but they may have the ability to inhibit several proteins crucial for the survival and expansion of neoplastic cells. Vascular endothelial growth factor receptor (VEGFR) and epidermal growth factor receptor (EGFR) are two examples. Inhibiting VEGFR blocks the growth of the tumor's endothelial cells, and inhibiting EGFR may deprive the tumor of one important growth factor, thus sustaining an aggressive phenotype. After promising in vitro experiments showed that these compounds are effective, some have been tested in clinical trials.[405-407] In a phase 2 trial of one of the first tyrosine kinase inhibitors, sorafenib, 6 of 41 patients showed a partial response by standard RECIST (Response Evaluation Criteria in Solid Tumors) criteria, and 56% had prolonged stable disease.[406] A dramatic response was observed by another group using sorafenib in a child with papillary cancer.[408] Responses to sunitinib in some patients with papillary and follicular cancer were sustained over 4 years.[409] Vandetanib, an inhibitor of VEGF, RET, and EGF tyrosine kinase activity is being tried alone and in combination with other agents such as docetaxel or pemetrexed.[410] Gefitinib[411] and axitinib[412] have also been effective in some cases of aggressive thyroid cancer nonresponsive to [131]I. These agents currently are used only in clinical trials, but it makes sense to offer participation in an ongoing trial to patients with aggressive or progressive thyroid cancers that have resisted standard treatments, including ^{131}I therapy.

It appears that all of the kinase inhibitors so far tested have a beneficial effect in some patients and not others; improved understanding of the individual tumor molecular defect is expected to help elucidate this problem. It is likely that multiple agents of different types will be combined for treatment, for instance, kinase inhibitors and valproic acid, a histone deacetylase inhibitor. Side effects of these drugs are very significant, which is not surprising because of the centrality of the functions of inhibited proteins. Rashes, nausea, weakness, mucosal damage, diarrhea, and hypertension often limit or prohibit treatment. It is interesting to note that hypothyroidism is commonly observed as a side effect, and the cause is not yet fully understood.

We are at the very beginning of the "era" of targeted therapy. Many additional trials are needed to guide the clinician in finding the most appropriate drug for an individual patient, and many issues need to be resolved. But there is now a legitimate basis for beneficial treatment of many patients who until this time have had no therapeutic options.

REFERENCES

1. Vander JB, Gaston EA, Dawber TR: Significance of solitary non-toxic thyroid nodules, N Engl J Med 251:970–973, 1954.
2. Vander JB, Gaston EA, Dawber TR: The significance of nontoxic thyroid nodules: final report of a 15-year study of the incidence of thyroid malignancy, Ann Intern Med 69:537–540, 1968.
3. Tunbridge WM, Evered DC, Hall R, et al: The spectrum of thyroid disease in an English community: the Wickham survey, Clin Endocrinol 7:481–493, 1977.
4. Liechty RD, Stoffel PT, Zimmerman DE, et al: Solitary thyroid nodules, Arch Surg 112:59–64, 1977.
5. Mortensen JD, Woolner LB, Bennett WA: Gross and microscopic findings in clinically normal thyroid glands, J Clin Endocrinol Metab 15:1270–1280, 1955.
6. Tan GH, Gharib H: Thyroid incidentalomas: management approaches to nonpalpable nodules discovered incidentally on thyroid imaging, Ann Intern Med 126:226–231, 1997.

7. Baldwin DB, Rowett D: Incidence of thyroid disorders in Connecticut, JAMA 239:742–744, 1978.

8. Pinchera A: Thyroid incidentalomas, Horm Res 68(Suppl 5):199–201, 2007.

9. Brander A, Viikinkoski P, Nickels J, et al: Thyroid gland: US screening in a random adult population, Radiology 181:683–687, 1991.

10. Brander A, Viikinkoski P, Nickels J, et al: Importance of thyroid abnormalities detected at US screening: a 5-year follow-up, Radiology 215:801–806, 2000.

11. Dean DS, Gharib H: Epidemiology of thyroid nodules, Best Pract Res Clin Endocrinol Metab 22:901–911, 2008.

12. Belfiore A, LaRosa GL, LaPorta GA, et al: Cancer risk in patients with cold thyroid nodules: relevance of iodine intake, sex, age, and multinodularity, Am J Med 93:363–369, 1992.

13. Davies L, Welch HG: Increasing incidence of thyroid cancer in the United States, 1973–2002, JAMA 295:2164–2167, 2006.

14. Leenhardt L, Grosclaude P, Cherie-Challine L: Increased incidence of thyroid carcinoma in France: a true epidemic or thyroid nodule management effect? Report from France Thyroid Cancer Committee, Thyroid 14:1056–1060, 2004.

15. Grodski S, Delbridge L: An update on papillary microcarcinoma, Curr Opin Oncol 21:1–4, 2008.

16. Pazaitou-Panayiotou K, Capezzone M, Pacini F: Clinical features and therapeutic implication of papillary thyroid microcarcinoma, Thyroid 17:1–8, 2007.

17. Namba H, Matsuo K, Fagin JA: Clonal composition of benign and malignant human thyroid tumors, J Clin Invest 86:120–125, 1990.

18. Namba H, Rubin SA, Fagin JA: Point mutations of Ras oncogenes are an early event in thyroid tumorigenesis, Mol Endocrinol 4:1474–1479, 1990.

19. Parma J, Duprez L, Van Sande J, et al: Somatic mutations in the thyrotropin receptor gene cause hyperfunctioning thyroid adenomas, Nature 365:649–651, 1993.

20. Tonacchera M, Chiovato L, Pinchera A, et al: Hyperfunctioning thyroid nodules in toxic multinodular goiter share activating thyrotropin receptor mutations with solitary toxic adenoma, J Clin Endocrinol Metab 83:492–498, 1998.

21. Tonacchera M, Vitti P, Agretti P, et al: Activating thyrotropin receptor mutations in histologically heterogeneous hyperfunctioning nodules of multinodular goiter, Thyroid 8:559–564, 1998.

22. Suarez HG, du Villard JA, Caillou B, et al: Gsp mutations in human thyroid tumors, Oncogene 6:677–679, 1991.

23. Masini-Repiso AM, Cabanillas A, Bonaterra M, et al: Dissociation of thyrotropin-dependent enzyme activities, reduced ioidide transport, and preserved iodide organification in nonfunctioning thyroid adenoma and multinodular goiter, J Clin Endocrinol Metab 79:39–44, 1994.

24. Field JB, Larsen PR, Yamashita K, et al: Demonstration of iodide transport defect but normal iodide organification in nonfunctioning nodules of human thyroid glands, J Clin Invest 52:2404–2410, 1973.

25. Fragu P, Nataf BM: Human thyroid peroxidase activity in benign and malign thyroid disorders, J Clin Endocrinol Metab 45:1089–1096, 1977.

26. Demeester-Mirkine N, Van Sande J, Corvilain H, et al: Benign thyroid nodule with normal iodide trap and defective organification, J Clin Endocrinol Metab 41:1169–1171, 1975.

27. Morris JC: Mutations and disorders involving the thyroid iodide transporter: the next wave in thyroid diseases, J Clin Endocrinol Metab 82:3964–3965, 1997.

28. Miller JM, Zafar SU, Karo JJ: The cystic thyroid nodule: recognition and management, Radiology 110:257–261, 1974.

29. Sipple JH: Association of pheochromocytoma with carcinoma of thyroid gland, Am J Med 31:163–166, 1961.

30. Schimke RN, Hartmann WH, Prout TE, et al: Syndrome of bilateral pheochromocytoma, medullary thyroid carcinoma, and multiple neuromas, N Engl J Med 279:1–7, 1968.

31. Sapira JD, Altman M, Vandyk K, et al: Bilateral adrenal pheochromocytoma and medullary thyroid carcinoma, N Engl J Med 273:140–143, 1965.

32. Capezzone M, Marchisotta S, Cantara S, et al: Familial non-medullary thyroid carcinoma displays the features of clinical anticipation suggestive of a distinct biological entity, Endocr Relat Cancer 15:1075–1081, 2008.

33. Loh K-C: Familial nonmedullary thyroid carcinoma: a meta-review of case series, Thyroid 7:107–113, 1997.

34. Refetoff S, Harrison J, Karanfilski BT, et al: Continuing occurrence of thyroid carcinoma after irradiation to the neck in infancy and childhood, N Engl J Med 292:171–175, 1975.

35. Kazakov VS, Demidchik EP, Astakhova LN: Thyroid cancer after Chernobyl, Nature 359:21, 1992.

36. Compagno J, Oertel JE: Malignant lymphoma and other lymphoproliferative disorders of the thyroid gland, Am J Clin Pathol 74:1–11, 1980.

37. Farbota LM, Calandra DB, Lawrence AM, et al: Thyroid carcinoma in Graves' disease, Surgery 98:1148–1152, 1985.

38. Pacini F, Elisei R, DiCoscio GC, et al: Thyroid carcinoma in thyrotoxic patients treated by surgery, J Endocrinol Invest 11:107–112, 1988.

39. Shapiro SJ, Friedmen NB, Perzik SL, et al: Incidence of thyroid carcinoma in Graves' disease, Cancer 26:1261–1270, 1970.

40. Belfiore A, Garofalo MR, Giuffrida D, et al: Increased aggressiveness of thyroid cancer in patients with Graves' disease, J Clin Endocrinol Metab 70:830–835, 1990.

41. Hales JB, McElduff A, Crummer P, et al: Does Graves' disease or thyrotoxicosis affect the prognosis of thyroid cancer? J Clin Endocrinol Metab 75:886–889, 1992.

42. Hay ID: Papillary thyroid carcinoma, Endocrinol Metab Clin North Am 19:545–576, 1990.

43. Hamming JF, Goslings BM, Van Steenis GJ, et al: The value of fine-needle aspiration biopsy in patients with nodular thyroid disease divided into groups of suspicion of malignant neoplasms on clinical grounds, Arch Intern Med 150:113–116, 1990.

44. Veith FJ, Brooks JR, Grigsby WP, et al: The nodular thyroid gland and cancer, N Engl J Med 270:431–436, 1964.

45. DeGroot LJ, Paloyan E: Thyroid carcinoma and radiation: a Chicago endemic, JAMA 225:487–491, 1973.

46. Hoffman GL, Thompson NW, Heffron C: The solitary thyroid nodule, Arch Surg 105:379–385, 1972.

47. Guarino E, Tarantini B, Pilli T, et al: Presurgical serum thyroglobulin has no prognostic value in papillary thyroid cancer, Thyroid 15:1041–1045, 2005.

48. Pacini F, Fontanelli M, Fugazzola L, et al: Routine measurement of serum calcitonin in nodular thyroid diseases allows the preoperative diagnosis of unsuspected sporadic medullary thyroid carcinoma, J Clin Endocrinol Metab 78:826–829, 1994.

49. Rieu M, Lame MC, Richard A, et al: Prevalence of sporadic medullary thyroid carcinoma: the importance of routine measurement of serum calcitonin in the diagnostic evaluation of thyroid nodules, Clin Endocrinol (Oxf) 42:453–457, 1995.

50. Niccoli P, Wion-Barbot N, Caron P, et al: Interest of routine measurement of serum calcitonin: study in a large series of thyroidectomized patients, J Clin Endocrinol Metab 82:338–341, 1997.

51. Vierhapper H, Raber W, Bieglmayer C, et al: Routine measurement of plasma calcitonin in nodular thyroid diseases, J Clin Endocrinol Metab 82:1589–1593, 1997.

52. Elisei R, Bottici V, Luchetti F, et al: Impact of routine measurement of serum calcitonin on the diagnosis and outcome of medullary thyroid cancer: experience in 10,864 patients with nodular thyroid disorders, J Clin Endocrinol Metab 89:163–168, 2004.

53. Pacini F, Schlumberger M, Dralle H, et al: European Thyroid Cancer Taskforce: European consensus for the management of patients with differentiated thyroid carcinoma of the follicular epithelium, Eur J Endocrinol 154:787–803, 2006.

54a. Cooper DS, Doherty GM, Kloos RT, et al: American Thyroid Association Guidelines Taskforce: management guideliness for patients with thyroid nodules and differentiated thyroid cancer, Thyroid 16:1324–1325, 2006.

54b. Bonnet S, Hartl D, Leboulleux S, et al: Prophylactic lymph node dissection for papillary thyroid cancer less than 2 cm: implications for radioiodine treatment, J Clin Endocrinol Metab 94:1162–1167, 2009.

55. Cheung K, Roman SA, Wang TS, et al: Calcitonin measurement in the evaluation of thyroid nodules in the United States: a cost effectiveness and decision analysis, J Clin Endocrinol Metab 93:2173–2180, 2008.

56. Clark OH, Okerlund MD, Cavalieri RR, et al: Diagnosis and treatment of thyroid, parathyroid, and thyroglossal duct cysts, J Clin Endocrinol Metab 48:983–988, 1979.

57. Rago T, Santini F, Scutari M, et al: Elastografia: new development in ultrasound for predicting malignancy in thyroid nodules, J Clin Endocrinol Metab 92:2917–2922, 2007.

58. Rago T, Vitti P, Chiovato L, et al: Role of conventional ultrasonography and colour flow-doppler sonography in predicting malignancy in "cold" thyroid nodules, Eur J Endocrinol 138:41–46, 1998.

59. Rojeski MT, Gharib H: Nodular thyroid disease: evaluation and management, N Engl J Med 313:428–436, 1985.

60. Sokal JE: The problem of malignancy in nodular goiter: recapitulation and a challenge, JAMA 170:405–412, 1959.

61. Van Herle AJ, Rich P, Ljung BM, et al: The thyroid nodule, Ann Intern Med 96:221–232, 1982.

62. Kendall LW, Condon RE: Prediction of malignancy in solitary thyroid nodules, Lancet 1:1071–1073, 1969.

63. Sebastianes FM, Cerci JJ, Zanoni PH, et al: Role of 18F-fluorodeoxyglucose positron emission tomography in preoperative assessment of cytologically indeterminate thyroid nodules, J Clin Endocrinol Metab 92:4485–4488, 2007.

64. Mitchell JC, Grant F, Evenson AR, et al: Preoperative evaluation of thyroid nodules with 18FDG-PET/CT, Surgery 138:1166–1174, 2005; discussion 1174–1175.

65. Walfish PG, Hazani E, Strawbridge HTG, et al: Combined ultrasound and needle aspiration cytology in the assessment and management of hypofunctioning thyroid nodule, Ann Intern Med 87:270–274, 1977.

66. Gershengorn MC, McClung MR, Chu WE, et al: Fine-needle aspiration cytology in the preoperative diagnosis of thyroid nodules, Ann Intern Med 87:265–269, 1977.

67. Hamlin E, Vickery AL: Needle biopsy of the thyroid gland, N Engl J Med 254:742–746, 1956.

68. Willems J-S, Lowhagen T: Fine needle aspiration cytology in thyroid disease, Clin Endocrinol Metab 2:247–256, 1981.

69. Morris LF, Ragavendra N, Yeh MW: Evidence-based assessment of the role of ultrasonography in the management of benign thyroid nodules, World J Surg 32:1253–1263, 2008.

70. Cai XJ, Valiyaparambath N, Nixon P, et al: Ultrasound-guided fine needle aspiration cytology in the diagnosis and management of thyroid nodules, Cytopathology 17:251–256, 2006.

71. Hatada T, Okada K, Ishii H, et al: Evaluation of ultrasound-guided fine-needle aspiration biopsy for thyroid nodules, Am J Surg 175:133–136, 1998.

72. Gharib H, Goellner JR, Johnson DA: Fine needle aspiration cytology of the thyroid: a 12-year experience with 11,000 biopsies, Clin Lab Med 13:699–709, 1993.

73. Miller JM, Hamburger JI, Kini S: Diagnosis of thyroid nodules: use of fine needle aspiration and needle biopsy, JAMA 241:481–484, 1979.

74. Hamburger JL, Husain M, Nishiyama R, et al: Increasing the accuracy of fine-needle biopsy for thyroid nodules, Arch Pathol Lab Med 113:1035–1041, 1989.

75. Caruso D, Mazzaferri EL: Fine-needle aspiration in the management of thyroid nodules, Endocrinologist 1:194–202, 1991.

76. Gharib H, Goellner JR: Fine-needle aspiration of the thyroid: an appraisal, Ann Intern Med 118:282–289, 1993.

77. Giuffrida D, Gharib H: Controversies in the management of cold, hot, and occult thyroid nodules, Am J Med 99:642–650, 1995.

78. Ridgway EC: Clinician's evaluation of a solitary thyroid nodule, J Clin Endocrinol Metab 74:231–235, 1992.

79. Bieche I, Ruffet E, Zweibaum A, et al: MUC1 mucin gene, transcripts, and protein in adenomas and papillary carcinomas of the thyroid, Thyroid 7:725–731, 1997.

80. Brousset P, Chaouche N, Leprat F, et al: Telomerase activity in human thyroid carcinomas originating from the follicular cells, J Clin Endocrinol Metab 82:4214–4216, 1997.

81. Bartolazzi A, Gasbarri A, Papotti M, et al: Thyroid Cancer Study Group: Application of an immunodiag-

nostic method for improving preoperative diagnosis of nodular thyroid lesions, Lancet 357:1644–1650, 2001.

82. Saggiorato E, Cappia S, De Giuli P, et al: Galectin-3 as a presurgical immunocytodiagnostic marker of minimally invasive follicular thyroid carcinoma, J Clin Endocrinol Metab 86:5152–5158, 2001.

83. Giannini R, Faviana P, Cavinato T, et al: Galectin-3 and oncofetal-fibronectin expression in thyroid neoplasia as assessed by reverse transcription-polymerase chain reaction and immunochemistry in cytologic and pathologic specimens, Thyroid 13:765–770, 2003.

84. Pagedar NA, Chen DH, Wasman JK, et al: Molecular classification of thyroid nodules by cytology, Laryngoscope 118:692–696, 2008.

85. Bartolazzi A, Orlandi F, Saggiorato E, et al: Italian Thyroid Cancer Study Group (ITCSG): Galectin-3-expression analysis in the surgical selection of follicular thyroid nodules with indeterminate fine-needle aspiration cytology: a prospective multicentre study, Lancet Oncol 9:543–549, 2008.

86. Caplan RH, Kisken WA, Strutt PJ, et al: Fine-needle aspiration biopsy of thyroid nodules: a cost-effective diagnostic plan, Postgrad Med 90:183–190, 1991.

87. Gollner JR, Gharib H, Grant CS, et al: Fine-needle aspiration cytology of the thyroid, 1980 to 1986, Acta Cytol 31:587–590, 1987.

88. Pacini F, Fugazzola L, Lippi F, et al: Detection of thyroglobulin in fine needle aspirates of nonthyroidal neck masses: a clue to the diagnosis of metastatic thyroid cancer, J Clin Endocrinol Metab 74:1401–1404, 1992.

89. Boi F, Maurelli I, Pinna G, et al: Calcitonin measurement in wash-out fluid from fine needle aspiration of neck masses in patients with primary and metastatic medullary thyroid carcinoma, J Clin Endocrinol Metab 92:2115–2118, 2007.

90. Esnaola NF, Cantor SB, Sherman SI, et al: Optimal treatment strategy in patients with papillary thyroid cancer: a decision analysis, Surgery 130:921–930, 2001.

91. Mazzaferri EL, Jhiang SM: Long-term impact of initial surgical and medical therapy on papillary and follicular thyroid cancer, Am J Med 97:418–428, 1994.

92. Machens A, Holzhausen HJ, Dralle H: The prognostic value of primary tumor size in papillary and follicular thyroid carcinoma, Cancer 103:2269–2273, 2005.

93. Baloch ZW, Fleisher S, LiVolsi VA, et al: Diagnosis of "follicular neoplasm": a gray zone in thyroid fine needle aspiration cytology, Diagn Cytopathol 26:41–44, 2002.

94. Sclabas GM, Staerkel GA, Shapiro SE, et al: Fine-needle aspiration of the thyroid and correlation with histopathology in a contemporary series of 240 patients, Am J Surg 186:702–709, 2003.

95. Goldstein RE, Netterville JL, Burkey B, et al: Implications of follicular neoplasms, atypia, and lesions suspicious for malignancy diagnosed by fine-needle aspiration of thyroid nodules, Ann Surg 235:656–662, 2002.

96. de los Santos ET, Keyhani-Rofagha S, Cunningham JJ, et al: Cystic thyroid nodules: the dilemma of malignant lesions, Arch Intern Med 150:1422–1427, 1990.

97. Gardner RE, Tuttle RM, Burman KD, et al: Prognostic importance of vascular invasion in papillary thyroid carcinoma, Arch Otolaryngol Head Neck Surg 126:309–312, 2000.

98. Tuttle RM, Lemar H, Burch HB: Clinical features associated with an increased risk of thyroid malignancy in patients with follicular neoplasia by fine-needle aspiration, Thyroid 8:377–383, 1998.

99. Smith SL, Rosales RF, Weaver AL: Factors that predict malignant thyroid lesions when fine-needle aspiration is "suspicious for follicular neoplasm." Mayo Clin Proc 72:913–916, 1997.

100. Rouxel A, Hejblum G, Bernier M, et al: Prognostic factors associated with the survival of patients developing loco-regional recurrences of differentiated thyroid carcinomas, J Clin Endocrinol Metab 89:5362–5368, 2004.

101. Gharib H, Goellner JR, Johnson DA: Fine-needle aspiration cytology of the thyroid: a 12-year experience with 11,000 biopsies, Clin Lab Med 13:699–709, 1993.

102. Randolph GW, Daniels GH: Radioactive iodine lobe ablation as an alternative to completion thyroidectomy

for follicular carcinoma of the thyroid, Thyroid 12:989–996, 2002.

103. DeGroot LJ, Kaplan EL: Second operations for "completion" of thyroidectomy in treatment of differentiated thyroid cancer, Surgery 110:936–940, 1991.

104. Zelmanovits F, Genro S, Gross JL: Suppressive therapy with levothyroxine for solitary thyroid nodules: a double-blind controlled clinical study and cumulative meta-analyses, J Clin Endocrinol Metab 83:3881–3885, 1998.

105. Bartalena L, Martino E, Pacchiarotti I, et al: Factors affecting suppression of endogenous thyrotropin secretion by thyroxine treatment: retrospective analysis in athyreotic and goitrous patients, J Clin Endocrinol Metab 64:849–855, 1987.

106. Papini E, Petrucci L, Guglielmi R, et al: Long-term changes in nodular goiter: a 5-year prospective randomized trial of levothyroxine suppressive therapy for benign cold thyroid nodules, J Clin Endocrinol Metab 83:780–783, 1998.

107. Marcocci C, Golia F, Bruno-Bossio G, et al: Carefully monitored levothyroxine suppressive therapy is not associated with bone loss in premenopausal women, J Clin Endocrinol Metab 78:818–823, 1994.

108. Tarantini B, Ciuoli C, Di Cairano G, et al: Effectiveness of radioiodine (131-I) as definitive therapy in patients with autoimmune and non-autoimmune hyperthyroidism, J Endocrinol Invest 29:594–598, 2006.

109. Lippi F, Ferrari C, Manetti L, et al: Treatment of solitary autonomous thyroid nodules by percutaneous ethanol injection: results of an Italian multicenter study, The Multicenter Study Group, J Clin Endocrinol Metab 81:3261–3264, 1996.

110. Martino E, Murtas ML, Loviselli A, et al: Percutaneous intranodular ethanol injection for treatment of autonomously functioning thyroid nodules, Surgery 112:1161–1165, 1992.

111. Zingrillo M, Modoni S, Conte M, et al: Percutaneous ethanol injection plus radioiodine versus radioiodine alone in the treatment of large toxic thyroid nodules, J Nucl Med 44:207–210, 2003.

112. Pacini F: Role of percutaneous ethanol injection in management of nodular lesions of the thyroid gland, J Nucl Med 44:211–212, 2003.

113. Monzani F, Lippi F, Goletti O, et al: Percutaneous aspiration and ethanol sclerotherapy for the thyroid cysts, J Clin Endocrinol Metab 78:800–804, 1994.

114. Pacini F, Antonelli A, Lari R, et al: Unsuspected parathyroid cysts diagnosed by measurement of thyroglobulin and parathyroid hormone concentrations in fluid aspirates, Ann Intern Med 102:793–794, 1985.

115. Enewold L, Zhu K, Ron E, et al: Rising thyroid cancer incidence in the United States by demographic and tumor characteristics, 1980–2005, Cancer Epidemiol Biomarkers Prev 18:784–791, 2009.

116. Annual Cancer Statistical Review, National Institutes of Health Publication No, 882789, 1987.

117. Sampson RJ, Woolner LB, Bahn RC, et al: Occult thyroid carcinoma in Olmsted County, Minnesota: prevalence at autopsy compared with that in Hiroshima and Nagasaki, Japan, Cancer 34:2072–2076, 1974.

118. Fukunaga FH, Yatani R: Geographic pathology of occult thyroid carcinomas, Cancer 36:1095–1099, 1975.

119. Verby JE, Woolner LB, Nobrega FT, et al: Thyroid cancer in Olmsted County, 1935–1965, J Natl Cancer Inst 43:813–820, 1969.

120. Vanderlaan WP: The occurrence of carcinoma of the thyroid gland in autopsy material, N Engl J Med 237:221–222, 1947.

121. Silverberg SG, Vidone RA: Carcinoma of the thyroid in surgical and postmortem material, Ann Surg 164:291–299, 1966.

122. Bisi H, Fernandes VSO, Asato de Camargo RY, et al: The prevalence of unsuspected thyroid pathology in 300 sequential autopsies, with special reference to the incidental carcinoma, Cancer 64:1888–1893, 1989.

123. Hedinger C, Williams ED, Sobin LH: Histological typing of thyroid tumours, vol 11. In: International Histological Classification of Tumors, ed 2, Berlin, Springer-Verlag, 1988.

124. Lang W, Borrush H, Bauer L: Occult carcinoma of the thyroid: evaluation of 1020 sequential autopsies, Am J Clin Pathol 90:72–76, 1988.

125. McConahey WM, Hay ID, Woolner LB, et al: Papillary thyroid cancer treated at the Mayo Clinic, 1946

through 1970: initial manifestation, pathologic findings, therapy, and outcome, Mayo Clin Proc 61:978–996, 1986.

126. Samaan NA, Schultz PN, Hickey RC, et al: The results of various modalities of treatment of well differentiated thyroid carcinoma: a retrospective review of 1599 patients, J Clin Endocrinol Metab 75:714–720, 1992.

127. Carcangiu ML, Zampi G, Pupi A, et al: Papillary carcinoma of the thyroid: a clinicopathologic study of 241 cases treated at the University of Florence, Italy, Cancer 55:805–828, 1985.

128. Iida F, Yonekura M, Miyakawa M: Study of intraglandular dissemination of thyroid cancer, Cancer 24:764–771, 1969.

129. Katoh R, Sasaki J, Kurihara H, et al: Multiple thyroid involvement (intraglandular metastasis) in papillary thyroid carcinoma: a clinicopathologic study of 105 consecutive patients, Cancer 70:1585–1590, 1992.

130. Pacini F, Elisei R, Capezzone M, et al: Contralateral papillary thyroid cancer is frequent at completion thyroidectomy with no difference in low- and high-risk patients, Thyroid 11:877–881, 2001.

131. Chan JKC, Saw D: The grooved nucleus: a useful diagnostic criterion of papillary carcinoma of the thyroid, Am J Surg Pathol 10:672–679, 1986.

132. Matsubayashi S, Kawai K, Matsumoto Y, et al: The correlation between papillary thyroid carcinoma and lymphocytic infiltration in the thyroid gland, J Clin Endocrinol Metab 80:3421–3424, 1995.

133. Pacini F, Cetani F, Miccoli P, et al: Outcome of 309 patients with metastatic differentiated thyroid carcinoma treated with radioiodine, World J Surg 18:600–604, 1994.

134. Rosai J, Zampi G, Carcangiu ML: Papillary carcinoma of the thyroid: a discussion of its several morphologic expressions, with particular emphasis on the follicular variant, Am J Surg Pathol 7:809–817, 1983.

135. Tielens ET, Sherman SI, Hruban RH, et al: Follicular variant of papillary thyroid carcinoma, Cancer 73:424–431, 1994.

136. Furmanchuk AW, Averkin JI, Egloff B, et al: Pathomorphological findings in thyroid cancers of children from the Republic of Belarus: a study of 86 cases occurring between 1986 (post Tchernobyl) and 1991, Histopathology 21:401–408, 1992.

137. Carcangiu ML, Bianchi S: Diffuse sclerosing variant of papillary thyroid carcinoma: clinicopathologic study of 15 cases, Am J Surg Pathol 13:1041–1049, 1989.

138. Johnson TL, Lloyd RV, Thompson NW, et al: Prognostic implications of the tall cell variant of papillary thyroid carcinoma, Am J Surg Pathol 12:22–27, 1988.

139. Sobrinho-Simoes M, Nesland JM, Johannessen JV: Columnar cell carcinoma: another variant of poorly differentiated carcinoma of the thyroid, Am J Clin Pathol 89:264–267, 1988.

140. Schroder S, Bocker W, Dralle H, et al: The encapsulated papillary carcinoma of the thyroid: a morphologic subtype of the papillary thyroid carcinoma, Cancer 54:90–93, 1984.

141. Lang W, Choritz H, Hundeshagen H: Risk factors in follicular thyroid carcinomas: a retrospective follow-up study covering a 14-year period with emphasis on morphological findings, Am J Surg Pathol 10:246–255, 1986.

142. Bronner MP, Livolsi VA: Oxyphilic (Askanazy/Hürthle cell) tumors of the thyroid: microscopic features predict biologic behaviour, Surg Pathol 1:137–150, 1988.

143. Carcangiu ML, Zampi G, Rosai J: Poorly differentiated "insular" thyroid carcinoma: a reinterpretation of Langhans "wuchernde Struma." Am J Surg Pathol 8:655–668, 1984.

144. Du Villard JA, Schlumberger M, Wicker R, et al: Role of ras and gsp oncogenes in human epithelial thyroid tumorigenesis, J Endocrinol Invest 18:124–126, 1995.

145. Fusco A, Grieco M, Santoro M, et al: A new oncogene in human thyroid papillary carcinomas and their lymph-nodal metastases, Nature 328:170–172, 1987.

146. Santoro M, Carlomagno F, Hay ID, et al: Ret oncogene activation in human thyroid neoplasms is restricted to the papillary cancer subtype, J Clin Invest 89:1517–1522, 1992.

147. Zou M, Shi Y, Farid NR: Low rate of ret proto-oncogene activation (PTC/ret TPC) in papillary thyroid carcinomas from Saudi Arabia, Cancer 73:176–180, 1994.

148. Wajjwalku W, Nakamura S, Hasegawa Y, et al: Low frequency of rearrangements of the ret and trk proto-oncogenes in Japanese thyroid papillary carcinomas, Jpn J Cancer Res 83:671–675, 1992.
149. Namba H, Yamashita S, Pei HC, et al: Lack of PTC gene (ret proto-oncogene rearrangement) in human thyroid tumors, Endocrinol Jpn 38:627–632, 1991.
150. Ito T, Seyama T, Iwamoto KS, et al: Activated RET oncogene in thyroid cancers of children from areas contaminated by Chernobyl accident, Lancet 344:259, 1994.
151. Fugazzola L, Pilotti S, Pinchera A, et al: Oncogenic rearrangements of the RET proto-oncogene in papillary thyroid carcinomas from children exposed to the Chernobyl nuclear accident, Cancer Res 55:5617–5620, 1995.
152. Klugbauer S, Lengfelder E, Demidchik EP, et al: High prevalence of RET rearrangement in thyroid tumors of children from Belarus after the Chernobyl reactor accident, Oncogene 11:2459–2467, 1995.
153. Elisei R, Romei C, Capezzone M, et al: Ret protooncogene rearrangements (RET/PTC) in malignant and benign thyroid nodular diseases, both spontaneous and radioinduced (abstract), J Endocrinol Invest 21:76, 1998.
154. Bounacer A, Wicker R, Caillou B, et al: High prevalence of activating ret proto-oncogene rearrangements, in thyroid tumors from patients who had received external radiation, Oncogene 15:1263–1273, 1997.
155. Nikiforov YE, Rowland JM, Bove KE, et al: Distinct pattern of ret oncogene rearrangements in morphological variants of radiation-induced and sporadic thyroid papillary carcinomas in children, Cancer Res 57:1690–1694, 1997.
156. Bongarzone I, Fugazzola L, Vigneri P, et al: Age-related activation of the tyrosine kinase receptor protooncogenes RET and NTRK1 in papillary thyroid carcinoma, J Clin Endocrinol Metab 81:2006–2009, 1996.
157. Elisei R, Ugolini C, Viola D, et al: BRAF(V600E) mutation and outcome of patients with papillary thyroid carcinoma: a 15-year median follow-up study, J Clin Endocrinol Metab 93:3943–3949. 2008.
158. Challeton C, Bounacer A, Du Villard JA, et al: Pattern of ras and gsp oncogene mutations in radiation-associated human thyroid tumors, Oncogene 11:601–603, 1995.
159. Russo D, Arturi F, Schlumberger M, et al: Activating mutations of the TSH receptor in differentiated thyroid carcinomas, Oncogene 11:1907–1911, 1995.
160. Fagin JA, Matsuo K, Karmakar A, et al: High prevalence of mutations of the p53 gene in poorly differentiated human thyroid carcinomas, J Clin Invest 91:179–184, 1993.
161. Yamashita S, Ong J, Fagin JA, et al: Expression of the myc cellular protooncogene in human thyroid tissue, J Clin Endocrinol Metab 63:1170–1173, 1986.
162. Matsuo K, Tang SH, Fagin JA: Allelotype of human thyroid tumors: loss of chromosome 11q13 sequences in follicular neoplasms, Mol Endocrinol 5:1873–1879, 1991.
163. Farid NR, Shi Y, Zou M: Molecular basis of thyroid cancer, Endocr Rev 15:202–228, 1994.
164. Nikiforova MN, Lynch RA, Biddinger PW, et al: RAS point mutations and PAX8-PPAR gamma rearrangement in thyroid tumors: evidence for distinct molecular pathways in thyroid follicular carcinoma, J Clin Endocrinol Metab 88:2318–2326, 2003.
165. Masago K, Asato R, Fujita S, et al: Epidermal growth factor receptor gene mutations in papillary thyroid carcinoma, Int J Cancer 124:2744–2749, 2009.
166. Lazar V, Bidart JM, Caillou B, et al: Exspession of the Na+/I– symporter gene in human thyroid tumors: a comparson study with other thyroid specific genes, J Clin Endocrinol Metab 84:3228–3234, 1999.
167. Ron E, Lubin JH, Shore RE, et al: Thyroid cancer after exposure to external radiation: a pooled analysis of seven studies, Radiat Res 141, 259–277, 1995.
168. Schneider AB, Ron E: Pathogenesis. In Braverman LE, Utiger RD, editors: Werner and Ingbar's The Thyroid: A Fundamental and Clinical Text, ed 7, Philadelphia, 1996, Lippincott-Raven, pp 902–909.
169. Favus MJ, Schneider AB, Stachyra ME: Thyroid cancer occurring as a late consequence of head-and-neck irradiation, N Engl J Med 294:1019–1025, 1976.
170. Franceschi S, Boyle P, Maissonneuve P: The epidemiology of thyroid carcinoma, Crit Rev Oncog 4:25–52, 1993.
171. Pacini F, Vorontsova T, Demidchik EP, et al: Post-Chernobyl thyroid carcinoma in Belarus children and adolescents: comparison with naturally occurring thyroid carcinoma in Italy and France, J Clin Endocrinol Metab 82:3563–3569, 1997.
172. Tronko N, Bogdanova T, Kommisarenko I, et al: Thyroid cancer in children and adolescents in Ukraine after the Chernobyl accident (1986–1995). In Karaoglou A, Desmet G, Kelly GN, et al, editors: The Radiological Consequences of the Chernobyl Accident. ERU 16544 EN, European Union, 1996, Luxembourg, p 683.
173. Dobyns BM, Hyrmer BA: The surgical management of benign and malignant thyroid neoplasms in Marshall Islanders exposed to hydrogen bomb fallout, World J Surg 16:126–140, 1992.
174. Baverstock K, Egloff B, Pinchera A, et al: Thyroid cancer after Chernobyl, Nature 359:21–22, 1992.
175. Cooper DS, Axelrod L, DeGroot LJ, et al: Congenital goiter and the development of metastatic follicular carcinoma with evidence for a leak of nonhormonal iodide: clinical, pathological, kinetic, and biochemical studies and a review of the literature, J Clin Endocrinol Metab 52:294–303, 1981.
176. Abe Y, Ichikawa Y, Muraki T, et al: Thyrotropin (TSH) receptor and adenylate cyclase activity in human thyroid tumors: absence of high affinity receptor and loss of TSH responsiveness in undifferentiated thyroid carcinoma, J Clin Endocrinol Metab 52:23–28, 1981.
177. Behar R, Arganini M, Wu TC, et al: Graves' disease and thyroid cancer, Surgery 100:1121–1127, 1986.
178. Hsu TC, Pathak S, Samaan N, et al: Chromosome instability in patients with medullary carcinoma of the thyroid, JAMA 246:2046–2048, 1981.
179. Panza N, Vecchio LD, Maio M, et al: Strong association between an HLA-DR antigen and thyroid carcinoma, Tissue Antigen 20:155–158, 1982.
180. Weissel M, Kainz H, Hoefer R, et al: HLA-DR and differentiated thyroid cancer: lack of association with the nonmedullary types and possible association with the medullary type, Cancer 62:2486–2488, 1988.
181. Sridama V, Hara Y, Fauchet R, et al: Association of differentiated thyroid carcinoma with HLA-DR7 antigen (abstract 24). In Proceedings of the 59th Meeting of the American Thyroid Association, New Orleans, October 6, 1983.
182. Lloyd KM II, Dennis M: Cowden's disease: a possible new symptom complex with multiple system involvement, Ann Intern Med 58:136–142, 1963.
183. de Mestier P: Thyroid cancer and familial rectocolonic polyposis, Chirurgie 116:514–516, 1990.
184. Plail RO, Bussey HJ, Glazer G, et al: Adenomatous polyposis: an association with carcinoma of the thyroid, Br J Surg 74:377–380, 1987.
185. Camiel MR, Mule JE, Alexander LL, et al: Association of thyroid carcinoma with Gardner's syndrome in siblings, N Engl J Med 278:1056–1058, 1968.
186. Albores-Saavedra J, Duran ME: Association of thyroid carcinoma in chemodectoma, Am J Surg 116:887–890, 1968.
187. Uchino S, Noguchi S, Kawamoto H, et al: Familial nonmedullary thyroid carcinoma characterized by multifocality and a high recurrence rate in a large study population, World J Surg 26:897–902, 2002.
188. Capezzone M, Cantara S, Marchisotta S, et al: Short telomeres, telomerase reverse transcriptase gene amplification, and increased telomerase activity in the blood of familial papillary thyroid cancer patients, J Clin Endocrinol Metab 93:3950–3957, 2008.
189. Leenhardt L, Grosclaude P, Chérié-Challine L: Thyroid Cancer Committee: increased incidence of thyroid carcinoma in France: a true epidemic or thyroid nodule management effects? Report from the French Thyroid Cancer Committee, Thyroid 14:1056–1060, 2004.
190. Lin JD, Huang BY, Chao TC, et al: Diagnosis of occult thyroid carcinoma by thyroid ultrasonography with fine needle aspiration cytology, Acta Cytol 41:1751–1756, 1997.
191. Elisei R, Bottici V, Luchetti F, et al: Impact of routine measurement of serum calcitonin on the diagnosis and outcome of medullary thyroid cancer: experience in 10,864 patients with nodular thyroid disorders, J Clin Endocrinol Metab 89:163–168, 2004.
192. McDermott WV Jr, Morgan WS, Hamlin E Jr, et al: Cancer of the thyroid, J Clin Endocrinol Metab 14:1336–1354, 1954.
193. DeGroot LJ, Kaplan EL, McCormick M, et al: Natural history, treatment, and course of papillary thyroid carcinoma, J Clin Endocrinol Metab 71:414–424, 1990.
194. Woolner LB, Lemmon ML, Beahrs OH, et al: Occult papillary carcinoma of the thyroid: study of 140 cases observed in a 30-year period, J Clin Endocrinol Metab 20:89–105, 1960.
195. Franssila K: Value of histologic classification of thyroid cancer, Acta Pathol Microbiol Scand [A] 225(suppl):1–76, 1971.
196. Schlumberger M, De Vathaire F, Travagli JP, et al: Differentiated thyroid carcinoma in childhood: long-term follow-up of 72 patients, J Clin Endocrinol Metab 65:1088–1094, 1987.
197. Hazard JB, Hawk WA, Crile G Jr: Medullary (solid) carcinoma of the thyroid: a clinicopathologic entity, J Clin Endocrinol Metab 19:152–161, 1959.
198. Wolfe HJ, Melvin KEW, Cervi-Skinner SJ, et al: C-cell hyperplasia preceding medullary thyroid carcinoma, N Engl J Med 289:437–441, 1973.
199. Donahower GF, Schumacher OP, Hazard JB: Medullary carcinoma of the thyroid: a cause of Cushing's syndrome: report of two cases, J Clin Endocrinol Metab 28:1199–1204, 1968.
200. Pacini F, Basolo F, Elisei R, et al: Medullary thyroid cancer: an immunohistochemical and humoral study using six separate antigens, Am J Clin Pathol 95:300–308, 1991.
201. Graze K, Spiler IJ, Tashjian AH Jr, et al: Natural history of familial medullary thyroid carcinoma: effect of a program for early diagnosis, N Engl J Med 299:980–985, 1978.
202. Melvin KEW, Miller HH, Tashjian AH: Early diagnosis of medullary carcinoma of the thyroid gland by means of calcitonin assay, N Engl J Med 285:1115–1120, 1971.
203. Wells SA Jr, Baylin SB, Linehan WM, et al: Provocative agents and the diagnosis of medullary carcinoma of the thyroid gland, Ann Surg 188:139–141, 1978.
204. Eng C, Clayton D, Schuffenecker I, et al: The relationship between specific RET proto-oncogene mutation and disease phenotype in multiple endocrine neoplasia type 2: International RET Mutation Consortium Analysis, JAMA 276:1575–1579, 1996.
205. Pacini F, Romei C, Miccolo P, et al: Early treatment of hereditary medullary thyroid carcinoma after attribution of multiple endocrine neoplasia type 2 gene carrier status by screening for ret gene mutations, Surgery 118:1031–1035, 1995.
206. Harada T, Ito K, Shimaoka K, et al: Fatal thyroid carcinoma: anaplastic transformation of adenocarcinoma, Cancer 39:2588–2596, 1977.
207. Justin EP, Seabold JE, Robinson RA, et al: Insular carcinoma: a distinct thyroid carcinoma with associated iodine-131 localization, J Nucl Med 32:1358–1363, 1991.
208. Romei C, Ciampi R, Faviana P, et al: BRAFV600E mutation, but not RET/PTC rearrangements, is correlated with a lower expression of both thyroperoxidase and sodium iodide symporter genes in papillary thyroid cancer, Endocr Relat Cancer 15:511–520, 2008.
209. Casara D, Rubello D, Saladini G, et al: Differentiated thyroid carcinoma in the elderly, Aging (Milano) 4:333–339, 1992.
210. Simpson WJ, McKinney SE, Carruthers JS, et al: Papillary and follicular thyroid cancer: prognostic factors in 1578 patients, Am J Med 83:479–488, 1987.
211. Tubiana M, Schlumberger M, Rougier P, et al: Long-term results and prognostic factors in patients with differentiated thyroid carcinoma, Cancer 55:794–804, 1985.
212. Akslen LA, Haldorsen T, Thoresen SO, et al: Survival and causes of death in thyroid cancer: a population-based study of 2479 cases from Norway, Cancer Res 51:1234–1241, 1991.
213. DeGroot LJ, Kaplan EL, Shukla MS, et al: Morbidity and mortality in follicular thyroid cancer, J Clin Endocrinol Metab 80:2946–2953, 1995.
214. Joensuu H, Klemi PJ, Paul R, et al: Survival and prognostic factors in thyroid carcinoma, Acta Radiol Oncol 25:243–248, 1986.

215. Mizukami Y, Noguchi M, Michigishi T, et al: Papillary thyroid carcinoma in Kanazawa, Japan: prognostic significance of histological subtypes, Histopathology 20:243–250, 1992.
216. Shah JP, Loree TR, Dharker D, et al: Prognostic factors in differentiated carcinoma of the thyroid gland, Am J Med 164:658–661, 1992.
217. Ceccarelli C, Pacini F, Lippi F, et al: Thyroid cancer in children and adolescents, Surgery 104:1143–1148, 1988.
218. La Quaglia MP, Corbally MT, Heller G, et al: Recurrence and morbidity in differentiated thyroid carcinoma in children, Surgery 104:1149–1156, 1988.
219. Thoresen S, Akslen LA, Glattre E, et al: Thyroid cancer in children in Norway, 1953–1987, Eur J Cancer 29A:365–366, 1993.
220. Akslen LA, Myking AO, Salvesen H, et al: Prognostic importance of various clinico-pathological features in papillary thyroid carcinoma, Eur J Cancer 29A:44–51, 1993.
221. Ahuja S, Ernst H: Hyperthyroidism and thyroid carcinoma, Acta Endocrinol (Copenh) 124:146–151, 1991.
222. Dobyns BM, Sheline GE, Workman JB, et al: Malignant and benign neoplasms of the thyroid in patients treated for hyperthyroidism: a report of the Cooperative Thyrotoxicosis Therapy Follow-up Study, J Clin Endocrinol Metab 38:976–998, 1974.
223. Soh EY, Park CS: Diagnostic approach to thyroid carcinoma in Graves' disease, Yonsei Med J 34:191–194, 1993.
224. Hay ID, Bergstralh EJ, Goellner JR, et al: Predicting outcome in papillary thyroid carcinoma: development of a reliable prognostic scoring system in a cohort of 1779 patients surgically treated at one institution during 1940 through 1989, Surgery 114:1050–1057, 1993.
225. Segal K, Ben-Bassat M, Avraham A, et al: Hashimoto's thyroiditis and carcinoma of the thyroid gland, Int Surg 70:205–209, 1985.
226. Pacini F, Mariotti S, Formica N, et al: Thyroid autoantibodies in thyroid cancer: incidence and relationship with tumour outcome, Acta Endocrinol (Copenh) 119:373–380, 1988.
227. Chiovato L, Latrofa F, Braverman LE, et al: Disappearance of humoral thyroid autoimmunity after complete removal of thyroid antigens, Ann Intern Med 139:346–351, 2003.
228. Hawk WA, Hazard JB: The many appearances of papillary carcinoma of the thyroid, Clev Clin Q 43:207–215, 1976.
229. Evans HL: Columnar-cell carcinoma of the thyroid: a report of two cases of an aggressive variant of thyroid carcinoma, Am J Clin Pathol 85:77–80, 1986.
230. Herrera MF, Hay ID, Wu PS-C, et al: Hürthle cell (oxyphilic) papillary thyroid carcinoma: a variant with more aggressive biologic behaviour, World J Surg 16:669–674, 1992.
231. Sobrinho-Simoes MA, Nesland JM, Holm R, et al: Hürthle cell and mitochondrion-rich papillary carcinomas of the thyroid gland: an ultrastructural and immunocytochemical study, Ultrastruct Pathol 8:131–142, 1985.
232. Carcangiu ML, Zampi G, Rosai J: Papillary thyroid carcinoma: a study of its many morphologic expressions and clinical correlates, Pathol Ann 20:1–44, 1985.
233. Evans HL: Encapsulated papillary neoplasms of the thyroid: a study of 14 cases followed for a minimum of 10 years, Am J Surg Pathol 11:592–597, 1987.
234. Soares J, Limbert E, Sobrinho-Simoes M: Diffuse sclerosing variant of papillary thyroid carcinoma: a clinicopathologic study of 10 cases, Pathol Res Pract 185:200–206, 1989.
235. Akslen LA, Myking AO: Differentiated thyroid carcinomas: the relevance of various pathological features for tumour classification and prediction of tumour progress, Virchows Arch 421:17–23, 1992.
236. Schlumberger M, Challeton C, De Vathaire F, et al: Radioactive iodine treatment and external radiotherapy for lung and bone metastases from thyroid carcinoma, J Nucl Med 37:598–605, 1996.
237. Schelfhout LJ, Creuzberg CL, Hamming JF, et al: Multivariate analysis of survival in differentiated thyroid cancer: the prognostic significance of the age factor, Eur J Cancer Clin Oncol 24:331–337, 1988.
238. Schroder S, Dralle H, Rehpenning W, et al: Prognostic criteria in papillary thyroid carcinoma, Langenbecks Arch Chir 371:263–280, 1987.
239. Joensuu H, Klemi PJ, Eerola E, et al: Influence of cellular DNA content on survival in differentiated thyroid cancer, Cancer 58:2462–2467, 1986.
240. Mazzaferri EL: Impact of initial tumor features and treatment selected on the long-term course of differentiated thyroid cancer, Thyroid Today 18:1–13, 1995.
241. Schindler AM, van Melle G, Evequoz B, et al: Prognostic factors in papillary carcinoma of the thyroid, Cancer 68:324–330, 1991.
242. Katoh R, Sasaki J, Kurihara H, et al: Multiple thyroid involvement (intraglandular metastasis) in papillary thyroid carcinoma: a clinicopathologic study of 105 consecutive patients, Cancer 70:1585–1590, 1992.
243. Tscholl-Ducommun J, Hedinger CE: Papillary thyroid carcinomas: morphology and prognosis, Virchows Arch 396:19–39, 1982.
244. Cody HS III, Shah JP: Locally invasive, well differentiated thyroid cancer: 22 years' experience at Memorial Sloan-Kettering Cancer Center, Am J Surg 142:480–483, 1981.
245. Salvesen H, Njolstad PR, Akslen LA, et al: Papillary thyroid carcinoma: a multivariate analysis of prognostic factors including an evaluation of the p-TNM staging system, Eur J Surg 158:583–589, 1992.
246. Noguchi M, Kinami S, Kinoshita K, et al: Risk of bilateral cervical lymph node metastases in papillary thyroid cancer, J Surg Oncol 52:155–159, 1993.
247. Rossi RL: Lymph node metastases in thyroid carcinoma: incidence, patterns of progression, and significance, Lahey Clin Found Bull 32:168, 1983.
248. Mazzaferri EL: Thyroid carcinoma: papillary and follicular. In Mazzaferri EL, Samaan N, editors: Endocrine Tumors, Cambridge, 1993, Blackwell, pp 278–804.
249. Coburn M, Wanebo HJ: Prognostic factors and management considerations in patients with cervical metastases of thyroid cancer, Am J Surg 164:671–676, 1992.
250. Scheumann GFW, Gimm O, Wegener G, et al: Prognostic significance and surgical management of locoregional lymph node metastases in papillary thyroid cancer, World J Surg 18:559–568, 1994.
251. Sellers M, Beenken S, Blankenship A, et al: Prognostic significance of cervical lymph node metastases in differentiated thyroid cancer, Am J Surg 164:578–581, 1992.
252. Coburn M, Teates D, Wanebo HJ: Recurrent thyroid cancer: role of surgery versus radioactive iodine (I^{131}), Ann Surg 219:587–593, 1994.
253. Hoie J, Stenwig AE, Kullmann G, et al: Distant metastases in papillary thyroid cancer: a review of 91 patients, Cancer 61:1–6, 1988.
254. Ozaki O, Ito K, Sugino K: Clinico-pathologic study of pulmonary metastasis of differentiated thyroid carcinoma: age-, sex-, and histology-matched case-control study, Int Surg 78:218–220, 1993.
255. Rodriquez-Cuevas S, Almendaro SL, Cardoso JMR, et al: Papillary thyroid cancer in Mexico: review of 409 cases, Head Neck 15:537, 1993.
256. Casara D, Rubello D, Saladini G, et al: Distant metastases in differentiated thyroid cancer: long-term results of radioiodine treatment and statistical analysis of prognostic factors in 214 patients, Tumori 77:432–436, 1991.
257. Casara D, Rubello D, Saladini G, et al: Different features of pulmonary metastases in differentiated thyroid cancer: natural history and multivariate analysis of prognostic variables, J Nucl Med 34:1626–1631, 1993.
258. Beierwaltes WH, Nishiyama RH, Thompson NW, et al: Survival time and "cure" in papillary and follicular thyroid carcinoma with distant metastases: statistics following University of Michigan therapy, J Nucl Med 23:561–568, 1982.
259. Rossi RL, Cady B, Silverman ML, et al: Surgically incurable well-differentiated thyroid carcinoma: prognostic factors and results of therapy, Arch Surg 123:569–574, 1988.
260. Elisei R, Pinchera A, Romei C, et al: Expression of thyrotropin receptor (TSH-R), thyroglobulin, thyroperoxidase, and calcitonin messenger ribonucleic acids in thyroid carcinomas: evidence of TSH-R gene transcript in medullary histotype, J Clin Endocrinol Metab 78:867–871, 1994.
261. Pollina L, Pacini F, Fontanini G, et al: Bcl-2, p53 and proliferating cell nuclear antigen expression is related to the degree of differentiation in thyroid carcinomas, Br J Cancer 73:139–143, 1996.
262. Basolo F, Pinchera A, Fugazzola L, et al: Expression of the p21 ras protein as a prognostic factor in papillary thyroid cancer, Eur J Cancer 30A:171–174, 1994.
263. Romano MI, Grattone M, Karner MP, et al: Relationship between the level of c-myc mRNA and histologic aggressiveness in thyroid tumors, Horm Res 39:161–165, 1993.
264. Basolo F, Molinaro E, Agate L, et al: RET protein expression has no prognostic impact on the long-term outcome of papillary thyroid carcinoma, Eur J Endocrinol 145:599–604, 2001.
265. Dvorakova S, Vaclavikova E, Sykorova V, et al: Somatic mutations in the RET proto-oncogene in sporadic medullary thyroid carcinomas, Mol Cell Endocrinol 284:21–27, 2008.
266. Romei C, Elisei E, Pinchera A, et al: Somatic mutations of the ret protooncogene in sporadic medullary thyroid carcinoma are not restricted to exon 16 and are associated with tumor recurrence, J Clin Endocrinol Metab 81:1619–1622, 1996.
267. Halnan KE: Influence of age and sex on incidence and prognosis of thyroid cancer: 344 cases followed for ten years, Cancer 19:1534–1541, 1966.
268. Mazzaferri EL, Young RL: Papillary thyroid carcinoma: a 10 year follow-up report of the impact of therapy in 576 patients, Am J Med 70:511–518, 1981.
269. Mazzaferri EL, Young RL, Oertel JE, et al: Papillary thyroid carcinoma: the impact of therapy in 576 patients, Medicine (Baltimore) 56:171–196, 1977.
270. Samaan NA, Mageshwari YK, Nadal S, et al: Impact of therapy for differentiated carcinoma of the thyroid: an analysis of 706 cases, J Clin Endocrinol Metab 56:1131–1138, 1983.
271. Massin JP, Savoie JP, Garnier H, et al: Pulmonary metastases in differentiated thyroid carcinoma: study of 58 cases with implications for the primary treatment, Cancer 53:982–987, 1984.
272. Mazzaferri EL: Papillary thyroid carcinoma: factors affecting prognosis and current therapy, Semin Oncol 14:315–332, 1987.
273. Pacini F, Ceccarelli C, Elisei R, et al: Serum thyroglobulin determination in thyroid cancer: a ten years experience. In Nagataki S, Torizuka K, editors: The Thyroid, New York, 1988, Elsevier, p 685.
274. Pacini F, Mari R, Mazzeo S, et al: Diagnostic value of a single serum tg determination on and off thyroid suppressive therapy in the follow-up of differentiated thyroid cancer, Clin Endocrinol (Oxf) 23:405–411, 1985.
275. Schlumberger M, Parmentier C, de Vathaire F, et al: 131-I and external radiation in the treatment of local and metastatic thyroid cancer. In Falk S, editor: Thyroid Disease, New York, 1990, Raven, p 537.
276. Pacini F, Lippi F, Formica N, et al: Therapeutic doses of iodine-131 reveal undiagnosed metastases in thyroid cancer patients with detectable serum thyroglobulin levels, J Nucl Med 28:1888–1891, 1987.
277. Byar DP, Green SB, Dor P, et al: A prognostic index for thyroid carcinoma: a study of the EORTC Thyroid Cancer Cooperative Group, Eur J Cancer 15:1033–1041, 1979.
278. Tennvall J, Biorklund A, Moller T, et al: Is the EORTC prognostic index of thyroid cancer valid in differentiated thyroid carcinoma? Retrospective multivariate analysis of differentiated thyroid carcinoma with long follow-up, Cancer 57:1405–1414, 1986.
279. Hermanek P, Henson DE, Hutter RVP, et al: TNM Supplement 1993: A Commentary on Uniform Use, International Union Against Cancer, Berlin, 1993, Springer-Verlag.
280. Hermanek P, Sobin LH: TNM Classification of Malignant Tumors: International Union Against Cancer, ed 4, New York, 1987, Springer-Verlag.
281. Cady B, Rossi R: An expanded view of risk-group definition in differentiated thyroid carcinoma, Surgery 104:947–953, 1988.
282. Pasieka JL, Zedenius J, Auer G, et al: Addition of nuclear DNA content to the AMES risk-group classification for papillary thyroid cancer, Surgery 112:1154–1159, 1992.
283. Allo MD, Christianson W, Koivunen D: Not all "occult" papillary carcinomas are "minimal." Surgery 104:971–976, 1988.

284. Clark OH, Levin K, Zeng QH, et al: Thyroid cancer: the case for total thyroidectomy, Eur J Cancer Clin Oncol 24:305–313, 1988.
285. Mazzaferri EL: Treating differentiated thyroid carcinoma: where do we draw the line? Mayo Clin Proc 66:105–111, 1991.
286. Snyder J, Gorman C, Scanlon P: Thyroid remnant ablation: questionable pursuit of an ill-defined goal, J Nucl Med 24:659–665, 1983.
287. Rustad WH, Lindsay S, Dailey ME: Comparison of the incidence of complications following total and subtotal thyroidectomy for thyroid carcinoma, Surg Gynecol Obstet 116:109–112, 1963.
288. Black B, Yadeau R, Woolner L: Surgical treatment of thyroid carcinomas, Arch Surg 88:610–618, 1964.
289. Shands WC, Gatling RR: Cancer of the thyroid: review of 109 cases, Ann Surg 171:735–745, 1970.
290. Tollefsen HR, Shah JP, Huvos AG: Papillary carcinoma of the thyroid: recurrence in the thyroid gland after initial surgical treatment, Am J Surg 124:468–472, 1972.
291. Tollefsen H, DeCosse J: Papillary carcinoma of the thyroid: the case for radical neck dissection, Am J Surg 108:547–551, 1964.
292. Duffield RGM, Lowe D, Burnand KG: Treatment of well-differentiated carcinoma of the thyroid based on initial staging, Br J Surg 69:426–428, 1982.
293. Young RL, Mazzaferri EL, Rahe AJ, et al: Pure follicular thyroid carcinoma: impact of therapy in 214 patients, J Nucl Med 21:733–737, 1980.
294. Pacini F, Schlumberger M, Harmer C, et al: Post-surgical use of radioiodine (131I) in patients with papillary and follicular thyroid cancer and the issue of remnant ablation: a consensus report, Eur J Endocrinol 153:651–659, 2005.
295. Pilli T, Brianzoni E, Capoccetti F, et al: A comparison of 1850 (50 mCi) and 3700 MBq (100 mCi) 131-iodine administered doses for recombinant thyrotropin-stimulated postoperative thyroid remnant ablation in differentiated thyroid cancer, J Clin Endocrinol Metab 92:3542–3546, 2007.
296. Block GE, Wilson SM: A modified neck dissection for carcinoma of the thyroid, Surg Clin North Am 51:139–148, 1971.
297. Mustard RA: Treatment of papillary carcinoma of the thyroid with emphasis on conservative neck dissection, Am J Surg 120:697–703, 1970.
298. Simpson WJ, Panzarella T, Carruthers JS, et al: Papillary and follicular thyroid cancer: impact of treatment in 1578 patients, Int J Radiat Oncol Biol Phys 14:1063–1075, 1988.
299. Devine RM, Edis AJ, Banks PM: Primary lymphoma of the thyroid: a review of the Mayo Clinic experience through 1978, World J Surg 5:33–38, 1981.
300. Butler JS Jr, Brady LW, Amendola BE: Lymphoma of the thyroid: report of five cases and review, Am J Clin Oncol 13:64–69, 1990.
301. Leedman PJ, Sheridan WP, Downey WF, et al: Combination chemotherapy as single modality therapy for stage IE and IIE thyroid lymphoma, Med J Aust 152:40–43, 1990.
302. Smedal MI, Messner WA: The results of x-ray treatment in undifferentiated carcinoma of the thyroid, Radiology 76:927, 1961.
303. Shimaoka K, Schoenfeld DA, DeWys WD: A randomized trial of doxorubicin versus doxorubicin plus cisplatin in patients with advanced thyroid carcinoma, Cancer 56:2155–2160, 1985.
304. Sokal M, Harmer GI: Chemotherapy for anaplastic carcinoma of the thyroid, Clin Oncol 4:3–10, 1978.
305. Pacini F, Pinchera A, Mancusi F, et al: Anaplastic thyroid carcinoma: a retrospective clinical and immunohistochemical study, Oncol Rep 1:921–925, 1994.
306. Tallroth E, Wallin G, Lundell G, et al: Multimodality treatment in anaplastic giant cell thyroid carcinoma, Cancer 60:1428–1431, 1987.
307. Werner B, Abele J, Alveryd A, et al: Multimodal therapy in anaplastic giant cell thyroid carcinoma, J World Surg 8:64–70, 1984.
308. Nel CJ, van Heerden JA, Goellner JR: Anaplastic carcinoma of the thyroid: a clinicopathological study of eighty-two cases, Mayo Clin Proc 60:51–58, 1985.
309. Venkatesh YS, Ordonez NG, Schultz PN, et al: Anaplastic carcinoma of the thyroid: a clinicopathological study of 121 cases, Cancer 66:321–330, 1990.
310. Tennvall J, Tallroth E, El Hassan A, et al: Anaplastic thyroid carcinoma: doxorubicin, hyperfractionated radiotherapy and surgery, Acta Oncol 29:1025–1028, 1990.
311. Tennvall J, Lundell G, Hallquist A, et al: Combined doxorubicin, hyperfractionated radiotherapy, and surgery in anaplastic thyroid carcinoma, Cancer 74:1348–1354, 1994.
312. Schlumberger M, Parmentier C, Delisle MJ, et al: Combination therapy for anaplastic giant cell thyroid carcinoma, Cancer 67:564–566, 1991.
313. Kim JH, Leeper RD: Treatment of anaplastic giant and spindle cell carcinoma of the thyroid gland with combination Adriamycin and radiation therapy: a new approach, Cancer 52:954–957, 1983.
314. Ito T, Seyama T, Mizuno T, et al: Unique association of p53 mutations with undifferentiated but not with differentiated carcinomas of the thyroid gland, Cancer Res 52:1369–1371, 1992.
315. Pacini F, Laderson W, Schlumberger M, et al: Radioiodine ablation of thyroid remnants after preparation with recombinant human thyrotropin in differentiated thyroid carcinoma: results of an international, randomized, controlled study, J Clin Endocrinol Metab 91:926–932, 2006.
316. Hänscheid H, Lassmann M, Luster M, et al: Iodine biokinetics and dosimetry in radioiodine therapy of thyroid cancer: procedures and results of a prospective international controlled study of ablation after rhTSH or hormone, J Nucl Med 47:648–654, 2006.
317. Pacini F, Molinaro E, Castagna MG, et al: Ablation of thyroid residues with 30 mCi (131)I: a comparison in thyroid cancer patients prepared with recombinant human TSH or thyroid hormone withdrawal, J Clin Endocrinol Metab 87:4063–4068, 2002.
317a. Mäenpää HO, Heikkonen J, Vaalavirta L, et al: Low vs, high radioiodine activity to ablate the thyroid after thyroidectomy for cancer: a randomized study, PLoS ONE 3:e1885, 2008.
318. Maxon HR III, Smith HS: Radioiodine-131 in the diagnosis and treatment of metastatic well differentiated thyroid cancer, Endocrinol Metab Clin North Am 19:685–718, 1990.
319. Schlumberger M, Tubiana M, De Vathaire F, et al: Long-term results of treatment of 238 patients with lung and bone metastases from differentiated thyroid carcinoma, J Clin Endocrinol Metab 63:960–967, 1986.
320. Brown AP, Greening WP, McCready VR, et al: Radioiodine treatment of metastatic thyroid carcinoma: the Royal Marsden Hospital experience, Br J Radiol 57:323–327, 1984.
321. Samaan NA, Schultz PN, Haynie TP, et al: Pulmonary metastasis of differentiated thyroid carcinoma: treatment results in 101 patients, J Clin Endocrinol Metab 60:376–380, 1985.
322. Ruegemer JJ, Hay ID, Bergstralh EJ, et al: Distant metastases in differentiated thyroid carcinoma: a multivariate analysis of prognostic variables, J Clin Endocrinol Metab 67:501–508, 1988.
323. Marcocci C, Pacini F, Elisei R, et al: Clinical and biological behaviour of bone metastases from differentiated thyroid carcinoma, Surgery 106:960–966, 1989.
324. Grunwald F, Menzel C, Bender H, et al: Comparison of 18 FDG-PET with 131 iodine and 99 Tc-sestamibi scintigtaphy in differentiated thyroid cancer, Thyroid 7:327–335, 1997.
325. Dietlen M, Scheidhauer K, Voth E, et al: Fluorine-18-fluorodesoxyglucose positron emission tomography and iodine-131 whole-body scintigraphy in the follow-up of differentiated thyroid cancer, Eur J Nucl Med 24:1342–1348, 1997.
326. Feine U, Lietzenmayer R, Hanke JP, et al: Fluorine-18-FDG abd iodine 131 uptake in thyroid cancer, J Nucl Med 37:1468–1472, 1996.
327. Sisson JC, Ackermann RJ, Meyer MA, et al: Uptake of 18-fluoro-2-deoxy-D-glucose by thyroid cancer: implications for diagnosis and therapy, J Clin Endocrinol Metab 77:1090–1094, 1993.
328. Plotkin M, Hautzel H, Krause BJ, et al: Implication of 2–18-fluoro-2-deoxyglucose positron emission tomography in the follow-up of Hürthle cell thyroid cancer, Thyroid 12:155–161, 2002.
329. Frilling A, Tecklenborg K, Gorges R, et al: Preoperative diagnostic value of (18)F-fluorodeoxyglucose positron emission tomography in patients with radioiodine-negative recurrent well-differentiated thyroid carcinoma, Ann Surg 234:804–811, 2001.
330. Helal BO, Merlet P, Toubert ME, et al: Clinical impact of (18)F-FDG PET in thyroid carcinoma patients with elevated thyroglobulin levels and negative (131)I scanning results after therapy, J Nucl Med 42:1464–1469, 2001.
331. Van Herle AJ, Uller RP: Elevated serum thyroglobulin: a marker of metastases in differentiated thyroid carcinomas, J Clin Invest 56:272–277, 1975.
332. Schlumberger M, Fragu P, Parmentier C, et al: Thyroglobulin assay in the follow-up of patients with differentiated thyroid carcinomas: comparison of its value in patients with or without normal residual tissue, Acta Endocrinol (Copenh) 98:215–221, 1981.
333. Ozata M, Suzuki S, Miyamoto T, et al: Serum thyroglobulin in the follow-up of patients with treated differentiated thyroid cancer, J Clin Endocrinol Metab 79:98–105, 1994.
334. Edmonds CJ, Smith T: The long-term hazard of the treatment of thyroid cancer with radioiodine, Br J Radiol 59:45–51, 1986.
335. Mariotti S, Barbesino G, Caturegli P, et al: Assay of thyroglobulin in serum with thyroglobulin autoantibodies: an unobtainable goal? J Clin Endocrinol Metab 80:468–472, 1995.
336. Pacini F, Pinchera A, Giani C, et al: Serum thyroglobulin concentrations and 131-I whole body scans in the diagnosis of metastases from differentiated thyroid carcinoma (after thyroidectomy), Clin Endocrinol (Oxf) 13:107–110, 1980.
337. Ashcraft MW, Van Herle AJ: The comparative value of serum thyroglobulin measurements and iodine-131 total body scans in the follow-up study of patients with treated differentiated thyroid cancer, Am J Med 71:806–814, 1981.
338. Schlumberger M, Arcangioli O, Piekarski JD, et al: Detection and treatment of lung metastases of differentiated thyroid carcinoma in patients with normal chest x-rays, J Nucl Med 29:1790–1794, 1988.
339. Pineda JD, Lee T, Ain K, et al: Iodine-131 therapy for thyroid cancer patients with elevated thyroglobulin and negative diagnostic scan, J Clin Endocrinol Metab 80:1488–1492, 1995.
340. Pacini F, Agate L, Elisei R, et al: Outcome of differentiated thyroid cancer with detectable serum Tg and negative diagnostic 131-I whole body scan: comparison of patients treated with high 131-I activities versus untreated patients, J Clin Endocrinol Metab 86:4092–4097, 2001.
341. Schlumberger M, Charbord P, Fragu P, et al: Circulating thyroglobulin and thyroid hormones in patients with metastases of differentiated thyroid carcinoma: relationship to serum thyrotropin levels, J Clin Endocrinol Metab 51:513–519, 1980.
342. Schneider AB, Line BR, Goldman JM, et al: Sequential serum thyroglobulin determinations, ^{131}I scans, and ^{131}I uptakes after triiodothyronine withdrawal in patients with thyroid cancer, J Clin Endocrinol Metab 53:1199–1206, 1981.
343. Ladenson PW, Braverman LE, Mazzaferri EL, et al: Comparison of administration of recombinant human thyrotropin with withdrawal of thyroid hormone for radioactive iodine scanning in patients with thyroid carcinoma, N Engl J Med 337:888–896, 1997.
344. Haugen BR, Pacini F, Reiners C, et al: A comparison of recombinant human thyrotropin and thyroid hormone withdrawal for the detection of thyroid remnant or cancer, J Clin Endocrinol Metab 84:3877–3885, 1999.
345. Jeevanram RK, Shah DH, Sharma SM, et al: Influence of initial large dose on subsequent uptake of therapeutic radioiodine in thyroid cancer patients, Nucl Med Biol 13:277–279, 1986.
346. Roy-Camille R, Leger FA, Merland JJ, et al: Perspectives actuelles dans le traitement des metastases osseuses des cancers thyroidiens, Chirurgie 106:32–36, 1980.
347. Hays MT, Solomon DH, Werner SC: The effect of purified bovine thyroid-stimulating hormone in man, II: loss of effectiveness with prolonged administration, J Clin Endocrinol Metab 21:1475–1482, 1961.
348. Wondisford FE, Radovick S, Moates JM, et al: Isolation and characterization of the human thyrotropin beta-subunit gene, J Biol Chem 263:12538–12542, 1988.
349. Robbins RJ, Tuttle RM, Sharaf RN, et al: Preparation by recombinant human thyrotropin or thyroid hormone withdrawal are comparable for the detection of residual

differentiated thyroid carcinoma, J Clin Endocrinol Metab 86:619–625, 2001.

350. Pacini F, Molinaro E, Lippi F, et al: Prediction of disease status by recombinant human TSH-stimulated serum Tg in the postsurgical follow-up of differentiated thyroid carcinoma, J Clin Endocrinol Metab 86:5686–5690, 2001.

351. Mazzaferri EL, Kloos RT: Is diagnostic iodine-131 scanning with recombinant human TSH useful in the follow-up of differentiated thyroid cancer after thyroid ablation? J Clin Endocrinol Metab 87:1490–1498, 2002.

352. Cailleux AF, Baudin E, Travagli JP, et al: Is diagnostic iodine-131 scanning useful after total thyroid ablation for differentiated thyroid carcinoma? J Clin Endocrinol Metab 85:175–178, 2000.

353. Pacini F, Capezzone M, Elisei R, et al: Diagnostic 131-Iodine whole-body scan may be avoided in thyroid cancer patients who have undetectable stimulated serum Tg levels after initial treatment, J Clin Endocrinol Metab 87:1499–1501, 2002.

354. Pacini F, Molinaro E, Castagna MG, et al: Recombinant human thyrotropin-stimulated serum thyroglobulin combined with neck ultrasonography has the highest sensitivity in monitoring differentiated thyroid carcinoma, J Clin Endocrinol Metab 88:3668–3673, 2003.

355. Robbins RJ, Larson SM, Sinha N, et al: A retrospective review of the effectiveness of recombinant human TSH as preparation for radioiodine thyroid remnant ablation, J Nucl Med 43:1482–1488, 2002.

356. Wartofsky L: Editorial: Using baseline and recombinant human TSH-stimulated Tg measurements to manage thyroid cancer without diagnostic 131-I scanning, J Clin Endocrinol Metab 87:1486–1489, 2002.

357. Mazzaferri EL, Robbins RJ, Spencer CA, et al: A consensus report of the role of serum thyroglobulin as a monitoring method for low-risk patients to papillary thyroid carcinoma, J Clin Endocrin Metab 88:1433–1441, 2003.

358. Rossi RL, Cady B, Silverman ML, et al: Current results of conservative surgery of differentiated thyroid carcinoma, World J Surg 10:612–622, 1986.

359. Kukkonen ST, Reijo KH, Kaarle OF, et al: Papillary thyroid carcinoma: the new, age-related TNM classification system in a retrospective analysis of 199 patients, World J Surg 14:837–841, 1990.

360. Grant MD, Hay MB, Gough IR, et al: Local recurrence in papillary thyroid carcinoma: is extent of surgical resection important? Surgery 104:654, 1988.

361. Ricard M, Tenenbaum F, Schlumberger M, et al: Intraoperative detection of pheochromocytoma with iodine-125 labelled meta-iodobenzylguanidine: a feasibility study, Eur J Nucl Med 20:426–430, 1993.

362. Tubiana M, Haddad E, Schlumberger M, et al: External radiotherapy in thyroid cancers, Cancer 55(suppl):2062–2071, 1985.

363. Niederle B, Roka R, Schemper M, et al: Surgical treatment of distant metastases in differentiated thyroid cancer: indication and results, Surgery 100:1088–1097, 1986.

364. Proye CAG, Dromer DHR, Carnaille BM, et al: It is still worthwhile to treat bone metastases from differentiated thyroid carcinoma with radioactive iodine? World J Surg 16:640–645, 1992.

365. Mazzaferri EL: Papillary and follicular thyroid cancer: a selective approach to diagnosis and treatment, Annu Rev Med 32:73–91, 1981.

366. Parker LN, Wu SY, Kim DD, et al: Recurrence of papillary thyroid carcinoma presenting as a focal neurological deficit, Arch Intern Med 146:1985–1987, 1986.

367. Hay ID: Brain metastases from papillary thyroid carcinoma, Arch Intern Med 147:607, 611, 1987.

368. Venkatesh A, Leavens ME, Samaan NA: Brain metastases in patients with well-differentiated thyroid carcinoma: study of 11 cases, Eur J Surg Oncol 16:448–450, 1990.

369. Rall JE, Alpers JB, Lewallen CG, et al: Radiation pneumonitis and fibrosis: a complication of radioiodine treatment of pulmonary metastases from cancer of the thyroid, J Clin Endocrinol Metab 17:1263–1276, 1957.

370. Durante C, Haddy N, Baudin E, et al: Long-term outcome of 444 patients with distant metastases from papillary and follicular thyroid carcinoma: benefits and limits of radioiodine therapy, J Clin Endocrinol Metab 91:2892–2899, 2006.

371. Leeper R: Controversies in the treatment of thyroid cancer: the New York Memorial Hospital approach, Thyroid Today 5:1–4, 1982.

372. Schober O, Gunter HH, Schwarzrock R, et al: Hamatologische langzeitveranderungen bei der schilddrusenkarzinoms, Strahlenther Onkol 163:464–474, 1987.

373. Pacini F, Gasperi M, Fugazzola L, et al: Testicular function in patients with differentiated thyroid carcinoma treated with radioiodine, J Nucl Med 35:1418–1422, 1994.

374. Raymond JP, Izembart M, Marliac V, et al: Temporary ovarian failure in thyroid cancer patients after thyroid remnant ablation with radioactive iodine, J Clin Endocrinol Metab 69:186–190, 1989.

375. Dottorini ME, Lomuscio G, Mazzucchelli L, et al: Assessment of female fertility and carcinogenesis after iodine-131 therapy for differentiated thyroid carcinoma, J Nucl Med 36:21–27, 1995.

376. Schlumberger M, De Vathaire F, Ceccarelli C, et al: Exposure to radioactive iodine-131 for scintigraphy or therapy does not preclude pregnancy in thyroid cancer patients, J Nucl Med 37:606–612, 1996.

377. Simpson WJ, Carruthers JS: The role of external radiation in the management of papillary and follicular thyroid cancer, Am J Surg 136:457–460, 1978.

378. Grauer A, Raue F, Gagel RF: Changing concepts in the management of hereditary and sporadic medullary thyroid carcinoma, Endocrinol Metab Clin North Am 19:613–635, 1990.

379. Shimaoka K: Adjunctive management of thyroid cancer: chemotherapy, J Surg Oncol 15:283–286, 1980.

380. Bukowski RM, Brown L, Weick JK, et al: Combination chemotherapy of metastatic thyroid cancer: phase II study, Am J Clin Oncol 6:579–581, 1983.

381. De Besi P, Busnardo B, Toso S, et al: Combined chemotherapy with bleomycin, Adriamycin, and platinum in advanced thyroid cancer, J Endocrinol Invest 14:475–480, 1991.

382. Droz JP, Schlumberger M, Rougier P, et al: Chemotherapy in metastatic nonanaplastic thyroid cancer: experience at the Institut Gustave-Roussy, Tumori 76:480–483, 1990.

383. Gottlieb JA, Hill CS: Adriamycin (NSC123127) therapy in thyroid carcinoma, Cancer Chemother Rep 6:283–296, 1975.

384. Hill CS: Chemotherapy of thyroid cancer. In Kaplan EL, editor: Surgery of the Thyroid and Parathyroid Glands, Edinburgh, 1983, Churchill Livingstone, pp 120–126.

385. Santini F, Bottici V, Elisei R, et al: Cytotoxic effects of carboplatinum and epirubicin in the setting of an elevated serum thyrotropin for advanced poorly differentiated thyroid cancer, J Clin Endocrinol Metab 87:4160–4165, 2002.

386. Lazar V, Bidart JM, Caillou B, et al: Expression of the Na⁺/I⁻ symporter gene in human thyroid tumors: a comparison study with other thyroid-specific genes, J Clin Endocrinol Metab 84:3228–3234, 1999.

387. Eigelberger MS, Wong MG, Duh QY, et al: Phenylacetate enhances the antiproliferative effect of retinoic acid in follicular thyroid cancer, Surgery 130:931–935, 2001.

388. Schmutzler C, Winzer R, Meissner-Weigl J, et al: Retinoic acid increases sodium/iodide symporter mRNA levels in human thyroid cancer cell lines and suppresses expression of functional symporter in nontransformed FRTL-5 rat thyroid cells, Biochem Biophys Res Commun 240:832–838, 1997.

389. Van Herle AJ, Agatep ML, Padua DN 3rd, et al: Effects of 13 cis-retinoic acid on growth and differentiation of human follicular carcinoma cells (UCLA RO 82 W-1) in vitro, J Clin Endocrinol Metab 71:755–763, 1990.

390. Havekes B, Schroder van der Elst JP, van der Pluijm G, et al: Beneficial effects of retinoic acid on extracellular matrix degradation and attachment behaviour in follicular thyroid carcinoma cell lines, J Endocrinol 167:229–238, 2000.

391. Grunwald F, Menzel C, Bender H, et al: Redifferentiation therapy-induced radioiodine uptake in thyroid cancer, J Nucl Med 39:1903–1906, 1998.

392. Simon D, Koehrle J, Reiners C, et al: Redifferentiation therapy with retinoids: therapeutic option for advanced follicular and papillary thyroid carcinoma, World J Surg 22:569–574, 1998.

393. Simon D, Koehrle J, Schmutzler C, et al: Redifferentiation therapy of differentiated thyroid carcinoma with retinoic acid: basics and first clinical results, Exp Clin Endocrinol Diabetes 104(suppl 4):13–15, 1996.

394. Schmutzler C, Koehrle J: Innovative strategies for the treatment of thyroid cancer, Eur J Endocrinol 143:15–24, 2001.

395. Battista S, Martelli ML, Fedele M, et al: A mutated p53 gene alters thyroid cell differentiation, Oncogene 11:2029–2037, 1995.

396. Fagin JA, Tang SH, Zeki K, et al: Reexpression of thyroid peroxidase in a derivative of an undifferentiated thyroid carcinoma cell line by introduction of wild-type p53, Cancer Res 56:765–771, 1996.

397. Moretti F, Farsetti A, Soddu S, et al: p53 re-expression inhibits proliferation and restores differentiation of human thyroid anaplastic carcinoma cells, Oncogene 14:729–740, 1997.

398. Velasco JA, Medina DL, Romero J, et al: Introduction of p53 induces cell-cycle arrest in p53-deficient human medullary-thyroid-carcinoma cells, Int J Cancer 73:449–455, 1997.

399. Zeki K, Tanaka Y, Morimoto I, et al: Induction of expression of MHC-class-II antigen on human thyroid carcinoma by wild-type p53, Int J Cancer 75:391–395, 1998.

400. Gallagher WM, Brown R: p53-oriented cancer therapies: current progress, Ann Oncol 10:139–150, 1999.

401. Nishihara E, Nagayama Y, Narimatsu M, et al: Treatment of thyroid carcinoma cells with four different suiide gene/prodrug in vitro, Anticancer Res 18:1521–1525, 1998.

402. Zhang R, Minemura K, DeGroot LJ: Immunotherapy for medullary thyroid carcinoma by a replication-defective adenovirus transducing murine interleukin-2, Endocrinology 139:601–608, 1998.

403. Zhang R, Straus FH, DeGroot LJ: Cell-specific viral gene therapy of a Hürthle cell tumor, J Clin Endocrinol Metab 87:1407–1414, 2002.

404. Zhang R, Straus FH, DeGroot LJ: Effective genetic therapy of established medullary thyroid carcinomas with murine interleukin-2: dissemination and cytotoxicity studies in a rat tumor model, Endocrinology 138:4493–4496, 1997.

405. Sherman SI, Wirth LJ, Droz J-P, et al: Motesanib diphosphate in progressive differentiated thyroid cancer, N Engl J Med 359:31–42, 2008.

406. Kloss RT, Ringel MD, Knopp MV, et al: Phase II trial of sorafenib in metastatic thyroid cancer, J Clin Oncol 27:1675–1684, 2009.

407. Pennel NA, Daniels GH, Haddad RI, et al: A phase II study of gefitinib in patient with advanced thyroid cancer, Thyroid 18:317–324, 2008.

408. Waguespack SG, Sherman SI, Williams MD, et al: The successful use of sorafenib to treat pediatric papillary thyroid carcinoma, Thyroid 19:407–412, 2009.

409. Dawson SJ, Conus NM, Toner GC, et al: Sustained clinical responses to tyrosine kinase inhibitor sunitinib in thyroid carcinoma, Anticancer Drugs 19:547–552, 2008.

410. Morabito A, Piccirillo MC, Falasconi F, et al: Vandetanib (ZD6474), a dual inhibitor of vascular endothelial growth factor receptor (VEGFR) and epidermal growth factor receptor (EGFR) tyrosine kinases: current status and future directions, Oncologist 14:378–390, 2009.

411. Matsumoto F, Itoh S, Ohba SI, et al: A case report of thyroid cancer showing a remarkable effect of gefitinib, Auris Nasus Larynx 36:623–626, 2009.

412. Cohen EE, Rosen LS, Vokes EE, et al: Axitinib is an active treatment for all histologic subtypes of advanced thyroid cancer: results from a phase II study, J Clin Oncol 26:4708–4713, 2008.

Chapter 19

MEDULLARY THYROID CARCINOMA AND MULTIPLE ENDOCRINE NEOPLASIA TYPE 2

DIANA L. LEAROYD, LYNDAL J. TACON, and BRUCE ROBINSON

Prevalence and Epidemiology

Medullary thyroid carcinoma (MTC) accounts for only 5% to 10% of all thyroid cancers, but its management can be very challenging, and early diagnosis is of vital importance. MTC arises from the calcitonin-secreting parafollicular cells of the thyroid known as the *C cells*. Seventy-five percent of MTC cases are sporadic, while the remaining 25% occur in several well-defined familial endocrine syndromes with autosomal dominant inheritance. *Multiple endocrine neoplasia type 2A* (MEN2A) refers to the occurrence of MTC in association with pheochromocytoma in 50% of cases, and in association with hyperparathyroidism in

20% to 30% of cases.[1] *Multiple endocrine neoplasia type 2B* (MEN2B) consists of MTC in conjunction with pheochromocytoma and several additional features, including mucosal neuromas, ganglioneuromatoses of the gastrointestinal tract, and a marfanoid habitus. Parathyroid disease is very rare in MEN2B. *Familial medullary thyroid carcinoma* (FMTC) describes the autosomal dominant inheritance of medullary thyroid carcinoma alone.

The overall prevalence of MEN2 is approximately 1:25,000.[2] The penetrance is approximately 70% at 70 years of age.[3] It has been reported that 90% of MEN2 carriers will eventually show evidence of MTC.[4] This contrasts with MEN1, in which penetrance is 94% by the age of 50 years.[5]

Table 19-1. The Most Common Germline RET Mutations

RET Mutation	Affected Exon	Affected Codon	Mutation Nucleotide	Amino Acid
C609R	10	609	TGC→CGC	Cys→Arg
C611Y	10	611	TGC→TAC	Cys→Tyr
C618				
C618F	10	618	TGC→TTC	Cys→Phe
C618G	10	618	TGC→GGC	Cys→Gly
C618R	10	618	TGC→CGC	Cys→Arg
C618S	10	618	TGC→AGC/TCC	Cys→Ser
C618Y	10	618	TGC→TAC	Cys→Tyr
C620				
C620F	10	620	TGC→TTC	Cys→Phe
C620R	10	620	TGC→CGC	Cys→Arg
C620S	10	620	TGC→AGC/TCC	Cys→Ser
C620Y	10	620	TGC→TAC	Cys→Tyr
C630R	11	630	TGC→CGC	Cys→Arg
C634				
C634F	11	634	TGC→TTC	Cys→Phe
C634G	11	634	TGC→GGC	Cys→Gly
C634R	11	634	TGC→CGC	Cys→Arg
C634S	11	634	TGC→AGC/TCC	Cys→Ser
C634W	11	634	TGC→TGG	Cys→Trp
C634Y	11	634	TGC→TAC	Cys→Tyr
E768D	13	768	GAG→GAC	Glu→Asp
L790F	13	790	TTG→TTC/TTT	Leu→Phe
Y791F	13	791	TAT→TTT	Tyr→Phe
V804M	14	804	GTG→ATG	Val→Met
S891A	15	891	TCG→GCG	Ser→Ala
M918T	16	918	ATG→ACG	Met→Thr

From Machens A, Niccoli-Sire P, Hoegel J et al: Early malignant progression of hereditary medullary thyroid cancer. N Engl J Med 349:1517–1525, 2003.

Molecular Pathogenesis: RET Proto-Oncogene

The causative gene for the MEN2 syndromes was identified in 1993.[6,7] The gene is the RET (REarranged during Transfection) proto-oncogene located on chromosome 10q11.2.[8]

The RET proto-oncogene encodes a tyrosine kinase cell surface receptor. Point mutations in RET segregating with the disease phenotype were identified in MEN2 and FMTC in 1993.[7] Germline mutations of RET were subsequently identified in MEN2B, at a different site.[9] Genetic screening has revolutionized the management of MEN2 families.

The International RET Mutation Consortium performed an extensive study of 477 MEN2 families around the world and established important phenotype/genotype correlations.[10] RET mutations have been characterized in approximately 97% of MEN2 families overall. In MEN2A and FMTC, approximately 96% of families will have an identifiable RET germline mutation, and in MEN2B, approximately 98% of families are mutation positive. The most common RET mutations are summarized in Table 19-1.[11]

RET STRUCTURE AND FUNCTION

The *RET* gene consists of over 20 exons spanning a minimum of 30 kilobases of genomic DNA. The protein product of the gene encodes a cell surface receptor. The gene consists of an extracellular domain (exons 1 to 10), a transmembrane domain (exon 11), and an intracellular domain (exons 12 onwards) (Fig. 19-1).[12]

The RET protein is membrane-bound, with its intracellular portion having tyrosine kinase activity. The extracellular domain

A *RET* PROTO-ONCOGENE

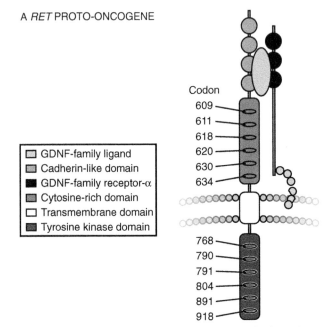

FIGURE 19-1. Structure of RET Proto-oncogene. (From Cote GJ, Gagel RF: Lessons learned from the management of a rare genetic cancer. N Engl J Med 349:1566–1568, 2003.)

extends for the initial 635 amino acids and includes an area of cadherin homology and a conserved cysteine-rich region immediately adjacent to the transmembrane domain.[13] The cysteine-rich domain is typical of the transforming growth factor beta (TGF-β) superfamily.[14] The protein is glycosylated to produce receptors with molecular weights of 150 and 170 kilodaltons. The 170-kD form is present in the cell membrane, while the 150-kD form is an immature form present in the cell cytoplasm.[15] Phosphorylation of RET tyrosine residues results in activation of several intracellular second messenger systems and signaling pathways.[16] These include phospholipase Cγ/protein kinase C (PLCγ/PKC), c-Jun N-terminal kinases (c-Jun/JNK), products of the proto-oncogene Src-related kinases, and nuclear factor κB (NF-κB). Other downstream targets include the Ras/Raf/ERK (extracellular regulated kinase) and phosphatidylinositol-3-kinase (P13-kinase)/Akt pathways. Through these signaling cascades, RET appears to have a central role in cellular proliferation, differentiation, and migration.[17-19] Interestingly, in addition to its role in endocrine neoplasia, aberrant RET signaling has been associated with distinct phenotypes. Hirschsprung's disease occurring with MEN2 is described in subjects with codon 609, 618, and 620 mutations,[20] and cutaneous lichen amyloidosis with codon 634 mutations.[21]

RET LIGANDS

There was intense interest in the early 1990s in identifying the ligand for RET. In 1996 the first ligand, glial cell line–derived neurotrophic factor (GDNF), was identified.[22] Other ligands were soon identified, including neurturin (NTN),[23] artemin,[24] and persephin.[25]

RET activation by ligand appears to occur via membrane-bound proteins that function as the ligand-binding domain of a ligand/receptor complex. The link between RET and its first ligand, GDNF, was suggested by the study of mice that were deficient in GDNF expression. These mice were very similar to RET knockout mice, with absent or limited development of the kidney and an absence of enteric neurons in the colon and small intestine.[26]

GDNF-family ligands bind to specific GDNF-family receptor proteins, all of which form receptor complexes and signal through the RET receptor, tyrosine kinase. Additional proteins, GDNF receptor alpha (GFRα) or GDNF-family receptor alpha 1 (GFRα-1), were found to be essential for the high-affinity binding of GDNF to RET and for its consequent functional effects.[27] A single molecule of ligand binds two GFRα-1 molecules, which interact with two molecules of RET and lead to activation of RET tyrosine kinase. Similarly, the other ligands such as neurturin, persephin, and artemin bind to different GFRαs before eventual receptor activation occurs, with consequent effects. It was suggested that MEN2 families with no identifiable RET mutations may have GDNF mutations, but so far no such mutations have been described in MEN2. However, somatic GDNF mutations have been found in sporadic pheochromocytomas.[28]

FUNCTIONAL EFFECTS OF RET MUTATIONS

Although the genotypes do overlap, in general, different codons are affected in either MEN2A or MEN2B. These mutations in different regions of the RET proto-oncogene increase the transforming activity of the kinase by distinct mechanisms. In MEN2A, the extracellular cysteine-rich or transmembrane domains are predominantly affected. Such mutations lead to a loss of cysteine residues. As a result, two RET molecules may undergo ligand-independent dimerization, with resultant constitutive activation of tyrosine kinase activity.[29] A mutation in codon 634, usually a cysteine-to-arginine substitution (TGC to CGC), occurs in 85% of cases of MEN2A.[17] In contrast, MEN2B is usually caused by a mutation in the intracellular tyrosine kinase domain. Codon 918 is involved in 95% of cases, in a methionine-to-threonine substitution (ATG to ACG).[17] This alters the kinase specificity, with alternative substrate phosphorylation and altered downstream signaling.[30] The rarer intracellular RET mutations in codons 768 and 804 have been shown to produce "gain of function" of the receptor, although the precise mechanism by which tumor formation occurs is unclear.[31]

Histogenesis

C CELLS

The calcitonin-secreting C cells of the thyroid originate from the neural crest. They are located mainly in the upper and middle thirds of the thyroid gland. They are members of the amine-precursor uptake and decarboxylation (APUD) family and express a variety of neuroendocrine markers, including calcitonin, chromogranin A, neuron-specific enolase, and serotonin.[32] Calcitonin is a very effective tumor marker for the monitoring of MTC. Carcinoembryonic antigen (CEA) is also a C-cell marker used in clinical practice. C cells usually display an endocrine phenotype but may revert to a neuronal phenotype following malignant transformation.[32] The alternately spliced calcitonin gene-related peptide (CGRP) is then the predominant protein expressed by the cells.

The biological role of C cells is not precisely clear. They are involved in calcium homeostasis, and they contribute to the thyroid follicle's microenvironment. Pharmacologically, calcitonin inhibits calcium resorption from bone, and this has been used therapeutically for treatment of Paget's disease, postmenopausal bone loss, and hypercalcemia.

C-CELL HYPERPLASIA

C-cell hyperplasia (CCH) is the pathologic description of an increase in C-cell numbers that can precede malignancy. Criteria for the diagnosis of CCH are variable in the literature, although consensus suggests that there should be more than 50 C cells per field at ×100 magnification.[33] C cells may increase in number with age, and CCH is a common finding in normal thyroids at autopsy.[34] CCH is no longer considered to be a specific marker of familial MTC. Multifocal CCH is regarded as a precursor lesion to hereditary MTC. Its progression to microscopic MTC is variable and may take many years.[35]

Clinical Relevance of Germline RET Mutations in MEN2A, FMTC, and MEN2B

MEN2A AND FMTC

Extensive studies of MEN2A families from around the world have now clarified that 97% will have a germline RET mutation, usually in the cysteine-encoding codons 609, 611, 618, 620, or 634. The codon 634 mutation in exon 10 predominates, usually with an arginine substitution, although other substitutions such as by tyrosine or glutamine are described.[10] In FMTC, 88% of families have a germline mutation in one of the listed cysteine codons or, more rarely, in intracellular codons including 768, 790, and 791. The common MEN2A C634R mutation of cysteine to arginine (TGC to CGC) is not found in FMTC.[36] RET mutations in the intracellular exons 13, 14, and 15 are less common in MEN2A, although they will be detected by routine sequencing of these exons. Isolated cases of kindreds with germline mutations in other exons (including exons 5 and 8) have been reported, and these may account for cases of apparently mutation-negative FMTC.[17]

MEN2B

In 95% of MEN2B families, the germline RET mutation at codon 918 in exon 16 occurs, causing mutation of methionine to threonine (ATG to ACG).[37] This mutation is in the tyrosine kinase domain and is specific to MEN2B.[9] Of note, this codon 918 RET mutation is also found somatically in the tumor tissue in some sporadic MTCs. A germline RET codon 918 mutation can also occur de novo, where MEN2B patients have no family history of the disease. However, they still have a 50% chance of passing this mutation on to their offspring.[38] Rarer tyrosine kinase domain mutations occur in codons 883[39] and 891.[12]

Specific Genotype/Phenotype Correlations

There has been much interest in the prediction of phenotypic behavior from genotype analysis. As published by the International RET Consortium, the presence of any codon 634 RET mutation correlates significantly with the presence of both pheochromocytoma and hyperparathyroidism. One study suggested more aggressive behavior of MTC with the common arginine substitution at codon 634 (C634R), compared to the C634Y mutation.[40] The C634R mutation has not been associated with FMTC. It has been suggested that FMTC is a milder variant of MEN2A, and that pheochromocytoma may eventually occur if the patient survives long enough.[10] In support of this concept, it had previously been believed that the codon 804 mutation was specific to FMTC. Subsequent reports have described pheochromocytoma occurring in these families, albeit at an older age than in other MEN2A kindreds.[41,42] The occurrence of different phenotypes in different families with the same germline RET mutation suggest a role for more complex gene interactions. The rarer phenotypes associated with MEN2 include Hirschsprung's disease with RET codon 609, 618, and 620 mutations[43] and cutaneous lichen amyloidosis with codon 634 mutations.[44] The codon 918 mutation is MEN2B specific.[17]

Clinical Presentation of MTC and MEN2

Patients with MTC may present with a palpable thyroid lump or with the symptoms of calcitonin excess—in particular, diarrhea and flushing. Diarrhea does not usually occur until the calcitonin level is very high (at least 10-fold above the upper limit of the normal range). Unfortunately it is very likely that the MTC will have spread to regional lymph nodes by the time diarrhea occurs. Familial cases of MTC will have different presentations depending on the specific RET mutation, as described earlier. Patients with MEN2B will have a more aggressive phenotype and may present in early childhood with diarrhea from very high calcitonin levels or with the other features of the MEN2B syndrome.[1] Mucosal neuromas can occur on the tongue, in the lips, and on the eyelids, giving a distinctive facial appearance. Neuromas in the gastrointestinal tract can cause abdominal pain, gaseous distension, and even pseudo-obstruction. Hirschsprung's disease can have a similar presentation in children and is due to inactivating mutations in the extracellular domain of RET, as distinct from the activating mutations of the tyrosine kinase domain seen in MEN2B patients.[1] MEN2B patients may also have a marfanoid body habitus and corneal nerve thickening. Some patients with MEN2A will also show corneal nerve thickening. Pheochromocytoma occurs in 50% of MEN2B patients, sometimes at a young age, but hyperparathyroidism is very rare.

The purpose of biochemical and genetic screening in MEN2 families is to detect MTC well before it becomes clinically apparent, because once clinically evident, it may have spread to lymph nodes.

Screening in MEN2 and FMTC

BIOCHEMICAL SCREENING

The pentagastrin (PG) stimulation test was used for many years to identify biochemically affected members of MEN2 families. The advent of genetic screening has dramatically reduced the need for this test, although it still has a role in follow-up and management. A number of limitations of the PG test have been uncovered since RET mutation analysis became available. It is possible for RET mutation-negative members of MEN2 families to have elevated calcitonin responses to pentagastrin stimulation.[45]

In the early literature, some of these positive PG tests led to thyroidectomy, and C-cell hyperplasia was found in some patients but not in others.[46] This is probably because CCH can be a normal variant.[34] PG testing can also be used to detect

hereditary MTC carriers in families where no RET mutation is identified, although these families are now rare. Adverse effects from the PG test include retrosternal discomfort, nausea, vomiting, metallic taste, abdominal cramps, esophageal spasm, and tachycardia.

GENETIC SCREENING

RET mutations are clustered tightly, and the analysis can be confined to specific exons. This compares favorably with genetic analysis in MEN1, where the mutations are scattered. Once a mutation is identified, other family members are screened with a straightforward analysis for that specific mutation. Various techniques have been used, and currently, direct polymerase chain reaction (PCR)-based sequencing is performed in most laboratories. Other methods include restriction enzyme digestion of PCR products[47] with subsequent sequencing,[48] single-strand conformation polymorphism, and denaturing gradient gel electrophoresis.[49] Denaturing high-performance liquid chromatography can also be used to identify mutations, provided that appropriate positive controls are available, since there are multiple polymorphisms in the RET gene in normal individuals.[50] Linkage analysis is not commonly performed, although it may rarely have a role if no RET mutation can be identified with other techniques.[51] Testing should be performed on two separate occasions on two different blood samples to avoid the risk of sample mix-ups. RET mutation-negative members of known MEN2 families (i.e., where RET mutation is identified in the family) can be reassured that their risk of developing MTC is no greater than for the general population.

Genetic screening must therefore be comprehensive and include sequencing of exons 10, 11, 13, 14, 15, and 16.[52]

Management Implications of Genetic Results

TIMING OF PROPHYLACTIC THYROIDECTOMY

The advent of genetic screening has allowed prophylactic thyroidectomy to be performed earlier than it would be by traditional biochemical screening. Logically, this would be expected to lead to an improvement in the prognosis of RET-mutation carriers. Long-term data is slowly accumulating to support the practice of prophylactic thyroidectomy based on genetic screening rather than on clinical or biochemical screening. Consensus was reached at the MEN '97 Workshop that the decision to perform thyroidectomy in MEN2 should be based predominantly on the result of RET-mutation testing rather than on calcitonin testing.[53]

The specific mutated RET codon may be correlated with the degree of aggressiveness of the MTC. A three-level risk stratification system has been adopted since its inception at the Seventh International Workshop on Multiple Endocrine Neoplasia in 1999.[52] Category 1, the highest risk group, includes all MEN2B-mutation carriers, because mutations in RET codon 883 and 918 are associated with the most aggressive MTC. Such patients should have thyroidectomy within the first 6 months of life because metastases within the first year of life have been described. Those with RET codon 611, 618, 620, or 634 are classified as category 2, having a high risk of MTC, and thyroidectomy before 5 years of age is recommended. MTC with the codon 634 mutation has been reported as early as age 2 years, although cases of MTC are generally rare before the age of 5 years

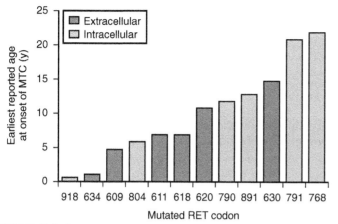

FIGURE 19-2. Earliest reported age at the onset of MTC, according to the RET mutation. (From Cote GJ, Gagel RF: Lessons learned from the management of a rare genetic cancer. N Engl J Med 349:1566–1568, 2003.)

in MEN2A and FMTC. Thyroidectomy at this age is technically possible without significant morbidity. Category 3 includes those with RET codon 609, 768, 790, 791, 804, and 891 mutations, having the lowest risk among the stratification categories. It should be noted that a single case of metastatic MTC in a 6-year-old was reported in a family with the codon 804 RET mutation.[54] Some have recommended thyroidectomy by age 5 years, whereas others have suggested it by age 10 years, for gene-positive members of category 3–risk families. If baseline calcitonin is elevated, then thyroidectomy should be performed immediately, regardless of the RET mutation found. Histology in this setting is likely to show MTC rather than C-cell hyperplasia, with the associated risk of lymph node spread.[55] Fig. 19-2 describes the earliest age of reported MTC for each of the known RET mutations. Early prophylactic surgery also alleviates the need for ongoing unpleasant PG stimulation testing being performed in a child.

STRATEGY AND EXTENT OF THYROIDECTOMY

Although there has been a general consensus regarding the timing of prophylactic thyroidectomy based on risk stratification, the strategy of central lymph node dissection at prophylactic thyroidectomy is controversial. Most advocate thyroid surgery with central node dissection for MEN2B. The practice of routine central-node clearance is most important in asymptomatic gene carriers with the higher-risk mutations but can be modified for lower-risk mutations with normal preoperative calcitonin.

The Role of Somatic RET Mutations

SPORADIC MTC

Somatic mutations of RET are observed in a proportion of sporadic MTC cases. The commonest somatic RET mutation is the codon 918 ATG-to-ACG (M918T) mutation. Its prevalence varies widely (from 28% to 86%) in different series.[56] This may reflect either geographic differences in population studies or perhaps methodological differences. Other somatic mutations reported in sporadic MTC include codon 883 in exon 15 and codon 634 in exon 11.[57] Although not a universal finding, smaller series had suggested that the somatic RET codon 918 mutation was associated with a poorer prognosis in sporadic MTC, correlating the mutation with distant metastases and

tumor recurrence.[58,59,60] A recent large study of 100 sporadic MTC patients with a 10-year follow-up period supported this concept.[57] This study reported increased lymph node metastases at diagnosis, increased likelihood of persistent disease, and lower overall survival in those subjects with a somatic RET mutation.[57]

SOMATIC MUTATIONS IN HEREDITARY MTC

Somatic RET mutations have also been described in hereditary MTC. The somatic codon 918 RET mutation has been reported, albeit rarely, in association with germline RET mutations in exon 10 or 11.[61] This important observation negated the theory that the codon 918 somatic RET mutation could be used as a specific marker of sporadic disease. Others have observed the somatic codon 918 RET mutation occurring in patients with a germline codon 768 RET mutation.[62] Microdissection techniques have uncovered the fact that somatic RET mutations may be found in some regions of an MTC tumor but not in others.[63] It has been suggested that the presence of a somatic mutation in addition to the germline RET mutation provides a "second hit" that may explain the more aggressive behavior of some familial cases of MTC.

ROUTINE GERMLINE SCREENING OF SPORADIC MTCS

It is now recommended that all new cases of sporadic MTC should have germline screening for RET mutations. Unsuspected familial cases are uncovered in approximately 6% of such patients despite an apparently negative family history.[64] This was confirmed in a recent series of apparently sporadic MTC, in which 7.3% of subjects were found to possess a germline mutation. Lower-risk RET mutations in the non-cysteine codons were most commonly discovered, including codons 804, 891, and 768, although cysteine codon mutations were also found. The majority of these unsuspected familial cases were diagnosed as FMTC, based on the absence of other endocrine neoplasia at follow up.[65] Of note, genetic screening of first-degree relatives should be undertaken if a germline RET mutation is identified in a subject with MTC.

Given that more than 97% of MEN2 families have identifiable RET mutations, a negative-germline RET-mutation test provides a high degree of certainty that a particular individual has sporadic MTC. This is assuming the genetic analysis is comprehensive. It is important to include exons 13, 14, and 15 because mutations in these exons are most likely to manifest late, with a lower prevalence of pheochromocytoma, and are more likely to escape detection as familial.[66]

Natural Progression and Behavior of MTC

HEREDITARY VERSUS SPORADIC MTC

Hereditary MTC is characterized by the early onset of bilateral and multifocal disease. Sporadic MTC may present as a palpable thyroid mass or a nodule on ultrasound, and lymph node involvement is present in 30% to 60% of cases at diagnosis.[67] Local lymph-node spread occurs early in the course of the disease in both hereditary and sporadic forms.

A study by Raue and colleagues evaluating prognostic factors in MTC found that the stage of disease at diagnosis, age, sex, and type of disease (sporadic versus hereditary) were relevant prognostic factors in a univariate analysis, with better prognosis for young female patients with familial disease diagnosed at an early stage. The difference in the survival rate of patients with hereditary disease versus those with the sporadic form disappeared in multivariate proportional hazards analysis, but the prognostic information provided by age and sex was still significant. The overall adjusted survival rate was 86.7% at 5 years and 64.2% at 10 years. These rates are comparable to those quoted by other studies.[68-70] A more recent study found only the stage of disease and presence of extrathyroidal growth at presentation with MTC to be independent predictors of clinical behavior and life expectancy. In this study, increased age at diagnosis was found to be associated with a reduction in overall survival; however, when adjusted for the baseline mortality rate of the general population on multivariate analysis, this effect was lost.[70]

Management

THE PRIMARY OPERATION FOR MTC

Current therapy for MTC is restricted to surgical removal of all neoplastic tissue, and alternative forms of treatment using radiotherapy or chemotherapy provide little benefit. Overall, 50% of MTC patients will have lymph node involvement at presentation.[71] Patients with MEN2B and sporadic MTC have a higher rate of extrathyroidal spread than do those with MEN2A.[72]

The primary operation should include total thyroidectomy and the removal of all lymph nodes in the central neck compartment bounded by the hyoid bone, sternal notch, and internal jugular veins. Lymph nodes in the upper mediastinum and lateral neck regions should also be examined and removed if macroscopically abnormal. Scollo and colleagues have advocated the routine performance of central and bilateral neck dissection for all sporadic and hereditary MTC cases. They showed that the ipsilateral, contralateral, and central compartments were involved with the same frequency in patients with either sporadic or hereditary MTC, even in the case of unilateral thyroid tumors. It was suggested that contralateral lymph node dissection could be avoided only in those with unilateral tumor involvement and no central or ipsilateral lymph node involvement.[73] It should be mentioned that whenever a patient is assessed for thyroid surgery, urinary catecholamines and metanephrines should be measured prior to undergoing general anesthesia to exclude unrecognized pheochromocytoma. Serum calcium and parathyroid hormone levels should also be measured preoperatively.

LOCALIZATION OF RECURRENT MTC

Persistent elevation of serum calcitonin is a useful marker of the presence of residual or recurrent MTC. CEA may also be useful if the tumor stains poorly for calcitonin. The most common sites of distant metastases from MTC are the liver, lung, bone, and brain. Regional spread in the neck and chest is very common and can occur early.

Localization of recurrence is often very difficult, particularly when calcitonin levels are only modestly elevated. One commonly faces the problem of failure of detection of metastatic disease even when its presence is suggested by persistently elevated serum calcitonin or CEA. The biological behavior of MTC varies between subjects. As well as being a tumor marker, calcitonin doubling time has been reported to be a prognostic factor for poor survival.[74,75] One recent study reported both calcitonin and CEA doubling times to be associated with progressive disease in most patients,[76] suggesting these could be used to guide the

frequency and intensity of serial imaging. Of note, calcitonin and CEA markers can fluctuate significantly in the short term, so caution in assessing trends is required.[77]

The large number of imaging modalities used to investigate persistently elevated calcitonin reflects the inadequacies of each modality. Reports in the literature are limited by the lack of use of a gold standard of histologic confirmation.

Ultrasonography/Computed Tomography/Magnetic Resonance Imaging

There is a paucity of systematic studies assessing various radiographic imaging protocols. One recent study compared ultrasonography, spiral computed tomography (CT) scan, magnetic resonance imaging (MRI) of the liver and whole body, as well as 18-fluoro-2-deoxy-D-glucose (FDG) positron emission tomography (PET) in a group of 55 patients with MTC and persistently elevated calcitonin.[78] They found neck ultrasound to be the most sensitive tool in detecting lymph node metastases. Chest CT was found to be superior in detecting lung lesions, and liver MRI the most sensitive in diagnosing hepatic metastases. Bone scan complemented MRI in the detection of axial skeletal metastases but was superior in assessing peripheral skeletal lesions. As discussed below, 18FDG PET was disappointing.

Nuclear Imaging

A variety of nuclear imaging methods have been used in an attempt to take advantage of the specific expression of hormonal receptors or transporters by endocrine tumors to allow disease localization. The radionuclide agents used in trials include ^{201}Tl-chloride, ^{131}I-meta-iodobenzylguanidine (MIBG), ^{99m}Tc pentavalent-dimercapto-succinic acid (DMSA), ^{131}I anti-CEA or anticalcitonin antibodies or fragments, labeled somatostatin receptors, and technetium-99m-sestamibi (^{99m}Tc-sestamibi).[79] PET scanning has also been investigated. Unfortunately, no single method is adequately sensitive or specific for definitive diagnosis.

Imaging with ^{131}I MIBG and ^{131}I anti-CEA is not sensitive but is specific. These tracers are therefore inappropriate for primary use in the early diagnosis or exclusion of MTC. Once MTC has been diagnosed, it is worthwhile establishing whether these tracers accumulate in the tumor to evaluate their potential therapeutic use. ^{201}Tl Chloride and ^{99m}Tc DMSA have slightly better sensitivity, with the advantage of no competitive tracer uptake by normal thyroid tissue, but neither is specific for MTC.[80]

The use of ^{99m}Tc-sestamibi can image differentiated thyroid carcinomas, parathyroid tumors, and cardiac muscles because of its avid mitochondrial uptake. The use of ^{99m}Tc-sestamibi in MTC has been limited. It was found to be useful in detecting MTC recurrence in the soft tissues of the neck and chest in patients with calcitonin values in excess of 6000 ng/L[81], and it complements other modalities such as CT in the overall assessment of patients with very high calcitonin levels. The drawback is that this radiopharmaceutical is excreted via the hepatic route, thereby confounding the identification of liver metastasis.

6-(18F)-Fluorodopamine is a positron-emitting analogue of dopamine used as a tracer for PET scanning. It has shown particular promise in imaging the sympathetic nervous system (e.g., in pheochromocytomas). In a case report, metastatic histologically proven MTC was unequivocally detected by 6-(18F)-fluorodopamine PET scanning.[82] However, the broader use of this agent remains to be evaluated, and its availability is limited. Results with 18-FDG PET have also been disappointing, with one recent study reporting a sensitivity of only 58% in imaging metastatic MTC. This study found a low standardized uptake value of FDG in the metastatic MTCs, possibly due to slow growth, small size, or the sclerotic, necrotic, or calcified nature of the tumors.[78]

Selective Venous Catheterization

Selective venous catheterization (SVC) has been regarded as the most sensitive tool for the localization of residual disease and for the early detection of distant metastases in MTC.[83] In this study, neck and/or mediastinal tumor foci were found in 12 out of 18 patients with calcitonin gradients in the neck and/or the mediastinum. Distant metastases emerged clinically in all five patients with significant gradients.

The procedure of SVC involves the insertion of catheters via the femoral vein into the main neck veins, a hepatic vein, and a peripheral vein. Sequential samples of calcitonin values are obtained at these sites and are expressed as a ratio with the mean peripheral value. A local/peripheral calcitonin gradient of 2.5, yielding a sensitivity of 100%, has been reported.[84] The invasive nature of this technique and need for angiographic expertise limits its widespread applicability.

In essence, there is no single imaging modality that can localize soft-tissue recurrence in the neck, liver metastases, and bony metastases together. Localization is enhanced with the use of combined modalities.

REOPERATION

Elevated levels of calcitonin persist after primary operation in many patients with MTC. Failure of normalization of calcitonin is more likely in subjects with a higher preoperative calcitonin level and in those in whom nodal metastases were confirmed at surgery.[85] Because of the lack of a highly sensitive and specific diagnostic tool to detect micrometastases postoperatively, one is often confronted with the unique situation of whether to reoperate without definite localization and, if so, to what extent. Gimm and Dralle found that lymph node metastases were found in 94% of those patients with elevated calcitonin levels after primary therapy. Four-compartment lymphadenectomy gives a chance of cure in 35% of patients without distant metastases.[86]

Reoperation is recommended if local disease in the neck and/or upper mediastinum is found without evidence of distant metastases. Exploration of the mediastinum is controversial because of the greater morbidity and the lower chance of cure. If distant metastases are found, there is no indication for surgical intervention unless the patient develops diarrhea, for which tumor debulking may be beneficial.[53]

OTHER MODALITIES OF TREATMENT

Somatostatin Analogues

Therapy with different formulations of octreotide and lanreotide does not seem to modify serum concentrations of calcitonin and CEA in patients with recurrent MTC. No significant decrease in the size of metastases has been found with the use of somatostatin analogues in patients with advanced MTC.[87] However, such agents do have a role in symptomatic control of diarrhea, flushing, weight loss, or bone pain.[88] Sandostatin has been used in practice, with some partial relief of symptoms.

Chemotherapy

Chemotherapy has been of limited value. Doxorubicin has been the most widely used single chemotherapeutic agent in the treatment of MTC and therefore is the one associated with most reported responses. Dacarbazine is the most widely used agent in combination therapy. Petursson reported a patient with metastatic MTC who demonstrated a complete response with combination chemotherapy of dacarbazine and 5-fluorouracil.[89] Combined chemotherapy has been tried in patients with advanced MTC using cyclophosphamide, vincristine, and dacarbazine; this yielded only moderate antitumor activity.[90] Trials of other combination therapy are ongoing. Small studies have investigated selective arterial chemoembolization to treat hepatic metastases, with some tumor response and symptom palliation.[91,92]

Radiotherapy

There is no demonstrable survival benefit of adjuvant external beam radiotherapy. A retrospective study by Brierley and colleagues in 73 patients demonstrated no overall difference in local or regional relapse-free rate between those who received external irradiation and those who did not.[93] Also of concern is the potential for radiation treatment to cause tissue damage, thus increasing the potential for complications from future surgery. Radiotherapy does have a role in controlling local disease and in alleviating symptoms such as bone pain.[94] If reoperation is deemed unfeasible, then the effect on local tumor shrinkage may be significant, particularly if there is concern about mass obstruction or extension of tumor into an important structure such as the trachea, esophagus, or carotid artery.[95]

Recent Advances in Treatment of Medullary Thyroid Carcinoma

Given the limited success with chemotherapy or radiotherapy, MTC has provided an attractive target for radionuclide treatment, immunomodulation, gene therapy, and small-molecule tyrosine kinase inhibitors. A perspective of the recent trials and research into novel treatments of MTC is summarized in the following.

RADIONUCLIDE TREATMENT

Radioactive iodine (^{131}I) has not demonstrated efficacy in treatment of MTC.[96] This is attributed to the fact that MTC arises from parafollicular C cells of the thyroid, which do not concentrate iodine. The therapeutic response of ^{131}I-MIBG in treatment has been poor in a limited experience.[95] Other attempts to deliver targeted radioactivity are under ongoing investigation. One approach has been to administer monoclonal antibodies coupled to radioisotopes. A recent non-randomized study reported disease stabilization and prolonged survival with two-part radio-immunotherapy against CEA in MTC patients with a high calcitonin doubling time.[97] Other groups have used yttrium-90-labeled somatostatin analogues for targeted radiotherapy, with some promise in early reports.[98] As yet these studies are preliminary.

IMMUNOTHERAPY

Immunotherapy for MTC has been studied with the rationale that stimulation of immune responses against tumor antigens may result in a clinical response. One study, by Schott and colleagues, explored immunization with calcitonin and/or CEA peptide-pulsed dendritic cells to induce T-cellular antigen-specific immune responses in patients with MTC to achieve a clinical response.[99] One of their seven patients had a regression of detectable liver metastases and pulmonary lesions. Other approaches have included genetic immunization using transfer of cytokines into tumor tissues to mount an immune response against tumor antigens. The cytokines investigated include interleukin 2 (IL-2) and 12 (IL-12).[100] IL-2, also known as T-cell growth factor, may exhibit antineoplastic capacity through activation of cytotoxic T lymphocytes, CD4+ and CD8+ lymphocytes, and natural killer cells. This was illustrated in a murine MTC study by Zhang and colleagues, who demonstrated some tumor response by in vivo delivery of adenoviral vectors expressing murine IL-2.[101] A follow-up study showed that the injection of adenovirus expressing murine IL-2 directly into rat MTC had antitumor effect.[102] IL-12 has also been studied by Zhang and DeGroot. They studied a rat MTC model to investigate murine IL-12 therapy using an adenoviral vector system, demonstrating tumor regression in 86% of treated animals and evidence of long-term immunity to tumor cells.[103] Studies of immunomodulation in MTC are ongoing.

GENE THERAPY

Targeting gene therapy to the inhibition of oncogenic "activated RET" is another attractive treatment modality for MTC, and several methods have been investigated.[104] The practical considerations in endocrine tumor gene therapy were well explored in a review by Messina and colleagues.[105] Adenoviral vectors expressing a dominant-negative RET mutant provide one potential mechanism by which endogenous RET signaling may be blocked.[104] Another approach has been the use of small interfering ribonucleic acid (siRNA) to silence RET gene expression.[17] Suicide gene therapy has also been investigated. This involves the gene transfer of prodrug activating enzymes, along with the prodrugs, to result in targeted antitumor effects.[106] Unfortunately, early promise in gene therapy has not yet been translated into clinical results.

MOLECULAR TARGETS

MTC expresses the constitutively active RET receptor, tyrosine kinase. This forms the basis of studies using tyrosine kinase inhibitors as potential therapeutic tools. Several small molecule inhibitors have been assessed in small, phase 2 clinical trials, and other agents are in preclinical development. These compounds have been designed to block the RET signaling cascade at varying levels.[17,18] Tyrosine kinase inhibitors such as imatinib block autophosphorylation. Despite success in treating chronic myeloid leukemia and gastrointestinal stromal tumors, imatinib appears disappointing in the treatment of MTC.[107,108] Another tyrosine kinase inhibitor, vandetanib (ZD6474), has shown promise in phase 2 studies,[109] with results of both the open-labeled study in hereditary MTC and the double-blind, randomized, phase 3 study in sporadic MTC patients awaited. Other potential molecular targets include inhibition of adaptor protein recruitment or of downstream pathways such as Ras/Raf/ERK, P13K/Akt, PLCγ/PKC and c-Jun/JNK.[17,18] Sorafenib (Bay43-9006) is an orally available kinase inhibitor that was initially developed to inhibit BRAF. It has subsequently been found to inhibit multiple other pathways including RET, and phase 2 clinical trials in MTC are ongoing.[18] Of note, the trial compounds to date also inhibit the vascular endothelial growth factor receptor (VEGFR), thereby potentially inhibiting tumor angiogenesis in addition to oncogenic RET signaling.[17,18] Indeed, no agent in clinical trial demonstrates specificity for the RET tyrosine kinase, creating the potential for multiple side effects. The toxicity with these agents is not insignificant, and photosensitive skin rashes, hypertension, fatigue, and diarrhea have been observed.[18,109] Also of interest is the potential for RET mutations at distinct codons to confer selective resistance to these compounds. In vitro work has suggested that the codon 804 mutation results in resistance to vandetinib.[110] Study into these compounds is ongoing, and with our increasing understanding of molecular oncology, these targeted biological agents will remain a prime area of investigation for medullary thyroid carcinoma therapy.

Conclusion

MTC, although uncommon, is an area of great research interest because current therapeutic modalities are suboptimal in advanced disease. Surgery is the mainstay of therapy, but its success depends on very early diagnosis. The advent of genetic screening for RET mutations has revolutionized the management of familial MTC and MEN2 by enabling prophylactic surgery or early diagnosis of established disease. The more common sporadic disease remains a much greater challenge. Novel therapies for MTC are being developed that may offer a better prognosis and quality of life for patients with MTC.

REFERENCES

1. Marsh DJ, Learoyd DL, Robinson BG: Medullary thyroid carcinoma: recent advances and management update, Thyroid 5:407–424, 1995.
2. Kidd KK, Simpson NE: Search for the gene for multiple endocrine neoplasia type 2A, Recent Prog Horm Res 46:305–343, 1990.
3. Komminoth P: The RET proto-oncogene in medullary and papillary thyroid carcinoma. Molecular features, pathophysiology and clinical implications, Virchows Arch 431:1–9, 1997.
4. Easton DF, Ponder MA, Cummings T, et al: The clinical and screening age-at-onset distribution for the MEN-2 syndrome, Am J Hum Genet 44:208–215, 1989.
5. Chandrasekharappa SC, Guru SC, Manickam P, et al: Positional cloning of the gene for multiple endocrine neoplasia-type 1, Science 276:404–407, 1997.
6. Donis-Keller H, Dou S, Chi D, et al: Mutations in the RET proto-oncogene are associated with MEN2A and FMTC, Hum Mol Genet 2:851–856, 1993.
7. Mulligan LM, Kwok JB, Healey CS, et al: Germ-line mutations of the RET proto-oncogene in multiple endocrine neoplasia type 2A, Nature 363:458–460, 1993.
8. Pasini B, Hofstra RM, Yin L, et al: The physical map of the human RET proto-oncogene, Oncogene 11:1737–1743, 1995.
9. Hofstra RM, Landsvater RM, Ceccherini I, et al: A mutation in the RET proto-oncogene associated with multiple endocrine neoplasia type 2B and sporadic medullary thyroid carcinoma, Nature 367:375–376, 1994.
10. Eng C, Clayton D, Schuffenecker I, et al: The relationship between specific RET proto-oncogene mutations and disease phenotype in multiple endocrine neoplasia type 2. International RET mutation consortium analysis, JAMA 276:1575–1579, 1996.
11. Machens A, Niccoli-Sire P, Hoegel J, et al: Early malignant progression of hereditary medullary thyroid cancer, N Engl J Med 349:1517–1525, 2003.
12. Cote GJ, Gagel RF: Lessons learned from the management of a rare genetic cancer, N Engl J Med 349:1566–1568, 2003.
13. Takahashi M, Buma Y, Iwamoto T, et al: Cloning and expression of the RET proto-oncogene encoding a tyrosine kinase with two potential transmembrane domains, Oncogene 3:571–578, 1988.
14. Ullrich A, Schlessinger J: Signal transduction by receptors with tyrosine kinase activity, Cell 61:203–212, 1990.
15. Takahashi M, Asai N, Iwashita T, et al: Characterization of the RET proto-oncogene products expressed in mouse L cells, Oncogene 8:2925–2929, 1993.
16. Salvatore D, Barone MV, Salvatore G, et al: Tyrosines 1015 and 1062 are in vivo autophosphorylation sites in RET and RET-derived oncoproteins, J Clin Endocrinol Metab 85:3898–3907, 2000.
17. de Groot JW, Links TP, Plukker JTM, et al: RET as a diagnostic and therapeutic target in sporadic and hereditary endocrine tumors, Endocrine Reviews 27:535–560, 2006.
18. Schlumberger M, Carlomagno F, Baudin E, et al: New therapeutic approaches to treat medullary thyroid carcinoma, Nat Clin Pract Endocrinol Metab 4:22–32, 2008.

19. Santoro M, Carlomagno F: Drug insight: small-molecule inhibitors of protein kinases in the treatment of thyroid cancer, Nat Clin Pract Endocrinol Metab 2:42–51, 2006.

20. Mulligan LM, Eng C, Attie T, et al: Diverse phenotypes associated with exon 10 mutations of the RET proto-oncogene, Hum Mol Genet 3:2163–2167, 1994

21. Donovan DT, Levy ML, Furst EJ, et al: Familial cutaneous lichen amyloidosis in association with multiple endocrine neoplasia type 2A: a new variant, Henry Ford Hosp Med J 37:147–150, 1989.

22. Jing S, Wen D, Yu Y, et al: GDNF-induced activation of the RET protein tyrosine kinase is mediated by GDNFR-alpha, a novel receptor for GDNF, Cell 85:1113–1124, 1996.

23. Klein RD, Sherman D, Ho WH, et al: A GPI-linked protein that interacts with Ret to form a candidate neurturin receptor, Nature 387:717–721, 1997.

24. Baloh RH, Tansey MG, Lampe PA, et al: Artemin, a novel member of the GDNF ligand family, supports peripheral and central neurons and signals through the GFRalpha3-RET receptor complex, Neuron 21:1291–1302, 1998.

25. Milbrandt J, de Sauvage FJ, Fahrner TJ, et al: Persephin, a novel neurotrophic factor related to GDNF and neurturin, Neuron 20:245–253, 1998.

26. Schuchardt A, D'Agati V, Larsson-Blomberg L, et al: Defects in the kidney and enteric nervous system of mice lacking the tyrosine kinase receptor RET, Nature 367:380–383, 1994.

27. Treanor JJ, Goodman L, de Sauvage F, et al: Characterization of a multicomponent receptor for GDNF, Nature 382:80–83, 1996.

28. Woodward ER, Eng C, McMahon R, et al: Genetic predisposition to phaeochromocytoma: Analysis of candidate genes GDNF, RET and VHL, Hum Mol Genet 6:1051–1056, 1997.

29. Asai N, Iwashita T, Matsuyama M, et al: Mechanism of activation of the ret proto-oncogene by multiple endocrine neoplasia 2A mutations, Mol Cell Biol 15:1613–1619, 1995.

30. Santoro M, Carlomagno F, Romano A, et al: Activation of RET as a dominant transforming gene by germline mutations of MEN-2A and MEN-2B, Science 267:381–383, 1995.

31. Pasini A, Geneste O, Legrand P, et al: Oncogenic activation of RET by two distinct FMTC mutations affecting the tyrosine kinase domain, Oncogene 15:393–402, 1997.

32. Russo AF, Clark MS, Durham PL: Thyroid parafollicular cells. An accessible model for the study of serotonergic neurons, Mol Neurobiol 13:257–276, 1996.

33. Rosai J, Carcangiu ML, De Lellis RA: Tumors of the thyroid gland. In Atlas of Tumor Pathology. Washington, DC, 1995, Armed Forces Institute of Pathology.

34. Guyetant S, Rousselet MC, Durigon M, et al: Sex-related C cell hyperplasia in the normal human thyroid: a quantitative autopsy study, J Clin Endocrinol Metab 82:42–47, 1997.

35. Papotti M, Botto Micca F, Favero A, et al: Poorly differentiated thyroid carcinomas with primordial cell component. A group of aggressive lesions sharing insular, trabecular, and solid patterns, Am J Surg Pathol 17:291–301, 1993.

36. Berndt I, Reuter M, Saller B, et al: A new hot spot for mutations in the ret protooncogene causing familial medullary thyroid carcinoma and multiple endocrine neoplasia type 2A, J Clin Endocrinol Metab 83:770–774, 1998.

37. Carlson KM, Dou S, Chi D, et al: Single missense mutation in the tyrosine kinase catalytic domain of the RET protooncogene is associated with multiple endocrine neoplasia type 2B, Proc Natl Acad Sci U S A 91:1579–1583, 1994.

38. Carlson KM, Bracamontes J, Jackson CE, et al: Parent-of-origin effects in multiple endocrine neoplasia type 2B, Am J Hum Genet 55:1076–1082, 1994.

39. Gimm O, Marsh DJ, Andrew SD, et al: Germline dinucleotide mutation in codon 883 of the RET proto-oncogene in multiple endocrine neoplasia type 2B without codon 918 mutation, J Clin Endocrinol Metab 82:3902–3904, 1997.

40. Punales MK, Graf H, Gross JL, et al: RET codon 634 mutations in multiple endocrine neoplasia type 2: variable clinical features and clinical outcome, J Clin Endocrinol Metab 88:2644–2649, 2003.

41. Nilson O, Tissell L, Janson S, et al: Adrenal and extra-adrenal pheochromocytomas in a family with germline RET V804L mutation, JAMA 281:1587, 1999.

42. Learoyd DL, Gosnell J, Elston MS, et al: Experience of prophylactic thyroidectomy in multiple endocrine neoplasia type 2A kindreds with RE codon 804 mutations, Clin Endocrinol 63:636–641, 2005.

43. Mulligan LM, Eng C, Attie T, et al: Diverse phenotypes associated with exon 10 mutations of the RET proto-oncogene, Hum Mol Genet 3:2163–2167, 1994.

44. Donovan DT, Levy ML, Furst EJ, et al: Familial cutaneous lichen amyloidosis in association with multiple endocrine neoplasia type 2A: a new variant, Henry Ford Hosp Med J 37:147–150, 1989.

45. Lips CJ, Landsvater RM, Hoppener JW, et al: Clinical screening as compared with DNA analysis in families with multiple endocrine neoplasia type 2A, N Engl J Med 331:828–835, 1994.

46. Marsh DJ, McDowall D, Hyland VJ, et al: The identification of false positive responses to the pentagastrin stimulation test in RET mutation negative members of MEN2A families, Clin Endocrinol (Oxf) 44:213–220, 1996.

47. Marsh DJ, Robinson BG, Andrew S, et al: A rapid screening method for the detection of mutations in the RET proto-oncogene in multiple endocrine neoplasia type 2A and familial medullary thyroid carcinoma families, Genomics 23:477–479, 1994.

48. Frilling A, Dralle H, Eng C, et al: Presymptomatic DNA screening in families with multiple endocrine neoplasia type 2 and familial medullary thyroid carcinoma, Surgery 118:1099–1103; discussion 1103–1104, 1995.

49. Decker RA, Peacock ML, Borst MJ, et al: Progress in genetic screening of multiple endocrine neoplasia type 2A: is calcitonin testing obsolete? Surgery 118:257–263; discussion 263–264, 1995.

50. Marsh DJ, Theodosopoulos G, Howell V, et al: Rapid mutation scanning of genes associated with familial cancer syndromes using denaturing high-performance liquid chromatography, Neoplasia 3:236–244, 2001.

51. Tsai MS, Ledger GA, Khosla S, et al: Identification of multiple endocrine neoplasia, type 2 gene carriers using linkage analysis and analysis of the RET proto-oncogene, J Clin Endocrinol Metab 78:1261–1264, 1994.

52. Brandi ML, Gagel RF, Angeli A, et al: Guidelines for diagnosis and therapy of MEN type 1 and type 2, J Clin Endocrinol Metab 86:5658–5671, 2001.

53. Lips CJ: Clinical management of the multiple endocrine neoplasia syndromes: results of a computerized opinion poll at the Sixth International Workshop on Multiple Endocrine Neoplasia and von Hippel-Lindau disease, J Intern Med 243:589–594, 1998.

54. Fronhauer MK, Decker RA: Update on MEN2A c804 RET mutation: is prophylactic thyroidectomy indicated? Surgery 128:1052–1058, 2000.

55. Learoyd DL, Robinson BG: Do all patients with RET mutations associated with multiple endocrine neoplasia type 2 require surgery? Nat Clin Pract Endocrinol Metab 1:60–61, 2005.

56. Learoyd DL, Capes AG, Robinson BG: Multiple endocrine neoplasia type 2 and glial cell line-derived neurotrophic factor, Curr Opin Endocrinol Diabetes 4:130–137, 1997.

57. Elisei R, Cosci B, Romei C, et al: Prognostic significance of somatic RET oncogene mutations in sporadic medullary thyroid cancer: a 10-year follow-up study, J Clin Endocrinol Metab 93:682–687, 2008.

58. Zedenius J, Larsson C, Bergholm U, et al: Mutations of codon 918 in the RET proto-oncogene correlate to poor prognosis in sporadic medullary thyroid carcinomas, J Clin Endocrinol Metab 80:3088–3090, 1995.

59. Romei C, Elisei R, Pinchera A, et al: Somatic mutations of the RET protooncogene in sporadic medullary thyroid carcinoma are not restricted to exon 16 and are associated with tumor recurrence, J Clin Endocrinol Metab 81:1619–1622, 1996.

60. Marsh DJ, Learoyd DL, Andrew SD, et al: Somatic mutations in the RET proto-oncogene in sporadic medullary thyroid carcinoma, Clin Endocrinol (Oxf) 44:249–257, 1996.

61. Marsh DJ, Andrew SD, Eng C, et al: Germline and somatic mutations in an oncogene: RET mutations in inherited medullary thyroid carcinoma, Cancer Res 56:1241–1243, 1996.

62. Miyauchi A, Egawa S, Futami H, et al: A novel somatic mutation in the RET proto-oncogene in familial medullary thyroid carcinoma with a germline codon 768 mutation, Jpn J Cancer Res 88:527–531, 1997.

63. Eng C, Mulligan LM, Healey CS, et al: Heterogeneous mutation of the RET proto-oncogene in subpopulations of medullary thyroid carcinoma, Cancer Res 56:2167–2170, 1996.

64. Wohllk N, Cote GJ, Bugalho MM, et al: Relevance of RET proto-oncogene mutations in sporadic medullary thyroid carcinoma, J Clin Endocrinol Metab 81:3740–3745, 1996.

65. Elisei R, Romei C, Cosci B, et al: RET genetic screening in patients with medullary thyroid cancer and their relatives: experience with 807 individuals at one center, J Clin Endocrinol Metab 92:4725–4729, 2007.

66. Eng C, Mulligan LM, Smith DP, et al: Low frequency of germline mutations in the RET proto-oncogene in patients with apparently sporadic medullary thyroid carcinoma, Clin Endocrinol (Oxf) 43:123–127, 1995.

67. Rougier P, Parmentier C, Laplanche A, et al: Medullary thyroid carcinoma: prognostic factors and treatment, Int J Radiat Oncol Biol Phys 9:161–169, 1983.

68. Saad MF, Ordonez NG, Rashid RK, et al: Medullary carcinoma of the thyroid. A study of the clinical features and prognostic factors in 161 patients, Medicine (Baltimore) 63:319–342, 1984.

69. Raue F, Kotzerke J, Reinwein D, et al: Prognostic factors in medullary thyroid carcinoma: evaluation of 741 patients from the German Medullary Thyroid Carcinoma Register, Clin Investig 71:7–12, 1993.

70. de Groot JWB, Plukker JTM, Wolffenbuttel BHR, et al: Determinants of life expectancy in medullary thyroid cancer: age does not matter, Clin Endocrinol 65:729–736, 2006.

71. Wells SA Jr, Baylin SB, Gann DS, et al: Medullary thyroid carcinoma: relationship of method of diagnosis to pathologic staging, Ann Surg 188:377–383, 1978.

72. Russell CF, Van Heerden JA, Sizemore GW, et al: The surgical management of medullary thyroid carcinoma, Ann Surg 197:42–48, 1983.

73. Scollo C, Baudin E, Travagli JP, et al: Rationale for central and bilateral lymph node dissection in sporadic and hereditary medullary thyroid cancer, J Clin Endocrinol Metab 88:2070–2075, 2003.

74. Miyauchi A, Onishi T, Morimoto S, et al: Relation of doubling time of plasma calcitonin levels to prognosis and recurrence of medullary thyroid carcinoma, Ann Surg 1999:461–466, 1984.

75. Barbet J, Campion L, Kraeber-Bodere L, et al: Prognostic impact of serum calcitonin and carcinoembryonic antigen doubling-times in patients with medullary thyroid carcinoma, J Clin Endocrinol Metab 90:6077–6084, 2005.

76. Giraudet AL, Ghulzan AA, Auperin A, et al: Progression of medullary thyroid carcinoma: assessment with calcitonin and carcinoembryonic antigen doubling times, Eur J Endocrinol 158:239–248, 2008.

77. de Groot JW, Kema IP, Breukelman H, et al: Biochemical markers in the follow-up of medullary thyroid cancer, Thyroid 16:1163–1170, 2006.

78. Giraudet AL, Vanel D, Leboulleux S, et al: Imaging medullary thyroid carcinoma with persistent elevated calcitonin levels, J Clin Endocrinol Metab 93:4185–4190, 2007.

79. Lebouthillier G, Morais J, Picard M, et al: Tc-99m sestamibi and other agents in the detection of metastatic medullary carcinoma of the thyroid, Clin Nucl Med 18:657–661, 1993.

80. Hoefnagel CA, Delprat CC, Zanin D, et al: New radionuclide tracers for the diagnosis and therapy of medullary thyroid carcinoma, Clin Nucl Med 13:159–165, 1988.

81. Learoyd DL, Roach PJ, Briggs GM, et al: Technetium-99m-sestamibi scanning in recurrent medullary thyroid carcinoma, J Nucl Med 38:227–230, 1997.

82. Gourgiotis L, Sarlis NJ, Reynolds JC, et al: Localization of medullary thyroid carcinoma metastasis in a multiple endocrine neoplasia type 2A patient by 6-[18F]-fluorodopamine positron emission tomography, J Clin Endocrinol Metab 88:637–641, 2003.

83. Abdelmoumene N, Schlumberger M, Gardet P, et al: Selective venous sampling catheterisation for localization of persisting medullary thyroid carcinoma, Br J Cancer 69:1141–1144, 1994.

84. Ben Mrad MD, Gardet P, Roche A, et al: Value of venous catheterization and calcitonin studies in the treatment and management of clinically inapparent medullary thyroid carcinoma, Cancer 63:133–138, 1989.

85. Machens A, Schneyer U, Holzhausen H-J, et al: Prospects of remission in medullary thyroid carcinoma according to basal calcitonin level, J Clin Endocrinol Metab 90:2029–2034, 2005.

86. Gimm O, Dralle H: Reoperation in metastasizing medullary thyroid carcinoma: is a tumor stage–oriented approach justified? Surgery 122:1124–1130; discussion 1130–1131, 1997.

87. Diez JJ, Iglesias P: Somatostatin analogs in the treatment of medullary thyroid carcinoma, J Endocrinol Invest 25:773–778, 2002.

88. Kebebew E, Clark OH: Medullary thyroid cancer, Curr Treat Options Oncol 1:359–367, 2000.

89. Petursson SR: Metastatic medullary thyroid carcinoma. Complete response to combination chemotherapy with dacarbazine and 5-fluorouracil, Cancer 62:1899–1903, 1988.

90. Wu LT, Averbuch SD, Ball DW, et al: Treatment of advanced medullary thyroid carcinoma with a combination of cyclophosphamide, vincristine, and dacarbazine, Cancer 73:432–436, 1994.

91. Lorenz K, Brauckhoff M, Behrmann C, et al: Selective arterial chemoembolization for hepatic metastases from medullary thyroid carcinoma, Surgery 138:986–993, 2005.

92. Fromigue J, De Baere T, Baudin E, et al: Chemoembolization for liver metastases from medullary thyroid carcinoma, J Clin Endocrinol Metab 91:2496–2499, 2006.

93. Brierley J, Tsang R, Simpson WJ, et al: Medullary thyroid cancer: analyses of survival and prognostic factors and the role of radiation therapy in local control, Thyroid 6:305–310, 1996.

94. Steinfield AD: The role of radiation therapy in medullary carcinoma of the thyroid, Radiology 123:745–746, 1977.

95. Gagel RF, Robinson MF, Donovan DT, et al: Clinical review 44: medullary thyroid carcinoma: recent progress, J Clin Endocrinol Metab 76:809–814, 1993.

96. Saad MF, Guido JJ, Samaan NA: Radioactive iodine in the treatment of medullary carcinoma of the thyroid, J Clin Endocrinol Metab 57:124–128, 1983.

97. Chatal J-F, Campion L, Kraeber-Bodere F, et al: Survival improvement in patients with medullary thyroid carcinoma who undergo pretargeted anti-carcinoembryonic-antigen radioimmunotherapy: a collaborative study with the French Endocrine Tumor Group, J Clin Oncol 24:1075–1711, 2006.

98. Iten F, Muller B, et al: Response to [90Yttrium-DOTA]-TOC treatment is associated with long-term survival benefit in metastasized medullary thyroid cancer: a phase II clinical trial, Clin Cancer Res 13:6696–6702, 2007.

99. Schott M, Seissler J, Lettmann M, et al: Immunotherapy for medullary thyroid carcinoma by dendritic cell vaccination, J Clin Endocrinol Metab 86:4965–4969, 2001.

100. Drosten M, Putzer BM: Gene therapeutic approaches for medullary thyroid carcinoma treatment, J Mol Med 81:411–419, 2003.

101. Zhang R, Baunoch D, DeGroot LJ: Genetic immunotherapy for medullary thyroid carcinoma: destruction of tumors in mice by in vivo delivery of adenoviral vector transducing the murine interleukin-2 gene, Thyroid 8:1137–1146, 1998.

102. Zhang R, Straus FH, DeGroot LJ: Effective genetic therapy of established medullary thyroid carcinomas with murine interleukin-2: dissemination and cytotoxicity studies in a rat tumor model, Endocrinology 140:2152–2158, 1999.

103. Zhang R, DeGroot LJ: Genetic immunotherapy of established tumors with adenoviral vectors transducing murine interleukin 12 (mIL-12) subunits in a rat medullary thyroid carcinoma model, Clin Endocrinol (Oxf) 52:687–694, 2000.

104. Drosten M, Frilling A, Stiewe T, et al: A new therapeutic approach in medullary thyroid cancer treatment: inhibition of oncogenic RET signaling by adenoviral vector-mediated expression of a dominant-negative RET mutant, Surgery 132:991–997; discussion 997, 2002.

105. Messina M, Learoyd DL, Both GW, et al: Gene therapy for endocrine tumors: strategies and progress, Curr Opin Endocrinol Diabetes 8:35–40, 2001.

106. Aghi M, Hochberg F, Breakefield XO: Prodrug activation enzymes in cancer gene therapy, J Gene Med 2:148–164, 2000.

107. Frank-Raue K, Fabel M, Delorme S, et al: Efficacy of imatinib mesylate in advanced medullary thyroid carcinoma, Eur J Endocrinol 157:215–220, 2007.

108. de Groot JWB, Zonnenberg BA, Ufford-Mannesse PQ, et al: A phase II trial of imatinib therapy for metastatic medullary thyroid carcinoma, J Clin Endocrinol Metab 92:3466–3469, 2007.

109. Wells SW, Gosnell JE, Gagel RF, et al: Vandetanib in metastatic hereditary medullary thyroid cancer: follow-up results of an open-label phase II trial. Abstract 6018 presented at the 43rd Annual Meeting of the American Society of Clinical Oncology (ASCO) 2007) ASCO Meeting Abstracts June 20, 2007.

110. Carlomagno F, Guida T, Anaganti S, et al: Disease-associated mutations at valine 804 in the RET receptor tyrosine kinase confer resistance to selective kinase inhibitors, Oncogene 23:6056–6063, 2004.

Chapter 20

THYROID-STIMULATING HORMONE RECEPTOR MUTATIONS

GILBERT VASSART

Gain-of-Function Mutations
Familial Nonautoimmune Hyperthyroidism or Hereditary
  Toxic Thyroid Hyperplasia
Sporadic Toxic Thyroid Hyperplasia
Somatic Mutations: Autonomous Toxic Adenomas
Structure-Function Relationships of the TSH Receptor, as
  Deduced from Activating Mutations
Familial Gestational Hyperthyroidism

Loss-of-Function Mutations
Clinical Cases With the Mutations Identified

Polymorphisms

Gain-of-Function Mutations

For a hormone receptor, "gain of function" may have three meanings: activation in the absence of ligand (constitutivity), increased sensitivity to its normal agonist, or broadening of its specificity. When the receptor is part of a chemostat, as is the case for the thyroid-stimulating hormone (TSH) receptor, the first situation is expected to lead to tissue "autonomy," whereas the second would be expected to simply cause adjustment of the agonist concentration to a lower value. In the third case, inappropriate stimulation of the gland is expected to occur because the promiscuous agonist is not expected to be subjected to the normal negative feedback. If a gain-of-function mutation of the first category occurs in a single cell normally expressing the receptor (somatic mutation), it will become symptomatic only if the regulatory cascade controlled by the receptor is mitogenic in this particular cell type. Autonomous activity of the receptor will cause clonal expansion of the mutated cell. If the regulatory cascade also positively controls function, the resulting tumor will progressively take over function of the normal tissue, ultimately resulting in autonomous hyperfunction. If the mutation is present in all cells of an organism (germline mutation), autonomy will be displayed by the whole tissue expressing the receptor. In cases in which the regulatory cascade is mitogenic and activates function, the expected result is hyperplasia associated with hyperfunction.

From what we know of thyroid cell physiology, it is easy to predict the phenotypes associated with gain-of-function muta-

tions of the cyclic adenosine monophosphate (cAMP)-dependent regulatory cascade. Two observations provide pertinent models of this situation. Transgenic mice made to ectopically express the adenosine A2a receptor in their thyroid display severe hyperthyroidism associated with thyroid hyperplasia.[1] Because the A2a adenosine receptor is coupled to G_s and displays constitutive activity as a result of continuous stimulation by ambient adenosine, this model closely mimics the situation expected for a gain-of-function germline mutation of the TSH receptor. Patients with the McCune-Albright syndrome are mosaic for mutations in G_s (*gsp* mutations), which also leads to constitutive stimulation of adenylyl cyclase.[2] Hyperfunctioning thyroid adenomas develop in these patients from cells harboring the mutation, which makes them a model for gain-of-function somatic mutations of the TSH receptor. A transgenic model in which *gsp* mutations are targeted for expression in the mouse thyroid has been constructed. Although with a less dramatic phenotype, this represents a pertinent model for a gain of function in the cAMP regulatory cascade.[3]

FAMILIAL NONAUTOIMMUNE HYPERTHYROIDISM OR HEREDITARY TOXIC THYROID HYPERPLASIA

The major cause of hyperthyroidism in adults is Graves' disease, in which an autoimmune reaction is mounted against the thyroid gland and autoantibodies are produced that recognize and stimulate the TSH receptor. This origin may explain why the initial description by the group of Leclère of a family showing segregation of thyrotoxicosis as an autosomal dominant trait in the absence of signs of autoimmunity was met with skepticism.[4] Reinvestigation of this family together with that of another family from Reims (France) identified two mutations of the *TSH receptor* gene that segregated in perfect linkage with the disease.[5] A series of additional families have been studied since, almost systematically with a different mutation of the *TSH receptor* gene[6-19] (Fig. 20-1). (For comprehensive lists of activating mutations, see http://gris.ulb.ac.be/ and http://www.ssfa-gphr.de/main/ssfa.php.) The functional characteristics of these mutant receptors confirm that they are constitutively stimulated (see below). Hereditary toxic thyroid hyperplasia (HTTH), sometimes called Leclère's disease, is characterized by the following clinical characteristics: autosomal dominant transmission; hyperthyroidism with a variable age of onset (from infancy to adulthood, even within a given family); hyperplastic goiter of variable size, but with steady growth; and absence of clinical or biological stigmata

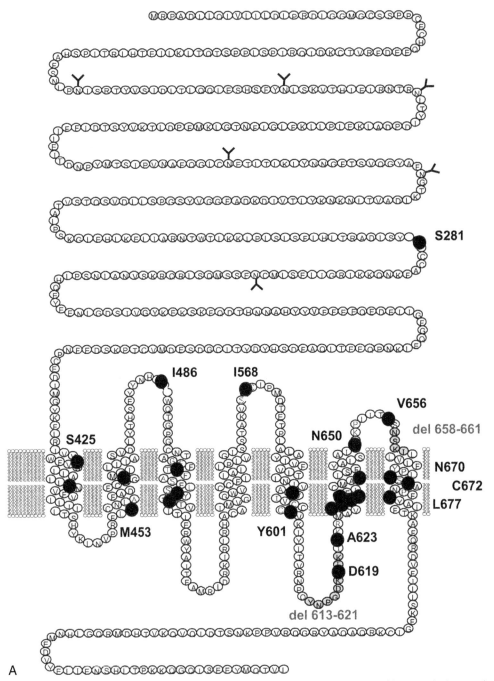

FIGURE 20-1. Schematic representation of the thyroid-stimulating hormone (TSH) receptor. **A,** The locations of known activating mutations are indicated.

Continued

of autoimmunity. An observation common to cases to date is the need for drastic ablative therapy (surgery or radioiodine) to control the disease once the patient has become hyperthyroid. The autonomous nature of the thyroid tissue from these patients has been elegantly demonstrated by grafting in nude mice.[20] In contrast to tissue from patients with Graves' disease, HTTH cells continue to grow in the absence of stimulation by TSH or thyroid-stimulating antibody.

The prevalence of hereditary toxic thyroid hyperplasia is difficult to estimate at the present time. It is likely that many cases have been (and still are) mistaken for Graves' disease. This may be explained by the high frequency of thyroid autoantibodies (antithyroglobulin, antithyroperoxidase) in the general population. It is expected that wider knowledge of the existence of the

disease will lead to better diagnosis. This is not a purely academic problem, in that presymptomatic diagnosis in children of affected families may prevent the developmental or psychological complications associated with infantile or juvenile hyperthyroidism. A country-wide screening for the condition has been performed in Denmark. It was found in 1 out of 121 patients with juvenile thyrotoxicosis (0.8%; 95% confidence interval [CI]: 0.02% to 4.6%), which corresponds to 1 in 17 patients with presumed nonautoimmune juvenile thyrotoxicosis (6%; 95% CI: 0.15% to 28.69%).[21]

SPORADIC TOXIC THYROID HYPERPLASIA

Cases of toxic thyroid hyperplasia have been described in children of unaffected parents.[7,22-29] Conspicuously, congenital

CODON	Substitution	Somatic mutation	Germline Neomutation	Germline Familial	Cancer	Stimulation of [cAMP]	Stimulation of [IP]
Ser 281	Asn	+				+	−
	Thr	+				+	−
	Ile		+			+	−
Ser 425	Ile	+				+	−
Gly 431	Ser			+		+	+
Met 453	Thr	+	+		+	+	−
Met 463	Val			+		+	−
Ile 486	Phe	+				+	+
	Met	+				+	+/−
Ser505	Arg			+		+	−
	Asn		+			+	−
Val509	Ala			+		+	−
Leu 512	Arg	+				+	nd
	Gln	+				+	nd
Ile568	Thr	+	+			+	+/−
Val 597	Leu		+			+	nd
	Phe		+			+	nd
Tyr 601	Asn	+				+	−
Del 613-631		+				+	−
Asp 619	Gly	+				+	−
Ala 623	Ile	+				+	+/−
	Val	+		+		+	−
	Ser	+			+	+	−
Leu 629	Phe	+		+		+	−
Ile 630	Leu	+				+	−
Phe 631	Leu	+	+			+	−
	Cys	+				+	−
	Ile				+	+	−
Thr 632	Ile	+	+			+	−
	Ala	+			+	+	nd
Asp 633	Tyr	+			+	+	−
	Glu	+				+	−
	His	+			+	+	−
	Ala	+				+	−
Pro 639	Ser	+		+		+	+
Asn 650	Tyr			+		+	−
Val 656	Phe	+				+	−
Del658-661		+				+	−
Asn670	Ser			+		+	−
Cys672	Tyr			+		+	−
Leu 677	Val				+	+	nd

B

FIGURE 20-1, cont'd. **B,** The nature of the mutations is indicated along with their origins (somatic, germline sporadic, germline familial, cancer) and effects on intracellular regulatory cascades. (For a complete list of activating mutations with their functional characteristics, see http://gris.ulb.ac.be/ and http://www.ssfa-gphr.de/main/ssfa.php.)

hyperthyroidism was present in most of the patients and required aggressive treatment. Mutations of one TSH receptor allele were identified in the children but were absent in the parents. Because paternity was confirmed by minisatellite or microsatellite testing, these cases qualify as true neomutations. When the amino acid substitutions implicated in hereditary and sporadic cases are compared, for the majority, they do not overlap (see Fig. 20-1). Although most of the sporadic cases harbor mutations that are also found in toxic adenomas, most of the hereditary cases have "private" mutations. Analysis of the functional characteristics of the individual mutant receptors in COS cells and the clinical course of individual patients suggests an explanation for this observation: "sporadic" mutations seem to have a stronger activating effect than "hereditary" mutations do. From their severe phenotypes, it is likely that newborns with neomutations would not have survived if not treated efficiently. On the contrary, from inspection of the available pedigrees, it seems that the milder phenotype of patients with hereditary mutations has only a limited effect on reproductive fitness. The fact that hereditary mutations are rarely observed in toxic adenomas is compatible with the suggestion that they would cause extremely slow tissue growth and, accordingly, would rarely cause thyrotoxicosis, if somatic. There is, however, no a priori reason for neomutations to cause stronger gain of function than hereditary mutations. Accordingly, an activating mutation of the TSH receptor gene has been found in a 6-month-old child with subclinical hyperthyroidism who presents with weight loss as the initial symptom.[30]

SOMATIC MUTATIONS: AUTONOMOUS TOXIC ADENOMAS

Soon after mutations of $G_s\alpha$ had been found in adenomas of the pituitary somatotrophs,[31] similar mutations (also called *gsp* mutations) were found in some toxic thyroid adenomas and follicular carcinomas.[32-35] The mutated residues (*Arg201, Glu227*) are homologous to those found mutated in the *ras* proto-oncogenes, that is, the mutations decrease the endogenous guanine triphosphatase activity of the G protein, thereby resulting in a constitutively active molecule.

Toxic adenoma was found to be a fruitful source of somatic mutations activating the TSH receptor, probably because the phenotype is very conspicuous and easy to diagnose. Whereas mutations are distributed all along the serpentine portion of the receptor[36-42] and even in the extracellular aminoterminal domain,[43] there is clearly a hotspot at the cytoplasmic side of the sixth transmembrane segment (see Fig. 20-1). (For a complete list of TSH receptor gene mutations with their functional characteristics, see http://gris.ulb.ac.be/ and http://www.ssfa-gphr.de/main/ssfa.php.) The clustering reflects the pivotal role of this portion of the molecule in activation mechanisms.[44-49]

Despite some dispute about the prevalence of TSH receptor mutations in toxic adenomas, which may be due to different origins among patients[50] or different sensitivities of methods, the current consensus is that activating mutations of the TSH receptor are the major cause of solitary toxic adenomas and account for about 60% to 80% of cases.[36,42,51-53] Contrary to initial suggestions, the same percentage of TSH receptor mutation is observed in Japan, an iodine-sufficient country with low prevalence of toxic adenomas.[54] In some patients with multinodular goiter and two zones of autonomy at scintigraphy, a different mutation of the TSH receptor was identified in each nodule.[55-58] This finding indicates that the pathophysiologic mechanism responsible for solitary toxic adenomas can be at work on a background of multinodular goiter. In agreement with this notion, activating mutations of the *TSH receptor* have been identified in hyperfunctioning areas of multinodular goiter.[57,59-61] The independent occurrence of two activating mutations in a patient may seem highly improbable at first. However, the multiplicity of the possible amino acid targets for activating mutations within the TSH receptor makes this event less unlikely. It is also possible that a mutagenic environment is created in glands exposed to chronic stimulation by TSH in which H_2O_2 is produced.[62,63] Finally, involvement of *TSH receptor* mutations in thyroid cancer has been implicated in a limited proportion of follicular thyroid carcinomas.[61,64-69]

STRUCTURE-FUNCTION RELATIONSHIPS OF THE TSH RECEPTOR, AS DEDUCED FROM ACTIVATING MUTATIONS

Most of the activating mutations of the *TSH receptor* have been studied by transient expression in *COS* or *HEK293T* cells. There is no guarantee that the mutants will function in an identical way in these artificial systems as they do in thyrocytes. Arguments have been obtained for such cell-type specific effects.[70] In thyrocytes, a better relation has been observed between adenylyl cyclase stimulation and differentiation than with growth.[70] However, the built-in amplification associated with transfection of constructs in *COS* or *HEK 293T* cells makes it possible to detect even slight increases in constitutive activity of *TSH receptor* mutants. An important observation has been that the wild-type receptor itself displays significant constitutive activity.[38,71] This characteristic is not unique to the TSH receptor, but it is interesting to note that it is not shared by its close relatives, the luteinizing hormone/chorionic gonadotropin (LH/

CG) receptor and the follitropin receptor (FSH). The effect of activating mutations accordingly must be interpreted in terms of "increase in constitutive activity." Most receptor mutants found in toxic adenomas and/or toxic thyroid hyperplasia share common characteristics: (1) they increase the constitutive activity of the receptor toward stimulation of adenylyl cyclase; (2) with a few notable exceptions (see Fig. 20-1),[72] they do not display constitutive activity toward the inositol phosphate/diacylglycerol pathway; (3) their expression at the cell surface is decreased (from slightly to severely); (4) most but not all of them keep responding to TSH for stimulation of cAMP and inositol phosphate generation, with a tendency to do so at decreased median effective concentrations; and (5) they bind ^{125}I-labeled bovine TSH with an apparent affinity higher than that of the wild-type receptor.

No simple relationship exists between the position of the mutations or the nature of the amino acid substitution and their functional characteristics. Mutations found in transmembrane segments 1, 2, 3, 6, and 7 and the third cytoplasmic loop all have similar phenotypes; they involve amino acids belonging to all classes (charged, polar, hydrophobic), with substitutions not necessarily involving a shift to another class. Mutations involving *Ile486* and *Ile568* in the first and second extracellular loops, respectively, and *Pro639* in transmembrane segment 6 are exceptional in that, in addition to stimulating adenylyl cyclase, they cause constitutive activation of the inositol phosphate pathway.

No direct relationship has been found between the level of cAMP achieved by different mutants in transfected *COS* cells and their level of expression at the cell membrane,[73] which means that individual mutants have widely different "specific constitutive activity" (measured as the stimulation of cAMP accumulation/receptor number at the cell surface). Although this specific activity may tell us something about the mechanisms of receptor activation, it is not a measure of the actual phenotypic effect of the mutation in vivo. Indeed, one of the relatively mild mutations, observed up until now only in a family with HTTH (*Cys672Tyr*), is among the strongest according to this criterion. It would be logical to expect the best correlation to be found between the phenotype and the actual level of cAMP achieved, irrespective of the level of receptor expression. However, differences between the effects of the mutants in transfected *COS* or *HEK293* cells and thyrocytes in vivo may render these correlations a difficult exercise.[70]

According to a current model of G protein–coupled receptor (GPCR) activation, the receptor would exist under at least two interconverting conformations: R (silent conformations) and R* (the active forms).[44] The unliganded receptor would shuttle between both forms, the equilibrium being in favor of R. Binding of the ligand to the slit between the transmembrane segments (for biogenic amines) and/or the residues of the N-terminal segment or extracellular loops (for neuropeptides) is believed to stabilize the R* conformations. The resulting R-to-R* transition is supposed to involve a conformational change that modifies the relative position of transmembrane helices, which in turn would translate into conformational changes in the cytoplasmic domains interacting with trimeric G proteins. Seminal studies with the adrenergic receptor α_{1b} have shown that a variety of amino acid substitutions in the C-terminal portion of the third intracellular loop lead to their constitutive activation.[74] The observation that all amino acid substitutions at *Ala293* were effective in activating the receptor led to the concept that the silent form of GPCRs would be submitted to a structural constraint requiring the wild-type primary structure of the third intracellular loop. This constraint could be released by a wide spectrum of amino acid substitutions in this segment.[44,75]

The observation that amino acid substitutions in a large number of residues scattered over the serpentine portion of the TSH receptor cause an increase in its constitutive activity is fully compatible with the above model and provided arguments for its extension. The fact that mutations in residues distributed over most of the serpentine portion of the receptor are equally effective in activating it (which does not seem to be a general characteristic in all GPCRs) suggests that the unliganded TSH receptor might be less constrained than others. The readily measurable constitutive activity of the wild-type receptor is compatible with this contention. Being already "noisy," the TSH receptor would be more prone to further destabilization by a variety of mutations.

The precise effects of individual mutations in structural terms are beginning to emerge from analogies with the limited list of GPCRs whose tridimensional structure has been solved.[76]

FAMILIAL GESTATIONAL HYPERTHYROIDISM

Some degree of stimulation of the thyroid gland by human chorionic gonadotropin (hCG) is commonly observed during early pregnancy. It is usually responsible for a decrease in serum thyrotropin with an increase in the concentration of free thyroxine (T_4), which remains within the normal range (for references, see 77). When concentrations of hCG are abnormally high, as in molar pregnancy, true hyperthyroidism may ensue. The pathophysiologic mechanism is believed to be promiscuous stimulation of the TSH receptor by excess hCG, as suggested by the rough direct or inverse relation between serum hCG and free T_4 or TSH concentrations, respectively.[77] A convincing rationale is provided by the close structural relationships and evolutionary origins of the glycoprotein hormones and their receptors.[78]

A new syndrome was described in 1998 in a family with dominant transmission of hyperthyroidism limited to pregnancy.[79] The proposita and her mother had severe thyrotoxicosis together with hyperemesis gravidarum during the course of each of their pregnancies. When nonpregnant, they were clinically and biologically euthyroid. Both patients were heterozygous for a *Lys183Arg* mutation in the extracellular aminoterminal domain of the TSH receptor. When tested by transient transfection in COS cells, the mutant receptor displayed normal characteristics toward TSH. However, a convincing explanation for the phenotype was provided in that it showed higher sensitivity to stimulation by hCG than the wild-type TSH receptor.

The amino acid substitution responsible in these patients for promiscuous stimulation of the TSH receptor by hCG is surprisingly conservative. Also surprising is the observation that residue 183 is a lysine in both the TSH and LH/CG receptors. When placed on the three-dimensional structure of the hormone-binding domain of the TSH receptor,[80] residue 183 belongs to one of the β sheets that constitute the surface of interaction with the hormones. Detailed analysis of the effect of the *K183R* mutation by site-directed mutagenesis indicated that any amino acid substitution at this position confers a slight increase in stability to the illegitimate hCG/TSH receptor complex.[81] This increase in stability would be enough to cause signal transduction by the hCG concentrations achieved in pregnancy, but not by the LH concentrations observed after menopause. Indeed, the mother of the proposita remained euthyroid after menopause. This finding is compatible with a relatively modest gain in function of the *Lys183Arg* mutant upon stimulation by hCG.

In contrast to other mammals, humans and primates rely on CG for maintenance of the corpus luteum in early pregnancy. The frequent partial suppression of TSH observed at peak hCG levels during normal pregnancy indicates that evolution has selected physiologic mechanisms operating very close to the border of thyrotoxicosis. This finding may provide a rationale for the observation that in comparison with other species, the glycoprotein hormones of primates display lower biological activity because of positive evolutionary selection of specific amino acid substitutions in their α subunits.[78] Up to now, no spontaneous mutation has been identified that would increase the bioactivity of hCG. An interesting parallel may be drawn between familial gestational hyperthyroidism and cases of spontaneous ovarian hyperstimulation syndrome (sOHSS).[82,83] In sOHSS, mutations of the *FSH receptor* gene render the receptor abnormally sensitive to hCG. The result is recurrent hyperstimulation of the ovary, on the occasion of each pregnancy.

Loss-of-Function Mutations

Loss-of-function mutations in the *TSH receptor* gene are expected to cause a syndrome of "resistance to TSH." The expected phenotype is likely to resemble that of patients with mutations in TSH itself. These mutations have been described early because of the prior availability of information on TSH α and β genes.[84] Mouse models of resistance to TSH are available as natural (*hyt/hyt mouse*)[85] or experimental TSH receptor mutant lines.[86,87] It is interesting to note and contrary to the situation in humans (see below) that the thyroid of newborn TSH receptor knockout mice is of normal size. As expected, the homozygote animals displayed profound hypothyroidism. Their thyroids did not express the sodium-iodide symporter but showed significant (noniodinated) thyroglobulin production. From this information, one would expect patients with two TSH receptor–mutated alleles to exhibit a degree of hypothyroidism in accordance with the extent of loss of function, going from mild, compensated hypothyroidism to profound neonatal hypothyroidism with absent iodide trapping. Heterozygous carriers are expected to be normal or to display minimal increase in plasma TSH (see below).

CLINICAL CASES WITH THE MUTATIONS IDENTIFIED

A few patients with convincing resistance to TSH had been described before molecular genetics permitted identification of the mutations.[88,89] The first cases described in molecular terms involved euthyroid siblings with elevated TSH.[90] Sequencing of the *TSH receptor* gene identified a different mutation in each allele of the affected individuals, which made them compound heterozygotes. The substitutions occurred in the extracellular aminoterminal portion of the receptor (maternal allele, *Pro-162Ala*; paternal allele, *Ile167Asn*). The functional characteristics of the mutant receptors showed that the paternal allele was virtually completely nonfunctional, whereas the maternal allele displayed an increase in the median effective TSH concentration for stimulation of cAMP production. Current knowledge of the tridimensional structure of part of the ectodomain of

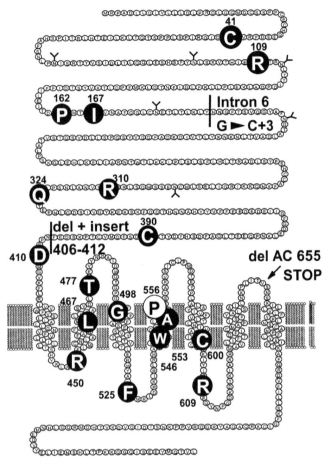

Position	Substitution	Loss-of-Function
Cys 41	Ser	partial (?)
Arg 109	Gln	partial
Pro 162	Ala	partial
Ile 167	Asn	complete
Arg 310	Cys	partial
Gln 324	Stop	complete
Cys 390	Trp	partial (?)
406-412	del + insert	complete
Asp 410	Asn	partial
Arg 450	His	partial
Leu 467	Pro	severe
Thr 477	Ile	complete
Gly 498	Ser	severe
Phe 525	Leu	partial (?)
Trp 546	Stop	complete
Ala 553	Thr	complete
Cys 600	Arg	complete
Arg 609	Stop	complete
655 del AC		complete
+3 IVS 6	G > C	complete
Pro 556 (hyt/hyt mouse)	Leu	complete

FIGURE 20-2. Loss-of-function mutations of the thyroid-stimulating hormone (TSH) receptor. The locations of known loss-of-function mutations are indicated (left) together with their nature and functional characteristics. (For a complete list of loss of function mutations with their functional characteristics, see http://gris.ulb.ac.be/ and http://www.ssfa-gphr.de/main/ssfa.php.)

the receptor[80,91] allows one to establish structure-function relationships for mutations affecting this portion of the receptor.[92]

A large number of familial cases with loss-of-function mutations of the *TSH receptor* have been identified in the course of screening programs for congenital hypothyroidism[93-106] (Fig. 20-2). (For a complete list of TSH receptor gene mutations with their functional characteristics, see http://gris.ulb.ac.be/ and http://www.ssfa-gphr.de/main/ssfa.php.) Some of the patients displayed the usual criteria for congenital hypothyroidism, including high TSH, low free T_4, and undetectable trapping of ^{99}Tc. In some cases, plasma thyroglobulin levels were normal or high. Patients can be compound heterozygotes for complete loss-of-function mutations,[94] or they may be homozygotes, born to consanguineous[93] or apparently unrelated parents.[100] In agreement with the phenotype of knockout mice with homozygous invalidation of the TSH receptor, patients with complete loss of function of the receptor display an in-place thyroid with completely absent iodide or ^{99}Tc trapping. However, in contrast to the situation in mice, the gland is hypoplastic. Activation of the cAMP pathway, although dispensable for the anatomic development of the gland and thyroglobulin production, thus is absolutely required for expression of the sodium-iodide-symporter (*NIS*) gene and, at least in humans, for normal growth of the tissue during fetal life. This explains how in the absence of thyroglobulin measurements or expert echography, loss-of-function mutations of the *TSH receptor* may easily be misdiagnosed as thyroid agenesis.

In the heterozygous state, complete loss-of-function mutation of the TSH receptor is a cause of moderate hyperthyrotropinemia (subclinical hypothyroidism), segregating as an autosomal dominant trait.[107] Finally, it must be stressed that an autosomal dominant form of partial resistance to TSH has been demonstrated in families in which linkage to the *TSH receptor* gene has been excluded.[108] A locus has been identified on chromosome 15q25.3–26.1, but the gene responsible for this phenotype has not been identified yet.[109]

Polymorphisms

A series of single-nucleotide polymorphisms affecting the coding sequence have been identified in the *TSH receptor* gene. After the initial suggestion that some of these (D36H, P52T, D727E) would be associated with susceptibility to autoimmune thyroid disease,[110-112] the current consensus is that they represent neutral alleles with no pathophysiologic significance.[113-116] However, a genome-wide study involving a large cohort of patients recently demonstrated an association between noncoding single nucleotide polymorphisms (SNPs) at the *TSH receptor* gene locus and Graves'disease.[117,118] The genetic substratum responsible for this association is still under study.[117]

One polymorphic residue deserves special mention: position 601 was found to be a tyrosine or a histidine in the two initial reports of TSH receptor cloning.[119,120] Characterization of the two alleles by transfection in *COS* cells indicated interesting functional differences: the Y601 allele displayed readily detectable constitutive activity, whereas H601 was completely silent; the Y601 allele responded to stimulation by TSH by activating the adenylyl cyclase– and phospholipase C–dependent regulatory cascades, when the H601 allele was active only on the cAMP pathway.[121] The Y601 allele is by far the most frequent among all populations tested, and a Y601N mutation was found in a toxic adenoma. Characterization of the mutant demonstrated increased constitutive activation of the cAMP regulatory cascade,[121] making the 601 residue an interesting target for structure-function studies.

REFERENCES

1. Ledent C, Dumont JE, Vassart G, et al: Thyroid expression of an A2 adenosine receptor transgene induces thyroid hyperplasia and hyperthyroidism, EMBO J 11:537–542, 1992.
2. Weinstein LS, Yu S, Warner DR, et al: Endocrine manifestations of stimulatory G protein alpha-subunit mutations and the role of genomic imprinting, Endocr Rev 22:675–705, 2001.
3. Michiels FM, Caillou B, Talbot M, et al: Oncogenic potential of guanine nucleotide stimulatory factor alpha subunit in thyroid glands of transgenic mice, Proc Natl Acad Sci U S A 91:10488–10492, 1994.
4. Thomas JS, Leclere J, Hartemann P, et al: Familial hyperthyroidism without evidence of autoimmunity, Acta Endocrinol Copenh 100:512–518, 1982.
5. Duprez L, Parma J, Van Sande J, et al: Germline mutations in the thyrotropin receptor gene cause non autoimmune autosomal dominant hyperthyroidism, Nat Genet 7:396–401, 1994.
6. Tonacchera M, Van Sande J, Cetani F, et al: Functional characteristics of three new germline mutations of the thyrotropin receptor gene causing autosomal dominant toxic thyroid hyperplasia, J Clin Endocrinol Metab 81:547–554, 1996.
7. Fuhrer D, Wonerow P, Willgerodt H, et al: Identification of a new thyrotropin receptor germline mutation (Leu629Phe) in a family with neonatal onset of autosomal dominant nonautoimmune hyperthyroidism, J Clin Endocrinol Metab 82:4234–4238, 1997.
8. Fuhrer D, Warner J, Sequeira M, et al: Novel TSHR germline mutation (Met463Val) masquerading as Graves' disease in a large Welsh kindred with hyperthyroidism, Thyroid 10:1035–1041, 2000.
9. Biebermann H, Schoneberg T, Hess C, et al: The first activating TSH receptor mutation in transmembrane domain 1 identified in a family with nonautoimmune hyperthyroidism, J Clin Endocrinol Metab 86:4429–4433, 2001.
10. Arturi F, Chiefari E, Tumino S, et al: Similarities and differences in the phenotype of members of an Italian family with hereditary non-autoimmune hyperthyroidism associated with an activating TSH receptor germline mutation, J Endocrinol Invest 25:696–701, 2002.
11. Alberti L, Proverbio MC, Costagliola S, et al: A novel germline mutation in the TSH receptor gene causes non-autoimmune autosomal dominant hyperthyroidism, Eur J Endocrinol 145:249–254, 2001.
12. Akcurin S, Turkkahraman D, Tysoe C, et al: A family with a novel TSH receptor activating germline mutation (p.Ala485Val), Eur J Pediatr 167:1231–1237, 2008.
13. Gozu HI, Mueller S, Bircan R, et al: A new silent germline mutation of the TSH receptor: coexpression in a hyperthyroid family member with a second activating somatic mutation, Thyroid 18:499–508, 2008.
14. Liu Z, Sun Y, Dong Q, et al: A novel TSHR gene mutation (Ile691Phe) in a Chinese family causing autosomal dominant non-autoimmune hyperthyroidism, J Hum Genet 53:475–478, 2008.
15. Ferrara AM, Capalbo D, Rossi G, et al: A new case of familial nonautoimmune hyperthyroidism caused by the M463V mutation in the TSH receptor with anticipation of the disease across generations: a possible role of iodine supplementation, Thyroid 17:677–680, 2007.
16. Nishihara E, Nagayama Y, Amino N, et al: A novel thyrotropin receptor germline mutation (Asp617Tyr) causing hereditary hyperthyroidism, Endocr J 54:927–934, 2007.
17. Nwosu BU, Gourgiotis L, Gershengorn MC, et al: A novel activating mutation in transmembrane helix 6 of the thyrotropin receptor as cause of hereditary nonautoimmune hyperthyroidism, Thyroid 16:505–512, 2006.
18. Claus M, Maier J, Paschke R, et al: Novel thyrotropin receptor germline mutation (Ile568Val) in a Saxonian family with hereditary nonautoimmune hyperthyroidism, Thyroid 15:1089–1094, 2005.
19. Vaidya B, Campbell V, Tripp JH, et al: Premature birth and low birth weight associated with nonautoimmune hyperthyroidism due to an activating thyrotropin receptor gene mutation, Clin Endocrinol (Oxf) 60:711–718, 2004.
20. Leclere J, Béné MC, Duprez A, et al: Behavior of thyroid tissue from patients with Graves' disease in nude mice, J Clin Endocrinol Metab 59:175–177, 1984.
21. Lavard L, Jacobsen BB, Perrild H, et al: Prevalence of germline mutations in the TSH receptor gene as a cause of juvenile thyrotoxicosis, Acta Paediatr 93:1192–1194, 2004.
22. Holzapfel HP, Wonerow P, von Petrykowski W, et al: Sporadic congenital hyperthyroidism due to a spontaneous germline mutation in the thyrotropin receptor gene, J Clin Endocrinol Metab 82:3879–3884, 1997.
23. Kopp P, Van Sande J, Parma J, et al: Congenital nonautoimmune hyperthyroidism caused by a neomutation in the thyrotropin receptor gene, N Engl J Med 332:150–154, 1995.
24. Kopp P, Jameson JL, Roe TF: Congenital nonautoimmune hyperthyroidism in a nonidentical twin caused by a sporadic germline mutation in the thyrotropin receptor gene, Thyroid 7:765–770, 1997.
25. Gruters A, Schoneberg T, Biebermann H, et al: Severe congenital hyperthyroidism caused by a germ-line neo mutation in the extracellular portion of the thyrotropin receptor, J Clin Endocrinol Metab 83:1431–1436, 1998.
26. Bircan R, Miehle K, Mladenova G, et al: Multiple relapses of hyperthyroidism after thyroid surgeries in a patient with long term follow-up of sporadic nonautoimmune hyperthyroidism, Exp Clin Endocrinol Diabetes 116:341–346, 2008.
27. Watkins MG, Dejkhamron P, Huo J, et al: Persistent neonatal thyrotoxicosis in a neonate secondary to a rare thyroid-stimulating hormone receptor activating mutation: case report and literature review, Endocr Pract 14:479–483, 2008.
28. Fricke-Otto S, Pfarr N, Muhlenberg R, et al: Mild congenital primary hypothyroidism in a Turkish family caused by a homozygous missense thyrotropin receptor (TSHR) gene mutation (A593 V). Exp Clin Endocrinol Diabetes 113:582–585, 2005.
29. Nishihara E, Fukata S, Hishinuma A, et al: Sporadic congenital hyperthyroidism due to a germline mutation in the thyrotropin receptor gene (Leu 512 Gln) in a Japanese patient, Endocr J 53:735–740, 2006.
30. Pohlenz J, Pfarr N, Kruger S, et al: Subclinical hyperthyroidism due to a thyrotropin receptor (TSHR) gene mutation (S505R). Acta Paediatr 95:1685–1687, 2006.
31. Landis CA, Masters SB, Spada A, et al: GTPase inhibiting mutations activate the alpha chain of Gs and stimulate adenylyl cyclase in human pituitary tumours, Nature 340:692–696, 1989.
32. Goretzki PE, Lyons J, Stacy Phipps S, et al: Mutational activation of RAS and GSP oncogenes in differentiated thyroid cancer and their biological implications, World J Surg 16:576–581, 1992.
33. Lyons J, Landis CA, Harsh G, et al: Two G protein oncogenes in human endocrine tumors, Science 249:655–659, 1990.
34. O'Sullivan C, Barton CM, Staddon SL, et al: Activating point mutations of the gsp oncogene in human thyroid adenomas, Mol Carcinog 4:345–349, 1991.
35. Suarez HG, du Villard JA, Caillou B, et al: GSP mutations in human thyroid tumours, Oncogene 6:677–679, 1991.
36. Fuhrer D, Holzapfel HP, Wonerow P, et al: Somatic mutations in the thyrotropin receptor gene and not in the Gs alpha protein gene in 31 toxic thyroid nodules, J Clin Endocrinol Metab 82:3885–3891, 1997.
37. Holzapfel HP, Scherbaum WA, Paschke R: Identification of two different somatic TSH receptor mutations in the same patient with hyperthyroidism due to multifocal thyroid autonomy. International Congress of Endocrinology San Francisco, 1996, Abstract 1:P2–P945, 1996.
38. Parma J, Duprez L, Van Sande J, et al: Somatic mutations in the thyrotropin receptor gene cause hyperfunctioning thyroid adenomas, Nature 365:649–651, 1993.
39. Paschke R, Tonacchera M, Van Sande J, et al: Identification and functional characterization of two new somatic mutations causing constitutive activation of the TSH receptor in hyperfunctioning autonomous adenomas of the thyroid, J Clin Endocrinol Metab 79:1785–1789, 1994.
40. Porcellini A, Ciullo I, Laviola L, et al: Novel mutations of thyrotropin receptor gene in thyroid hyperfunctioning adenomas, J Clin Endocrinol Metab 79:657–661, 1994.
41. Wonerow P, Schoneberg T, Schultz G, et al: Deletions in the third intracellular loop of the thyrotropin receptor. A new mechanism for constitutive activation, J Biol Chem 273:7900–7905, 1998.
42. Parma J, Duprez L, Van Sande J, et al: Diversity and prevalence of somatic mutations in the TSH receptor and Gs alpha genes as a cause of toxic thyroid adenomas, J Clin Endocrinol Metab 82, 2695–2701. 1997.
43. Duprez L, Parma J, Costagliola S, et al: Constitutive activation of the TSH receptor by spontaneous mutations affecting the N-terminal extracellular domain, FEBS Lett 409:469–474, 1997.
44. Gether U: Uncovering molecular mechanisms involved in activation of G protein-coupled receptors, Endocr Rev 21:90–113, 2000.
45. Govaerts C, Lefort A, Costagliola S, et al: A conserved ASN in TM7 is an on/off switch in the activation of the TSH receptor, J Biol Chem 276:22991–22999, 2001.
46. Neumann S, Krause G, Chey S, et al: A free carboxylate oxygen in the side chain of position 674 in transmembrane domain 7 is necessary for TSH receptor activation, Mol Endocrinol 15:1294–1305, 2001.
47. Jaeschke H, Kleinau G, Sontheimer J, et al: Preferences of transmembrane helices for cooperative amplification of G(alpha)s and G (alpha)q signaling of the thyrotropin receptor, Cell Mol Life Sci 65:4028–4038, 2008.
48. Kleinau G, Claus M, Jaeschke H, et al: Contacts between extracellular loop two and transmembrane helix six determine basal activity of the thyroid-stimulating hormone receptor, J Biol Chem 282:518–525, 2007.
49. Vassart G, Pardo L, Costagliola S: A molecular dissection of the glycoprotein hormone receptors, Trends Biochem Sci 29:119–126, 2004.
50. Takeshita A, Nagayama Y, Yokoyama N, et al: Rarity of oncogenic mutations in the thyrotropin receptor of autonomously functioning thyroid nodules in Japan, J Clin Endocrinol Metab 80:2607–2611, 1995.
51. Georgopoulos NA, Sykiotis GP, Sgourou A, et al: Autonomously functioning thyroid nodules in a former iodine-deficient area commonly harbor gain-of-function mutations in the thyrotropin signaling pathway, Eur J Endocrinol 149:287–292, 2003.
52. Trulzsch B, Krohn K, Wonerow P, et al: Detection of thyroid-stimulating hormone receptor and Gs alpha

mutations: in 75 toxic thyroid nodules by denaturing gradient gel electrophoresis, J Mol Med 78:684–691, 2001.

53. Palos-Paz F, Perez-Guerra O, Cameselle-Teijeiro J, et al: Prevalence of mutations in TSHR, GNAS, PRKAR1A and RAS genes in a large series of toxic thyroid adenomas from Galicia, an iodine-deficient area in NW Spain, Eur J Endocrinol 159:623–631, 2008.

54. Vanvooren V, Uchino S, Duprez L, et al: Oncogenic mutations in the thyrotropin receptor of autonomously functioning thyroid nodules in the Japanese population, Eur J Endocrinol 147:287–291, 2002.

55. Duprez L, Hermans J, Van Sande J, et al: Two autonomous nodules of a patient with multinodular goiter harbor different activating mutations of the thyrotropin receptor gene, J Clin Endocrinol Metab 82:306–308, 1997.

56. Holzapfel HP, Fuhrer D, Wonerow P, et al: Identification of constitutively activating somatic thyrotropin receptor mutations in a subset of toxic multinodular goiters, J Clin Endocrinol Metab 82:4229–4233, 1997.

57. Tonacchera M, Vitti P, Agretti P, et al: Activating thyrotropin receptor mutations in histologically heterogeneous hyperfunctioning nodules of multinodular goiter, Thyroid 8:559–564, 1998.

58. Tonacchera M, Chiovato L, Pinchera A, et al: Hyperfunctioning thyroid nodules in toxic multinodular goiter share activating thyrotropin receptor mutations with solitary toxic adenoma, J Clin Endocrinol Metab 83:492–498, 1998.

59. Tonacchera M, Agretti P, Chiovato L, et al: Activating thyrotropin receptor mutations are present in nonadenomatous hyperfunctioning nodules of toxic or autonomous multinodular goiter, J Clin Endocrinol Metab 85:2270–2274, 2000.

60. Georgopoulos NA, Sykiotis GP, Sgourou A, et al: Autonomously functioning thyroid nodules in a former iodine-deficient area commonly harbor gain-of-function mutations in the thyrotropin signaling pathway, Eur J Endocrinol 149:287–292, 2003.

61. Gozu H, Avsar M, Bircan R, et al: Mutations in the thyrotropin receptor signal transduction pathway in the hyperfunctioning thyroid nodules from multinodular goiters: a study in the Turkish population, Endocr J 52:577–585, 2005.

62. Krohn K, Fuhrer D, Bayer Y, et al: Molecular pathogenesis of euthyroid and toxic multinodular goiter, Endocr Rev 26:504–524, 2005.

63. Maier J, van Steeg H, van Oostrom C, et al: Deoxyribonucleic acid damage and spontaneous mutagenesis in the thyroid gland of rats and mice, Endocrinology 147:3391–3397, 2006.

64. Russo D, Arturi F, Schlumberger M, et al: Activating mutations of the TSH receptor in differentiated thyroid carcinomas, Oncogene 11:1907–1911, 1995.

65. Spambalg D, Sharifi N, Elisei R, et al: Structural studies of the TSH receptor and Gsa in human thyroid cancers: low prevalence of mutations predicts infrequent involvement in malignant transformation, J Clin Endocrinol Metab 81:3898–3901, 1996.

66. Camacho P, Gordon D, Chiefari E, et al: A Phe 486 thyrotropin receptor mutation in an autonomously functioning follicular carcinoma that was causing hyperthyroidism, Thyroid 10:1009–1012, 2000.

67. Fuhrer D, Tannapfel A, Sabri O, et al: Two somatic TSH receptor mutations in a patient with toxic metastasising follicular thyroid carcinoma and non-functional lung metastases, Endocr Relat Cancer 10:591–600, 2003.

68. Mircescu H, Parma J, Huot C, et al: Hyperfunctioning malignant thyroid nodule in an 11-year-old girl: pathologic and molecular studies, J Pediatr 137:585–587, 2000.

69. Niepomniszcze H, Suarez H, Pitoia F, et al: Follicular carcinoma presenting as autonomous functioning thyroid nodule and containing an activating mutation of the TSH receptor (T620I) and a mutation of the Ki-RAS (G12C) genes, Thyroid 16:497–503, 2006.

70. Fuhrer D, Lewis MD, Alkhafaji F, et al: Biological activity of activating thyroid-stimulating hormone receptor mutants depends on the cellular context, Endocrinology 144:4018–4030, 2003.

71. Kosugi S, Okajima F, Ban T, et al: Mutation of Alanine 623 in the third cytoplasmic loop of the rat TSH receptor results in a loss in the phosphoinositide but not cAMP signal induced by TSH and receptor autoantibodies, J Biol Chem 267:24153–24156, 1992.

72. Parma J, Van Sande J, Swillens S, et al: Somatic mutations causing constitutive activity of the thyrotropin receptor are the major cause of hyperfunctioning thyroid adenomas: identification of additional mutations activating both the cyclic adenosine 3′,5′-monophosphate and inositol phosphate-Ca2+ cascades, Mol Endocrinol 9:725–733, 1995.

73. Van Sande J, Parma J, Tonacchera M, et al: Somatic and germline mutations of the TSH receptor gene in thyroid diseases, J Clin Endocrinol Metab 80:2577–2585, 1995.

74. Kjelsberg MA, Cotecchia S, Ostrowski J, et al: Constitutive activation of the alpha 1B-adrenergic receptor by all amino acid substitutions at a single site, Evidence for a region which constrains receptor activation, J Biol Chem 267:1430–1433, 1992.

75. Lefkowitz RJ, Cotecchia S, Samama P, et al: Constitutive activity of receptors coupled to guanine nucleotide regulatory proteins, TiPS 14:303–307, 1994.

76. Mustafi D, Palczewski K: Topology of class A G protein-coupled receptors: insights gained from crystal structures of rhodopsins, adrenergic and adenosine receptors, Mol Pharmacol 75:1–12, 2009.

77. Glinoer D: The regulation of thyroid function in pregnancy: pathways of endocrine adaptation from physiology to pathology, Endocr Rev 18:404–433, 1997.

78. Grossmann M, Weintraub BD, Szkudlinski MW: Novel insights into the molecular mechanisms of human thyrotropin action: structural, physiological, and therapeutic implications for the glycoprotein hormone family, Endocr Rev 18:476–501, 1997.

79. Rodien P, Bremont C, Sanson ML, et al: Familial gestational hyperthyroidism caused by a mutant thyrotropin receptor hypersensitive to human chorionic gonadotropin, N Engl J Med 339:1823–1826, 1998.

80. Sanders J, Chirgadze DY, Sanders P, et al: Crystal structure of the TSH receptor in complex with a thyroid-stimulating autoantibody, Thyroid 17:395–410, 2007.

81. Smits G, Govaerts C, Nubourgh I, et al: Lysine 183 and glutamic acid 157 of the thyrotropin receptor: two interacting residues with a key role in determining specificity towards TSH and hCG. Mol Endocrinol 16:722–735, 2002.

82. Smits G, Olatunbosun O, Delbaere A, et al: Ovarian hyperstimulation syndrome due to a mutation in the follicle-stimulating hormone receptor, N Engl J Med 349:760–766, 2003.

83. Vasseur C, Rodien P, Beau I, et al: A chorionic gonadotropin-sensitive mutation in the follicle-stimulating hormone receptor as a cause of familial gestational spontaneous ovarian hyperstimulation syndrome, N Engl J Med 349:753–759, 2003.

84. Szkudlinski MW, Fremont V, Ronin C, et al: Thyroid-stimulating hormone and thyroid-stimulating hormone receptor structure-function relationships, Physiol Rev 82:473–502, 2002.

85. Stein SA, Oates EL, Hall CR, et al: Identification of a point mutation in the thyrotropin receptor of the hyt/hyt hypothyroid mouse, Mol Endocrinol 8:129–138, 1994.

86. Marians RC, Ng L, Blair HC, et al: Defining thyrotropin-dependent and -independent steps of thyroid hormone synthesis by using thyrotropin receptor-null mice, Proc Natl Acad Sci U S A 99:15776–15781, 2002.

87. Postiglione MP, Parlato R, Rodriguez-Mallon A, et al: Role of the thyroid-stimulating hormone receptor signaling in development and differentiation of the thyroid gland, Proc Natl Acad Sci U S A 99:15462–15467, 2002.

88. Codaccioni JL, Carayon P, Michel Bechet M, et al: Congenital hypothyroidism associated with thyrotropin unresponsiveness and thyroid cell membrane alterations, J Clin Endocrinol Metab 50:932–937, 1980.

89. Stanbury JB, Rocmans P, Buhler UK, et al: Congenital hypothyroidism with impaired thyroid response to thyrotropin, N Engl J Med 279:1132–1136, 1968.

90. Sunthornthepvarakul T, Gottschalk ME, Hayashi Y, et al: Resistance to thyrotropin caused by mutations in the thyrotropin-receptor gene, N Engl J Med 332:155–160, 1995.

91. Smits G, Campillo M, Govaerts C, et al: Glycoprotein hormone receptors: determinants in leucine-rich repeats responsible for ligand specificity, EMBO J 22:2692–2703, 2003.

92. Kleinau G, Krause G: Thyrotropin and homologous glycoprotein hormone receptors: structural and functional aspects of extracellular signaling mechanisms, Endocr Rev 30:133–151, 2009.

93. Abramowicz MJ, Duprez L, Parma J, et al: Familial congenital hypothyroidism due to inactivating mutation of the thyrotropin receptor causing profound hypoplasia of the thyroid gland, J Clin Invest 99:3018–3024, 1997.

94. Biebermann H, Schoneberg T, Krude H, et al: Mutations of the human thyrotropin receptor gene causing thyroid hypoplasia and persistent congenital hypothyroidism, J Clin Endocrinol Metab 82:3471–3480, 1997.

95. Clifton-Bligh RJ, Gregory JW, Ludgate M, et al: Two novel mutations in the thyrotropin (TSH) receptor gene in a child with resistance to TSH, J Clin Endocrinol Metab 82:1094–1100, 1997.

96. De Roux N, Misrahi M, Brauner R, et al: Four families with loss of function mutations of the thyrotropin receptor, J Clin Endocrinol Metab 81:4229–4235, 1996.

97. Gagne N, Parma J, Deal C, et al: Apparent congenital athyreosis contrasting with normal plasma thyroglobulin levels and associated with inactivating mutations in the thyrotropin receptor gene: are athyreosis and ectopic thyroid distinct entities? J Clin Endocrinol Metab 83:1771–1775, 1998.

98. Park SM, Clifton-Bligh RJ, Betts P, et al: Congenital hypothyroidism and apparent athyreosis with compound heterozygosity or compensated hypothyroidism with probable hemizygosity for inactivating mutations of the TSH receptor, Clin Endocrinol (Oxf) 60:220–227, 2004.

99. Bretones P, Duprez L, Parma J, et al: A familial case of congenital hypothyroidism caused by a homozygous mutation of the thyrotropin receptor gene, Thyroid 11:977–980, 2001.

100. Jordan N, Williams N, Gregory JW, et al: The W546X mutation of the thyrotropin receptor gene: potential major contributor to thyroid dysfunction in a Caucasian population, J Clin Endocrinol Metab 88:1002–1005, 2003.

101. Tonacchera M, Agretti P, Pinchera A, et al: Congenital hypothyroidism with impaired thyroid response to thyrotropin (TSH) and absent circulating thyroglobulin: evidence for a new inactivating mutation of the TSH receptor gene, J Clin Endocrinol Metab 85:1001–1008, 2000.

102. Sura-Trueba S, Aumas C, Carre A, et al: An inactivating mutation within the first extracellular loop of the thyrotropin receptor impedes normal posttranslational maturation of the extracellular domain, Endocrinology 150:1043–1050, 2009.

103. Yuan ZF, Mao HQ, Luo YF, et al: Thyrotropin receptor and thyroid transcription factor-1 genes variant in Chinese children with congenital hypothyroidism, Endocr J 55:415–423, 2008.

104. Kanda K, Mizuno H, Sugiyama Y, et al: Clinical significance of heterozygous carriers associated with compensated hypothyroidism in R450H, a common inactivating mutation of the thyrotropin receptor gene in Japanese, Endocrine 30:383–388, 2006.

105. Tsunekawa K, Onigata K, Morimura T, et al: Identification and functional analysis of novel inactivating thyrotropin receptor mutations in patients with thyrotropin resistance, Thyroid 16:471–479, 2006.

106. Tenenbaum-Rakover Y, Grasberger H, Mamanasiri S, et al: Loss-of-function mutations in the thyrotropin receptor gene as a major determinant of hyperthyrotropinemia in a consanguineous community, J Clin Endocrinol Metab 94:1706–1712, 2009.

107. Alberti L, Proverbio MC, Costagliola S, et al: Germline mutations of TSH receptor gene as cause of nonautoimmune subclinical hypothyroidism, J Clin Endocrinol Metab 87:2549–2555, 2002.

108. Xie J, Pannain S, Pohlenz J, et al: Resistance to thyrotropin (TSH) in three families is not associated with mutations in the TSH receptor or TSH [see comments], J Clin Endocrinol Metab 82:3933–3940, 1997.

109. Grasberger H, Vaxillaire M, Pannain S, et al: Identification of a locus for nongoitrous congenital hypothyroidism on chromosome 15q25.3–26.1, Hum Genet 118:348–355, 2005.

110. Bohr UR, Behr M, Loos U: A heritable point mutation in an extracellular domain of the TSH receptor involved

in the interaction with Graves' immunoglobulins, Biochim Biophys Acta 1216:504–508, 1993.

111. Bahn RS, Dutton CM, Heufelder AE, et al: A genomic point mutation in the extracellular domain of the thyrotropin receptor in patients with Graves' ophthalmopathy, J Clin Endocrinol Metab 78:256–260, 1994.

112. Gabriel EM, Bergert ER, Grant CS, et al: Germline polymorphism of codon 727 of human thyroid-stimulating hormone receptor is associated with toxic multinodular goiter, J Clin Endocrinol Metab 84:3328–3335, 1999.

113. Ban Y, Greenberg DA, Concepcion ES, et al: A germline single nucleotide polymorphism at the intracellular domain of the human thyrotropin receptor does not have a major effect on the development of Graves' disease, Thyroid 12:1079–1083, 2002.

114. Muhlberg T, Herrmann K, Joba W, et al: Lack of association of nonautoimmune hyperfunctioning thyroid disorders and a germline polymorphism of codon 727 of the human thyrotropin receptor in a European Caucasian population, J Clin Endocrinol Metab 85:2640–2643, 2000.

115. Simanainen J, Kinch A, Westermark K, et al: Analysis of mutations in exon 1 of the human thyrotropin receptor gene: high frequency of the D36H and P52T polymorphic variants, Thyroid 9:7–11, 1999.

116. Ho SC, Goh SS, Khoo DH: Association of Graves' disease with intragenic polymorphism of the thyrotropin receptor gene in a cohort of Singapore patients of multi-ethnic origins, Thyroid 13:523–528, 2003.

117. Brand OJ, Barrett JC, Simmonds MJ, et al: Association of the thyroid stimulating hormone receptor gene (TSHR) with Graves' disease (GD), Hum Mol Genet 18:1704–1713, 2009.

118. Burton PR, Clayton DG, Cardon LR, et al: Association scan of 14,500 nonsynonymous SNPs in four diseases identifies autoimmunity variants, Nat Genet 39:1329–1337, 2007.

119. Libert F, Lefort A, Gerard C, et al: Cloning, sequencing and expression of the human thyrotropin (TSH) receptor: evidence for binding of autoantibodies, Biochem Biophys Res Commun 165:1250–1255, 1989.

120. Nagayama Y, Kaufman KD, Seto P, et al: Molecular cloning, sequence and functional expression of the cDNA for the human thyrotropin receptor, Biochem Biophys Res Commun 165:1184–1190, 1989.

121. Arseven OK, Wilkes WP, Jameson JL, et al: Substitutions of tyrosine 601 in the human thyrotropin receptor result in increase or loss of basal activation of the cyclic adenosine monophosphate pathway and disrupt coupling to Gq/11, Thyroid 10:3–10, 2000.

Chapter 21

GENETIC DEFECTS IN THYROID HORMONE SYNTHESIS AND ACTION

PAOLO EMIDIO MACCHIA and GIANFRANCO FENZI

Defects in Thyroid Hormone Synthesis
Hyporesponsiveness to Thyroid-Stimulating Hormone
Thyroid Dysgenesis
Dyshormonogenesis
Central Congenital Hypothyroidism

Peripheral Congenital Hypothyroidism
Defects in Transmembrane Transport of Thyroid Hormone

Clinical Manifestations of Congenital Hypothyroidism

Neonatal Screening and Diagnosis
Transient Congenital Hypothyroidism

Treatment

Congenital hypothyroidism (CH) is the most frequent endocrine-metabolic disease in infancy, with an incidence of about 1 in 3000 to 4000 newborns.[1,2] With the exception of rare cases due to hypothalamic or pituitary defects, CH is characterized by elevated thyroid-stimulating hormone (TSH) in response to reduced thyroid hormone (TH) levels.

Thyroid hormones play critical roles in differentiation, growth, and metabolism. Therefore, THs are required for the normal function of nearly all tissues, with major effects on oxygen consumption and metabolic rate.[3]

TH is synthesized exclusively by the thyroid gland. Its synthesis, storage, and secretion require a sequence of finely tuned reactions in which several proteins and factors are involved. Disturbances in these reactions may lead to abnormalities in thyroid function, ending in hypothyroidism.

Defects in Thyroid Hormone Synthesis

In the majority of cases (80% to 85%), primary permanent CH is due to alterations occurring during the gland organogenesis, resulting either in a thyroid that is absent (thyroid agenesis, or athyreosis), hypoplastic (thyroid hypoplasia), or located in an unusual position (thyroid ectopy). All these entities are grouped under the term *thyroid dysgenesis* (TD).[4] TD occurs mostly as a sporadic disease, but a genetic cause of the disease has been demonstrated in about 5% of reported cases. Genes associated with TD (Table 21-1) include several thyroid transcription factors expressed in the early phases of thyroid organogenesis (*NKX2.1/TITF1*, *FOXE1/TITF2*, *PAX8*, *NKX2.5*), as well as genes like the thyrotropin receptor gene (*TSHR*) expressed later during gland morphogenesis.

In the remaining 15% of cases, the disease is caused by inborn errors in the molecular steps required for the biosynthesis of thyroid hormones, and generally it is characterized by enlargement of the gland (goiter), presumably due to elevated TSH levels.[5] Thyroid dyshormonogenesis shows classical Mendelian recessive inheritance (Table 21-2).

Rarely, CH of central origin is due to hypothalamic and/or pituitary diseases, with reduced production and/or effect of thyrotropin-releasing hormone (TRH) or of the thyrotropin hormone (TSH).[6]

HYPORESPONSIVENESS TO THYROID-STIMULATING HORMONE

Hyporesponsiveness to TSH may be due to alterations in the TSH stimulation pathway, unresponsive TSH receptor (TSHR), or mutation in the modulating proteins downstream in the signaling pathway, such as G proteins, adenylate cyclase, or the various kinases. To date, only defects in the TSHR and $G_s\alpha$ have been described.

Defects in the Thyroid-Stimulating Hormone Receptor

The *TSHR* gene maps to human chromosome 14q31 and to mouse chromosome 12; it is encoded by 10 exons producing a 1.8-kb mRNA. The TSHR belongs to the superfamily of G protein–coupled receptors. It contains an extracellular N-terminal domain with a repetitive leu-rich motif, seven transmembrane helices, three intracellular and three extracellular loops, and an intracellular C-terminal part. The TSHR is responsible for mediating TSH action on thyroid follicular cell growth, metabolism, and function, ultimately resulting in TH synthesis and secretion.

Table 21-1. Genetic Basis of Thyroid Dysgenesis

Thyroid Alteration	Genes	Clinical Manifestations	References
Athyreosis	*FOXE1*	Bamforth-Lazarus syndrome	16, 17
	NKX2-5	Athyreosis, no cardiac alterations	19
Thyroid ectopy	*NKX2-5*	Athyreosis, no cardiac alterations	19
	FOXE1	Bamforth-Lazarus syndrome	21
Thyroid hypoplasia	*NKX2-1*	Choreoathetosis, hypothyroidism, and pulmonary alterations	23–40
	TSHR	Resistance to thyroid-stimulating hormone (TSH)	6, 10
	PAX8	Hypothyroidism	18, 41–46

Table 21-2. Genes Causing Defects in Thyroid Hormone Synthesis

Gene	Protein Function	Inheritance	Human Phenotype
Sodium-iodide symporter (*NIS*)	Transports iodine across basal membrane	AR	CH (moderate to severe) Euthyroid goiter
Thyroperoxidase (*TPO*)	Catalyses the oxidation, organification, and coupling reactions	AR	Goiter and CH due to total iodide organification defect
Dual oxidases (*DUOX1* and *DUOX2*)	H_2O_2 generation in the follicle	AD and AR	Permanent hypothyroidism (from mild to severe) Transient and moderate hypothyroidism
Dual oxidase maturation factor 2 (*DUOXA2*)	Required to express DUOX2 enzymatic activity	AR	Goiter and CH due to partial iodide organification defect
Pendrin (*PDS*)	Transport iodine across apical membrane	AR	Goiter, moderate hypothyroidism, and deafness
Thyroglobulin (*TG*)	Support for thyroid hormone synthesis	AD and AR	Goiter and CH (from moderate to severe)
Iodotyrosine deiodinase (*IYD*)	Nitroreductase-related enzyme capable of deiodinating iodotyrosines	AR	Hypothyroidism with variable age of diagnosis

The role of the *TSHR* gene in CH with TSH unresponsiveness and absence of goiter was hypothesized almost 40 years ago. Useful models for studying this autosomal recessive form of CH were offered through (1) identification of *hyt/hyt* mice that were affected by primary hypothyroidism with elevated TSH and hypoplastic thyroid due to a loss-of-function mutation in the *Tshr* gene[7,8] and (2) the production of *Tshr*^−/−^ mice.[9]

TSHR mutations in humans were identified for the first time in three siblings with CH associated with high serum TSH and normal thyroid hormone.[10] The siblings were compound heterozygous, carrying a different mutation in each of the two alleles. Since this report, other mutations in the *TSHR* gene have been identified in several patients with thyroid hypoplasia and increased TSH secretion. All the affected individuals are homozygous or compound heterozygous for loss-of-function mutations, and consistently in the familial forms, the disease is inherited as an autosomal recessive trait. This form of CH is characterized by a "small" thyroid gland in normal position. In the case of total failure of TSHR function, the patient is severely hypothyroid because the complete lack of TSH stimulation almost completely represses the metabolic activity of the thyroid gland.[11] When the TSHR has a diminished affinity to its ligand, the effect may largely be compensated for by high plasma TSH concentrations. The high TSH level in these cases does not result in an exaggerated stimulation of thyroid metabolism, and goitrogenesis is not observed.

Abnormalities in the G$_s$ Protein Subunit

Hyporesponsiveness to TSH is found in patients with pseudohypoparathyroidism type 1a (Albright's hereditary osteodystrophy),[12] a variably expressed disorder with autosomal-dominant inheritance. The cause is a defect in the G$_s\alpha$ subunit (gene map locus 20q13). G$_s\alpha$ is involved in the stimulatory pathways of TSH and TRH as well as pathways of other hormones binding to a G$_s\alpha$-coupled receptor (parathyroid hormone [PTH], gonadotropin-releasing hormone [GnRH], follicle-stimulating hormone [FSH], luteinizing hormone [LH], etc.). Several mutations have been found in these cases.[13,14] Patients tend to have only mild manifestations of hypothyroidism, with normal or slightly decreased plasma free thyroxine (FT$_4$) levels and slightly elevated TSH levels. Detection of patients with pseudohypoparathyroidism type 1a by neonatal CH screening has been reported, but it is likely that most affected newborns would be missed because their blood TSH and thyroxine (T$_4$) concentrations would not reach the cutoff levels used in the screening programs. Otherwise, the mild hypothyroidism is just a minor component of the syndrome, and early T$_4$ supplementation therapy is unable to prevent mental and growth retardation.

Other Causes

Hyporesponsiveness to TSH may also be caused by factors other than mutations in the TSHR or G proteins. Many families express the phenotype of resistance to TSH in the absence of a TSHR defect. In many subjects, the inheritance is dominant and the genetic cause has not yet been clarified.[15] Possible candidates are factors located downstream of the TSHR/G-protein/cAMP cascade or other thyroid developmental genes.

THYROID DYSGENESIS

Athyreosis

The absence of thyroid follicular cells is called *athyreosis* or *agenesis* of the thyroid. The term *agenesis* should be used to define the absence of the gland due to a defective initiation of thyroid morphogenesis, whereas *athyreosis* indicates a dysgenesis characterized by the disappearance of the thyroid following any step after the thyroid anlage specification. Athyreosis accounts for 22% to 44% of the cases of primitive permanent CH (Fig. 21-1). So far, the absence of thyroid was reported in patients with CH associated with *FOXE1* gene defects (Bamforth-Lazarus syndrome),[16,17] in one subject carrying a mutation in *PAX8*[18] and in one patient with *NKX2-5* mutation.[19]

The Bamforth-Lazarus syndrome[20] is a clinical entity characterized by cleft palate, bilateral choanal atresia, spiky hair, and athyreosis. Two homozygous mutations in the *FOXE1* gene have been described in two pairs of siblings affected by this syndrome[16,17] and in one patient with syndromic congenital hypothyroidism but not athyreosis.[21] All affected members carry homozygous missense mutations in conserved amino acids within the FOXE1 forkhead domain. The mutant proteins were tested in vitro and have shown a reduction in both DNA binding and transcriptional activity.

Ectopic Thyroid

An ectopic thyroid is due to a failure in the descent of the developing thyroid from the thyroid anlage region to its definitive location in front of the trachea, therefore an ectopic thyroid can be found in any location along the path of migration from the foramen caecum to the mediastinum.

In humans, more than 50% of TD cases are associated with an ectopic thyroid (see Fig. 21-1); however, up to now, only three heterozygous mutations in the *NKX2-5* gene have been linked to human ectopic thyroid.[19] The functional studies of the mutant NKX2-5 demonstrated a significant functional impairment, with reduction of transactivation properties and a dominant-negative effect. The patients described were all heterozygous, and the mutations were inherited from one of the parents, suggesting that *NKX2-5* mutations have variable penetrance and clinical significance.

Hypoplasia

The presence of hypoplastic thyroid has been reported in 24% to 36% of cases of CH (see Fig. 21-1). Thyroid hypoplasia is a genetically heterogeneous disease, since mutations in *NKX2-1*, *PAX8*, or *TSHR* genes have been reported in patients with thyroid hypoplasia.

Patients with *NKX2-1* loss-of-function mutations are affected by choreoathetosis, hypothyroidism, and pulmonary alterations, with incomplete penetrance and a variability of the phenotype.[22]

So far, 22 loss-of-function mutations in the *NKX2-1* gene have been identified in patients with this clinical picture.[23-40] The unfavorable outcome in the case of impaired NKX2-1 expression, regardless of early T₄ supplementation, is most likely caused by defects in the central nervous system rather than fetal hypothyroidism.

The involvement of *PAX8* has been described in sporadic and familial cases of CH with TD.[18,41-46] In vitro transfection assays demonstrated that the mutated proteins are unable to bind DNA and to drive transcription of the *TPO* promoter. All affected individuals are heterozygous for the mutations, and in the familial cases, transmission is autosomal dominant with a variable penetrance and expressivity.

Hemiagenesis

Thyroid hemiagenesis is a dysgenesis in which one thyroid lobe fails to develop. The prevalence of this morphologic abnormality ranges from 0.05% to 0.2% in healthy children, with the absence of the left lobe in almost all the cases. In these subjects, thyroid function tests are within the normal range.[47]

The molecular mechanisms leading to the formation of the two symmetrical thyroid lobes are still unclear, and in humans, candidate genes responsible for hemiagenesis of the thyroid have not yet been described. Indeed, *Shh*[−/−] mice embryos can display either a nonlobulated gland[48] or hemiagenesis of thyroid.[49] Hemiagenesis of the thyroid is also frequent in mice double heterozygous for *Titf1*[+/−] and *Pax8*[+/−].[50]

DYSHORMONOGENESIS

As mentioned before, in about 15% of cases, CH is due to hormonogenesis defects (see Fig. 21-1) caused by mutations in genes involved in thyroid hormone synthesis, secretion, or recycling. These cases are clinically characterized by the presence of goiter, and the molecular mechanisms in most of these forms have been identified.

In thyroid follicular cells, iodide is actively transported and concentrated by the sodium-iodide symporter present in the basolateral membrane. Subsequently it is oxidized by a hydrogen peroxide–generation system (thyroperoxidase, pendrin) and bound to tyrosine residues in thyroglobulin to form iodotyrosine (iodide organification). Some of these iodotyrosine residues (monoiodotyrosine and diiodotyrosine) are coupled to form the hormonally active iodotyronines T₄ and triiodothyronine (T₃), and when needed, thyroglobulin is hydrolyzed and hormones are released in the blood. A small part of the iodotyronines are hydrolyzed into the gland, and iodine is recovered by the action of specific enzymes, namely the intrathyroidal dehalogenases.

Defects in any of these steps lead to reduced circulating thyroid hormone, resulting in congenital hypothyroidism and goiter. With the exception of rare cases, all mutations in these genes appear to be inherited in autosomal-recessive fashion (see Table 21-2).

Sodium-Iodide Symporter

The sodium-iodide symporter (NIS) is a member of the sodium/solute symporter family that actively transports iodide across the membrane of the thyroid follicular cells. In 1996, NIS mRNAs from rats[51] and humans[52] were isolated. The human gene (*SLC5A5*) maps to chromosome 19p13.2-p12. It has 15 exons and encodes a 643-amino-acid protein expressed primarily in thyroid but also in salivary glands, gastric mucosa,

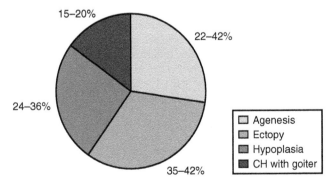

FIGURE 21-1. Prevalence of the various causes of primary congenital hypothyroidism.

15–20%

22–42%

24–36%

35–42%

☐ Agenesis
☐ Ectopy
☐ Hypoplasia
☐ CH with goiter

small intestinal mucosa, lacrimal gland, nasopharynx, thymus, skin, lung tissue, choroid plexus, ciliary body, uterus, lactating mammary tissue and mammary carcinoma cells, and placenta.[53,54] Only in thyroid cells iodide transport is regulated by TSH.

The inability of the thyroid gland to accumulate iodine was one of the early known causes of CH, and before the cloning of NIS, a clinical diagnosis of hereditary iodide transport defect had been made on the basis of goitrous hypothyroidism and absent thyroidal radioiodine uptake. To date, several mutations inherited in an autosomal-recessive manner have been described, with a clinical picture characterized by hypothyroidism of variable severity (from severe to fully compensated) and goiter.[55,56] Thyroid morphology is heterogeneous in patients with the same NIS mutation.[57]

In the neonatal period, infants with iodide transport defects are found to have a normal-size or slightly enlarged thyroid gland by ultrasonography and elevated serum thyroglobulin levels.[58] Radioactive iodide uptake is absent. Measurement of the saliva-to-plasma ^{123}I ratio is around one. The degree of hypothyroidism is variable and ranges from mild to severe, possibly depending on the amount of iodide in the diet. These children are severely hypothyroid if maintained with a normal iodine diet, but addition of high amounts of iodide to the diet tends to compensate for the iodide transport failure.

Thyroperoxidase

The most frequent cause of dyshormonogenesis is thyroperoxidase (TPO) deficiency. TPO is the enzyme that catalyses the oxidation, organification, and coupling reactions.

Accumulation of iodine in the thyroid gland reaches a steady state between active influx, protein binding, and efflux, resulting in a relatively low free intracellular iodide concentration in normal conditions, but increased in the presence of TPO defects. The kinetics of iodide uptake and release can be traced by administration of radioiodide, and iodide reuptake can be inhibited by anions of similar molecular size and charge, such as perchlorate or thiocyanate. Radioiodide uptake and perchlorate inhibition give an idea of the intrathyroidal iodide concentration in relation to the circulating iodine. Iodine organification defects can be quantified as total or partial: total iodide organification defects are characterized by discharge of more than 90% of the radioiodide taken up by the gland within 1 hour after administration of sodium perchlorate, usually given 2 hours after radioiodide. A total disappearance of the thyroid image is also observed. Partial iodide organification defects are characterized by discharge of 20% to 90% of the accumulated radioiodine.[59]

The human TPO gene is located on chromosome 2p25 and spans approximately 150 kb; the coding sequence of 3048 bp is divided over 17 exons[60] and encodes for a 933-amino-acid, membrane-bound, glycated, heme-containing protein located on the apical membranes of the thyroid follicular cell.

Defects in the TPO gene have been reported to cause congenital hypothyroidism by a total iodide organification defect, and mutations have been identified in all exons of the TPO gene. Most mutations are found in exons 8, 9, or 10, encoding the active center and heme-binding portion of the enzyme. Nonsense, splice-site, and frameshift mutations have been also described by several groups.[56,61,62]

If untreated, patients with organification defects show variable degrees of mental retardation, very large goiter, and hypothyroidism. In some cases with partial defects, hypothyroidism appears compensated.

DUOX1 and DUOX2

The generation of H_2O_2 is a crucial step in thyroid hormonogenesis. Recently two new proteins involved in the H_2O_2 generation in the apical membrane of the follicular thyroid cell have been identified.[60] These proteins, initially named THOX1 and THOX2 (for thyroid oxidase), map to chromosome 15q15.3, only 16 kb apart from each other and in opposite transcriptional orientation. In 2001, since these proteins contain two distinct functional domains, it was suggested that they be called DUOX (for dual oxidase).

DUOX1 and DUOX2 are glycoproteins with seven putative transmembrane domains. Their function remained unclear until a factor named DUOXA2, which allows the transition of DUOX2 from the endoplasmic reticulum to the Golgi, was identified.[63] The coexpression of this factor with DUOX2 in HeLa cells is able to reconstitute the H_2O_2 production in vitro. A similar protein (DUOXA1) is necessary for the complete maturation of the DUOX1. Interestingly, both DUOXA genes map in the 16 kb that separate the DUOX1 and DUOX2 genes on chromosome 15.

Several mutations in DUOX genes have been reported in patients with congenital hypothyroidism showing very variable phenotypes.[64-67] To produce congenital permanent hypothyroidism, a severe alteration of both alleles of the DUOX2 gene is required. The presence of some residual activity in one of the alleles may produce a less severe phenotype, whereas monoallelic severe inactivation of the DUOX2 gene is associated with transient CH. In addition, the phenotype of monoallelic inactivation seems to be modulated by other factors, including environmental conditions (such as iodine insufficiency) or lifetime events (pregnancy, immediate postnatal life).

So far, no mutation in the DUOX1 gene has been identified in patients with CH. In contrast, very recently a biallelic inactivation in the dual oxidase maturation factor 2 (DUOXA2) gene has been identified in a patient with congenital hypothyroidism.[68]

Pendrin

In 1896, Vaughan Pendred described a syndrome characterized by congenital neurosensorial deafness and goiter.[69] The disease is transmitted as an autosomal-recessive disorder. Patients have a moderately enlarged thyroid gland, are usually euthyroid, and show only a partial discharge of iodide after the administration of thiocyanate or perchlorate. The impaired hearing characteristic of the condition is not constant and is due to a cochlear defect that corresponds to the Mondini's type of developmental abnormality of the cochlea.

In 1997, the PDS gene was cloned, and the predicted protein of 780 amino acids (86 kD) was called pendrin.[70] The PDS gene maps to human chromosome 7q31, contains 21 exons, and is expressed both in the cochlea and in the thyroid. Pendrin has been localized into the apical membrane of thyroid follicular cells.[71,72] In thyroid follicular cells and in transfected oocytes, pendrin is able to transport iodide.

Patients with Pendred's syndrome are subclinically hypothyroid, with goiter, and show moderate to severe sensorineural hearing impairment. Discharge of radioiodide after administration of sodium perchlorate is moderately increased (>20%). The prevalence varies between 1:15,000 and 1:100,000.

A number of mutations in the *PDS* gene have been described in patients with Pendred's syndrome.[73] Despite the goiter, individuals are likely to be euthyroid and only rarely present congenital hypothyroidism. However, TSH levels are often in the upper limit of the normal range, and hypothyroidism of variable severity may eventually develop.[74]

Thyroglobulin

Thyroglobulin is a homodimer protein synthesized exclusively in the thyroid. The human gene is located on chromosome 8q24, and the coding sequence, containing 8307 bp,[75] is divided into 42 exons.[76] Following a signal peptide of 19 amino acids, the polypeptide chain is composed of 2750 amino acids containing 66 tyrosine residues. Thyroglobulin is a dimer with identical 330-kD subunits containing 10% carbohydrate residues.

Patients with disorders of thyroglobulin synthesis are moderately to severely hypothyroid. Usually, plasma thyroglobulin concentration is low, especially in relation to the TSH concentrations, and does not change after T_4 treatment or injection of TSH. Patients classified in the category "thyroglobulin synthesis defects" often have abnormal iodoproteins, mainly iodinated plasma albumin, and they excrete iodopeptides of low molecular weight in the urine.[77]

Several mutations in the thyroglobulin gene have been reported in patients with CH[78,79] and in animals, including Afrikander cattle (p.R697X),[80] Dutch goats (p.Y296X),[81] *cog/cog* mice (p.L2263P),[82] and *rdw* rats (p.G2300R).[83]

Mutations in the human thyroglobulin gene are associated with congenital goiter and with moderate to severe hypothyroidism.

IYD

In addition to the active transport from the blood due to the NIS, iodine in the thyroid follicular cells derives also from the deiodination of monoiodotyrosine and diiodotyrosine.[84] The gene encoding for this enzymatic activity was recently identified and named *IYD* (or *DEHAL1*).[85,86] The human gene maps to chromosome 6q24-q25 and consists of 6 exons encoding a protein of 293 amino acids, with a nitroreductase-related enzyme capable of deiodinating iodotyrosines.

In the past, it was suggested that *IYD* mutations could be responsible for congenital hypothyroidism, but only very recently, four patients with three mutations in the *IYD* gene have been reported.[87,88] The disease was transmitted either as an autosomal-recessive[87] or an autosomal-dominant pattern of inheritance with incomplete penetration.[88] Patients were hypothyroid and goitrous, with a high phenotypic variability, depending on the time of expression of the disease manifestations. The patients born after the introduction of the screening program for CH were not identified by the screening. There is also a variable severity in the clinical picture, and this can derive either from the molecular effects of the mutation (complete absence or partial activity of the protein) or from environmental factors, such as iodine diet content.

CENTRAL CONGENITAL HYPOTHYROIDISM

Central hypothyroidism is the less frequent form of CH. It occurs with an incidence of 1 in 50,000 newborns and is generally associated with alterations in hypothalamus or pituitary development.

Most patients with central CH are mildly to moderately hypothyroid. The accompanying pituitary hormonal deficiencies, especially the lack of cortisol, may be responsible for high morbidity and mortality.

Developmental Defects of the Pituitary

The pituitary gland is formed from an invagination of the floor of the third ventricle and from Rathke's pouch, developing into the thyrotropic cell lineage and the four other neuroendocrine cell types, each defined by the hormone produced: TSH, growth hormone (GH), prolactin (PRL), gonadotropins (LH and FSH), and adrenocorticotropic hormone (ACTH).

The ontogeny of the pituitary gland depends on numerous developmental genes that guide differentiation and proliferation. These genes are highly conserved among species, suggesting crucial evolutionary roles for the associated proteins (PIT1 and PROP1, HESX1, LHX3, LHX4, and SOX3).

Lhx3 and *Lhx4* belong to the LIM family of homeobox genes that are expressed early in Rathke's pouch. In *Lhx3* knockout mice, the thyrotrope, somatotrope, lactotrope, and gonadotrope cell lineages are depleted, whereas the adrenocorticotropic cell lineage fails to proliferate. This murine model shows that pituitary organ fate commitment depends on *Lhx3*. *Lhx4* null mutants show Rathke's pouch formation with expression of α-glycoprotein subunit, TSH-β, GH, and Pit1 transcripts, although cell numbers are reduced.

Recent studies have identified a variety of mutations in the *LHX3* and *LHX4* genes in patients with combined pituitary hormone deficiency diseases. These patients have complex and variable syndromes involving short stature, metabolic disorders, reproductive system deficits, and nervous system developmental abnormalities.[89]

Hesx1 (also called *Rpx*), a member of the paired-like class of homeobox genes, is one of the earliest markers of the pituitary primordium.[90] Extinction of *Hesx1* is important for activation of downstream genes such as *Prop1*, suggesting that both proteins act as opposing transcription factors.[91] Targeted disruption of *Hesx1* in the mouse revealed a reduction in the prospective forebrain tissue, absent optic vesicles, markedly decreased head size, and severe microphthalmia reminiscent of the syndrome of septo-optic dysplasia (SOD) in humans.

SOD is a rare heterogeneous anomaly hypoplasia of the optic nerves, various types of forebrain defects, and a variety of pituitary hormone deficiencies. Endocrine dysfunction ranges from isolated GH deficiency to complete pituitary hormonal deficiency. The human *HESX1* gene maps to chromosome 3p21.-3p21.2, and its coding region spans 1.7 kb, with a highly conserved genomic organization consisting of 4 coding exons. The first homozygous missense mutation (Arg160Cys) was found in the homeobox of *HESX1* in two siblings with SOD.[90] Subsequently, several other homozygous and heterozygous mutations have been shown to present with varying phenotypes characterized by pituitary hormone deficiency and SOD.[91]

Defects in the *TRH* Gene and the Thyrotropin-Releasing Hormone Receptor

In mice, homozygous deletion of the *TRH* gene produced a phenotype characterized by hypothyroidism and hyperglycemia.[92] Only a few patients with reduced TRH production have been described in the literature,[93,94] but no human mutations have been described so far.

Similarly, mice lacking the TRH receptor appear almost normal, with some growth retardation and a considerable decrease in serum T_3, T_4, and PRL levels but not in serum TSH.[95] Thus far, only one family with a compound heterozygous[96] and one family with a homozygous[97] loss-of-function mutation of the TRH receptor have been described.

Defects in Thyroid-Stimulating Hormone Synthesis

TSH is a heterodimer synthesized in the pituitary gland under the control of local thyroid hormone and TRH. TSH consists of two different subunits (α and β) noncovalently linked. The TSH α subunit is in common with LH, FSH, and chorionic gonadotropin; the β subunit is unique for TSH. The β subunit (gene map locus 1p13) synthesis is under the control of several transcription factors, including POU1F1 and PROP1. These transcription factors are the main stimulators of TSH, GH, and PRL synthesis.

Pit1/POU1F1

Pit1 (called POU1F1 in humans) is a pituitary-specific transcription factor belonging to the POU homeodomain family. The human POU1F1 maps to chromosome 3p11 and consists of 6 exons spanning 17 kb encoding for a 291-amino-acid protein. After the initial report,[98] several heterozygous, compound heterozygous, and homozygous POU1F1 deletions and missense and nonsense mutations have been reported to cause this type of hereditary CH.[99] Deficiency of GH, PRL, and TSH is generally severe in patients harboring mutations in POU1F1.

PROP1

Prop1 (Prophet of Pit1) is a pituitary-specific paired-like homeodomain transcription required for the expression of Pit1 and also important in regulating Hesx1 expression. Dwarf mice harboring a homozygous missense mutation in Prop1 exhibit GH, TSH, and PRL deficiency and an anterior pituitary gland reduced in size by about 50%. Additionally, these mice have reduced gonadotropin expression.[100]

The human PROP1 maps to chromosome 5q. The gene consists of 3 exons encoding for a 226-amino-acid protein. After the first report of mutations in PROP1 in four unrelated pedigrees with GH, TSH, PRL, LH, and FSH deficiencies,[101] several distinct mutations have been identified in over 170 patients,[91] suggesting that PROP1 mutations account for most cases of familial multiple pituitary hormone deficiency. Affected individuals exhibit recessive inheritance. The timing of initiation and the severity of hormonal deficiency in patients with PROP1 mutations is highly variable; diagnosis of GH deficiency preceded that of TSH deficiency in 80%. Following the deficiencies in GH and TSH, there is a delayed onset of gonadotropin insufficiency. Although most patients fail to enter puberty spontaneously, some start puberty before deficiencies in LH and FSH evolve. ACTH deficiency is a relatively late manifestation of PROP1 mutation, often evolving several decades after birth. The degree of prolactin deficiency and pituitary morphologic alterations are variable.[91]

Structural Thyroid-Stimulating Hormone Defects

The TSH α subunit has the amino acid sequence in common with LH, FSH, and chorionic gonadotropin. The β subunit is different for each of these hormones and carries specific information for receptor binding and expression of hormonal action. For biological activity, the heterodimer configuration is required.[102]

Mutations in the TSH-β gene are a rare cause of congenital hypothyroidism, and in all the reported cases, the mutations were homozygous or compound heterozygous. Available data have been recently reviewed by Miyai.[103] The phenotype is quite variable, and it may range from a very mild hypothyroidism to severe forms associated with mental retardation in cases of delayed treatment. Patients with mutations in TSHB are characterized by the presence of low levels of circulating TSH that will not be stimulated by TRH. Finally, cases of immunologically reactive but biologically inactive TSH have also been reported.[103]

Peripheral Congenital Hypothyroidism

DEFECTS IN TRANSMEMBRANE TRANSPORT OF THYROID HORMONE

Although T_3 is the major receptor-active form of thyroid hormone, T_4 is the predominant iodothyronine secreted by the thyroid gland under normal conditions. As consequence, target tissues need to convert T_4 into T_3 by so-called outer-ring deiodination (ORD). Alternatively, T_4 is metabolized by inner-ring deiodination (IRD) to receptor-inactive reverse T_3 (rT_3), and by the same reaction, T_3 is inactivated to T_2.[104] The latter is also produced by ORD from rT_3. Three iodothyronine deiodinases (D1–3) are involved in these reactions. These selenoproteins, each with a different catalytic preference and tissue distribution pattern, not only regulate the basic metabolic activity in the various tissues but are also involved in processes that adapt the body to extraordinary conditions such as fasting and illness.

Endemic selenium deficiency may potentially affect iodothyronine activity in large populations, but until now, no clinicopathologic entity that could be ascribed with certainty to genetic defects in any of the iodothyronine deiodinases has been described. Furthermore, mice knockouts for D1 and D2 have a surprisingly mild phenotype, their serum T_3 level is normal (probably due to enhanced secretion and formation of T_3 from the thyroid gland), and their general health and reproductive capacity are unimpaired.[105]

Besides secretion of the prohormone T_4 and its deiodination to T_3, transmembrane transport of thyroid hormone (T_4, T_3, or both) into the cells of the peripheral tissues is a prerequisite for binding of T_3 to its nuclear receptors and the subsequent protein synthesis. It has been thought for a long time that the lipophilic iodothyronines are capable of crossing the plasma membrane by simple diffusion, but it has become increasingly clear that for such crossing, transporters are needed.[106]

More recently, monocarboxylate transporter 8 (MCT8) has been shown to be an active and specific thyroid hormone transporter.[107,108] The gene encoding for MCT8 (named SLC16A2) is located on human chromosome Xq13.2 and consists of 6 exons and 5 introns, the first of which is about 100,000 kb in size.[109,110] The mature mRNA is about 4.4 kb large and contains two possible translation start sites (TLSs). Depending on which of these TLSs is used, proteins are generated consisting of 613 or 539 amino acids, respectively. The human MCT8 protein contains 12 putative transmembrane domains, and both the N and C terminus are located intracellularly. The important role of MCT8 in maintaining euthyroidism, especially in brain tissues, is demonstrated by the identification of several male subjects with a particular combination of severe neurologic deficits and abnormal serum thyroid hormone levels.[111-125] The neurologic phenotype includes central hypotonia with poor head control; peripheral hypotonia that evolves into spastic quadriplegia; inability to sit, stand, or walk independently; severe mental retardation; and absence of speech.[113,126]

To date, more than 40 different mutations have been identified in *MCT8*,[127] including large deletions with loss of one or more exons, smaller frame-shift deletions, 3-nucleotide deletions or insertions, and nonsense and missense mutations. Most of these mutations resulted in a complete inactivation of MCT8 function, although some residual activity has been associated with certain *MCT8* mutations, ending in a milder clinical phenotype.[119,127] Of note, mouse mutants deficient in MCT8 exhibit a marked increase in serum T_3 and a decrease in serum T_4 and rT_3, but in contrast to the human phenotype, *Mct8*-null animals do not have any overt neurologic abnormalities.[128,129]

Clinical Manifestations of Congenital Hypothyroidism

In the absence of an adequate treatment, severe CH results in serious mental retardation, motor handicaps, and the signs and symptoms of impaired metabolism. Before the introduction of neonatal screening programs, CH was one of the most frequent causes of mental retardation, and sooner or later the patients needed institutionalization.

TH concentrations are low in the fetus during the first half of pregnancy. During this time, the fetus is entirely dependent on maternal TH. The fetal hypothalamic-pituitary-thyroid axis begins to function by mid-gestation and is mature in term infants at delivery. Despite the critical importance of TH to multiple organ systems, especially the brain, most infants with CH appear normal at birth because of the protective effects of a substantial maternal-fetal transfer of T_4[130] and in consequence of the increased intracerebral conversion of T_4 to T_3, resulting in greater local availability of T_3 despite its low serum concentration.[131,132] The cerebral damage is mainly due to lack of TH after birth. The introduction of screening programs allowing the early identification of affected patients and prompt treatment with L-thyroxine prevent mental and neuromotor damage.

The clinically detectable consequences of CH strongly depend on severity and duration of thyroid hormone deprivation, but there is also a large individual variability in treatment response. In the first 4 to 6 months after birth, only untreated patients with severe CH have clinical manifestations. Milder cases can remain undiscovered for years. The only characteristic sign of CH is goiter, but this is present only in the few patients with a defect of hormonogenesis. Thus, the most common feature in young infants with CH is the *absence* of specific signs.

Finally, it should be remembered that infants with CH appear to be at increased risk of other congenital anomalies, mostly cardiac (approximately 10% of infants with CH, compared with 3% in the general population).[133]

Neonatal Screening and Diagnosis

As mentioned, most newborns with CH have normal appearance and no detectable physical signs. Delayed diagnosis leads to the most severe outcome of CH, such as mental retardation, and this emphasizes the importance of neonatal screening and immediately starting T_4 therapy to prevent cerebral damage. Pilot screening programs for CH were developed in Quebec, Canada, and Pittsburgh, Pennsylvania, in 1974 and have now been established in Western Europe, North America, Japan, Australia, and parts of Eastern Europe, Asia, South America, and Central America.[134-136] Since then, the apparent overall incidence of CH has increased considerably as a consequence of the detection of mild disorders that previously remained undetected or were not recognized as congenital problems.

International studies show that the incidence of permanent (thyroidal) CH is approximately 1 in 3500 newborns (in iodine-sufficient areas). There is considerable ethnic variation in incidence, ranging from 1 in 30,000 in the African American population in the United States[137] to 1 in 900 in Asian populations in the United Kingdom.[138] With few exceptions, the international screening programs do not detect patients with permanent central CH.

CH is usually sporadic, with a 2:1 female-to-male ratio. Familial cases occur with a frequency that is 15-fold higher than by chance alone[139]; the genetic basis of these familial cases has been established in some but not all pedigrees.[140] On the other hand, more than 90% of monozygotic twin pairs are discordant for thyroid dysgenesis, suggesting that postzygotic events play a major role in the developmental abnormality.[141]

Certainly, the main objective of screening, the eradication of severe mental retardation after CH, has been achieved. In addition to the great clinical benefit, it has been estimated that the cost of screening for CH is much lower than the cost of diagnosis at an older age. Finally, newborn screening has also shown the prevalence of the various causes of CH (see Fig. 21-1), including transient disorders found predominantly in preterm infants.[142]

Population-based newborn screening measures TSH or TSH and total T_4 in dried blood spots obtained in the first 3 days of life. In newborns with a screening result suspicious for hypothyroidism, the diagnosis of primary CH is confirmed when serum TSH levels are above and FT_4 levels are below the age-related reference ranges. Hypothalamic-pituitary hypothyroidism is more difficult to diagnose. Most infants with this diagnosis are missed in screening programs unless FT_4 and TSH or TSH, T_4, and thyroxine-binding globulin (TBG) are simultaneously measured.

If hypothyroidism is confirmed by laboratory analysis, imaging studies should be performed, but it is not acceptable to delay hormone replacement therapy if imaging studies are not readily available.[143]

Tests commonly used to determine the underlying cause of congenital hypothyroidism are presented in Table 21-3.

In the cases of thyroid dysgenesis, thyroid scintigraphy, with ^{99m}technetium or ^{123}I, is the most informative diagnostic procedure.[144] Although thyroid ultrasonography is useful in demonstrating enlarged or absent glands, it is less accurate than scintigraphy in showing ectopic glands.[145] Large thyroid glands may be due to inborn errors of thyroid hormone synthesis or to diseases produced by maternal TSHR autoantibodies. More specialized tests, such as perchlorate discharge; evaluation of serum, salivary, and urinary radioiodine; and measurement of serum T_4 precursors, such as diiodothyronine, may be necessary to delineate specific inborn errors of thyroid hormone biosynthesis (Table 21-4).[61]

TRANSIENT CONGENITAL HYPOTHYROIDISM

A small number of infants with abnormal screening values will have transient hypothyroidism as demonstrated by normal serum T_4 and TSH concentrations at the confirmatory laboratory tests. Transient hypothyroidism is more frequent in iodine-deficient areas of the world, and it is much more common in preterm infants.

Transient hypothyroidism may be the consequence of intrauterine exposure to maternal antithyroid drugs, maternal TSHR-blocking antibodies (TSHRBAb), or heterozygous $DUOX2$[64] or $TSHR$ germline mutations.[146] Endemic iodine deficiency or prenatal or postnatal exposure to iodides excess are also frequent causes of transient CH.[147,148]

Transplacental passage of potent maternal TSHBAb is a very rare cause of transient CH, but can be suspected in presence of a maternal history of autoimmune thyroid disease. The half-life of maternal TSHBAb in the neonate is approximately 3 to 4 weeks,[149] and disappearance from serum lasts from 3 to 6 months of age.

Because the transient nature of the hypothyroidism will not be recognized clinically or through laboratory tests, initial treatment will be similar to that of the infant with permanent CH; however, at a later age, interruption of therapy allows transient hypothyroidism to be distinguished from permanent hypothyroidism.[142]

Treatment

Treatment of a patient with CH is similar to the treatment of any other hypothyroid patient. At a young age, the primary goal of treatment is prevention of brain damage.

All infants with hypothyroidism, with or without goiter, should be rendered euthyroid as promptly as possible by replacement therapy with TH.[150-153] An optimal cognitive outcome

Table 21-3. Tests to Complete the Diagnosis of Congenital Hypothyroidism

1. Imaging studies (to determine thyroid location and size)
   a. Scintigraphy (^{99m}Tc or ^{123}I)
   b. Ultrasonography
2. Functional studies
   a. ^{123}I uptake
   b. Serum thyroglobulin
3. Suspected inborn errors of thyroid hormone synthesis
   a. ^{123}I uptake and perchlorate discharge
   b. Serum/salivary/urine iodine studies
4. Suspected autoimmune thyroid disease
   a. Maternal and neonatal serum thyroid antibodies determination
5. Suspected iodine exposure (or deficiency)
   a. Urinary iodine measurement

Table 21-4. Diagnostic Features in Congenital Hypothyroidism

Causes		Manifestations
Thyroid dysgenesis	Athyreosis	Hypothyroidism (severe)
		Absent circulating Tg
		No radioiodine uptake in the neck
	Ectopy of the thyroid	Hypothyroidism (from moderate to severe)
		Presence of thyroid uptake in abnormal position
	Hypoplasia	Hypothyroidism (variable)
		Normal or reduced radioiodine uptake
		Normal or reduced serum Tg
Dyshormonogenesis	Sodium-iodide symporter mutations	Hypothyroidism (from severe to fully compensated)
		Goiter
		Absence of thyroid on scintigraphy and low iodine uptake
		Serum Tg normal or elevated
	Thyroperoxidase mutations	Hypothyroidism (from severe to fully compensated)
		Goiter
		Positive perchlorate discharge test
	$DUOX1$ and $DUOX2$ mutations	Hypothyroidism (from transient to severe)
		Goiter
		Positive perchlorate discharge test
	Pendrin mutations	Usually euthyroid
		Moderately enlarged thyroid gland
		Impaired hearing (not constant)
		Partial positive perchlorate discharge test
	Thyroglobulin mutations	Hypothyroidism (moderate to severe)
		Goiter
		Low serum thyroglobulin
		Abnormal circulating iodoproteins (iodinated plasma albumin)
		Presence of iodopeptides of low molecular weight in the urine
	IYD mutations	Hypothyroidism (mild to moderate)
		Absence of goiter
		Low circulating TSH
		Reduced response to TRH (in case of pituitary defects)
		Possibly association with reduction in other pituitary hormone
Central hypothyroidism		Hypothyroidism (mild to moderate)
		Absence of goiter
		Low circulating TSH
		Reduced response to TRH (in case of pituitary defects)
		Possibly association with reduction in other pituitary hormones

Tg, Thyroglobulin; *TRH,* thyrotropin-releasing hormone; *TSH,* thyroid-stimulating hormone.

depends on both the adequacy and timing of postnatal therapy, particularly in severe cases of CH. The goal of therapy is to normalize T_4 within 2 weeks and TSH within 1 month. An initial dosage of 10 to 15 $\mu g/kg$ of L-thyroxine (LT_4) has been recommended.[142]

Administration of LT_4 is the treatment of choice. Although T_3 is the more biologically active TH, most brain T_3 comes from local deiodination of T_4, thus T_3 should not be used. The pill should be crushed and suspended in few milliliters of formula, breast milk, or water. Very recently, a new preparation of T_4 in drops became available in several countries. Breastfeeding can be continued.

Clinical examination, including assessment of growth and development, should be performed every few months during the first 3 years of life. The aim of therapy is to ensure normal growth and development by maintaining the serum total T_4 or FT_4 concentration in the upper half of the reference range during the first year of life, with a serum TSH in the reference range. Parental counseling is of great importance: poor compliance or noncompliance may produce major sequelae.

Growth rate and adult height are normal in children with CH who received adequate treatment.[154-156] The best reported outcome occurred with L-thyroxine therapy started within 2 weeks of age with 9.5 $\mu g/kg$ or more per day.[142,153]

Guidelines for treatment of patients with central CH do not exist. Because the use of plasma TSH evaluation, essential for establishing thyroid hormone state, requires an intact hypothalamic-pituitary unit, the optimal dose of T_4 for central CH patients can be adjusted only by determination of plasma FT_4, which should be kept in the upper limit of the normal range.

After 3 years of age, LT_4 administration should be discontinued for 30 to 45 days if no definite cause of CH was found by scan or if there was no TSH increase after the newborn period.[157] After this withdrawal period, serum FT_4 and TSH should be measured. Low FT_4 and elevated TSH values indicate permanent hypothyroidism, and TH therapy should be started again. If the FT_4 and TSH concentrations remain within the normal range, the diagnosis of transient hypothyroidism is confirmed. Nevertheless, these children need to continue follow-up to detect a later increase in TSH.

Patients with CH receiving early treatment with TH show only minor differences in intelligence, school achievement, and neuropsychological tests when compared with classmates and siblings.[158-162] If treatment is started within the first 2 months of life, although physical recovery is good and stature is normal,[156] patients may still have a low to normal IQ.[163] Similarly, although more than 80% of infants receiving replacement therapy before 3 months of age have an IQ greater than 85, 77% show some signs of minimal brain damage, including impairment of arithmetic ability, speech, or fine motor coordination. Even in early-treated patients with CH, auditory brainstem evoked potentials were abnormal in 25% of the children studied. The reason for this is unknown, but it may suggest that prenatal maternal T_4 production does not provide complete protection to alterations in the developing central nervous system.[164]

Transplacental transfer of maternal T_4 in the first trimester may protect the brain during early development.[165] For the same reason, maternal hypothyroidism during fetal development can have persistent effects on the child's neural development.[165-167]

Finally, in the case of severe CH due to genetic defects diagnosed before birth, starting intrauterine treatment with L-thyroxine should be considered. This may offer definite short-term and possible long-term beneficial effects for the patient.[168-173]

REFERENCES

1. Toublanc JE: Comparison of epidemiological data on congenital hypothyroidism in Europe with those of other parts in the world, Horm Res 38:230–235, 1992.
2. Klett M: Epidemiology of congenital hypothyroidism, Exp Clin Endocrinol Diabetes 105(Suppl 4):19–23, 1997.
3. Oppenheimer JH, Schwartz HL, Mariash CN, et al: Advances in our understanding of thyroid hormone action at the cellular level, Endocr Rev 8:288–308, 1987.
4. Fisher DA, Klein A: Thyroid development and disorders of thyroid function in the newborn, New Engl J Med 304:702–712, 1981.
5. Medeiros-Neto G, Stanbury JB: Inherited Disorders of the Thyroid System, Boca Raton, FL, 1994, CRC Press.
6. Grüters A, Krude H, Biebermann H: Molecular genetic defects in congenital hypothyroidism, Eur J Endocrinol 151(Suppl 3):U39–U44, 2004.
7. Stuart A, Oates E, Hall C, et al: Identification of a point mutation in the thyrotropin receptor of the hyt/hyt hypothyroid mouse, Mol Endocrinol 8:129–138, 1994.
8. Beamer WJ, Cresswell LA: Defective thyroid ontogenesis in fetal hypothyroid (hyt/hyt) mice, Anat Rec 202:387–393, 1982.
9. Marians RC, Ng L, Blair HC, et al: Defining thyrotropin-dependent and -independent steps of thyroid hormone synthesis by using thyrotropin receptor-null mice, Proc Natl Acad Sci U S A 99:15776–15781, 2002.
10. Sunthornthepvarakui T, Gottschalk M, Hayashi Y, Refetoff S: Brief report: resistance to thyrotropin caused by mutations in the thyrotropin-receptor gene, N Engl J Med 332:155–160, 1995.
11. Biebermann H, Schoneberg T, Krude H, et al: Mutations of the human thyrotropin receptor gene causing thyroid hypoplasia and persistent congenital hypothyroidism, J Clin Endocrinol Metab 82:3471–3480, 1997.
12. Albright F, Burnett C, Smith P, Parson W: Pseudohypoparathyroidism: An example of "Seabright-Bantam syndrome": Report of three cases, Endocrinology 30:922, 1942.
13. Spiegel AM, Shenker A, Weinstein LS: Receptor-effector coupling by G proteins: implications for normal and abnormal signal transduction, Endocr Rev 13:536–565, 1992.
14. Weinstein LS, Liu J, Sakamoto A, et al: Minireview: GNAS: normal and abnormal functions, Endocrinology 145:5459–5464, 2004.
15. Refetoff S: Resistance to thyrotropin, J Endocrinol Invest 26:770–779, 2003.
16. Clifton-Bligh RJ, Wentworth JM, Heinz P, et al: Mutation of the gene encoding human TTF-2 associated with thyroid agenesis, cleft palate and choanal atresia, Nat Genet 19:399–401, 1998.
17. Castanet M, Park SM, Smith A, et al: A novel loss-of-function mutation in TTF-2 is associated with congenital hypothyroidism, thyroid agenesis and cleft palate, Hum Mol Genet 11:2051–2059, 2002.
18. Macchia PE, Lapi P, Krude H, et al: PAX8 mutations associated with congenital hypothyroidism caused by thyroid dysgenesis, Nat Genet 19:83–86, 1998.
19. Dentice M, Cordeddu V, Rosica A, et al: Missense mutation in the transcription factor NKX2-5: a novel molecular event in the pathogenesis of thyroid dysgenesis, J Clin Endocrinol Metab 91:1428–1433, 2006.
20. Bamforth JS, Hughes IA, Lazarus JH, et al: Congenital hypothyroidism, spiky hair, and cleft palate, J Med Genet 26:49–60, 1989.
21. Baris I, Arisoy AE, Smith A, et al: A novel missense mutation in human TTF-2 (FKHL15) gene associated with congenital hypothyroidism but not athyreosis, J Clin Endocrinol Metab 91:4183–4187, 2006.
22. De Felice M, Di Lauro R: Thyroid development and its disorders: genetics and molecular mechanisms, Endocr Rev 25:722–746, 2004.
23. Devriendt K, Vanhole C, Matthijs G, de Zegher F: Deletion of Thyroid Transcription Factor-1 gene in an infant with neonatal thyroid dysfunction and respiratory failure, N Engl J Med 338:1317–1318, 1998.
24. Iwatani N, Mabe H, Devriendt K, et al: Deletion of NKX2.1 gene encoding thyroid transcription factor-1 in two siblings with hypothyroidism and respiratory failure, J Pediatr 137:272–276, 2000.
25. de Vries BB, Arts WF, Breedveld GJ, et al: Benign hereditary chorea of early onset maps to chromosome 14q, Am J Hum Genet 66:136–142, 2000.
26. Guala A, Nocita G, Di Maria E, et al: Benign hereditary chorea: a rare cause of disability, Riv Ital Pediatr 27:150–152, 2001.
27. Pohlenz J, Dumitrescu A, Zundel D, et al: Partial deficiency of thyroid transcription factor 1 produces predominantly neurological defects in humans and mice, J Clin Invest 109:469–473, 2002.
28. Krude H, Schutz B, Biebermann H, et al: Choreoathetosis, hypothyroidism, and pulmonary alterations due to human NKX2-1 haploinsufficiency, J Clin Invest 109:475–480, 2002.
29. Breedveld GJ, Percy AK, MacDonald ME, et al: Clinical and genetic heterogeneity in benign hereditary chorea, Neurology 59:579–584, 2002.
30. Kleiner-Fisman G, Rogaeva E, Halliday W, et al: Benign hereditary chorea: clinical, genetic, and pathological findings, Ann Neurol 54:244–247, 2003.
31. Doyle DA, Gonzalez I, Thomas B, Scavina M: Autosomal dominant transmission of congenital hypothyroid-

ism, neonatal respiratory distress, and ataxia caused by a mutation of NKX2-1, J Pediatr 145:190–193, 2004.

32. Asmus F, Horber V, Pohlenz J, et al: A novel TITF-1 mutation causes benign hereditary chorea with response to levodopa, Neurology 64:1952–1954, 2005.

33. do Carmo Costa M, Costa C, Silva AP, et al: Nonsense mutation in TITF1 in a Portuguese family with benign hereditary chorea, Neurogenetics 6:209–215, 2005.

34. Willemsen MA, Breedveld GJ, Wouda S, et al: Brain-thyroid-lung syndrome: a patient with a severe multi-system disorder due to a de novo mutation in the thyroid transcription factor 1 gene, Eur J Pediatr 164:28–30, 2005.

35. Kleiner-Fisman G, Calingasan NY, Putt M, et al: Alterations of striatal neurons in benign hereditary chorea, Mov Disord 20:1353–1357, 2005.

36. Devos D, Vuillaume I, de Becdelievre A, et al: New syndromic form of benign hereditary chorea is associated with a deletion of TITF-1 and PAX-9 contiguous genes, Mov Disord 21:2237–2240, 2006.

37. Moya CM, Perez de Nanclares G, Castano L, et al: Functional study of a novel single deletion in the TITF1/NKX2.1 homeobox gene that produces congenital hypothyroidism and benign chorea but not pulmonary distress, J Clin Endocrinol Metab 91:1832–1841, 2006.

38. Provenzano C, Veneziano L, Appleton R, et al: Functional characterization of a novel mutation in TITF-1 in a patient with benign hereditary chorea, J Neurol Sci 264:56–62, 2008.

39. Nagasaki K, Narumi S, Asami T, et al: Mutation of a gene for thyroid transcription factor-1 (TITF1) in a patient with clinical features of resistance to thyrotropin, Endocr J 55:875–888, 2008.

40. Ferrara AM, De Michele G, Salvatore E, et al: A novel NKX2.1 mutation in a family with hypothyroidism and benign hereditary chorea, Thyroid 18:1005–1009, 2008.

41. Vilain C, Rydlewski C, Duprez L, et al: Autosomal dominant transmission of congenital thyroid hypoplasia due to loss-of-function mutation of PAX8, J Clin Endocrinol Metab 86:234–238, 2001.

42. Congdon T, Nguyen LQ, Nogueira CR, et al: A novel mutation (Q40P) in PAX8 associated with congenital hypothyroidism and thyroid hypoplasia: evidence for phenotypic variability in mother and child, J Clin Endocrinol Metab 86:3962–3967, 2001.

43. Komatsu M, Takahashi T, Takahashi I, et al: Thyroid dysgenesis caused by PAX8 mutation: the hypermutability with CpG dinucleotides at codon 31, J Pediatr 139:597–599, 2001.

44. de Sanctis L, Corrias A, Romagnolo D, et al: Familial PAX8 small deletion (c.989_992delACCC) associated with extreme phenotype variability, J Clin Endocrinol Metab 89:5669–5674, 2004.

45. Al Taji E, Biebermann H, Limanova Z, et al: Screening for mutations in transcription factors in a Czech cohort of 170 patients with congenital and early-onset hypothyroidism: identification of a novel PAX8 mutation in dominantly inherited early-onset non-autoimmune hypothyroidism, Eur J Endocrinol 156:521–529, 2007.

46. Esperante SA, Rivolta CM, Miravalle L, et al: Identification and characterization of four PAX8 rare sequence variants (p.T225M, p.L233L, p.G336S and p.A439A) in patients with congenital hypothyroidism and dysgenetic thyroid glands, Clin Endocrinol (Oxf) 68:828–835, 2008.

47. Maiorana R, Carta A, Floriddia G, et al: Thyroid hemiagenesis: prevalence in normal children and effect on thyroid function, J Clin Endocrinol Metab 88:1534–1536, 2003.

48. Alt B, Elsalini OA, Schrumpf P, et al: Arteries define the position of the thyroid gland during its developmental relocalisation, Development 133:3797–3804, 2006.

49. Fagman H, Grande M, Gritli-Linde A, Nilsson M: Genetic deletion of sonic hedgehog causes hemiagenesis and ectopic development of the thyroid in mouse, Am J Pathol 164:1865–1872, 2004.

50. Amendola E, De Luca P, Macchia PE, et al: A mouse model demonstrates a multigenic origin of congenital hypothyroidism, Endocrinology 146:5038–5047, 2005.

51. Dai G, Levy O, Carrasco N: Cloning and characterization of the thyroid iodide symporter, Nature 379:458–460, 1996.

52. Smanik PA, Ryu KY, Theil KS, et al: Expression, exon-intron organization, and chromosome mapping of the human sodium iodide symporter, Endocrinology 138:3555–3558, 1997.

53. Caillou B, Troalen F, Baudin E, et al: Na⁺/I⁻ symporter distribution in human thyroid tissues: an immunohistochemical study, J Clin Endocrinol Metab 83:4102–4106, 1998.

54. Lazar V, Bidart J, Caillou B, et al: Expression of the Na⁺/I⁻ symporter gene in human thyroid tumors: a comparison study with other thyroid-specific genes, J Clin Endocrinol Metab 84:3228–3234, 1999.

55. Dohan O, De la Vieja A, Paroder V, et al: The sodium/iodide symporter (NIS): characterization, regulation, and medical significance, Endocr Rev 24:48–77, 2003.

56. Park SM, Chatterjee VK: Genetics of congenital hypothyroidism, J Med Genet 42:379–389, 2005.

57. De la Vieja A, Dohan O, Levy O, Carrasco N: Molecular analysis of the sodium/iodide symporter: Impact on thyroid and extrathyroid pathophysiology, Physiol Rev 80:1083–1105, 2000.

58. Vulsma T, Rammeloo J, Gons M, de Vijlder J: The role of serum thyroglobulin concentration and thyroid ultrasound imaging in the detection of iodide transport defects in infants, Acta Endocrinol (Copenh) 124:405–410, 1991.

59. de Vijlder J: Primary congenital hypothyroidism: Defects in iodine pathways, Eur J Endocrinol 149:247–256, 2003.

60. De Deken X, Wang D, Many M, et al: Cloning of two human thyroid cDNAs encoding new members of the NADPH oxidase family, J Biol Chem 275:23227–23233, 2000.

61. LaFranchi S: Congenital hypothyroidism: etiologies, diagnosis, and management, Thyroid 9:735–740, 1999.

62. Bakker B, Bikker H, Vulsma T, et al: Two decades of screening for congenital hypothyroidism in The Netherlands: TPO gene mutations in total iodide organification defects (an update), J Clin Endocrinol Metab 85:3708–3712, 2000.

63. Grasberger H, Refetoff S: Identification of the maturation factor for dual oxidase. Evolution of an eukaryotic operon equivalent, J Biol Chem 281:18269–18272, 2006.

64. Moreno JC, Visser TJ: New phenotypes in thyroid dyshormonogenesis: hypothyroidism due to DUOX2 mutations, Endocr Dev 10:99–117, 2007.

65. Johnson KR, Marden CC, Ward-Bailey P, et al: Congenital hypothyroidism, dwarfism, and hearing impairment caused by a missense mutation in the mouse dual oxidase 2 gene, Duox2, Mol Endocrinol 21:1593–1602, 2007.

66. Ohye H, Fukata S, Hishinuma A, et al: A novel homozygous missense mutation of the dual oxidase 2 (DUOX2) gene in an adult patient with large goiter, Thyroid 18:561–566, 2008.

67. Maruo Y, Takahashi H, Soeda I, et al: Transient congenital hypothyroidism caused by biallelic mutations of the dual oxidase 2 gene in Japanese patients detected by a neonatal screening program, J Clin Endocrinol Metab 93:4261–4267, 2008.

68. Zamproni I, Grasberger H, Cortinovis F, et al: Biallelic inactivation of the dual oxidase maturation factor 2 (DUOXA2) gene as a novel cause of congenital hypothyroidism, J Clin Endocrinol Metab 93:605–610, 2008.

69. Pendred V: Deaf mutism and goitre, Lancet 2:532, 1896.

70. Gausden E, Coyle B, Armour JA, et al: Pendred syndrome: evidence for genetic homogeneity and further refinement of linkage, J Med Genet 34:126–129, 1997.

71. Royaux I, Suzuki K, Mori A, et al: Pendrin, the protein encoded by the Pendred syndrome gene (PDS), is an apical porter of iodide in the thyroid and is regulated by thyroglobulin in FRTL-5 cells, Endocrinology 141:839–845, 2000.

72. Yoshida A, Taniguchi S, Hisatome I, et al: Pendrin is an iodide-specific apical porter responsible for iodide efflux from thyroid cells, J Clin Endocrinol Metab 87:3356–3361, 2002.

73. Kopp P: Pendred's syndrome and genetic defects in thyroid hormone synthesis, Rev Endocr Metab Disord 1:109–121, 2000.

74. Glaser B: Pendred syndrome, Pediatr Endocrinol Rev 1(Suppl 2):199–204, 2003.

75. Van de Graaf S, Pauws E, de Vijlder J, Ris-Stalpers C: The revised 8307 base pair coding sequence of human thyroglobulin transiently expressed in eukaryotic cells, Eur J Endocrinol 136:508–515, 1997.

76. Mendive F, Rivolta C, Vassart G, Targovnik H: Genomic organization of the 3' region of the human thyroglobulin gene, Thyroid 9:903–912, 1999.

77. Gons M, Kok J, Tegelaers W, de Vijlder J: Concentration of plasma thyroglobulin and urinary excretion of iodinated material in the diagnosis of thyroid disorders in congenital hypothyroidism, Acta Endocrinol (Copenh) 104:27–34, 1983.

78. Rivolta CM, Targovnik HM: Molecular advances in thyroglobulin disorders, Clin Chim Acta 374:8–24, 2006.

79. Caputo M, Rivolta CM, Esperante SA, et al: Congenital hypothyroidism with goitre caused by new mutations in the thyroglobulin gene, Clin Endocrinol (Oxf) 67:351–357, 2007.

80. Ricketts MH, Simons MJ, Parma J, et al: A nonsense mutation causes hereditary goiter in the Afrikander cattle and unmasks alternative splicing of thyroglobulin transcripts, Proc Natl Acad Sci U S A 84:3181–3184, 1987.

81. Veenboer G, de Vijlder J: Molecular basis of the thyroglobulin synthesis defect in Dutch goats, Endocrinology 132:377–381, 1993.

82. Kim PS, Hossain SA, Park YN, et al: A single amino acid change in the acetylcholinesterase-like domain of thyroglobulin causes congenital goiter with hypothyroidism in the cog/cog mouse: a model of human endoplasmic reticulum storage diseases, Proc Natl Acad Sci U S A 95:9909–9913, 1998.

83. Hishinuma A, Furudate S, Oh-Ishi M, et al: A novel missense mutation (G2320R) in thyroglobulin causes hypothyroidism in rdw rats, Endocrinology 141:4050–4055, 2000.

84. Roche J, Michel R, Michel O, Lissitzky S: Enzymatic dehalogenation of iodotyrosine by thyroid tissue; on its physiological role, Biochim Biophys Acta 9:161–169, 1952.

85. Moreno JC, Pauws E, van Kampen AH, et al: Cloning of tissue-specific genes using serial analysis of gene expression and a novel computational subtraction approach, Genomics 75:70–76, 2001.

86. Moreno JC: Identification of novel genes involved in congenital hypothyroidism using serial analysis of gene expression, Horm Res 60(Suppl 3):96–102, 2003.

87. Moreno JC, Klootwijk W, van Toor H, et al: Mutations in the iodotyrosine deiodinase gene and hypothyroidism, N Engl J Med 358:1811–1818, 2008.

88. Afink G, Kulik W, Overmars H, et al: Molecular characterization of iodotyrosine dehalogenase deficiency in patients with hypothyroidism, J Clin Endocrinol Metab 93:4894–4901, 2008.

89. Colvin SC, Mullen RD, Pfaeffle RW, Rhodes SJ: LHX3 and LHX4 transcription factors in pituitary development and disease, Pediatr Endocrinol Rev 6(Suppl 2):283–290, 2009.

90. Dattani MT, Martinez-Barbera JP, Thomas PQ, et al: Mutations in the homeobox gene HESX1/Hesx1 associated with septo-optic dysplasia in human and mouse, Nat Genet 19:125–133, 1998.

91. Mehta A, Dattani MT: Developmental disorders of the hypothalamus and pituitary gland associated with congenital hypopituitarism, Best Pract Res Clin Endocrinol Metab 22:191–206, 2008.

92. Yamada M, Saga Y, Shibusawa N, et al: Tertiary hypothyroidism and hyperglycemia in mice with targeted disruption of the thyrotropin-releasing hormone gene, Proc Natl Acad Sci U S A 94:10862–10867, 1997.

93. Niimi H, Inomata H, Sasaki N, Nakajima H: Congenital isolated thyrotrophin releasing hormone deficiency, Arch Dis Child 57:877–878, 1982.

94. Katakami H, Kato Y, Inada M, Imura H: Hypothalamic hypothyroidism due to isolated thyrotropin-releasing hormone (TRH) deficiency, J Endocrinol Invest 7:231–233, 1984.

95. Rabeler R, Mittag J, Geffers L, et al: Generation of thyrotropin-releasing hormone receptor 1-deficient

mice as an animal model of central hypothyroidism, Mol Endocrinol 18:1450–1460, 2004.

96. Collu R, Tang J, Castagne J, et al: A novel mechanism for isolated central hypothyroidism: inactivating mutations in the thyrotropin-releasing hormone receptor gene, J Clin Endocrinol Metab 82:1561–1565, 1997.

97. Bonomi M, Busnelli M, Beck-Peccoz P, et al: A family with complete resistance to thyrotropin-releasing hormone, N Engl J Med 360:731–734, 2009.

98. Tatsumi K, Miyai K, Notomi T, et al: Cretinism with combined hormone deficiency caused by a mutation in the PIT1 gene, Nat Genet 1:56–58, 1992.

99. Cohen LE, Radovick S: Molecular basis of combined pituitary hormone deficiencies, Endocr Rev 23:431–442, 2002.

100. Ward RD, Raetzman LT, Suh H, et al: Role of PROP1 in pituitary gland growth, Mol Endocrinol 19:698–710, 2005.

101. Wu W, Cogan JD, Pfaffle RW, et al: Mutations in PROP1 cause familial combined pituitary hormone deficiency, Nat Genet 18:147–149, 1998.

102. Cohen R, Weintraub B, Wondisford F: Thyrotropin: Chemistry and biosynthesis of thyrotropin. In Braverman L, Utiger R, editors: Werner and Ingbar's the Thyroid, Philadelphia, 2000, Lippincott Williams & Wilkins, pp 202–218.

103. Miyai K: Congenital thyrotropin deficiency–from discovery to molecular biology, postgenome and preventive medicine, Endocr J 54:191–203, 2007.

104. Gereben B, Zavacki AM, Ribich S, et al: Cellular and molecular basis of deiodinase-regulated thyroid hormone signaling, Endocr Rev 29:898–938, 2008.

105. Galton VA, Schneider MJ, Clark AS, St Germain DL: Life without thyroxine to 3,5,3′-triiodothyronine conversion: Studies in mice devoid of the 5′-deiodinases, Endocrinology 150:2502–2504, 2009.

106. Hennemann G, Docter R, Friesema EC, et al: Plasma membrane transport of thyroid hormones and its role in thyroid hormone metabolism and bioavailability, Endocr Rev 22:451–476, 2001.

107. Friesema EC, Ganguly S, Abdalla A, et al: Identification of monocarboxylate transporter 8 as a specific thyroid hormone transporter, J Biol Chem 278:40128–40135, 2003.

108. Friesema EC, Kuiper GG, Jansen J, et al: Thyroid hormone transport by the human monocarboxylate transporter 8 and its rate-limiting role in intracellular metabolism, Mol Endocrinol 20:2761–2772, 2006.

109. Lafreniere RG, Carrel L, Willard HF, Lafreniere RG, Carrel L, Willard HF: A novel transmembrane transporter encoded by the XPCT gene in Xq13.2, Hum Mol Genet 3:1133–1139, 1994.

110. Halestrap AP, Meredith D: The SLC16 gene family-from monocarboxylate transporters (MCTs) to aromatic amino acid transporters and beyond, Pflugers Arch 447:619–628, 2004.

111. Dumitrescu AM, Liao XH, Best TB, et al: A novel syndrome combining thyroid and neurological abnormalities is associated with mutations in a monocarboxylate transporter gene, Am J Hum Genet 74:168–175, 2004.

112. Biebermann H, Ambrugger P, Tarnow P, et al: Extended clinical phenotype, endocrine investigations and functional studies of a loss-of-function mutation A150V in the thyroid hormone specific transporter MCT8, Eur J Endocrinol 153:359–366, 2005.

113. Brockmann K, Dumitrescu AM, Best TT, et al: X-linked paroxysmal dyskinesia and severe global retardation caused by defective MCT8 gene, J Neurol 252:663–666, 2005.

114. Friesema EC, Grueters A, Biebermann H, et al: Association between mutations in a thyroid hormone transporter and severe X-linked psychomotor retardation, Lancet 364:1435–1437, 2004.

115. Friesema EC, Jansen J, Heuer H, et al: Mechanisms of disease: psychomotor retardation and high T_3 levels caused by mutations in monocarboxylate transporter 8, Nat Clin Pract Endocrinol Metab 2:512–523, 2006.

116. Frints SG, Lenzner S, Bauters M, et al: MCT8 mutation analysis and identification of the first female with Allan-Herndon-Dudley syndrome due to loss of MCT8 expression, Eur J Hum Genet 16:1029–1037, 2008.

117. Fuchs O, Pfarr N, Pohlenz J, Schmidt H: Elevated serum triiodothyronine and intellectual and motor disability with paroxysmal dyskinesia caused by a monocarboxylate transporter 8 gene mutation, Dev Med Child Neurol 51:240–244, 2009.

118. Herzovich V, Vaiani E, Marino R, et al: Unexpected peripheral markers of thyroid function in a patient with a novel mutation of the MCT8 thyroid hormone transporter gene, Horm Res 67:1–6, 2007.

119. Jansen J, Friesema EC, Kester MH, et al: Functional analysis of monocarboxylate transporter 8 mutations identified in patients with X-linked psychomotor retardation and elevated serum triiodothyronine, J Clin Endocrinol Metab 92:2378–2381, 2007.

120. Jansen J, Friesema EC, Kester MH, et al: Genotype-phenotype relationship in patients with mutations in thyroid hormone transporter MCT8, Endocrinology 149:2184–2190, 2008.

121. Maranduba CM, Friesema EC, Kok F, et al: Decreased cellular uptake and metabolism in Allan-Herndon-Dudley syndrome (AHDS) due to a novel mutation in the MCT8 thyroid hormone transporter, J Med Genet 43:457–460, 2006.

122. Namba N, Etani Y, Kitaoka T, et al: Clinical phenotype and endocrinological investigations in a patient with a mutation in the MCT8 thyroid hormone transporter, Eur J Pediatr 167:785–791, 2008.

123. Vaurs-Barriere C, Deville M, Sarret C, et al: Pelizaeus-Merzbacher-like disease presentation of MCT8 mutated male subjects, Ann Neurol 65:114–118, 2009.

124. Visser WE, Friesema EC, Jansen J, Visser TJ: Thyroid hormone transport in and out of cells, Trends Endocrinol Metab 19:50–56, 2008.

125. Wemeau JL, Pigeyre M, Proust-Lemoine E, et al: Beneficial effects of propylthiouracil plus L-thyroxine treatment in a patient with a mutation in MCT8, J Clin Endocrinol Metab 93:2084–2088, 2008.

126. Holden KR, Zuniga OF, May MM, et al: X-linked MCT8 gene mutations: characterization of the pediatric neurologic phenotype, J Child Neurol 20:852–857, 2005.

127. Heuer H, Visser TJ: Pathophysiological importance of thyroid hormone transport, Endocrinology 150:1078–1083, 2009.

128. Dumitrescu AM, Liao XH, Weiss RE, et al: Tissue-specific thyroid hormone deprivation and excess in monocarboxylate transporter (mct) 8-deficient mice, Endocrinology 147:4036–4043, 2006.

129. Trajkovic M, Visser TJ, Mittag J, et al: Abnormal thyroid hormone metabolism in mice lacking the monocarboxylate transporter 8, J Clin Invest 117:627–635, 2007.

130. Vulsma T, Gons MH, de Vijlder JJ: Maternal-fetal transfer of thyroxine in congenital hypothyroidism due to a total organification defect or thyroid agenesis, N Engl J Med 321:13–16, 1989.

131. Ruiz de Ona C, Obregon MJ, Escobar del Rey F, Morreale de Escobar G: Developmental changes in rat brain 5′-deiodinase and thyroid hormones during the fetal period: the effects of fetal hypothyroidism and maternal thyroid hormones, Pediatr Res 24, 1988.

132. Kester MH, Martinez de Mena R, Obregon MJ, et al: Iodothyronine levels in the human developing brain: major regulatory roles of iodothyronine deiodinases in different areas, J Clin Endocrinol Metab 89:3117–3128, 2004.

133. Olivieri A, Stazi MA, Mastroiacovo P, et al: A population-based study on the frequency of additional congenital malformations in infants with congenital hypothyroidism: Data from the Italian Registry for Congenital Hypothyroidism, 1991–1998, J Clin Endocrinol Metab 87:557–562, 2002.

134. Dussault JH, Coulombe P, Laberge C, et al: Preliminary report on a mass screening program for neonatal hypothyroidism, J Pediatr 86:670–674, 1975.

135. Revised guidelines for neonatal screening programmes for primary congenital hypothyroidism, Working Group on Neonatal Screening of the European Society for Paediatric Endocrinology, Horm Res 52:49–52, 1999.

136. LaFranchi SH, Snyder DB, Sesser DE, et al: Follow-up of newborns with elevated screening T_4 concentrations, J Pediatr 143:296–301, 2003.

137. Brown AL, Fernhoff PM, Milner J, et al: Racial differences in the incidence of congenital hypothyroidism, J Pediatr 99:934–936, 1981.

138. Rosenthal M, Addison GM, Price DA: Congenital hypothyroidism: increased incidence in Asian families, Arch Dis Child 63:790–793, 1988.

139. Castanet M, Polak M, Bonaiti-Pellie C, et al: Nineteen years of national screening for congenital hypothyroidism: familial cases with thyroid dysgenesis suggest the involvement of genetic factors, J Clin Endocrinol Metab 86:2009–2014, 2001.

140. Castanet M, Sura Trueba S, Chauty A, et al: Linkage and mutational analysis of familial thyroid dysgenesis suggest genetic heterogeneity, Eur J Hum Genet 13:232–239, 2005.

141. Perry R, Heinrichs C, Bourdoux P, et al: Discordance of monozygotic twins for thyroid dysgenesis: implications for screening and for molecular pathophysiology, J Clin Endocrinol Metab 87:4072–4077, 2002.

142. Rose SR, Brown RS, Foley T, et al: Update of newborn screening and therapy for congenital hypothyroidism, Pediatrics 117:2290–2303, 2006.

143. Gruters A, Krude H: Update on the management of congenital hypothyroidism, Horm Res 68(Suppl 5):107–111, 2007.

144. Muir A, Daneman D, Daneman A, Ehrlich R: Thyroid scanning, ultrasound, and serum thyroglobulin in determining the origin of congenital hypothyroidism, Am J Dis Child 142:214–216, 1988.

145. Takashima S, Nomura N, Tanaka H, et al: Congenital hypothyroidism: assessment with ultrasound, AJNR Am J Neuroradiol 16:1117–1123, 1995.

146. Calaciura F, Motta RM, Miscio G, et al: Subclinical hypothyroidism in early childhood: a frequent outcome of transient neonatal hyperthyrotropinemia, J Clin Endocrinol Metab 87:3209–3214, 2002.

147. Glinoer D: Pregnancy and iodine, Thyroid 11:471–481, 2001.

148. Bartalena L, Bogazzi F, Braverman LE, Martino E: Effects of amiodarone administration during pregnancy on neonatal thyroid function and subsequent neurodevelopment, J Endocrinol Invest 24:116–130, 2001.

149. van Der Zwet WC, Vandenbroucke-Grauls CM, van Elburg RM, et al: Neonatal antibody titers against varicella-zoster virus in relation to gestational age, birth weight, and maternal titer, Pediatrics 109:79–85, 2002.

150. de Escobar GM, Obregon MJ, del Rey FE: Maternal thyroid hormones early in pregnancy and fetal brain development, Best Pract Res Clin Endocrinol Metab 18:225–248, 2004.

151. Bakker B, Kempers MJ, De Vijlder JJ, et al: Dynamics of the plasma concentrations of TSH, FT_4 and T_3 following thyroxine supplementation in congenital hypothyroidism, Clin Endocrinol (Oxf) 57:529–537, 2002.

152. Cassio A, Cacciari E, Cicognani A, et al: Treatment for congenital hypothyroidism: thyroxine alone or thyroxine plus triiodothyronine? Pediatrics 111:1055–1060, 2003.

153. Bongers-Schokking JJ, Koot HM, Wiersma D, et al: Influence of timing and dose of thyroid hormone replacement on development in infants with congenital hypothyroidism, J Pediatr 136:292–297, 2000.

154. Ohnishi H, Inomata H, Watanabe T, et al: Clinical utility of thyroid ultrasonography in the diagnosis of congenital hypothyroidism, Endocr J 49:293–297, 2002.

155. Salerno M, Micillo M, Di Maio S, et al: Longitudinal growth, sexual maturation and final height in patients with congenital hypothyroidism detected by neonatal screening, Eur J Endocrinol 145:377–383, 2001.

156. Morin A, Guimarey L, Apezteguia M, et al: Linear growth in children with congenital hypothyroidism detected by neonatal screening and treated early: a longitudinal study, J Pediatr Endocrinol Metab 15:973–977, 2002.

157. Eugster EA, LeMay D, Zerin JM, Pescovitz OH: Definitive diagnosis in children with congenital hypothyroidism, J Pediatr 144:643–647, 2004.

158. Bongers-Schokking JJ: Pre- and postnatal brain development in neonates with congenital hypothyroidism, J Pediatr Endocrinol Metab 14(Suppl 6):1463–1468, 2001.

159. Gruters A, Jenner A, Krude H: Long-term consequences of congenital hypothyroidism in the era of screening programmes, Best Pract Res Clin Endocrinol Metab 16:369–382, 2002.

160. Oerbeck B, Sundet K, Kase BF, Heyerdahl S: Congenital hypothyroidism: influence of disease severity and L-thyroxine treatment on intellectual, motor, and school-associated outcomes in young adults, Pediatrics 112:923–930, 2003.

161. Rovet J, Daneman D: Congenital hypothyroidism: a review of current diagnostic and treatment practices in

relation to neuropsychologic outcome, Paediatr Drugs 5:141–149, 2003.

162. Rovet JF: Congenital hypothyroidism: an analysis of persisting deficits and associated factors, Child Neuropsychol 8:150–162, 2002.

163. Mirabella G, Feig D, Astzalos E, et al: The effect of abnormal intrauterine thyroid hormone economies on infant cognitive abilities, J Pediatr Endocrinol Metab 13:191–194, 2000.

164. Chou YH, Wang PJ: Auditory brainstem evoked potentials in early-treated congenital hypothyroidism, J Child Neurol 17:510–514, 2002.

165. Haddow JE, Palomaki GE, Allan WC, et al: Maternal thyroid deficiency during pregnancy and subsequent neuropsychological development of the child, N Engl J Med 341:549–555, 1999.

166. Lavado-Autric R, Auso E, Garcia-Velasco JV, et al: Early maternal hypothyroxinemia alters histogenesis and cerebral cortex cytoarchitecture of the progeny, J Clin Invest 111:1073–1082, 2003.

167. Morreale de Escobar G, Obregon MJ, Escobar del Rey F: Is neuropsychological development related to maternal hypothyroidism or to maternal hypothyroxinemia? J Clin Endocrinol Metab 85:3975–3987, 2000.

168. Perelman AH, Johnson RL, Clemons RD, et al: Intra-uterine diagnosis and treatment of fetal goitrous hypothyroidism, J Clin Endocrinol Metab 71:618–621, 1990.

169. Abuhamad AZ, Fisher DA, Warsof SL, et al: Antenatal diagnosis and treatment of fetal goitrous hypothyroidism: case report and review of the literature, Ultrasound Obstet Gynecol 6:368–371, 1995.

170. Caron P, Moya CM, Malet D, et al: Compound heterozygous mutations in the thyroglobulin gene (1143delC and 6725G→A [R2223H]) resulting in fetal goitrous hypothyroidism, J Clin Endocrinol Metab 88:3546–3553, 2003.

171. Gruner C, Kollert A, Wildt L, et al: Intrauterine treatment of fetal goitrous hypothyroidism controlled by determination of thyroid-stimulating hormone in fetal serum. A case report and review of the literature, Fetal Diagn Ther 16:47–51, 2001.

172. Borgel K, Pohlenz J, Holzgreve W, Bramswig JH: Intra-uterine therapy of goitrous hypothyroidism in a boy with a new compound heterozygous mutation (Y453D and C800R) in the thyroid peroxidase gene. A long-term follow-up, Am J Obstet Gynecol 193:857–858, 2005.

173. Miyata I, Abe-Gotyo N, Tajima A, et al: Successful intrauterine therapy for fetal goitrous hypothyroidism during late gestation, Endocr J 54:813–817, 2007.

Chapter 22

THYROID HORMONE BINDING AND VARIANTS OF TRANSPORT PROTEINS

JIM STOCKIGT

More than 60 years ago, it was shown that circulating thyroid hormones are noncovalently bound to plasma proteins.[1] Well over 99% of circulating thyroxine (T_4) and triiodothyronine (T_3) is protein bound in the circulation, with bound and free moieties in constant rapid equilibrium. An understanding of thyroid hormone binding allows the clinician to better appreciate tissue delivery and interconversion of thyroid hormones, especially when these phenomena change as a result of illness or drug therapy, or when treatment is given to alter thyroid status. This knowledge aids the interpretation of (1) atypical thyroid function tests, in particular unusual relationships between serum thyroid-stimulating hormone (TSH) and circulating thyroid hormones

that may indicate hereditary or acquired abnormalities of the three major thyroid hormone–binding proteins; (2) aberrant estimates of serum free T_4 that may be due to analytic artifact that results from abnormal tracer binding by a variant protein, and (3) the effects of medications and critical illness on protein binding of the thyroid hormones.

The evolution of thyroid hormone binding to plasma proteins can be traced from fish, which show only albumin binding, through birds, in which T_4 binds to both albumin and transthyretin (TTR, previously known as prealbumin). Most larger mammals, with the exception of felines, have in addition a low capacity, high-affinity protein, termed thyroxine-binding globulin (TBG) that carries well over half the total circulating T_3 and T_4. In humans, only 0.02% to 0.03% (about 1 part in 4000) of T_4 and 0.2% to 0.3% (1 part in 400) of T_3 circulate in the free or unbound state in undiluted normal human serum or plasma at equilibrium at 37°C. Other iodothyronines, whether synthetic analogues or metabolites, also are generally highly protein bound.[2] Numerous other hydrophobic ligands that are unrelated to thyroid hormones can also compete for the various plasma protein–binding sites (see below).

In normal human serum, about 75% of the total circulating T_4 concentration of 60 to 140 nmol/L or 4 to 11 µg/dL is carried on TBG, with about 10% to 15% attached to TTR and 10% to 15% bound to albumin. The electrophoretic techniques used to make these estimates allow some dissociation of labeled hormone during separation and thus tend to underestimate proportional carriage on lower-affinity sites. A minor fraction (<5%) of circulating T_4 and T_3 is associated with lipoprotein.[3]

Binding to plasma proteins is noncovalent and rapidly reversible; it is important to emphasize that the much larger bound moiety of hormone acts, in effect, as a reservoir. Dissociation of bound hormone almost instantaneously replenishes the free hormone concentration, as this fraction is taken up by tissues or diminished by sample dilution in vitro. A rigid distinction between bound and free hormone moieties may be artificial in light of studies that suggest dissociation and reassociation so rapid that the free and bound moieties interchange several million times per day.[4]

Marked hereditary differences in the protein binding of iodothyronines lead to wide variations in the total T_4 concentration in humans (Fig. 22-1), while the free hormone concentration

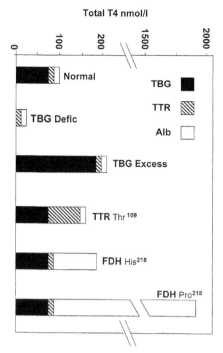

FIGURE 22-1. Estimated proportional carriage of thyroxine (T$_4$) on the three major plasma binding proteins is shown for euthyroid subjects with normal or variant T$_4$ binding proteins. In the face of normal free T$_4$ and thyroid-stimulating hormone (TSH) concentrations, the concentration of total T$_4$ can vary from about 25 nmol/L in total TBG deficiency to about 1800 nmol/L in the Pro^{218} variant of familial dysalbuminemic hyperthyroxinemia (FDH) described in several Japanese kindreds.

Table 22-1. Properties of the Major Human Thyroid Hormone–Binding Proteins

	Thyroxine	Transthyretin Binding Globulin	Albumin
Molecular weight, kD	54	55	66
Structure	Glycoprotein	Peptide tetramer	Single peptide chain
Concentration, M	3×10^{-7}	2×10^{-6}	6×10^{-4}
Half-life, days	5	2	15
Degradation rate, mg/day	15	650	17,000
Proportion of T$_4$ carried	75%	10%-15%	10%-15%
Occupancy by T$_4$	30%	0.5%	<0.01%
Dissociation constant*			
T$_4$ K_d M/L	10^{-10}	10^{-8}	$10^{-6\dagger}$
T$_3$ K_d M/L	2×10^{-9}	6×10^{-8}	$10^{-5\dagger}$
Off rate‡			
T$_4$ $t_{1/2}$ sec	20-40	8	<2
T$_3$ $t_{1/2}$ sec	5-10	<2	<1

T_3, Triiodothyronine; T_4, thyroxine.
*Free hormone concentration at half occupancy of binding site at equilibrium.
†Highest-affinity site.
‡Unidirectional dissociation rate.

remains within much narrower limits. This finding supports the free hormone hypothesis (see below), which proposes that the minute free fraction of the total circulating T$_4$ and T$_3$ pool is the major determinant of hormone action, clearance, and negative feedback. Even when different species are compared, the concentration of free hormone varies much less than total concentration.[5]

Concentrations of the binding proteins can vary independent of thyroid status. When the concentration of TBG changes, the total serum T$_4$ and T$_3$ concentrations tend to alter to restore the preexisting concentration of free hormone, as determined by the set point of the feedback relationship with TSH. Hence, in theory, free hormone estimates will give a more accurate reflection of thyroid status than will measurement of total hormone. However, sample storage and dilution and the presence of competitors can alter the relationship between free and total hormone concentration, so that an analytically correct free hormone estimate may not reflect the in vivo situation (see below).

Characteristics of Hormone Binding

The definition of a number of terms assists the understanding of thyroid hormone binding. *Capacity* expresses the molar concentration of a specific class of ligand-binding site; if one binding site is present per protein molecule, capacity and protein concentration will be identical in molar terms. When about half the binding sites are empty, the free and hormone concentrations will change to about the same extent (i.e., the free fraction will show little change). However, as the total concentration of ligand approaches the binding protein capacity, the free hormone concentration will rise disproportionately, as occurs in thyrotoxico-

sis as the total T$_4$ serum concentration approaches the capacity of TBG.[6]

Proportional carriage, the distribution of total hormone between a number of heterogeneous binding proteins, is influenced by the concentration of binding protein, the affinity of binding, and the free hormone concentration, but it is not directly influenced by the total hormone concentration.[7] In a heterogeneous mixture of binding proteins, as in serum, proportional carriage can change as the free hormone concentration alters in response to dilution or hormone loading (see below).

Free fraction describes the percentage of the total hormone that is unbound. When serum that contains a highly bound ligand is progressively diluted, bound hormone will dissociate, so that the free hormone concentration at first is well maintained, with an increase in free fraction.

Occupancy, the proportion of a particular class of binding site that is filled with hormone, is a direct function of the free hormone concentration and is fundamental to the definition of affinity or kD. TBG is normally about one third occupied by T$_4$; TTR is <1% occupied by T$_4$, and albumin shows negligible occupancy (Table 22-1).

Affinity or dissociation constant (kD, mol/L) describes the free hormone concentration at which a particular binding site is half occupied. The association constant (kA, L/mol) is the inverse of kD. (kA is a theoretical concept of the number of liters at which 1 mole of ligand would occupy half the sites on 1 mole of binding protein.) By definition, a binding protein is 50% occupied when the free hormone concentration is the inverse of kA.

Dissociation rate (TΩ, sec) or rate constant (sec-1) defines the rate of unidirectional dissociation or delivery of hormone from a binding site.[4] The unidirectional maximum rate of hormone delivery is relevant under non–steady state conditions, as, for example, when free hormone is rapidly removed from the circulation during tissue transit. The dissociation rate, as well as kA and kD, are highly temperature dependent. The free T$_4$ fraction is higher at 37°C than at room temperature by a factor of up to two[8] and dissociation of ligand is much faster.[4]

The reversible interaction between free T_4 (fT4) and the unoccupied TBG-binding sites (uTBG) can be represented by the following:

$$fT_4 + uTBG \rightleftharpoons TBG \cdot T_4$$

When represented in terms of the association constant, kTBG, this relationship becomes

$$kTBG = \frac{[TBG \cdot T_4]}{[fT_4][uTBG]}$$

It follows that

$$[fT_4] = \frac{[TBG \cdot T_4]}{KTBG[uTBG]}$$

At half occupancy of the binding site, $[TBG \cdot T_4]$ will equal $[uTBG]$ and

$$[fT_4] = \frac{1}{Ka} = K_d$$

For the total hormone concentration to have a regulatory influence on tissue function, it is appropriate for the kD of the dominant binding protein and the physiologic concentration of free hormone to be of the same order, as is the case for the relationship between normal serum free T_4 (10 to 25 pM) and the kD of TBG (100 pM). A wide disparity between the kD of the dominant binding protein and the free hormone concentration would require relatively large changes in total hormone concentration to achieve regulatory variation. In effect, TBG stabilizes the tissue distribution of T_4, while allowing normal regulatory variation over an approximately twofold range of total hormone concentration. In the absence of TBG, a greater proportional change in total hormone concentration would be necessary to achieve regulatory variation.

Free Hormone Hypothesis

According to this hypothesis, it is the free or unbound equilibrium concentration of a hormone that determines biological activity. The validity of this hypothesis, which generally is well sustained for the thyroid hormones, has been analyzed in detail.[9,10] Earlier liver perfusion experiments that showed the loosely albumin-bound moiety of the total circulating hormone pool to be virtually as readily available as the free hormone[11] have now been refuted.[9] No conclusive evidence suggests that any particular class of binding protein facilitates tissue uptake of thyroid hormones. When isolated rat liver was perfused with T_4 bound to various normal and variant binding proteins,[12] tissue uptake of T_4 was proportional to the spontaneous dissociation of T_4 from each protein.[12]

Under some circumstances, especially when capillary transit is slow, or when mixing of layers across the diameter of a vessel is incomplete, tissue uptake of hormone may be limited by dissociation of bound hormone.[9] Under these circumstances, the local concentration of free hormone at a particular site may be lower than the equilibrium concentration. The albumin-bound moiety with the fastest rate of unidirectional dissociation (see Table 22-1) will then make a large contribution in replenishing the free concentration.[9]

As formulated by Mendel,[9,10] the unmodified free hormone hypothesis will be valid when tissue uptake of hormone is limited by influx or elimination. When flow or dissociation is the limiting condition, for example, when flow is slow and clearance is rapid in a tissue such as the liver, the free hormone hypothesis still holds, with hormone dissociation as an additional critical variable.

Structure and Binding Characteristics of Normal and Variant Transport Proteins

The characteristics of the three normal major iodothyronine-binding proteins, thyroxine-binding globulin, transthyretin and albumin, are summarized in Table 22-1. The numerous structural variants of the three major thyroid hormone–binding proteins that have been described (Table 22-2) were initially recognized from the investigation of euthyroid subjects who showed markedly abnormal levels of total serum T_4 or T_3, but recently, additional variants have been identified from population screening and genetic studies. The total concentrations of serum T_4 and T_3 range widely in association with variant binding proteins, but none of the multiple hereditary binding alterations has been shown to confer any advantage or disadvantage, or to disturb thyroid hormone action, unless thyroid disease is associated. Plasma TSH concentrations remain normal, as do free T_4 and T_3 concentrations, provided the method of estimation is free of artifact. In general, TBG abnormalities tend to affect T_4 and T_3 similarly; by contrast, some albumin variants lead to selective abnormalities of T_4 or T_3 binding.

Variants of iodothyronine-binding proteins have attracted the attention of clinicians and basic scientists for numerous reasons, including the following:

- *Effect on diagnostic tests.* In euthyroid subjects, abnormal total T_4 or T_3 concentrations occur in association with normal free hormone concentrations. Particularly with the albumin variants, method-dependent artifacts may compromise measurements of free, occasionally total, T_4 or T_3.
- *Modes of inheritance.* TBG variants are X-linked, whereas TTR and albumin variants show autosomal dominant inheritance.
- *Structure-function relationships.* Structure-function relationships of specific hormone-binding sites can be studied by using the large amounts of material available in serum. Albumin variants have shown how structural changes can increase the binding affinity for a particular ligand. In

Table 22-2. Known Human Variants of Thyroid Hormone–Binding Proteins

Protein	Circulating Protein Concentration	T_4 Binding Affinity	Number of Variants
TBG	Undetectable	—	17
	Low	Low	8
	Normal	Normal	1
	Normal	Undetectable	1
	High	Normal	1
TTR*	?Normal	Undetectable	1
	?Normal	Low	5
	?Normal	Normal	3
	Normal/High	Increased	4
Albumin	Normal	Increased	3†
	Undetectable	—	1

Compiled from references 14, 15, 16, 17, 21, 22, 23, 32, 38, and 53.
T_3, Triiodothyronine; *T_4*, thyroxine; *TBG*, thyroxine-binding globulin; *TTR*, transthyretin.
*The T_4 binding affinity of more than 30 additional variants remains undefined.
†One variant has selective affinity for T_3.

contrast, TBG mutants show either normal or diminished binding affinity, often associated with abnormal heat lability.

- *Effects of variant binding proteins.* The effects of variant binding proteins on T_4 and T_3 distribution, clearance, and delivery to tissues can test the hypothesis that it is the free hormone concentration, as determined at equilibrium, that determines hormone clearance and action.
- *Changes in binding protein configuration.* The recent demonstration that TBG, a member of the serine protease inhibitor (SERPIN) class of proteins, can undergo cleavage or change in configuration at local tissue sites has led to important speculation that changes in binding protein configuration may facilitate tissue-specific hormone delivery (see below).
- *Tissue effects of abnormal proteins.* Other associated pathology, for example, the familial amyloidosis associated with some TTR variants, can elucidate tissue effects of abnormal proteins.

In contrast to the multitude of clearly defined plasma protein–binding variants, the possibility of genetically determined abnormalities of cell membrane transport, cytoplasmic binding, or deiodination of iodothyronines is less clearly defined (see below).

THYROXINE-BINDING GLOBULIN (TBG)

TBG is a single polypeptide chain α globulin, with molecular weight of about 54 kD synthesized as a 415 amino acid protein.[13-15] The first 20 amino acid residues of the TBG peptide are hydrophobic in nature and probably represent the signal peptide, which is removed in the endoplasmic reticulum, leaving a mature protein of 395 amino acids in a single chain with a molecular weight of about 44 kD. Multiple glycosylation sites allow an average of 10 terminal sialic acid moieties. The carbohydrate portions of TBG influence protein half-life in blood, stability in vitro, and microheterogeneity on electrophoresis, with only minor effects noted on immunoreactivity or T_4 binding. Although TBG is stable in stored serum at 4°C, it gradually loses its binding affinity for T_4 at 37°C or above. Differences in the rate of loss of binding affinity at raised temperature have been important in identifying TBG variants. Of particular interest are a variant with markedly increased heat stability (TBG-Chicago)[16] and a variant with an extremely heat-labile protein with an abnormally high concentration of denatured TBG and subnormal total T_4 (TBG-Gary).[17]

The amino acid sequence of human TBG shows homology with rat TBG (70%), human cortisol-binding globulin (55%) and members of the serum protease inhibitor family (SERPINS), which includes α-antitrypsin (53% homology) and a 1-antichymotrypsin (58% homology).[18] The significance of the structural similarity between human TBG, CBG, and the SERPINS remains unclear, because the hormone-binding proteins do not exhibit antiprotease activity.

Susceptibility to cleavage and change in configuration may modulate hormone delivery from the SERPIN family of binding proteins. The study of Zhou et al.[19] confirms that the binding of thyroxine to TBG can alter in response to changes in configuration of the binding protein. Using nonglycosylated recombinant human TBG, investigators reported that thyroxine is carried in a surface pocket and not within the beta barrel of the TBG molecule. With this structural model, conformational changes that result from relocation of a mobile peptide loop within the TBG molecule can favor binding or release of thyroxine. The demonstration of labile interaction between TBG and thyroxine raises the important possibility of modulated or tissue-specific delivery

of thyroxine that could vary in response to changes in local pH, temperature, or redox status. The details of how local tissue factors may enhance or limit local hormone release from SERPIN binding proteins remain to be studied (see later section, "Function of Iodothyronine Binding Proteins").

The normal concentration of human plasma TBG measured by radioimmunoassay is between 10 and 30 mg/L (0.2 to 0.6 μmol/L). TBG is normally 20% to 40% occupied by T_4 and <1% occupied by T_3. Occupancy may increase markedly in hyperthyroidism owing to increased total T_4 and decreased TBG concentrations, leading to a disproportionate rise in free T_4 relative to total T_4.[6] The T_4-binding affinity (kD), is about 50 pmol/L at 37°C, consistent with the estimate that TBG is approximately 30% occupied by T_4 at the normal free T_4 concentration of about 20 pmol/L.[20]

HEREDITARY TBG VARIANTS

The single 8 kilobase human *TBG* gene has been localized to the long arm of the X chromosome at site Xq21-q22.[14] Male hemizygotes who express a single mutant allele can show one of three variant phenotypes for T_4 binding to TBG: increase, decrease, or absolute deficiency. Despite the presence of two X chromosomes, normal females have TBG levels similar to those of males. Females heterozygous for complete TBG deficiency usually show less than the anticipated 50% reduction in serum TBG, a phenomenon attributed to selective inactivation of the mutant allele.[14,15] However, selective inactivation of the normal allele occasionally may result in females showing complete deficiency of TBG.[21]

Multiple inherited TBG variants, often designated geographically, can result in partial or complete deficiency of immunoreactive TBG in serum. Of at least 24 known X-linked TBG mutants, 15 may cause complete TBG deficiency, and eight other variants are associated with subnormal concentrations of immunoreactive serum TBG, often with reduced affinity for T_4.[13-15,22] The structural basis of numerous variants is summarized in Fig. 22-2. Several variants of TBG show decreased heat lability in vitro, which generally correlates with accelerated clearance in vivo. TBG deficiency (complete or partial) results from missense or nonsense mutations in the coding exons or in donor or acceptor splice sites.[14,15] Thus, single nucleotide deletions or substitutions can lead to a frame shift with premature termination of translation, resulting in a truncated protein that is retained and degraded intracellularly.[13-15] In some reports no mutations could be demonstrated in the TBG gene.[23]

In general, the various methods for serum free T_4 estimation, as well as binding corrections based on T_3–uptake measurements, give a useful semi-quantitative correction for TBG abnormalities, whether hereditary or acquired.

In total TBG deficiency, total T_4 is about 25 nmol/L (see Fig. 22-1), associated with normal free T_4 and TSH. By contrast, in hemizygous TBG excess, the total T_4 concentration is typically over 200 nmol/L, of which over 80% is carried on TBG (see Fig. 22-1).

From newborn screening studies, the prevalence of complete TBG deficiency in males is about 1 : 5000, with 1 : 15,000 showing complete deficiency,[15] but marked ethnic differences are noted in the frequency of hereditary TBG deficiency, with complete deficiency being highest in the Japanese.[14] Diminished TBG binding of T_4 is especially prevalent in Australian aborigines, up to 30% of whom have subnormal serum concentrations of total T_4, associated with subnormal serum concentrations of an abnormally heat-labile TBG that shows subnormal affinity for T_4.[24] Owing to a very high gene frequency in this population, the

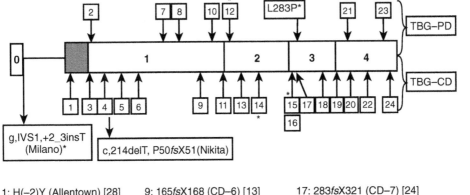

1: H(−2)Y (Allentown) [28]
2: S23T (San Diego) [16]
3: S23X (Portogues) [25]
4: 28fsX51 (Yonago) [20]
5: 38fsX51 (Negev) [23]
6: S52N (TBG–CDTI) [27]
7: I96N (Gary) [8]
8: A113P (Montreal) [14]

9: 165fsX168 (CD–6) [13]
10: D171N (TBG–Slow) [11]
11: 188fsX195 (Katakee) [22]
12: T191A (TBG–Aborigine) [9]
13: Q223X (Portogues) [25]
14: L227P (CD–5) [10]
15: W280X (Buffalo) [21]
16: W280X (TBG–CDT2) [27]

17: 283fsX321 (CD–7) [24]
18: Y309P (Chicago) [19]
19: 280fsX325 (Jackson) [26]
20: 329fsX374 (CD–8) [24]
21: H331Y (Quebec) [12]
22: 352fsX374 (CD–Japan) [15]
23: P363L (PD–J/Kumamoto) [17,18]
24: 382fsX384 (CDH or Harwichport) [24]

FIGURE 22-2. Summary of reported thyroxine-binding globulin (TBG) deficiency mutations. The numbered panel designates the five exons of TBG. Mutations above that panel refer to partial deficiency of TBG, and those below refer to total TBG deficiency. Polymorphisms are designated by an asterisk. Below the figure, details of each mutation are given, together with geographic designation and literature reference, as in Mannavola et al.[14] (From Mannavola et al., 2006.[14])

pattern of inheritance was initially thought to be autosomal dominant.[25] Abnormal heat lability at 37°C was found in both male and female subjects from affected families, but the pattern of intermediate heat lability was found exclusively in female subjects,[26] demonstrating that inheritance must be X-linked (Fig. 22-3). Hereditary TBG excess, probably due to gene duplication,[27] appears to have a prevalence of about 1:25,000 in newborn males.[15] The binding of T_4 to TBG in inherited X-linked TBG excess is indistinguishable from the common type of TBG. In contrast to the albumin variants, no known TBG mutant shows increased T_4-binding affinity.

ALBUMIN

Human serum albumin, a highly conserved 66 kD nonglycoprotein,[28] has a molar plasma concentration of approximately 600 μmol/L, corresponding to about 40 g/L. As well as being the principal carrier of numerous hydrophobic compounds in serum, albumin binds T_4 in its region 2, with an affinity about four orders of magnitude less than that of normal TBG. Albumin normally carries 10% to 15% of circulating T_4, but the proportion of albumin occupied by T_4 is less than 0.002%.

HEREDITARY ALBUMIN VARIANTS

Hyperthyroxinemia can result from variant albumins with increased affinity for T_4 or T_3, the total albumin concentration being normal (Table 22-3). In familial dysalbuminemic hyperthyroxinemia (FDH), the total T_4 concentration in affected individuals is about 200 nM,[29,30] with over 50% of T_4 carried on the variant albumin (see Fig. 22-1). FDH appears to be the most common hereditary T_4-binding abnormality, with a prevalence as high as 1:1000 in some Latin American populations.[31] As with other variants that show enhanced binding affinity or capacity, the increased concentration of total circulating T_4 appears to be an appropriate response to maintain a normal free T_4 concentration in feedback relationships with TSH.[30]

In FDH, Scatchard analysis of albumin binding shows two T_4-binding sites: a normal site with kD 4.3 mmol/L and an

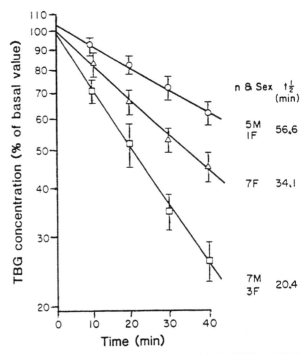

FIGURE 22-3. Heat stability of thyroxine-binding globulin (TBG) at 56°C in sera from Australian aborigines. Both male and female subjects showed either normal (*upper line*) or markedly reduced stability (*lower line*). No male subject showed the intermediate affinity (*middle line*) that demonstrates the heterozygous state, thereby confirming X-linked inheritance. (From Refetoff S, Murata Y: X-chromosome-linked inheritance of the variant thyroxine-binding globulin in Australian Aborigines. J Clin Endocrinol Metab 1985;60:356-360.)

abnormal site with 50- to 100-fold higher affinity, kD 50 nmol/L.[32] The capacity of the higher-affinity T_4-binding site is approximately 200 μmol/L, suggesting that relative to the molar concentration of albumin, at least one third of albumin molecules have the abnormal binding site.[32] As a result, the occupancy of albumin

Table 22-3. Abnormal Albumin Binding of Iodothyronines

	*Total Hormone (nmol/L)		Relative Affinity			
	T_4	T_3	T_4	T_3	Mutation	References
Normal serum	100	2.0	1	1	—	—
FDH	200	2.2	50-60	1.5	Arg 218 His	32, 34
FDH Japan	1800	4.0	>1000†	1	Arg 218 Pro	37
FDH Thailand	120	5.0	1.5	40	Leu 66 Pro	38

FDH, Familial dysalbuminemic hyperthyroxinemia; T_3, triiodothyronine; T_4, thyroxine.
*Free T_4 and free T_3 are normal by valid methods.
†Predicted.

by T_4 increases about fivefold to about 0.01%. The common FDH variant is due to Arg-His substitution at position 218 of human albumin,[33] with a T_4 affinity 65-fold greater than normal,[34] similar to the affinity reported for the natural protein more than a decade before.[32] Kinetic studies in vivo show altered distribution of T_4 in favor of the extracellular compartment and a reduced metabolic clearance rate of T_4.[35]

In FDH, because of a markedly increased affinity of the variant protein for numerous T_4-analogue tracers, serum free T_4 estimated by early analogue-tracer methods yielded results suggestive of thyrotoxicosis.[36] Greater albumin binding of tracer in FDH samples than in normal serum standards made less tracer available for binding to the assay antibody; the spurious decrease in bound counts resulted in a falsely high free T_4 estimate.

A related autosomal dominant albumin variant at the same site *(Arg 218 Pro)*, so far reported only in the Japanese,[37] shows an even higher selective T_4 affinity than the common FDH phenotype found in Caucasians. In euthyroid subjects with normal TSH, total T_4 is almost 20-fold elevated at about 1800 nmol/L (see Fig. 22-1), whereas total T_3 is only about twofold elevated. Free T_4 estimates using analogue tracer also show spurious elevations in this variant.[37]

To explain the mechanism of increased T_4 affinity in both types of FDH, it has been suggested that the guanidine group of arginine 218 normally may give an unfavorable binding interaction with T_4. Histidine and proline, which lack the guanidine group, allow higher-affinity binding than is seen with wild-type albumin.[37]

A recent report described a mutation of the albumin gene at a different site *(Leu 66 Pro)* with selective affinity for T_3 rather than T_4.[38] Eight euthyroid members of a Thai family showed total T_3 levels of 4 to 8 nmol/L (normal, 1.0 to 2.6) when measured by radioimmunoassay with the use of I^{125} T_3. Free T_3 and free T_4 were normal. This mutant albumin was estimated to have a 40-fold higher T_3 affinity than normal albumin, but only a 1.5-fold higher affinity for T_4. However, spuriously low total T_3 values were found when T_3 conjugates were used as tracer in enzyme-linked immunosorbent (ELISA) assays.[38] The conjugate tracer, linked to alkaline phosphatase or to peroxidase, showed less binding to the variant albumin than to the natural protein, making more tracer available for binding to antibody in sample than in standard, the opposite artifact to that found with analogue-tracer free T_4 estimates in the common type of FDH.

Only a few cases of total hereditary analbuminemia have been described in man, but in one kindred,[39] evidence of mild TSH excess was found, consistent with impaired thyroid hormone delivery. In contrast, the Nagase strain of analbuminemic rat showed no evidence of any abnormality of thyroid hormone action or distribution.[40]

TRANSTHYRETIN

Transthyretin (TTR, previously known as prealbumin), a protein of approximately 55 kD that circulates in the serum of a wide range of vertebrates, is a tetramer consisting of four identical polypeptide chains held together by noncovalent bonds. Each monomer is a 127 amino acid chain regulated by a single gene on chromosome 18. The tetramer is symmetrical about a central cavity that completely penetrates the molecule and contains two T_4-binding sites, one at each end of the central cavity.[41]

The normal serum concentration of TTR in healthy humans (2 to 8 μmol/L, 100 to 400 mg/L) can decrease rapidly during acute illness or malnutrition as a result of reduced hepatic synthesis.[42] At normal concentrations, TTR is <1% occupied by T_4, with a T_4 affinity (kD $\approx$ 10 nmol/L) lower than TBG and higher than albumin. TTR has about 10-fold lower affinity for T_3 than for T_4. The liver is the principal site of synthesis of TTR, but the choroid plexus[43] and the pancreatic islets[44] are additional sites of TTR synthesis. In evolutionary terms, TTR synthesis at the choroid plexus long preceded the ontogeny of TTR synthesis in the liver.[45] The T_4-binding domain of TTR appears to have been conserved over the past 350 million years.[45]

HEREDITARY TRANSTHYRETIN VARIANTS

Many autosomal dominant TTR variants characterized by single amino acid substitutions have been described in man, some found in association with familial amyloidosis due to formation of abnormal amyloid fibrils (see reference 46 for review). Complete deficiency of TTR has never been described in humans, suggesting that a deficiency of this protein might be lethal. However, transthyretin-null mice produced by gene knockout show no obvious abnormality of thyroid hormone metabolism or action.[47]

The Thr[109] TTR variant[48] can give rise to mild hyperthyroxinemia with a total concentration of T_4 of 160 to 200 nmol/L,[49] associated with some increase in the total concentration of TTR.[49] Kinetic studies with this variant protein show a T_4-binding affinity about sevenfold higher than normal TTR.[50] In the face of normal TBG and albumin concentrations, Thr[109] TTR probably binds about 50% of circulating T_4 in euthyroid subjects (see Fig. 22-1). The Val[109] and Met[119] variants of TTR also have increased affinity for T_4, but serum total T_4 is outside the reference range only in the former.[51,52] TTR variants are not known to cause spurious assay values for total or free T_4.

Of at least 30 mutations described for TTR, many have now been examined for T_4 affinity. A study that compared the interaction of T_4 with 10 different naturally occurring human TTR variants showed a wide range of T_4 affinities.[53] Relative to the wild-type TTR, three show increased affinity for T_4—the Thr[109] and Val[109] variants of sufficient affinity to cause euthyroid hyperthyroxinemia—and three have approximately normal affinity, with five TTR variants showing reduced affinity for T_4.[54]

Function of Iodothyronine-Binding Proteins

The large pool of extracellular thyroxine that is maintained as a result of plasma protein binding is equivalent to 10 to 15 days of hormone secretion from the normal thyroid. Avid protein binding is the basis for the long plasma half-life of about 7 days and the slow metabolic clearance rate of thyroxine, both of which favor sustained thyroid hormone action. A high degree of protein binding also serves to protect against iodine loss from urinary excretion of unbound iodothyronines. It is notable that Ekins had pointed out that protein binding of T_4 may have a key role in T_4 delivery to the fetus in early pregnancy[55] (see below), well before the homology of TBG with the serine antiproteases was demonstrated in 1986.[16]

Autoradiographic studies suggest that binding proteins facilitate even tissue distribution of iodothyronines[56] but indicate that multiple binding protein classes are redundant in this respect. When rat liver lobules were perfused with ^{125}I T_4 in the absence of binding protein, almost all of the T_4 was taken up by the periportal cells. When 4% human serum albumin or human serum was added to the perfusate, the labeled hormone was taken up uniformly by all cells within the lobule. When a competitor was added to displace T_4 from albumin, uptake was again predominantly periportal.[56]

Interest is increasing in the possibility that selective cleavage or change in the configuration of TBG, as occurs with other SERPIN proteins, may facilitate selective delivery of T_4, for example, at sites of inflammation or in the placenta.[57,58] Rapid clearance of TBG has been reported in the early postoperative phase after coronary artery surgery,[59] and a truncated circulating form of the molecule, with lower affinity for T_4, has been reported in sera from patients with sepsis[60] and after cardiopulmonary bypass.[61] Cleavage of TBG with decreased T_4-binding affinity has been demonstrated to result from leukocyte elastase activity.[62] These findings have renewed interest in the earlier suggestion[63] that high local tissue T_4 concentrations might allow release of iodine in concentrations sufficient to enhance leukocyte bactericidal activity. However, it is notable that males who are completely deficient in TBG appear to suffer no disadvantage in terms of their response to infection.

It is speculated that selective placental TBG cleavage with local release of free T_4 could facilitate transfer of iodine to the fetus.[64] If additional studies confirm these mechanisms, it will become relevant to consider TBG as a selective delivery protein, rather than a molecule that simply prevents rapid T_4 clearance and ensures uniform tissue delivery of the hormone. Although TBG does not appear to have a role in targeted hormone delivery via specific cellular receptors for this protein, as shown for corticosteroid-binding globulin,[65] a similar effect may be achieved through selective tissue-specific dissociation of thyroid hormone.

Thus, accumulating evidence suggests that the thyroid hormone–binding proteins are more than simply passive reservoirs of bound hormone. Based on cross-species differences and ontogeny, as well as the tissue perfusion study cited above, the trend is to designate the serum carriers of thyroid hormone as "distributor proteins" rather than passive carriers.[66] Nevertheless,

none of the many human variants in any of the three major binding proteins appears to confer any survival advantage or disadvantage.

Acquired Alterations in the Concentration of Transport Proteins

Numerous drugs can influence the concentrations of TBG and TTR (Table 22-4) through effects that alter protein synthesis or influence degradation; in many instances, the mechanism has not yet been clearly defined. The most common acquired change in TBG is an increase in concentration due to exogenous or endogenous estrogens that result in TBG with a greater proportion of bands with anodal mobility on isoelectric focusing, caused by an increase in sialic acid content of the side chains.[67] Reduced TBG degradation due to this oligosaccharide modification appears to be the major mechanism of estrogen-induced TBG excess.[68] Transdermal estrogens without predominant effect on the liver do not have this effect.[69]

Serum concentrations of TBG are reduced in thyrotoxicosis and increased in hypothyroidism in humans[70] and in experimental primate studies.[71] Serum TBG concentrations are decreased by glucocorticoid excess.[72] Unlike human TBG, rat TBG is strongly repressed during adult life but actively expressed during postnatal development, in senescence, in the face of malnutrition, and in hypothyroidism,[73] and also after adrenalectomy,[74] possibly as part of an adaptive response.

If the concentration of TBG were to increase acutely, a number of changes would result in reequilibration of the pituitary-thyroid axis. First, a shift of T_4 from tissues to blood would decrease T_4 clearance, and this would be followed by activation of pituitary TSH secretion in response to lower tissue levels of free T_4, with increased T_4 production until the original concentration of serum free T_4 is restored at a higher total T_4. At the new steady state, the intravascular T_4 pool would increase with a decrease in the fractional turnover rate, but the rate of T_4 secretion and degradation would return to baseline. Opposite changes would follow an abrupt decrease in the concentration of TBG, similar to the changes in occupancy of TBG by an alternative ligand, for example, a drug competitor (see below).

Acquired changes in TTR concentration are common but have relatively minor effects on the total serum concentrations of T_4 and T_3 because of the low occupancy of this protein.

Table 22-4. Drug Effects on Serum TBG and TTR Concentrations in Humans

Increase TBG	Decrease TBG
Estrogens	Thyroid hormones
Tamoxifen	Androgens, anabolic steroids
Heroin	Glucocorticoids
Methadone	L-asparaginase
5-Fluorouracil	Interleukin-6
Perphenazine	
Clofibrate	
Mitotane	

Increase TTR	Decrease TTR
Androgens	Estrogens
Glucocorticoids	

TBG, Thyroxine-binding globulin; TTR, transthyretin.

Androgens[75] and glucocorticoids[72] increase, while estrogens decrease the concentrations of TTR[76]; these agents have the opposite effect on TBG. Hepatic synthesis of TTR decreases abruptly during any major illness. Some islet cell carcinomas can directly synthesize and release sufficient TTR to cause euthyroid hyperthyroxinemia.[77]

Competition for Thyroid Hormone Transport Sites

In contrast to binding proteins for corticosteroids, vitamin D, and sex hormones, which are highly specific for a single family of ligands, the iodothyronine-binding proteins show wide cross-reactivity with unrelated hydrophobic ligands, such as nonesterified fatty acids (NEFAs) and numerous drugs (Table 22-5). Each of these substances itself is highly bound to albumin; the unbound rather than the total concentrations of each ligand determine competition.

COMPETITION IN SERUM

When competition is studied by examining displacement of labeled T_4 or T_3 from an isolated binding protein, using the unlabeled hormone as reference, the affinities of important drug competitors for TBG range from three orders of magnitude less (furosemide) to almost seven orders of magnitude less than T_4 itself, in the case of aspirin.[78] However, such direct studies do not reflect in vivo competition, because the free serum concentration of a competitor is determined by its binding to sites other than TBG, in particular albumin. Many highly bound drugs circulate in micromolar concentrations and may occupy 5% to 50% of albumin-binding sites; the concentration of albumin, or its occupancy by other ligands, then becomes an important determinant of the free drug concentration. Because of differences in albumin binding, the hierarchy of drug competitor potency at relevant therapeutic concentrations in undiluted serum differs markedly from the affinity of drugs for TBG in isolation.[25,26] The data shown in Table 22-5 are influenced by the total concentration of each drug and its free fraction, as well as by its affinity for T_4-binding proteins.

Table 22-5. Principal Drugs That Displace T_4 from TBG Binding in Normal Human Serum

Drug	Mean Percent Increase in Free T_4 Fraction*
Salicylates	
Acetyl salicylic acid (aspirin)	62
Salicyl salicylic acid (salsalate)	>100
Furosemide[†]	5-30
Fenclofenac	90
Mefenamic acid	31
Flufenamic acid	10
Diclofenac	7
Diflunisal	37
Phenytoin	45
Carbamazepine	30

Data from references 78, 80, 83, 87, and 88.
T_4, Thyroxine; *TBG*, thyroxine-binding globulin.
*Equilibrium dialysis or ultrafiltration of undiluted serum at 37°C in vitro, at appropriate therapeutic concentrations of each drug.
†Wide therapeutic range.

DILUTION EFFECTS

When working with a highly bound ligand, such as T_4, it is technically easier to study binding in diluted serum. In the absence of competitors, such measurements give useful comparisons between samples with high, normal, and low free hormone concentrations. However, it is difficult to establish a system in which the concentrations of free hormone, competitors, and unoccupied binding sites are maintained in the relationships that apply in vivo. Existing literature on competitor effects has become confused because details such as dilution and albumin concentration are often poorly defined. The terms "pre-dilution" and "co-dilution" are useful in defining potential artifacts.[7]

Pre-dilution occurs when the concentration of binding proteins is progressively decreased before particular concentrations of competitor are added (Fig. 22-4). The lower the concentration of albumin, the higher is the occupancy of available binding sites; this leads to a disproportionate increase in the free competitor concentration, which magnifies apparent competitor potency.[79] For example, in the case of a highly albumin-bound competitor, the T_4-displacing effect of 5 mM oleic acid added to undiluted serum could be matched almost exactly by 0.5 mM oleic acid in serum diluted 1:10.[80] In general, pre-dilution of the sample magnifies apparent competition.

Co-dilution occurs when whole serum is serially diluted so that total concentrations of binding proteins, hormone, and competitors diminish in parallel. Notably, the **free** ligand concentrations do not decrease in parallel. The difference becomes clear when a hormone such as T_4, with a free fraction of about 1:4000, is compared with a drug that has a free fraction in serum of 1:50. Progressive dissociation will sustain the free T_4 concentration at 1:100 dilution (although the free fraction rises sharply as a result of dissociation). In contrast, the free drug concentration decreases markedly after a dilution of only 1:10. Hence, co-dilution effects

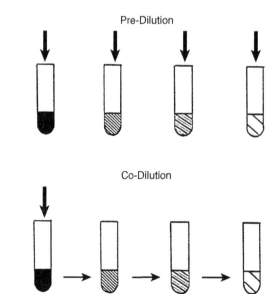

FIGURE 22-4. Pre-dilution: serum is diluted, followed by addition of a particular concentration of competitor. The effect of the competitor will be overestimated as albumin occupancy increases. Co-dilution: The competitor is added to serum, followed by identical simultaneous dilution of binding proteins, hormone, and competitors. If the competitor is less highly bound than the hormone, its effect will be progressively underestimated. (From Stockigt et al: Thyroid hormone transport. In Weetman AP, Grossman A [eds]: Pharmacotherapeutics of the thyroid gland, pp 119–150. Springer, Berlin, 1997.)

lead to underestimation of the potency of competitors that are less highly protein bound than the hormone itself.

A co-dilution effect was the clue that led to the recognition of furosemide as an important inhibitor of T_4 binding in serum.[81] When T_4 binding was studied in serial dilution in critically ill hypothyroxinemic patients, those who had received high-dose furosemide showed a marked increase in free T_4 fraction that became less obvious with progressive dilution.[81] When the abilities of three commercial free T_4 assays to detect the T_4-displacing effect of furosemide were compared, the effect was most obvious in the method with least sample dilution[82] (Fig. 22-5).

The importance of a pre-dilution effect was demonstrated for therapeutic concentrations of phenytoin and carbamazepine, which increased the free fraction of T_4 by 40% to 50% with the use of ultrafiltration of undiluted serum.[83] However, no increase in T_4 free fraction was seen with a commercial single-step free T_4 assay after 1:5 serum dilution.[83] During continuing drug therapy, total T_4 was lowered by 25% to 50%, resulting in calculated free concentrations within the normal range.

KINETICS OF THE COMPETITOR

The kinetics of the competitor itself will determine how it influences hormone binding in vivo (Fig. 22-6). A competitor of short half-life such as furosemide or salsalate will show fluctuating effects on hormone binding so that free hormone estimates may vary widely, depending on the time between dosage and sampling.[84,85] In contrast, a competitor of long half-life will result in a new steady state with a normal free hormone concentration and a lowered total hormone concentration (i.e., an increased free fraction). It is not yet known whether intermittent competitor-induced increases in free hormone concentration can augment hormone action in humans, but it has been shown that a T_3- and T_4-displacing synthetic flavonoid has a transient thyromimetic effect in rats.[86]

INTERACTION BETWEEN COMPETITORS

Increasing concentrations of any substance that shares albumin-binding sites with a competitor can increase the free concentration of that competitor. Two substances that show potential to exert such a "cascade" effect on T_4 binding in serum are oleic acid[87] and 3-carboxy-4-methyl-5-propyl-2-furanpropanoic acid

(CMPF),[88] a naturally occurring furanoid acid that accumulates in renal failure. At concentrations that had only a minimal direct effect on the binding of T_4 in undiluted normal serum, oleic acid and CMPF can augment the T_4-displacing effect in undiluted serum of several drug competitors for T_4 binding.[88] Through such a mechanism, free hormone concentrations can be influenced by substances that have little direct interaction with hormone-binding sites.

SPURIOUS COMPETITION

The effect of heparin in increasing the apparent free T_4 concentration can be misleading owing to another in vitro artifact. As summarized in Fig. 22-7, increases in free T_4 that result from heparin treatment may cause in vivo release of lipase, followed by in vitro generation of NEFA, during assay incubation or storage.[89] As a result of this artifact, serum NEFA concentrations at the time of assay can be much higher than they were in vivo.[90] This effect may account for some reports of apparent increases in free T_4 and free T_3 fractions in critically ill subjects, although selective degradation of TBG at the site of sepsis or inflammation[60,62] would provide an alternative explanation. In cases where heparin has been given, assays of total T_4 and T_3 are likely to be more informative than assays of free T_4 and T_3, unless special precautions are taken to avoid in vitro generation of NEFA.[90]

Studies of Specific Binding Sites

If the capacity and affinity of each of the heterogeneous thyroid hormone–binding sites in serum are known, it is possible to manipulate hormone concentration and sample dilution to

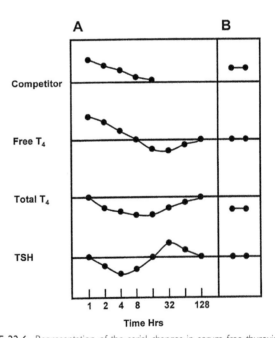

FIGURE 22-6. Representation of the serial changes in serum free thyroxine (T_4), total T_4, and thyroid-stimulating hormone (TSH) that follow ingestion of a single dose of a potent competitor for T_4 binding to thyroxine-binding globulin (TBG) *(panel A)*. An initial increase in free T_4 is followed by a decrease in TSH and accelerated T_4 clearance, resulting in a decrease in total and free T_4, followed by a rebound increase in TSH. Note logarithmic time scale. *Panel B* shows the effect of a competitor of long half-life, or frequent dosage of a short half-life competitor, with stabilization at a new steady state with normal serum free T_4 and TSH concentrations, but a decrease in total T_4. (Compiled from data in Newnham et al.[84] and Wang et al.[85])

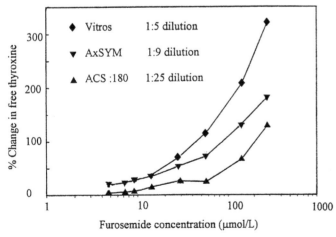

FIGURE 22-5. Effect of addition of furosemide to serum on estimates of free thyroxine (T_4) using three commercial free T_4 methods that involve varying degrees of sample dilution. The effect of the competitor is progressively obscured with increasing sample dilution. (Data from Hawkins RC. Furosemide interference in newer free thyroxine assays, Clin Chem 1998;44:2550-2551.)

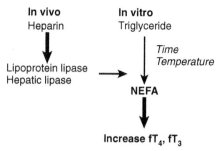

FIGURE 22-7. Summary of the heparin-induced changes that can markedly increase the apparent concentration of serum free thyroxine (T_4). Heparin acts in vivo *(left)* to liberate lipoprotein lipase from vascular endothelium. Lipase acts in vitro *(right)* to increase the concentration of nonesterified fatty acids (NEFA) to levels >3 mmol/L, resulting in displacement of T_4 and triiodothyronine (T_3) from thyroxine-binding globulin (TBG). In vitro generation of NEFA is increased by sample storage at room temperature or incubation at 37°C and by high concentration of serum triglyceride. The T_4-displacing effect of NEFA is accentuated at low albumin concentrations.[80,89]

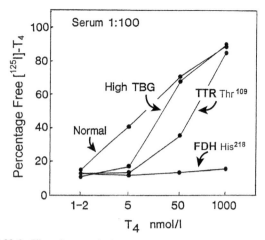

FIGURE 22-8. Effect of progressive increase in the load of unlabeled thyroxine (T_4) on dextran-charcoal uptake of ^{125}I T_4 at 4°C in sera (diluted in phosphate buffer) from normal, thyroxine-binding globulin (TBG) excess, transthyretin (TTR) Thr,[109] and familial dysalbuminemic hyperthyroxinemia (FDH) His[218] subjects. In the presence of 1000-fold T_4 excess, FDH shows unique persistence of ^{125}I T_4 binding at 4°C (low charcoal uptake) characteristic of a high-capacity site of increased affinity. Data from reference 92. (Modified from Stockigt JR: Serum TSH and thyroid hormone measurements and assessment of thyroid hormone transport. In Braverman LE and Utiger RD, eds: Werner and Ingbar's The Thyroid, 1996, Seventh Edition, pp 377–396. JB Lippincott, Philadelphia.)

effectively isolate a single class of binding site.[7] In this way, binding and competition can be characterized without isolating the protein. Similar approaches ultimately may be applicable to studies of heterogeneous hormone-binding sites in the intracellular milieu.

Because the affinity (kD) of any binding site is defined as the free hormone concentration that achieves half occupancy, it follows that change in bound/total or bound/free hormone is analytically optimal when the concentration of binding sites is approximately double the kD (i.e., when bound/free ratio is about unity and bound/total hormone about 50%).

Because the T_4-binding affinities of TBG and albumin differ by about four orders of magnitude, high-affinity binding can be "dissected" from low-affinity sites by manipulating the free hormone concentration via high sample dilution or hormone loading. For example, if normal serum with a total T_4 concentration of 100 nM is diluted 5000 fold, the total T_4 concentration will be 20 pM—close to the affinity of TBG. When ^{125}I-T4 of high specific activity is used, the effects of drug competitors on specific T_4 binding to TBG can be studied in such a system without the need to isolate the protein. The effects of TTR and albumin are negligible under these conditions.[7] Such a method can be used to measure the minute amounts of TBG produced by cultured cells.[91] Conversely, low-affinity binding is best examined after hormone loading to achieve a free concentration close to the affinity of that site; at high free hormone concentrations, the low-capacity sites are saturated and are not altered by changes in free hormone concentration. At artificially high hormone concentrations, the abnormally avid binding of T_4 to albumin in familial dysalbuminemic hyperthyroxinemia can be readily demonstrated in the presence of 1000-fold relative excess of unlabeled T_4[92] (Fig. 22-8).

Cell Membrane and Intracellular Transport

Until recently, it has been assumed that thyroid hormones move passively from the extracellular fluid through the cell membrane and cytoplasm to their nuclear receptors, but numerous studies have shown apparently specific binding or transport at both these locations. It is not yet clear whether the apparent

competition between T_3 or T_4 and other ligands is truly specific, or whether apparent saturability and competition merely reflect interaction between intensely lipophilic molecules.[93,94] Hennemann and Visser have reviewed the evidence for active cell membrane transport,[95] and studies from their group suggest that bilirubin[96] and fatty acids[97] in sera from critically ill patients may limit the rate of T_4 uptake by hepatocytes, thus limiting the amount of substrate available for conversion to T_3.

Numerous substances, including calmodulin antagonists and calcium channel blockers, have been shown to inhibit cellular uptake of T_3 by mechanisms that appear to be competitive.[98] The demonstration in a cultured cell line of a saturable, stereospecific, verapamil-inhibitable mechanism that mediates T_3 efflux[99] raises the possibility that variable exit of T_3 may modify thyroid hormone action. A putative transport protein was identified by photoaffinity labeling.[99]

Cytoplasmic T_3 binding can be competitively inhibited by some anti-inflammatory agents and non–bile acid cholephils,[100] but interpretation of these interactions is uncertain because the relevant free concentrations of hormone and competitor at cytoplasmic binding sites are not known. A nicotinamide adenine dinucleotide phosphate (NADPH)-dependent cytosolic T_3-binding protein has been reported to limit efflux of T_3 from the nucleus[101] and has been shown to be expressed mainly in cardiac and neural tissue.[102] Numerous possible nongenomic actions of thyroid and steroid hormones have been described,[103] but it is not known how novel binding sites or transport proteins might be involved in these effects.

Of the numerous cell membrane proteins that bind thyroid hormone, only monocarboxylate transporter 8 (MCT8) and organic anion-transporting polypeptide 1C1 (OATP-1C1) show sufficient specificity toward thyroid hormone to suggest a physiologic role.[104] It is now established that MCT8 is critical to the availability of thyroid hormone for intracellular deiodination and receptor binding, particularly in neural tissues and in placenta.[104]

The relative importance of these transport systems for inward and outward transit of thyroid hormone remains uncertain.[104]

Abnormalities of thyroid hormone transport across cell membranes of neural tissues, particularly those related to *MCT8* mutations, may be associated with severe disease.[105] The demonstration[106,107] that various *MCT8* mutations are associated with severe X-linked psychomotor retardation defines a new mechanism of disease. In this disorder, known by the eponym Allan-Herndon-Dudley syndrome, affected boys show serum T_3 concentrations two- to fourfold in excess of normal, without a clear-cut abnormality of serum T_4 or TSH. No deiodinase or thyroid hormone receptor abnormalities have been identified, and affected subjects appear to be euthyroid in tissues other than the brain. This uncommon hereditary disorder demonstrates that active transit of thyroid hormone into cells is crucial for normal brain development in humans.[106,107] Thyroid hormone action did not appear to be impaired in tissues such as liver, muscle, or fat. Treatment of this disorder remains unsatisfactory.[104-107]

REFERENCES

1. Trevorrow V: Studies on the nature of the iodine in blood, J Biol Chem 127:737–750, 1939.
2. Robbins J, Cheng S-Y, Gershengorn MC, et al: Thyroxine transport proteins of plasma, molecular properties and biosynthesis, Rec Prog Horm Res 34:477–519, 1978.
3. Benvenga S, Cahnmann HJ, Robbins J: Characterization of thyroid hormone binding to apolipoprotein-E: localization of the binding site in the exon 3-coded domain, Endocrinology 133:1300–1305, 1993.
4. Hillier AP: Thyroxine dissociation in human plasma: measurement of its rate by a continuous-flow dialysis method, Acta Endocrinologica 78:32–38, 1975.
5. Refetoff S, Robin NI, Fang VS: Parameters of thyroid function in serum from 16 selected vertebrate species, Endocrinology 86:793–805, 1970.
6. Nauman JA, Nauman A, Werner SC: Total and free triiodothyronine in human serum, J Clin Invest 46:1346–1355, 1967.
7. Stockigt JR, Lim C-F, Barlow JW, et al: Thyroid hormone transport. In Weetman AP, Grossman A, editors: Pharmacotherapeutics of the thyroid gland, Berlin, 1997, Springer, pp 119–150.
8. Korcek L, Tabachnick M: Thyroxine-protein interactions, interaction of thyroxine and triiodothyronine with human TBG, J Biol Chem 251:3558–3562, 1976.
9. Mendel CM: The free hormone hypothesis: a physiologically based mathematical model, Endocr Rev 10:232–274, 1989.
10. Mendel CM: The free hormone hypothesis and free hormone transport hypothesis: Update 1994 Endocrine Reviews monographs. In Braverman LE, Refetoff S, editors: Clinical and molecular aspects of diseases of the thyroid. Endocr Reviews Monographs, Vol 3, Chevy Chase, Md, 1994, The Endocrine Society, pp 208–209.
11. Pardridge WM: Transport of protein-bound hormones into tissue in vivo, Endocr Rev 2:103–123, 1981.
12. Mendel CM, Weisiger RA: Thyroxine uptake by perfused rat liver: no evidence for facilitation by five different thyroxine-binding proteins, J Clin Invest 86:1840–1847, 1990.
13. Refetoff S: Inherited thyroxine-binding globulin abnormalities in man, Endocr Rev 10:275–293, 1989.
14. Mannavola D, Vannucchi G, Fugazzola L, et al: TBG deficiency: description of two novel mutations associated with complete TBG deficiency and review of the literature, J Mol Med 84:864–871, 2006.
15. Refetoff S, Murata Y, Mori Y, et al: Thyroxine-binding globulin: organisation of the gene and variants, Horm Res 45:128–138, 1996.
16. Janssen OE, Chen B, Büttner C, et al: Molecular and structural characterization of the heat-resistant thyroxine-binding globulin—Chicago, J Biol Chem 270:28234–28238, 1995.
17. Murata Y, Takamatsu J, Refetoff S: Inherited abnormality of thyroxine-binding globulin with no demonstrable thyroxine-binding activity and high serum levels of denatured thyroxine-binding globulin, N Engl J Med 314:694–699, 1986.
18. Flink IL, Bailey TJ, Gustafson TA, et al: Complete amino acid sequence of human thyroxine-binding globulin deduced from cloned DNA: Close homology to the serine antiproteases, Proc Natl Acad Sci U S A 83:7708–7712, 1986.
19. Zhou A, Wei Z, Read RJ, et al: Structural mechanism for the carriage and release of thyroxine in the blood, Proc Nat Acad Sci U S A 103:13321–13326, 2006.
20. Robbins J, Bartalena L: Plasma transport of thyroid hormones. In Hennemann G, editor: Thyroid Hormone Metabolism, New York, 1986, Marcel Dekker, pp 3–38.
21. Okamoto H, Mori Y, Tani Y, et al: Molecular analysis of females manifesting thyroxine-binding globulin (TBG) deficiency: selective X-chromosome inactivation responsible for the difference between phenotype and genotype in TBG-deficient females, J Clin Endocrinol Metab 81:2204–2208, 1996.
22. Carvalho GA, Weiss RE, Refetoff S: Complete thyroxine-binding globulin (TBG) deficiency produced by a mutation in acceptor splice site causing frameshift and early termination of translation (TBG-Kankakee), J Clin Endocrinol Metab 83:3604–3608, 1998.
23. Retrakul A, Dimitrescu A, Macchia PE, et al: Complete TBG deficiency in two families without mutations in coding or promoter regions of the TBG genes: in vitro demonstration of exon skipping, J Clin Endocrinol Metab 87:1045–1051, 2002.
24. Murata Y, Refetoff S, Sarne DH, et al: Variant thyroxine-binding globulin in serum of Australian aborigines: its physical, chemical and biological properties, J Endocrinol Invest 8:225–232, 1985.
25. Watson F, Dick M: Distribution and inheritance of low serum thyroxine-binding globulin levels in Australian Aborigines, Med J Aust 2:385–387, 1980.
26. Refetoff S, Murata Y: X-chromosome-linked inheritance of the variant thyroxine-binding globulin in Australian Aborigines, J Clin Endocrinol Metab 60:356–360, 1985.
27. Mori Y, Miura Y, Takeuchi H, et al: Gene amplification as a cause of inherited thyroxine-binding globulin excess in two Japanese families, J Clin Endocrinol Metab 80:3758–3762, 1995.
28. Peters T Jr: Serum albumin, Adv Protein Chem 37:161–245, 1985.
29. Hennemann G, Docter R, Krenning EP, et al: Raised total thyroxine and free thyroxine index but normal free thyroxine, Lancet 1:639–642, 1979.
30. Stockigt JR, Topliss DJ, Barlow JW, et al: Familial euthyroid thyroxine excess: an appropriate response to abnormal thyroxine binding associated with albumin, J Clin Endocrinol Metab 53:353–359, 1981.
31. Arevalo G: Prevalence of familial dysalbuminemic hyperthyroxinemia in serum samples received for thyroid testing, Clin Chem 37:1430–1431, 1991.
32. Barlow JW, Csicsmann JM, White EL, et al: Familial euthyroid thyroxine excess: characterisation of abnormal intermediate-affinity thyroxine binding to albumin, J Clin Endocrinol Metab 55:244–250, 1982.
33. Petersen CE, Scottolini AG, Cody LR, et al: A point mutation in the human serum albumin gene results in familial dysalbuminaemic hyperthyroxinaemia, J Med Genet 31:355–359, 1994.
34. Petersen CE, Ha CE, Mandel M, et al: Expression of a human serum albumin variant with high affinity for thyroxine, Biochem Biophys Res Commun 214:1121–1129, 1995.
35. Mendel CM, Cavalieri RR: Thyroxine distribution and metabolism in familial dysalbuminemic hyperthyroxinemia, J Clin Endocrinol Metab 59:499–504, 1984.
36. Stockigt JR, Stevens V, White EL, et al: "Unbound analog" radioimmunoassays for free thyroxin measure the albumin-bound hormone fraction, Clin Chem 29:1408–1410, 1983.
37. Wada N, Chiba H, Shimizu C, et al: A novel missense mutation in codon 218 of the albumin gene in a distinct phenotype of familial dysalbuminemic hyperthyroxinemia in a Japanese kindred, J Clin Endocrinol Metab 82:3246–3250, 1997.
38. Sunthornthepvarakul T, Likitmaskul S, Ngowngarmratana S, et al: Familial dysalbuminemic hypertriiodothyroninemia: a new, dominantly inherited albumin defect, J Clin Endocrinol Metab 83:1448–1454, 1998.
39. Kallee E: Bennhold's analbuminemia: a follow-up study of the first two cases (1953–1992), J Lab Clin Med 127:470–480, 1996.
40. Mendel CM, Cavalieri RR, Gavin LA, et al: Thyroxine transport and distribution in Nagase analbuminemic rats, J Clin Invest 83:143–148, 1989b.
41. Robbins J, Cheng S-Y, Gershengorn MC, et al: Thyroxine transport proteins of plasma, molecular properties and biosynthesis, Rec Prog Horm Res 34:477–519, 1978.
42. Schreiber G: Synthesis, processing and secretion of plasma proteins by the liver and other organs and their regulation. In Putnam PW, editor: The plasma proteins: structure, function and genetic control, ed 2, Vol V, Orlando, Fl, 1987, Academic Press, pp 293–363.
43. Schreiber G, Aldred AR, Jaworowski A, et al: Thyroxine transport from blood to brain via transthyretin synthesis in choroid plexus, Am J Physiol 258:R338–R345, 1990.
44. Jacobsson B, Carlstrom A, Plotz A, et al: Transthyretin messenger ribonucleic acid expression in the pancreas and in endocrine tumors of the pancreas and gut, J Clin Endocrinol Metab 71:875–880, 1990.
45. Richardson SJ, Bradley AJ, Duan W, et al: Evolution of marsupial and other vertebrate thyroxine-binding plasma proteins, Am J Physiol 266:R1359–R1370, 1994.
46. Saraiva MJM: Transthyretin mutations in health and disease, Human Mutation 5:191–196, 1995.
47. Palha JA, Episkopou V, Maede S, et al: Thyroid hormone metabolism in a transthyretin-null mouse strain, J Biol Chem 269:33135–33139, 1994.
48. Moses AC, Rosen HN, Moller DE, et al: A point mutation in transthyretin increases affinity for thyroxine and produces euthyroid hyperthyroxinaemia, J Clin Invest 86:2025–2033, 1990.
49. Moses AC, Lawlor J, Haddow J, et al: Familial euthyroid hyperthyroxinemia resulting from increased thyroxine binding to thyroxine-binding prealbumin, N Engl J Med 306:966–969, 1982.
50. Lalloz MRA, Byfield PGH, Himsworth RL: A prealbumin variant with an increased affinity for T_4 and reverse-T_3, Clin Endocrinol 21:331–338, 1984.
51. Refetoff S, Marinov VSZ, Tunca H, et al: A new family with hyperthyroxinemia caused by transthyretin Val[109] misdiagnosed as thyrotoxicosis and resistance to thyroid hormone—a clinical research centre study, J Clin Endocrinol Metab 81:3335–3340, 1996.
52. Curtis AJ, Scrimshaw BJ, Topliss DJ, et al: Thyroxine binding by human transthyretin variants: mutations at position 119, but not position 54, increase thyroxine binding affinity, J Clin Endocrinol Metab 78:459–462, 1994.
53. Rosen HN, Moses AC, Murrell JR, et al: Thyroxine interactions with transthyretin: a comparison of 10 different naturally occurring human transthyretin variants, J Clin Endocrinol Metab 77:370–374, 1993.
54. Bartalena L: Thyroid hormone-binding proteins: Update 1994. In Braverman LE, Refetoff S, editors: Clinical and molecular aspects of diseases of the thyroid. Endocrine Review monographs, vol 3,

Chevy Chase, Md, 1994, The Endocrine Society, pp 140–142.

55. Ekins RP: Roles of serum thyroxine-binding proteins and maternal thyroid hormones in foetal development, Lancet 1:1129–1132, 1985.

56. Mendel CM, Weisiger RA, Jones AL, et al: Thyroid hormone-binding proteins in plasma facilitate uniform distribution of thyroxine within tissues: a perfused rat liver study, Endocrinology 120:1742–1749, 1987.

57. Schussler GC: Review: the thyroxine-binding proteins, Thyroid 10:141–149, 2000.

58. Robbins J: Editorial: New ideas in thyroxine-binding globulin biology, J Clin Endocrinol Metab 85:3994–3995, 2000.

59. Afandi B, Schussler GC, Arafeh AH, et al: Selective consumption of thyroxine-binding globulin during cardiac by-pass surgery, Metabolism 49:270–274, 2000.

60. Jirasakuldech B, Schussler GC, Yap MG, et al: A characteristic serpin cleavage product of thyroxine-binding globulin appears in sepsis sera, J Clin Endocrinol Metab 85:3996–3999, 2000.

61. Jirasakuldech B, Schussler GC, Yap MG, et al: Cleavage of thyroxine-binding globulin during cardiac bypass, Metabolism 50:1113–1116, 2001.

62. Janssen OE, Golcher HM, Grasberger H, et al: Characterization of T4-binding globulin cleaved by human elastase, J Clin Endocrinol Metab 87:1217–1222, 2002.

63. Klebanoff SJ, Green WL: Degradation of thyroid hormones by phagocytosing human leukocytes, J Clin Invest 52:60–72, 1973.

64. Khan NS, Schussler GC, Holden JB, et al: Thyroxine-binding globulin cleavage in cord blood, J Clin Endocrinol Metab 87:3321–3323, 2002.

65. Rosner W: The functions of corticosteroid-binding globulin and sex hormone-binding globulin: recent advances, Endocr Rev 11:80–91, 1990.

66. Richardson SJ, Monk JA, Shepherdley CA, et al: Developmentally regulated thyroid hormone distributor proteins in marsupials, a reptile and fish, Am J Physiol Regul Integr Comp Physiol 288:R1364–R1372, 2005.

67. Ain KB, Mori Y, Refetoff S: Reduced clearance rate of thyroxine-binding globulin (TBG) with increased sialylation: a mechanism for estrogen-induced elevation of serum TBG concentration, J Clin Endocrinol Metab 65:689–696, 1987.

68. Ain KB, Refetoff S: Relationship of oligosaccharide modification to the cause of serum thyroxine-binding globulin excess, J Clin Endocrinol Metab 66:1037–1043, 1988.

69. Chetkowski RJ, Meldrum DR, Steingold KA, et al: Biologic effects of transdermal estradiol, N Engl J Med 314:1615–1620, 1986.

70. Konno N, Kakinoki K, Hagiwara K: Serum concentrations of unsaturated thyroxine-binding globulin in hyper- and hypothyroidism, Clin Chem 22:249–255, 1985.

71. Glinoer D, McGuire R, Dubois A, et al: Thyroxine-binding globulin metabolism in Rhesus monkeys: effects of hyper- and hypothyroidism, Endocrinology 104:175–183, 1979.

72. Oppenheimer J, Werner S: Effect of prednisone on thyroxine-binding proteins, J Clin Endocrinol Metab 26:715–721, 1966.

73. Rouaze-Romet M, Savu L, Vranckx R, et al: Re-expression of thyroxine-binding globulin in post-weaning rats during protein or energy malnutrition, Acta Endocrinologica 127:441–448, 1992.

74. Emerson CH, Seiler CM, Alex S, et al: Gene expression and serum thyroxine-binding globulin are regulated by adrenal status and corticosterone in the rat, Endocrinology 133:1192–1196, 1993.

75. Arafah BM: Decreased levothyroxine requirement in women with hypothyroidism during androgen therapy for breast cancer, Ann Intern Med 121:247, 1994.

76. Man EB, Reid WA, Hellegers AE: Thyroid function in human pregnancy. III. Serum thyroxine binding prealbumin (TBPA) and thyroxine-binding globulin (TBG) of pregnant women, Am J Obstet Gynecol 103:338–347, 1969.

77. Maye P, Bisetti A, Burger A, et al: Hyperprealbuminemia, euthyroid hyperthyroxinemia, Zollinger-Ellison-like syndrome and hypercorticism in a pancreatic endocrine tumour, Acta Endocrinol 120:87–91, 1989.

78. Munro SL, Lim C-F, Hall JG, et al: Drug competition for thyroxine binding to transthyretin (prealbumin): comparison with effects on thyroxine-binding globulin, J Clin Endocrinol Metab 68:1141–1147, 1989.

79. Mendel CM, Frost PH, Cavalieri RR: Effect of free fatty acids on the concentration of free thyroxine in human serum: the role of albumin, J Clin Endocrinol Metab 63:1394–1399, 1986.

80. Lim C-F, Bai Y, Topliss DJ, et al: Drug and fatty acid effects on serum thyroid hormone binding, J Clin Endocrinol Metab 67:682–688, 1988.

81. Stockigt JR, Lim C-F, Barlow JW, et al: High concentrations of furosemide inhibit plasma binding of thyroxine, J Clin Endocrinol Metab 59:62–66, 1984.

82. Hawkins RC: Furosemide interference in newer free thyroxine assays, Clin Chem 44:2550–2551, 1998.

83. Surks MI, Defesi CR: Normal serum free thyroid hormone concentrations in patients treated with phenytoin or carbamazepine: a paradox resolved, JAMA 275:1495–1498, 1996.

84. Newnham HH, Hamblin PS, Long F, et al: Effect of oral furosemide on diagnostic indices of thyroid function, Clin Endocrinol 26:423–431, 1987.

85. Wang R, Nelson JC, Wilcox RB: Salsalate administration in a potential pharmacological model of the sick euthyroid syndrome, J Clin Endocrinol Metab 83:3095–3099, 1998.

86. Lueprasitsakul W, Alex S, Fang SL, et al: Flavonoid administration immediately displaces thyroxine (T4) from serum transthyretin, increases serum free T4 and decreases serum thyrotropin in the rat, Endocrinology 126:2890–2895, 1990.

87. Lim C-F, Curtis AJ, Barlow JW, et al: Interactions between oleic acid and drug competitors influence specific binding of thyroxine in serum, J Clin Endocrinol Metab 73:1106–1110, 1991.

88. Lim C-F, Stockigt JR, Curtis AJ, et al: Influence of a naturally-occurring furanoid acid on the potency of drug competitors for specific thyroxine binding in serum, Metabolism 42:1468–1474, 1993.

89. Mendel CM, Frost PH, Kunitake ST, et al: Mechanism of the heparin-induced increase in the concentration of free thyroxine in plasma, J Clin Endocrinol Metab 65:1259–1264, 1987.

90. Zambon A, Hashimoto SI, Brunzell JD: Analysis of techniques to obtain plasma for measurement of levels of free fatty acids, J Lipid Res 34:1021–1028, 1993.

91. Crowe TC, Cowen NL, Loidl NM, et al: Down-regulation of thyroxine-binding globulin messenger ribonucleic acid by 3,5,3′-triiodothyronine in human

hepatoblastoma cells, J Clin Endocrinol Metab 80:2233–2237, 1995.

92. Stockigt JR, Dyer SA, Mohr VS, et al: Specific methods to identify plasma binding abnormalities in euthyroid hyperthyroxinemia, J Clin Endocrinol Metab 62:230–233, 1986.

93. Hulbert AJ: Thyroid hormones and their effects: a new perspective, Biological Reviews of the Cambridge Philosophical Society 75:519–631, 2000.

94. Scholz GH, Vieweg S, Uhlig M, et al: Inhibition of thyroid hormone uptake by calcium antagonists of the dihydropyridine class, J Med Chem 40:1530–1538, 1997.

95. Hennemann G, Visser TJ: Thyroid hormone synthesis, plasma membrane transport and metabolism. In Weetman AP, Grossman A, editors: Pharmacotherapeutics of the thyroid gland, Berlin, 1997, Springer, pp 75–117.

96. Lim C-F, Docter E, Visser TJ, et al: Inhibition of thyroxine transport into cultured rat hepatocytes by serum of nonuremic critically ill patients: effects of bilirubin and nonesterified fatty acids, J Clin Endocrinol Metab 76:1165–1172, 1993.

97. Lim C-F, Bernard BF, de Jong M, et al: A furan fatty acid and indoxyl sulfate are the putative inhibitors of thyroxine hepatocyte transport in uremia, J Clin Endocrinol Metab 76:318–324, 1993.

98. Topliss DJ, Kolliniatis E, Barlow JW, et al: Uptake of T3 cultured rat hepatoma cells is inhibitable by non-bile acid cholephils, diphenylhydantoin and non-steroidal anti-inflammatory drugs, Endocrinology 124:980–986, 1989.

99. Cavalieri RR, Simeoni LA, Park SW, et al: Thyroid hormone export in rat FRTL-5 thyroid cells and mouse NIH-3T3 cells is carrier mediated, verapamil sensitive and stereospecific, Endocrinology 130:4948–4954, 1994.

100. Barlow JW, Curtis AJ, Raggatt LE, et al: Drug competition for intracellular triiodothyronine-binding sites, Eur J Endocrinol 130:417–421, 1994.

101. Mori J, Suzuki S, Kobayashi M, et al: Nicotine adenine nucleotide phosphate-dependent cytosolic T3 binding protein as a regulator for T3 mediated transactivation, Endocrinology 143:1538–1544, 2002.

102. Suzuki S, Mori J, Kobayashi M, et al: Cell-specific expression of NADPH-dependent cytosolic 3,5,3′-triiodothyronine-L-thyroxine binding protein (p38CTBP), Eur J Endocrinol 148:259–268, 2003.

103. Davis PJ, Tillmann HC, Davis FB, et al: Comparison of the mechanisms of nongenomic actions of thyroid hormones and steroid hormones, J Endocrinol Invest 25:377–388, 2002.

104. Visser WE, Friesema ECH, Jansen J, et al: Thyroid hormone transport in and out of cells, Trends in Endocrinology and Metabolism 19:50–56, 2007.

105. Friesema EC, Ganguly S, Abdalla A, et al: Identification of monodecarboxylate transporter 8 as a specific thyroid hormone transporter, J Biol Chem 278:40128–40135, 2003.

106. Dumitrescu AM, Liao XH, Best TB, et al: A novel syndrome combining thyroid and neurological abnormalities is associated with mutations in a monocarboxylate transporter gene, Am J Hum Genet 74:168–175, 2004.

107. Friesema EC, Grueters A, Biebermann H, et al: Association between mutations in a thyroid hormone transporter and severe X-linked psychomotor retardation, Lancet 364:1435–1437, 2004.

Chapter 23

RESISTANCE TO THYROID HORMONE

MARK GURNELL, THEO J. VISSER, PAOLO BECK-PECCOZ, and V. KRISHNA CHATTERJEE

Thyroid Hormone Action

It is now recognized that entry of thyroid hormones (thyroxine [T_4] and triiodothyronine [T_3]) into cells is not a passive process. Monocarboxylate transporter 8 (MCT8), a membrane protein, has been shown to mediate cellular thyroid hormone transport, particularly in the central nervous system (CNS). Intracellularly, deiodinase enzymes (DIOs) mediate hormone metabolism, with a high-affinity type 2 enzyme (DIO2) mediating T_4-to-T_3 conversion in the CNS, including the pituitary and hypothalamus, type 1 deiodinase (DIO1) in peripheral tissues generating T_3, and type 3 deiodinase (DIO3) mediating catabolism of thyroid hormones to inactive metabolites. The effects of thyroid hormones on physiologic processes are mediated principally by a receptor protein, the thyroid receptor (TR), belonging to the steroid/nuclear receptor superfamily of ligand-inducible transcription factors, which modulates target gene expression in different tissues (Fig. 23-1). TR binds preferentially to regulatory DNA sequences (thyroid response elements [TREs]) in target gene promoters as a heterodimer with the retinoid X receptor (RXR), although the receptor can bind some TREs as a homodimer or monomer. In the absence of hormone, unliganded receptor homodimers/heterodimers recruit corepressors (e.g., nuclear receptor corepressor [NCoR], silencing mediator for retinoic acid and thyroid receptors [SMRT]) to repress or "silence" gene transcription. Hormone binding results in corepressor dissociation and relief of repression together with ligand-dependent transcriptional activation, mediated by a complex of coactivators (e.g., steroid receptor coactivator 1 [SRC-1], CREB-binding protein [CBP], and CBP-associated factor [pCAF]).[1] In humans, two highly homologous thyroid hormone receptors, TRα and TRβ, are encoded by genes on chromosomes 17 and 3, respectively. Two different proteins are generated from the TRα gene locus by alternate splicing: TRα1 is a ubiquitously expressed receptor isoform with particular abundance in the CNS, myocardium, and skeletal muscle; TRα2, which exhibits a modified carboxy-terminal region such that it is unable to bind hormone, is expressed in a variety of tissues (e.g., brain and testis) where it may act as a functional antagonist of TR signaling pathways. The TRβ gene generates two major receptor isoforms, TRβ1 and TRβ2, which differ in their amino-terminal regions. TRβ1, which is widely expressed, is the predominant isoform in liver and kidney; TRβ2 expression is limited principally to the hypothalamus, pituitary, inner ear, and retina.[2]

Differential Diagnosis of Elevated T₄, T₃ With Nonsuppressed TSH

A number of genetic disorders and clinical contexts are associated with elevated thyroid hormones and nonsuppressed thyroid-stimulating hormone (TSH) levels (Table 23-1). The first step in making a diagnosis is to verify the validity of hormone measurements. Confirmation of elevated free thyroid hormone levels in two-step or equilibrium dialysis assays excludes abnormal circulating binding proteins or antiiodothyronine antibodies. Preservation of linearity when TSH is assayed in dilution suggests this measurement is not artifactual. Many causes (non-thyroidal illness, psychiatric disorder, neonatal period, drugs) can be excluded by clinical context.

Genetic disorders associated with elevated thyroid hormone levels can also be distinguished on the basis of different patterns of abnormal thyroid function (Table 23-2). The basis for such distinct biochemical profiles in each disorder is described later.

Resistance to Thyroid Hormone

CLINICAL FEATURES

The syndrome of resistance to thyroid hormone (RTH) is characterized by elevated circulating levels of free thyroid hormones

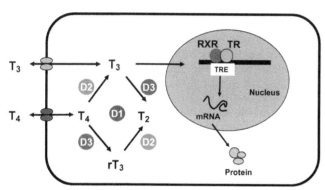

FIGURE 23-1. Transport, deiodination, and nuclear action of thyroid hormones. Transporters are required for passage of T_3 and T_4 across the plasma membrane, facilitating hormone uptake, efflux, or both. Deiodinases catalyze conversion of T_4 to T_3 (D1, D2) or inactivation of T_4 to rT_3 and T_3 to T_2 (D3). T_3 interaction with its nuclear receptor (TR), usually part of a heterodimer with RXR, modulates target gene transcription and protein synthesis.

Table 23-1. Causes of Elevated Thyroid Hormones With Detectable TSH

Raised serum binding proteins
Familial dysalbuminemic hyperthyroxinemia
Antiiodothyronine antibodies
Heterophile and anti–thyroid-stimulating hormone (TSH) antibodies
Nonthyroidal illness
Acute psychiatric disorders
Neonatal period
Drugs (e.g., amiodarone, heparin)
Thyroxine replacement therapy (including noncompliance)
TSH-secreting pituitary adenoma
Resistance to thyroid hormone
Disorder of thyroid hormone transport
Disorder of thyroid hormone metabolism

together with nonsuppressed pituitary TSH secretion. It reflects resistance to thyroid hormone action in the hypothalamic-pituitary-thyroid (HPT) axis and is accompanied by variable refractoriness in peripheral tissues.

RTH was first described in 1967 in two siblings who were clinically euthyroid despite high circulating thyroid hormone levels. The siblings exhibited several other abnormalities, including deaf-mutism, stippled femoral epiphyses with delayed bone maturation and short stature, and dysmorphic facies, winging of the scapulae, and pectus carinatum.[3] It is now clear that some of these features are unique to this kindred in whom the disorder was recessively inherited. The majority of RTH cases that have been subsequently described are dominantly inherited, with a highly variable clinical phenotype. Affected subjects are either asymptomatic or have nonspecific symptoms and may be noted to have a goiter, prompting thyroid function tests that suggest the diagnosis. In these individuals, classified as exhibiting generalized resistance to thyroid hormone (GRTH), the high thyroid hormone levels are thought to compensate for ubiquitous tissue resistance, resulting in a euthyroid state. In contrast, a smaller number of individuals (around 15%) who share the same biochemical phenotype exhibit clinical features of thyrotoxicosis. In adults, these can include weight loss, tremor, palpitations, insomnia, and heat intolerance; in children, failure to thrive, accelerated growth, and hyperkinetic behavior have also been noted. When this clinical entity was first described, patients were thought to exhibit "selective" pituitary resistance to thyroid hormone (PRTH) action, with preservation of normal hormonal responses in peripheral tissues,[4] but it is now recognized that peripheral resistance (typically hepatic) to hormone action is present even in these subjects. Less commonly, hypothyroid features such as growth retardation, delayed dentition, and bone age in children or asthenia and hypercholesterolemia in adults have been observed in RTH and may even coexist with thyrotoxic symptoms in the same individual.[5] Taken together, these observations suggest that the clinical features of this disorder are influenced by the degree of refractoriness of peripheral tissues to high circulating levels of free thyroid hormones.

The estimated prevalence of RTH is 1 in 50,000 live births; the disorder can be diagnosed neonatally by screening with a combination of TSH and free T_4 measurements.[6] Over 700 cases of RTH (from more than 250 families) have now been described worldwide, enabling clinical characteristics of this disorder to be defined more precisely.

Goiter

A palpable goiter has been documented in 65% of individuals, particularly adult females. The enlargement is usually diffuse, with multinodular glands being typical of recurrent goiters fol-

Table 23-2. Genetic Disorders Associated With Elevated Thyroid Hormones

Disorder	Familial Dysalbuminemic Hyperthyroxinemia (FDH)	Resistance to Thyroid Hormone (RTH)	Allan-Herndon-Dudley Syndrome	SBP2 Deficiency
GENE	ALB	THRB	MCT8	SBP2
Free T_4	Raised	Raised	Normal or low	Raised
Free T_3	Normal*	Raised	Raised	Normal or low
TSH	Normal	Normal	Normal (or raised)	Normal (or raised)
Reverse T_3	Raised	Raised	Low	Raised
SHBG	Normal	Normal	Raised	Normal

SBP2, SECIS-binding protein 2; *SHBG*, sex hormone–binding globulin; T_3, triiodothyronine; T_4, thyroxine; *TSH*, thyroid-stimulating hormone.
*Free T_3 is raised in a rare form of FDH.

lowing partial thyroidectomy. Development of toxic multinodular goiter on the background of RTH has been documented in a single case.[7] Interestingly, it has been noted that fewer children with RTH born to affected mothers exhibit thyroid enlargement (35%) compared to offspring of unaffected mothers (87%), suggesting that maternal hyperthyroxinemia with transplacental passage of thyroid hormones during development might protect against goitrogenesis.[8] The bioactivity of circulating TSH has been shown to be significantly enhanced in RTH, perhaps accounting for the goiter and markedly elevated serum thyroid hormones, despite the normal immunoreactive TSH levels observed in many cases.[9]

Cardiovascular System

Palpitations and resting tachycardia have been reported in approximately 75% of those with GRTH and almost all cases of PRTH, with a particular predisposition to atrial fibrillation in older subjects.[8] The incidence of these symptoms is notably higher in RTH patients than in unaffected relatives or in the general population, although still less frequent when compared to patients with classic hyperthyroidism.[10] In one study, although resting heart rates were comparable to unaffected family members, 30% of RTH subjects showed echocardiographic features of increased myocardial contractility and impaired diastolic relaxation, with a greater incidence of mitral valve prolapse.[8] In a prospective study of cardiovascular involvement in a large cohort of children and adults with RTH, resting heart rate was significantly higher. Some indices of cardiac systolic and diastolic function (e.g., stroke volume, cardiac output, maximal aortic flow velocity) were intermediate between values in normal and hyperthyroid subjects. Other parameters (e.g., ejection and shortening fractions of the left ventricle, systolic diameter, and left ventricle wall thickness) were not different, indicating a partially hyperthyroid response of the heart in this disorder.[10] Systemic vascular resistance and arterial stiffness are increased in RTH.[11,12]

Musculoskeletal System

Stippled epiphyses and winged scapulae were noted in the original RTH kindred but have not been observed in other cases. These features may represent a specific manifestation of the known gene deletion (TRβ) or an unrelated genetic abnormality in this consanguineous kindred.[3] In contrast, growth retardation and delayed skeletal maturation are more common in childhood RTH patients, with height below the fifth percentile in 18% and delayed bone age (>2 SD) in 29%,[8] with no significant differences between GRTH and PRTH cases. Despite these abnormalities, final adult height is often unaffected.[13]

Bearing in mind the known adverse effects of untreated hyperthyroidism on bone mineralization, we have conducted a cross-sectional survey of approximately 80 adult subjects with RTH and observed a reduction in bone mineral density in the femoral neck (mean Z score −0.71) and lumbar spine (mean Z score −0.73) but with normal markers of bone turnover (Chatterjee and Beck-Peccoz, unpublished observations).

Basal Metabolic Rate

The basal metabolic rate (BMR) is variably affected in RTH, being normal in some cases.[14] In keeping with others,[8] we have observed an elevated BMR, particularly in childhood RTH (Gurnell, Chatterjee, and Beck-Peccoz, unpublished observation), which may account for the abnormally low body mass index seen in approximately a third of children.

Central Nervous System

Two studies have documented neuropsychological abnormalities in RTH. First, a history of attention deficit hyperactivity disorder (ADHD) in childhood was elicited more frequently in patients with RTH (75%) compared to their unaffected relatives (15%).[15] A second study showed that both children and adults with RTH exhibited problems with language development, manifested by poor reading skills and problems with articulation (e.g., speech delay, stuttering).[16] Frank mental retardation (IQ < 60) is relatively uncommon (3%), although 30% of patients show mild learning disability (IQ < 85), probably due to uncompensated CNS hypothyroidism.[14] A direct comparison of individuals with ADHD and RTH versus ADHD alone indicates an association with lower nonverbal intelligence and academic achievement in the former group.[17] In detailed analysis of one family, RTH cosegregated with lower IQ rather than ADHD,[18] so it is possible that low IQ facilitates the manifestation of ADHD. However, two different surveys of unselected children with ADHD failed to detect any cases of RTH by biochemical screening, suggesting that the latter disorder is unlikely to be a common cause of hyperactivity.[19,20] Although magnetic resonance imaging (MRI) shows that anomalies of the sylvian fissure or Heschl's gyri are more frequent in RTH, these features do not correlate with ADHD.[21]

Hearing and Vision

Significant hearing loss has been documented in 21% of RTH cases, similar to the prevalence reported in congenital hypothyroidism.[8] In the majority, audiometric tests indicated a conductive defect, probably related to the increased incidence of recurrent ear infections in childhood RTH (67% in RTH versus 28% in normal controls). Abnormal otoacoustic emissions, consistent with cochlear dysfunction, have also been documented in those with hearing deficit,[8,22] and cochlear expression of TRβ has been shown.[23] The single kindred with deaf-mutism and recessively inherited RTH harbored a complete deletion of the TRβ gene,[3] which correlates with the finding that TRβ knockout (KO) mice are deaf.[24,25] Together, these observations underscore the importance of TRβ in auditory development and function. Deletion of the TRβ2 isoform in mice is associated with selective loss of M-cone photoreceptors and abnormal color vision,[26] but monochromatic color vision has only been reported in the rare human kindred with recessively inherited RTH and a complete TRβ gene deletion.[3] Detailed assessment of 10 subjects with TRβ point mutations and dominantly inherited RTH showed no common color-vision abnormalities (Gurnell and Chatterjee, unpublished observations).

Other Associated Disorders

Rarely, cases of RTH have been described where coexistent autoimmune thyroid disease has also been documented,[27-29] raising the possibility of a pathogenic association between these disorders. Coexistence of Pendred syndrome and RTH has been documented in a single case.[30] Pituitary enlargement, as a consequence of impaired negative-feedback regulation of TSH secretion, is another potential association with RTH. While pituitary hyperplasia has been reported in a single case, it occurred in the context of massively elevated TSH levels with suboptimal thyroxine replacement therapy following inappropriate thyroid ablation and regressed once TSH levels normalized.[31] Only a few cases of RTH associated with pituitary adenomas have been described,[32,33] suggesting that pituitary hyperplasia or adenoma

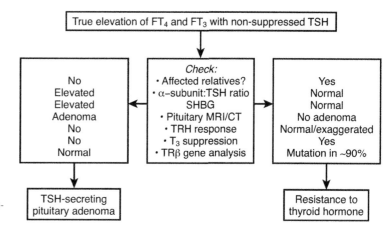

FIGURE 23-2. Algorithm for differentiation of RTH from TSH-secreting pituitary adenoma.

formation are uncommon clinical sequelae in RTH, provided the altered set-point of the HPT axis is not perturbed. A greater frequency of recurrent upper respiratory tract and pulmonary infections has been reported in RTH, and affected individuals have reduced serum immunoglobulin levels.[8] A retrospective study of a large Azorean kindred has shown a higher rate of miscarriage in mothers affected by RTH, with unaffected offspring being of lower birth weight, suggesting that intrauterine exposure to high TH levels does have adverse fetal effects.[34]

Differential Diagnosis

Differentiation of RTH, particularly the form associated with hyperthyroid features from a TSH-secreting pituitary tumor, can be difficult (Fig. 23-2). Similar abnormalities in thyroid function tests in first-degree relatives strongly suggest RTH, together with normal pituitary imaging and serum α-glycoprotein subunit levels.

The development of Graves' disease in RTH is suggested by atypical features such as ophthalmopathy, severe thyrotoxic symptoms, and a further rise in thyroid hormones leading to a subnormal or suppressed TSH. Following antithyroid drug treatment, TSH levels become elevated despite normalization of thyroid hormones. Similarly, normalization of TSH but elevated thyroid hormones following supraphysiologic doses of thyroxine replacement in primary hypothyroidism suggests coexistent RTH.

In addition to clinical features, the measurement of various tissue markers of thyroid hormone action has been suggested to be a useful method for evaluating the differing responses of various target organs and tissues to elevated circulating thyroid hormones (Table 23-3). These measurements are most useful in assessing the tissue effects of marked thyroid hormone excess (as typically found in overt thyrotoxicosis) but may be less discriminatory in borderline hyperthyroidism or in hypothyroidism. To improve the sensitivity and specificity of these parameters, it has been suggested that individuals with RTH be assessed by measuring tissue responses dynamically following the administration of graded supraphysiologic doses of T_3 (50, 100, and 200 μg/day, each given for a period of 3 days), with comparison of any change in indices from baseline values to those observed in normal subjects.[35]

Table 23-3 Tissue Indices of Thyroid Hormone Action

Pituitary:	Thyroid-stimulating hormone (TSH)
General:	Basal metabolic rate (BMR)
Hepatic:	Sex hormone–binding globulin (SHBG), ferritin, cholesterol
Muscle:	Creatine kinase, ankle jerk relaxation time
Bone:	Height, bone age, bone density, osteocalcin, alkaline phosphatase, pyridinium crosslinks, type I collagen telopeptide
Cardiac:	Sleeping pulse rate, systolic time interval, diastolic isovolumic relaxation time
Hematologic:	Soluble interleukin 2 receptor (sIL-2R)
Lung:	Angiotensin-converting enzyme (ACE)

MOLECULAR GENETICS

TRβ RTH

Following the cloning of TRα and TRβ, RTH was shown to be tightly linked to the TRβ gene locus in a single family.[36] This prompted analysis of the TRβ gene in other cases, and a large number of receptor defects have since been associated with this disorder. Eighty percent of RTH is familial, dominantly inherited, and associated with heterozygous mutations in the TRβ gene[14,37-39]; de novo receptor mutations occur in the remaining 20% of sporadic cases. Over 100 different defects including point mutations, in-frame deletions, and frameshift insertions have been documented to date, which localize to three mutation clusters within the ligand-binding domain of the receptor (Fig. 23-3). Within each cluster, some codon changes (e.g., R243W, R338W, R438H) representing transitions in mutation-prone CpG dinucleotides occur more frequently and are overrepresented.[40]

Based on the supposition that PRTH was associated with selective pituitary resistance, it had been hypothesized that this disorder might be associated with defects in DIO2 or the TRβ2 receptor isoform, but a number of reports have documented TRβ mutations in PRTH.[38,41,42] Receptor mutations found in individuals with PRTH have also been associated with GRTH in unrelated kindreds. Furthermore, even within a single family, the same receptor mutation can be associated with abnormal thyroid function and thyrotoxic features consistent with PRTH in some individuals but similar biochemical abnormalities and a lack of symptoms indicative of GRTH in other members. Overall, these

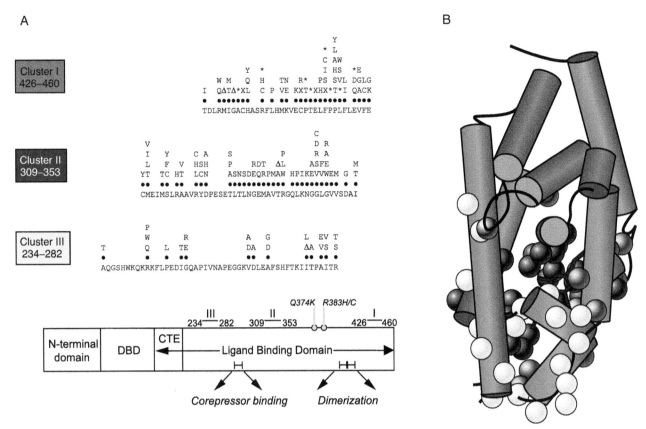

FIGURE 23-3. A, A schematic representation of the domains of TR-β showing that with two exceptions (Q374K, R383H/C), RTH receptor mutations localize to three clusters within the ligand-binding domain (LBD). The receptor defects described include different missense substitutions at each codon, in-frame codon deletions (Δ), premature termination codons (X), and frameshift mutations (*). The mutations shown include those listed in a public database (HGMD) together with our unpublished data. No RTH receptor mutations have been described in the zinc-finger DNA-binding domain (DBD) or its carboxy-terminal extension (CTE), which together mediate interaction with DNA, or regions in the LBD important for corepressor binding or dimerization with RXR. **B,** The crystal structure of the TR-β ligand-binding domain (LBD) (Protein Data Bank accession no. 1BSX) composed of 12 α helices is shown, with the location of missense mutations associated with RTH superimposed. As predicted from their functional properties, the majority of mutations involve residues surrounding the ligand-binding (T_3) cavity.

findings indicate that GRTH and PRTH represent the phenotypic spectrum associated with a single genetic entity.

Non-TRβ RTH

In a small but significant number of cases (10% to 15%), clear-cut biochemical evidence of RTH is not associated with a mutation in the coding region of TRβ—so-called non-TRβ RTH. One explanation for this is somatic mosaicism, with occurrence of a TRβ mutation whose expression is selective, being detectable in some tissues but not peripheral blood leukocyte DNA.[43] Alternatively, defects in other proteins involved in TR signaling have also been postulated. This latter hypothesis is supported by the description of kindreds with thyroid function tests and resistance to exogenous T_3 similar to subjects with TRβ RTH, but in whom linkage and sequence analyses have excluded defects in TRβ and TRα genes.[44,45] While it is theoretically possible that defects at any point in the pathway of thyroid hormone action could manifest as an RTH phenotype, evidence exists to favor some candidate genes such as RXR or the cofactors (e.g., corepressors, coactivators, TR-associated proteins) that regulate thyroid hormone–dependent gene transcription.

Mice harboring a deletion of the SRC-1 gene show abnormalities in thyroid function tests suggestive of RTH, together with subtle evidence of resistance in other steroid receptor axes.[46] Similar findings were noted in mice doubly heterozygous for knockouts of the SRC-1 and transcriptional intermediary factor 2 (TIF-2) coactivator genes.[47] To date, no homologous human disorder has been described, with linkage studies and direct sequence analysis of several cofactor genes (e.g., SRC-1, SRC-3, SMRT) in non-TRβ RTH kindreds or individuals failing to identify any abnormality.[49] In one case, wild-type TRβ was found to exhibit aberrant binding to a unique 84-kD protein from patient but not control fibroblast nuclear extracts, suggesting abnormal receptor interaction with a cofactor[44] whose identity has not been elucidated. It is known that patients with Rubinstein-Taybi syndrome, a disorder associated with heterozygous defects in the nuclear receptor coactivator CBP, exhibit a number of somatic abnormalities (broad thumbs, mental retardation, short stature) yet have normal circulating free T_4 and TSH levels,[50] indicating that mutations in this cofactor are not a cause of non-TRβ RTH. Several lines of evidence favor RXR as a candidate gene in non-TRβ RTH. First, knockout mice lacking the RXRγ isoform, whose tissue expression is limited but includes pituitary thyrotrophs, exhibit thyroid hormone resistance together with an increased metabolic rate.[51] Second, the administration of RXR-selective agonists in humans inhibits pituitary TSH secretion, resulting in central hypothyroidism.[52] Finally, in two kindreds with non-TRβ RTH, possible linkage to the RXRγ gene locus was noted,[45,48] but in another study, no RXRγ gene mutations were identified in four non-TRβ RTH subjects.[53] Together, these observations suggest that defects in pituitary-expressed RXRγ might also impair negative feedback in the pituitary-thyroid axis and manifest as RTH. Finally, it is tempting to speculate that a combination of "less functionally deleterious" mutations or even polymorphisms in several genes involved in thyroid hormone action could result in an RTH phenotype, representing an oligogenic basis for the disorder.

PROPERTIES OF MUTANT RECEPTORS

Consonant with their location in the hormone-binding domain, the majority of receptor mutants identified in RTH exhibit moderate or markedly reduced T_3 binding; consequently, their ability to activate or repress target gene expression is impaired.[54,55] A subset of RTH mutations associated with markedly abnormal thyroid function in vivo and altered transcriptional function in vitro (but little impairment in ligand binding) have been described. Such natural mutations involve residues that mediate receptor interaction with transcriptional coactivators.[39,56] In the first RTH family described, with the recessively inherited form of the disorder, the two affected siblings were found to be homozygous for a complete deletion of both alleles of the TRβ receptor gene.[57] Importantly, the obligate heterozygotes in this family harboring a deletion of one TRβ allele were completely normal with no evidence of thyroid dysfunction. This suggested that simple deficiency of a functional β receptor, as a consequence of the single deleted TRβ allele, was insufficient to generate the resistance phenotype. This led to the hypothesis that the heterozygous mutant receptors in dominantly inherited RTH were not simply functionally impaired but also capable of inhibiting wild-type receptor action. Studies confirmed that when coexpressed, the mutant proteins are able to inhibit the function of their wild-type counterparts in a dominant-negative manner.[58,59] Further clinical and genetic evidence supporting this notion have been provided by two rare examples of RTH. In the first, a childhood case, severe resistance with marked developmental delay and growth retardation associated with cardiac hyperthyroidism was ultimately fatal due to heart failure following septicemia; this individual was homozygous for a mutation (Δ337T) in both alleles of the TRβ gene.[60] In the second more recently reported case, the affected subject also exhibited a particularly severe clinical phenotype and was found to be either homozygous or hemizygous for a TRβ mutation (I280S).[61] Presumably, the extreme phenotype observed in both cases reflected not only the absence of normally functioning TRβ but the added dominant-negative inhibitory effect of mutant β receptors.

Functional studies of mutant receptors indicate that although they are transcriptionally impaired and dominant-negative inhibitors, their ability to bind DNA and form heterodimers with RXR is preserved.[54,55] Conversely, it has been shown that the introduction of additional artificial mutations that abolish DNA binding or heterodimer formation abrogates the dominant-negative activity of mutant receptors in vitro.[55,62,63] Mice heterozygous for a TRβ mutation lacking DNA binding do not exhibit RTH.[64] It has also been suggested that the ability of mutant receptors in RTH to repress or "silence" basal gene transcription is likely to be an important factor contributing to their dominant-negative potency. Non-T_3-binding mutants exhibit constitutive silencing function, particularly when bound to DNA as homodimers, which cannot be relieved by ligand. Conversely, RTH mutants with impaired homodimerization properties are weaker dominant-negative

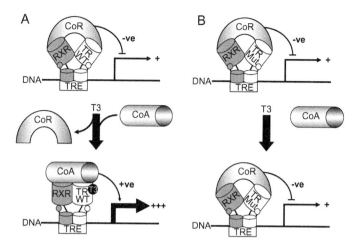

FIGURE 23-4. A model for dominant-negative inhibition by mutant receptors in RTH. Left panel **(A)** depicts current understanding of wild-type TR action on target genes. The unliganded TR-RXR heterodimer or homodimer (not shown) recruits a corepressor (CoR) complex to inhibit or silence basal gene transcription. Receptor occupancy by T_3 promotes corepressor dissociation and derepression, followed by binding of coactivators (CoA), which leads to target gene activation. Right panel **(B)** shows RTH mutant receptor action. In comparison to wild-type TR, the primary defect in mutant receptors may be impaired hormone-dependent corepressor dissociation and coactivator recruitment. For the majority of receptor mutants, this functional alteration is a consequence of their reduced ability to bind ligand, but a subset of mutants exhibit enhanced corepressor binding, delayed corepressor release, or impaired coactivator recruitment, with relative preservation of hormone binding. Mutant receptor-CoR complexes compete with their wild-type counterparts for occupancy of promoter thyroid response elements (TREs), resulting in inhibition of target gene expression. In this model, DNA binding, dimerization, and corepressor interaction are functional properties preserved in mutant receptors and required for their dominant-negative activity.

inhibitors.[65] With the identification of corepressors, these observations have been extended to show that some RTH mutants either bind corepressor more avidly when unliganded or fail to dissociate fully from corepressor upon T_3 binding.[66] Furthermore, artificial mutations that abolish corepressor binding abrogate the dominant-negative activity of RTH receptor mutants.[66] It has also been suggested that corepressors mediate basal activation of negatively regulated gene promoters (e.g., thyrotropin-releasing hormone [TRH], TSH-α, TSH-β) by unliganded TR.[67] An unusual RTH receptor mutant (R383H) exhibits both delayed T_3-dependent corepressor release and impaired hormone-dependent negative transcriptional regulation.[68] Given the pivotal role of negatively regulated target genes in the pathogenesis of RTH, aberrant corepressor recruitment or release may well prove to be the critical receptor abnormality in this disorder.

Together, these observations allow a model to be constructed (Fig. 23-4) in which occupancy of target gene binding sites by mutant receptor-corepressor complexes mediates dominant-negative inhibition by RTH mutants. Mapping of the three clusters of RTH receptor mutations identified hitherto on the crystal structure of the ligand-binding domain of TRβ[69] provides insights into structure-function relationships in TR (see Fig. 23-3). As expected from their impaired ligand-binding properties, most mutations are located around the hormone-binding cavity, and receptor regions mediating DNA binding, dimerization, and corepressor interaction are devoid of naturally occurring mutations, possibly because they lack dominant-negative activity and therefore elude discovery—being biochemically and clinically silent.

PATHOGENESIS OF VARIABLE RESISTANCE

Genetic and functional evidence suggests that the ability to exert a dominant-negative effect on target genes within the HPT axis is a fundamental property of RTH receptor mutants, generating the abnormal thyroid function characteristic of the disorder. Indeed, some studies indicate that for a subset of RTH mutants, there is a correlation between their functional impairment in vitro and the degree of central pituitary resistance, as measured by the magnitude of elevation in serum-free T_4 in vivo.[70,71] On this biochemical background, the heterogeneous clinical phenotype may be due to differing degrees of peripheral resistance in different individuals as well as variable resistance in different tissues within a single subject. A number of factors may contribute to such variable tissue resistance.

One important contributory element may be the differing tissue distributions of receptor isoforms. The hypothalamus/pituitary, and liver express predominantly TRβ2 and TRβ1 receptors, respectively, and TRα1 is the major species detected in myocardium. Mutations in the TRβ gene are likely to be associated with pituitary and liver resistance, as exemplified by non-suppressed TSH and normal sex hormone–binding globulin (SHBG) levels seen in patients, whereas the tachycardia and cardiac hyperthyroidism in some cases may represent retention of myocardial sensitivity to high circulating thyroid hormones acting via a normal α receptor. Another factor that may influence the degree of tissue resistance is the relative expression of mutant versus wild-type TRβ alleles. One study has suggested that both alleles are equally expressed[72]; another showed marked differences in the relative levels of wild-type and mutant receptor messenger RNA in skin fibroblasts from two RTH cases.[73] In one of these individuals, a temporal variation in expression of the mutant allele in fibroblasts appeared to correlate with the degree of skeletal tissue resistance. The dominant-negative inhibitory potency of mutant receptors has been shown to differ depending on target gene promoter context[55,74] and is a further variable that may influence the degree of resistance. Finally, factors unrelated to the TRβ gene might influence the phenotype. For example, a deleterious R316H mutation was associated with normal thyroid hormone levels in some members of one kindred[75] but clearly abnormal thyroid function in an unrelated family,[38] suggesting that other genetic variables can modulate the effect of receptor mutations.

While the absence or presence of overt thyrotoxic features allows patients to be classified as either GRTH or PRTH—a clinical definition that will probably remain useful as a guide to the most appropriate form of treatment—studies indicate that there is some overlap of features between the two forms of the disorder. For example, there are no significant differences in age, sex ratio, frequency of goiter, thyroid function, or clinical features between patients with GRTH or PRTH.[76] Importantly, features such as tachycardia, hyperkinetic behavior, and emotional disturbance have been documented in individuals with GRTH.[76] Conversely, serum SHBG, a hepatic index of thyroid hormone action, is almost invariably normal in patients with PRTH, suggesting that tissue resistance is not solely confined to the HPT axis in this group of patients.[77]

Attempts to correlate the phenotype of RTH with the nature of the underlying TRβ mutation have been confounded by three factors: (1) the relative imprecision of clinical criteria used to define GRTH and PRTH; (2) the apparent temporal variation in hyperthyroid features in some RTH cases, such that thyrotoxic symptoms and signs can develop and disappear spontaneously when individuals are followed over several years[76]; and (3) the relatively small number of patients with any given mutation that have been identified. Nevertheless, some interesting correlations have emerged from the published literature. The first patient reported to have PRTH[4] was found to harbor an R338W receptor mutation,[41] and the same phenotype has been described in the majority of individuals with this or similar substitutions at this codon.[38,42] Interestingly, when tested in vitro, this mutant exhibits dominant-negative activity with the negatively regulated pituitary TSH α subunit gene promoter, but it is a relatively poor inhibitor of wild-type receptor action in other promoter contexts.[55] When introduced into other RTH receptor–mutant backgrounds, this mutation weakens their dominant-negative potency on positively regulated reporter genes.[78] A patient with the R383H receptor defect, which is impaired mainly in regulation of TRH and TSH genes, exhibited predominant central resistance following T_3 administration,[79] and the R429Q mutation, with similar functional properties, may also occur more frequently in association with PRTH. Some receptor mutants (R338W or L, V349M, R429Q, I431T) associated with PRTH are either more deleterious[80] or exert a greater dominant-negative inhibitory effect in a TRβ2 than a TRβ1 context.[81] A receptor mutation that selectively fails to bind NCoR but not SMRT is associated with PRTH.[82]

ANIMAL MODELS

The generation of various receptor knockout mice has greatly enhanced our understanding of the physiologic roles of individual TR isoforms, particularly in regulation of the HPT axis. For example, homozygous TRβ gene deletion (TRβ KO), leading to absence of both TRβ1 and TRβ2 isoforms, increased circulating thyroid hormone levels approximately threefold,[24] whereas deletion of the TRα1 isoform had no effect.[83] When only the TRβ2 isoform was deleted, the biochemical phenotype was similar to that of TRβ KO, suggesting that TRβ2 is the key isoform mediating feedback regulation of hypothalamic TRH and pituitary TSH output.[84] Importantly, many of the features in the recessively inherited cases of RTH associated with a deletion encompassing the human TRβ gene were recapitulated in TRβ KO mice.[24] Homozygous animals exhibited elevated serum thyroid hormones and an inappropriately elevated TSH, while their heterozygous littermates were biochemically normal. To explore the properties of mutant TRβs in RTH in vivo, several groups have developed transgenic mice in which dominant-negative TRβ mutants have been overexpressed either ubiquitously[85] or selectively in tissues.[86,87] These models have provided valuable insights into mutant receptor function and pathophysiologic mechanisms that mediate RTH. For example, selective targeting of an RTH mutant to the pituitary using a tissue-specific promoter generated transgenic mice with elevated TSH but only marginally raised T_4 levels. This suggests that the additional dominant-negative effect of mutant receptors on the hypothalamic TRH gene might be required to produce the full biochemical phenotype.[87] In contrast, ubiquitous transgenic mutant TRβ expression resulted in an animal model with more generalized tissue resistance; these mice displayed decreased body weight, hyperactivity, and learning deficit, which are recognized features of the human syndrome.[85] An important limitation of these animal models is that expression of the mutant receptor transgene is not controlled by the TRβ gene promoter, so the pattern of mutant receptor expression or the resulting phenotype might not correspond with that of human RTH. Transgenic mice in which either a frameshift mutation involving 14 carboxy-terminal amino acids (TRβ PV)[88] or an in-frame deletion of a threonine residue (Δ337T)[89] have been introduced into the TRβ gene locus have also been generated. Both these TRβ mutations have been identified in human RTH, and the mutant receptors exhibit markedly impaired transcriptional activation and potent dominant-negative activity in vitro. Extensive characterization of the phenotype of TRβ PV[88,90] and Δ337T mice has indicated that these animal models recapitulate the human RTH phenotype, with heterozygous mice exhibiting mild to moderate resistance and homozygous littermates severe resistance in the HPT axis. Interestingly, when compared with TRβ KO mice, thyroid hormone and TSH levels were significantly more elevated in the Δ337T knock-in animals, supporting the notion that dominant-negative inhibition by the mutant receptor antagonizes residual TRβ1 activity in the HPT axis. Both heterozygous and homozygous Δ337T mice exhibited abnormalities of vestibulomotor function which correlated with an overall reduction in cerebellar size and in the area of the Purkinje cell layer.

Studies with TRβ PV mice have provided insights into the molecular basis for dominant-negative activity in vivo, confirming that mutant receptor homodimers and heterodimers compete with wild-type TRβ for binding to target gene TREs. The interplay of receptor isoform predominance (e.g., TRβ1 in liver, TRα1 in heart) together with the promoter context of target gene TREs can influence the degree of dominant-negative inhibition observed in different tissues.[90] Interestingly, crossing TRβ PV mice with SRC-1 KO animals enhanced the degree of resistance in the HPT axis in heterozygous TRβ PV mice, providing evidence that coactivator "availability" can also modulate mutant TRβ action in vivo.[91] Metastatic thyroid carcinoma was an unexpected finding in older, homozygous TRβ PV mutant mice but has not been observed in their heterozygous counterparts.[92] Mice harboring a TRβ mutation (R429Q) associated with PRTH exhibit greater dysregulation of negative versus positively regulated target genes, providing a mechanism for correlation of some TRβ genotypes with phenotype.[93]

Finally, it is appropriate to include a brief description of mice harboring mutations in the TRα gene locus. Selective knockout of the TRα1 isoform was associated with low or normal serum thyroid hormones, a decreased heart rate, and lower body temperature—a phenotype quite dissimilar to RTH.[83] Knock-in mice with heterozygous point mutations in TRα that correspond to naturally occurring TRβ mutations in RTH have either normal or mildly reduced thyroid hormone levels,[95-98] with additional features including bradycardia, growth retardation, CNS abnormalities,[95,98] and insulin resistance,[96] which may provide important clues to the probable phenotype of a homologous human disorder.[97]

MANAGEMENT

The management of RTH is difficult, since variable resistance makes it difficult to maintain euthyroidism in all tissues. In general, the presence or absence of hyperthyroid features is a useful guide to the need for therapy. In most individuals, the receptor defect is compensated by high circulating thyroid hormone levels, leading to a euthyroid state not associated with abnormalities other than a small goiter. Attempts to treat the biochemical abnormality with surgery or radioiodine are usually unsuccessful, with recrudescence of the goiter (often nodular in nature) and disruption of the thyroid axis.[14] Certain circumstances such as hypercholesterolemia in adults or developmental delay and growth retardation in young children may warrant the administration of supraphysiologic doses of L-T$_4$ to overcome a

higher degree of resistance in certain tissues. Although successful in some cases,[14] such therapy needs careful monitoring of indices of thyroid hormone action (e.g., SHBG, heart rate, BMR, bone markers) to avoid the adverse cardiac effects or excess catabolism associated with thyroxine overtreatment. Inappropriate thyroid ablation also renders the RTH patient hypothyroid, with elevated TSH levels and risk of thyrotroph hyperplasia,[31] and is another context in which supraphysiologic thyroxine replacement is indicated. Alternate-day administration of L-T$_3$ in supraphysiologic dosage led to significant regression of goiter without inducing thyrotoxic symptoms in one case.[99]

In contrast, a general reduction in thyroid hormone levels may be of benefit in the management of patients with thyrotoxic symptoms. However, the administration of conventional antithyroid drugs usually causes a further rise in serum TSH levels that stimulates thyroid enlargement and may also induce thyrotroph hyperplasia, with a theoretic risk of developing autonomous neoplasms at either site. Accordingly, agents that inhibit pituitary TSH secretion but are relatively devoid of peripheral thyromimetic effects are administered to reduce thyroid hormone levels. The most widely used example is the thyroid hormone analog 3,5,3′-triiodothyroacetic acid (TRIAC), which has been shown to be beneficial in both childhood and adult cases.[100-102] This compound has a number of interesting properties that make it an attractive therapeutic option in RTH: (1) it exerts predominantly pituitary and hepatic thyromimetic effects in vivo,[103] target tissues that are relatively refractory to thyroid hormones in RTH; (2) it has greater affinity, potency, and activity than T$_3$ for TRβ[104]; and (3) it exhibits a higher affinity for TRβ than TRα in vitro.[105] A daily dose of 1.4 to 2.8 mg is generally used, and one study has suggested that twice daily administration might be optimal in inhibiting TSH secretion.[106] TRIAC has been successfully used in pregnancy to control maternal thyrotoxic symptoms but may have induced fetal goiter.[107] Treatment with TRIAC is not always effective, however,[108] and dextrothyroxine is another agent that has been shown to be useful in some cases.[109,110] If these compounds fail, the dopaminergic agent, bromocriptine,[111] or the somatostatin analog, octreotide,[112] may be administered, but past experience indicates that TSH secretion escapes the inhibitory effects of both bromocriptine[100,111] and octreotide.[113] In view of the spontaneous variation in thyrotoxic symptoms in RTH, periodic cessation of thyroid hormone–lowering therapy and reevaluation of the clinical status of the patient is advisable. In rare circumstances such as severe thyrotoxic cardiac failure associated with RTH, thyroid ablation followed by subphysiologic thyroxine replacement may be indicated.

The treatment of thyrotoxic features (e.g., failure to thrive) in childhood RTH also requires careful monitoring to ensure that any reduction in thyroid hormone levels is not associated with growth retardation or adverse neurologic sequelae. Indeed, control of cardiac and sympathomimetic manifestations with β-blockade may be the safest course in this context. One study reported that L-T$_3$ therapy improved hyperactivity in nine children with ADHD and RTH, including three individuals who were unresponsive to methylphenidate.[114]

The therapeutic potential of TRIAC in RTH could be limited by the nature of the TRβ mutation, with some mutant receptors being less responsive, such that the dose of TRIAC required to activate mutant TRβ function is associated with unwanted TRα-mediated toxicity (e.g., tachycardia). Accordingly, the identification of compounds with higher affinity and selective agonist activity for mutant TRβ than for normal TRβ or TRα would represent a major therapeutic advance: TRβ-selective thyromimetics (e.g., GC1, KB2115) are being developed and may have utility in treating some abnormalities (e.g., dyslipidemia) in RTH.[115,116] HY1, an analog of GC1, is five times more potent with an R320C TRβ mutant than wild-type TRβ, suggesting that it may indeed be feasible to design hormone analogs that selectively overcome abnormal mutant receptor function without further activating normal β or α receptors.[117] Rational molecular design has also led to the development of TR isoform–selective antagonists that may also be useful in, for example, controlling TRα-mediated toxic symptoms in RTH.[118]

Disorder of Thyroid Hormone Transport

CLINICAL FEATURES

Worldwide, at least 50 families have been reported in which males are affected by severe psychomotor retardation associated with a particular combination of abnormal serum thyroid hormone levels. In 1944, long before thyroid involvement was suspected, the first description of this syndrome of X-linked mental retardation (XLMR) in a large family was published by Allan, Herndon, and Dudley.[119] Since then, this disorder has been typically referred to as the *Allan-Herndon-Dudley syndrome* (AHDS). Only 60 years later was it realized that patients with AHDS also have abnormal thyroid function tests.[120-122]

Usually, patients with AHDS are born at term after an uncomplicated pregnancy, with a normal birthweight, body length, and head circumference. During the first 6 months, general hypotonia is noticed. During development, truncal hypotonia persists, resulting in poor head control, whereas distal hypotonia progresses into spasticity. Growth is relatively normal, but final body length is reduced, and body weight is usually extremely low with obvious signs of muscle wasting. There is also progressive microcephaly. In the first 2 years of life, brain MRI shows delayed myelination, but this normalizes in subsequent years. Based on the delayed myelination, this combination of clinical features has also been referred to as *Pelizaeus-Merzbacher-like disorder* (PMLD).[123]

Although the clinical phenotype is somewhat milder in some families, AHDS patients are usually incapable of sitting, standing, or walking independently and do not develop any speech. They are severely mentally retarded, with IQ values below 40. Feeding is a problem in AHDS patients; they have swallowing difficulties, and aspiration is a frequent cause of pneumonia. Patients with AHDS usually have a friendly nature. Recent reviews provide a detailed description of the clinical features of patients with AHDS.[123-126]

In addition to severe psychomotor retardation, AHDS patients have a characteristic combination of abnormal serum thyroid hormone levels.[125] This is also observed in a subset of patients with PMLD.[123] Both T_4 and free T_4 levels are either low-normal or clearly reduced, whereas serum T_3 and free T_3 are markedly elevated, and rT_3 is always low. Consequently, circulating T_3/T_4 and T_3/rT_3 ratios are markedly elevated. Although within the normal range, mean serum TSH levels in AHDS patients are about twice that in healthy controls. Serum SHBG levels are markedly elevated, and several studies have reported raised serum lactate in young patients.[127,128]

MOLECULAR GENETICS

In all male patients with the characteristic combination of psychomotor retardation and abnormal serum thyroid hormone

Table 23-4. Mutations in the MCT8 Gene

MCT8 Mutation	
Nucleotide	**Protein**
exon1del	
exon3-4del	
exon2-6del	
565insATC	189insI
575A>G	H192R
581C>T	S194F
630insA	N210fs30X
631-644del	R211fs25X
661G>A	G221R
671C>T	A224V
689-691delTCT	230delF
703G>A	V235M
706insGTG	236insV
733C>T	R245X
798-1G>C	267-370del
812G>A	R271H
962C>T	P321L
1003C>T	Q335X
1201G>A	G401R
1212delT	A405fs12X
1301T>G	L434W
1306delT	C436fs
1333C>T	R445C
1343C>A	S448X
1412T>C	L471P
1500-1502delCTT	501delF
1535T>C	L512P
1558C>T	Q520X
1610C>T	P537L
1649delA	Y550fs17X
1673G>A	G558D
1690G>A	G564R
1703T>C	L568P
1826delC	P609fs71X
1835delC	P612fs68X

levels, different mutations in the monocarboxylate transporter 8 (*MCT8*) gene have been identified (Table 23-4). Both MCT8 and the highly homologous protein, MCT10, have been shown to be specific and active thyroid hormone transporters, although MCT10 is also capable of transporting aromatic amino acids.[129-131] These proteins belong to a wider family of MCT transporters, so named because MCTs 1 to 4 have been shown to facilitate transport of monocarboxylates such as lactate and pyruvate.[132] The function of most other MCTs is as yet unknown.

MCT8 and *MCT10* have identical gene structures; both consist of six exons and five introns, with a particularly long first intron (~100 kb). The *MCT10* gene is located on chromosome 6q21-q22, encoding a protein of 515 amino acids. The *MCT8* gene is located on chromosome Xq13.2 and has two possible translation start sites, generating either 613 (long) or 539 (short) amino acid protein products (Fig. 23-5). The significance of the N-terminal extension in the long form of the MCT8 protein (shown in light gray in Fig. 23-5) remains to be elucidated. All in vitro studies of the function of wild-type and mutated MCT8 have been carried out in the short protein context. Like MCT10, MCT8 has 12 putative transmembrane domains (TMDs), with both the N-terminal and C-terminal ends of the protein being located intracellularly. The amino acids that are identical and occupy corresponding positions in MCT8 and MCT10 are highlighted

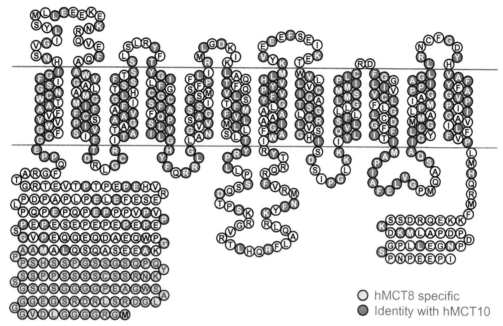

FIGURE 23-5. Predicted topology of human MCT8, showing the 12 putative transmembrane domains and the extended N-terminal domain (shaded light gray) in the long form of the protein. Residues that are conserved in identity and location with human MCT10 are also highlighted (shaded dark gray).

(see Fig. 23-5), showing that homology between these proteins is particularly high in their TMDs.

MCT8 mutations have now been identified in over 50 families with AHDS, and the majority of them are listed in Table 23-4. These mutations include (1) rather large deletions affecting one or more exons; (2) smaller deletions or insertions which result in a shift in the reading frame, leading to altered peptide sequence and/or truncation of proteins; (3) nonsense mutations resulting in truncated proteins; (4) three-nucleotide changes causing single codon deletions or insertions; (5) single nucleotide changes causing amino acid substitutions; and (6) a splice site mutation resulting in deletion of 94 amino acids and 3 TMDs.

The larger deletions and frameshift and nonsense mutations are obviously deleterious for MCT8 function. The functional consequences of single amino acid substitutions, deletions, or insertions have been investigated in cells transfected with wild-type or mutated MCT8. Most mutations were found to result in an almost complete loss of thyroid hormone transport by MCT8. However, the extent to which these mutations affect MCT8 function depends on the cell type used for functional studies, for reasons which need to be fully explored.[133-136]

ANIMAL MODELS

Studies in humans and animals have indicated that MCT8 is expressed in a variety of tissues, including brain, liver, kidney, heart, skeletal muscle, and thyroid. The distribution of MCT8 expression in mouse brain has been examined in detail by Heuer et al.,[137] indicating that MCT8 is predominantly found in neurons in different brain areas, including hippocampus, cerebral cortex, striatum, hypothalamus, and cerebellum. Significantly, MCT8 is also expressed in capillary endothelial cells, the choroid plexus, and tanycytes which line the third ventricle.[137,138] MCT8 expression in neurons coincides with expression of DIO3, which catalyzes the degradation of T_3. DIO2, which catalyzes the conversion of T_4 to T_3, is largely expressed in adjacent astrocytes. Another transporter involved specifically in brain T_4 uptake, OATP1C1, is expressed in capillaries and the choroid plexus.[137,138]

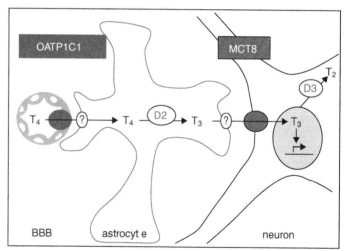

FIGURE 23-6. A pathway which regulates T_3 supply to neuronal target cells. OATP1C1 mediates T_4 transport through the blood-brain barrier (BBB), with T_4 uptake into astrocytes via an unidentified transporter, conversion to T_3 by DIO2, and release of T_3 by another unidentified transporter. Neuronal uptake of T_3 is mediated by MCT8, and the cells also express DIO3 which catabolizes and may therefore terminate hormone action.

Based on studies by Heuer et al.[137] and Bernal,[139] a pathway which regulates T_3 supply to neuronal target cells is shown in Fig. 23-6. The steps involved in this process include: (1) transport of T_4 by OATP1C1 through the blood-brain barrier, (2) uptake of T_4 into astrocytes by an unidentified transporter, (3) conversion of T_4 to T_3 by DIO2 in astrocytes, (4) release of T_3 from the astrocytes by another unidentified transporter, and (5) neuronal uptake of T_3 mediated by MCT8. Neurons may also express DIO3 to catabolize and terminate T_3 action, but this schema is an oversimplification. It ignores the importance of thyroid hormone transport across the blood-brain barrier by MCT8 and across the blood-CSF barrier by both MCT8 and

OATP1C1, as well as the importance of other target cells for thyroid hormone in the brain, such as oligodendrocytes.

MCT8 KO mice have been studied by Trajkovic et al.,[140] Dumitrescu et al.,[141] and Wirth et al.[142] In contrast to the severe neurologic features in male patients with MCT8 mutations, neither hemizygous MCT8 null male mice nor homozygous MCT8 KO female mice show an obvious neurologic phenotype. However, they do exhibit the same biochemical thyroid abnormalities as patients with MCT8 mutations: a large decrease in T_4, a large increase in serum T_3, and slightly elevated TSH levels. In addition, MCT8 KO mice show the following features: (1) normal brain T_4 uptake but impaired brain T_3 uptake, (2) decreased brain T_4 and T_3 content, (3) increased DIO2 and decreased DIO3 activities in brain, (4) normal liver T_4 and T_3 uptake, (5) increased kidney T_4 and T_3 uptake, (6) increased kidney T_4 and T_3 content, and (7) increased type 1 deiodinase (DIO1) activity in both liver and kidney.

The paradoxical increase in renal T_4 and T_3 uptake in MCT8 KO mice is unexplained, but the combination of increased renal T_4 content and DIO1 expression may lead to enhanced renal T_4-to-T_3 conversion, thus contributing to the observed decrease in serum T_4 and increase in serum T_3 levels.[143] There is also evidence suggesting that thyroidal hormone synthesis is affected by MCT8 inactivation, leading to preferential T_3 secretion (Trajkovic et al., unpublished observations). Since MCT8 is expressed in the hypothalamus, its inactivation is associated with impaired feedback action of thyroid hormone, presumably contributing to slightly increased serum TSH levels.[140] The lack of an obvious neurologic phenotype in MCT8 KO mice remains to be explained.

PATHOGENESIS

The known essential role of thyroid hormone in brain development requires optimal spatiotemporal regulation of T_3 supply to CNS target cells, and MCT8 is critical for T_3 transport into central neurons. Inactivation of MCT8 and neuronal T_3 deprivation results in impaired CNS development, leading to severe psychomotor retardation. It is also conceivable that MCT8 is more important for T_3 uptake in a subset of neurons, resulting in an imbalance of T_3 supply to different neuronal populations and defective coordinated development of neuronal networks in the brain.

Depending on the importance of MCT8 for T_3 transport across the blood-brain barrier and choroid plexus, MCT8 inactivation may also result in an overall reduction in brain T_3 uptake, as seen in MCT8 KO mice. It is also possible that the abnormal circulating T_4 and T_3 levels in MCT8 deficiency are directly detrimental for brain development. Elucidation of pathogenic mechanisms responsible for psychomotor retardation may have important implications for the management of patients with MCT8 mutations.

In addition to dysregulated thyroid hormone action in the brain, the effects of MCT8 mutations on the thyroid status of peripheral tissues should also be considered. Despite exposure to highly elevated circulating T_3 levels, the heart usually appears to function normally in MCT8 patients, suggesting partially impaired cardiac T_3 uptake and implying the involvement of additional thyroid hormone transporters in the heart. MCT8 patients exhibit profound muscle wasting and increased serum SHBG levels, which likely reflect a hyperthyroid state of skeletal muscles and liver, respectively. This indicates that MCT8 inactivation does not impair muscle and liver T_3 uptake and suggests that other transporters may be more important in these tissues. Finally, findings in MCT8 KO mice also suggest renal hyperthy-

roidism in MCT8 patients, but there is no direct clinical evidence to support this notion.

MANAGEMENT

Two types of treatment have been evaluated in MCT8 deficiency. One is normalization of serum T_4 and T_3 levels with a block-and-replace regimen using a combination of PTU and T_4. Treatment of a 16-year-old boy with markedly low body mass (25 kg) and tachycardia did not result in major neurologic improvement but had a marked beneficial effect on body weight and heart rate.[144] Perhaps neurologic benefit can only occur if such therapy is initiated soon after birth.

An alternative treatment could involve the administration of a thyroid hormone analog that is taken up by the brain independently of MCT8. Promising results using diiodothyropropionic acid (DITPA)[145] have been observed in MCT8 KO mice. Clinical trials in patients with MCT8 mutations have been initiated, and the results are eagerly awaited.

Disorder of Thyroid Hormone Metabolism

CLINICAL FEATURES

Three families (A, B, C) with affected individuals exhibiting a disorder of thyroid hormone metabolism have been described.[146,147] In each instance, childhood growth retardation was a common feature that brought probands to clinical attention. Affected individuals showed a distinctive abnormal pattern of thyroid function tests, with elevated free T_4, low free T_3, raised reverse T_3, and normal or slightly high TSH levels. This pattern was suggestive of a defect in iodothyronine metabolism. Consistent with this hypothesis, affected siblings in family A required higher-than-normal amounts of exogenous T_4 to suppress TSH levels, whereas their response to T_3 administration was normal.[146] We have identified additional adult and childhood cases of this disorder with a similar pattern of thyroid function tests and growth retardation in childhood (Gurnell, Beck-Peccoz, and Chatterjee, unpublished observations).

MOLECULAR GENETICS

The biochemical phenotype in affected cases suggested a defect in T_4-to-T_3 conversion, but linkage studies ruled out defects at *DIO* loci or in genes involved in posttranslational modification (ubiquitination/de-ubiquitination) of *DIO2*. However, affected subjects in family A shared homozygous haplotypes at the *SECISBP2/SBP2* locus.[146] Subsequent analyses of this gene have identified a homozygous missense mutation (R540Q) in cases from family A, compound heterozygous abnormalities (nonsense mutation K438X plus missplicing of ~50% of transcripts from the other allele) in the proband from family B, and a homozygous stop mutation (R128X) in the propositus from family C.[147]

There are 25 known human proteins which contain the amino acid selenocysteine (Sec), and SECIS-binding protein 2 (SBP2) is a factor required for the cotranslational incorporation of Sec during their biosynthesis. The mechanism of selenoprotein synthesis and role of SBP2 is further described in Fig 23-7. Recent studies also indicate that the architecture of *SBP2* is complex, with alternative splicing of the gene generating multiple transcripts and internal methionine residues directing synthesis of shorter protein isoforms.[148] Indeed, there is evidence (albeit in

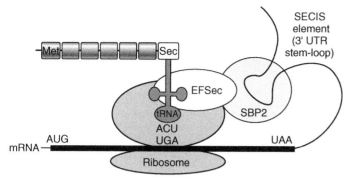

SECIS element (3' UTR stem-loop)

FIGURE 23-7. Mechanism of selenoprotein biosynthesis. The 3'-untranslated region of selenoprotein mRNA contains a stem-loop RNA structure (SECIS element) which interacts with a protein complex that includes SBP2 and Sec-specific elongation factor (EFSec) to enable ribosomal recruitment of selenocysteyl-transfer RNA to the UGA codon and selenocysteine (Sec) incorporation into the nascent polypeptide. Failure of this mechanism results in miscoding of the UGA as a stop codon, terminating protein synthesis.

pattern in this disorder is likely to be mediated by combined, partial deficiency of all three DIOs rather than lack of a single enzyme.

Targeted disruption of the murine *SBP2* gene has not been described, so no animal model of this disorder exists, but cellular knockdown of SBP2 has been achieved and is associated with variable but global reduction in levels of many selenoproteins.[149] Consistent with this notion, deficiencies of other selenoproteins have been documented in affected cases: glutathione peroxidase (GPx) activity in cells (mainly GPx type1) and serum (mainly GPx type 3) is markedly reduced, and circulating levels of hepatic selenoprotein P (SEPP) are low.[146,147] Such deficiency of the major circulating selenoproteins (SEPP, GPx3) is also likely to be the basis of low serum selenium levels recorded in cases.[146] Furthermore, functional characterization of the mutant SBP2 protein identified in family A indicates that its ability to bind Sec insertion sequence (SECIS) elements in other selenoprotein genes (e.g., *GPx4*) is impaired,[150] suggesting the possibility of more widespread selenoprotein deficiencies in patients with this disorder.

MANAGEMENT

Trials of oral selenium supplementation, either in the form of selenomethionine-rich yeast which can be incorporated generally into circulating proteins or sodium selenite, a substrate for selenocysteine incorporation, have been undertaken in affected cases. Although selenomethionine treatment raised circulating selenium concentrations, there was no change in thyroid function, GPx3 activity or SEPP levels.[147,151] However, T$_3$ treatment was clearly beneficial for growth in one published report[147] and our childhood case (Gurnell and Chatterjee, unpublished observations).

vitro) to suggest that usage of methionines downstream of a homozygous null mutation (e.g., in proband of family C) might generate shorter but functional SBP2 protein to ameliorate the phenotype of this disorder.[147]

PATHOGENESIS

Selenocysteine is a component of all three deiodinase enzymes, and DIO2 activity was indeed reduced in fibroblasts from family A.[146] However, based on the biochemical phenotype of DIO null mice, it is likely that the abnormal thyroid function test

REFERENCES

1. Horlein AJ, Heinzel T, Rosenfeld MG: Gene regulation by thyroid hormone receptors, Curr Opin Endocrinol Diabetes 3:412–416, 1996.
2. Lazar MA: Thyroid hormone receptors: multiple forms, multiple possibilities, Endocr Rev 14:184–193, 1993.
3. Refetoff S, De Wind LT, De Groot LJ: Familial syndrome combining deaf-mutism, stippled epiphyses, goiter and abnormally high PBI: possible target organ refractoriness to thyroid hormone, J Clin Endocrinol Metab 27:279–294, 1967.
4. Gershengorn MC, Weintraub BD: Thyrotropin-induced hyperthyroidism caused by selective pituitary resistance to thyroid hormone. A new syndrome of inappropriate secretion of TSH, J Clin Invest 56:633–642, 1975.
5. Magner JA, Petrick P, Menezes-Ferreira M, et al: Familial generalized resistance of thyroid hormones: a report of three kindreds and correlation of patterns of affected tissues with the binding of [¹²⁵I]triiodothyronine to fibroblast nuclei, J Endocrinol Invest 9:459–469, 1986.
6. Snyder D, Sesser D, Skeels M, et al: Thyroid disorders in newborn infants with elevated screening T4, Thyroid 2(suppl 1):S-29 (abstract), 1997.
7. Taniyama M, Ishikawa N, Momotani N, et al: Toxic multinodular goiter in a patient with generalized resistance to thyroid hormone who harbours the R429Q mutation in the thyroid hormone receptor β gene, Clin Endocrinol 54:121–124, 2001.
8. Brucker-Davis F, Skarulis MC, Grace MB, et al: Genetic and clinical features of 42 kindreds with resistance to thyroid hormone, Ann Intern Med 123:572–583, 1995.
9. Persani L, Asteria C, Tonacchera M, et al: Evidence for the secretion of thyrotropin with enhanced bioactivity in syndromes of thyroid hormone resistance, J Clin Endocrinol Metab 78:1034–1039, 1994.

10. Kahaly JG, Matthews CH, Mohr-Kahaly S, et al: Cardiac involvement in thyroid hormone resistance, J Clin Endocrinol Metab 87:204–212, 2002.
11. Pulcrano M, Palmieri EA, Ciulla DM, et al: Impact of resistance to thyroid hormone on the cardiovascular system in adults, J Clin Endocrinol Metab 94:2812–2816, 2009.
12. Owen PJD, Chatterjee VK, John R, et al: Augmentation index in resistance to thyroid hormone (RTH), Clin Endocrinol 70:650–654, 2009.
13. Weiss RE, Refetoff S: Effect of thyroid hormone on growth: lessons from the syndrome of resistance to thyroid hormone, Endocrinol Metab Clin North Am 25:719–730, 1996.
14. Refetoff S, Weiss RE, Usala SJ: The syndromes of resistance to thyroid hormone, Endocr Rev 14:348–399, 1993.
15. Hauser P, Zametkin AJ, Martinez P, et al: Attention deficit-hyperactivity disorder in people with generalized resistance to thyroid hormone, N Engl J Med 328:997–1001, 1993.
16. Mixson AJ, Parrilla R, Ransom SC, et al: Correlation of language abnormalities with localization of mutations in the β-thyroid hormone receptor in 13 kindreds with generalized resistance to thyroid hormone: identification of four new mutations, J Clin Endocrinol Metab 75:1039–1045, 1992.
17. Stein MA, Weiss RE, Refetoff S: Neurocognitive characteristics of individuals with resistance to thyroid hormone: comparisons with individuals with attention-deficit hyperactivity disorder, J Dev Behav Pediatr 16:406–411, 1995.
18. Weiss RE, Stein MA, Duck SC, et al: Low intelligence but not attention deficit hyperactivity disorder is associated with resistance to thyroid hormone caused by mutation R316H in the thyroid hormone receptor

β gene, J Clin Endocrinol Metab 78:1525–1528, 1994.
19. Weiss RE, Stein MA, Trommer B, et al: Attention-deficit hyperactivity disorder and thyroid function, J Paediatr 123:539–545, 1993.
20. Valentine J, Rossi E, O'Leary P, et al: Thyroid function in a population of children with attention deficit hyperactivity disorder, J Paediatr Child Health 33:117–120, 1997.
21. Leonard CM, Martinez P, Weintraub BD, et al: Magnetic resonance imaging of cerebral anomalies in subjects with resistance to thyroid hormone, Am J Med Genet 60:238–243, 1995.
22. Brucker-Davis F, Skarulis MC, Pikus A, et al: Prevalence and mechanism of hearing loss in patients with resistance to thyroid hormone, J Clin Endocrinol Metab 81:2768–2772, 1996.
23. Bradley DJ, Twole HC, Young WS: A and b thyroid hormone receptor (TR) gene expression during auditory neurogenesis: evidence for TR isoform specific transcriptional regulation in vivo, Proc Natl Acad Sci U S A 91:439–443, 1994.
24. Forrest D, Hanebuth E, Smeyne RJ, et al: Recessive resistance to thyroid hormone in mice lacking thyroid hormone receptor beta: evidence for tissue-specific modulation of receptor function, EMBO J 15:3006–3015, 1996.
25. Forrest D, Erway LC, Ng L, et al: Thyroid hormone receptor beta is essential for development of auditory function, Nat Genet 13:354–357, 1996.
26. Ng L, Hurley JB, Bierks B, et al: A thyroid hormone receptor that is required for the development of green cone photoreceptors, Nat Genet 27:94–98, 2001.
27. De Meirleir K, Golstein J, Jonckheer MH, et al: Hypothyroidism with normal thyroid hormone levels as a consequence of autoimmune thyroiditis and peripheral

resistance to thyroid hormone, Acta Clin Belg 35:107–109, 1980.

28. Aksoy DY, Gurlek A, Ringkananont U, et al: Resistance to thyroid hormone associated with autoimmune thyroid disease in a Turkish family, J Endocrinol Invest; 28:379–383, 2005.
29. Fukata S, Brent GA, Sugawara M: Resistance to thyroid hormone in Hashimoto's thyroiditis, N Engl J Med 352:517–518, 2005.
30. Borck G, Seewi O, Jung A, et al: Genetic causes of goiter and deafness: Pendred syndrome in a girl and cooccurrence of Pendred syndrome and resistance to thyroid hormone in her sister, J Clin Endocrinol Metab 94:2106–2109, 2009.
31. Gurnell M, Rajanayagam O, Barbar I, et al: Reversible pituitary enlargement in the syndrome of resistance to thyroid hormone, Thyroid 8:679–682, 1998.
32. Watanabe K, Kameya T, Yamauchi A, et al: Thyrotropin-producing adenoma associated with pituitary resistance to thyroid hormone, J Clin Endocrinol Metab 76:1025–1030, 1993.
33. Safer JD, Colan SD, Fraser LM, et al: A pituitary tumour in a patient with thyroid hormone resistance: a diagnostic dilemma, Thyroid 11:281–291, 2001.
34. Anselmo J, Cao D, Karrison T, et al: Fetal loss associated with excess thyroid hormone exposure, J Am Med Assoc 292:691–695, 2004.
35. Sarne DH, Refetoff S, Rosenfield RL, et al: Sex hormone-binding globulin in the diagnosis of peripheral tissue resistance to thyroid hormone: the value of changes after short term triiodothyronine administration, J Clin Endocrinol Metab 66:740–746, 1988.
36. Usala SJ, Bale AE, Gesundheit N, et al: Tight linkage between the syndrome of generalized thyroid hormone resistance and the human c-erbA β gene, Mol Endocrinol 2:1217–1220, 1988.
37. Parrilla R, Mixson AJ, McPherson JA, et al: Characterization of seven novel mutations of the c-erbA β gene in unrelated kindreds with generalized thyroid hormone resistance: evidence for two "hot spot" regions of the ligand binding domain, J Clin Invest 88:2123–2130, 1991.
38. Adams M, Matthews CH, Collingwood TN, et al: Genetic analysis of twenty-nine kindreds with generalised and pituitary resistance to thyroid hormone, J Clin Invest 94:506–515, 1994.
39. Collingwood TN, Wagner R, Matthews CH, et al: A role of helix 3 of the TRβ ligand binding domain in coactivator recruitment identified by characterization of a third cluster of mutations in resistance to thyroid hormone, EMBO J 17:4760–4770, 1998.
40. Weiss RE, Weinberg M, Refetoff S: Identical mutations in unrelated families with generalized resistance to thyroid hormone occur in cytosine-guanine-rich areas of the thyroid hormone receptor β gene, J Clin Invest 91:2408–2415, 1993.
41. Mixson AJ, Renault JC, Ransom S, et al: Identification of a novel mutation in the gene encoding the β-triiodothyronine receptor in a patient with apparent selective pituitary resistance to thyroid hormone, Clin Endocrinol 38:227–234, 1993.
42. Sasaki S, Nakamura H, Tagami T, et al: Pituitary resistance to thyroid hormone associated with a base mutation in the hormone-binding domain of the human 3,5,3′-triiodothyronine receptor β, J Clin Endocrinol Metab 76:1254–1258, 1993.
43. Mamanasiri S, Yesil S, Dumitrescu AM, et al: Mosaicism of a thyroid hormone receptor-beta gene mutation in resistance to thyroid hormone, J Clin Endocrinol Metab 91:3471–3477, 2006.
44. Weiss RE, Hayashi Y, Nagaya T, et al: Dominant inheritance of resistance to thyroid hormone not linked to defects in the thyroid hormone receptor alpha or beta genes may be due to a defective cofactor, J Clin Endocrinol Metab 81:4196–4203, 1996.
45. Pohlenz J, Weiss RE, Macchia PE, et al: Five new families with resistance to thyroid hormone not caused by mutations in the thyroid hormone receptor β gene, J Clin Endocrinol Metab 84:3919–3928, 1999.
46. Weiss RE, Xu J, Ning G, et al: Mice deficient in the steroid receptor coactivator 1 (SRC-1) are resistant to thyroid hormone, EMBO J 18:1900–1904, 1999.
47. Weiss RE, Gehin M, Xu J, et al: Thyroid function in mice with compound heterozygous and homozygous disruptions of SRC-1 and TIF-2 coactivators: evidence for haploinsufficiency, Endocrinology 143:1554–1557, 2002.
48. Refetoff S, Sadow PM, Reutrakul S, et al: Resistance to thyroid hormone in the absence of mutations in the thyroid hormone receptor genes. In Beck-Peccoz, editor: Syndromes of hormone resistance on the hypothalamic-pituitary-thyroid axis, ed 1, Boston, 2004, Kluwer Academic Publishers, pp 89–107.
49. Hamon B, Hamon P, Bovier-Lapierre M, et al: A child with resistance to thyroid hormone without thyroid hormone receptor gene mutation: a 20-year follow-up, Thyroid 18:35–44, 2008.
50. Olson DP, Koenig RJ: Thyroid function in Rubinstein-Taybi syndrome, J Clin Endocrinol Metab 82:3264–3266, 1997.
51. Brown NS, Smart A, Sharma V, et al: Thyroid hormone resistance and increased metabolic rate in the RXR-γ-deficient mouse, J Clin Invest 106:73–79, 2000.
52. Sherman SI, Gopal J, Haugen BR, et al: Central hypothyroidism associated with retinoid X receptor-selective ligands, N Engl J Med 340:1075–1079, 1999.
53. Romeo S, Menzaghi C, Rocco B, et al: Search for genetic variants in the retinoid X receptor-γ gene by polymerase chain reaction-single strand conformation polymorphism in patients with resistance to thyroid hormone without mutations in the thyroid hormone receptor β gene, Thyroid 14:355–358, 2004.
54. Meier CA, Dickstein BM, Ashizawa K, et al: Variable transcriptional activity and ligand binding of mutant b1 3,5,3′-triiodothyronine receptors from four families with generalised resistance to thyroid hormone, Mol Endocrinol 6:248–258, 1992.
55. Collingwood TN, Adams M, Tone Y, et al: Spectrum of transcriptional dimerization and dominant negative properties of twenty different mutant thyroid hormone β receptors in thyroid hormone resistance syndrome, Mol Endocrinol 8:1262–1277, 1994.
56. Collingwood TN, Rajanayagam O, Adams M, et al: A natural transactivation mutation in the thyroid hormone β receptor: impaired interaction with putative transcriptional mediators, Proc Natl Acad Sci U S A 94:248–253, 1997.
57. Takeda K, Sakurai A, De Groot LJ, et al: Recessive inheritance of thyroid hormone resistance caused by complete deletion of the protein-coding region of the thyroid hormone receptor-β gene, J Clin Endocrinol Metab 74:49–55, 1992.
58. Sakurai A, Miyamoto T, Refetoff S, et al: Dominant negative transcriptional regulation by a mutant thyroid hormone receptor β in a family with generalised resistance to thyroid hormone, Mol Endocrinol 4:1988–1994, 1990.
59. Chatterjee VKK, Nagaya T, Madison LD, et al: Thyroid hormone resistance syndrome: inhibition of normal receptor function by mutant thyroid receptors, J Clin Invest 87:1977–1984, 1991.
60. Ono S, Schwartz ID, Mueller OT, et al: Homozygosity for a dominant negative thyroid hormone receptor gene responsible for generalized resistance to thyroid hormone, J Clin Endocrinol Metab 73:990–994, 1991.
61. Frank-Raue K, Lorenz A, Haag C, et al: Severe form of thyroid hormone resistance in a patient with homozygous/hemizygous mutation of T3 receptor gene, Eur J Endocrinol 150:819–823, 2004.
62. Nagaya T, Madison LD, Jameson JL: Thyroid hormone receptor mutants that cause resistance to thyroid hormone: evidence for receptor competition for DNA sequences in target genes, J Biol Chem 267:13014–13019, 1992.
63. Nagaya T, Jameson JL: Thyroid hormone receptor dimerization is required for dominant negative inhibition by mutations that cause thyroid hormone resistance, J Biol Chem 268:15766–15771, 1993.
64. Shibusawa N, Hashimoto K, Nikrodhanond AA, et al: Thyroid hormone action in the absence of thyroid hormone receptor DNA-binding in vivo, J Clin Invest 112:588–597, 2003.
65. Kitajima K, Nagaya T, Jameson JL: Dominant negative and DNA-binding properties of mutant thyroid hormone receptors that are defective in homodimerization but not heterodimerization, Thyroid 5:343–353, 1995.
66. Yoh SM, Chatterjee VKK, Privalsky ML: Thyroid hormone resistance syndrome manifests as an aberrant interaction between mutant T3 receptors and transcriptional corepressors, Mol Endocrinol 11:470–480, 1997.
67. Tagami T, Madison LD, Nagaya T, et al: Nuclear receptor corepressors activate rather than suppress basal transcription of genes that are negatively regulated by thyroid hormone, Mol Cell Biol 17:2642–2648, 1997.
68. Clifton-Bligh RJ, de Zegher F, Wagner RL, et al: A novel TRβ mutation (R383H) in resistance to thyroid hormone predominantly impairs corepressor release and negative transcriptional regulation, Mol Endocrinol 12:609–621, 1998.
69. Wagner RL, Huber BR, Shiau AK, et al: Hormone selectivity in thyroid hormone receptors, Mol Endocrinol 15:398–410, 2001.
70. Hayashi Y, Weiss RE, Sarne DH, et al: Do clinical manifestations of resistance to thyroid hormone correlate with the functional alteration of the corresponding mutant thyroid hormone b receptors? J Clin Endocrinol Metab 80:3246–3256, 1995.
71. Gurnell M, Rajanayagam O, Agostini M, et al: Three novel mutations at codon 314 in the thyroid hormone receptor β differentially impair ligand binding in the syndrome of resistance to thyroid hormone, Endocrinology 140:5901–5906, 1999.
72. Hayashi Y, Janssen OE, Weiss RE, et al: The relative expression of mutant and normal thyroid hormone receptor genes in patients with generalized resistance to thyroid hormone determined by estimation of their specific messenger ribonucleic acid products, J Clin Endocrinol Metab 76:64–69, 1993.
73. Mixson AJ, Hauser P, Tennyson G, et al: Differential expression of mutant and normal β T3 receptor alleles in kindreds with generalized resistance to thyroid hormone, J Clin Invest 91:2296–2300, 1993.
74. Zavacki AM, Harney JW, Brent GA, et al: Dominant negative inhibition by mutant thyroid hormone receptors is thyroid response element and receptor isoform specific, Mol Endocrinol 7:1319–1330, 1993.
75. Geffner ME, Su F, Ross NS, et al: An arginine to histidine mutation in codon 311 of the c-erbA β gene results in a mutant thyroid hormone receptor that does not mediate a dominant negative phenotype, J Clin Invest 91:538–546, 1993.
76. Beck-Peccoz P, Chatterjee VKK: The variable clinical phenotype in thyroid hormone resistance syndrome, Thyroid 4:225–232, 1994.
77. Beck-Peccoz P, Roncoroni R, Mariotti S, et al: Sex hormone-binding globulin measurement in patients with inappropriate secretion of thyrotropin (IST): evidence against selective pituitary thyroid hormone resistance in nonneoplastic IST, J Clin Endocrinol Metab 71:19–25, 1990.
78. Ando S, Nakamura H, Sasaki S, et al: Introducing a point mutation identified in a patient with pituitary resistance to thyroid hormone (Arg 338 to Trp) into other mutant thyroid hormone receptors weakens their dominant negative activities, J Endocrinol 151:293–300, 1996.
79. Safer JD, O'Connor MG, Colan SD, et al: The thyroid hormone receptor-β gene mutation R383H is associated with isolated central resistance to thyroid hormone, J Clin Endocrinol Metab 84:3099–3109, 1999.
80. Wan W, Farboud B, Privalsky ML: Pituitary resistance to thyroid hormone syndrome is associated with T3 receptor mutants that selectively impair beta2 isoform function, Mol Endocrinol 19:1529–1542, 2005.
81. Safer JD, Langlois MF, Cohen R, et al: Isoform variable action among thyroid hormone receptor mutants provides insight into pituitary resistance to thyroid hormone, Mol Endocrinol 11:16–26, 1997.
82. Wu SY, Cohen RN, Simsek E, et al: A novel thyroid hormone receptor-beta mutation that fails to bind nuclear receptor corepressor in a patient as an apparent cause of severe, predominantly pituitary resistance to thyroid hormone, J Clin Endocrinol Metab 91:1887–1895, 2006.
83. Wikstrom L, Johansson C, Salto C, et al: Abnormal heart rate and body temperature in mice lacking thyroid hormone receptor α1, EMBO J 17:455–461, 1998.
84. Abel ED, Boers ME, Pazos-Moura C, et al: Divergent roles for thyroid hormone beta receptor isoforms in the endocrine axis and auditory system, J Clin Invest 104:291–300, 1999.

85. Wong R, Vasilyev VV, Ting Y-T, et al: Transgenic mice bearing a human mutant thyroid hormone β1 receptor manifest thyroid function anomalies, weight reduction and hyperactivity, Mol Med 3:303–314, 1997.

86. Hayashi Y, Xie J, Weiss RE, et al: Selective pituitary resistance to thyroid hormone produced by expression of a mutant thyroid hormone receptor beta gene in the pituitary gland of transgenic mice, Biochem Biophys Res Commun 245:204–210, 1998.

87. Abel ED, Kaulbach HC, Campos-Barros A, et al: Novel insight from transgenic mice into thyroid hormone resistance and the regulation of thyrotropin, J Clin Invest 103:271–279, 1999.

88. Kaneshige M, Kaneshige K, Zhu X, et al: Mice with a targeted mutation in the thyroid hormone beta receptor gene exhibit impaired growth and resistance to thyroid hormone, Proc Natl Acad Sci U S A 97:13209–13214, 2000.

89. Hashimoto K, Curty FH, Borges PP, et al: An unliganded thyroid hormone receptor causes severe neurological dysfunction, Proc Natl Acad Sci U S A 98:3998–4003, 2001.

90. Cheng S-Y: Multi-factorial regulation of in vivo action of TRβ mutants. Lessons learned from RTH mice with a targeted mutation in the TRβ gene. In Beck-Peccoz P editor: Syndromes of hormone resistance on the hypothalamic-pituitary-thyroid axis, ed 1, Boston, 2004, Kluwer Academic Publishers, pp 137–148.

91. Kamiya Y, Zhang XY, Ying H, et al: Modulation by steroid receptor coactivator-1 of target-tissue responsiveness in resistance to thyroid hormone, Endocrinology 144:4144–4153, 2003.

92. Suzuki H, Willingham MC, Cheng SY, et al: Mice with mutation in the thyroid hormone receptor β gene spontaneously develop thyroid carcinoma: A mouse model of thyroid carcinogenesis, Thyroid 12:963–969, 2002.

93. Machado DS, Sabet A, Santiago LA, et al: a thyroid hormone receptor mutation that dissociates thyroid hormone regulation of gene expression in vivo, Proc Natl Acad Sci U S A 106:9441–9446, 2009.

94. Deleted in proofs.

95. Kaneshige M, Suzuki H, Kaneshige K, et al: A targeted dominant negative mutation of the thyroid hormone α1 receptor causes increased mortality, infertility, and dwarfism in mice, Proc Natl Acad Sci U S A 98:15095–15100, 2001.

96. Liu YY, Schultz JJ, Brent GA: A thyroid hormone receptor alpha gene mutation (P398H) is associated with visceral adiposity and impaired catecholamine-stimulated lipolysis in mice, J Biol Chem 278:38913–38920, 2003.

97. Vennstrom B, Mittag J, Wallis K. Severe psychomotor and metabolic damages caused by a mutant thyroid hormone receptor alpha 1 in mice: can patients with a similar mutation be found and treated? Acta Paediatr 97:1605–1610, 2008.

98. Tinnikov A, Nordstrom K, Thoren P: Retardation of post-natal development caused by a negatively acting thyroid hormone receptor alpha1, EMBO J 21:5079–5087, 2002.

99. Anselmo J, Refetoff S: Regression of a large goiter in a patient with resistance to thyroid hormone by every other day treatment with triiodothyronine, Thyroid 14:71–74, 2004.

100. Beck Peccoz P, Piscitelli G, Cattaneo MG, et al: Successful treatment of hyperthyroidism due to nonneoplastic pituitary TSH hypersecretion with 3,5,3'-triiodothyroacetic acid (TRIAC), J Endocrinol Invest 6:217–223, 1983.

101. Crino A, Borrelli P, Salvatori R, et al: Anti-iodothyronine autoantibodies in a girl with hyperthyroidism due to pituitary resistance to thyroid hormones, J Endocrinol Invest 15:113–120, 1992.

102. Radetti G, Persani L, Molinaro G, et al: Clinical and hormonal outcome after two years of TRIAC treatment in a child with thyroid hormone resistance, Thyroid 7:775–778, 1997.

103. Bracco D, Morin O, Schutz Y, et al: Comparison of the metabolic and endocrine effects of 3,5,3'-triiodothyroacetic acid and thyroxine, J Clin Endocrinol Metab 77:221–228, 1993.

104. Schueler PA, Schwartz HL, Strait KA, et al: Binding of 3,5,3'-triiodothyronine (T3) and its analogues to the in vitro translational products of c-erbA protooncogenes—differences in the affinity of the alpha forms and beta forms for the acetic-acid analogue and failure of the human testis and kidney alpha-2 products to bind T3, Mol Endocrinol 4:227–234, 1990.

105. Takeda T, Suzuki S, Liu R-T, et al: Triiodothyroacetic acid has unique potential for therapy of resistance to thyroid hormone, J Clin Endocrinol Metab 80:2033–2040, 1995.

106. Ueda S, Takamatsu J, Fukata S, et al: Differences in response of thyrotropin to 3,5,3'-triiodothyronine and 3,5,3'-triiodothyroacetic acid in patients with resistance to thyroid hormone, Thyroid 6:563–570, 1996.

107. Asteria C, Rajanayagam O, Collingwood TN, et al: Prenatal diagnosis of thyroid hormone resistance, J Clin Endocrinol Metab 84:405–410, 1999.

108. Kunitake JM, Hartman N, Henson LC, et al: 3,5,3'-triiodothyroacetic acid therapy for thyroid hormone resistance, J Clin Endocrinol Metab 69:461–466, 1989.

109. Hamon P, Bovier-LaPierre M, Robert M, et al: Hyperthyroidism due to selective pituitary resistance to thyroid hormones in 15-month-old boy: efficacy of D-thyroxine therapy, J Clin Endocrinol Metab 67:1089–1093, 1988.

110. Dorey F, Strauch G, Gayno JP: Thyrotoxicosis due to pituitary resistance to thyroid hormones. Successful control with D-thyroxine; a study in three patients, Clin Endocrinol 32:221–227, 1990.

111. Dulgeroff AJ, Geffner ME, Koyal SN, et al: Bromocriptine and TRIAC therapy for hyperthyroidism due to pituitary resistance to thyroid hormones, J Clin Endocrinol Metab 75:1071–1075, 1992.

112. Williams G, Kraenzlin M, Sandler L, et al: Hyperthyroidism due to non-tumoural inappropriate TSH secretion: effect of long-acting somatostatin analogue (SMS 201-995), Acta Endocr (Copenh) 113:42–46, 1986.

113. Beck-Peccoz P, Mariotti S, Guillausseau PJ, et al: Treatment of hyperthyroidism due to inappropriate secretion of thyrotropin with the somatostatin analog SMS 201-995, J Clin Endocrinol Metab 68:208–214, 1989.

114. Weiss RE, Stein MA, Refetoff S: Behavioral effects of liothyronine (L-T3) in children with attention deficit hyperactivity disorder in the presence and absence of resistance to thyroid hormone, Thyroid 7:389–393, 1997.

115. Chiellini G, Apriletti JW, Yoshihara HA, et al: A high-affinity subtype-selective agonist ligand for the thyroid hormone receptor, Chem Biol 5:299–306, 1998.

116. Berkenstam A, Kristensen J, et al: The thyroid hormone mimetic compound KB2115 lowers plasma LDL cholesterol and stimulates bile acid synthesis without cardiac effects in humans, Proc Natl Acad Sci U S A 105:663–667, 2008.

117. Koh JT, Putnam MC: Towards the rational design of hormone analogues which complement receptor mutations. In Beck-Peccoz P, editor: Syndromes of hormone resistance on the hypothalamic-pituitary-thyroid axis, ed 1, Boston, 2004, Kluwer Academic Publishers, pp 119–136.

118. Schapira M, Raaka BM, Das S, et al: Discovery of diverse thyroid hormone receptor antagonists by high-throughput docking, Proc Natl Acad Sci U S A 100:7354–7359, 2003.

119. Allan W, Herndon CN, Dudley FC: Some examples of the inheritance of mental deficiency: apparently sex-linked idiocy and microcephaly, Am J Mental Defic 48:325–334, 1944.

120. Dumitrescu AM, Liao XH, Best TB, et al: A novel syndrome combining thyroid and neurological abnormalities is associated with mutations in a monocarboxylate transporter gene, Am J Hum Genet 74:168–173, 2004.

121. Friesema EC, Grueters A, Biebermann H, et al: Association between mutations in a thyroid hormone transporter and severe X-linked psychomotor retardation, Lancet 364:1435–1437, 2004.

122. Schwartz CE, May MM, Carpenter NJ, et al: Allan-Herndon-Dudley syndrome and the monocarboxylate transporter 8 (MCT8) gene, Am J Hum Genet 77:41–53, 2005.

123. Vaurs-Barriere C, Deville M, Sarret C, et al: Pelizaeus-Merzbacher-like disease presentation of MCT8 mutated male subjects, Ann Neurol 65:114–118, 2009.

124. Brockmann K, Dumitrescu AM, Best TT, et al: X-linked paroxysmal dyskinesia and severe global retardation caused by defective MCT8 gene, J Neurol 252:663–666, 2005.

125. Friesema EC, Jansen J, Heuer H, et al: Mechanisms of disease: psychomotor retardation and high T3 levels caused by mutations in monocarboxylate transporter 8, Nat Clin Pract Endocrinol Metab 2:512–523, 2006.

126. Holden KR, Zuniga OF, May MM, et al: X-linked MCT8 gene mutations: characterization of the pediatric neurologic phenotype, J Child Neurol 20:852–857, 2005.

127. Herzovich V, Vaiani E, Marino R, et al: Unexpected peripheral markers of thyroid function in a patient with a novel mutation of the MCT8 thyroid hormone transporter gene, Horm Res 67:1–6, 2007.

128. Namba N, Etani Y, Kitaoka T, et al: Clinical phenotype and endocrinological investigations in a patient with a mutation in the MCT8 thyroid hormone transporter, Eur J Pediatr 167:785–791, 2008.

129. Friesema EC, Ganguly S, Abdalla A, et al: Identification of monocarboxylate transporter 8 as a specific thyroid hormone transporter, J Biol Chem 278:40128–40135, 2003.

130. Friesema EC, Jansen J, Jachtenberg JW, et al: Effective cellular uptake and efflux of thyroid hormone by human monocarboxylate transporter 10, Mol Endocrinol 22:1357–1369, 2008.

131. Friesema ECH, Kuiper GGJM, Jansen J, et al: Thyroid hormone transport by the human monocarboxylate transporter 8 and its rate-limiting role in intracellular metabolism, Mol Endocrinol 20:2761–2772, 2006.

132. Halestrap AP, Meredith D: The SLC16 gene family-from monocarboxylate transporters (MCTs) to aromatic amino acid transporters and beyond, Pflugers Arch 447:619–628, 2004.

133. Jansen J, Friesema EC, Kester MH, et al: Functional analysis of monocarboxylate transporter 8 mutations identified in patients with x-linked psychomotor retardation and elevated serum triiodothyronine, J Clin Endocrinol Metab 92:2378–2381, 2007.

134. Jansen J, Friesema EC, Kester MH, et al: Genotype-phenotype relationship in patients with mutations in thyroid hormone transporter MCT8, Endocrinology 149:2184–2190, 2008.

135. Kinne A, Roth S, Biebermann H, et al: Surface translocation and T3 uptake of mutant MCT8 proteins are cell type-dependent, J Mol Endocrinol (ahead of print), 2009.

136. Visser WE, Jansen J, Friesema EC, et al: Novel pathogenic mechanism suggested by ex vivo analysis of MCT8 (SLC16A2) mutations, Hum Mutat 30:29–38, 2009.

137. Heuer H, Maier MK, Iden S, et al: The monocarboxylate transporter 8 linked to human psychomotor retardation is highly expressed in thyroid hormone-sensitive neuron populations, Endocrinology 146:1701–1706, 2005.

138. Roberts LM, Woodford K, Zhou M, et al: Expression of the thyroid hormone transporters MCT8 (SLC16A2) and OATP14 (SLCO1C1) at the blood-brain barrier, Endocrinology 149:6251–6261, 2008.

139. Bernal J: Thyroid hormones and brain development, Vitam Horm 71:95–122, 2005.

140. Trajkovic M, Visser TJ, Mittag J, et al: Abnormal thyroid hormone metabolism in mice lacking the monocarboxylate transporter 8, J Clin Invest 117:627–635, 2007.

141. Dumitrescu AM, Liao XH, Weiss RE, et al: Tissue-specific thyroid hormone deprivation and excess in monocarboxylate transporter (MCT) 8-deficient mice, Endocrinology 147:4036–4043, 2006.

142. Wirth EK, Roth S, Blechschmidt C, et al: Neuronal 3',3,5-triiodothyronine (T3) uptake and behavioral phenotype of mice deficient in Mct8, the neuronal T3 transporter mutated in Allan-Herndon-Dudley syndrome, J Neurosci 29:9439–9449, 2009.

143. Trajkovic M, Visser TJ, Darras WM, et al: Consequences of MCT8 deficiency for renal transport and metabolism of thyroid hormones in mice, Endocrinology 2009. In press.

144. Wemeau JL, Pigeyre M, Proust-Lemoine E, et al: Beneficial effects of propylthiouracil plus L-thyroxine treatment in a patient with a mutation in MCT8, J Clin Endocrinol Metab 93:2084–2088, 2008.

145. Di Cosmo C, Liao XH, Dumitrescu AM, et al: A thyroid hormone analog with reduced dependence on the monocarboxylate transporter 8 for tissue transport, Endocrinology 150:4450–4458, 2009.

146. Dumitrescu AM, Liao X, Abdullah MSY, et al: Mutations in SECISBP2 result in abnormal thyroid hormone metabolism, Nat Genet 37:1247–1252, 2005.

147. Di Cosmo C, McLellan N, Liao X, et al: Clinical and molecular characterization of a novel selenocysteine insertion sequence-binding protein 2 (SBP2) gene mutation (R128X), J Clin Endocrinol Metab 94:4003–4009, 2009.

148. Papp LV, Wang J, Kennedy D et al: Functional characterization of alternatively spliced human SECISBP2 transcript variants, Nucleic Acids Research 36:7192–7206, 2008.

149. Squires J, Stoytchev I, Forry EP, et al: SBP2 binding affinity is a major determinant in differential selenoprotein mRNA translation and sensitivity to nonsense-mediated decay, Mol Cell Biol 27:7848–7855, 2007.

150. Bubenik JL, Driscoll DM: Altered RNA binding activity underlies abnormal thyroid hormone metabolism linked to a mutation in selenocysteine insertion sequence-binding protein 2, J Biol Chem 282:34653–34662, 2007.

151. Schomburg L, Dumitrescu AM, Liao X, et al: Selenium supplementation fails to correct the selenoprotein synthesis defect in subjects with SBP2 gene mutations, Thyroid 19:277–281, 2009.

Chapter 24

SURGERY OF THE THYROID

EDWIN L. KAPLAN and PETER ANGELOS

Modern thyroid surgery, as we know it today, began in the 1860s in Vienna with the school of Billroth.[1] The mortality associated with thyroidectomy was high, recurrent laryngeal nerve injuries were common, and tetany was thought to be caused by "hysteria." The parathyroid glands in humans were not discovered until 1880 by Sandstrom,[2] and the fact that hypocalcemia was the definitive cause of tetany was not wholly accepted until several decades into the twentieth century. Kocher,[3] a master thyroid surgeon who operated in the late nineteenth and early twentieth centuries in Bern, practiced meticulous surgical technique and greatly reduced the mortality and operative morbidity of thyroidectomy for goiter. He described "cachexia strumipriva" in patients years after thyroidectomy[3] (Fig. 24-1). Kocher recognized that this dreaded syndrome developed only in patients who had undergone total thyroidectomy. As a result, he stopped performing total resection of the thyroid. We now know, of course, that cachexia strumipriva was surgical hypothyroidism. Kocher received the Nobel Prize for this very important contribution, which proved beyond a doubt the physiologic importance of the thyroid gland.

By 1920, advances in thyroid surgery had reached the point that Halsted referred to this operation as a "feat which today can be accomplished by any competent operator without danger of mishap."[1] Unfortunately, decades later, complications still occur. In the best of hands, however, thyroid surgery can be performed today with a mortality that varies little from the risk of general anesthesia alone, as well as with low morbidity. To obtain such enviable results, however, surgeons must have a thorough understanding of the pathophysiology of thyroid disorders; must be versed in the preoperative and postoperative care of patients; must have a clear knowledge of the anatomy of the neck region; and, finally, must use an unhurried, careful, and meticulous operative technique.

Important Surgical Anatomy

The thyroid (which means "shield") gland is composed of two lobes connected by an isthmus that lies on the trachea approximately at the level of the second tracheal ring (Fig. 24-2). The gland is enveloped by the deep cervical fascia and is attached firmly to the trachea by the ligament of Berry. Each lobe resides in a bed between the trachea and larynx medially and the carotid sheath and sternocleidomastoid muscles laterally. The strap muscles are anterior to the thyroid lobes, and the parathyroid glands and recurrent laryngeal nerves are associated with the posterior surface of each lobe. A pyramidal lobe is often present. This structure is a long, narrow projection of thyroid tissue that extends upward from the isthmus and lies on the surface of the thyroid cartilage. It represents a vestige of the embryonic thyroglossal duct, and it often becomes palpable in cases of thyroiditis

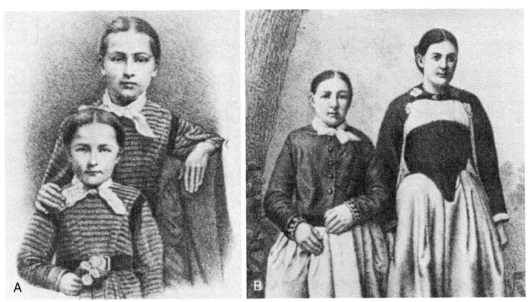

FIGURE 24-1. The dramatic case of Maria Richsel, the first patient with postoperative myxedema to have come to Kocher's attention. **A,** The child and her younger sister before the operation. **B,** Changes 9 years after the operation. The younger sister, now fully grown, contrasts vividly with the dwarfed and stunted patient. Also note Maria's thickened face and fingers, which are typical of myxedema. (From Kocher T: Uber Kropfextirpation und ihre Folgen, Arch Klin Chir 29:254, 1883.)

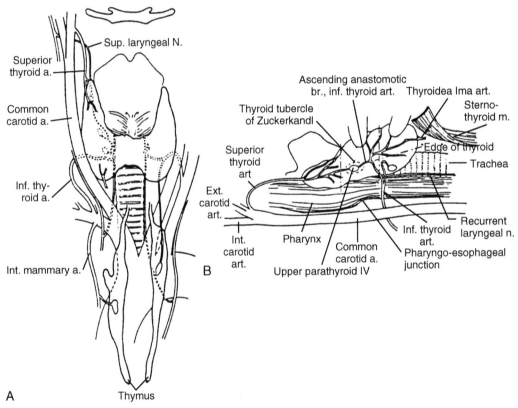

FIGURE 24-2. Anatomy of the thyroid and parathyroid glands. **A,** Anterior view. **B,** Lateral view with the thyroid retracted anteriorly and medially to show the surgical landmarks (the head of the patient is to the left). (From Kaplan EL: Thyroid and parathyroid. In Schwartz SI [ed]: Principles of Surgery, 5th ed. New York, McGraw-Hill, 1989, pp 1613–1685. Copyright © by McGraw-Hill, Inc. Used by permission of McGraw-Hill Book Company.)

or Graves' disease. The normal thyroid varies in size in different parts of the world, depending on the iodine content in the diet. In the United States, it weighs about 15 g.

VASCULAR SUPPLY

The thyroid has an abundant blood supply (see Fig. 24-2). The arterial supply to each thyroid lobe is twofold. The superior thyroid artery arises from the external carotid artery on each side and descends several centimeters in the neck to reach the upper pole of each thyroid lobe, where it branches. The inferior thyroid artery, each of which arises from the thyrocervical trunk of the subclavian artery, crosses beneath the carotid sheath and enters the lower or midpart of each thyroid lobe. The thyroidea ima is sometimes present; it arises from the arch of the aorta and enters the thyroid at the midline. A venous plexus forms under the thyroid capsule. Each lobe is drained by the superior thyroid vein at the upper pole, which flows into the internal jugular vein; and by the middle thyroid vein at the middle part of the lobe, which enters the internal jugular or the innominate vein. Arising from each lower pole is the inferior thyroid vein, which drains directly into the innominate vein.

NERVES

The thyroid gland's relationship to the recurrent laryngeal nerve and to the external branch of the superior laryngeal nerve is of major surgical significance because damage to these nerves leads to disability in phonation or to difficulty in breathing.[4] Both nerves are branches of the vagus nerve.

Recurrent Laryngeal Nerve

The right recurrent laryngeal nerve arises from the vagus nerve, loops posteriorly around the subclavian artery, and ascends behind the right lobe of the thyroid (Fig. 24-3). It enters the larynx behind the cricothyroid muscle and the inferior cornu of the thyroid cartilage and innervates all the intrinsic laryngeal muscles except the cricothyroid. The left recurrent laryngeal nerve comes from the left vagus nerve, loops posteriorly around the arch of the aorta, and ascends in the tracheoesophageal groove posterior to the left lobe of the thyroid, where it enters the larynx and innervates the musculature in a similar fashion as the right nerve. Several factors make the recurrent laryngeal nerve vulnerable to injury, especially in the hands of inexperienced surgeons[4,6]

1. *The presence of a nonrecurrent laryngeal nerve (Fig. 24-4).* Nonrecurrent nerves occur more often on the right side (0.6%) than on the left (0.04%).[5] They are associated with vascular anomalies such as an aberrant takeoff of the right subclavian artery from the descending aorta (on the right) or a right-sided aortic arch (on the left). In these abnormal positions, each nerve is at greater risk of being divided.

2. *Proximity of the recurrent nerve to the thyroid gland.* The recurrent nerve is not always in the tracheoesophageal groove where it is expected to be. It often can be posterior or anterior to this position, or it may even be surrounded by thyroid parenchyma. Thus, the nerve is vulnerable to injury if it is not visualized and traced up to the larynx during thyroidectomy.

3. *Relationship of the recurrent nerve to the inferior thyroid artery.* The nerve often passes anterior, posterior, or through the branches of the inferior thyroid artery. Medial traction of the lobe often lifts the nerve anteriorly, thereby making it more vulnerable. Likewise, ligation of this artery, practiced by many surgeons, may be dangerous if the nerve is not identified first.

4. *Deformities from large thyroid nodules.*[6] In the presence of large nodules, the laryngeal nerves may not be in their "correct" anatomic location but may be found even anterior to the thyroid (Fig. 24-5). Once more, there is no substitute for identification of the nerve in a gentle and careful manner.

External Branch of the Superior Laryngeal Nerve

On each side, the external branch of the superior laryngeal nerve innervates the cricothyroid muscle. In most cases, this nerve lies close to the vascular pedicle of the superior poles of the thyroid lobe,[7] which requires that the vessels be ligated with care to avoid injury to it (Fig. 24-6). In 21%, the nerve is intimately associated with the superior thyroid vessels. In some patients, the external branch of the superior laryngeal nerve lies on the anterior surface of the thyroid lobe, making the possibility of damage during thyroidectomy even greater.[8] In only 15% of patients is the superior laryngeal nerve sufficiently distant from the superior pole vessels to be protected from manipulation by the surgeon. Unfortunately, many surgeons do not even attempt to identify this nerve before performing ligation of the upper pole of the thyroid.[9,9a]

PARATHYROID GLANDS

The parathyroids are small glands that secrete parathyroid hormone, the major hormone that controls serum calcium homeostasis in humans. Usually, four glands are present, two on each side, but three to six glands have been found. Each gland normally weighs 30 to 40 mg, but glands may be heavier if more

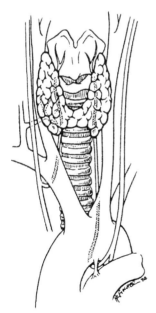

FIGURE 24-3. Anatomy of the recurrent laryngeal nerves. (From Thompson NW, Demers M: Exposure is not necessary to avoid the recurrent laryngeal nerve during thyroid operations. In Simmons RL, Udekwu AO [eds]: Debates in Clinical Surgery, Chicago, Year Book, 1990.)

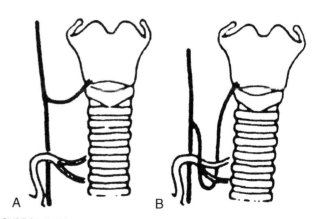

FIGURE 24-4. "Nonrecurrent" right laryngeal nerves coursing **(A)** near the superior pole vessels or **(B)** around the inferior thyroid artery. Because of the abnormal location of "nonrecurrent" nerves, they are much more likely to be damaged during surgery. (From Skandalakis JE, Droulis C, Harlaftis N, et al: The recurrent laryngeal nerve, Am Surg 42:629–634, 1976.)

fat is present. Because of their small size, their delicate blood supply, and their usual anatomic position adjacent to the thyroid gland, these structures are at risk of being accidentally removed, traumatized, or devascularized during thyroidectomy.[10]

The upper parathyroid glands arise embryologically from the fourth pharyngeal pouch (Figs. 24-7 and 24-8). They descend only slightly during embryologic development, and their position in adult life remains constant. This gland is usually found adjacent to the posterior surface of the middle part of the thyroid lobe, often just anterior to the recurrent laryngeal nerve as it enters the larynx.

The lower parathyroid glands arise from the third pharyngeal pouch, along with the thymus; hence, they often descend with the thymus. Because they travel so far in embryologic life, they have a wide range of distribution in adults, from just beneath the mandible to the anterior mediastinum[11] (see Fig. 24-8). Usually, however, these glands are found on the lateral or posterior surface of the lower part of the thyroid gland or within several centimeters of the lower thyroid pole within the thymic tongue.

Parathyroid glands can be recognized by their tan appearance; their small vascular pedicle; the fact that they bleed freely when a biopsy is performed, as opposed to fatty tissue; and their darkening color of hematoma formation when they are traumatized. With experience, one becomes much more adept at recognizing these very important structures and in differentiating them from lymph nodes or fat. Frozen section examination during surgery can be helpful in their identification.

LYMPHATICS

A practical description of the lymphatic drainage of the thyroid gland for the thyroid surgeon has been proposed by Taylor.[12] The results of his studies, which are clinically very relevant to the lymphatic spread of thyroid carcinoma, are summarized in the following section.

Central Compartment of the Neck

1. The most constant site to which dye goes when injected into the thyroid is the trachea, the wall of which contains a rich network of lymphatics. This fact probably accounts for the frequency with which the trachea is involved by thyroid carcinoma, especially when it is anaplastic. This involvement is sometimes the limiting factor in surgical excision.
2. A chain of lymph nodes lies in the groove between the trachea and the esophagus.

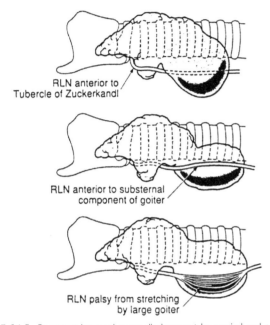

FIGURE 24-5. Recurrent laryngeal nerve displacement by cervical and substernal goiters. Such nerves are at risk during lobectomy unless the surgeon anticipates the unusual locations and is very careful. Rarely, the nerves are so stretched that spontaneous palsy results. After careful dissection and preservation, functional recovery may occur postoperatively. (From Thompson NW, Demers M: Exposure is not necessary to avoid the recurrent laryngeal nerve during thyroid operations. In Simmons RL, Udekwu AO [eds]: Debates in Clinical Surgery. Chicago, Year Book, 1990.)

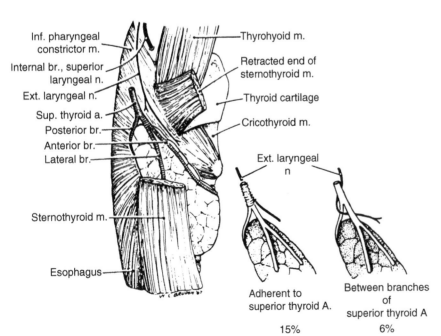

FIGURE 24-6. Proximity of the external branch of the superior laryngeal nerve to the superior thyroid vessels. (From Moosman DA, DeWeese MS: The external laryngeal nerve as related to thyroidectomy, Surg Gynecol Obstet 127:1101, 1968.)

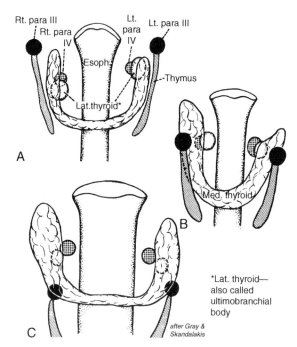

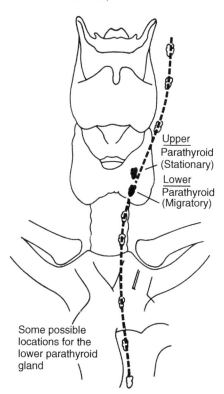

FIGURE 24-7. **A** and **B,** Shifts in location of the thyroid, parafollicular, and parathyroid tissues. **C** approximates the adult location. Note that what has been called the lateral thyroid is now commonly referred to as the ultimobranchial body, which contains both C cells and follicular elements. (From Sedgwick CE, Cady B: Surgery of the Thyroid and Parathyroid Gland, 2nd ed. Philadelphia, WB Saunders, 1980; adapted from Norris EH: Parathyroid glands and lateral thyroid in man: their morphogenesis, histogenesis, topographic anatomy and prenatal growth, Contrib Embryol Carnegie Inst Wash 26:247–294, 1937.)

FIGURE 24-8. Descent of the lower parathyroid. Whereas the upper parathyroid occupies a relatively constant position in relation to the middle or upper third of the lateral thyroid lobe, the lower parathyroid normally migrates in embryonic life and may end up anywhere along the course of the *dotted line.* When this gland is in the chest, it is nearly always in the anterior mediastinum. (From Kaplan EL: Thyroid and parathyroid. In Schwartz SI [ed]: Principles of Surgery, 5th ed. New York, McGraw-Hill, 1989, pp 1613–1685. Copyright © by McGraw-Hill, Inc. Used by permission of McGraw-Hill Book Company.)

3. Lymph can always be shown to drain toward the mediastinum and to the nodes intimately associated with the thymus.
4. One or more nodes lying above the isthmus, and therefore in front of the larynx, are sometimes involved. These nodes have been called the Delphian nodes (named for the oracle of Delphi), because it has been said that if palpable, they are diagnostic of carcinoma. However, this clinical sign is often misleading.
5. Central lymph node dissection clears out all these lymph nodes from one carotid artery to the other carotid artery and down into the superior mediastinum as far as possible.[12a]

Lateral Compartment of the Neck

A constant group of nodes lies along the jugular vein on each side of the neck. The lymph glands found in the supraclavicular fossae may also be involved in more distant spread of malignant disease from the thyroid gland. Finally, it should not be forgotten that the thoracic duct on the left side of the neck, a lymph vessel of considerable size, arches up out of the mediastinum and passes forward and laterally to drain into the left subclavian vein, usually just lateral to its junction with the internal jugular vein. If the thoracic duct is damaged, the wound is likely to fill with lymph; in such cases, the duct should always be sought and tied. A wound that discharges lymph postoperatively should always raise suspicion of damage to the thoracic duct or a major tributary. A lateral lymph node dissection encompasses removal of these lateral lymph nodes. Rarely, the submental nodes are involved by metastatic thyroid cancer as well.

The lymph node regions of the neck are divided into levels I through VII: (1) level I nodes are the submental and submandibular nodes; (2) level II are the upper jugular nodes; (3) level III are the midjugular nodes; (4) level IV are the lower jugular nodes; (5) level V are the posterior triangle and supraclavicular nodes; (6) level VI or central compartment nodes incorporate the Delphian/prelaryngeal, pretracheal, and paratracheal lymph nodes; and (7) level VII nodes are those within the superior mediastinum (see Fig. 24-12).[12a]

Indications for Thyroidectomy

Thyroidectomy is usually performed for the following reasons:
1. As therapy for some individuals with thyrotoxicosis, both those with Graves' disease and others with hot nodules
2. To establish a definitive diagnosis of a mass within the thyroid gland, especially when cytologic analysis after fine-needle aspiration (FNA) is nondiagnostic or equivocal
3. To treat benign and malignant thyroid tumors
4. To alleviate pressure symptoms or respiratory difficulties associated with a benign or malignant process
5. To remove an unsightly goiter
6. To remove large substernal goiters, especially when they cause respiratory difficulties

SOLITARY THYROID NODULES

Solitary thyroid nodules are present in 4% to 9% of patients by clinical examination, and in 22% of patients by ultrasound in the United States; most are benign.[13] Therefore, rather than operating on every patient with a thyroid nodule, the physician or surgeon should select patients for surgery who are at high risk for thyroid cancer. Furthermore, each surgeon must know the complications of thyroidectomy and must be able to perform a proper operation for thyroid cancer in a safe and effective manner or must refer the patient to a center where it can be done.

LOW-DOSE EXTERNAL IRRADIATION OF THE HEAD AND NECK

A history of low-dose external irradiation of the head or neck is probably the most important historical fact that can be obtained in a patient with a thyroid nodule because it indicates that cancer of the thyroid is more likely (in up to 35% of cases), even if the gland is multinodular.[14,15] Fortunately, treatments of low-dose radiation for thymic enlargement, tonsils, and acne have long been discontinued. However, patients who had this therapy in childhood are still seen and are still at greater risk for cancer.

HIGH-DOSE EXTERNAL IRRADIATION THERAPY

High-dose external irradiation therapy, that is, more than 2000 rad, does not confer safety from thyroid carcinoma, as was previously thought.[16] Rather, an increased prevalence of thyroid carcinoma, usually papillary cancer, has been found, particularly in patients with Hodgkin's disease and other lymphomas who received upper mantle irradiation that included the thyroid gland. Usually, a dose of about 4000 to 5000 rads was given. Both benign and malignant thyroid nodules are being recognized, now that these persons survive for longer periods.[17] If a thyroid mass appears, it should be treated aggressively. These patients should also be observed carefully for the development of hypothyroidism.

RISK OF IONIZING RADIATION

Children in the area of the Chernobyl nuclear accident have been shown to have at least a 30-fold increase in papillary thyroid cancer.[18] This cancer also may be more aggressive than the usual papillary carcinoma. It is thought to result from exposure to iodine isotopes that were inhaled or that entered the food chain. The mechanism of radiation-induced thyroid cancer is thought to be caused primarily by chromosomal rearrangements such as RET/PTC.[19]

DIAGNOSIS OF THYROID NODULES

A number of diagnostic modalities have been used in the past, but currently most have been superseded by FNA of the mass with cytologic analysis. In the hands of a good thyroid cytologist, more than 90% of nodules can be categorized histologically. Approximately 65% to 70% are found to be compatible with a colloid nodule. Twenty percent demonstrate sheets of follicular cells with little or no colloid. Five percent to 10% are malignant, and less than 10% are nondiagnostic. To improve the diagnostic ability of FNA, researchers are adding biomarkers to the cytologic analyses.[20,21]

All patients who have malignant cytologic results should be operated on. False-positive diagnoses are rare. All patients with sheets of follicular cells with little or no colloid also should undergo surgery, because their findings are compatible with a follicular neoplasm. This nodule is called a follicular nodule or an indeterminate nodule. Most, up to 90%, prove to be benign; however, a follicular carcinoma or a follicular variant of papillary cancer may exhibit the same cytologic characteristics and cannot be differentiated by FNA. Only by careful histologic examination, after operative removal of the nodule, can follicular carcinoma and adenoma be differentiated, because follicular cancers exhibit capsular and/or vascular invasion.

When the diagnosis of colloid nodule is made cytologically, the patient should be observed and not operated on unless tracheal compression or a substernal goiter is present, or unless the patient desires the benign mass to be removed. Finally, if an inadequate specimen is obtained, FNA with cytologic examination should be repeated. With small, nonpalpable masses, FNA should be performed under ultrasound guidance. Thus, FNA with cytologic assessment is the most powerful tool in our armamentarium for the diagnosis of a thyroid nodule.

In summary, the algorithm for the diagnosis of a thyroid nodule with isotope scintigraphy and ultrasonography as initial steps (Fig. 24-9) has been replaced in most hospitals, including our own, by an emphasis on the importance of early cytologic examination of the needle aspirate (Fig. 24-10). Far fewer isotope scans are currently being done because carcinomas represent only 5% to 10% of all cold nodules. This test usually is reserved for diagnosis of a "hot" nodule.

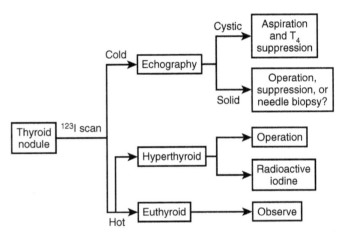

FIGURE 24-9. Algorithm for the diagnosis of a thyroid nodule that uses needle aspiration with cytologic examination of each nodule. Greater accuracy is obtained by using this diagnostic scheme. (Courtesy Dr. Jon van Heerden.)

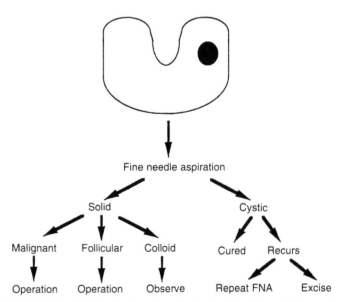

FIGURE 24-10. Algorithm for the diagnosis of a thyroid nodule with fine-needle aspiration (FNA) and cytologic examination of each nodule. Greater accuracy is obtained by using this diagnosis scheme. (Courtesy Dr. Jon van Heerden.)

Preparation for Surgery

Most patients undergoing a thyroid operation are euthyroid and require no specific preoperative preparation related to their thyroid gland. Determination of the serum calcium level may be helpful, and endoscopic or indirect laryngoscopy definitely should be performed in those who are hoarse and in others who have had a prior thyroid, parathyroid, or cervical disc operation in order to detect the possibility of a recurrent laryngeal nerve injury.

HYPOTHYROIDISM

Modest hypothyroidism is of little concern when one is treating a surgical patient; however, severe hypothyroidism can be a significant risk factor. Severe hypothyroidism can be diagnosed clinically by myxedema, as well as by slowness of affect, speech, and reflexes.[22] Circulating thyroxine and triiodothyronine values are low. The serum thyroid-stimulating hormone (TSH) level is high in all cases of hypothyroidism that are not caused by pituitary insufficiency, and it is the best test of thyroid function. In the presence of severe hypothyroidism, both the morbidity and the mortality of surgery are increased as a result of the effects of both the anesthesia and the operation. Such patients have a higher incidence of perioperative hypotension, cardiovascular problems, gastrointestinal hypomotility, prolonged anesthetic recovery, and neuropsychiatric disturbances. They metabolize drugs slowly and are very sensitive to all medications. Therefore, when severe myxedema is present, it is preferable to defer elective surgery until a euthyroid state is achieved.

If urgent surgery is necessary, it should not be postponed simply for repletion of thyroid hormone. Endocrine consultation is imperative, and an excellent anesthesiologist is mandatory for success. In most cases, intravenous thyroxine can be started preoperatively and continued thereafter. In general, small doses of thyroxine are given initially to patients who are severely hypothyroid, and then the dose is gradually increased.

HYPERTHYROIDISM

In the United States, most patients with thyrotoxicosis have Graves' disease. In the United States, about 90% of all patients with Graves' disease are treated with radioiodine therapy. Young patients, those with very large goiters, some pregnant women, and those with thyroid nodules or severe ophthalmopathy are commonly operated upon.

Persons with Graves' disease or other thyrotoxic states should be treated preoperatively to restore a euthyroid state and to prevent thyroid storm, a severe accentuation of the symptoms and signs of hyperthyroidism that can occur during or after surgery. Thyroid storm results in tachycardia or cardiac arrhyth-

mias, fever, disorientation, coma, and even death. In the early days of thyroid surgery, operations on the toxic gland were among the most dangerous surgical procedures because of the common occurrence of severe bleeding, as well as all the symptoms and signs of thyroid storm. Now, with proper preoperative preparation,[23] operations on the thyroid gland in Graves' disease can be performed with about the same degree of safety as operations for other thyroid conditions.

In mild cases of Graves' disease with thyrotoxicosis, iodine therapy alone has been used for preoperative preparation, although we do not recommend this approach routinely.[22] Lugol's solution or a saturated solution of potassium iodide is given for 8 to 10 days. Although only several drops per day are needed to block the release of thyroxine from the toxic thyroid gland, it is our practice to administer two drops two or three times daily. This medication is taken in milk or orange juice to make it more palatable.

Most of our patients with Graves' disease are treated initially with the antithyroid drugs propylthiouracil or methimazole (Tapazole) until they approach a euthyroid state. Then iodine is added to the regimen for 8 to 10 days before surgery. The iodine decreases the vascularity and increases the firmness of the gland. Sometimes thyroxine is added to this regimen to prevent hypothyroidism and to decrease the size of the gland. β-Adrenergic blockers such as propranolol (Inderal) have increased the safety of thyroidectomy for patients with Graves' disease.[23] We use them commonly with antithyroid drugs to block β-adrenergic receptors and to ameliorate the major signs of Graves' disease by decreasing the patient's pulse rate and eliminating the tremor. Some surgeons recommend preoperative use of propranolol alone or with iodine.[24] These regimens, they believe, shorten the preparation time of patients with Graves' disease for surgery and make the operation easier because the thyroid gland is smaller and less friable than it would otherwise be.[24] We do not favor these regimens for routine preparation because they do not appear to offer the same degree of safety as do preoperative programs that restore a euthyroid state before surgery. Instances of fever and tachycardia have been reported in persons with Graves' disease who were taking only propranolol. We have used propranolol therapy alone or with iodine without difficulty in some patients who are allergic to antithyroid medications. In such patients, it is essential to continue the propranolol for several weeks postoperatively. Remember that they are still in a thyrotoxic state immediately after surgery, although the peripheral manifestations of their disease have been blocked.

The advantages and disadvantages of radioiodine versus thyroidectomy as definitive treatment for Graves' disease are listed in Table 24-1. Among our patients, we have never had a death from thyroidectomy for Graves' disease in over 35 years. Surgical

Table 24-1. Ablative Treatment for Graves' Disease With Thyrotoxicosis

Method	Dose or Extent of Surgery	Onset of Response	Complications	Remarks
Surgery	Subtotal excision of gland (leaving about 2 g remnant or less)	Immediate	Mortality: <1% Permanent hypothyroidism: 20%-30% Recurrent hyperthyroidism: <15% Vocal cord paralysis: ≈1% Hypoparathyroidism: ≈1%	Applicable in younger patients and pregnant women
Radioiodine	5-10 mCi	Several weeks to months	Permanent hypothyroidism: 50%-70%, often with delayed onset; multiple treatments sometimes necessary; recurrence possible	Avoid in children or pregnant women

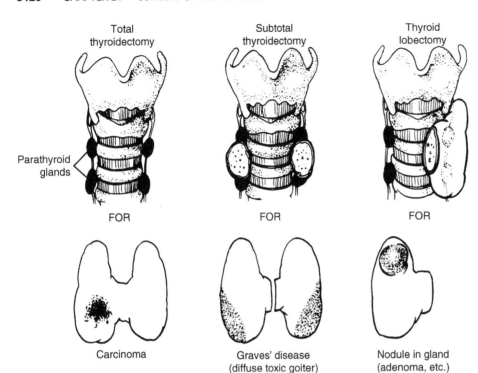

Total thyroidectomy

Subtotal thyroidectomy

Thyroid lobectomy

Parathyroid glands

FOR

FOR

FOR

Carcinoma

Graves' disease (diffuse toxic goiter)

Nodule in gland (adenoma, etc.)

FIGURE 24-11. Common operations on the thyroid. In near-total thyroidectomy, a small amount of thyroid tissue is left to protect the recurrent laryngeal nerve and the upper parathyroid gland. (From Kaplan EL: Surgical endocrinology. In Polk HC, Stone HH, Gardner B [eds]: Basic Surgery, 4th ed. St. Louis, Quality Medical Publishing, 1993, pp 162–195.)

resection involves subtotal or near-total thyroidectomy (Fig. 24-11) or lobectomy with contralateral subtotal or near-total lobectomy. Currently we leave less than 2 g of thyroid tissue in the neck at the end of the operative procedure. Leaving more leads to a higher rate of recurrence.[25] In children and adolescents, one should consider leaving smaller remnants because the incidence of recurrence of thyrotoxicosis appears to be greater in this group. Finally, when operating for severe ophthalmopathy, we try to perform near-total or total thyroidectomy. The major benefits of thyroidectomy appear to be the speed with which normalization is achieved and a lower rate of hypothyroidism than is seen after radioiodine therapy.

Surgical Approach to Thyroid Nodules

NONIRRADIATED PATIENTS

Any nodule suspected of being a carcinoma should be completely removed, along with surrounding tissue; this means that a total lobectomy (or lobectomy with isthmectomy) is the initial operation of choice in most patients (see Fig. 24-11). A frozen section should be obtained intraoperatively. If a colloid nodule is diagnosed, the operation is terminated. If a follicular neoplasm is diagnosed, treatment is more controversial. Differentiating follicular adenoma from follicular carcinoma, or a benign Hürthle cell tumor from Hürthle cell carcinoma, with the use of frozen section is usually very difficult. These diagnoses require careful assessment of capsular and vascular invasion, which are often difficult to evaluate on frozen section. To aid in the diagnosis, enlarged lymph nodes of the central compartment are often sampled, and a biopsy of the jugular nodes is performed. If the result is negative, two options are available: (1) stopping the operation after lobectomy, with the understanding that a second

operation may be necessary to complete the thyroidectomy if a carcinoma is ultimately diagnosed; or (2) performing a resection of most of the thyroid on the contralateral side. We treat most patients with benign neoplasms with thyroxine replacement anyway, even if only one lobe has been removed. Furthermore, a second operation usually is eliminated if the lesion is later diagnosed as malignant, because the remaining small thyroid remnant can be ablated with radioiodine therapy. We discuss these options with the patient preoperatively.

IRRADIATED PATIENTS

In patients with multiple thyroid nodules who have been exposed to low-dose, external irradiation of the head and neck during infancy, childhood, or adolescence, a near-total resection of the thyroid gland with biopsy of the jugular nodes is usually performed, even if a frozen section of the dominant nodule is benign. Reasons for this include the frequency of bilaterality of the disease, the known coincidence of benign and malignant nodules in the same gland, and the prevalence of papillary carcinoma in up to 35% of such patients.[15] This therapy is thought to be advantageous, because small cancers can be present in the same gland, and the remaining small thyroid remnant of these patients can usually be ablated with radioiodine if a carcinoma is found on permanent section analysis. In any event, these patients require therapy with thyroid hormone. In patients with single nodules, however, we use FNA with cytology to determine the need for operation.

Patients who have received high-dose radiation to their thyroid bed (e.g., those treated with mantle irradiation for Hodgkin's disease) are at greater risk for the development of thyroid carcinoma years later and should be monitored carefully.[16] Once more, if they are operated on for nodular disease, most of the thyroid tissue should be removed, even if the dominant mass is thought to be benign.

Surgical Approach to Thyroid Cancer

PAPILLARY CARCINOMA

Surgical treatment for papillary carcinoma is best divided into two groups based on the clinical characteristics and virulence of these lesions.

Treatment for Minimal Papillary Carcinoma

The term *minimal papillary carcinoma* refers to a small papillary cancer, less than 1 cm in diameter, that demonstrates no local invasiveness through the thyroid capsule, that is not associated with lymph node metastases, and that often is found in a young person as an occult lesion when thyroidectomy has been performed for another benign condition. In such instances, especially when the cancer is unicentric and smaller than 5 mm, lobectomy is sufficient and reoperation is unnecessary. Thyroid hormone is given to suppress serum TSH levels, and the patient is monitored at regular intervals.

Standard Treatment for Most Papillary Carcinomas

Most papillary carcinomas are neither minimal nor occult. These tumors are known to be microscopically multicentric in up to 80% of patients; they also are known occasionally to invade locally into the trachea or esophagus, to metastasize commonly to lymph nodes and later to the lungs and other tissues, and to recur clinically in the other thyroid lobe in 7% to 18% of patients if treated only by thyroid lobectomy.[26,26a]

The authors firmly believe that the best treatment for papillary cancer is near-total or total thyroidectomy (see Fig. 24-11), with appropriate central and lateral neck dissection when nodes are involved. So-called cherry-picking operations, which remove only the enlarged lymph nodes, should not be performed. Rather, when tumor is found in the lateral triangle, a modified radical neck dissection should be performed[27] (Fig. 24-12). At the conclusion of a modified radical neck dissection, the lymph node–bearing tissue from the lateral triangle is removed, whereas the carotid artery, jugular vein, phrenic nerve, sympathetic ganglia, brachial plexus, and spinal accessory nerve are spared and left in place. Many times sensory nerves can be retained as well. Prophylactic neck dissection of the lateral triangle should not be performed for papillary cancer; such dissections should be done only when enlarged nodes with tumor are found.

In recent years, for clarity and uniformity of reporting, the location of lymph nodes in the neck and upper mediastinum has been defined as shown in Fig. 24-12B. Central lymph nodes (level VI) are frequently involved with metastases from ipsilateral thyroid cancers, as are levels III, IV, and V, which are removed in most lateral neck dissections. Although prophylactic lateral neck dissections are no longer performed, Delbridge and his group suggest that routine removal of level VI nodes (ipsilateral central compartment) should be done with total thyroidectomy to decrease the recurrence of papillary cancers postoperatively.[12a] They autotransplant one parathyroid as part of this procedure. We do not routinely perform this procedure because of the increased risk for hypoparathyroiditism, but we reserve it for cases in which ipsilateral central lymph nodes are clearly involved with tumor.

Surgeons with limited experience probably should not perform total or near-total thyroidectomy unless they are capable

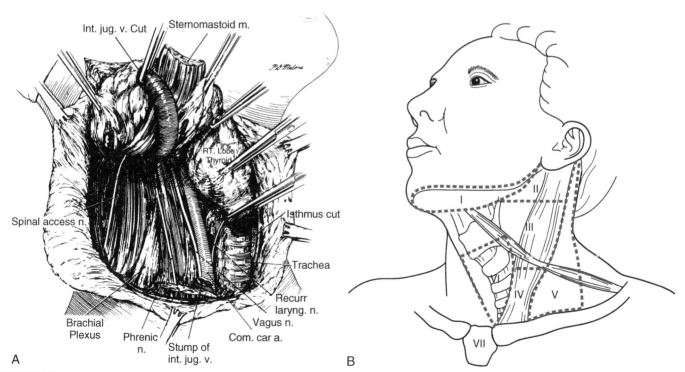

FIGURE 24-12. A, Lateral neck dissection. Note that during this procedure, the vagus nerve, sympathetic ganglia, phrenic nerve, brachial plexus, and spinal accessory nerve are preserved. In a modified neck dissection, the sternocleidomastoid muscle is not usually divided, and the jugular vein is not removed unless lymph nodes with tumor are adherent to it. (From Sedgwick CE, Cady B: Surgery of the Thyroid and Parathyroid Glands. Philadelphia, WB Saunders, 1980, p 180.) **B,** The lymph node regions of the neck are divided into levels I through VII: (1) level I nodes are the submental and submandibular nodes; (2) level II are the upper jugular nodes; (3) level III are the midjugular nodes; (4) level IV are the lower jugular nodes; (5) level V are the posterior triangle and supraclavicular nodes; (6) level VI or central compartment nodes incorporate the Delphian/prelaryngeal, pretracheal, and paratracheal lymph nodes; and (7) level VII nodes are those within the superior mediastinum.

of doing so with a low incidence of recurrent laryngeal nerve injury and permanent hypoparathyroidism, because these complications are serious. Otherwise, it may be advisable to refer such patients to a major medical center where such expertise is available.

After surgery, radioiodine scanning and treatment are commonly used.[28,28a] [131]I is taken up by most metastatic papillary cancers, but only if the TSH level is very high and normal thyroid tissue has been removed or ablated. If all or a substantial part of a lobe of normal thyroid remains, radioiodine treatment for metastases cannot be performed effectively. Usually, reoperative completion thyroidectomy is done, and then radioiodine is given. In low-risk patients, recombinant TSH preparation is sometimes used.[28a]

Controversies

Because randomized prospective studies have not been performed, controversy still exists over proper treatment for papillary cancer in some patients. Many clinicians now accept that patients with this disease can be separated into different risk groups according to a set of prognostic factors. With use of the AGES (age, tumor grade, extent, and size),[29] AMES (age, metastases, extent, and size),[30] or MACIS (metastasis, age, completeness of resection, local invasion, and tumor size)[31] criteria, which evaluate risk by age, distant metastases, extent of local involvement, and size (MACIS adds completeness of excision), almost 80% of patients fall into a low-risk group. Treatment for this low-risk group is most controversial, perhaps because the cure rate is so good, certainly in the high 90% range. Should a lobectomy be done, or is bilateral thyroid resection more beneficial?

Low-Risk Papillary Cancer

Hay and associates studied 1685 patients treated at the Mayo Clinic between 1940 and 1991; the mean follow-up period was 18 years.[32] Of the total, 98% had complete tumor resection, and 38% had initial nodal involvement. Twelve percent had unilateral lobectomy, whereas 88% had bilateral lobar resection; total thyroidectomy was done in 18%, and near-total thyroidectomy was performed in 60%. Cause-specific mortality at 30 years was 2%, and distant metastases occurred in 3%. These indices did not differ between surgical groups; however, local recurrence and nodal metastases in the lobectomy group (14% and 19%, respectively) were significantly higher than the 2% and 6% rates seen after near-total or total thyroidectomy.

This study is excellent. Although no differences in mortality were reported, a threefold increase in tumor recurrence rates in the thyroid bed and lymph nodes was reported in the lobectomy group. In addition, this study recognizes patients' anxiety about tumor recurrence and their strong desire to face an operation only once and to be cured of their disease. If the operation can be done safely with low morbidity, this study supports the use of near-total or total thyroidectomy for patients with low-risk papillary cancer.

High-Risk Papillary Cancer

For high-risk patients, it is agreed that bilateral thyroid resection improves survival[29] and reduces recurrence rates[33] when compared with unilateral resection.

At the University of Chicago, most patients also receive radioiodine ablation or treatment with radioiodine as indicated.[34] In general, our studies[34,35] and those of Mazzaferri and Jhiang[36] have demonstrated a decrease in mortality and in recurrence after

near-total or total thyroidectomy followed by radioiodine ablation or therapy.

FOLLICULAR CARCINOMA

True follicular carcinomas are far less common than papillary cancer and now are rather uncommon. Remember that the "follicular variant" of papillary cancer should be classified and treated as a papillary carcinoma. Patients with follicular carcinoma are usually older than those with papillary cancer, and once more, females predominate. Microscopically, the diagnosis of follicular cancer is made when vascular and/or capsular invasion is present. Tumor multicentricity and lymph node metastases are far less common than in papillary carcinoma. Metastatic spread of tumor often occurs by hematogenous dissemination to the lungs, bones, and other peripheral tissues.

A follicular cancer that demonstrates only microinvasion of the capsule has a very good prognosis.[37] In this situation, ipsilateral lobectomy is probably sufficient. However, for most patients with follicular cancer that demonstrates gross capsular invasion or vascular invasion, the ideal operation is similar to that for papillary cancer, although the rationale for its performance differs. Near-total or total thyroidectomy should be performed not because of multicentricity but rather to facilitate later treatment with radioiodine.[36] Remnants of normal thyroid in the neck are ablated by radioiodine, and if peripheral metastases are detected (Fig. 24-13), they should be treated with high-dose radioiodine therapy. Although lymph node metastases in the lateral region of the neck are not commonly found, a modified radical neck dissection should be performed if large palpable metastatic nodes are present.

Finally, regardless of the operation, all patients with papillary or follicular cancer should be treated for life with levothyroxine therapy in doses sufficient to suppress TSH to the appropriate level.[36] Care should be taken to not cause cardiac or other problems from thyrotoxicosis, however.

HÜRTHLE CELL TUMORS AND CANCER

Hürthle cell tumors are thought to be variants of follicular neoplasms. They are more difficult to treat than the usual follicular neoplasms, however, for several reasons[38]: (1) the incidence of carcinoma varies from 5.3% to 62% in different clinical series; (2) benign-appearing tumors later metastasize in up to 2.5% of patients; and (3) Hürthle cell cancers are far less likely to concentrate radioiodine than are the usual follicular carcinomas, which makes treatment of metastatic disease particularly difficult.

Of 54 patients with Hürthle cell tumors whom we treated,[38] 4 had grossly malignant lesions, 10 had questionable diagnoses ("intermediate" lesions) because of partial penetration of their capsule by tumor, and 40 (74%) had lesions that were thought to be benign. About half the patients had a history of low-dose external irradiation; many had separate papillary or follicular cancers in the same thyroid gland.

During a mean follow-up period of 8.4 years, three additional Hürthle cell tumors were recognized as malignant after metastases were discovered: two were originally classified as intermediate lesions, and one was in the benign-appearing group. Thus, 7 of 54 (13%) of our patients who had a Hürthle cell tumor had Hürthle cell carcinoma. One of the 7 patients with Hürthle cell cancer died of widespread metastases after 35 years, and the other 6 are currently free of disease.

We believe that treatment for these lesions should be individualized.[38,39] Total thyroid ablation is appropriate for frankly

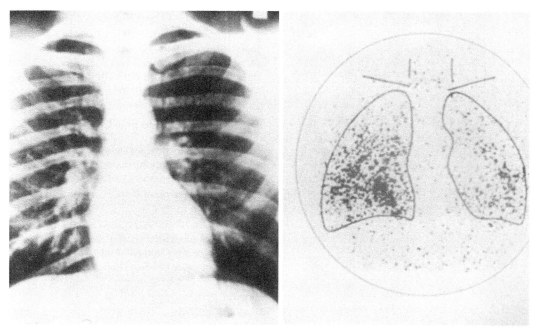

FIGURE 24-13. Despite the fact that the chest radiograph was read as normal, a total body scan using radioiodine demonstrated uptake in both lung fields, thus signifying the presence of unknown metastatic disease. Note that the thyroid has been removed surgically because no uptake of isotope is present in the neck.

malignant Hürthle cell cancers, for all Hürthle cell tumors in patients who received low-dose childhood irradiation, for patients with associated papillary or follicular carcinomas, for all large tumors, and for patients whose tumors exhibit partial capsular invasion. On the other hand, single, well-encapsulated, benign-appearing Hürthle cell tumors that are small may be treated by lobectomy and careful follow-up because the chance that they will later exhibit malignant behavior is low (2.5% in our series and 1.5% among patients described in the literature).[38] Nuclear DNA analysis may aid the surgeon in recognizing tumors that are potentially aggressive, because such tumors usually demonstrate aneuploidy.[40] Furthermore, increased genetic abnormalities have been shown in Hürthle cell carcinomas when compared with Hürthle cell adenomas.[41]

In a review of follicular cancers at the University of Chicago,[39] the overall mortality was 16%—twice that of papillary carcinomas. However, in non–Hürthle cell follicular cancers, the mortality was 12%, whereas in Hürthle cell cancers, it was 24%, thus demonstrating the difficulty involved in treating metastatic disease, which cannot be resected in the latter group.

ANAPLASTIC CARCINOMA

Anaplastic thyroid carcinoma remains one of the most virulent of all cancers in humans. The tumor grows very rapidly, and systemic symptoms are common. Survival for most patients is measured in months. The previously so-called small cell type, now known to be a lymphoma, is most often treated by a combination of external radiation and chemotherapy. The large cell type may be manifested as a solitary thyroid nodule early in its clinical course. If it is operated on at that time, near-total or total thyroidectomy should be performed, with appropriate central and lateral neck dissection. However, anaplastic cancer is almost always advanced when the patient is first evaluated. In such patients, surgical cure is unlikely no matter how aggressively it is pursued. In particularly advanced cases, diagnosis by needle biopsy or by small open biopsy may be all that is appropriate. Sometimes the isthmus must be divided to relieve tracheal com-

pression, or a tracheostomy might be beneficial. Most treatment, however, has been provided by external radiation therapy, chemotherapy, or both. Hyperfractionated external radiation therapy that uses several treatments per day has some enthusiasts, but complications may be high.[42] Radioiodine treatment is almost always ineffective because tumor uptake is absent. Although some success has been observed with doxorubicin, prolonged remissions are rarely achieved, and multidrug regimens and combinations of chemotherapy with radiation therapy are being tried.[43] Although remissions do occur, cures have rarely been achieved in advanced cases and new experimental techniques with tissue cultures following FNA are being tried,[44] as are new experimental drugs.

MEDULLARY THYROID CARCINOMA

Medullary thyroid carcinoma is a C cell, calcitonin-producing tumor that contains amyloid or an amyloid-like substance. In addition to calcitonin, it may elaborate or secrete other peptides and amines such as carcinoembryonic antigen, serotonin, neurotensin, and a high-molecular-weight adrenocorticotropic hormone–like peptide. These substances may result in a carcinoid-like syndrome with diarrhea and Cushing's syndrome, especially when widely metastatic tumor is present. Most medullary cancer of the thyroid is sporadic (about 70% to 80%), but it can be transmitted in a familial pattern. This tumor or its precursor, C cell hyperplasia, occurs as part of the multiple endocrine neoplasia type 2A (MEN2A) and type 2B (MEN2B) syndromes[45] (Fig. 24-14 and Table 24-2), or, rarely, as part of the familial medullary thyroid cancer syndrome. The MEN2 syndromes are transmitted as an autosomal dominant trait, so 50% of the offspring would be expected to have this disease. Mutations of the *ret* oncogene on chromosome 10 have been found to be the cause of the MEN2 syndromes.[46] These defects are germline mutations and therefore can be found in blood samples. All patients with medullary thyroid carcinoma should be screened for hyperparathyroidism and pheochromocytoma.[47] If a pheochromocytoma (or its precursor, adrenal medullary

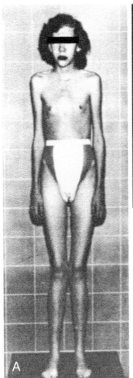
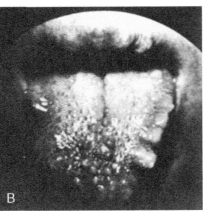

FIGURE 24-14. An 18-year-old female who demonstrates the appearance typically associated with multiple endocrine neoplasia type 2B (MEN2B) was found to have bilateral medullary carcinoma of the thyroid gland at surgery. **A,** The Marfan-like body habitus and facial features typically present in patients with MEN2B are clearly seen. **B,** Multiple neuromas of the tongue and lips are demonstrated. (Courtesy Glen W. Sizemore.)

Table 24-2. Diseases Included in the MEN2 Syndromes

MEN2A	MEN2B
Medullary carcinoma	Medullary carcinoma
Pheochromocytoma	Pheochromocytoma
Hyperparathyroidism	Hyperparathyroidism—unlikely
	Ganglioneuroma phenotype

MEN, Multiple endocrine neoplasia.

hyperplasia) is present, this growth should be operated on first because it presents the greatest immediate risk to the patient. Family members (including children) of a patient with medullary cancer of the thyroid should be screened for medullary cancer of the thyroid, especially if the tumor is bilateral or if C cell hyperplasia is present. Genetic testing for *ret* mutations has largely replaced screening by calcitonin in family members. However, calcitonin measurement is still useful for screening patients with a thyroid mass when FNA analysis raises the possibility of medullary thyroid cancer.

Medullary cancer spreads to the lymph nodes of the neck and mediastinum, and later disseminates to the lungs, bone, liver, and elsewhere. The tumor is relatively radioresistant, does not take up radioiodine, and is not responsive to thyroid hormone suppression. Hence, an aggressive surgical approach is mandatory. The operation of choice for medullary cancer is total thyroidectomy coupled with aggressive resection of the central, lateral, and mediastinal lymph nodes.[46] If lymph nodes of the lateral neck area contain tumor, careful and extensive modified

radical neck dissection is required. Reoperations for metastatic tumor were rarely considered to be rewarding until the work of Tisell and Jansson.[48] Their work and that of others[49] demonstrated that 25% to 35% of patients with elevated circulating calcitonin levels could be rendered eucalcitoninemic after extensive, meticulous, reoperative neck dissection under magnification to remove all tiny lymph nodes. In other patients, computed tomography (CT) and magnetic resonance imaging (MRI) have localized some sites of tumor recurrence, whereas octreotide and meta-iodobenzylguanidine scanning sometimes have been helpful. Recently, positron emission tomography combined with computed tomography (PET-CT) has been successful in some patients.[49a] Laparoscopic evaluation of the liver is helpful before a reoperation in that small metastatic lesions on its surface sometimes can be identified.

Cure is most likely in young children who are found by genetic screening to have a mutated *ret* oncogene. One hopes to operate on them when C cell hyperplasia is present and before medullary cancer has started.[49b] Patients with MEN2A syndrome have a better prognosis than do those with sporadic tumor.[45] Patients with MEN2B syndrome have very aggressive tumors and rarely survive to middle age. Thus, in recent years, children 5 years of age or younger who are found by genetic screening to have MEN2A have received prophylactic total thyroidectomy to prevent the development of medullary cancer. In children with MEN2B and with a mutated *ret* oncogene, total thyroidectomy should be done at an earlier age, often by age 2 years, because this cancer develops at a younger age than does MEN2A.[49] With these prophylactic operations, cures are expected.

Long-term studies of medullary cancer from the Mayo Clinic group have shown that in patients without initial distant metastatic involvement and with complete resection of their medullary cancer, the 20-year survival rate, free of distant metastatic lesions, was 81%.[50] Overall 10 and 20 year survival rates were 63% and 44%, respectively. Thus, early diagnosis and complete initial resection of tumor are very important. A number of new therapies that use tyrosine kinase inhibition are now being evaluated for metastatic disease.[50a] Treatment for pheochromocytoma and hyperparathyroidism is discussed elsewhere.

Operative Technique for Thyroidectomy

Under general endotracheal anesthesia, the patient is placed in a supine position with the neck extended. A low collar incision is made and is carried down through the subcutaneous tissue and platysma muscle (Fig. 24-15A). Currently, small incisions are the rule unless a goiter is present. Superior and inferior subplatysmal flaps are developed, and the strap muscles are divided vertically in the midline and retracted laterally (Fig. 24-15B).

LOBECTOMY OR TOTAL THYROIDECTOMY

The thyroid isthmus usually is divided early in the course of the operation. The thyroid lobe is bluntly dissected free from its investing fascia and is rotated medially. The middle thyroid vein is ligated (Fig. 24-15C). The superior pole of the thyroid is dissected free, and care is taken to identify and preserve the external branch of the superior laryngeal nerve (see Fig. 24-7). The superior pole vessels are ligated adjacent to the thyroid lobe, rather than cephalic to it, to prevent damage to this nerve (Fig. 24-15D). This nerve can be visualized in over 90% of patients if it is carefully dissected.[51] The inferior thyroid artery and the recurrent laryngeal nerve are identified (Fig. 24-15E). To preserve blood

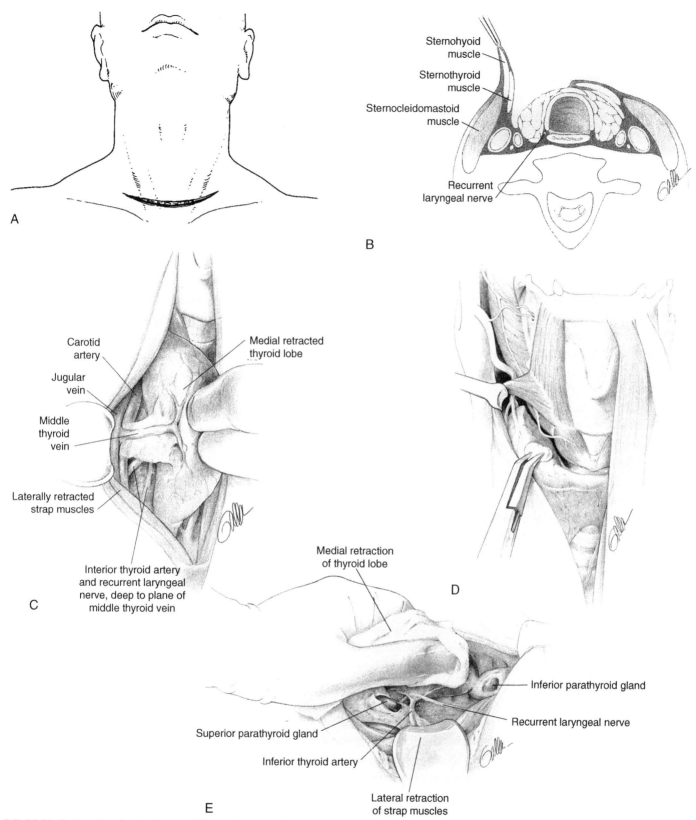

FIGURE 24-15. **A,** Incision for thyroidectomy. The neck is extended, and a symmetrical, gently curved incision is made 1 to 2 cm above the clavicle. In recent years, the author has used a much smaller incision except when a large goiter is present. **B,** The sternohyoid and sternothyroid muscles are retracted to expose the surface of the thyroid lobe. **C,** The surgeon's hand retracts the gland anteriorly and medially to expose the posterior surfaces of the thyroid gland. The middle thyroid vein is identified, ligated, and divided. **D,** The superior thyroid vessels are ligated on the thyroid capsule of the superior pole to avoid inadvertent injury to the external branch of the superior laryngeal nerve. This nerve can be seen in many cases. **E,** With careful retraction of the lobe medially, the inferior thyroid artery is placed under tension. This facilitates exposure of the recurrent laryngeal nerve and the parathyroid glands.

Continued

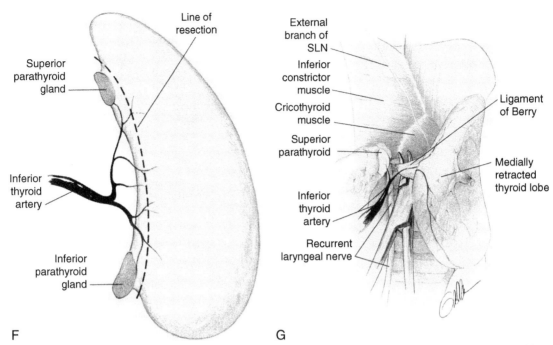

FIGURE 24-15, cont'd. **F,** The inferior thyroid artery is not ligated as a single trunk, but rather its tertiary branches are ligated and divided on the thyroid capsule. This preserves the blood supply to the parathyroid glands, which can be moved away from the thyroid lobe. **G,** The ligament of Berry is then ligated and divided and the thyroid lobe is removed. (Courtesy Drs. Alan P. B. Dackiw and Orlo H. Clark.)

supply to the parathyroid glands, the inferior thyroid artery should not be ligated laterally; rather, its branches should be ligated individually on the capsule of the lobe after they have supplied the parathyroid glands (Fig. 24-15, F). The parathyroid glands are identified, and an attempt is made to leave each with an adequate blood supply while moving the gland off the thyroid lobe. Any parathyroid gland that appears to be devascularized can be minced and implanted into the sternocleidomastoid muscle after a frozen section biopsy has confirmed that it is in fact a parathyroid gland. Care is taken to try to identify the recurrent laryngeal nerve along its course if a total lobectomy is to be done. The nerve is gently unroofed from surrounding tissue, with care taken to avoid trauma to it. The nerve is in greatest danger near the junction of the trachea with the larynx, where it is adjacent to the thyroid gland. Once the nerve and parathyroid glands have been identified and preserved, the thyroid lobe can be removed from its tracheal attachments by dividing the ligament of Berry (Fig. 24-15G). The contralateral thyroid lobe is removed in a similar manner when total thyroidectomy is performed. A near-total thyroidectomy means that a small amount of thyroid tissue is left on the contralateral side to protect the parathyroid glands and recurrent nerve. Careful hemostasis and visualization of all important anatomic structures are mandatory for success. Some surgeons utilize the harmonic scalpel and believe that this decreases the time of operation. However, one must be careful not to cause damage.[51a]

When closing, we do not tightly approximate the strap muscles in the midline; this allows drainage of blood superficially and thus prevents a hematoma in the closed deep space. Furthermore, we obtain better cosmesis by not approximating the platysmal muscle. Rather, the dermis is approximated by interrupted 4-0 sutures, and the epithelial edges are approximated with a running subcuticular 5-0 absorbable suture. Sterile paper tapes (Steri-Strips) then are applied and left in place for

about a week. When it is needed, a small suction catheter is inserted through a small stab wound; generally it is removed within 12 hours.

SUBTOTAL THYROIDECTOMY

Bilateral subtotal or near-total lobectomy is the usual operation for Graves' disease. An alternative operation, which is equally good, combines lobectomy on one side and subtotal or near-total lobectomy on the other side. Once more, the parathyroid glands and recurrent nerves should be identified and preserved. Great care should be taken to not damage the recurrent laryngeal nerve when cutting across or suturing the thyroid lobe. At the end of the operation, several grams or less of thyroid tissue is usually left in place. The aim is to try to achieve a euthyroid state without a high recurrence of hyperthyroidism. When the operation is done for severe ophthalmopathy, however, near-total or total thyroidectomy is performed.

After thyroidectomy, even if a modified neck dissection is done for carcinoma, the patient can almost always be safely discharged on the first postoperative day. Others are kept longer if the need arises. The author does not think that it is safe to discharge a patient on the day of surgery because of the risk for bleeding; however, same-day discharge is being practiced at some centers.[52]

ALTERNATIVE TECHNIQUE OF THYROIDECTOMY

An alternative technique of thyroidectomy is practiced by some excellent surgeons[6,53] and is used by the author in some operations. With this technique, the dissection is begun on the thyroid lobe and the parathyroids are moved laterally as described previously. However, the recurrent laryngeal nerve is not dissected along its length, but rather small bites of tissue are carefully divided along the thyroid capsule until the nerve is encountered near the ligament of Berry. Proponents of this technique believe that visualization of the recurrent laryngeal nerve by its early dissection may lead to greater nerve damage; however, the author believes that in many instances, seeing the nerve and knowing its pathway is safer and facilitates the dissection.

MINIMALLY INVASIVE OPTIONS FOR THYROIDECTOMY

Over recent years, the development of ultrasonic shears for hemostasis and small endoscopes has allowed surgeons to perform thyroidectomies through much smaller incisions than with the use of traditional techniques. Two different approaches have been taken to minimally invasive thyroidectomies. One technique, largely popularized in areas of the Far East such as Japan, China, and Korea, involves making incisions away from the neck in hidden areas such as in the axillae or chest, or in the areola of the breast. The surgeon then creates a tunnel up to the neck, where the thyroidectomy is performed with endoscopic instruments while the endoscope is used for visualization. Approaches such as this generally are performed with low-pressure insufflation and can completely avoid any incisions on the neck itself.[54-57] Although some authors utilizing such approaches have described removing large thyroid glands, most reports suggest significantly longer operative times. Perhaps of greatest concern to many American surgeons regarding these approaches is that if bleeding problems are encountered in the course of the thyroid dissection, a separate neck incision may have to be made to solve the problem. Additionally, recent reports have suggested the possibility that recurrent thyroid cancer can develop in the subcutaneous tunnel after the performance of an endoscopic thyroidectomy.[57a] Such complications will have to be carefully evaluated before wide acceptance of this technique can be recommended in cases of malignancy.

An alternative technique, developed by Dr. Paolo Miccoli and more widely utilized in Europe and to a less extent in the United States, utilizes a smaller incision than usual, but it is placed in the conventional location in the neck.[58,59] In general, a 1.5 to 2.0 cm incision is made in a conventional location in the neck, and after the strap muscles have been retracted from the thyroid gland, a 5-mm, 30-degree endoscope is introduced into the incision. The scope is utilized to visualize the tissue along the lateral aspect of the thyroid gland, especially for the superior pole vessels. Usually after the superior and lateral aspects of the thyroid gland have been dissected free, the parathyroid glands and the recurrent nerve are visualized, and then the thyroid lobe is delivered through the neck incision and the remainder of the operation is performed in the conventional manner through the small cervical incision. Several authors in the United States have reported good results in small series with this video-assisted approach.[60,61,61a] A significant benefit of this approach is that the incision is made in the usual location, so that if any bleeding results in difficulty with visualization during the procedure, the incision can be enlarged and a conventional thyroidectomy can be completed readily. Most authors have found this approach to be similar to conventional thyroidectomy in operative time, although the small neck incision does limit the size of the thyroid gland that could be resected with the use of this technique. At this time in the United States, minimally invasive video-assisted thyroidectomy is offered in a few specialized centers for selected patients with small thyroid nodules (usually less than 3 cm) and without evidence of thyroiditis. Except in the hands of surgeons very experienced in the technique, it should not be utilized for the treatment of patients with most thyroid cancers.

Postoperative Complications

Many authors have reported large series of thyroidectomies with no deaths. In other reports, mortality does not differ greatly from that with anesthesia alone. Five major complications are associated with thyroid surgery: (1) thyroid storm, (2) wound hemorrhage, (3) wound infection, (4) recurrent laryngeal nerve injury, and (5) hypoparathyroidism.

THYROID STORM

Thyroid storm reflects an exacerbation of a thyrotoxic state; it is seen most often in Graves' disease, but it occurs less commonly in patients with toxic adenoma or toxic multinodular goiter. Clinical manifestations and management of thyroid storm are discussed elsewhere in this text.

WOUND HEMORRHAGE

Wound hemorrhage with hematoma is an uncommon complication reported in 0.3% to 1.0% of patients in most large series. However, it is a well-recognized and potentially lethal complication.[52] A small hematoma deep to the strap muscles can compress the trachea and cause respiratory distress. A small suction drain placed in the wound is not usually adequate for decompression, especially if bleeding occurs from an arterial vessel. Swelling of the neck and bulging of the wound can be followed quickly by respiratory impairment.

Wound hemorrhage is an emergency situation, especially if any respiratory compromise is present. Treatment consists of immediately opening the wound and evacuating the clot, even at the bedside. Pressure should be applied with a sterile sponge and the patient returned to the operating room. Later, the bleeding vessel can be ligated in a careful and more leisurely manner under optimal sterile conditions with good lighting in the operating room. The urgency of treating this condition as soon as it is recognized cannot be overemphasized if respiratory compromise is present.

INJURY TO THE RECURRENT LARYNGEAL NERVE

Injuries to the recurrent laryngeal nerve occur in 1% to 2% of thyroid operations when performed by experienced neck surgeons, and at a higher prevalence when thyroidectomy is done by a less experienced surgeon. They occur more commonly when thyroidectomy is done for malignant disease. Sometimes the nerve is purposely sacrificed if it runs into an aggressive thyroid cancer. Nerve injuries can be unilateral or bilateral and temporary or permanent, and they can be deliberate or accidental. Loss of function can be caused by transaction, ligation, clamping, traction, or handling of the nerve. Tumor invasion can also involve the nerve. Occasionally, vocal cord impairment occurs as a result of pressure from the balloon of an endotracheal tube as the recurrent nerve enters the larynx. In unilateral recurrent nerve injuries, the voice becomes husky because the vocal cords do not approximate one another. Shortness of breath and aspiration of liquids sometimes occur. Usually, vocal cord function returns within several months; it certainly returns within 9 to 12 months if it is to return at all. If no function returns by that time, the voice can be improved by operative means. The choice is insertion of a piece of Silastic to move the paralyzed cord to the midline; this procedure is called a laryngoplasty.

Bilateral recurrent laryngeal nerve damage is much more serious, because both vocal cords may assume a medial or paramedian position and may cause airway obstruction and difficulty with respiratory toilet. Most often, tracheostomy is required. In the authors' experience, permanent injury to the recurrent laryngeal nerve is best avoided by identifying and carefully tracing the path of the recurrent nerve. Accidental transaction occurs most often at the level of the upper two tracheal rings, where the nerve closely approximates the thyroid lobe in the area of Berry's ligament. If recognized, many believe that the transected nerve should be reapproximated by microsurgical techniques, although this is controversial. A number of procedures to later reinnervate the laryngeal muscles have been attempted with only limited success.[62]

Injury to the external branch of the superior laryngeal nerve may occur when the upper pole vessels are divided (see Fig. 24-6) if the nerve is not visualized.[9] This injury results in impairment of function of the ipsilateral cricothyroid muscle, a fine tuner of the vocal cord. This injury causes an inability to forcefully project one's voice or to sing high notes because of loss of function of the cricothyroid muscle. Often, this disability improves during the first few months after surgery.

RECURRENT LARYNGEAL NERVE MONITORING

In recent years, many surgeons have sought to try to further diminish the low incidence of recurrent laryngeal nerve (RLN) injury by using nerve monitoring devices during surgery. Although several devices have been utilized, all have in common some means of detecting vocal cord movement when the recurrent laryngeal nerve is stimulated. Many small series reported in the literature have assessed the potential benefits of monitoring to decrease the incidence of nerve injury.[63-65] Given the low incidence of RLN injury, it is not surprising that no study has shown a statistically significant decrease in RLN injury when using a nerve monitor. The largest series in the literature by Dralle reported on a multi-institutional German study of 29,998 nerves at risk in thyroidectomy.[66] Even with a study this large, no statistically significant decrease in rates of RLN injury could be showed with nerve monitoring.

Among the problems of nerve monitoring technology are that the devices can malfunction so that the surgeon cannot depend on the device to always identify the nerve.[67] Proponents of nerve monitoring suggest that the technology might be helpful even if a statistically significant decrease in the rate of RLN cannot be shown. Although some authors have suggested that RLN monitors may be most helpful in difficult reoperative cases when significant scar tissue is encountered, this has not been shown to be the case, and some authors have advocated more routine use.[67a] At this time, nerve monitoring technology in thyroid surgery should never take the place of meticulous dissection. Surgeons may choose to use the technology, but the data do not support the suggestion that nerve monitors allow thyroid surgery to be performed in a safer fashion than that performed by a good surgeon who utilizes careful technique.

HYPOPARATHYROIDISM

Postoperative hypoparathyroidism can be temporary or permanent. The incidence of permanent hypoparathyroidism has been reported to be as high as 20% when total thyroidectomy and radical neck dissection are performed, and as low as 0.9% for subtotal thyroidectomy. Other excellent neck surgeons have reported a lower incidence of permanent hypoparathyroidism.[66] Postoperative hypoparathyroidism is rarely the result of inadvertent removal of all of the parathyroid glands but is more commonly caused by disruption of their delicate blood supply.

Devascularization can be minimized during thyroid lobectomy by dissecting close to the thyroid capsule, by carefully ligating the branches of the inferior thyroid artery on the thyroid capsule distal to their supply of the parathyroid glands (rather than ligating the inferior thyroid artery as a single trunk), and by treating the parathyroids with great care. If a parathyroid gland is recognized to be nonviable during surgery, it can be autotransplanted after identification by frozen section. The gland is minced into 1 to 2 mm cubes and is placed into pockets in the sternocleidomastoid muscle.

Postoperative hypoparathyroidism results in hypocalcemia and hyperphosphatemia; it is manifested by circumoral numbness, tingling of the fingers and toes, and intense anxiety that occurs soon after surgery. Chvostek's sign appears early, and carpopedal spasm can occur. Symptoms develop in most patients when the serum calcium level is less than 7.5 to 8 mg/dL. The parathyroid hormone is low or absent in hyopoparathyroidism.

We measure the serum calcium level every 12 hours while the patient is in the hospital. Most patients are able to leave the hospital on the morning after surgery if they are asymptomatic and their serum calcium level is 7.8 mg/dL or above. Oral calcium pills are used liberally. Patients with severe symptomatic hypocalcemia are treated in the hospital with 1 g (10 mL) of 10% calcium gluconate infused intravenously over several minutes, and then with 5 g of this calcium solution placed in each 500 mL intravenous bottle to run continuously, starting with about 30 mL/hr. Oral calcium, usually as calcium carbonate (1250 mg to 2500 mg four times per day), should be started. With this treatment regimen, most patients become asymptomatic. Intravenous therapy is tapered and stopped as soon as possible, and the patient is sent home and told to take oral calcium pills. This condition is referred to as transient hypocalcemia or transient hypoparathyroidism. Serum calcium, phosphorus, and parathyroid hormone determinations are helpful.

Management of more persistent severe hypocalcemia requires the addition of a vitamin D preparation to facilitate the absorption of oral calcium. We prefer the use of 1,25-dihydroxyvitamin D (calcitriol) because it is the active metabolite of vitamin D, and it has a more rapid action. Calcitriol (0.5 mcg to 1.0 mcg) with oral calcium carbonate therapy is given four times daily for the first several days, then this priming dose of vitamin D is reduced. The usual maintenance dose for most patients with permanent hypoparathyroidism is calcitriol 0.25 to 0.5 µg daily, along with calcium carbonate, 500 mg Ca^{2+} once or twice daily, although some patients require larger doses. Serum calcium levels must be monitored carefully after discharge, and the dosage of the medications is adjusted promptly to prevent hypercalcemia and hypocalcemia. Finally, the serum parathyroid hormone level should be analyzed periodically to determine whether permanent hypoparathyroidism is truly present, because the authors and others have seen cases of postoperative tetany, perhaps caused by "bone hunger," that later resolved completely. In such cases, circulating parathyroid hormone is normal and all therapy could be stopped. Remember that in bone hunger, serum calcium and phosphorus values are low, whereas in hypoparathyroidism, the serum calcium value is low but the phosphorus level is elevated.

McHenry[66a] has shown that the incidence of complications following thyroidectomy varies greatly. In general, those surgeons with excellent training and a large experience with this operation have fewer complications, particularly after cancer procedures and reoperative surgery.

Developmental Abnormalities of the Thyroid

To understand the different thyroid anomalies, it is important to briefly review normal development of this gland. The thyroid is embryologically an offshoot of the primitive alimentary tract, from which it later becomes separated[67-70] (Figs. 24-16 and 24-17). During the third to fourth week in utero, a median anlage of epithelium arises from the pharyngeal floor in the region of the foramen cecum of the tongue (i.e., at the junction of the anterior two thirds and the posterior third of the tongue). The main body of the thyroid, referred to as the median lobe or the median thyroid component, follows the descent of the heart and great vessels and moves caudally into the neck from this origin. It divides into an isthmus and two lobes, and by 7 weeks it forms a "shield" over the front of the trachea and thyroid cartilage. It is joined by a pair of lateral thyroid lobes originating from the fourth and fifth branchial pouches[3,4] (see Fig. 24-7). From these lateral thyroid components, now commonly called the ultimobranchial bodies, C cells (parafollicular cells) enter the thyroid lobes. C cells contain and secrete calcitonin and are the cells that give rise to medullary carcinoma of the thyroid gland. Williams and associates have described cystic structures in the neck near the upper parathyroid glands in cases in which thyroid tissue was totally lingual in location.[71] These cysts contained both cells staining for calcitonin and others staining for thyroglobulin. This study, they believe, offers evidence that the ultimobranchial body contributes both C cells and follicular cells to the thyroid gland of humans.

As the gland moves downward, it leaves behind a trace of epithelial cells known as the thyroglossal tract. From this structure, both thyroglossal duct cysts and the pyramidal lobe of the thyroid develop. The mature thyroid gland may take on many different configurations, depending on the embryologic development of the thyroid and its descent (Fig. 24-18).

THYROID ABNORMALITIES

The median thyroid anlage, on rare occasions, may fail to develop. The resultant athyrosis, or absence of the thyroid gland, is associated with cretinism. The anlage also may differentiate in locations other than the isthmus and lateral lobes. The most

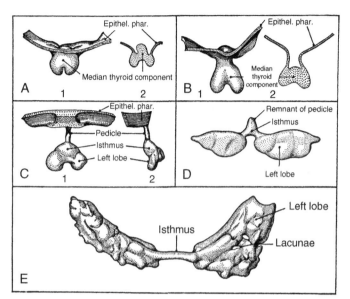

FIGURE 24-17. Stages in the development of the thyroid gland. **A,** _1,_ Thyroid primordium and pharyngeal epithelium of a 4.5-mm human embryo; _2,_ section through the same structure showing a raised central portion. **B,** _1,_ Thyroid primordium of a 6.5-mm embryo; _2,_ section through the same structure. **C,** _1,_ Thyroid primordium of an 8.2-mm embryo beginning to descend; _2,_ lateral view of the same structure. **D,** Thyroid primordium of an 11-mm embryo. The connection with the pharynx is broken, and the lobes are beginning to grow lateral. **E,** Thyroid gland of a 13.5-mm embryo. The lobes are thin sheets curving around the carotid arteries. Several lacunae, which are not to be confused with follicles, are present in the sheets. (From Weller GL: Development of the thyroid, parathyroid and thymus glands in man, Contrib Embryol Carnegie Inst Wash 24:93–142, 1933.)

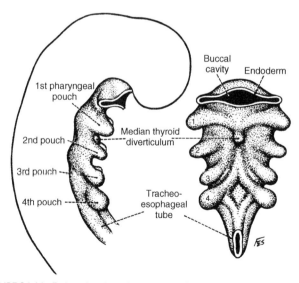

FIGURE 24-16. Early embryologic development of the pharyngeal anlage in a 4-mm embryo. Note the beginning of thyroid development in the median thyroid diverticulum. (From Sedgwick CE, Cady B: Surgery of the Thyroid and Parathyroid Glands, 2nd ed. Philadelphia, WB Saunders, 1980, p 7; adapted from Weller GL: Development of the thyroid, parathyroid and thymus glands in man, Contrib Embryol Carnegie Inst Wash 24:93–142, 1933.)

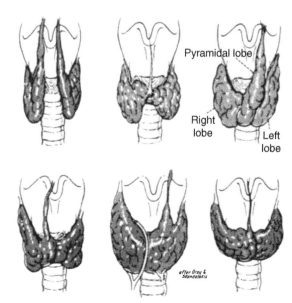

FIGURE 24-18. Variations of normal adult thyroid anatomy resulting from embryologic descent and division of the thyroid gland. (From Sedgwick CE, Cady B: Surgery of the Thyroid and Parathyroid Glands, 2nd ed. Philadelphia, WB Saunders, 1980; adapted from Gray SW, Skandalakis JE: Embryology for surgeons. Philadelphia, WB Saunders, 1972.)

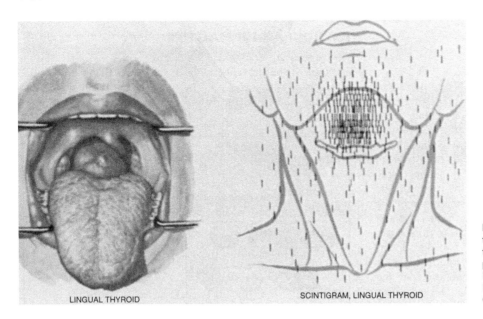

LINGUAL THYROID

SCINTIGRAM, LINGUAL THYROID

FIGURE 24-19. *Left,* The appearance of a large lingual thyroid. *Right,* A radioiodine scan demonstrating all activity to be above the hyoid bone, with no evidence of the presence of normally placed thyroid tissue. (From Netter RA: Endocrine system and selected metabolic diseases. In Ciba Collection of Medical Illustrations. Summit, NJ, Ciba-Geigy, 1974, p 45.)

common developmental abnormality, if looked on as such, is the pyramidal lobe, which has been reported to be present in as many as 80% of patients in whom the gland was surgically exposed. Usually, the pyramidal lobe is small; however, in Graves' disease or in lymphocytic thyroiditis, it is often enlarged and is commonly clinically palpable. The pyramidal lobe generally lies in the midline but can arise from either lobe. Origin from the left lobe is more common than is origin from the right lobe.[72]

THYROID HEMIAGENESIS

More than 100 cases have been reported in which only one lobe of the thyroid is present.[73] The left lobe is absent in 80% of these patients. Often, the thyroid lobe that is present is enlarged, and both hyperthyroidism and hypothyroidism have been reported at times. Females are affected three times as often as males. Both benign and malignant nodules have been reported in this condition.[74]

Other variations involving the median thyroid anlage represent an arrest in the usual descent of part or all of the thyroid-forming material along the normal pathway. Ectopic thyroid development can result in a lingual thyroid or in thyroid tissue in a suprahyoid, infrahyoid, or intratracheal location. Persistence of the thyroglossal duct as a sinus tract or as a cyst (called a thyroglossal duct cyst) is the most common of the clinically important anomalies of thyroid development. Finally, the entire gland or part of it may descend more caudally; this results in thyroid tissue located in the superior mediastinum behind the sternum, adjacent to the aortic arch or between the aorta and pulmonary trunk, within the upper portion of the pericardium, and even within the interventricular septum of the heart. Most intrathoracic goiters, however, are not true anomalies, but rather are extensions of pathologic elements of a normally situated gland into the anterior or posterior mediastinum. Each of these abnormalities is discussed in greater depth.

ECTOPIC THYROID
Lingual Thyroid

A lingual thyroid is relatively rare and is estimated to occur in 1 in 3000 cases of thyroid disease. However, it represents the most common location for functioning ectopic thyroid tissue. Lingual thyroid tissue is associated with an absence of the normal cervical thyroid in 70% of cases. It occurs much more commonly in women than in men.

The diagnosis usually is made by the discovery of an incidental mass on the back of the tongue in an asymptomatic patient (Fig. 24-19). The mass may enlarge and cause dysphagia, dysphonia, dyspnea, or a sensation of choking.[75] Hypothyroidism is often present and may cause the mass to enlarge and become symptomatic, but hyperthyroidism is very unusual. In women, symptomatic lingual thyroid glands develop during puberty or early adulthood in most cases. Buckman, in his review of 140 cases of symptomatic lingual thyroids in females, reported that 30% occurred in puberty, 55% between the ages of 18 and 40 years, 10% at menopause, and 5% in old age.[76] He attributed this distribution to hormonal disturbances, which are more apparent in female subjects during puberty and may be precipitated by pregnancy. The incidence of malignancy in lingual thyroid glands is low.[77] The diagnosis of a lingual thyroid should be suspected when a mass is detected in the region of the foramen cecum of the tongue, and it is definitively established by radioisotope scanning (see Fig. 24-19).

The usual treatment for this condition is thyroid hormone therapy to suppress the lingual thyroid and reduce its size. Only rarely is surgical excision necessary. Indications for extirpation include failure of suppressive therapy to reduce the size, ulceration, hemorrhage, and suspicion of malignancy.[78] Autotransplantation of thyroid tissue has been tried on rare occasions when no other thyroid tissue is present, and it has apparently been successful. A lingual thyroid was reported in two brothers, which suggests that this condition may be inherited.[79]

Suprahyoid and Infrahyoid Thyroid

In these cases, thyroid tissue is present in a midline position above or below the hyoid bone. Hypothyroidism with elevation of thyrotropin (TSH) secretion is commonly present because of the absence of a normal thyroid gland in most instances. An enlarging mass commonly occurs during infancy, childhood, or later life. Often, this mass is mistaken for a thyroglossal duct cyst, because it is usually located in the same anatomic position.[80] If it is removed, all thyroid tissue may be ablated, a

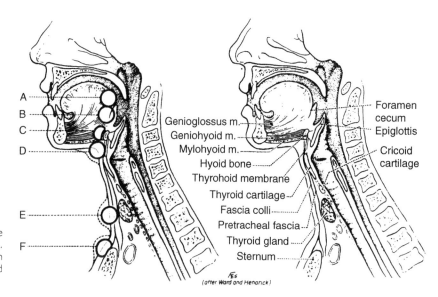

FIGURE 24-20. Location of thyroglossal cysts. A, In front of the foramen cecum. B, At the foramen cecum. C, Suprahyoid. D, Infrahyoid. E, Area of the thyroid gland. F, Suprasternal. (From Sedgwick CE, Cady B: Surgery of the Thyroid and Parathyroid Glands, 2nd ed. Philadelphia, WB Saunders, 1980.)

consequence that has definite physiologic as well as possible medicolegal implications. To prevent total thyroid ablation, many recommend that a thyroid scan or ultrasound examination be performed in all cases of thyroglossal duct cyst before its removal to ensure that a normal thyroid gland is present. Furthermore, before removing what appears to be a thyroglossal duct cyst, a prudent surgeon should be certain that no solid areas are present. If any doubt exists, the normal thyroid gland should be explored and palpated. Finally, if ectopic thyroid tissue rather than a thyroglossal duct cyst is encountered during surgery in an infant, its blood supply should be preserved; the ectopic gland divided vertically; and each half translocated laterally, deep to the strap muscles, where it is no longer manifested as a mass. If normal thyroid tissue is demonstrated to be present elsewhere or in the adult, it may be better to remove the ectopic tissue rather than transplant it, because carcinoma arising from these developmental abnormalities, although rare, has been reported.

THYROGLOSSAL DUCT CYSTS

Both cysts and fistulas can develop along the course of the thyroglossal duct[81] (Fig. 24-20). These cysts are the most common anomaly in thyroid development seen in clinical practice.[82] Normally, the thyroglossal duct becomes obliterated early in embryonic life, but occasionally it persists as a cyst. Such lesions occur equally in males and females. They are seen at birth in about 25% of cases; most appear in early childhood; and the rest, about one third, become apparent only after age 30 years.[83] Cysts usually appear in the midline or just off the midline between the isthmus of the thyroid and the hyoid bone. They commonly become repeatedly infected and may rupture spontaneously. When this complication occurs, a sinus tract or fistula persists. Removal of a thyroglossal cyst or fistula requires excision of the central part of the hyoid bone and dissection of the thyroglossal tract to the base of the tongue (the Sistrunk procedure) if recurrence is to be minimized. This procedure is necessary because the thyroglossal duct is intimately associated with the central part of the hyoid bone (Fig. 24-21). Recurrent cysts are very common if this operative procedure is not followed.

At least 115 cases of thyroid carcinoma have been reported to originate from the thyroglossal duct.[82] Often, in such cases, an association is noted with low-dose external irradiation of the

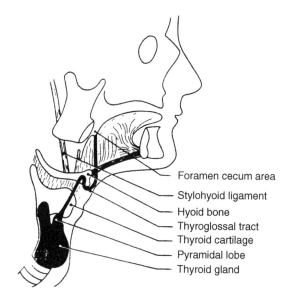

FIGURE 24-21. Diagram of the course of the thyroglossal tract. Note its proximity to the hyoid bone. (From Allard RHB: The thyroglossal cyst, Head Neck Surg 5:134–146, 1982.)

head and neck in infancy or childhood. Almost all carcinomas have been papillary, and their prognosis is excellent. If a carcinoma is recognized, at the time of surgery the thyroid gland should be inspected for evidence of other tumor nodules, and the lateral lymph nodes should be sampled. Our practice and that of many others is to perform near-total or total thyroidectomy with appropriate nodal resection when a thyroglossal duct carcinoma is found and resected. In one series of 35 patients with papillary carcinoma arising in a thyroglossal duct cyst, the thyroid gland of 4 patients (11.4%) also contained papillary cancer.[82] This operative procedure permits later radioiodine therapy as well.

In addition to papillary cancer, about 5% of all carcinomas arising from a thyroglossal duct cyst are squamous; rare cases of Hürthle cell and anaplastic cancer have also been reported. Finally, three families have been reported in which a total of 11 members had a thyroglossal duct cyst.[84]

LATERAL ABERRANT THYROID

Small amounts of histologically normal thyroid tissue are occasionally found separate from the thyroid. If these tissue elements are near the thyroid, not in lymph nodes, and are entirely normal histologically, it is possible that they represent developmental abnormalities. True lateral aberrant thyroid tissue or embryonic rests of thyroid tissue in the lymph nodes of the lateral neck region are very rare. Most agree that the overwhelming number of cases of what in the past was called "lateral aberrant thyroid" actually represent well-differentiated, metastatic thyroid cancer within cervical lymph nodes, or replacing them, rather than an embryonic rest. In such cases, we favor near-total or total thyroidectomy with a modified radical neck dissection on the side of the lymph node, probably followed by radioiodine therapy.

Several lateral thyroid masses have been reported that are said to be benign adenomas in lateral ectopic sites.[85,86] The authors of these studies suggest that they may develop ectopically because of failure of fusion of the lateral thyroid component with the median thyroid. However, before this explanation is accepted, it is important to make certain that each of these lesions does not represent a well-differentiated metastasis that has totally replaced a lymph node, and in which the primary thyroid carcinoma is small or even microscopic and was not recognized.

SUBSTERNAL GOITERS

Developmental abnormalities may lead to the finding of thyroid tissue in the mediastinum or, rarely, even within the tracheal or esophageal wall. However, most substernal goiters undoubtedly originate in the neck and then "fall" or are "swallowed" into the mediastinum and are not embryologically determined at all.

Intrathoracic goiters have been reported to occur in 0.1% to 21% of patients in whom thyroidectomies were performed. This large variability undoubtedly is caused partly by a difference in classification among the authors, but it also may be caused by the incidence of endemic goiter. More recent series report an incidence of 2% or less.[87]

Many substernal goiters are found on routine chest radiography in patients who are completely asymptomatic. Other patients may have dyspnea or dysphagia from tracheal or esophageal compression or displacement. Superior vena caval obstruction occasionally can occur with edema and cyanosis of the face,[88] and venous engorgement of the arms and face is present (Fig. 24-22). Most individuals with substernal goiters are euthyroid or hypothyroid; however, hyperthyroidism occurs as well. Although the goiters of Graves' disease are rarely intrathoracic, single or multiple "hot" nodules may occur within an intrathoracic goiter, resulting in hyperthyroidism as part of a toxic nodular goiter.

Intrathoracic goiters are usually found in the anterior mediastinum and, less commonly, in the posterior mediastinum. In either instance, the diagnosis is suggested if a goiter can be palpated in the neck and if it appears to continue below the sternum. Rarely, however, no thyroid enlargement in the cervical area is present, and instead of being in continuity, the intrathoracic component may be attached to the cervical thyroid only by a narrow bridge of thyroid or fibrous tissue. The diagnosis of an intrathoracic thyroid mass can be made with certainty by the use of a thyroid isotope scan; however, CT or MRI also may be helpful.

Regarding therapy, we generally agree with the recommendation made by Lahey and Swinton more than 50 years ago that goiters that are definitely intrathoracic usually should be removed

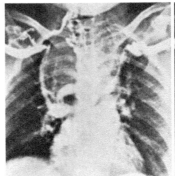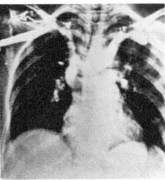

FIGURE 24-22. Large substernal goiter resulting in superior vena caval syndrome. *Left,* A venogram demonstrated complete obstruction of the superior vena cava, displacement of the innominate veins, and marked collateral circulation. *Right,* Three weeks after thyroidectomy, patency of the vena cava was restored. Some displacement of the innominate veins remained at that time. (From Lesavoy MA, Norberg HP, Kaplan EL: Substernal goiter with superior vena caval obstruction, Surgery 77:325–329, 1975.)

if the patient is a good operative risk.[89] Because of the cone-shaped anatomy of the upper thoracic outlet, once part of a thyroid goiter has passed into the superior mediastinum, it can increase its size only by descending farther into the chest. Thus, delay in surgical management may lead to increased size of the lesion, a greater degree of symptoms, and perhaps a more difficult or hazardous operative procedure.

Substernal goiters should be operated on initially through a cervical incision, because the blood supply to the substernal thyroid almost always originates in the neck and can be readily controlled in this area. Only rarely does an intrathoracic goiter receive its blood supply from mediastinal vessels; however, such a finding favors a developmental cause. Thus, in most instances, good hemostasis can be obtained by control of the superior and inferior thyroid arteries in the neck. Thus, most substernal goiters can be removed through the neck.

The authors like to divide the isthmus and the upper pole vessels early in the dissection. The affected thyroid lobe then is carefully dissected along its capsule by blunt dissection into the superior mediastinum. While gentle traction is exerted from above, the mass is elevated by the surgeon's fingers or by blunt, curved clamps (Fig. 24-23). Often these maneuvers suffice to permit extraction of a mass from the mediastinum and into the neck area. Any fluid-filled cysts may be aspirated to reduce the size of the mass and permit its egress through the thoracic outlet. Piecemeal morcellation of the thyroid gland should not be practiced, because this occasionally has led to severe bleeding. Furthermore, several substernal goiters have been found to contain carcinoma, and this technique violates all principles of cancer surgery.

With the use of this method, the great majority of substernal thyroid glands can be removed transcervically. If the thyroid gland cannot be extracted easily from the mediastinum, however, a partial or complete sternotomy should be performed. This procedure affords direct control of any mediastinal vessels and permits resection of the thyroid gland to be carried out safely.

As in all thyroid surgery, the recurrent laryngeal nerves must be preserved and treated with care. The parathyroid glands should be identified and preserved, and the inferior thyroid artery's branches should be ligated close to the thyroid capsule

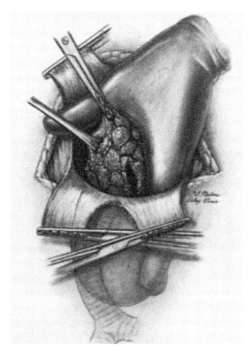

FIGURE 24-23. Finger dissection of a substernal goiter. Note that the index finger is inserted into the mediastinum outside the thyroid capsule and is swept around until the gland is freed from the pleura and other tissue in the mediastinum. Occasionally, despite traction, a substernal goiter does not pass out through the superior thoracic outlet because of its size. In such cases, it may be necessary to evacuate some of the colloid material from within the goiter. Then, with gentle upward traction on the capsule, the mass can be elevated into the neck wound and resected. Occasionally, a sternotomy is necessary. (From Sedgwick CE, Cady B: Surgery of the Thyroid and Parathyroid Glands, 2nd ed. Philadelphia, WB Saunders, 1980.)

to prevent ischemia of the parathyroid glands, which might result in hypoparathyroidism.

STRUMA OVARII

Ectopic development of thyroid tissue far from the neck area can lead to difficulties in rare instances. Dermoid cysts or teratomas, which are uncommon ovarian germ cell tumors, occur in female subjects of all age groups. About 3% can be classified as an ovarian struma, because they contain functionally significant thyroid tissue or thyroid tissue that occupies more than 50% of the volume of the tumor. Many more such tumors contain small amounts of thyroid tissue. Some strumae ovarii are associated with carcinoid-appearing tissue. These strumal-carcinoid tumors secrete or contain thyroid hormones as well as somatostatin, chromogranin, serotonin, glucagon, insulin, gastrin, or calcitonin.[90] Some are associated with carcinoid syndromes.

Struma ovarii sometimes is manifested as an abdominal mass lesion, often with peritoneal or pleural effusion that may be bloody. Most of these lesions synthesize and iodinate thyroglobulin poorly, and thus, despite growth of the mass, thyrotoxicosis does not develop. However, perhaps one fourth to one third of ovarian strumae are associated with thyrotoxicosis.[91,92] Many of these lesions may be contributing to autoimmune hyperthyroidism in response to a common stimulator such as thyroid-stimulating immunoglobulins. In other instances, the struma alone is clearly responsible for the thyrotoxicity. An elevated free thyroxine index, a suppressed TSH value, and uptake of radioiodine in a mass in the pelvis are the obvious prerequisites for making the diagnosis.[93] Often, in ovarian struma, symptoms and findings of thyrotoxicosis are present in patients who have low uptake of radioiodine in their thyroid glands. Thus, a "high index of suspicion" is most important. Usually, operative resection of an ovarian tumor is indicated. After surgery, transient postoperative hypothyroidism and "thyroid storm" occasionally have been reported.

Benign thyroid adenomas in strumae are common, and about 5% manifest evidence of carcinoma.[94] Usually, these lesions are resectable, but external radiation therapy and/or ^{131}I ablation has been advised after resection of the malignant tumors to avoid the tendency for late recurrence or metastatic disease, which sometimes has been fatal. Metastatic disease occurs in about 5% of these malignant tumors. The condition is best treated with ^{131}I therapy, and TSH suppression should be given as for thyroid cancer originating in the usual location.

STRUMA CORDIS

Functioning, apparently normal intracardiac thyroid tissue has been reported a few times and has been visualized by radioiodine imaging.[95] The clinical finding is usually a right ventricular mass, and the diagnosis typically has been made after operative removal.

Acknowledgment

Supported in part by a generous grant from the Nathan and Frances Goldblatt Society for Cancer Research.

REFERENCES

1. Halsted WS: The operative story of goiter, Johns Hopkins Hosp Rep 19:71, 1920.
2. Thompson NW: The history of hyperparathyroidism, Acta Chir Scand 156:5–21, 1990.
3. Kocher T: Uber Kropfextirpation und ihre Folgen, Arch Klin Chirurgie 29:254, 1883.
4. Kaplan EL, Kadowaki MH, Schark C: Routine exposure of the recurrent laryngeal nerve is important during thyroidectomy. In Simmons RL, Udekwu AO, editors: Debates in Clinical Surgery, vol 1, Chicago, 1990, Year Book, pp 191–206.
5. Henry JF, Audriffe J, Denizot A, et al: The non-recurrent inferior laryngeal nerve: review of 33 cases including 2 on the left side, Surgery 104:977–984, 1988.
6. Thompson NW, Demers M: Exposure is not necessary to avoid the recurrent laryngeal nerve during thyroid operations. In Simmons RL, Udekwu AO, editors: Debates in Clinical Surgery, vol 1, Chicago, 1990, Year Book, pp 207–219.

7. Moosman DA, DeWeese JS: The external laryngeal nerve as related to thyroidectomy, Surg Gynecol Obstet 127:1011, 1968.
8. Cernea CR, Ferraz AR, Nishio S, et al: Surgical anatomy of the external branch of the superior layrngeal nerve, Head Neck 14:380–383, 1992.
9. Lennquist S, Cahlin C, Smeds S: The superior laryngeal nerve in thyroid surgery, Surgery 102:999, 1987.
9a. Friedman M, LoSavio P, Ibrahim H: Superior laryngeal nerve identification and preservation during surgery, Arch Otolaryngol Head Neck Surg 128:296–303, 2002.
10. Kaplan EL, Sugimoto J, Yang H, et al: Postoperative hypoparathyroidism: Diagnosis and management. In Kaplan EL, editor: Surgery of the Thyroid and Parathyroid Glands, New York, 1983, Churchill Livingstone, pp 262–274.
11. Gilmour JR: The embryology of the parathyroid glands, the thymus and certain associated rudiments, J Pathol 45:507, 1937.

12. Taylor S: Surgery of the thyroid gland. In DeGroot LJ, Stanbury JB, editors: The Thyroid and its Diseases, ed 4, New York, 1975, John Wiley & Sons, pp 776–779.
12a. Grodski S, Cornford L, Sywak M, et al: Routine level VI lymph node dissection for papillary thyroid cancer: Surgical technique, ANZ J Surg 77:203–208, 2007.
13. Ezzat S, Sarti DA, Cain DR, et al: Thyroid incidentalomas. Prevalence by palpation and ultrasonography, Arch Intern Med 154:1838–1840, 1994.
14. DeGroot LJ: Clinical features and management of radiation-associated thyroid carcinoma. In Kaplan EL, editor: Surgery of the Thyroid and Parathyroid Glands, Edinburgh, 1983, Churchill Livingstone, p 940.
15. Kaplan EL: An operative approach to the irradiated thyroid gland with possible carcinoma: criteria technique and results. In DeGroot LJ, Frohman LA, Kaplan EL, et al, editors: Radiation Associated Carcinoma of the Thyroid, New York, 1977, Grune & Stratton, p 371.

16. Naunheim KS, Kaplan EL, Straus FH II, et al: High dose external radiation to the neck and subsequent thyroid carcinoma. In Kaplan EL, editor: Surgery of the Thyroid and Parathyroid Glands, New York, 1983, Churchill Livingstone, pp 51–62.

17. Shafford EA, Kingston JE, Healy JC, et al: Thyroid nodular disease after radiotherapy to the neck for childhood Hodgkin's disease, Br J Cancer 80:808–814, 1999.

18. Ron E: Thyroid cancer incidence among people living in areas contaminated by radiation from the Chernobyl accident, Health Physics 93:502–511, 2007.

19. Nikiforov YE: Radiation-induced thyroid cancer: What have we learned from Chernobyl, Endocr Pathol 17:307–317, 2006.

20. Shibru D, Chung K-W, Kebebew E: Recent developments in the clinical application of thyroid cancer biomarkers, Curr Opinion Oncol 20:13–18, 2008.

21. Xing M: BRAF mutation in papillary thyroid cancer: Pathogenic role, molecular bases, and clinical implications, Endocr Rev 28:742–762, 2007.

22. Becker C: Hypothyroidism and atherosclerotic heart disease: Pathogenesis, medical management, and the role of coronary artery bypass surgery, Endocr Rev 6:432, 1985.

23. Klementschitsch P, Shen K-L, Kaplan EL: Reemergence of thyroidectomy as treatment for Graves' disease, Surg Clin North Am 59:35, 1979.

24. Lennquist S, Jortso E, Anderberg B, et al: Beta-blockers compared with antithyroid drugs as preoperative treatment of hyperthyroidism: Drug tolerance, complications and postoperative thyroid function, Surgery 98:1141, 1985.

25. Sridama V, Reilly M, Kaplan EL, et al: Long-term follow up study of compensated low dose ¹³¹I therapy for Graves' disease, N Engl J Med 311:426, 1984.

26. Clark OH: Total thyroidectomy: The treatment of choice for patients with differentiated thyroid cancer, Ann Surg 196:361–370, 1982.

26a. Cobin RH, Gharib H, Bergman DA, et al: AACE/AAES medical/surgical guidelines for clinical practice: management of thyroid cancer, Endocr Pract 7:203–220, 2001.

27. Attie JN: Modified neck dissection in treatment of thyroid cancer: A safe procedure, Eur J Cancer Clin Oncol 2:315–324, 1988.

28. Beierwaltes WH: Treatment of metastatic thyroid cancer with radioiodine and external radiation therapy. In Kaplan EL editor: Surgery of the Thyroid and Parathyroid Glands, Clinical Surgery International, vol 4, Edinburgh, 1983, Churchill Livingstone, p 103.

28a. Pacini F, Ladenson PW, Schlumberger M, et al: Radioiodine ablation of thyroid remnants after preparation with recombinant human thyrotropin in differentiated thyroid carcinoma, J Clin Endocrinol 91:926–932, 2006.

29. Hay ID, Grant CS, Taylor WF, et al: Ipsilateral lobectomy versus bilateral lobar resection in papillary thyroid carcinoma: a retrospective analysis of surgical outcome using a novel prognostic scoring system, Surgery 102:1088, 1988.

30. Cady B, Rossi R: An expanded view of risk-group definition in differentiated thyroid carcinoma, Surgery 104:947, 1988.

31. Hay ID, Bergstralh EJ, Goellner JR, et al: Predicting outcome in papillary thyroid carcinoma: Development of a reliable scoring system in a cohort of 1779 patients surgically treated at one institution during 1940 through 1989, Surgery 114:1050–1058, 1993.

32. Hay ID, Grant CS, Bergstralh MS, et al: Unilateral lobectomy: is it sufficient surgical treatment for patients with AMES low-risk papillary thyroid carcinoma? Surgery 124:958–964, 1998.

33. Grant CS, Hay ID, Gough IR, et al: Local recurrence in papillary thyroid carcinoma. Is extent of surgical resection important? Surgery 104:954–962, 1988.

34. DeGroot LJ, Kaplan EL, McCormick M, et al: Natural history, treatment and course of papillary thyroid carcinoma, J Clin Endocrinol Metab 71:414–424, 1990.

35. DeGroot LJ, Kaplan EL, Straus FH II, et al: Does the method of management of papillary thyroid carcinoma make a difference in outcome? World J Surg 18:123–130, 1994.

36. Mazzaferri EL, Jhiang SM: Long-term impact of initial surgical and medical therapy on papillary and follicular thyroid cancer, Am J Med 97:418–428, 1994.

37. van Heerden JA, Hay ID, Goellner JR, et al: Follicular thyroid carcinoma with capsular invasion alone: a non-threatening malignancy, Surgery 112:1130–1136, 1992.

38. Arganini M, Behar R, Wu FL, et al: Hürthle cell tumors: A twenty-five year experience, Surgery 100:1108, 1986.

39. DeGroot LJ, Kaplan EL, McCormick M, et al: Morbidity and mortality in follicular thyroid cancer, J Clin Endocrinol Metab 80:2946–2952, 1995.

40. Schark C, Fulton N, Yashiro T, et al: The value of measurement of ras oncogenes and nuclear DNA analysis in the diagnosis of Hürthle cell tumors of the thyroid, World J Surg 16:745–752, 1992.

41. Segev DL, Saji M, Phillips GS, et al: Polymerase chain reaction-based microsatellite polymorphism analysis of follicular and Hurthle cell neoplasms of the thyroid, J Clin Endocrinol Metab 83:2036–2042, 1998.

42. Mitchell G, Huddart R, Harmer C: Phase II evaluation of high dose accelerated radiotherapy for anaplastic thyroid carcinoma, Radiother Oncol 50:33–38, 1999.

43. Agiris A, Agarwala SS, Karamouzis MV, et al: A phase II trial of doxorubicin and interferon alpha 2b in advanced, non-medullary thyroid cancer. Investigation New Drugs 26:183–188, 2008.

44. Antonelli A, Ferrari SM, Fallahi P, et al: Primary cell cultures from anaplastic thyroid cancer obtained by fine-needle aspiration used for chemosensitivity tests, Clin Endocrin 69:148–152, 2008.

45. Sizemore GW, van Heerden JA, Carney JA: Medullary carcinoma of the thyroid gland and the multiple endocrine neoplasia type 2 syndrome. In Kaplan EL, editor: Surgery of the Thyroid and Parathyroid Glands, Clinical Surgery International, vol 4, Edinburgh, 1983, Churchill Livingstone, p 75.

46. Hofstra RM, Landsvater RM, Ceccherini I, et al: A mutation in the RET proto oncogene associated with multiple endocrine neoplasia type 2B and sporadic medullary thyroid carcinoma, Nature 367:375–376, 1994.

47. Goretzki PE, Hoppner W, Dotzenrath C, et al: Genetic and biochemical screening for endocrine disease, World J Surg 22:1202–1207, 1998.

48. Tisell LE, Jansson S: Recent results of reoperative surgery in medullary carcinoma of the thyroid, Wien Klin Wochenschr 100:347–348, 1988.

49. Skinner MA, DeBenedetti MK, Moley JF, et al: Medullary thyroid carcinoma in children with multiple endocrine neoplasia types 2A and 2B, J Pediatr Surg 31:177–181, 1996.

49a. Iagaru A, Kalinyak JE, McDougall Ir: F-18 FDG PET/CT in the management of thyroid cancer, Clin Nucl Med 32:690–695, 2007.

49b. Machens A, Niccoli-Sire P, Hoegel J, et al: Early malignant progression of hereditary medullary thyroid cancer, N Engl J Med 349:1517–1525, 2003.

50. Gharib H, McConahey WM, Tiego RD, et al: Medullary thyroid carcinoma: clinicopathologic features and long term follow up of 65 patients treated during 1946 through 1970, Mayo Clin Proc 67:934–940, 1992.

50a. Ball DW: Medullary thyroid cancer: therapeutic targets and molecular markers, Curr Opinion in Oncol 19:18–23, 2007.

51. Aina EN, Hisham A: The external laryngeal nerve in thyroid surgery: recognition and implication, ANZ J Surg 71:212–214, 2001.

51a. Manouras A, Markogiannakis H, Koutras AS, et al: Thyroid surgery: comparison between the electrothermal bipolar vessel sealing system, harmonic scalpel, and classic suture ligation, Am J Surg 195(1):48–52, 2008.

52. Schwartz AE, Clark O, Ituarte P, et al: Therapeutic controversy. Thyroid surgery: the choice, J Clin Endocrinol Metab 83:1097–1105, 1998.

53. Delbridge L: Total thyroidectomy: the evolution of surgical technique, ANZ J Surg 73:761–768, 2003.

54. Chung YS, Choe JH, Kang KH, et al: Endoscopic thyroidectomy for thyroid malignancies: comparison with conventional open thyroidectomy, World J Surg 31:2302–2306, 2007.

55. Miccoli P, Berti P, Raffaelli M, et al: Minimally invasive video-assisted thyroidectomy, Am J Surg 181:567–570, 2001.

56. Ferzli G, Sayad P, Abdo Z, et al: Minimally invasive, nonendoscopic thyroid surgery, J Am Coll Surg 192:665–668, 2001.

57. Park CS, Chung WY, Chang HS: Minimally invasive open thyroidectomy, Surg Today 31:665–669, 2001.

57a. Kim JH, Choi YJ, Kim JA, et al: Thyroid cancer that developed around the operative bed and subcutaneous tunnel after endoscopic thyroidectomy via a breast approach, Surg Laparosc, Endosc & Percutaneous Tech 18:197–201, 2008.

58. Miccoli P, Elisei R, Materazzi G, et al: Minimally invasive video-assisted thyroidectomy for papillary carcinoma: a prospective study of its completeness, Surgery 132:1070–1074, 2002.

59. Duh QY: Recent advances in minimally invasive endocrine surgery, Asian J Surg 26:62–63, 2003.

60. Ikeda Y, Takami H, Sasaki Y, et al: Comparative study of thyroidectomies. Endoscopic surgery vs. conventional open surgery, Surg Endosc 16:1741–1745, 2002.

61. Ng JWT: Minimally invasive thyroid surgery: where are we now? ANZ J Surg 73:769–770, 2003.

61a. Terris DJ, Angelos P, Steward DL, et al: Minimally invasive video-assisted thyroidectomy: a multi-institutional North American experience, Arch Otolaryngol, Head and Neck Surg 134:81–84, 2008.

62. Yeung GHC, Wong HWY: Videoscopic thyroidectomy: The uncertain path to practicality, Asian J Surg 26:133–138, 2003.

63. Delbridge L: Minimally invasive parathyroidectomy: The Australian experience, Asian J Surg 26:76–81, 2003.

64. Brunaud L, Zarnegar R, Wada N, et al: Incision length for standard thyroidectomy and parathyroidectomy. When is it minimally invasive? Arch Surg 138:1140–1143, 2003.

65. Miyauchi A, Matsusaka K, Kihara M, et al: The role of ansa to recurrent laryngeal nerve anastomosis in operations for thyroid cancer, Eur J Surg 164:927–933, 1998.

66. Pattou F, Combemale F, Fabre S, et al: Hypocalcemia following thyroid surgery: Incidence and prediction of outcome, World J Surg 22:718–724, 1998.

66a. McHenry CR: Patient volumes and complications in thyroid surgery, Brit J Surg 89:821–823, 2002.

67. Sedgwick CE, Cady B: Surgery of the Thyroid and Parathyroid Glands, ed 2, Philadelphia, 1980, WB Saunders.

67a. Dralle H, Sekulla C, Lorenz K, et al: Intraoperative monitoring of the recurrent laryngeal nerve in thyroid surgery, World J Surg 32:1358–1366, 2008.

68. Weller GL: Development of the thyroid, parathyroid and thymus glands in man, Contrib Embryol Carnegie Inst Wash 24:93–142, 1933.

69. Gray SW, Skandalakis JE: Embryology for Surgeons, Philadelphia, 1972, WB Saunders.

70. Norris EH: Parathyroid glands and lateral thyroid in man: their morphogenesis, histogenesis, topographic anatomy and prenatal growth, Contrib Embryol Carnegie Inst Wash 26:247–294, 1937.

71. Williams ED, Toyn CE, Harach HR: The ultimobranchial gland and congenital thyroid abnormalities in man, J Pathol 159:135–141, 1989.

72. Siraj QH, Aleem N, Inam-Ur-Rehman A, et al: The pyramidal lobe: a scintigraphic assessment, Nucl Med Commun 10:685–693, 1989.

73. Vasquez-Chavez C, Acevedo-Rivera K, Sartorius C, et al: Thyroid hemiagenesis: report of 3 cases and review of the literature, Gac Med Mex 125:395–399, 1989.

74. Khatri VP, Espinosa MH, Harada WA: Papillary adenocarcinoma in thyroid hemiagenesis, Head Neck 14:312–315, 1992.

75. Netter RA: Endocrine system and selected metabolic diseases. In Ciba Collection of Medical Illustrations. Summit, NJ, 1974, Ciba Pharmaceutical Company, p 45.

76. Buckman LT: Lingual thyroid, Laryngoscope 46:765–784, 878–897, 935–955, 1936.

77. Zink A, Rave F, Hoffmann R, et al: Papillary carcinoma in ectopic thyroid, Horm Res 35:86–88, 1991.

78. Elprana D, Manni JJ, Smals AGH: Lingual thyroid, ORL J Otorhinolaryngol Relat Spec 46:147–152, 1984.

79. Defoer FY, Mahler C: Lingual thyroid in two natural brothers, J Endocrinol Invest 13:65–67, 1990.

80. Conklin WT, Davis RM, Dabb RW, et al: Hypothyroidism following removal of a "thyroglossal duct cyst," Plast Reconstr Surg 68:930–932, 1981.

81. Allard RHB: The thyroglossal cyst, Head Neck 5:134–146, 1982.

82. Weiss SD, Orlich CC: Primary papillary carcinoma of a thyroglossal duct cyst: report of a case and review of the literature, Br J Surg 78:87–89, 1991.

83. Katz AD, Hachigian M: Thyroglossal duct cysts: a thirty-year experience with emphasis on occurrence in older patients, Am J Surg 155:741–744, 1988.

84. Issa MM, de Vries P: Familial occurrence of thyroglossal duct cyst, J Pediatr Surg 26:30–31, 1991.

85. Zieren J, Paul M, Scharfenberg M, et al: Submandibular ectopic thyroid gland, J Craniofacial Surg 17:1194–1198, 2006.

86. Stanton A, Allen-Mersh TG: Is laterally situated ectopic thyroid tissue always malignant? J R Soc Med 77:333–334, 1984.

87. Wychulis AR, Payne WS, Clagett OT, et al: Surgical treatment of mediastinal tumors, J Thorac Cardiovasc Surg 62:379, 1971.

88. Lesavoy MA, Norberg HP, Kaplan EL: Substernal goiter with superior vena caval obstruction, Surgery 77:325–329, 1975.

89. Lahey FH, Swinton NW: Intrathoracic goiter, Surg Gynecol Obstet 59:627, 1934.

90. Stagno PA, Petras RE, Hart WR: Strumal carcinoids of the ovary: an immunohistologic and ultrastructural study, Arch Pathol Lab Med 111:440–446, 1987.

91. Ramagopal E, Stanbury JB: Studies of the distribution of iodine and protein in a struma ovarii, J Clin Endocrinol Metab 25:526, 1965.

92. Kempers RD, Dockerty MB, Hoffman DL, et al: Struma ovarii—ascitic, hyperthyroid, and asymptomatic syndromes, Ann Intern Med 72:883, 1970.

93. March DE, Desai AG, Park CH, et al: Struma ovarii: Hyperthyroidism in a postmenopausal woman, J Nucl Med 29:263–265, 1988.

94. Thomas RD, Batty VB: Metastatic malignant struma ovarii: two case reports, Clin Nucl Med 17:577–578, 1992.

95. Rieser GD, Ober KP, Cowan RJ, et al: Radioiodide imaging of struma cordis, Clin Nucl Med 13:421, 1988.

Chapter 25

DIAGNOSIS AND TREATMENT OF THYROID DISEASE DURING PREGNANCY

ERIK K. ALEXANDER and SUSAN J. MANDEL

Background and Historical Perspective

Thyroid Disease and Reproductive Health
Hypothyroidism
Thyrotoxicosis
Reproductive Status and Thyroid Disease Risk

Maternal and Fetal Thyroid Physiology in Pregnancy
Maternal Thyroid Physiology
Serum Thyroid Hormones and Protein Binding
Fetal Thyroid Function
Goiter and Pregnancy

Pathology of Thyrotoxicosis in Pregnancy
Incidence and Etiology
Diagnosis
Treatment
Pregnancy Outcome
Lactation

Pathology of Hypothyroidism in Pregnancy
Maternal Hypothyroidism
Neonatal Hypothyroidism

Postpartum Thyroid Disease
Postpartum Thyroiditis

Thyroid Nodules and Carcinoma During Pregnancy

Background and Historical Perspective

Thyroid diseases occur commonly in women of reproductive age and are well-described complications of reproductive dysfunction, pregnancy, and the puerperium.[1] Historically, in Egyptian and Roman times, an enlarging thyroid gland was viewed as a positive sign of pregnancy in younger women,[2] but it remains controversial whether significant goiter is an acceptable physiologic accompaniment of pregnancy. Regardless, increasing numbers of women are referred to physicians for clinical evaluation of thyroid illness during pregnancy. The spectrum of thyroid disease in pregnancy is similar to that in the normal female population (Table 25-1), although the prevalence of thyroid disease is likely higher in this subpopulation because many cases of thyrotoxicosis can be attributed to the physiologic, thyroid-stimulating effects of human chorionic gonadotropin (hCG) or related molecules.[3] Furthermore, an estimated 1 in 20 women experience postpartum thyroiditis (PPT).[4] The clinical manifestations of thyroid disease overlap those of normal pregnancy, and results of traditional tests of thyroid and metabolic status may be abnormal because of pregnancy itself.[5,6] Fetal considerations influence thyroid diagnostic protocols and therapeutic options for women of reproductive age or those currently pregnant.[7,61] Fortunately, improved assays for thyroid-stimulating hormone (TSH)[7,8,117] have recently permitted better assessment of thyroid status in pregnancy. The availability of effective therapy, in conjunction with close clinical follow-up and monitoring, generally ensures a safe pregnancy for the mother and can reduce the fetal morbidity and mortality caused by spontaneous abortion, intrauterine growth retardation, stillbirth, and neonatal death.[7]

Pregnancy itself may be viewed as a clinically euthyroid state amid the complex changes in endocrine and cardiovascular physiology that characterize gestation.[9,10] Pregnancy can have a favorable effect on the course of maternal autoimmune thyroid disorders, although the tendency is for exacerbation postpartum.[11,74] This favorable effect is due to generalized suppression of humoral and cell-mediated immunity during gestation, which is itself an example of a successful allograft bearing a complement of maternal antigens.[12,13] The loss of immune suppression with delivery often results in a rebound during the postpartum period.

Herein, we focus on thyroid physiology associated with human reproduction. Following a review of maternal and fetal changes that occur during 40 weeks of pregnancy, we turn our attention to the diagnosis, treatments, and outcomes associated with maternal hypothyroidism and maternal hyperthyroidism during pregnancy, as well as the postpartum period thereafter. We conclude by discussing the evaluation and management of thyroid neoplasia in this complex setting.

Thyroid Disease and Reproductive Health

Thyroid disease has been implicated in several reproductive disorders, including menstrual abnormalities, infertility, hyper-

Table 25-1. Thyroid Disorders in Pregnancy

Hyperthyroidism

Common
Graves' disease
Subacute (painful) thyroiditis
Lymphocytic (painless) thyroiditis
Toxic adenoma or "hot" nodule
Toxic multinodular goiter
Hyperemesis gravidarum

Rare
Iodine-induced thyrotoxicosis
Thyrotoxicosis factitia
Gestational trophoblastic neoplasia
Inappropriate thyroid-stimulating hormone secretion
Metastatic follicular carcinoma

Hypothyroidism

Common
Hashimoto's thyroiditis
Postablative hypothyroidism
Surgical hypothyroidism

Rare
Pituitary dysfunction (central hypothyroidism)

Postpartum Thyroiditis

Common
Thyrotoxicosis
Hypothyroidism

Goiter and Thyroid Nodules

Common
Simple (nontoxic) goiter
Solitary thyroid nodule
Multinodular goiter
Papillary carcinoma

prolactinemia, and pregnancy wastage.[1] Whether reproductive status has an effect on the risk of thyroid disease for women is not clear.

HYPOTHYROIDISM

Effects on Menstruation, Fertility, and Maternal Health

Overt hypothyroidism may be accompanied by oligomenorrhea and anovulation and is sometimes associated with elevated concentrations of prolactin (PRL), galactorrhea, or an enlarged sella turcica.[14] Increased production of thyrotropin-releasing hormone (TRH) is often responsible for elevations in thyroid-stimulating hormone (TSH) and PRL. Another proposed mechanism is a defect in hypothalamic dopamine turnover, which would also explain the observation of increased luteinizing hormone levels.[15-17] Ovulatory defects, increased PRL, and galactorrhea are thought to be reversible with thyroxine replacement therapy in most cases. Mild hypothyroidism may be associated with menorrhagia.[18] Anovulatory cycles and luteal phase dysfunction contribute to infertility and may accompany mild or subclinical hypothyroidism.[19,20] Subclinical hypothyroidism may also be associated with slight elevations in serum PRL.[21] Studies in infertile women with mild hypothyroidism have also found increased PRL responses to metoclopramide challenge.[19,22] Contrary to earlier reports,[19] treatment of latent hyperprolactinemia in hypothyroidism with dopamine agonists is not effective in improving pregnancy rates.[22] At present, normalization of thyroid function remains the recommended therapeutic intervention. An ovarian hyperstimulation syndrome (multiple giant follicular cysts) with normal PRL and gonadotropin levels has been reported in a

patient with primary hypothyroidism[23]; thyroxine therapy resulted in cyst involution. Specific to maternal health, a study investigating the effects of subclinical and overt hypothyroidism on maternal health documented a two- to threefold increase in gestational hypertension (eclampsia, preeclampsia, and pregnancy-induced hypertension) in affected women compared with euthyroid controls.[24]

Effects on Miscarriage and Pregnancy

In some patients, recurrent abortions have been attributed to the presence of hypothyroidism.[25] Up to a fourfold increase in fetal death has been reported with overt hypothyroidism compared with control women.[26] Lower serum total thyroxine (T_4) levels may be due to a fall in thyroxine-binding globulin (TBG) associated with declining estrogen levels in a nonviable pregnancy rather than to the presence of hypothyroidism.[7] Adequate thyroxine replacement for women with mild or overt hypothyroidism in early pregnancy results in term deliveries in more than 90%. However, failure to achieve a normal serum TSH level during pregnancy has been reported to be associated with term deliveries in only 20% of women.[27] These and other studies suggest that thyroxine replacement therapy increases the chance of a successful pregnancy outcome even when known thyroid dysfunction is present. Finally, several studies have associated an increased risk of pregnancy complications with maternal hypothyroidism, even if delivery of a live infant occurs. Casey and colleagues investigated a cohort of 17,298 pregnant women, detecting a 2.3% overall prevalence of subclinical or overt hypothyroidism. Placental abruption was approximately three times more likely in women with subclinical hypothyroidism compared with controls. Preterm birth (delivery before 34 weeks' gestation) was almost twice as likely in the women with subclinical hypothyroidism. Although not all parameters differed between groups, these findings suggest a subtle but important adverse effect on maternal and fetal health resulting from even mild thyroid dysfunction.[28]

Recent studies have reported a doubling of the spontaneous miscarriage rate early in gestation among women who have serum antithyroid antibodies (either anti–thyroid peroxidase [TPO] or antithyroglobulin) detected in the first trimester.[29-32] Most of these antibody-positive women who miscarry have normal thyroid function. Furthermore, the presence of antithyroid antibodies in the first trimester is not correlated with that of anticardiolipin antibodies, which are known to be associated with pregnancy loss. The mechanism linking thyroid autoimmunity and miscarriage is not known. It may be a marker for more generalized activation of the immune system or for subtle changes in maternal/fetal thyroid metabolism. In addition, among women undergoing in vitro fertilization, although the presence of antithyroid antibodies does not alter pregnancy rate, the miscarriage rate is significantly higher, as reported in a study by Poppe and colleagues.[33] Separately, a report investigating more than 1500 Pakistani women also reported a threefold higher rate of preterm delivery in women with known antithyroid antibodies compared with antibody-negative women.[34] The authors speculate that the high levels of preterm delivery in antibody-positive women may contribute to a high rate of low birth rate nationally. A recent meta-analysis on this subject confirms a consistent pattern of higher rates of preterm delivery in women who have serum antithyroid antibodies.[35]

Most recently, a randomized, prospective study has suggested that levothyroxine replacement in women with serum thyroid antibodies can reduce the risk of both miscarriage and premature deliveries.[36] The authors prospectively treated a cohort of 57 TPO antibody–positive women with a low dose of levothyroxine beginning in the first trimester of pregnancy. Adverse events were compared with a cohort of 58 antibody-positive women who were not treated, as well as with 869 antibody-negative women. Results confirmed that TPO antibody–positive women who received levothyroxine therapy were about four times less likely to miscarry, and overall risk approximated that of the antibody-negative cohort. Similar reductions in preterm delivery were also documented. Confirmation of these data is awaited; however, the prospective, randomized nature of this trial suggests that adoption of such an intervention is reasonable at this time. In extrapolating from these data, it can be seen that most thyroid antibody–positive pregnant women (if euthyroid or subclinically hypothyroid) are reasonable candidates for 25 to 50 mcg of levothyroxine administration daily. Such therapy may also be reasonable for thyroid antibody–positive women with repeated miscarriages, although the benefit is less clear for those with persistent infertility.

Premenstrual Syndrome

It had been suggested that mild hypothyroidism, defined by isolated elevation of serum TSH levels or even an exaggerated TSH response to TRH, is associated with premenstrual syndrome (PMS) in a significant proportion of cases.[37,38] This finding was not confirmed in a prospective study of patients with PMS and age-matched controls.[39] There now would seem to be little basis for associating PMS with thyroid dysfunction or for recommending thyroxine replacement therapy in this condition.

THYROTOXICOSIS

Mild to moderate thyrotoxicosis does not necessarily affect fertility.[7] Such thyrotoxic women remain ovulatory and have a normal chance of becoming pregnant. Severe thyrotoxicosis, however, may be accompanied by oligoamenorrhea or amenorrhea.[1] The exact mechanism is not known. Hyperthyroidism is a hyperestrogenic state, in part caused by increased conversion of weak androgens to estrogen.[40] Gonadotropin levels may be elevated with loss of the midcycle luteinizing hormone surge[41] yet may remain responsive to exogenous gonadotropin-releasing hormone (GnRH).[42] Nutritional, weight, and psychological changes in thyrotoxicosis may also contribute to menstrual dysfunction.[43] Recent data suggest that only severe thyrotoxicosis is likely to be associated with an increased risk of spontaneous abortion.[44] Studies of this complex subject are often confounded, as women with thyrotoxicosis in early pregnancy are usually already treated, and adequate control data for untreated thyrotoxicosis during gestation are lacking. The appearance of biochemical hyperthyroidism can be mimicked by the physiologic effects of maternal hCG upon the thyroid. Differentiation between the physiologic effects of hCG and pathologic hyperthyroid illness can be difficult. Adequate treatment of thyrotoxicosis should restore fertility and menstruation and reduce early pregnancy wastage.

REPRODUCTIVE STATUS AND THYROID DISEASE RISK

Epidemiologic studies of thyroid disease, including autoimmune thyroid disease, nodular thyroid disease, and thyroid carcinoma, indicate a high prevalence among women, typically those in their late-reproductive or postreproductive years.[45,46] This high prevalence may suggest possible influences of sex hormones on the development of thyroid disease. Experimentally, autoimmune thyroiditis in rats and chickens is modulated by exposure

to estrogens and androgens, with androgens having a protective effect.[47] Estrogen exposure leads to a reduction in suppressor/cytotoxic T cells that may permit an increase in autoantibody synthesis.[48] A case-control study of 89 patients with autoimmune thyroiditis (Hashimoto's disease) found no association of thyroiditis with parity.[49] However, a longer reproductive span (early menarche and/or late menopause) was associated with a twofold to threefold increased relative risk of euthyroid or hypothyroid Hashimoto's disease. A prospective study in pregnancy from an area of marginally low iodine intake reported that a greater number of pregnancies and increased parity were associated with an increased prevalence of nodular thyroid disease and goiter in women with thyroid autoimmunity, or in women with a past history of thyroid disease, compared with controls.[50] These changes were independent of maternal age, biochemical thyroid status, or evidence of thyroid autoimmunity. Iodide levels in the population may have played a role.

Maternal and Fetal Thyroid Physiology in Pregnancy

MATERNAL THYROID PHYSIOLOGY

Basal Metabolic Rate

The basal metabolic rate increases from 15% to 20% between 4 and 8 months' gestation.[5] Most of this increase is due to oxygen consumption by the fetoplacental unit; the balance is accounted for by changes in cardiovascular physiology that accompany pregnancy. Difficulty distinguishing the true basal metabolic rate, which could be a useful indicator of thyroid function status, from total metabolism in the setting of pregnancy mitigates against its use for diagnosis or measurement of therapeutic response to treatment.

Maternal Iodine Economy

Glomerular filtration rates increase by 50% in pregnancy, resulting in a sustained increase in iodide clearance.[5] Reduced tubular reabsorption of iodide by the kidneys may also contribute to increased renal clearance.[51] Plasma inorganic iodide levels may fall as a result. Similar changes in renal iodide clearance have been observed in women treated postpartum with diethylstilbestrol.[51] Additionally, iodide readily crosses the placenta with a reported fetal-maternal gradient of 5:1, suggesting an active transport process.[52] Iodide accumulates in the fetal thyroid primarily after 90 days' gestation. Lactation is another source of iodide loss in the mother.[53] This iodide loss during pregnancy has implications for maternal and fetal thyroid hormone economy in view of the major problems still encountered with endemic iodine deficiency disorders on a global basis.[54] In many geographic areas outside North America, iodide intake is marginal, that is, average intake is less than 100 µg/day.[50,51,55] Goiter is unlikely to develop unless plasma inorganic iodide levels are less than 0.08 µg/dL.[56] Levels are considerably higher in North America, with no differences in iodide balance reported in pregnant versus nonpregnant women.[57] Although such studies are now contraindicated, previous measurements of thyroid radioiodine uptake have shown increases in pregnancy that depend on changes in plasma inorganic iodide and thyroid-stimulating activity.[5,58,59] These studies used [123]I. In some cases, ^{131}I treatment was inadvertently given to thyrotoxic pregnant women.

Therefore, to compensate for this increased iodine loss during pregnancy, increased daily intake of iodine is required during pregnancy. Initial recommendations favored daily iodine intake of at least 150 μg/day.[60] More recently, expert consensus favors maternal daily iodine intake of 250 mcg/day or more.[61] The World Health Organization has also adopted this recommendation. This supplementation should continue throughout pregnancy, as well as during lactation. The most recent National Health and Nutrition Examination Survey in the United States reported a substantial increase in the number of women with a low urinary iodine excretion (<50 μm per gram of creatinine) over the last 20 years (from <1% to 5%).[62] In this survey, very low urine iodine concentrations were documented in nearly 7% of pregnant women and in nearly 15% of women of childbearing age. A recent survey conducted by one of the authors found that about 50% of prescription prenatal vitamins may not contain iodine, although recent campaigns have lobbied drug makers to address this shortcoming. Together, the above data support a recommendation that aggressive assessment of iodine nutritional status should be performed on every woman of childbearing age (or actively pregnant). Physicians should have a low threshold for recommending iodine supplementation as needed to reach the goal of 250 mcg/day.

SERUM THYROID HORMONES AND PROTEIN BINDING

Circulating TBG concentrations double in pregnancy as a result of estrogen stimulation of hepatic production[63] and reduction in clearance of TBG secondary to sialylation.[64] Transthyretin (prealbumin) and albumin levels are reduced. As a result, total serum thyroxine (T_4), triiodothyronine (T_3), and reverse T_3 levels are frankly elevated in pregnancy because of increased hormone-TBG binding[65-67]; binding to transthyretin and albumin is paradoxically reduced. The increase in total T_4 during gestation is predictable, with a suggested adjustment of the nonpregnant reference range by a factor of 1.5.[68] Indirect estimates of free thyroid hormone status using the resin T_3 uptake test may be reduced as the result of increased TBG, and the free thyroxine (FT_4) index calculated from the resin T_3 uptake test and total serum T_4 generally remains within normal limits. However, this technique does not yield a particularly accurate estimate of free hormone status when TBG concentrations are greatly increased.[69] Women with congenital TBG deficiency show little TBG rise or change in serum T_4 in pregnancy.[70] Hypothyroid patients receiving low-dose replacement therapy fail to increase protein-bound iodine (T_4) after estrogen therapy even though T_4-binding capacity, or TBG, is increased. This finding indicates that an increase in T_4 production is required during normal pregnancy, along with increased binding capacity.

It is now well recognized that many hypothyroid women require an increase of 25% to 40% in thyroxine dosage during pregnancy.[71,83] A prospective study of 19 women demonstrated that thyroid hormone demand increases early in the first half of pregnancy, climbs through 20 weeks' gestation, and plateaus thereafter. If mothers do not have adequate endogenous thyroid function, the increased hormone demand of pregnancy will induce a hypothyroid state in most individuals unless their levothyroxine dose is increased. Separate retrospective analysis supports this conclusion. Serum thyrotropin has long been assumed to be the major stimulus for the necessary increase in thyroxine production from the thyroid. However, recent data suggest the importance of hCG in this physiologic process as well.[72] Serum thyroglobulin levels also increase during pregnancy and in some studies returned to normal by 6 weeks' postpartum.[50,73] In euthyroid women with no known thyroid dysfunction, early studies

of free thyroid hormone concentrations during pregnancy suggest that they remain within normal limits.[66,74] Results from longitudinal studies reveal significant fluctuations in free thyroid hormone levels throughout pregnancy, although these concentrations also generally remain within normal reference limits.[8,73-75] FT_4 and FT_3 levels may be slightly increased in the first trimester at between 6 and 12 weeks and may fall progressively throughout gestation, often to levels below the nonpregnant assay-specific reference ranges; TBG saturation is reduced (Figs. 25-1, 25-2). This pattern is consistent regardless of the FT_4 assay method used (dialysis, ultrafiltration, gel filtration and adsorption, or free hormone immunoassay).[8,76,79] Thus, reductions in free thyroid hormone levels in late pregnancy seem to be a real phenomenon that cannot be accounted for by changes in serum albumin, nonesterified fatty acids, or TBG. The

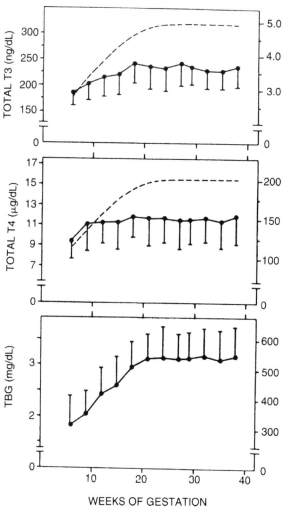

FIGURE 25-1. Serum thyroxine (T_4), triiodothyronine (T_3), and thyroxine-binding globulin (TBG) as a function of gestational age. Each point gives the mean value (±1 standard deviation [SD]) of determinations performed at the initial evaluation, pooled for 3 weeks, between 5 and 28 weeks (n = 510), and again for samples obtained between 28 and 39 weeks (n = 355). The latter samples include both late initial evaluations and the second series of determinations at 30 to 33 weeks. Each point represents an average of 72 individual determinations. The dashed lines illustrate the theoretical curves of T_3 and T_4 concentrations required to yield the average molar ratios of T_4/TBG and T_3/TBG that correspond to nonpregnant reference subjects (0.37 for T_4/TBG and 0.0089 for T_3/TBG with a molecular weight of 57 kDa for TBG). (Data from Glinoer D, De Nayer P, Bourdoux P, et al: Regulation of maternal thyroid during pregnancy, J Clin Endocrinol Metab 71:276. ©1990 by The Endocrine Society.)

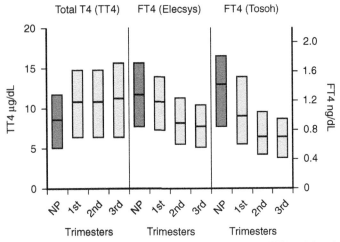

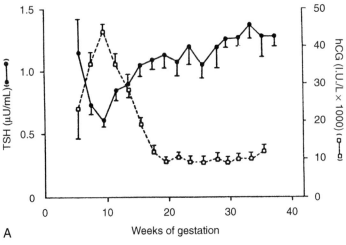

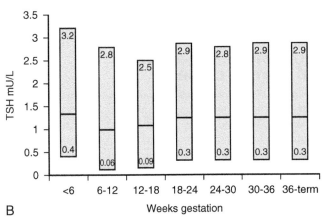

FIGURE 25-2. Serum total thyroxine (TT₄) and free thyroxine (FT₄) levels by trimester. Interquartile ranges are shown by the shaded boxes, with the median value indicated by the line. Serum TT₄ levels rise to approximately 1.5 times the normal nonpregnant reference range. Although serum FT₄ ranges were method dependent, as shown by differences in measurement by the Elecsys system, Roche Diagnostic and Tosoh, Tosoh Corporation methods, both methods show a consistent decrease in FT₄ as pregnancy progresses. (*NP,* Nonpregnant [n = 62]; *1st,* first trimester [n = 105]; *2nd,* second trimester [n = 39]; *3rd,* third trimester [n = 64].) (Data courtesy of Carole Spencer, PhD.) (From Chan GW, Mandel SJ: Therapy insight: management of Graves' disease during pregnancy, Nat Clin Pract Endocrinol Metab 3:470. © 2007.)

physiologic relevance of these observations is unclear, especially for patients with no evidence of thyroid pathology.

In pregnant women, the T_3/T_4 ratio is increased in the third trimester. Increased binding of T_4 and T_3 to monocyte nuclear receptors has also been reported in human pregnancy.[77] Unfortunately, except for the equilibrium dialysis FT₄ assay, none of the other commercial assays has reported trimester-specific and method-specific FT₄ reference ranges during pregnancy. The commercially available automated FT₄ assays that use two-step or labeled antibody methods are protein sensitive and therefore are affected by pregnancy-induced changes in serum albumin or TBG.[78,79] Consequently, no universal absolute FT₄ value can be used to define a low serum FT₄ level across methods. It has been suggested that the normal range for the serum total T_4 level during pregnancy is 1.5 times the nonpregnant reference range.[68] Until validated pregnancy reference ranges are available for serum FT₄ assays, the serum total T_4 level (adjusted for protein binding) may be more reliable for use during pregnancy.

Because serum free thyroid hormone measurements are difficult to assess during pregnancy, serum TSH measurements remain the best assessment of a pregnant woman's thyroid status. However, population-specific normal ranges for serum TSH are derived primarily from healthy, nonpregnant individuals. Recently, some have advocated "trimester-specific" reference ranges for TSH.[80,81,117] These data derive from analysis of serum TSH in healthy euthyroid women who then are assessed during pregnancy (Fig. 25-3). Serum TSH values in the first trimester range much lower than would be expected in a nonpregnant individual, generally between 0.03 mIU/L and 2.5 mIU/L. In the second and third trimesters, greater variance is seen, although the lower limit of "normal" remains below what would be expected for nonpregnant individuals.[80] Debate on how these data should be translated into clinical practice is ongoing. Regardless, these data suggest that, compared with nonpregnant reference ranges, mildly suppressed TSH in a pregnant woman should be viewed as safe, and perhaps physiologically normal.

FIGURE 25-3. Serum thyroid-stimulating hormone (TSH) and human chorionic gonadotropin (hCG) as a function of gestational age. **A,** Serum hCG was determined at the initial evaluation and TSH at the initial evaluation and during late gestation. The symbols give the mean value (±standard error [SE]) for samples pooled for 2 weeks' gestation. Each point corresponds to an average of 33 determinations for hCG and 49 for TSH. (From Glinoer D, De Nayer P, Bourdoux P, et al: Regulation of maternal thyroid during pregnancy, J Clin Endocrinol Metab 71:276. © 1990 by The Endocrine Society.) **B,** Gestational age–specific serum TSH concentrations in women without thyroid autoimmunity. The shaded areas represent the 2.5th to the 97.5th percentile values, with the median value indicated by the line. (Data graphed from Stricker R, Echenard M, Eberhart R, et al: Evaluation of maternal thyroid function during pregnancy: the importance of using gestational age-specific reference intervals, Eur J Endocrinol 157:509, 2007.)

Thyroid Stimulation and Regulation

The histologic picture of the thyroid gland during pregnancy is one of active stimulation. Columnar epithelium can be seen lining hyperplastic follicles.[82] The increase in maternal T_4 production that occurs during normal gestation is most evident from clinical observations of thyroxine-replaced hypothyroid women who require a 25% to 40% dosage increase to maintain normal serum TSH levels in pregnancy.[71,83] Furthermore, findings of relative hypothyroxinemia and slightly increased serum TSH levels during pregnancy in women from areas of borderline iodine sufficiency (<100 mcg/day) support the view that pregnancy constitutes a stress for the maternal thyroid by stimulating thyroid hormone production.[84]

Several factors are known to tax gravid thyroid economy, and each may have relative importance at a different time in gestation. In early pregnancy, the serum concentration of TBG increases rapidly and more thyroid hormone may be needed to saturate binding sites. Glomerular filtration rate increases, resulting in increased iodide clearance. Later, with placental growth, metabolism of T_4 to its inactive metabolite reverse T_3 is increased by the high levels of placental type III deiodinase.[85] In addition, transplacental passage of maternal T_4 may occur.[86] Finally, alterations in the volume of distribution of thyroid hormone may occur because of both gravid physiology and the fetal/placental unit.

Human Chorionic Gonadotropin

Serum hCG has thyromimetic effects and is responsible for the hyperthyroidism associated with trophoblastic disease.[87-94] In normal pregnancy, hCG is a physiologic regulator of thyroid function early in gestation.[73,74,95-100] Clinically, hCG levels peak in pregnancy at 50 to 100 times 100,000-200,000 IU/L at between 9 and 14 weeks; this peak correlates with reduced TSH levels in the first trimester[73,98] (see Fig. 25-3). Levels decline thereafter and are undetectable by a few weeks postpartum. An overall increase in thyromimetic activity in the sera of women during early pregnancy may be due to hCG, as determined by immunoadsorption studies using hCG monoclonal antibodies.[99,100]

Ekins and colleagues have effectively argued that an alternative control system such as hCG may regulate maternal thyroid activity in early pregnancy, when the most important changes in TBG and T_4 secretion occur, to ensure an adequate supply of thyroid hormones to the placenta and embryo (Fig. 25-4).[98,101,102] Experimentally, in vitro studies show that hCG binds to the TSH receptor (TSHR), as assessed by radioreceptor assays using porcine and human thyroid membranes incubated with ^{125}I-TSH,[103-106] stimulates adenylate cyclase activity and cyclic adenosine monophosphate (cAMP) generation, and enhances T_3 secretion in human and porcine thyroid slices.[107] More recently, hCG has been shown to stimulate growth, iodide uptake, and cAMP generation in the rat thyroid cell line FRTL5.[99,100,108-110] Species differences[111,112] and microheterogeneity of hCG molecules through pregnancy and in gestational trophoblastic diseases may account for the variable thyrotropic activities reported.[98-100,106-108,113-115] However, with reported TSH bioactivity of up to 0.7 μU/U hCG,[106,108] the hCG levels obtained in early pregnancy could produce a noticeable thyrotropic effect, and it has been reported that up to 9% of pregnant women may have an isolated subnormal serum TSH level in the first trimester.[116] A recent study reported greater susceptibility to hCG-associated suppression of serum TSH in pregnant women whose serum TSH levels were in the lowest 25th percentile in early pregnancy.[72] Overall, maternal serum TSH concentrations decrease in the first half of pregnancy compared with the nonpregnant state and remain lower until term (see Fig. 25-3B).[117] Consequently, in healthy pregnant women at between 6 and 18 weeks' gestation, the lower limit of the 95% confidence interval for serum TSH levels is between 0.03 and 0.09 mIU/L, which then rises to 0.3 mIU/L as pregnancy progresses.[80,117]

FETAL THYROID FUNCTION

The fetal hypothalamic-pituitary-thyroid axis develops autonomously and has been extensively studied in the human, sheep, and rat.[52,118-120] A number of agents and maternal factors may affect fetal thyroid function, depending on whether they cross the placenta (Table 25-2).

Placental Transfer

The placenta is impermeable to TSH but permeable to TRH, although endogenous maternal levels are probably too low to

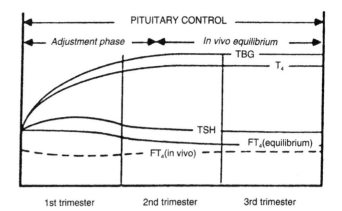

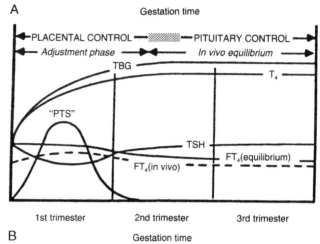

FIGURE 25-4. A, Conventional model of maternal thyroid gland control throughout pregnancy if based on the traditional hypothalamic-pituitary feedback mechanism. **B,** Hypothetical model of maternal thyroid gland control throughout pregnancy if a putative "placental thyroid stimulator" (PTS), possibly human chorionic gonadotropin, assumes regulatory control over maternal thyroid secretion. FT_4, Free T_4; T_4, thyroxine; *TBG*, thyroxine-binding globulin; *TSH*, thyroid-stimulating hormone. (From Ballabio M, Poshyachinda M, Ekins RP: Pregnancy-induced changes in thyroid function: role of human chorionic gonadotropin as a putative regulator of maternal thyroid, J Clin Endocrinol Metab 73:824. © 1991 by The Endocrine Society.)

Table 25-2. Placental Transfer and Fetal Thyroid Function

Without Difficulty	Some Transfer	Little or No Transfer
Iodides	T_4	TSH
Thionamides	T_3	
Thyroid autoantibodies		
TRH		

T_3, Triiodothyronine; T_4, thyroxine; *TRH*, thyrotropin-releasing hormone; *TSH*, thyroid-stimulating hormone.
Modified from Burrow GN: Thyroid diseases in pregnancy. In Burrow GN, Oppenheimer JH, Volp JR (eds): Thyroid function and disease, Philadelphia, 1989, WB Saunders, p 292.

influence fetal thyroid function.[121] Pituitary and serum TSH in the fetus may be under the control of pancreatic TRH before the maturation of hypothalamic TRH after 20 weeks' gestation.[122-126] Injection of TRH in the mother is accompanied by increased cord serum TSH, T_4, and T_3 levels, thus indicating that endogenous TSH stimulates the fetal thyroid.[127]

Before the onset of human fetal thyroid gland function at 10 to 12 weeks' gestation,[128-132] any requirement for thyroid hormone would be met by the maternal supply. The presence of human fetal tissue thyroid hormones and receptors before 12 to 18 weeks, when fetal serum T_4 production increases, is consistent with an early requirement for thyroid hormones from the mother.[133] The placenta has generally been viewed as a substantial barrier to thyroid hormone transfer, in part because of preferential 5'-monodeiodination of T_4 to reverse T_3.[119,121] Studies in rats have provided good evidence for transfer of maternal thyroid hormones to the fetus in early and late pregnancy, which may be important for early brain development and later brain growth and neuronal differentiation.[134-139] In the rat, maternal T_4 is the principal source of intracellular T_3 in the early developing brain.[139] The local intracellular generation of T_3 from T_4 of maternal origin protects the fetal brain from T_3 deficiency in cases of fetal thyroid failure, because cerebral 5' type 2 deiodinase activity increases markedly in response to a minor decrease in T_4.[140] In humans and sheep, maternal thyroid hormones have more limited access to the fetal circulation.[119] Recent human studies have confirmed the presence of T_4 and T_3 in coelomic and amniotic fluid in the first trimester. Although the concentrations of total T_4 and T_3 are 100-fold lower than those in maternal serum, because of the lack of binding protein in these fetal compartment fluids, the concentration of FT_4 is biologically relevant.[141]

The apparent normality of sporadic congenitally hypothyroid infants at birth indicates the role of maternal thyroid hormones. The devastating effects of maternal and fetal/neonatal thyroid hormone deficiency in endemic cretinism in humans underscore the overall importance of thyroid hormones to the fetus.[54,142,143] Fortunately, this problem does not seem to occur in areas where iodine intake is just marginal,[55] but concern remains with respect to any effect of maternal hypothyroxinemia on early fetal brain development and its effects on progeny.[101,102,133,144-146] Early studies suggested limited transfer of T_4 and T_3 across the placenta in humans in the later part of pregnancy and at term,[147-153] with T_3 crossing more readily than T_4. Vulsma and colleagues have convincingly demonstrated maternal-to-fetal T_4 transfer in neonates born with a complete organification defect. These infants have subnormal fetal T_4 concentrations when compared with normal newborns, but their levels are approximately 40% of the maternal concentration.[86] Because of their absolute inability to produce thyroid hormone, this T_4 must be maternal in origin.

Iodide is actively transported to the fetus.[121] The fetal and neonatal thyroid is susceptible to iodine-induced hypothyroidism and goiter with excessive exposure.[119,154,155] This complication can occur after intravenous, oral, mucosal, or topical exposure and absorption in the mother,[156] after amniography,[157] and as a result of postnatal topical absorption,[158] as well as through breast milk.[159] A number of pregnant women have been treated with amiodarone, an antiarrhythmic drug containing 75 mg of iodine per 200-mg dose that partially crosses the placenta and increases maternal and fetal iodide levels.[160] Although thyroid function may remain normal, case reports have described fetal or neonatal goiter, hypothyroidism, or hyperthyroxinemia in association with maternal amiodarone therapy.[161-163]

Diagnosis of Fetal Thyroid Disorders In Utero

The possibility of thyroid disease in the fetus is usually considered because of maternal thyroid disease. Fetal hyperthyroidism is generally encountered in the setting of maternal active or previously ablated Graves' disease via the transplacental passage of maternal TSH receptor–stimulating antibodies. Fetal hypothyroidism is associated with fetal thyroid maldevelopment, iodine deficiency disorders, thyroid autoimmunity, and excessive maternal antithyroid drug therapy.[164-166] In fetal hyperthyroidism, ultrasound usually demonstrates a fetal goiter with increased vascularity, and fetal bone maturation is accelerated.[167] In hypothyroidism, a fetal goiter may be visible on ultrasound,[167,168] or the radiographic appearance of distal femoral or proximal tibial epiphyses may be delayed.[169,170] The latter has limited clinical application. Although the fetus incurs serious risk, measurement of T_4 and TSH in serum collected by percutaneous umbilical cord sampling (cordocentesis)[120] is currently the most reliable means of diagnosing hypothyroidism[167,171] or hyperthyroidism in utero.[167,172] This technique has advantages over measurement of thyroid hormones or TSH in amniotic fluid, which has not been shown to reliably predict fetal thyroid status.[173,174] Fortunately, the diagnosis of fetal thyroid dysfunction can usually be inferred from the clinical scenario presented by the maternal thyroid disease status (see "Fetal and Neonatal Thyrotoxicosis"). The fetus can absorb thyroid hormones injected into amniotic fluid, and such therapy has been used successfully in the treatment of hypothyroidism and goiter in utero.[171,175]

GOITER AND PREGNANCY

Goiter has historically been associated with pregnancy, but its incidence and prevalence vary with the geographic area and iodine status of the general population. Up to 70% of pregnant women in Scotland and Ireland were considered on clinical grounds (visible and palpable thyroid gland) to have a goiter versus 38% of nonpregnant controls.[176] No cumulative influence of successive pregnancies was observed, inasmuch as goiters were seen in 39% of nulliparous women and 35% of nonpregnant parous women. These studies were conducted in areas of relatively low iodine intake. A comparative study in Iceland, an area of iodine sufficiency, showed a lower basal prevalence of goiter (20%) and no increase in the incidence of goiter in pregnancy.[177] Similar results have been reported in studies from North America,[178] which has led some authors to suggest that goiter in pregnancy is a myth.[179] Most goiters during pregnancy in North America are related to autoimmune thyroid disease, colloid nodular disease, or thyroiditis.

Ultrasonography has added a quantitative perspective to the assessment of goiter in pregnancy. In Denmark, an area of marginal iodine intake, a 30% increase in thyroid volume has been documented at between 18 and 36 weeks' gestation.[180] Volume returned to baseline postpartum, and no evidence of thyroid dysfunction or thyroid autoimmunity was apparent. Only 25% of the women actually had a goiter on clinical grounds. Serum thyroglobulin levels were also increased during pregnancy.[181] Only a 13% increase in thyroid volume was reported in a North American study.[182] The largest longitudinal and cross-sectional study of thyroid volume in pregnancy involved more than 600 women from Belgium, another area of marginal iodine intake.[73] Seventy percent of the women had a 20% or greater increase in thyroid volume during pregnancy, although only 9% had a significant goiter as defined by thyroid volume in excess of 23 mL. Thyroid volume showed positive correlations with higher serum thyroglobulin levels and an increased serum T_3/T_4 ratio. No correlation was seen with urine iodide excretion, and a negative correlation with serum TSH levels was noted. The latter may have been due to the influence of hCG during pregnancy. The same authors from Belgium prospectively studied preexisting mild thyroid abnormalities through pregnancy and noted a significant goitrogenic effect as well as an increase in the incidence and prevalence of thyroid nodules.[50] Many of these nodules were subclinical and were detected only on thyroid ultrasound. Serum thyroglobulin levels were disproportionately increased in women with goiters and nodules when compared with controls and pregnant women with autoimmune thyroid disease or a history of previous thyroid abnormalities. The authors further suggested that previous pregnancies were a significant risk factor for goiter and thyroid nodules. This same risk was also suggested in a study from the Netherlands.[183] It should be noted that an increase in thyroid volume during pregnancy does not necessarily denote increased mitotic activity because increased colloid volume, cell hypertrophy, inflammation, or increased thyroid blood flow could account for some of the enlargement.

No evidence of adverse effects on fetal development or neonatal thyroid function has been seen in these studies from areas of marginal iodine uptake.[50,55,73] Nor does there appear to be an increase in risk of neonatal thyroid dysfunction in goitrous, iodine-sufficient areas.[184] This finding contrasts with results from areas with endemic iodine deficiency.[54,185] Maternal smoking has been shown to be a risk factor for neonatal thyroid enlargement, as determined ultrasonographically.[186] Neonatal thyroid volume correlated with cord serum thyroglobulin and thiocyanate levels, but no evidence of neonatal thyroid dysfunction was found.

Pathology of Thyrotoxicosis in Pregnancy

INCIDENCE AND ETIOLOGY

All forms of thyroid disease are more common in women than in men, and thyrotoxicosis is not a rare event during pregnancy. It occurs in about 2 of every 1000 pregnancies. Autoimmune thyrotoxicosis, or Graves' disease, the most common cause of thyrotoxicosis in pregnant women, accounts for about 90% of cases. Toxic adenomas or nodular goiters are much less common in this age group. Other causes of thyrotoxicosis in pregnancy include gestational trophoblastic neoplasia[93] and hyperemesis gravidarum (see Table 25-1).

Gestational Thyrotoxicosis

A spectrum of hCG-induced hyperthyroidism occurs during pregnancy, and this entity has been referred to recently as "gestational thyrotoxicosis."[187-189] This disorder differs from Graves' disease in several ways: (1) nonautoimmune origin, with negative antithyroid and anti–TSH receptor antibodies (TRAbs); (2) absence of large goiter; and (3) resolution in almost all patients after 20 weeks.[187]

Findings range from an isolated subnormal serum TSH concentration (approximately 9% of pregnancies[116]) to elevations of free thyroid hormone levels in the clinical setting of hyperemesis gravidarum. Systematic screening of 1900 consecutive pregnant women in Belgium demonstrated low TSH and elevated FT_4 in 2.4%, half of whom had weight loss, lack of weight gain, or unexplained tachycardia.[189]

Hyperemesis gravidarum, or pernicious nausea and vomiting in pregnancy, is usually associated with weight loss and fluid and electrolyte disturbances. Its manifestation and diagnosis can be complicated because other causes of severe nausea and vomiting in pregnancy must be excluded. Suppressed TSH levels may occur in 60% of women with hyperemesis gravidarum, along with elevated FT_4 levels in almost 50%.[188-192] Serum hCG concentrations correlate with FT_4 levels and inversely with TSH determinations. The magnitude of the deviation from normal values increases with the severity of nausea and vomiting.[116,193] Only 12% of such women have an elevated free T_3 index, which

may help to differentiate this entity from Graves' disease.[116] Furthermore, thyroid-stimulating activity, as measured by adenylate cyclase activity per international unit of hCG, is reported to be greater in women with hyperemesis gravidarum than in those with occasional or no vomiting.[187]

Similar thyroid hormone changes and emetic symptoms may be present in multiple gestations, which are associated with higher peak and more sustained hCG levels.[194] In addition, a recent case report further supports the concept of hCG-induced thyrotoxicosis. A woman with recurrent gestational thyrotoxicosis and her mother with the same obstetric history were found to have a missense mutation in the extracellular domain of the TSH receptor. When this receptor was studied in transfected COS-7 cells, it caused a twofold to threefold increase in cAMP generation when exposed to hCG as compared with wild-type receptor.[192] This genetic mutation induced hyperresponsiveness to hCG as well as thyrotoxicosis.

Gestational thyrotoxicosis is transient and usually resolves within 10 weeks of diagnosis.[195] Treatment with antithyroid drugs is not recommended[61] but may be needed if there is concomitant Graves' disease. The clinician may consider antithyroid drug therapy for patients with hyperemesis who remain symptomatic after 20 weeks' gestation and continue to have elevated thyroid hormone concentrations and suppressed TSH levels, or who have evidence of significant clinical thyrotoxicosis.

DIAGNOSIS

The clinical diagnosis of mild to moderate hyperthyroidism is not easy and may be much more difficult to confirm during pregnancy. Hyperdynamic symptoms and signs, which are common in normal pregnant women, include anxiety, heat intolerance, tachycardia, and warm, moist skin. Laboratory tests may support a suspicion of thyrotoxicosis, but confirmation may be difficult. The ocular changes of thyroid ophthalmopathy or pretibial myxedema do not indicate whether Graves' thyrotoxicosis is active. A resting pulse above 100 that is not decreased by Valsalva's maneuver and a goiter with a palpable thrill are strongly suggestive of thyrotoxicosis.

Despite the difficulty associated with interpretation of thyroid function tests because of the elevated TBG concentration during pregnancy, the diagnosis of hyperthyroidism in pregnant women depends on laboratory testing. A sensitive TSH determination with a value less than 0.01 mU/L[196,197] and an elevated serum FT_4 (or total T_4 concentration above pregnancy reference values) is generally diagnostic. This illustrates the need for the manufacturers of commercial FT_4 assays to report trimester-specific and method-specific reference ranges during pregnancy. As noted, during the first trimester, the serum TSH may be below the nonpregnant reference range in response to an increase in serum hCG concentration.[73] The delay in TRAb measurement renders it generally impractical for routine diagnostic use in this clinical scenario. If the diagnosis is not clearcut, one can usually wait 3 to 4 weeks and then can repeat the thyroid function tests because most pregnant women tolerate mild to moderate thyrotoxicosis without difficulty.[224]

TREATMENT

Once the diagnosis of thyrotoxicosis has been established in a pregnant woman, therapy should be instituted. Treatment of a pregnant woman with thyrotoxicosis is limited to antithyroid drug therapy or surgery because radioactive iodine is absolutely contraindicated.[198-200] After the 10th to the 12th week of gestation, once the fetal thyroid has the ability to concentrate iodine, congenital hypothyroidism may be induced by ^{131}I treatment. In one study, in which 182 fetuses were inadvertently exposed to ^{131}I therapy during the first trimester, pregnancy resulted in two (1.1%) spontaneous abortions, two (1.1%) intrauterine deaths, six (3.3%) hypothyroid children, and four (2.2%) mentally retarded children. If ^{131}I treatment is inadvertently administered to a woman in early pregnancy, the effects on the thyroid could be blocked by iodide administration, but the optimal dosing of iodide has not been studied.

Thionamide Therapy

The thionamides propylthiouracil, methimazole, and carbimazole have all been prescribed for the treatment of thyrotoxicosis during pregnancy. Carbimazole, which is metabolized to methimazole, is used mainly in Europe. All these agents cross the placenta and are also secreted in breast milk.[201] The serum half-lives of propylthiouracil and methimazole are 1 hour and 5 hours, respectively.[202-206] These two antithyroid drugs have been used interchangeably. Thionamides block the synthesis but not the release of thyroid hormone. Propylthiouracil does have the potential additional advantage of partially blocking the conversion of T_4 to T_3. With propylthiouracil or methimazole, the typical patient will note some improvement after 1 or 2 weeks and may approach euthyroidism after 6 to 8 weeks of treatment, with no difference in the median time to lowering the FT_4 index to appropriate pregnant levels.[207]

If minor drug reactions occur, the thionamides may be interchanged, but cross-sensitivity is seen in about half of patients.[208] The most common reactions include fever, nausea, skin rash, pruritus, and metallic taste.[209] Transient leukopenia, not an uncommon reaction to thionamide therapy, occurs in about 12% of adults.[209,210] This association may be complicated because mild leukopenia is not uncommon in untreated Graves' disease.[202] This mild leukopenia is not a sign of agranulocytosis, which occurs in about 0.5% of patients, usually within 12 weeks of initiation of therapy, and may be an autoimmune phenomenon.[211-214] Hepatitis and vasculitis have also been reported as rare side effects of thionamide therapy, specifically with propylthiouracil[215-217]; these complications have not been reported to affect the fetus, although they have occurred in the pregnant mother.

Additionally, the possibility has been raised that methimazole is associated with the development of aplasia cutis of the scalp in the treated mother's offspring.[218-220] Some endocrinologists nonetheless recommend propylthiouracil as initial therapy during pregnancy because no cases of aplasia cutis have been reported in babies born to propylthiouracil-treated mothers.[61,220] In addition, perhaps of greater concern than aplasia cutis are recent descriptions of a methimazole embryopathy, which may include findings of choanal atresia, tracheal-esophageal fistulas, and hypoplastic nipples.[126] A recent case-control study raised the possibility that maternal hyperthyroidism itself, rather than methimazole treatment, might be the causal factor for this embryopathy, specifically choanal atresisa.[221] When the significance of all these reports is considered, it must be emphasized that no case reports of aplasia cutis or other congenital anomalies have been associated with propylthiouracil exposure. This generally remains the preferred drug therapy of maternal hyperthyroidism, in pregnancy. However, some have recently advocated propylthiouracil use only during the first trimester. Thereafter, methimazole may be substituted for propylthiouracil and continued until delivery.

The goal of antithyroid drug therapy is to gain control of the maternal thyrotoxicosis to ensure favorable gestational outcomes and to minimize the impact on the fetus.[61,222] Studies show a strong correlation between maternal and neonatal levels of free T_4, indicating that maternal thyroid status is the most clinically practical index of fetal thyroid status.[199,223] To optimize neonatal thyroid function and minimize the incidence of transient newborn hypothyroidism, maternal serum FT_4 should be maintained at or slightly higher than (<10%) the nonpregnant reference range.[61,223] An alternative approach would be to keep the total T_4 concentration in the high normal range for pregnancy (1.5 times the nonpregnant reference range).[61,68] When detectable, serum TSH concentrations at or just below the trimester-specific 95% confidence interval are acceptable.

Therefore, the therapeutic target for maternal thyroid hormone levels is actually very mild hyperthyroidism as compared with true "normal" levels for gestational physiology. Fortunately, subclinical and mild hyperthyroidism during pregnancy is not associated with adverse maternal gestational outcomes.[224]

Propylthiouracil (PTU) usually is started at doses sufficient to control the hyperthyroidism; the dose may be increased after 4 weeks if necessary to gain control of the thyrotoxicosis. Some women may require high doses (up to 450 mg/day of PTU) for this purpose and must be carefully monitored. Doses of this magnitude may cause fetal hypothyroidism and may justify a change in therapy to surgery. The need for larger doses may correlate with low serum concentrations of PTU[225] and could be caused by documented individual variability in serum propylthiouracil levels after an oral dose[226] or poor compliance with the medication. Methimazole should be used if PTU is not available, the side effect profile of PTU is deemed unacceptable, or if there is difficulty with adherence to a multidose, multi-pill PTU regimen. Free or total T_4 and sensitive TSH measurements should be performed monthly during pregnancy and the dose of thionamide decreased to maintain the therapeutic targets for FT_4, total T_4, and TSH indicated above. If a requirement for higher doses of PTU (>450 mg/day) or methimazole (>30 mg/day) continues and effects on the fetus are a concern, the clinician should consider thyroid surgery.

β-Adrenergic Blockers

If it is necessary to give drugs to a pregnant woman, they should be the least toxic agents possible. For this reason, the use of β-adrenergic blocking drugs has been advocated for the treatment of pregnant women with hyperthyroidism.[227] β-Blockers have been used in large numbers of pregnant women to treat hypertension without apparent significant side effects.[228] However, intrauterine growth retardation with a small placenta, impaired response to anoxic stress, postnatal bradycardia, and hypoglycemia have been reported in the offspring of mothers receiving these agents, indicating the need for caution in their use.[229] β-Blockers are particularly useful for rapid control of the β-adrenergic manifestations of thyrotoxicosis such as tremor and tachycardia. Propranolol, 20 to 40 mg three or four times a day, or atenolol, 50 to 100 mg/day, is usually adequate to control the maternal heart rate at 80 to 90 beats per minute. Esmolol, an ultra–short-acting cardioselective β-blocker given intravenously, controlled the heart rate in a pregnant woman with hyperthyroidism who required emergency surgery and was unresponsive to large doses of propranolol.[230] Current practice is to control hyperthyroidism with antithyroid drugs and to add β-blockers only in exceptional cases.

Surgery

In pregnant thyrotoxic women with poor compliance or for whom maternal or fetal toxicity from antithyroid drug therapy is a concern, subtotal thyroidectomy may be advised.[61] Thyrotoxicosis needs to be controlled medically before subtotal thyroidectomy can be performed. This treatment includes antithyroid drugs, β-blockers, and, rarely, possible short-term use of oral iodides.[231] A useful clinical parameter of control is a resting heart rate of 80 to 90 beats per minute. Because of concern about spontaneous abortion, surgery is often delayed until after the first trimester. The small but real anesthetic and surgical risk is probably greater than the risks associated with thionamide therapy.[232,233]

Iodide

Iodide has not been recommended in the routine treatment of hyperthyroidism during pregnancy because of its association with neonatal goiter and hypothyroidism when given in conjunction with thionamides. One study in which gravidas with mild Grave's disease (GD) were treated with low-dose iodine alone (6 to 40 mg daily) showed that 6% of neonates had elevated serum TSH levels, but none had a goiter.[231] With such little evidence, iodide should not be considered as primary therapy but may be used short term for control of thyrotoxicosis prior to thyroidectomy, or in the management of thyroid storm.

PREGNANCY OUTCOME

Severe maternal thyrotoxicosis significantly increases morbidity in both the fetus and the mother. The prevalence of low birth weight offspring is higher, with a trend toward increased neonatal mortality.[26,234] Whether fetal wastage is increased in established pregnancy is not clear. In one study of 57 thyrotoxic pregnancies, the fetal wastage rate was 8.4%, which compares favorably with the estimated overall fetal wastage rate of 17% in normal women, including those undergoing spontaneous abortion.[44] Very early spontaneous abortions could easily be missed in thyrotoxic women. A recent study reported a higher miscarriage rate in mothers affected by resistance to thyroid hormone. The inference is that these miscarriages may have predominantly involved genetically unaffected fetuses who therefore were exposed to high maternal thyroid hormone levels with resultant fetal thyrotoxicosis that proved toxic. This study provides valuable insight about the effects of in utero thyrotoxicosis without accompanying maternal gestational hyperthyroid physiology.[235] A higher incidence of minor congenital malformations has been suggested to occur in the children of thyrotoxic women who were untreated during the first trimester of pregnancy,[236] but this finding has not been confirmed by others.[207] Only one study has reported Down syndrome to occur more frequently in children born to women with hyperthyroidism.[237] Preterm delivery, perinatal mortality, and maternal congestive heart failure were markedly increased in untreated and inadequately treated thyrotoxic patients in a retrospective study of 60 pregnant women with hyperthyroidism admitted to an inner-city hospital over a 12-year period.[238] Women with newly diagnosed thyrotoxicosis during pregnancy had a higher incidence of morbidity and mortality than did women in whom the condition was diagnosed and treated before conception. Socioeconomic conditions might have played a role in the severity of hyperthyroidism or poor outcomes, but treatment of thyrotoxicosis is indicated nonetheless. These patients are at risk for congestive heart failure because the hyperdynamic state of thyrotoxicosis is superimposed on the increased cardiac output of normal pregnancy.[239] Management of diseases such as diabetes mellitus is also complicated in a pregnant woman with thyrotoxicosis, causing erratic glycemic control and a need for increased insulin.[240] Fortunately, these adverse outcomes are observed only with untreated overt or poorly controlled hyperthyroidism, not with subclinical hyperthyroidism.[224] In addition, successful treatment of overt hyperthyroidism with antithyroid drugs by the third trimester reduces the risk of low birth weight newborns to that of a control euthyroid populaton.[241]

Fetal and Neonatal Thyrotoxicosis

Fetal hyperthyroidism complicates pregnancy in 1% of women with active or treated Graves' disease, including those who have become hypothyroid after radioactive iodine therapy. These women have thyroid-stimulating immunoglobulins that, similar to other immunoglobulins such as IgG, cross the placenta.[242] In high enough concentrations, they may cause fetal or neonatal thyrotoxicosis. Maternal IgG antibodies, particularly subclasses 1 and 3, and thyroid autoantibodies are able to cross the placenta after 20 weeks' gestation[242,243] by micropinocytosis after IgG binding to Fc receptors on the syncytiotrophoblast. Maternal levels are indicative of the degree of fetal exposure and the potential for fetal thyroid stimulation.[244]

Measurement of maternal TSH receptor antibody (TRAb) levels may provide prognostic information about the development of fetal Graves' disease.[245-247] At present, TSH receptor antibodies can be measured by two techniques: an immunoassay (TSH binding inhibitory immunoglobulin [TBII]) or a functional assay of biological stimulation (thyroid-stimulating immunoglobulin [TSI]).[119,248] These antibodies may exhibit stimulating or blocking activity, resulting in fetal/neonatal hyperthyroidism or hypothyroidism.[166,245,249,250] Alternating neonatal hyperthyroidism and hypothyroidism have been described in infants born to the same mother.[251]

TSH receptor antibodies should be measured by the end of the second trimester in mothers with current Graves' disease, a history of Graves' disease and treatment with ^{131}I or thyroidectomy, or birth of a previous neonate with Graves' disease.[61] Women who have a negative TRAb and do not require antithyroid drug therapy have a very low risk of fetal or neonatal thyroid dysfunction.

In a woman with active or previously ablated Graves' disease, the diagnosis of fetal hyperthyroidism should be considered if persistent fetal tachycardia (>180 beats per minute) without beat-to-beat variation and advanced bone maturation are present, sometimes with fetal growth restriction.[167] The diagnosis is strengthened by the ultrasound documentation of a goiter with diffusely increased vascularity.[167] Diagnosis can be confirmed by cordocentesis if considered necessary after discussion of the potential risks, but this usually is not needed.[252] The pathology of fetal thyrotoxicosis includes goiter, visceromegaly, adenopathy, and pulmonary hypertension.[253] If fetal thyrotoxicosis occurs in the setting of active maternal Graves' disease, usually the mother is overtly hyperthyroid. Appropriate maternal antithyroid therapy will treat both the mother and the fetus because, as in the mother, fetal thyroid hormone synthesis represents the balance between the transplacental passage of inhibitory maternal antithyroid drug and stimulating maternal TRAb concentrations.

Levothyroxine replacement in women with a history of Graves' disease and prior ^{131}I ablation or thyroidectomy antedating pregnancy may still produce TRAb, causing fetal thyrotoxicosis. In this scenario, maternal therapy with propylthiouracil, 150 mg/day, may decrease the fetal heart rate to the normal range (140 to 160 beats per minute) within 2 weeks.[244,254] Maternal thyroid hormone levels should be monitored regularly, with thyroxine supplementation given if hypothyroxinemia occurs.

TSH receptor antibody levels usually decline progressively toward term,[13,251,255] and the PTU drug dose can be lowered to 50 to 75 mg/day or even discontinued with titration to the fetal heart rate and growth. In women with persistent elevations of TSH receptor antibodies at term (more than threefold elevated above reference values),[167,256,257] neonatal hyperthyroidism may occur, requiring continued antithyroid drug therapy after birth. In addition, the presence of cord blood TSH receptor antibodies is highly predictive of the development of neonatal hyperthyroidism.[256-259] If the mother has been treated with antithyroid drugs during pregnancy, the manifestations of neonatal thyrotoxicosis may be delayed until 5 to 10 days of life, when the pharmacologic effect of the transplacentally acquired antithyroid drug has cleared.[258] The neonate may become irritable and have feeding problems. Other manifestations include proptosis, goiter, and failure to thrive. In severe cases, congestive heart failure, jaundice, and thrombocytopenia may occur and can cause significant mortality.[260] Usually, the disease runs a self-limited course over a period of several months.[119] Temporary treatment with iodides, β-blockers, and antithyroid drugs is indicated. As maternal antibody levels decrease over the first 3 months of life, treatment generally can be discontinued.[259]

In addition, it has been reported that infants with central hypothyroidism have been born to mothers with uncontrolled Graves' disease. The hypothesis is that these infants are exposed to high levels of thyroid hormone in utero, which results in impaired development of the fetal hypothalamic-pituitary-thyroid axis and eventual central hypothyroidism.[258,261] The incidence of such central congenital hypothyroidism is estimated to be 1 in 35,000 live births.[262]

LACTATION

Until the last decade, lactation was strongly discouraged in women receiving thionamide therapy. The doctrine against lactation in women receiving antithyroid drug therapy originated in a 1948 report, which stated that the concentration of thiouracil measured 2 hours after ingestion was three times higher in breast milk than in serum.[263] Over the last 20 years, several studies have examined the extent of secretion of propylthiouracil and methimazole in breast milk and have evaluated the thyroid function of infants nursed by mothers taking these drugs. Propylthiouracil is more tightly protein bound than methimazole; therefore, the mean milk-to-serum concentration ratio is lower for propylthiouracil, at approximately 0.67,[264] than for methimazole, for which the ratio is 1.0.[265,266] Therefore, the mean total amount of methimazole excreted in breast milk is greater than that of propylthiouracil (0.14% versus 0.025%[264,265]).

Several studies have prospectively evaluated whether maternal antithyroid therapy affects the thyroid function of breastfed infants. Thyroid function remained unaffected in 171 infants whose mothers received daily doses of 50 to 300 mg of propylthiouracil, 5 to 20 mg of methimazole, or 5 to 15 mg of carbimazole for periods ranging from 3 weeks to 8 months.[264,267-269] In fact, serum TSH and T4 levels remained normal even in six women in whom elevated serum TSH levels (19 mU/L and 120 mU/L) had developed while they were receiving propylthiouracil.[269] Therefore, although the number of infants monitored is small, breastfeeding with continued antithyroid drugs may be contemplated as

long as the doses are less than 300 mg daily for propylthiouracil and 20 mg daily for methimazole. It is important to remember that these antithyroid drugs have other nonthyroidal effects such as agranulocytosis; no data are available on the possible occurrence of such effects in infants nursed by mothers taking these drugs.

Pathology of Hypothyroidism in Pregnancy

MATERNAL HYPOTHYROIDISM

Incidence and Etiology

Hypothyroidism is encountered more often in pregnancy than is hyperthyroidism. The most recent epidemiologic data have been obtained through the analysis of banked serum obtained at approximately 16 weeks' gestation in healthy pregnant women. In these women (without prior thyroid disease), two independent studies documented a 2% to 3% incidence of an elevated serum TSH concentration in midpregnancy.[26,28] In industrialized societies, the main causes of maternal hypothyroidism in pregnancy are related to thyroid autoimmunity: Hashimoto's thyroiditis and postablative hypothyroidism in Graves' disease (see Table 25-1, Fig. 25-5). A third cause that has been noted increasingly is primary hypothyroidism due to surgical thyroidectomy. In most women, the hypothyroidism has already been diagnosed and treated before pregnancy. Worldwide, the main cause of maternal hypothyroidism is iodine deficiency, which has been

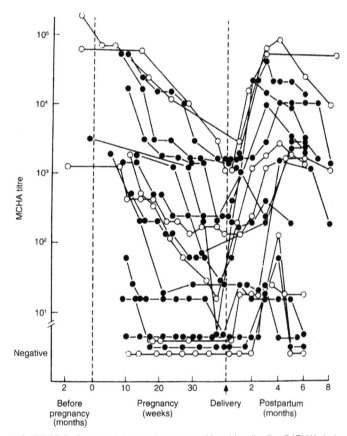

FIGURE 25-5. Sequential changes in serum antithyroid antibodies (MCHA) during pregnancy and after delivery in patients with Graves' disease *(black dots)* and autoimmune thyroiditis *(open dots).* (From Amino N, Kuro R, Tanizawa O, et al: Changes in serum antithyroid antibodies during and after pregnancy in autoimmune thyroid diseases, Clin Exp Immunol 31:30, 1978.)

estimated to affect more than one billion individuals. Population screening programs have documented that a substantial proportion of women of child-bearing age may also have mild TSH elevations. Furthermore, even those hypothyroid women treated to a goal TSH within the normal range, often are found to have abnormal hormone levels.[270,271] The former point is notable in that the average maternal age at pregnancy has been increasing in the United States over the past three decades. In summary, it is estimated that between 4% and 7% of women of child-bearing age in the United States are hypothyroid and unaware of it, or are at risk for hypothyroidism during pregnancy if their levothyroxine dose is not adjusted upon conception. This impressive number draws attention to the importance of this medical problem.

Evidence of thyroid autoimmunity is seen in other autoimmune endocrine disorders such as insulin-dependent (type 1) diabetes mellitus,[272] including that occurring during pregnancy.[273] Up to 40% of diabetic women are thyroid antibody positive, and up to 10% are mildly hypothyroid with elevated TSH levels. Hypothyroidism does not appear to progress in diabetic pregnancy unless proteinuria develops, in which case overt hypothyroidism may ensue.[274] Hypothyroidism may result from increased urinary loss of thyroid hormones as occurs with proteinuria, combined with the preexisting impaired thyroid reserve. Thyroxine therapy in this situation is appropriate but may result in an increase in insulin requirements.

Diagnosis and Screening

Clinical assessment of thyroid status during pregnancy is important, but it can be imprecise. Normal pregnancy symptoms such as lethargy and weight gain may be suggestive of hypothyroidism. Paresthesias resulting from median nerve compression (carpal tunnel syndrome) are seen in both hypothyroidism and pregnancy. Delayed relaxation of deep tendon reflexes (pseudomyotonia) is a good clinical sign of severe hypothyroidism, if present, but is rarely seen in mild thyroid failure. If present, signs of myxedema such as decreased body temperature, periorbital edema, swelling, thick tongue, and hoarse voice should be apparent in pregnancy but may be confused with the features of preeclampsia.[275] Goiter may be present, but its absence does not detract from a diagnosis of hypothyroidism. The most sensitive indicator of primary hypothyroidism in pregnancy is an elevated serum TSH level.[276] Serum TSH values during pregnancy are lower than those seen in healthy nonpregnant individuals.[80,81] Presently, serum TSH values greater than 4.5 to 5 mIU/L should be considered abnormal, warranting further evaluation and possible intervention. Some authors argue that TSH values greater than 3 to 3.5 mIU/L are abnormal and suggest the diagnosis of thyroid dysfunction. While further research findings are awaited, however, no data currently demonstrate the clinical superiority of using trimester-specific data. In contrast, TSH values between 3.0 and 5.0 mIU/L in pregnant women should indicate that repeat laboratory studies are required because the risk of overt hypothyroidism may be increased. When treating patients with levothyroxine for a known thyroid disorder, it is generally accepted that the therapeutic target is a TSH within the normal range. The presence of TPO antibodies indicates a probable autoimmune origin. Hypothalamic or pituitary hypothyroidism is rarely encountered; its presence is suggested by low FT_4 or total T_4 for gestational age with normal or slightly elevated TSH.

Currently, no recommendations have been put forth regarding universal screening of women for thyroid dysfunction before

or during pregnancy.[61] This type of screening program has both political and medical implications, which remain under active discussion by numerous public health and professional societies. Extensive published data have provided insight into the harmful effects of maternal hypothyroidism on the cognitive and neurologic development of offspring. Most often cited is an investigation by Haddow and colleagues, in which a case-control study demonstrated a decrement in intelligence quotient (IQ) among children born to untreated hypothyroid mothers.[277] In this study, 62 children born to untreated hypothyroid mothers (average age, approximately 8 years) were studied prospectively and compared with 124 children born to euthyroid mothers. IQ scores averaged seven points lower in children of hypothyroid mothers. Furthermore, nearly three times as many children had IQ scores lower than 85, in comparison with those born to euthyroid women. Although the lack of randomization has been acknowledged, these data provide the strongest evidence yet suggesting that maternal hypothyroidism is harmful to neurocognitive development and should be prevented. However, many argue that recommendations for universal screening of a population should be implemented only if data also confirm the benefit of a particular treatment intervention (such as levothyroxine replacement). No investigation to date has yet fulfilled this criterion in a prospective, randomized fashion, although several studies are ongoing. In the absence of recommendations for universal screening, it is presently believed that women deemed at high risk for development of hypothyroidism during pregnancy should undergo measurement of serum TSH before pregnancy or during early gestation. This would include women with a history of autoimmune thyroid disease or positive antithyroid antibodies, women with symptoms that are suggestive of hypothyroidism, women with other autoimmune disorders (such as type 1 diabetes mellitus) or a family history of autoimmune thyroid disease, women with a goiter on clinical examination, and women who have undergone previous thyroid surgery or who have a history of head or neck irradiation (including ^{131}I ablation).[61] Additionally, women 35 years of age and older are considered at higher risk for undiagnosed hypothyroidism, warranting evaluation. If a "case-finding" approach is followed, data suggest that nearly 70% of hypothyroid women can be identified in a general population.[278] However, these data also demonstrate that 30% of pregnant women may have elevated TSH during gestation and may avoid detection, even if clinical profiling is instituted.

Separate from consideration of universal screening, clinicians must identify and monitor all thyroxine-replaced hypothyroid women during pregnancy and must adjust levothyroxine early in gestation (Fig. 25-6).[61] A study of 20 pregnancies in 19 women prospectively assessed thyroid function every 2 to 4 weeks throughout gestation and adjusted levothyroxine doses to maintain normal TSH values.[71] Results demonstrated an increased demand for levothyroxine during pregnancy, primarily in the first 16 to 20 weeks. At 20 weeks' gestation, the increased requirement for levothyroxine persisted, although it had plateaued. To prevent abnormal elevations in maternal serum TSH, this study strongly suggests that pregnant women receiving levothyroxine therapy be required to undergo initial biochemical evaluation as early as 6 weeks' gestation. Women who become pregnant via assisted reproductive techniques appear to require the earliest adjustment in thyroid hormone doses, although further validation of this finding is required. These findings have important implications for populations. Because nearly 2% to 4% of women of child-bearing age currently require levothyroxine to maintain normal thyroid function, physicians must actively

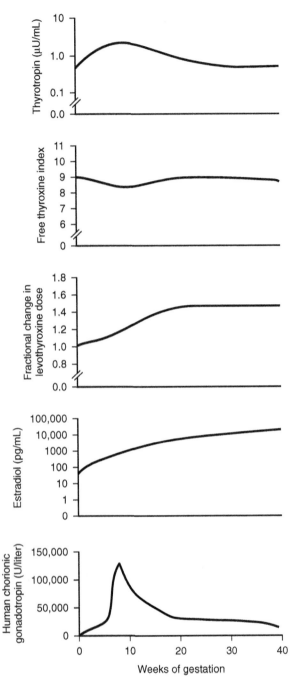

FIGURE 25-6. Changes in maternal hormone concentrations and the levothyroxine dose during gestation. The graphs depict the best-fit curves for serum thyrotropin (range, 0.5 to 5.0 µU per milliliter), the free thyroxine index (range, 5 to 11), the fractional increase in the dose of levothyroxine, the maternal estradiol concentration (range, 10 to 80 pg per milliliter), and the concentration of human chorionic gonadotropin (range, less than 5 U per liter) throughout pregnancy in the 14 women who required an increase in the levothyroxine dose during a full-term pregnancy. To convert the values for estradiol to picomoles per liter, multiply by 3.67. (Data from Alexander EK, Marqusee E, Lawrence J, et al: Timing and magnitude of increases in levothyroxine requirements during pregnancy in women with hypothyroidism, N Engl J Med 351:241, 2004.)

counsel such women to immediately notify a health care professional upon suspicion of a possible pregnancy. Confirmatory testing should then be performed, in conjunction with evaluation of thyroid status. If biochemical testing is delayed until the time of the first obstetric visit, serum TSH values may already be elevated, thus exposing the developing fetus to a period of mater-

nal hypothyroxinemia. Some have advocated that hypothyroid women treated with levothyroxine should be instructed to proactively increase their levothyroxine dosage (by two extra tablets per week) once pregnancy is suspected, while they await further medical testing. This recommendation has not been universally adopted.

Treatment

If hypothyroidism is diagnosed during pregnancy, thyroxine therapy should be initiated. When no endogenous thyroid function remains, full thyroxine replacement can be accomplished with a dosage of approximately 2 mcg/kg/day, a dose slightly higher than the replacement dose for a nonpregnant woman.[61] This usually is well tolerated in otherwise healthy individuals. However, in women with mild hypothyroidism who retain limited endogenous thyroid function, a lesser dose of thyroxine (1 mcg/kg/day) is often initiated and successfully achieves an adequate treatment response. Regardless of initial dose, serum TSH determinations should be repeated at 1 month and the levothyroxine dose adjusted accordingly, with the goal of maintaining TSH within normal limits for pregnancy, which translates practically to a serum TSH level ≤2.5 to 3.0 mIU/L. Women in whom subclinical hypothyroidism is diagnosed may be treated with lower thyroxine dosages. Although many advocate that subclinical hypothyroidism need not be treated in the general population, consensus indicates that even mild hypothyroidism during pregnancy can be harmful, and therefore levothyroxine therapy should be initiated.[279]

Women for whom levothyroxine is initiated or adjusted during pregnancy should be advised by their clinician to have serum TSH concentration tested every 4 weeks during the first half of pregnancy, with dosage adjusted as needed to maintain a normal TSH level. Even if the initial serum TSH concentration is normal, it should be retested at 4-week intervals because as many as 30% of patients may later require a dose change, and data confirm a dynamic physiology of increasing thyroxine requirements over 20 weeks' gestation, as was noted previously. After delivery, the thyroxine dosage should be lowered to the preconception level, with serum TSH testing conducted at 6 weeks' postpartum. Patients should be instructed to separate thyroxine ingestion by 4 hours from ingestion of prenatal vitamins containing iron and iron supplements, calcium supplements, and soy milk, all of which can interfere with thyroxine absorption.[280,281]

Pregnancy Outcome

Although hypothyroidism has long been known to negatively affect pregnancy, numerous reports over the past 100 years have documented hypothyroid women carrying their pregnancies to term.[282-284] Early studies reported up to a 20% incidence of perinatal mortality and congenital malformations associated with maternal hypothyroxinemia[25] (i.e., untreated or inadequately treated hypothyroidism), with up to 60% of surviving children having evidence of impaired mental or physical development. An increase in congenital malformations was seen even in the infants of women considered to have adequate thyroxine replacement therapy, although details from these early reports are difficult to fully evaluate because the biochemical assessment of thyroid hormone status in these studies was imprecise. In more recent studies, patients were well characterized with respect to degree of hypothyroidism and the adequacy of thyroxine replacement therapy.[284] Still, untreated or inadequately treated overtly hypothyroid women experienced up to a 40% incidence of anemia, preeclampsia, placental abruption, and postpartum hemorrhage;

30% of the neonates were small for gestational age; and a 10% incidence of perinatal mortality and congenital anomalies was noted. Women with untreated subclinical hypothyroidism (elevated serum TSH only) had approximately one-third the incidence of these problems, and in both groups it appeared that maternal and fetal outcomes were improved by adequate thyroxine therapy. Other studies confirm a pattern of increased pregnancy complications and maternal morbidity.[28]

A separate study focusing on gestational hypertension reported a 15% incidence in women with subclinical hypothyroidism and a 22% incidence in those with overt disease versus 7.6% in the general population. Preeclampsia occurred in 66% of women who were inadequately treated and remained hypothyroid, resulting in premature delivery.[24] Two investigations have suggested that fetal distress and fetal death may occur more frequently in hypothyroid women.[26,285] Wasserstrum and coworkers found that the likelihood of fetal distress, defined as an abnormal heart rate during labor, was significantly higher in women with overt hypothyroidism (56%) detected during gestation, especially if the serum TSH level remained elevated at term, than it was in women with only mild TSH elevations (3%).[285] In a screening study from Maine in the United States, an elevated serum TSH greater than 6 mIU/L at 15 to 18 weeks' gestation was associated with a higher rate of fetal death (3.8%) than occurred in euthyroid women (0.9%).[26] Many studies reporting gestational complications of hypothyroidism have consisted of populations in which, on average, the initial antenatal visit occurred at between 16 and 20 weeks' gestation—less than optimal prenatal care. These women often had other medical problems that could be associated with adverse fetal outcomes. However, the consistency of findings across several studies supports a contributing causal role of hypothyroidism.

Separate from maternal complications related to hypothyroidism, substantial interest has shifted toward assessing possible neurocognitive decline among the offspring of hypothyroid women. As was noted previously, a case-control study reported a 7-point IQ deficit in children born to untreated, hypothyroid mothers compared with euthyroid controls.[277] Beyond cognitive deficits, significantly worse attention, behavior, and motor skills were demonstrated in these children. Detailed anatomic brain imaging of offspring born to hypothyroid mothers has revealed that anatomic abnormalities are also detected in the visual, hippocampal, and other important areas of the brain.[24] Together, these data strongly suggest that maternal and fetal complications are increased during pregnancy in untreated, hypothyroid women. Even if the pregnancy remains uncomplicated, the data support long-term adverse effects on the fetus' cognitive abilities and development if maternal thyroid status remains undertreated.

A common finding throughout these observational studies is that complication rates (for both the mother and the fetus) may be related to the severity of maternal hypothyroidism at presentation, as well as to the duration of hypothyroidism itself. It appears that severe iodine deficiency (which significantly affects both maternal and fetal thyroid function) may be among the most harmful causes, especially if it occurs for a prolonged period of the pregnancy. Mild thyroid insufficiency, however, does contribute to adverse pregnancy outcomes. Even so, Casey and colleagues recently studied 25,765 women with no known thyroid disorder, who were followed for prenatal care and delivered a singleton infant. Blood was analyzed for TSH concentration from banked serum obtained at 16 to 20 weeks' gestation; 2.3% of women were found to have subclinical hypothyroidism. These pregnancies nonetheless continued to demonstrate a twofold to threefold increase in complications, including placental abruption and preterm birth.

An article by Abalovich confirms the importance of adequate thyroxine replacement during the remainder of the gestational period, once maternal hypothyroidism has been detected. Abalovich and colleagues correlated the pregnancy outcomes of 51 hypothyroid women (diagnosed in the first trimester) with the adequacy of subsequent thyroxine therapy.[27] Regardless of whether the initial diagnosis was overt or subclinical hypothyroidism, those with normalization of serum TSH levels had term pregnancies (93%), except for two preterm deliveries (7%). However, only 21% of those with inadequate thyroxine therapy had term deliveries; 67% had spontaneous abortions and 12% had preterm deliveries. In this as in other studies,[24,284] appropriate thyroxine therapy may ameliorate some of the adverse outcomes even if thyroid hormone deficiency is detected early during pregnancy. These data support the current belief that any degree of maternal hypothyroidism should be actively treated with levothyroxine replacement, with the goal of normalizing serum TSH. Presently, no available data support an adverse effect on the pregnancy or the fetus if mild hypothyroidism of short duration is effectively treated. However, further research is required.

NEONATAL HYPOTHYROIDISM

The incidence of congenital hypothyroidism is 1 per 3000 to 4000 live births, with most cases involving primary hypothyroidism.[119] Any delay in thyroxine treatment beyond 4 to 6 weeks of life reduces the chance of normal development and future intellectual performance of the offspring.[286,287] Because clinical diagnosis is imprecise, the solution has been to institute a neonatal screening program to measure heel-prick blood samples drawn between 3 and 5 days' postpartum for TSH alone or thyroxine. As needed, subsequent TSH measurements are performed on samples with the lowest decile T_4 values.[83,275] Most cases of congenital hypothyroidism are considered sporadic and likely to be permanent. A proportion of cases may be due to maternal autoimmunization or may be associated with maternal TSH receptor antibodies that inhibit thyroid growth or function[288,289] or with cytotoxic antibodies.[290] Antibodies to thyroglobulin or TPO probably are not causal in hypothyroidism. Maternal thyroid autoimmunity may play a role in transient neonatal hypothyroidism that results from transplacental passage of TSH receptor antibodies that block thyroid function or growth, or both, in utero or postpartum.[291] This transient hypothyroidism accounts for up to 10% of cases of congenital hypothyroidism. Familial forms are also recognized.[245] The main risk seems to involve a maternal history of primary myxedema rather than goitrous Hashimoto's disease.[165] Endemic cretinism has also been associated with the finding of maternal thyroid growth-blocking antibodies,[292] but this association has yet to be confirmed.

In any event, patients with neonatal hypothyroidism, including transient cases, must be treated with thyroxine. The risk of developmental problems may already be increased if maternal hypothyroxinemia has occurred during pregnancy. Treatment in cases of suspected transient hypothyroidism may be withdrawn after 1 to 3 years to assess for thyroid recovery.

Postpartum Thyroid Disease

Thyroid dysfunction is a well-recognized complication of the puerperium, and it follows that close surveillance of mothers with thyroid disease or a history of thyroid disease should be continued after delivery. Although Graves' thyrotoxicosis and Hashimoto's thyroiditis tend to improve (or remit) in later pregnancy, a relapse often occurs postpartum[11,293] and may be transient or protracted. The reason for relapse at this time is most likely the rebound in immune surveillance that occurs postpartum.[12] TPO antibodies often are increased postpartum in Hashimoto's disease and Graves' disease, but correlation of TSHR antibody status and the onset or relapse of thyrotoxicosis has been relatively weak.[294] Rarely, postpartum thyroid dysfunction is associated with hypothalamic-pituitary disease as part of pituitary failure in Sheehan's syndrome or lymphocytic hypophysitis.[295-297] Transient isolated thyrotropin deficiency in the postpartum period has been described.[297] Most often, thyroid dysfunction in the puerperium is part of the spectrum of postpartum thyroiditis (PPT), which differs significantly from the aforementioned disorders in terms of its pathogenesis, treatment, and outcome. Otherwise, diagnosis and treatment of thyroid disease in the postpartum period proceed as outlined earlier and are subject to the usual precautions relevant to pregnancy or breastfeeding.

POSTPARTUM THYROIDITIS

PPT is now well recognized as a distinct variant of silent (painless) thyroiditis[298-300] associated with thyroid autoimmunity and transient thyroid dysfunction (hypothyroidism and/or hyperthyroidism). Since the first modern descriptions of PPT more than 25 years ago, much has been learned about the pathophysiology, clinical course, treatment, and outcome of this disorder. The incidence of PPT averages 5%,[4] with a range as low as 1% to 2%, to as high as 20%. The prevalence of PPT appears to be higher in those with separate autoimmune disorders. For example, patients with type 1 diabetes mellitus appear to have a prevalence of PPT of 25% to 30%.[301,302]

Thyrotoxic Phase

Typically, 70% of women experience a transient period of thyrotoxicosis with onset between 6 weeks' and 3 months' postpartum and lasting 1 to 2 months before spontaneously resolving. A goiter develops in 50% of cases. Thyrotoxic symptoms usually are milder than in Graves' disease and may be overlooked or attributed to the adjustment to motherhood. Fatigue and palpitations may be prominent. Hypertension is seen occasionally.[303] Specific tests to detect biochemical thyrotoxicosis are the same as those generally used in pregnancy (Table 25-3). A caveat is that some patients in whom PPT develops have antibodies to T_4 and T_3, which may lead to spuriously high or low results for total or free thyroid hormone levels, depending on the immunoassay method used.[304] TPO antibodies usually are present in women with PPT. Higher TPO antibody titers are associated with more severe disease and a greater risk of subsequent hypothyroidism. In one study, nearly 40% of patients who had TPO antibody

positivity developed postpartum thyroid dysfunction, in contrast to <1% of patients who were TPO antibody negative. In this series, nearly 90% of patients who developed postpartum thyroid dysfunction were TPO antibody positive.[305] Overall, the risk of developing postpartum thyroid dysfunction for mothers who are TPO antibody negative appears to be 100-fold lower than in TPO antibody–positive women.[306]

Upon evaluating a patient who is thyrotoxic postpartum, it is important to distinguish between thyrotoxicosis caused by PPT and that caused by Graves' disease. Radioactive iodine uptake in the thyroid readily differentiates the two, with elevation seen in Graves' disease and reduction or absence noted in thyrotoxic PPT. However, this test is contraindicated in actively lactating mothers. If such testing is required, mothers should interrupt breastfeeding, while continuing to express and discard milk, for 1 to 3 days after receiving tracer doses of technetium 99m or ^{123}I.[307] Thereafter, lactation can be resumed. Rarely other causes of reduced radioactive iodine uptake include iodine-induced thyrotoxicosis and iatrogenic thyrotoxicosis secondary to thyroid hormone administration.

When symptoms of PPT are more severe, the differential diagnosis includes postpartum psychotic depression (postpartum psychosis). Typically, this condition occurs earlier than PPT, 1 to 2 weeks after delivery, and is less common, often reported in 1 per 1000 deliveries.[308] Although hyperthyroxinemia and impaired TSH responses to TRH may be seen in patients with acute psychiatric disorders, thyrotoxicosis has not been confirmed in women with postpartum psychosis. Thyroid antibodies are typically negative in those with postpartum psychosis.

Hypothyroid Phase

Most commonly, with or without symptoms or documentation of a preceding episode of thyrotoxicosis, primary hypothyroidism occurs 3 to 6 months' postpartum. Symptoms of lethargy, cold intolerance, and impaired memory and concentration are typically mild. Fatigue can be indistinguishable from that related to poor sleep patterns commonly experienced by mothers in the postpartum state. An increase in depressive symptoms and depression scores has been reported in patients with PPT hypothyroidism as compared with euthyroid postpartum controls.[309] Up to 20% of patients were considered mildly depressed on the basis of symptom scores, although the results did not achieve statistical significance. Moreover, depressed mood related to the course of hypothyroidism and to positive thyroid antibodies was seen more often in women with postpartum depression.[309] It has not yet been proven that postpartum hypothyroidism is a major cause of postpartum depression, however. The largest trial investigating this question enrolled nearly 750 women who were 6 months' postpartum.[310] Biochemical testing for thyroid dysfunction and TPO antibody status was complemented by a self-administered questionnaire for depression. Both the patient and the physician scoring the questionnaire were blinded regarding test data. Although nearly 12% of patients were found to have postpartum thyroid dysfunction, this trial failed to show any relation between thyroid status and the incidence of depression. The prevalence rate of depression was 9.4% among all women, as tested at 6 months' postpartum. However, hypothyroidism should be considered in patients with postpartum depression because treatment with thyroid hormone may result in clinical improvement when identified.

Although spontaneous recovery is usual by 10 to 12 months' postpartum, 15% to 20% of women remain permanently hypothyroid. The development of permanent hypothyroidism is cor-

Table 25-3. Diagnostic Measures in Postpartum Thyroiditis

Investigation	Results
Thyroid function tests	TSH suppressed, FT_4 or FT_3 elevated in thyrotoxicosis; TSH increased, FT_4 normal or low in hypothyroidism
Thyroid autoantibodies	Positive result indicates autoimmune thyroid disorder; higher titers associated with increased risk of hypothyroidism
Isotope uptake and scan (thyrotoxicosis only)	Low or absent uptake and scan in PPT; increased uptake and scan in Graves' disease

FT_3, Free triiodothyronine; FT_4, free thyroxine; PPT, postpartum thyroiditis; TSH, thyroid-stimulating hormone.

related with antibody titer and severity of the hypothyroid phase of PPT.[311,312] A high prevalence of organification defects and susceptibility to iodine-induced hypothyroidism is observed after PPT.[313] The risk of recurrence after subsequent pregnancies is up to 70%.[314] Even with full biochemical recovery, women with a history of postpartum thyroid dysfunction have a markedly increased risk of developing permanent primary hypothyroidism in the years thereafter. For this reason, it is recommended that these women receive annual testing of serum TSH, even if asymptomatic.[61]

Predisposing Factors

The major risk factor for the development of PPT is, of course, the postpartum state. The condition may also occur after miscarriage or abortion[300,315] and has been described after pregnancy losses as early as 5 to 6 weeks' gestation.[316] Women with a personal or family history of autoimmune thyroid disease are also at increased risk, specifically those with Hashimoto's thyroiditis. The presence of TPO antibodies in the first trimester is associated with a 30% to 35% incidence of PPT,[317] whereas PPT may develop in two thirds of women who remain TPO antibody positive 2 days' postpartum. White and Asian women, as opposed to blacks, may be at increased risk of PPT, as are cigarette smokers.[318] Maternal age, parity, presence of a goiter, breastfeeding, and infant birth weight have not been associated with an increased risk of PPT.[318] It is controversial whether the sex of the infant has any association with PPT.[315,318] On the other hand, a lower ponderal index[272] and a reduced early neonatal growth rate have been reported in association with maternal thyroid-antibody positivity in pregnancy and the subsequent development of PPT. Maternal thyroid function was normal in the women during these pregnancies. Iodide exposure may also be a risk factor for the development of PPT,[319,320] although a similar incidence of PPT is seen in geographic areas with high[315] and low iodine intake.

It has been suggested that all pregnant women be screened for thyroid antibodies during pregnancy to predict the risk of PPT. Whether such a practice would truly be cost-effective is unclear. It would seem reasonable to screen those with a previous episode of PPT or with known thyroid predisposition (such as separate autoimmune disorders). It also seems prudent to screen those women with a history of postpartum psychiatric disturbance. Finally, women known to be TPO antibody positive should have a TSH performed between 3 and 6 months' postpartum, even if no signs of clinical abnormalities are present, given the substantially increased risk for thyroid dysfunction in this population.

Genetic, Humoral, and Cellular Mechanisms

Immune injury to the thyroid gland in PPT is mediated by humoral and cellular mechanisms. A rebound in the immune response is thought to exacerbate autoimmune thyroid disease postpartum.[12,321] A decline in serum cortisol levels at this time may also be important.[322] The risk of development of PPT has been associated with HLA haplotypes B8, DR3, DR4, DR5, DRW3, DRW8, and DRW9.[311,323-326] The relative risk is increased twofold to fivefold. The risk of PPT is reduced in association with the HLA-DR2 haplotype.[311] Variability in HLA haplotypes associated with PPT risk may be due to geographic and population differences. Also, as proposed by DeGroot and Quintans, it is the interaction of genetics along with immune dysfunction and environmental factors that contributes to the clinical expression of autoimmune thyroid disorders.[327] TPO antibodies reflect disease

activity in PPT. Total IgG concentrations are elevated in women with PPT.[328] Thyroid antibodies are predominantly associated with IgG subclasses 1 and 4.[328,329] A nonspecific increase in anti-DNA antibodies is seen in postpartum relapses of thyroid autoimmune disorders, including the thyrotoxic phase of PPT.[330]

Thyroid cytolytic activity resulting from T cell or killer cell attack[320,327] may be important in the release of thyroid hormones in PPT, as opposed to thyroid antibodies, which serve as markers of the disease process.[329] A significant increase in circulation of large peripheral granular lymphocytes with killer cell and cytotoxic activity has been reported in women with PPT as opposed to euthyroid controls or patients with Graves' disease.[331] Others have found no differences in natural killer cell activity between postpartum euthyroid controls and patients with PPT,[332] although both groups showed a relative increase when compared with the reduced killer cell activity noted immediately postpartum. Similarly, these and other investigators showed no change in antibody-dependent cell-mediated cytotoxicity in PPT.[331,332] Analysis of circulating lymphocyte subsets showed an increase in activated T cells with helper-inducer activity in PPT,[333] opposite the findings in Graves' thyrotoxicosis. Stagnaro-Green and colleagues prospectively studied T cell phenotypes during pregnancy and postpartum and found that women in whom PPT developed had higher ratios of CD4⁺ to CD8⁺ T cells throughout gestation than did unaffected women, and therefore exhibited a lesser degree of immunosuppression.[317] Another study reported no change in peripheral blood lymphocytes in PPT but observed an increase in intrathyroidal activated B lymphocytes and T cells with helper-inducer activity.[334] Overall, the cellular mechanisms involved in the pathogenesis of PPT, although undoubtedly important, remain only partially defined.

Treatment and Prevention

Treatment in the hyperthyroid phase of PPT is often unnecessary in that spontaneous normalization may occur. The thyrotoxic phase of PPT is typically mild and self-limited. In more severe cases, β-blockers may provide symptomatic relief of tremor, hyperkinesis, palpitations, and anxiety symptoms. Antithyroid drugs and radioactive iodine have no role in the treatment of PPT during the hyperthyroid phase because thyrotoxicosis results from hormone release rather than from synthesis by the thyroid gland. (PTU could be used to decrease T_4 to T_3 conversion in severe hyperthyroidism.) Patients with symptomatic or severe (TSH >20 mIU/L) hypothyroidism should be considered for treatment with thyroid hormone replacement, but this therapy can often be withdrawn after 6 months. In such cases, patients must be followed with reevaluation of thyroid function after 6 weeks via measurement of serum TSH. Thyroid hormone therapy may also be useful in patients with PPT and depression who have evidence of hypothyroidism.

A recent investigation by Negro and colleagues suggested that selenium supplementation during pregnancy may reduce the risk of PPT in women who are TPO antibody positive.[335] In a prospective, randomized fashion, 2143 euthyroid pregnant women were screened for TPO antibody. Approximately 8% were found to have TPO antibody positivity. Women in this cohort were randomized to selenomethionine (200 μg/day) or placebo. A separate group of TPO antibody–negative women without intervention served as a dual control. TPO antibody–positive women who received selenium supplementation had a significant reduction in the prevalence of PPT (49%) compared with those receiving placebo (29%). These data are notable, although most clinicians have not incorporated selenium supplementation into clinical practice, in part because of lack of confirmatory data. Safety data regarding administration of this vitamin supplement throughout gestation are also limited. Notably, selenium administration has been associated recently with an increased risk of diabetes mellitus.

Thyroid Nodules and Carcinoma During Pregnancy

Ultrasonographic data suggest that thyroid nodules appear more frequently in multiparous women.[50,183,336] However, these studies have been conducted in areas with lower iodine intake than is found in the United States. Thyroid radioisotope scanning is contraindicated in the workup of a patient with a thyroid nodule during pregnancy, and although ultrasound provides excellent definition of anatomy, it is relatively nonspecific in terms of thyroid histology or pathology. If a nodule is clinically palpable, the diagnosis can be made most specifically by fine-needle aspiration (FNA) biopsy.

For this reason, FNA (with ultrasound guidance) should be considered the recommended diagnostic intervention for any pregnant women with a thyroid nodule larger than 1.0 to 1.5 cm in maximal diameter.[337,338] Generally, FNA is a safe procedure that is easily tolerated, with few contraindications. Because the primary risk is hematoma formation, the major relative contraindication is the concomitant use of anticoagulants such as heparin. Local anesthesia in the form of subcutaneous lidocaine is generally accepted.

Cancer per se is relatively uncommon in pregnancy. It is generally believed that pregnancy has little effect on the development or progression of thyroid carcinoma, and that thyroid carcinoma has little effect on pregnancy outcome.[337,339] Although some authors have reported an increased prevalence of neoplasia in thyroid nodules initially discovered during pregnancy, these reports fail to demonstrate a causative association between pregnancy and increased cancer risk. Of a series of 39 patients who underwent FNA biopsy during pregnancy, more than 60% had benign cytologic results and histology confirmed neoplasia in only 20%, half of whom had benign adenomas and the others, papillary thyroid cancer.[339] These data are similar to expected distributions in nonpregnant cohorts. Although theoretically important, the roles of estrogens, thyroid stimulators, and other growth factors, as well as of immunosuppression, in the development or progression of thyroid neoplasia during pregnancy remain uncertain. In addition, several authors have reported that the prognosis of patients with papillary and follicular cancers diagnosed during pregnancy does not differ from that of nonpregnant women with respect to disease stage, recurrence, or mortality.[340,341]

Although surgery during the second trimester is often considered for nodules that are suspicious for or diagnostic of thyroid cancer, some authors recommend delay until the postpartum period.[342] This is generally considered a reasonable approach, although patients must be evaluated on a case-by-case basis. For example, one might consider surgery to remove a cancerous nodule during pregnancy if the thyroid cancer was diagnosed early in gestation and if the nodule is enlarging by midpregnancy. Conversely, a small tumor identified late in pregnancy would likely warrant consideration of treatment following delivery. Very often, the anxiety caused by the cytologic diagnosis of possible cancer drives the patient's desire for operation in the near term. Among pregnant women in whom thyroid cancer is diagnosed, long-term outcomes do not differ between those undergoing surgery during pregnancy and those operated on postpartum.[340,343]

Surgery remains the initial therapy for thyroid cancer. As was previously noted, radioisotope administration (such as ^{131}I) is contraindicated in any patient with thyroid cancer who is currently pregnant or is actively breastfeeding. Although no studies have systematically investigated the appropriate timing of future pregnancy after high-dose radioactive iodine therapy is received for ablation of thyroid tissue, most endocrinologists recommend waiting 6 months or longer before attempting conception.[344] For patients with a known history of thyroid cancer (and on suppressive levothyroxine therapy) who become pregnant, it is prudent to maintain close clinical follow-up and ensure adequate thyroid hormone replacement (and possible TSH suppression) throughout gestation (Fig. 25-7). No standard recommendation has been put forth with regard to continued TSH suppression throughout gestation in patients with cancer. For low-risk patients, many physicians target a TSH value of approximately 0.5 mIU/L; high-risk patients often remain on levothyroxine doses that maintain prepregnancy levels of TSH suppression. No data presently support benefit or harm associated with either approach. Mild TSH suppression during pregnancy is considered safe.[224]

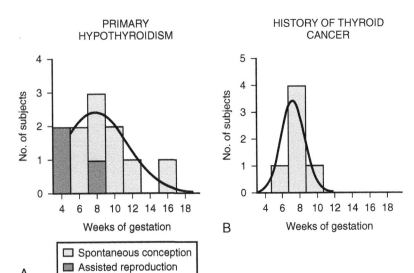

FIGURE 25-7. Gestational week of the initial increase in the levothyroxine dose. **A** shows the week at which the levothyroxine dose was first increased in 11 women with primary hypothyroidism; in these women, the dose was increased when the thyrotropin concentration was greater than 5.0 μU per milliliter. **B** shows the week at which the levothyroxine dose was first increased in women with a history of thyroid cancer; in these women, the dose was increased when the thyrotropin concentration was greater than 0.5 μU per milliliter. (Data from Alexander EK, Marqusee E, Lawrence J, et al: Timing and magnitude of increase in levothyroxine requirements during pregnancy in women with hyperthyroidism, N Engl J Med 351:241, 2004.)

REFERENCES

1. Thomas R, Reid RL: Thyroid disease and reproductive dysfunction: a review, Obstet Gynecol 70:789, 1987.
2. Medvei VC: A history of endocrinology, Boston, 1982, MTP, p 58.
3. Lazarus JH, Othman S: Thyroid disease in relation to pregnancy, Clin Endocrinol 34:91, 1991.
4. Gerstein HC: How common is postpartum thyroiditis? A methodological overview of the literature, Arch Intern Med 150:1397, 1990.
5. Abdoul-Khair SA, Crooks J, Turnbull AC, et al: The physiologic changes in thyroid function during pregnancy, Clin Sci 27:195, 1964.
6. Wong TK, Pekary AE, Hoo GS, et al: Comparison of methods for measuring free thyroxin in nonthyroidal illness, Clin Chem 38:720, 1992.
7. Burrow GN: Thyroid diseases in pregnancy. In Burrow GN, Oppenheimer JH, Volp JR, editors: Thyroid function and disease, Philadelphia, 1989, WB Saunders, p 292.
8. Wiersinga WM, Vet T, Berghout A, et al: Serum free thyroxine during pregnancy: a meta-analysis. In Beckers C, Reinwein D, editors: The thyroid and pregnancy, Stuttgart, Germany, 1991, Shattauer, p 79.
9. Burrow GN: Pituitary and adrenal disorders. In Burrow GN, Ferris TF, editors: Medical complications during pregnancy, ed 3, Philadelphia, 1988, WB Saunders, p 254.
10. Burrow GN, Fisher DA, Larsen PR: Maternal and fetal thyroid function, N Engl J Med 331:1072, 1994.
11. Salvi M, How J: Pregnancy and autoimmune thyroid disease, Endocrinol Metab Clin North Am 16:431, 1987.
12. Lewis JE, Coulam CB, Moore SB: Immunologic mechanisms in the maternal-fetal relationship, Mayo Clin Proc 61:655, 1986.
13. Amino N, Izumi Y, Hidaka Y, et al: No increase of blocking type anti-thyrotropin receptor antibodies during pregnancy in patients with Graves' disease, J Clin Endocrinol Metab 88:5871, 2003.
14. Goldsmith R, Sturgis S, Lerman J, et al: Menstrual pattern in thyroid disease, J Clin Endocrinol Metab 12:846, 1952.
15. Feek CM, Sawers JSA, Brown NS, et al: Influence of thyroid status on dopaminergic inhibition of thyrotropin and prolactin secretion, J Clin Endocrinol Metab 51:585, 1980.
16. Kramer M, Kauschansky A, Genel M: Adolescent secondary amenorrhea: association with hypothalamic hypothyroidism, Pediatrics 94:300, 1979.
17. Scanlon MF, Chan V, Heath M, et al: Dopaminergic control of thyrotropin α-subunit, thyrotropin, β-subunit, and prolactin in euthyroidism and hypothyroidism: dissociated responses to dopamine receptor blockade with metoclopramide in hypothyroid subjects, J Clin Endocrinol Metab 53:360, 1981.
18. Willansky DL, Greisman B: Early hypothyroidism in patients with menorrhagia, Am J Obstet Gynecol 160:673, 1989.
19. Bohnet HG, Fieldler K, Leidenberger FA: Subclinical hypothyroidism and infertility, Lancet 2:1278, 1981.
20. Gerhard I, Becker T, Eggert-Kruse W, et al: Thyroid and ovarian function in infertile women, Hum Reprod 6:338, 1991.
21. Seki K, Kato K: Increased thyroid-stimulating hormone response to thyrotropin-releasing hormone in hyperprolactinemic women, J Clin Endocrinol Metab 61.1130, 1985.
22. Gerhard I, Eggert-Kruse W, Merzoug K, et al: Thyrotropin-releasing hormone (TRH) and metoclopramide testing in infertile women, Gynecol Endocrinol 5:15, 1991.
23. Rotmensch S, Scommegna A: Spontaneous ovarian hyperstimulation syndrome associated with hypothyroidism, Am J Obstet Gynecol 160:1220, 1989.
24. Rovet J, Simic N: The role of transient hypothyroxinemia of prematurity in development of visual abilities, Semin Perinatol 32:431, 2008.
25. Greenman GW, Gabrielson MA, Howard-Flanders I, et al: Thyroid dysfunction in pregnancy: fetal loss and follow-up of evaluation of surviving infants, N Engl J Med 267:426, 1962.
26. Allan WC, Haddow JE, Palomaki GE, et al: Maternal thyroid deficiency and pregnancy complications: implications for population screening, J Med Screen 7:127, 2000.
27. Abalovich M, Gutierrez S, Alcaraz G, et al: Overt and subclinical hypothyroidism complicating pregnancy, Thyroid 12:63, 2002.
28. Casey B, Dashe JS, Wells CE, et al: Subclinical hypothyroidism and pregnancy outcomes, Obstet Gynecol 105:239, 2005.
29. Glinoer D, Fernandez-Soto D, Bourdoux P, et al: Pregnancy in patients with mild thyroid abnormalities: maternal and neonatal repercussions, J Clin Endocrinol Metab 73:421, 1991.
30. Iijima T, Tada H, Hidaka Y, et al: Effects of autoantibodies on the course of pregnancy and fetal growth, Obstet Gynecol 90:364, 1997.
31. Bagis T, Gokcel A, Saygili ES: Autoimmune thyroid disease in pregnancy and the postpartum period: relationship to spontaneous abortion, Thyroid 11:1049, 2001.
32. Prummel MF, Wiersinga WM: Thyroid autoimmunity and miscarriage, Eur J Endocrinol 150:751, 2004.
33. Poppe K, Glinoer D, Tournaye H, et al: Assisted reproduction and thyroid autoimmunity: an unfortunate combination? J Clin Endocrinol Metab 88:4149, 2003.
34. Ghafoor F, Mansoor M, Malik T, et al: Role of thyroid peroxidase antibodies in the outcome of pregnancy, J Coll Physicians Surg Pak 16:468, 2006.
35. Stagnaro-Greene A: Maternal thyroid disease and preterm delivery, J Clin Endocrinol Metab 94:21, 2009.
36. Negro R, Formoso G, Mangieri T, et al: Levothyroxine treatment in euthyroid pregnant women with autoimmune thyroid disease: effects on obstetrical complications, J Clin Endocrinol Metab 91:2587, 2006.
37. Brayshaw ND, Brayshaw DD: Thyroid hypofunction in premenstrual syndrome, N Engl J Med 315:1486, 1986.
38. Roy-Byrne PP, Rubinow DR, Hoban MC, et al: TSH and prolactin response to TRH in patients with premenstrual syndrome, Am J Psychiatry 144:480, 1987.
39. Casper RF, Patel-Christopher A, Powell AM: Thyrotropin and prolactin responses to thyrotropin releasing hormone in premenstrual syndrome, J Clin Endocrinol Metab 68:608, 1989.
40. Southern AL, Olivio J, Gorelon GG, et al: The conversion of androgens to estrogen in hyperthyroidism, J Clin Endocrinol Metab 38:207, 1974.
41. Akande E, Hockaday T: Plasma luteinizing hormone levels in women with thyrotoxicosis, J Endocrinol 53:173, 1972.
42. Tanaka T, Tamai H, Kuma K, et al: Gonadotropin response to luteinizing hormone releasing hormone in hyperthyroid patients with menstrual disturbances, Metabolism 30:323, 1981.
43. Roger J: Menstruation and systemic disease, N Engl J Med 259:676, 1958.
44. Anselmo J, Cao D, Karrison T, et al: Fetal loss associated with excess thyroid hormone exposure, JAMA 292:691, 2004.
45. Amino N: Autoimmunity and hypothyroidism. In Lazarus JH, Hall R, editors: Hypothyroidism and goiter, London, 1988, WB Saunders, p 591.
46. Rojeski MT, Gharib H: Nodular thyroid disease: evaluation and management, N Engl J Med 313:428, 1985.
47. Ansar Ahmed S, Young PR, Penhale WJ: Beneficial effect of testosterone in the treatment of chronic autoimmune thyroiditis in rats, J Immunol 136:143, 1986.
48. Talal N, Ansar Ahmed S: Immunomodulation by hormones: an area of growing importance, J Rheumatol 14:191, 1987.
49. Phillips DIW, Lazarus JH, Butland BK: The influence of pregnancy and reproductive span on the occurrence of autoimmune thyroiditis, Clin Endocrinol 32:301, 1990.
50. Glinoer D, Fernandez Soto M, Bourdoux P, et al: Pregnancy in patients with mild thyroid abnormalities: maternal and neonatal repercussions, J Clin Endocrinol Metab 73:421, 1991.
51. Beckers C: Iodine economy in and around pregnancy. In Beckers C, Reinwein D, editors: The thyroid and pregnancy, Stuttgart, Germany, 1991, Schattauer, p 25.
52. Roti E: Regulation of thyroid-stimulating hormone (TSH) secretion in the fetus and neonate, J Endocrinol Invest 11:145, 1988.
53. Gushurst CA, Mueller JA, Green JA, et al: Breast milk iodide: reassessment in 1980, Pediatrics 73:354, 1984.
54. Hetzel BS: Iodine deficiency disorders and their eradication, Lancet 2:1136, 1983.
55. Delange F, Burgi H: Iodine deficiency disorders in Europe, Bull World Health Organ 67:317, 1989.
56. Alexander WD, Koutras DA, Crooks J, et al: Quantitative studies of iodine metabolism in thyroid disease, Q J Med 31:281, 1966.
57. Dworkin HJ, Jacquez JA, Beirewaltes WH: Relationship of iodine ingestion to iodine excretion in pregnancy, J Clin Endocrinol Metab 26:1329, 1966.
58. Halnan KE: Radioiodine uptake of the human thyroid in pregnancy, Clin Sci 17:281, 1958.
59. Pochin EE: The iodine uptake of the human thyroid throughout the menstrual cycle and in pregnancy, Clin Sci 11:441, 1952.
60. Delange F: Optimal iodine nutrition during pregnancy, lactation and the neonatal period, Int J Endocrinol Metab 2:1, 2004.
61. Abalovich M, Nobuyuki A, Barbour LA, et al: Management of thyroid dysfunction during pregnancy and postpartum: an Endocrine Society clinical practice guideline, J Clin Endocrinol Metab 92:S1, 2007.
62. Hollowell JG, Staehling NW, Hannon WH, et al: Iodine nutrition in the United States. Trends and public health implications: iodine excretion data from National Health and Nutrition Examination Surveys I and III, J Clin Endocrinol Metab 83:3401, 1998.
63. Glinoer D, Gershengorn MC, Dubois A, et al: Stimulation of thyroxine-binding globulin synthesis by isolated rhesus monkey hepatocytes after in vivo 8-estradiol administration, Endocrinology 100:807, 1977.
64. Ain KB, Mori Y, Refetoff S: Reduced clearance of thyroxine binding globulin (TBG) with increased sialylation: a mechanism for estrogen-induced elevation of serum TBG concentration, J Clin Endocrinol Metab 65:686, 1987.
65. Oppenheimer JH: Role of plasma proteins in the binding, distribution and metabolism of thyroid hormones, N Engl J Med 278:1153, 1968.
66. Osathanondh R, Tulchinsky D, Chopra IJ: Total and free thyroxine and triiodothyronine in normal and complicated pregnancy, J Clin Endocrinol Metab 42:98, 1976.
67. Whitworth AS, Midgley JEM, Wilkins TA: A comparison of free T4 and the ratio of total T4 to T4-binding globulin in serum through pregnancy, Clin Endocrinol 17:307, 1982.
68. Demers LM, Spencer CA: NACB guidelines: laboratory medicine practice guidelines: laboratory support for the diagnosis and monitoring of thyroid disease, Thyroid 13:11, 2003.
69. Wilke TJ: A challenge of several concepts of free thyroxine index for assessing thyroid status in patients with altered thyroid-binding protein capacity, Clin Chem 29:56, 1983.
70. Premachandra BN, Gossain VV, Perlstein IB: Effect of pregnancy on thyroxine binding globulin (TBG) in partial TBG deficiency, Am J Med Sci 274:189, 1977.
71. Alexander EK, Marqusee E, Lawrence J, et al: Timing and magnitude of increases in levothyroxine requirements during pregnancy in women with hypothyroidism, N Engl J Med 351:241, 2004.
72. Haddow JE, McClain MR, Lambert-Messerlain G, et al: Variability in thyroid-stimulating hormone suppression by human chorionic gonadotropin during early pregnancy, J Clin Endocrinol Metab 93:3341, 2008.
73. Glinoer D, De Nayer P, Bourdoux P, et al: Regulation of maternal thyroid during pregnancy, J Clin Endocrinol Metab 71:276, 1990.
74. Yamamoto T, Amino N, Tanizawa O, et al: Longitudinal study of serum thyroid hormones, chorionic gonadotropin and thyrotropin during and after normal pregnancy, Clin Endocrinol 10:459, 1979.
75. Pachiarotti A, Martino E, Bartalena L, et al: Serum thyrotropin by ultrasensitive immunoradiometric assay and free thyroid hormones in pregnancy, J Endocrinol Invest 9:185, 1986.

76. Gow SM, Kellett HA, Seth J, et al: Limitations of new thyroid function tests in pregnancy, Clin Chim Acta 152:325, 1985.

77. Kvetny J, Poulsen HK: Nuclear thyroxine and 3,5,3'-triiodothyronine receptors in human mononuclear blood cells during pregnancy, Acta Endocrinol 105:19, 1984.

78. Calvo R, Obregon MJ, Riuz de Ona C, et al: Thyroid hormone economy in pregnant rats near term: a physiological animal model of non-thyroidal illness? Endocrinology 126:10, 1990.

79. Sapin R, d'Herbomez M: Free thyroxine measured by equilibrium dialysis and nine immunoassays in sera with various serum thyroxine-binding capacities, Clin Chem 49:1531, 2003.

80. Soldin OP, Tractenberg RE, Hollowell JG, et al: Trimester-specific changes in maternal thyroid hormone, TSH, and thyroglobulin concentrations during gestation: trends and associations across trimesters in iodine sufficiency, Thyroid 14:1084, 2004.

81. Dashe JS, Casey BM, Wells CE, et al: Thyroid-stimulating hormone in singleton and twin pregnancy: importance of gestational age-specific reference ranges, Obstet Gynecol 106:753, 2005.

82. Stoffer RP, Koeneke IA, Chesky VE, et al: The thyroid in pregnancy, Am J Obstet Gynecol 74:300, 1957.

83. Mandel SJ, Larsen PR, Seely EW, et al: Increased need for thyroxine during pregnancy in women with primary hypothyroidism, N Engl J Med 323:91, 1990.

84. Glinoer D, Delange F, Laboureur I, et al: Maternal and neonatal thyroid function at birth in an area of marginally low iodine intake, J Clin Endocrinol Metab 75:800, 1992.

85. Burrow GN, Fisher DA, Larsen PR: Maternal and fetal thyroid function, N Engl J Med 331:1072, 1994.

86. Vulsma T, Gous MH, De Vijlder JJM: Maternal-fetal transfer of thyroxine in congenital hypothyroidism due to a total organification defect or thyroid agenesis, N Engl J Med 321:13, 1989.

87. Rajatanavin R, Chailurkit L, Srisupandit S, et al: Trophoblastic hyperthyroidism: clinical and biochemical features in five cases, Am J Med 85:237, 1988.

88. Kenimer JC, Hershman JM, Higgins HP: The thyrotropin in hydatidiform moles in human chorionic gonadotropin, J Clin Endocrinol Metab 40:482, 1975.

89. Valdalem JL, Pirens G, Hennen G, et al: Thyroliberin and gonadoliberin tests during pregnancy and the puerperium, Acta Endocrinol 86:695, 1977.

90. Ylikorkala O, Kivinen S, Reinila M: Serial prolactin and thyrotropin responses to thyrotropin-releasing hormone throughout normal human pregnancy, J Clin Endocrinol Metab 48:288, 1979.

91. Burrow GN, Polackwich R, Donabedian R: The hypothalamic-pituitary-thyroid axis in normal pregnancy. In Fisher DA, Burrow GN, editors: Perinatal thyroid physiology and disease, New York, 1975, Raven, p 1.

92. Chan BY, Swaminanthan R: Serum thyrotropin concentration measured by sensitive assays in normal pregnancy, Br J Obstet Gynaecol 95:1332, 1988.

93. Desai RK, Norman RJ, Jialal I, et al: Spectrum of thyroid function abnormalities in gestational trophoblastic neoplasia, Clin Endocrinol 29:583, 1988.

94. Cave WT Jr, Dunn JT: Choriocarcinoma with hyperthyroidism: probable identity of the thyrotropin with human chorionic gonadotropin, Ann Intern Med 85:60, 1976.

95. Guillaume J, Schussler GC, Goldman J, et al: Components of the total serum thyroxine during pregnancy: high free thyroxine and blunted thyrothropin (TSH) response to TSH-releasing hormone in the first trimester, J Clin Endocrinol Metab 60:678, 1985.

96. Harada A, Hershman JM, Reed AW, et al: Comparison of thyroid stimulators and thyroid hormone concentrations in the sera of pregnant women, J Clin Endocrinol Metab 48:793, 1979.

97. Pekonen F, Alfthan H, Stenman UH, et al: Human chorionic gonadotropin (HCG) and thyroid function in early human pregnancy: circadian variation and evidence for intrinsic thyrotropic activity of HCG, J Clin Endocrinol Metab 66:853, 1988.

98. Ballabio M, Poshyachinda M, Ekins RP: Pregnancy-induced changes in thyroid function: role of human chorionic gonadotropin as a putative regulator of maternal thyroid, J Clin Endocrinol Metab 73:824, 1991.

99. Yoshikawa N, Nishikawa M, Horimoto M, et al: Thyroid stimulating activity in sera of normal pregnant women, J Clin Endocrinol Metab 69:891, 1989.

100. Kinmura M, Amino N, Tamaki H, et al: Physiologic thyroid activation in normal pregnancy is induced by circulating HCG, Obstet Gynecol 75:775, 1990.

101. Ekins R: Roles of serum thyroxine binding proteins and maternal thyroid hormones in fetal development, Lancet 1:1129, 1985.

102. Ekins R, Sinha A, Ballabio M, et al: Role of maternal carrier proteins in the supply of thyroid hormones to the feto-placental unit: evidence of a feto-placental requirement for thyroxine. In Delange F, Fisher DA, Glinoer D, editors: Research in congenital hypothyroidism, New York, 1989, Plenum, p 45.

103. Carayon P, Lefort G, Nisula B: Interaction of human chorionic gonadotropin and human luteinizing hormone with human thyroid membranes, Endocrinology 106:1907, 1980.

104. Davies TF, Taliadouros GS, Catt KJ, et al: Assessment of urinary thyrotropin-competing activity in choriocarcinoma and thyroid disease: further evidence for human chorionic gonadotropin interacting at the thyroid cell membrane, J Clin Endocrinol Metab 49:353, 1979.

105. Silverberg J, O'Donnel J, Sugenaya A, et al: Effect of human chorionic gonadotropin on human thyroid tissue in vitro, J Clin Endocrinol Metab 46:420, 1978.

106. Carayon P, Amir S, Nisula B, et al: Effect of carboxypeptidase digestion of the human chorionic gonadotropin molecule on its thyrotropic activity, Endocrinology 108:1891, 1981.

107. Mann K, Schneider N, Hoermann R: Thyrotropic activity of acidic isoelectric variants of human chorionic gonadotropin from trophoblastic tumors, Endocrinology 118:1558, 1986.

108. Hershman JM, Lee HY, Sugawara M, et al: Human chorionic gonadotropin stimulates iodide uptake, adenylate cyclase and deoxyribonucleic acid synthesis in cultured rat thyroid cells, Endocrinology 67:74, 1988.

109. Davies TF, Platzer M: HCG-induced TSH receptor activation and growth acceleration in FRTL-5 cells, Endocrinology 118:2149, 1986.

110. Ballabio M, Sinha AK, Ekins RP: Thyrotropic activity of crude HCG in FRTL-5 rat thyroid cells, Acta Endocrinol 116:479, 1987.

111. Amir SM, Eudo K, Osathanoudh R, et al: Divergent responses by human and mouse thyroids to human chorionic gonadotropin in vitro, Mol Cell Endocrinol 39:31, 1985.

112. Pekary AE, Azukizawa M, Hershman JM: Thyroidal responses to human chorionic gonadotropin in the chicken and rat, Horm Res 17:36, 1983.

113. Uchimura H, Nagataki S, Ito K, et al: Inhibition of the thyroid adenylate cyclase response to thyroid-stimulating immunoglobulin G by crude and asialo-human choriogonadotropin, J Clin Endocrinol Metab 55:347, 1982.

114. Amir S, Shimohigahsi Y, Carayon P, et al: Role of carbohydrate moiety of the human chorionic gonadotropin molecule in its thyrotropic activity, Arch Biochem Biophys 229:170, 1984.

115. Fein HG, Rosen SW, Weintraub BD: Increased glycosylation of serum human chorionic gonadotropin and subunits from eutopic and ectopic sources: comparison with placental and urinary forms, J Clin Endocrinol Metab 50:1111, 1980.

116. Goodwin TM, Montoro M, Mestman JH, et al: The role of chorionic gonadotropin in transient hyperthyroidism of hyperemesis gravidarum, J Clin Endocrinol Metab 75:1333, 1992.

117. Stricker R, Echenard M, Eberhart R, et al: Evaluation of maternal thyroid function during pregnancy: the importance of using gestational age-specific reference intervals, Eur J Endocrinol 157:509, 2007.

118. Fisher DA, Dussault JH, Sack J, et al: Ontogenesis of hypothalamic-pituitary-thyroid function in man, sheep and rat, Recent Prog Horm Res 33:59, 1977.

119. Fisher DA, Polk DH: Development of the thyroid, Baillieres Clin Endocrinol Metab 3:627, 1989.

120. Thorpe-Beeston JG, Nicolaides KH, Felton CV, et al: Maturation of the secretion of thyroid hormone and thyroid-stimulating hormone in the fetus, N Engl J Med 324:532, 1991.

121. Roti E, Gnudi A, Braverman LE: The placental transport, synthesis and metabolism of hormones and drugs which affect thyroid function, Endocr Rev 4:131, 1983.

122. Greenberg AH, Czernichow P, Reba RC, et al: Observations on the maturation of thyroid function in early fetal life, J Clin Invest 49:1790, 1970.

123. Koivusalo F: Evidence of thyrotropin releasing hormone activity in autopsy pancreata from newborns, J Clin Endocrinol Metab 5:734, 1981.

124. Leduque P, Aratan-Spire S, Czernichow P, et al: Ontogenesis of thyrotropin releasing hormone in human fetal pancreas, J Clin Invest 78:1028, 1986.

125. Polk DH, Reviczky AL, Lam RW, et al: Thyrotropin releasing hormone: effect of thyroid status on tissue concentrations in fetal sheep, Clin Res 36:203, 1988.

126. DiGianantonio E, Schaefer C, Mastroiacova PP, et al: Adverse effects of prenatal methimazole exposure, Teratology 64:262, 2001.

127. Roti E, Gundi A, Braverman LE, et al: Human cord blood concentrations of thyrotropin, thyroglobulin and iodothyronines after maternal administration of thyrotropin-releasing hormone, J Clin Endocrinol Metab 53:813, 1981.

128. Evans TC, Kretschmar RM, Hodges RE, et al: Radioiodine uptake studies of the human fetal thyroid, J Nucl Med 8:157, 1967.

129. Johnson JR: Fetal thyroid dose from intake of radioiodine by the mother, Health Physics 43:573, 1955.

130. Hodges RE, Evans TC, Bradbury JT, et al: The accumulation of radioactive iodine by human fetal thyroid, J Clin Endocrinol Metab 15:661, 1955.

131. Chapman EM, Corner GW, Robinson D, et al: The collection of radioactive iodine by human fetal thyroid, J Clin Endocrinol 8:717, 1948.

132. Fisher DA, Dussault J: Development of the mammalian thyroid gland. In Greer MA, Solomon DH, editors: Handbook of physiology: endocrinology. III, Baltimore, 1974, Williams & Wilkins, p 21.

133. Bernal J, Pekonen F: Ontogenesis of the nuclear 3,5,3'-triiodothyronine receptor in the human fetal brain, Endocrinology 114:677, 1984.

134. Calvo R, Obregon MJ, Ruiz de Ona C, et al: Congenital hypothyroidism as studied in rats: crucial role of maternal thyroxine but not 3,5,3'-triiodothyronine in the protection of the fetal brain, J Clin Invest 86:889, 1990.

135. Morreale de Escobar G, Obregon MJ, Escobar del Rey F: Maternal-fetal thyroid hormone relationships and the fetal brain, Acta Med Austriaca 15:66, 1988.

136. Morreale de Escobar G, Obregon MJ, Ruiz de Ona C, et al: Comparison of maternal to fetal transfer of 3,5,3'-triiodothyronine versus thyroxine in rats, Acta Endocrinol 120:20, 1989.

137. Ruiz de Ona C, Obregon MJ, Escobar del Rey F, et al: Developmental changes in rat brain 5'-deiodinase and thyroid hormones in the fetal period, Pediatr Res 24:588, 1988.

138. Vaccari A: Teratogenic mechanisms of dysthyroidism in the central nervous system, Prog Brain Res 73:71, 1988.

139. Morreale de Escobar G, Calvo R, Obregon MJ, et al: Contribution of maternal thyroxine to fetal thyroxine pools in normal rats near term, Endocrinology 126:2765, 1990.

140. Calvo R, Obregon MJ, Ruiz de Oña C, et al: Congenital hypothyroidism, as studied in rats: crucial role of maternal thyroxine but not of 3,5,3'-triiodothyronine in the protection of the fetal brain, J Clin Invest 86:889, 1990.

141. Calvo RM, Jauniaux E, Gulbis B, et al: Fetal tissues are exposed to biologically relevant free thyroxine concentrations during early phases of development, J Clin Endocrinol Metab 87:1768, 2002.

142. Hetzel BS: Progress in the prevention and control of iodine-deficiency disorders, Lancet 2:266, 1987.

143. Hetzel BS, Mano MT: A review of experimental studies of iodine deficiency in fetal development, J Nutr 119:145, 1989.

144. Ferreiro B, Bernal J, Goodyear G, et al: Estimation of nuclear thyroid hormone receptor saturation in human fetal brain and lung during early gestation, Endocrinology 67:853, 1988.

145. Man EB, Jones WS, Holden RH, et al: Thyroid function in human pregnancy. VIII. Retardation of progeny aged 7 years: relationships to maternal age and maternal thyroid function, Am J Obstet Gynecol 111:905, 1971.

146. Man EB, Brown JF, Serunian SA: Maternal hypothyroxinemia: psychoneurological deficits of progeny, Ann Clin Lab Sci 21:227, 1991.

147. Raiti S, Holsman GB, Scott RL, et al: Evidence for placental transfer of triiodthyronine in human beings, N Engl J Med 277:456, 1967.

148. Dussault J, Row VV, Lickrish G, et al: Studies of serum triiodothyronine concentration in maternal and cord blood, J Clin Endocrinol Metab 29:595, 1969.

149. Fisher DA, Lehman H, Lackey C: Placental transport of thyroxine, J Clin Endocrinol Metab 24:393, 1964.

150. Grumbach MM, Werner SC: Transfer of thyroid hormones across the human placenta at term, J Clin Endocrinol Metab 16:1392, 1956.

151. Carr EA, Bierwaltes WH, Raman G, et al: The effect of maternal thyroid function on fetal thyroid function and development, J Clin Endocrinol Metab 19:1, 1959.

152. Kearns JE, Hutson W: Tagged isomers and analogs of thyroxine: Their transmission across the human placenta and other studies, J Nucl Med 4:453, 1963.

153. Myant NB: Passage of thyroxine and triiodothyronine from mother to fetus in pregnant women, Clin Sci 17:75, 1958.

154. Penel C, Rognoni JB, Pastiani P: Thyroid autoregulation, Am J Physiol 16:E165, 1987.

155. Theodoropoulos T, Braverman LE, Vagenakis AG: Iodine-induced hypothyroidism, Science 205:502, 1979.

156. Mahillon I, Peers W, Bourdoux P, et al: Effects of vaginal douching with povidone-iodine during early pregnancy on the iodine supply to mother and fetus, Biol Neonate 56:210, 1989.

157. Stubbe P, Heidemann P, Schurnbrand P, et al: Transient congenital hypothyroidism after amniofetography, Eur J Pediatr 135:97, 1980.

158. Smerdley P, Boyages SC, Wu D, et al: Topical iodine-containing antiseptics and neonatal hypothyroidism in very low birth weight infants, Lancet 2:661, 1989.

159. Danziger Y, Pertzelan A, Mimouni M: Transient congenital hypothyroidism after topical iodine in pregnancy and lactation, Arch Dis Child 62:295, 1987.

160. Rey E, Bachrach LK, Burrow GN: Effects of amiodarone during pregnancy, Can Med Assoc J 136:959, 1987.

161. DeWolf D, DeSchepper J, Verhaaren H, et al: Congenital hypothyroid goiter and amiodarone, Acta Paediatr Scand 77:616, 1988.

162. Tubman R, Jenkins J, Lim J: Neonatal hyperthyroxinemia associated with maternal amiodarone therapy, Ir J Med Sci 157:243, 1988.

163. Widehorn J, Bhandari AK, Bughi S, et al: Fetal and neonatal adverse effects profile of amiodarone treatment during pregnancy, Am Heart J 122:1162, 1991.

164. Dussault JH, Rousseau F: Immunologically mediated hypothyroidism, Endocrinol Metab Clin North Am 16:417, 1987.

165. Tamaki H, Amino N, Aozasa M, et al: Effective method for prediction of transient neonatal hypothyroidism in infants born to mothers with chronic thyroiditis, Am J Perinatol 6:296, 1989.

166. Matsuura N, Konishi J: Transient hypothyroidism in infants born to mothers with chronic thyroiditis: a nationwide study of 23 cases, Endocrinol Jpn 37:369, 1990.

167. Luton D, Le Gac I, Vuillard E, et al: Management of Graves' disease during pregnancy: the key role of fetal thyroid gland monitoring, J Clin Endocrinol Metab 90:6093, 2005.

168. Perelman AH, Johnston RL, Clemons RD, et al: Intrauterine diagnosis and treatment of fetal goitrous hypothyroidism, J Clin Endocrinol Metab 71:618, 1990.

169. Glorieux J, Desjardins M, Letarte J, et al: Useful parameters to predict eventual mental outcome of hypothyroid children, Pediatr Res 24:6, 1988.

170. Virtanen M, Perheentupa J: Bone age at birth: method and effect of hypothyroidism, Acta Paediatr Scand 78:412, 1989.

171. Davidson KM, Richards DS, Schatz DA, et al: Successful in utero treatment of fetal goiter and hypothyroidism, N Engl J Med 324:543, 1991.

172. Wenstrom KD, Weiner CP, Williamson RA, et al: Prenatal diagnosis of fetal hyperthyroidism using funipuncture, Obstet Gynecol 76:513, 1990.

173. Yoshida K, Sakurada T, Takahashi T, et al: Measurement of TSH in human amniotic fluid, Clin Endocrinol 25:313, 1986.

174. Hollingsworth DR, Alexander NM: Amniotic fluid concentrations of iodothyronines and thyrotropin do not reliably predict fetal thyroid status in pregnancies complicated by maternal thyroid disorders or anencephaly, J Clin Endocrinol Metab 57:349, 1983.

175. Lightner ES, Fisher DA, Giles H, et al: Intra-amniotic injections of thyroxine to a human fetus, Am J Obstet Gynecol 127:487, 1977.

176. Drury MI: Hyperthyroidism in pregnancy, J R Soc Med 79:317, 1986.

177. Crooks J, Tulloch MI, Turnbull AC, et al: Comparative incidence of goiter in pregnancy in Iceland and Scotland, Lancet 2:625, 1964.

178. Long TJ, Felice ME, Hollingsworth DR: Goiter in pregnant teenagers, Am J Obstet Gynecol 152:670, 1985.

179. Levy RP, Newman DM, Rejali LS, et al: The myth of goiter in pregnancy, Am J Obstet Gynecol 137:701, 1980.

180. Rasmussen NG, Hornnes PJ, Hegedus L: Ultrasonographically determined thyroid size in pregnancy and postpartum: the goitrogenic effect of pregnancy, Am J Obstet Gynecol 160:1216, 1989.

181. Pedersen KM, Borlum KG, Knudson PR, et al: Urinary iodine excretion is low and serum thyroglobulin high in pregnant women in parts of Denmark, Acta Obstet Gynecol Scand 67:413, 1988.

182. Nelson M, Wickus GG, Caplan RH, et al: Thyroid gland size in pregnancy, J Reprod Med 32:888, 1987.

183. Struve C, Ohlen S: The influence of previous pregnancies on the prevalence of goitre and thyroid nodules in women without clinical evidence of thyroid disease, Dtsch Med Wochenschr 115:1050, 1990.

184. Gaitan E, Cooksey RC, Meydrech EF, et al: Thyroid function in neonates from goitrous and non-goitrous iodine-sufficient areas, J Clin Endocrinol Metab 69:359, 1989.

185. Liu JL, Zhuang ZJ, Cao XM: Changes in thyroid, cerebral cortex and bones of therapeutically aborted fetuses from endemic goiter region supplied with iodized salt for 5 years, Chin Med J 101:133, 1988.

186. Chanoine JP, Toppet V, Bourdoux P, et al: Smoking during pregnancy: a significant cause of neonatal thyroid enlargement, Br J Obstet Gynaecol 98:65, 1991.

187. Kimura M, Amino N, Tamaki H, et al: Gestational thyrotoxicosis and hyperemesis gravidarum: possible role of HCG with higher stimulating activity, Clin Endocrinol 38:345, 1993.

188. Goodwin TM, Hershman JM: Hyperthyroidism due to inappropriate production of human chorionic gonadotropin, Clin Obstet Gynecol 40:32, 1997.

189. Glinoer D, Merck AG, European Thyroid Symposium: Thyroid hyperfunction during pregnancy, Thyroid 8:859, 1998.

190. Chin RKH, Lao TTH: Thyroxine concentration and outcome of hyperemetic pregnancies, Br J Obstet Gynaecol 95:507, 1988.

191. Lao TT, Chin RKH, Panesar NS, et al: Observations on thyroid hormones in hyperemesis gravidarum, Asia Oceania J Obstet Gynaecol 14:449, 1988.

192. Rodien P, Bremont C, Sanson ML, et al: Familial gestational hyperthyroidism caused by a mutant thyrotropin receptor hypersensitive to human chorionic gonadotropin, N Engl J Med 339:1823, 1998.

193. Mori M, Amino N, Tamaki H, et al: Morning sickness and thyroid function in normal pregnancy, Obstet Gynecol 72:355, 1988.

194. Grun JP, Meuris S, De Nayer P, et al: The thyrotrophic role of human chorionic gonadotrophin (HCG) in the early stages of twin (versus single) pregnancies, Clin Endocrinol 46:719, 1997.

195. Goodwin TM, Montoro M, Mestman JH: Transient hyperthyroidism and hyperemesis gravidarum: Clinical aspects, Am J Obstet Gynecol 167:648, 1992.

196. de los Santos ET, Mazzaferri EL: Sensitive thyroid-stimulating hormone assays: clinical applications and limitations, Compr Ther 14:26, 1988.

197. Bassett F, Cresswell J, Eastman CJ, et al: Diagnostic value of thyrotropin concentrations in serum as measured by a sensitive immunoradiometric assay, Clin Chem 32:461, 1986.

198. Burrow GN: The management of thyrotoxicosis in pregnancy, N Engl J Med 313:562, 1985.

199. Momotani N, Noh J, Oyanagi H, et al: Antithyroid drug therapy for Graves' disease during pregnancy, optimal regimen for fetal thyroid status, N Engl J Med 315:24, 1986.

200. Pekonen F, Lamberg B-A: Thyrotoxicosis during pregnancy, Ann Chir Gynaecol 67:165, 1978.

201. Mutjaba Q, Burrow GN: Treatment of hyperthyroidism in pregnancy with propylthiouracil and methimazole, Obstet Gynecol 46:282, 1975.

202. Cooper DS, Saxe VC, Meskell M, et al: Acute effects of propylthiouracil (PTU) on thyroidal iodide organification and peripheral iodothyronine deiodination: correlation with serum PTU levels measured by radioimmunoassay, J Clin Endocrinol Metab 54:101, 1982.

203. Cooper DS, Bode HH, Nath B, et al: Methimazole pharmacology in man: studies using a newly developed radioimmunoassay for methimazole, J Clin Endocrinol Metab 58:473, 1984.

204. Sitar DS, Abu-Bakare A, Gardiner RJ: Propylthiouracil disposition in pregnancy and postpartum women, Pharmacology 25:57, 1982.

205. Skellern GG, Knight BI, Otter M, et al: The pharmacokinetics of methimazole in pregnant patients after oral administration of carbimazole, Br J Clin Pharmacol 9:145, 1980.

206. Marchant B, Brownlie BEW, Hart DM, et al: The placental transfer of propylthiouracil, methimazole and carbimazole, J Clin Endocrinol Metab 45:1187, 1977.

207. Wing DA, Millar LK, Koonings PP, et al: A comparison of propylthiouracil versus methimazole in the treatment of hyperthyroidism in pregnancy, Am J Obstet Gynecol 170:90, 1994.

208. Amrhein JA, Kenny FM, Ross D: Granulocytopenia, lupus-like syndrome, and other complications of propylthiouracil therapy, J Pediatr 76:54, 1970.

209. Jackson IMD: Management of thyrotoxicosis, J Maine Med Assoc 66:224, 1975.

210. Wing ES Jr, Asper SP Jr: Observations on the use of propylthiouracil in hyperthyroidism with special reference to long-term treatment, Bull Johns Hopkins Hosp 90:152, 1952.

211. Bilezikian SB, Lalei U, Tsan M-F, et al: Immunological reactions involving leukocytes. III. Agranulocytosis induced by antithyroid drugs, Johns Hopkins Med J 138:124, 1976.

212. Wall JR, Fang SL, Kuroki T, et al: In vitro immunoactivity to propylthiouracil, methimazole, and carbimazole in patients with Graves' disease: a possible cause of antithyroid drug–induced agranulocytosis, J Clin Endocrinol Metab 58:868, 1984.

213. Weitzman SA, Stossel TP, Desmond M: Drug-induced immunological neutropenia, Lancet 1:1068, 1978.

214. Tajiri J, Noguchi S, Murakami T, et al: Antithyroid drug–induced agranulocytosis, Arch Intern Med 150:621, 1990.

215. Romaldini JH, Bromberg N, Werner RS, et al: Comparison of effects of high and low dosage regimens of antithyroid drugs in the management of Graves' hyperthyroidism, J Clin Endocrinol Metab 57:563, 1983.

216. Safani MM, Tatro DS, Rudd P: Fatal propylthiouracil-induced hepatitis, Arch Intern Med 142:838, 1982.

217. Vasily DB, Tyler WB: Propylthiouracil-induced cutaneous vasculitis: case presentation and review of the literature, JAMA 23:458, 1980.

218. Milham S: Scalp defects in infants of mothers treated for hyperthyroidism with methimazole or carbimazole during pregnancy, Teratology 32:231, 1985.

219. Van Dijke CP, Heydendael RJ, De Kleine MJ: Methimazole, carbimazole and congenital skin defects, Ann Intern Med 106:60, 1987.

220. Mandel SJ, Brent GA, Larsen PR: Review of antithyroid drug use during pregnancy and report of a case of aplasia cutis, Thyroid 4:129, 1994.

221. Barbero P, Valdez R, Rodriguez H, et al: Choanal atresia associated with maternal hyperthyroidism treated with methimazole: a case-control study, Am J Med Genet A 146A:2390, 2008.

222. Chan GW, Mandel SJ: Therapy insight: management of Graves' disease during pregnancy, Nat Clin Pract Endocrinol Metab 3:470, 2007.

223. Momotani N, Iwama S, Noh JY, et al: Anti–thyroid drug therapy for Graves' disease during pregnancy: mildest thyrotoxic maternal free thyroxine concentrations to avoid fetal hypothyroidism. In 77th Annual Meeting of the American Thyroid Association, Phoenix, AZ, 2006.

224. Casey BM, Dashe JS, Wells CE, et al: Subclinical hyperthyroidism and pregnancy outcomes, Obstet Gynecol 107(2 Pt 1):337, 2006.
225. Sato K, Mimura H, Kato S, et al: Serum propylthiouracil concentration in patients with Graves' disease with various clinical courses, Acta Endocrinol 104:189, 1983.
226. Gardner DF, Cruikshank DP, Hays PM, et al: Pharmacology of propylthiouracil (PTU) in pregnant hyperthyroid women: correlation of maternal PTU concentrations with cord serum thyroid function tests, J Clin Endocrinol Metab 62:217, 1986.
227. Bullock JL, Harris RL, Young R: Treatment of thyrotoxicosis during pregnancy with propranolol, Am J Obstet Gynecol 121:242, 1975.
228. Rubin PC: Current concepts: beta-blockers in pregnancy, N Engl J Med 305:1323, 1981
229. Pruyn SC, Phelan JP, Buchanan GC: Long-term propranolol therapy in pregnancy: maternal and fetal outcome, Am J Obstet Gynecol 135:485, 1979.
230. Isley WL, Dahl S, Gibbs H: Use of esmolol in managing a thyrotoxic patient needing emergency surgery, Am J Med 89:122, 1990.
231. Momotani N, Hisaoka T, Noh J, et al: Effects of iodine on thyroid status of fetus versus mother in treatment of Graves' disease complicated by pregnancy, J Clin Endocrinol Metab 75:738, 1992.
232. Brodsky JF, Cohen EN, Brown BW Jr, et al: Surgery during pregnancy and fetal outcome, Am J Obstet Gynecol 138:1165, 1980.
233. Weingold AB: Surgical diseases in pregnancy, Clin Obstet Gynecol 26:793, 1983.
234. Mitsuda N, Tamaki H, Amino N, et al: Risk factors for developmental disorders in infants born to women with Graves' disease, Obstet Gynecol 80:359, 1992.
235. Anselmo J, Cao D, Karrison T, et al: Fetal loss associated with excess thyroid hormone exposure, JAMA 292:691, 2004.
236. Momotani N, Ito K, Hamada N, et al: Maternal hyperthyroidism and congenital malformation in the offspring, Clin Endocrinol 20:695, 1984.
237. Dinani S, Carpenter S: Down's syndrome and thyroid disorder, J Ment Defic Res 34:187, 1990.
238. Davis LE, Lucas MJ, Hankins GDV, et al: Thyrotoxicosis complicating pregnancy, Am J Obstet Gynecol 160:63, 1989.
239. Easterling TR, Schmucker BC, Carlson KL, et al: Maternal hemodynamics in pregnancies complicated by hyperthyroidism, Obstet Gynecol 78:348, 1991.
240. Bruner JP, Landon MB, Gabbe SG: Diabetes mellitus and Graves' disease complicated by maternal allergies to antithyroid drugs, Obstet Gynecol 72:443, 1988.
241. Phoojaroenchanachai M, Sriussadaporn S, Peerapatdit T, et al: Effect of maternal hyperthyroidism during late pregnancy on the risk of neonatal low birth weight, Clin Endocrinol (Oxf) 54:365, 2001.
242. Pitcher-Willmott RW, Hindocha P, Wood CBS: The placental transfer of IgG subclasses in human pregnancy, Clin Exp Immunol 41:308, 1980.
243. Ewin DL, McGregor AM: Pregnancy and autoimmune thyroid disease, Trends Endocrinol Metab 1:296, 1990.
244. Fisher DA: Fetal thyroid function: diagnosis and management of fetal thyroid disorders, Clin Obstet Gynecol 40:16, 1997.
245. Matsuura N, Yamada Y, Nohara Y, et al: Familial neonatal transient hypothyroidism due to maternal TSH-binding inhibitor immunoglobulins, N Engl J Med 303:738, 1980.
246. Mitsuda N, Tamaki H, Amino N, et al: Risk factors for developmental disorders in infants born to women with Graves' disease, Obstet Gynecol 80:359, 1992.
247. Tamajki H, Amino N, Aozasa M, et al: Universal predictive criteria for neonatal overt thyrotoxicosis requiring treatment, Am J Perinatol 5:152, 1988.
248. McKenzie JM, Zakarija M: The clinical use of thyrotropin receptor antibody measurements, J Clin Endocrinol Metab 69:1093, 1989.
249. Clavel S, Madec AM, Bornet H, et al: Anti–TSH-receptor antibodies in pregnant patients with autoimmune thyroid disorder, Br J Obstet Gynaecol 97:1003, 1990.
250. Iseki M, Shimizu YM, Oikawa T, et al: Sequential serum measurements of thyrotropin binding inhibition immunoglobulin G in transient familial neonatal hypothyroidism, J Clin Endocrinol Metab 57:384, 1983.
251. Zakarija M, McKenzie JM, Hoffman WH: Prediction and therapy of intrauterine and late onset neonatal hyperthyroidism, J Clin Endocrinol Metab 62:368, 1986.
252. Bruinse HW, Vermeulen-Meiners C, Wit JM: Fetal therapy for thyrotoxicosis in nonthyrotoxic pregnant women, Fetal Ther 3:152, 1988.
253. Page DV, Brady K, Mitchell J, et al: The pathology of intrauterine thyrotoxicosis: two case reports, Obstet Gynecol 72:479, 1988.
254. Wallace C, Couch R, Ginsberg J: Fetal thyrotoxicosis: a case report and recommendations for prediction, diagnosis, and treatment, Thyroid 5:125, 1995.
255. Mortimer RH, Tyack SA, Galligan JP, et al: Graves' disease in pregnancy: TSH receptor binding inhibiting immunoglobulins and maternal and neonatal thyroid function, Clin Endocrinol 32:141, 1990.
256. Tamaki H, Amino N, Takeoka K, et al: Prediction of later development of thyrotoxicosis or central hypothyroidism from the cord serum TSH level in neonates born to mothers with Graves' disease, J Pediatr 115:318, 1989.
257. Zakarija M, McKenzie JM: Pregnancy-associated changes in the thyroid-stimulating antibody of Graves' disease and the relationship to neonatal hyperthyroidism, J Clin Endocrinol Metab 57:1036, 1983.
258. Tamaki H, Amino N, Takeoka K, et al: Prediction of later development of thyrotoxicosis of central hypothyroidism from the cord serum thyroid-stimulating hormone level in neonates born to mothers with Graves' disease, J Pediatr 115:318, 1989.
259. Skuza KA, Sills IN, Stene M, et al: Prediction of neonatal hyperthyroidism in infants born to mothers with Graves' disease, J Pediatr 128:264, 1996.
260. Delange F: Effect of maternal thyroid function during pregnancy on fetal development. In Beckers C, Reinwein D, editors: The thyroid and pregnancy, Stuttgart, Germany, 1991, Schattauer, p 7.
261. Mandel S, Hanna C, LaFranchi S: Thyroid function of infants born to mother with Graves' disease, J Pediatr 117:169, 1990.
262. Kempers MJ, van Tijn DA, van Trotsenburg JA, et al: Central congenital hypothyroidism due to gestational hyperthyroidism: detection where prevention failed, J Clin Endocrinol Metab 88:5851, 2003.
263. Williams RH, Kay GA, Jandorf BJ: Thiouracil, its absorption, distribution, and excretion, J Clin Invest 23:613, 1943.
264. Kampmann JP, Hansen JM, Johansen K, et al: Propylthiouracil in human milk: revision of a dogma, Lancet 1:736, 1980.
265. Johansen K, Andersen AN, Kampmann JP, et al: Excretion of methimazole in human milk, Eur J Clin Pharmacol 23:39, 1982.
266. Cooper DS, Bode HH, Nath B, et al: Methimazole pharmacology in man: studies using a newly developed radioimmunoassay for methimazole, J Clin Endocrinol Metab 58:473, 1984.
267. Lamberg BA, Ikonen E, Österlund K, et al: Antithyroid treatment of maternal hyperthyroidism during lactation, Clin Endocrinol 21:81, 1984.
268. Momotani N, Yamashita R, Yoshimoto M, et al: Recovery from foetal hypothyroidism: evidence for the safety of breast-feeding while taking propylthiouracil, Clin Endocrinol 31:591, 1989.
269. Azizi F, Khoshniat M, Bahrainian M, et al: Thyroid function and intellectual development of infants nursed by mothers taking methimazole, J Clin Endocrinol Metab 85:3233, 2000.
270. Canaris GJ, Manowitz NR, Mayor G, et al: The Colorado Thyroid Disease Prevalence Study, Arch Intern Med 160:526, 2000.
271. Hollowell JG, Staehling NW, Flanders WD, et al: Serum TSH, T4, and thyroid antibodies in the United States population (1988 to 1994): National Health and Nutrition Examination Survey (NHANES III), J Clin Endocrinol Metab 87:489, 2002.
272. Gray RS, Dorsey DQ, Seth J, et al: Prevalence of subclinical thyroid failure in insulin dependent diabetes, J Clin Endocrinol Metab 50:1034, 1980.
273. Bech K, Hoier-Madsen M, Feldt-Rasmussen U, et al: Thyroid function and autoimmune manifestations in insulin-dependent diabetes mellitus during and after pregnancy, Acta Endocrinol 124:534, 1991.
274. Jovanovic-Peterson L, Peterson CM: De novo clinical hypothyroidism in pregnancies complicated by type I diabetes, subclinical hypothyroidism and proteinuria, Am J Obstet Gynecol 104:909, 1989.
275. Patel S, Robinson S, Bidgood RJ, et al: A pre-eclampsia-like syndrome associated with hypothyroidism during pregnancy, Q J Med 79:435, 1991.
276. Klein RZ, Haddow JE, Faix JD, et al: Prevalence of thyroid deficiency in pregnant women, Clin Endocrinol 35:41, 1995.
277. Haddow JE, Palomaki GE, Allan WC, et al: Maternal thyroid deficiency during pregnancy and subsequent neuropsychological development of the child, N Engl J Med 341:549, 1999.
278. Vaidya B, Anthony S, Bilous M, et al: Detection of thyroid dysfunction in early pregnancy: universal screening or targeted high-risk case finding? J Clin Endocrinol Metab 92:203, 2007.
279. Surks MI, Ortiz E, Daniels GH, et al: Subclinical thyroid disease: scientific review and guidelines for diagnosis and management, JAMA 291:228, 2004.
280. Singh N, Singh PN, Heshman JM: Effect of calcium carbonate on the absorption of levothyroxine, JAMA 283:2822, 2000.
281. Bell DS, Ovalle F: Use of soy protein supplement and resultant need for increased dose of levothyroxine, Endocr Pract 7:193, 2001.
282. Tamaki H, Amino N, Takeoka K, et al: Thyroxine requirement during pregnancy for replacement therapy of hypothyroidism, Obstet Gynecol 76:230, 1990.
283. Balen AH, Kurtz AB: Successful outcome of pregnancy with severe hypothyroidism: case report and literature review, Br J Obstet Gynaecol 97:536, 1990.
284. Montoro M, Collea JV, Frasier SD, et al: Successful outcome of pregnancy in hypothyroid women, Ann Intern Med 94:31, 1986.
285. Wasserstrum N, Anania CA: Perinatal consequences of maternal hypothyroidism in early pregnancy and inadequate replacement, Clin Endocrinol 42:353, 1995.
286. New England Congenital Hypothyroidism collaborative: Neonatal hypothyroidism screening: status of patients at six years of age, J Pediatr 107:915, 1985.
287. New England Congenital Hypothyroidism Collaborative: Elementary school performance of children with congenital hypothyroidism, J Pediatr 116:27, 1990.
288. Van der Gaag RD, Drexhage HA, Dussault JH: Role of maternal immunoglobulin blocking TSH-induced growth in sporadic forms of congenital hypothyroidism, Lancet 1:246, 1985.
289. Brown RS, Keating P, Mitchell E: Maternal thyroid-blocking immunoglobulins in congenital hypothyroidism, J Clin Endocrinol Metab 70:1341, 1990.
290. Bogner U, Graters AH, Sigle B, et al: Cytotoxic antibodies in congenital hypothyroidism, J Clin Endocrinol Metab 68:671, 1989.
291. Takasu N, Mori T, Koizumi Y, et al: Transient neonatal hypothyroidism due to maternal immunoglobulins that inhibit thyrotropin-binding and post-receptor processes, J Clin Endocrinol Metab 59:142, 1984.
292. Boyages SC, Halpern JP, Maberly GF, et al: Endemic cretinism: possible role for thyroid autoimmunity, Lancet 2:529, 1989.
293. Jansson R, Dahlberg PA, Winsa B, et al: The postpartum period constitutes an important risk for the development of clinical Graves' disease in young women, Acta Endocrinol 116:321, 1987.
294. Tamaki H, Amino N, Aozasa M, et al: Serial changes in thyroid-stimulating antibody and thyrotropin binding inhibitor immunoglobulin at the time of postpartum occurrence of thyrotoxicosis in Graves' disease, J Clin Endocrinol Metab 65:324, 1988.
295. Asa SL, Bilbao JM, Kovacs K, et al: Lymphocytic hypophysitis of pregnancy resulting in hypopituitarism: a distinct clinicopathologic entity, Ann Intern Med 96:166, 1981.
296. Kumar S: Isolated thyroid stimulating hormone deficiency following childbirth, Proc R Soc Med 59:1281, 1966.
297. Merenich JA, McDermott MT, Kidd GS: Transient isolated thyrotropin deficiency in the postpartum period, Am J Med 86:361, 1989.
298. Papetrou PD, Jackson IMD: Thyrotoxicosis due to silent thyroiditis, Lancet 1:361, 1975.
299. Muller AF, Drexhage HA, Berghout A: Postpartum thyroiditis and autoimmune thyroiditis in women of childbearing age: recent insights and consequences for antenatal and postnatal care, Endocr Rev 22:605, 2001.
300. Stagnaro-Green A: Clinical review 152: postpartum thyroiditis, J Clin Endocrinol Metab 87:4042, 2002.

301. Alvarez-Marfany M, Roman SH, Drexler AJ, et al: Long-term prospective study of postpartum thyroid dysfunction in women with insulin dependent diabetes mellitus, J Clin Endocrinol Metab 79:10, 1994.

302. Gerstein HC: Incidence of postpartum thyroid dysfunction in patients with type 1 diabetes mellitus, Ann Intern Med 118:419, 1993.

303. White WB, Andreoli JW: Severe, accelerated postpartum hypertension associated with hyperthyroxinemia, Br J Obstet Gynaecol 93:1297, 1986.

304. Rhys J, Othman S, Parkes AB, et al: Interference in thyroid function tests in postpartum thyroiditis, Clin Chem 37:1397, 1991.

305. Amino N, Nori H, Iwatani Y, et al: High prevalence of transient post-partum thyrotoxicosis and hypothyroidism, N Engl J Med 306:849, 1982.

306. Amino N, Tada H, Hidaka Y: Postpartum autoimmune thyroid syndrome: a model of aggravation of autoimmune disease, Thyroid 9:705, 1999.

307. Dydek GJ, Blue PW: Human breast milk excretion of iodine-131 following diagnostic and therapeutic administration to a lactating patient with Graves' disease, J Nucl Med 29:407, 1988.

308. Robinson GE, Stewart DE: Postpartum psychiatric disorders, Can Med Assoc J 134:31, 1986.

309. Pop VJM, de Rooy HAM, Vadar HL, et al: Postpartum thyroid dysfunction and depression in an unselected population, N Engl J Med 324:1815, 1991.

310. Kent GN, Stuckey BG, Allen JR, et al: Postpartum thyroid dysfunction: clinical assessment and relationship to psychiatric affective morbidity, Clin Endocrinol (Oxf) 51:429, 1999.

311. Tachi J, Amino N, Tamaki H, et al: Long-term follow-up and HLA association in patients with postpartum hypothyroidism, J Clin Endocrinol Metab 66:480, 1988.

312. Othman S, Phillips DIW, Parkes AB, et al: A long-term follow-up of postpartum thyroiditis, Clin Endocrinol 32:559, 1990.

313. Roti E, Minelli R, Gardini E, et al: Impaired intrathyroidal organification and iodine-induced hypothyroidism in euthyroid women with a previous episode of postpartum thyroiditis, J Clin Endocrinol Metab 73:958, 1991.

314. Lazarus JH: Postpartum thyroiditis, Thyroid Int 5:3, 1996.

315. Amino N, Mori H, Iwatani Y, et al: High prevalence of transient post-partum thyrotoxicosis and hypothyroidism, N Engl J Med 306:849, 1982.

316. Marqusee E, Hill JA, Mandel SJ: Thyroiditis after pregnancy loss, J Clin Endocrinol Metab 82:2455, 1997.

317. Stagnaro-Green A, Roman SH, Cobin RH, et al: A prospective study of lymphocyte-initiated immunosuppression in normal pregnancy: evidence of a T-cell etiology for postpartum thyroid dysfunction, J Clin Endocrinol Metab 74:645, 1992.

318. Fung HYM, Kologlu M, Collison K, et al: Postpartum thyroid dysfunction in Mid Glamorgan, Br Med J 296:241, 1988.

319. Kampe O, Jansson R, Karlsson FA: Effects of L-thyroxine and iodide on the development of autoimmune postpartum thyroiditis, J Clin Endocrinol Metab 70:1014, 1990.

320. Bech K: Importance of cytolytic activity and dietary iodine in the pathogenesis of postpartum thyroiditis, Allergy 43:161, 1988.

321. Sridama V, Pacini F, Yan SL, et al: Decreased levels of helper T cells: a possible cause of immunodeficiency in pregnancy, N Engl J Med 307:352, 1982.

322. Takasu N, Komiya I, Nagasawa Y, et al: Exacerbation of autoimmune thyroid dysfunction after unilateral adrenalectomy in patients with Cushing's syndrome due to an adrenocortical adenoma, N Engl J Med 322:1708, 1990.

323. Vargas MT, Briones-Urbina R, Gladman D, et al: Antithyroid microsomal autoantibodies and HLA-DR5 are associated with postpartum thyroid dysfunction: evidence supporting an autoimmune pathogenesis, J Clin Endocrinol Metab 67:327, 1988.

324. Kologlu M, Fung H, Darke C, et al: Postpartum thyroid dysfunction and HLA status, Eur J Clin Invest 20:56, 1990.

325. Jansson R, Safwenberg J, Dahlberg PA: Influence of the HLA-DR4 antigen and iodine status on the development of autoimmune postpartum thyroiditis, J Clin Endocrinol Metab 60:168, 1985.

326. Pryds O, Lervang HH, Ostergaard-Kristensen HP, et al: HLA-DR factors associated with postpartum hypothyroidism: an early manifestation of Hashimoto's thyroiditis? Tissue Antigens 30:34, 1987.

327. DeGroot LJ, Quintans J: The causes of autoimmune thyroid disease, Endocr Rev 10:537, 1989.

328. Weetman AP, Fung HYM, Richards CJ, et al: IgG subclass distribution and relative functional affinity of thyroid microsomal antibodies in postpartum thyroiditis, Eur J Clin Invest 20:133, 1990.

329. Briones-Urbina R, Parkes AB, Bogner U, et al: Increase in antimicrosomal antibody–related IgG1 and IgG4 and titers of antithyroid peroxidase antibodies but not antibody dependent cell-mediated cytotoxicity in postpartum thyroiditis with transient hyperthyroidism, J Endocrinol Invest 13:879, 1990.

330. Tachi J, Amino N, Iwatani Y, et al: Increase in anti-deoxyribonucleic acid antibody titer in postpartum aggravation of autoimmune thyroid disease, J Clin Endocrinol Metab 67:1049, 1988.

331. Iwatani Y, Amino N, Tamaki H, et al: Increase in peripheral large granular lymphocytes in postpartum autoimmune thyroiditis, Endocrinol Jpn 35:447, 1988.

332. Hayslip CC, Baker JR, Wartofsky L, et al: Natural killer cell activity and serum autoantibodies in women with postpartum thyroiditis, J Clin Endocrinol Metab 66:1089, 1988.

333. Chan JYC, Walfish PG: Activated (Ia+) T-lymphocytes and their subsets in autoimmune thyroid diseases: analysis by dual laser flow microfluorocytometry, J Clin Endocrinol Metab 62:403, 1986.

334. Jansson R, Totterman TH, Sallstrom J, et al: Intrathyroidal and circulating lymphocyte subsets in different stages of autoimmune postpartum thyroiditis, J Clin Endocrinol Metab 58:942, 1984.

335. Negro R, Greco G, Mangieri T, et al: The influence of selenium supplementation on postpartum thyroid status in pregnant women with thyroid peroxidase autoantibodies, J Clin Endocrinol Metab 92:1263, 2007.

336. Struve CW, Haupt S, Ohlen S: Influence of frequency of previous pregnancies on the prevalence of thyroid nodules in women without clinical evidence of thyroid disease, Thyroid 3:7, 1993.

337. Cooper DS, Doherty GM, Haugen B, et al: Management guidelines for patients with thyroid nodules and differentiated thyroid cancer, Thyroid 16:109, 2006.

338. Pacini F, Schlumberger M, Dralle H, et al: European consensus for the management of patients with differentiated thyroid carcinoma of the follicular epithelium, Eur J Endocrinol 154:787, 2006.

339. Tan GH, Gharib H, Goellner JR, et al: Management of thyroid nodules in pregnancy, Arch Intern Med 156:2317, 1996.

340. Moosa M, Mazzaferri EL: Outcome of differentiated thyroid cancer diagnosed on pregnant woman, J Clin Endocrinol Metab 82:2862, 1997.

341. McTiernan AM, Weiss NS, Daling JR: Incidence of thyroid cancer in women in relation to reproductive and hormonal factors, Am J Epidemiol 120:423, 1984.

342. Rosen IB, Walfish PG, Nikore V: Pregnancy and surgical thyroid disease, Surgery 98:1135, 1985.

343. Herzon FS, Morris DM, Segal MN, et al: Coexistent thyroid cancer and pregnancy, Arch Otolaryngol Head Neck Surg 120:1191, 1994.

344. Balan KK, Critchley M: Outcome of pregnancy following treatment of well-differentiated thyroid cancer with [131]iodine, Br J Obstet Gynaecol 99:1021, 1992.

Index

Page numbers followed by 'f' indicate figures and 't' indicate tables

Printed and bound by CPI Group (UK) Ltd, Croydon, CR0 4YY

03/10/2024

01040364-0016